Perioperative Nursing Care Planning

The material contained in this book is endorsed by AORN as a useful component in the ongoing education process of perioperative nurses.

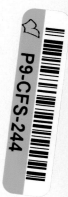

Perioperative Nursing Care Planning

Jane C. Rothrock, RN, DNSc, CNOR

Director of R.N. First Assistant and
Perioperative Nursing Programs
Delaware County Community College
Media, Pennsylvania

SECOND EDITION
with 180 *illustrations*

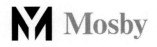 Mosby

St. Louis Baltimore Boston Carlsbad Chicago Naples New York Philadelphia Portland
London Madrid Mexico City Singapore Sydney Tokyo Toronto Wiesbaden

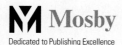

Mosby
Dedicated to Publishing Excellence

A Times Mirror
Company

Publisher: Nancy L. Coon
Editor: Michael S. Ledbetter
Senior Developmental Editor: Teri Merchant
Project Manager: John Rogers
Production Editor: Kathleen L. Teal
Designer: Renée Duenow
Manufacturing Supervisor: Theresa Fuchs

A NOTE TO THE READER
The author and the publisher have made every attempt to check dosages and
nursing content for accuracy. Because the science of pharmacology is continually
advancing, our knowledge base continues to expand. Therefore we recommend
that the reader always check product information for changes in dosage or
administration before administering any medication. This is particularly
important with new or rarely used drugs.

Printed in the United States of America
Composition by The Clarinda Company
Printing/binding by The Maple-Vail Book Manufacturing Group

Mosby–Year Book, Inc.
11830 Westline Industrial Drive
St. Louis, Missouri 63146

International Standard Book Number 0-8151-7147-1

96 97 98 99 00 / 9 8 7 6 5 4 3 2 1

Contributors

JOANNE D. CIMORELLI, RN, BS, CNOR, RNFA
RN First Assistant with Stephen H. Sinclair, MD, PC
Upland, Pennsylvania

BRENDA S. GREGORY DAWES, RN, BSN, CNOR
Director, Surgical Services
St. Anthony's Hospital, St. Petersburg, Florida

VICKI J. FOX, RN, MSN, CNS, CRNFA
Clinical Nurse Specialist
Trauma/General Surgery Care Coordinator
Mother Frances Hospital, Tyler, Texas

NANCY J. GIRARD, PhD, RN, CS
Associate Professor
University of Texas Health Science Center at San
  Antonio
School of Nursing, San Antonio, Texas

ELIZABETH W. GONZALEZ, PhD
Assistant Professor, Department of Nursing
College of Allied Health Sciences
Thomas Jefferson University
Philadelphia, Pennsylvania

DONNA N. HERSHEY, RN, MSN, CNOR
Staff Nurse, Operating Room
Lancaster General Hospital, Lancaster, Pennsylvania

CHRISTY R. JOHNSON, RN, BA, CNOR, CRNFA
Certified RN First Assistant
HCA Coliseum Medical Centers,
Macon, GA

JANE HERSHEY JOHNSON, RN, MSN, CNOR
Perioperative Faculty
Delaware County Community College
Media, Pennsylvania

JOANN MARSHALL, RN, CNOR
Registered Nurse First Assistant
Paoli Memorial Hospital, Paoli, Pennsylvania

GLORIA J. McNEAL, RN, MSN, CS
Assistant Professor, Department of Nursing
College of Allied Health Sciences
Thomas Jefferson University
Philadelphia, Pennsylvania

GRATIA M. NAGLE, RN, BA, CNOR, CRNFA
Nursing Director, Paoli Surgery Center
Paoli, Pennsylvania

CHERYL NYGREN, RN, CNOR, RNFA
Staff Nurse, Cardiothoracic Surgery
Children's Hospital of Philadelphia
Philadelphia, Pennsylvania

DENISE D. O'BRIEN, RN, BSN, CPAN, CAPA
Educational Nurse Coordinator/Clinical Nurse III
Ambulatory Surgery Unit
Department of Operating Rooms/PACU
University of Michigan Hospitals
Ann Arbor, Michigan

IRIS GAUTIER PEREZ, RN, MS
Assistant Professor, Department of Nursing
Cumberland County College, Vineland, New Jersey

ELIZABETH PETIT de MANGE, RN, MSN
Instructor, Department of Nursing
College of Allied Health Sciences
Thomas Jefferson University
Philadelphia, Pennsylvania

JEANETTE X. POLASCHEK, RN, MS
Clinical Information Systems Project Manager
Cedars-Sinai Medical Center, Los Angeles, California

KAREN L. RITCHEY, RN, MSN, CNOR
Clinical Nurse Specialist, Nelson 2 Operating Room
Johns Hopkins Hospital, Baltimore, Maryland;
Faculty Member, Delaware County Community College
Media, Pennsylvania

PATRICIA C. SEIFERT, RN, MSN, CRNFA, CNOR
Operating Room Coordinator, Cardiac Surgery
The Arlington Hospital, Arlington, Virginia

CHRISTINE E. SMITH, RN, MSN, CNOR
Clinical Educator, Perioperative Nursing
The Graduate Hospital, Philadelphia, Pennsylvania

SANDRA SMYTH, RN, CPSN, CNOR
Staff Nurse, Surgical Services
Williamsburg Community Hospital
Williamsburg, Virginia

KATIE STEUER, RN, BSN, CNOR
Core Nurse, General Surgery
Dartmouth-Hitchcock Medical Center
Hanover, New Hampshire

SHERI J. VOSS, RN, BS, CNOR
Director, Tower Surgical Services
Centennial Medical Center, Nashville, Tennessee

DIANA L. WADLUND, RN, MSN, CNOR
Registered Nurse First Assistant
Paoli Memorial Hospital, Paoli, Pennsylvania

Reviewer/Consultant Panel

BECKY W. ARMSTRONG, RN, MEd, CNOR

JAYNA INEZ BANNER, RN

JOHN R. BEETLE, RN, MSN, CNOR

KENNETH A. BROWN, MD

JUSTINE K. BUSCH, RN, BSN, CNOR

ROSEMARIE T. CEVALLOS, RN, CNOR, RNFA

MARY SMALLWOOD DALE, RN, CNOR

ANN B. DeMELLO, RN, BS, CNOR

CHRISTINE C. ESPERSEN, RN, CNOR, CRNFA

PATRICIA A. FIRTH, RN, MPH, ARNP, RNFA

JEAN M. REEDER, PhD, RN, CNOR, FAAN

JACQUELINE SAUNDERS, RN, MSN, CNOR

MARIA L. TALAMO, MA, RN, CNA, CCRN

KIMBERLY MROWIEC TOTER, RN, BS, CNOR

NATHALIE FORTINI WALKER, RN, CNOR

To my dear, departed friend,

NANCY CAMISHION,

whose caring nature embraced those she nursed

and those she loved. The constancy of her caring,

which is the core and heart of perioperative nursing, will keep us safe

from the blowing winds of change and the test of time,

making us stronger than we were before.

Preface

Florence Nightingale, whose legacy continues to inspire and amaze me, wrote of nursing, "Nursing is an art, it requires as exclusive a devotion, as hard a preparation, as any painter's or sculptor's work; for what is the having to do with dead canvas or cold marble, compared with having to do with the living body—the temple of God's spirit? It is one of the finest arts; I had almost said, the finest of the Fine Arts."

What was true over a hundred years ago remains true in 1996—nursing requires devotion and hard preparation. And, just as Nightingale had to "prove" the worth and value of the nurse in the Crimea, overcoming obstacles, collecting data, showing outcomes that were irrefutable in terms of improving life and death, so does the nurse in 1996. Like Nightingale, we must continue identifying what we do and relate it to having an effect on improving patient outcomes. Without a common framework to accurately describe "what we do," our efforts are thwarted. Dr. Norma Lang, Margaret Bond Simon Dean and Professor at the University of Pennsylvania School of Nursing and Chair of the American Nurses Association's Steering Committee on Data Bases to Support Clinical Nursing Practice has frequently reminded us that, if we cannot name it (what it is we do), we cannot control it, finance it, teach it, research it, or put it into public policy.

And so, this book, like the first edition, attempts to make perioperative nursing visible in terms of identifying the things we do to help effect safe, affordable, quality outcomes for our patients. Unit One contains content important to a framework for exploring nursing care processes in 1996 and beyond. Because the book is written for (and by) practicing nurses, we have added chapters on computerized patient records and case management. Both of these activities will be part of our future, as will the nursing process framework, quality and performance improvement efforts, means of documenting care provided, and external regulatory influences such as those of the Joint Commission. Unit One sets the background for exploring what it is we do in operative and other invasive procedure settings.

Unit Two begins with quantifying perioperative nursing's contributions to generic desirable outcomes for all perioperative patients; it provides the answer, in part, to the "what does the perioperative nurse do to (1) prevent infection; (2) educate the patient; (3) prevent injury; (4) maintain skin integrity; (5) maintain fluid and electrolyte balance; and (6) assist the patient in self-care and home care as he or she rehabilitates from the intervention?" Here the reader will find our best effort in describing perioperative nursing activities that effect these outcomes and making the outcomes themselves quantifiable. How do we determine that the patient is free from infection? If we all use different criteria, we will never be able to do large-scale outcomes research, for the data we use to describe that outcome will differ. That is not to say that this book is the final and absolute source for proposing ways to measure these outcomes, but it is seriously intended to set us on a course for the journey into outcomes measurement. Following the chapter on generic outcomes, you will find population-specific chapters and plans of care. With these chapters, we continue to attempt to move away from examining the success of, for example, hip surgery by focusing only on the role of the physician or whether the surgery was a success. To do that completely ignores the fact that a nurse prepared the patient for that surgery, got him or her through that surgery, and recovered and rehabilitated him or her from that surgery. In each of the population-specific chapters, we have tried to describe in some detail the elements of preparing the patient, with key assessment factors for the perioperative nurse, and what it is that we do to get a patient safely through the surgery and recovered from it. The contributors to this book believe, as do I, that we must continue to explicate this or we will continue to be lumped into the charge for the OR room. Since we believe that is important to all perioperative nurses, we have worked to make each of these chapters a fill in the gap for "patient to OR . . . patient returned from OR." In that, we intend to provide a description of the missing link in establishing just what the perioperative nurse does that contributes to "a successful surgery."

Unit Three addresses ambulatory surgery, trauma, pediatric patient populations, and the aging patient. For each of these patient populations, a general plan of care is presented that encompasses their special needs. The chapter on multiculturally diverse patients and their care is written by experts in cultural competence. As in the first edition, we continue to review unexpected events in surgery such as hemorrhage, malignant hyperthermia, cardiac arrest, and shock. We follow the patient into the postanesthesia unit, and posit important information to be shared between nurse caregivers to continue the achievement of desired patient outcomes. Finally, we conclude with a chapter on research considerations, because much of our future effort will continue to be directed at generating, using, and recommending perioperative research.

In all of this, we have attempted to recognize the "burden" that writing a care plan can be for the nurse intensivist, and that is who the perioperative nurse is. Thus, we present you with care plans that are intended to allow you to adapt them as standardized care plans, individualize them, and "chart" on them only when you need to represent an element of care that isn't captured in the care plan we have proposed. If you are able to use them that way, modified as you see fit to become preprinted or computerized standards of care specific to your perioperative practice setting, then you will have taken us a long way to meeting our mission in doing this book. You will be defined by what you know and what you do for perioperative patients, and that is the best way for us to be known. Early in nursing's history, we were known for giving special consideration to a patient's needs, desires, and comforts. Our process of caring then and now involves humanistic attention to all aspects of a perioperative patient's personhood; we attend to the science of our work and to the art of nursing as we provide care that is competent and compassionate. The spiritual meaning of being with another person during one of the most lonely and fearful events in his or her life is not our occupation, it is our sacred place, to be valued, given with gentleness, and fiercely protected as part of the essence of perioperative nursing.

From the contributors to this book, all of whom are colleagues or former students, and with whom I am honored to be listed,

Jane C. Rothrock

Contents

Unit **III**

Special Considerations in Care Planning

Perioperative Nursing Care Planning

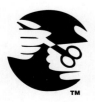

The material contained in this book is endorsed by AORN as a useful component in the ongoing education process of perioperative nurses.

Basic Principles of Perioperative Care Planning

Chapter 1

Introduction to the Nursing Process

Jane C. Rothrock

Florence Nightingale created the structure that spirited nursing out of the neighbor-helping-neighbor phase of history into a neophyte profession whose practitioners were educated in formal training schools and taught principles of care. A century later the nursing process was developed, a scientific problem-solving approach to patient care that today remains the profession's model of clinical inquiry. The nursing process components of assessing, diagnosing, identifying desired patient outcomes, planning, implementing, and evaluating are now integrated into the standards of care and recommendations for documentation by each of the nursing specialties. The systematic, rational, deliberate nursing process supports the premise that nurses function intellectually and with purpose. Nursing is a thinking, caring, doing profession that is evolving a specialized body of knowledge based on the basic sciences and nursing research. The nursing process is the clinical inquiry model that links scientific knowledge, research, theory, and applications of knowledge (Koldjeski, 1993).

Nursing is defined as the diagnosis and treatment of human responses to health and illness (ANA, 1994). The nursing process describes the methods used by the nurse to undertake the important work of nursing care. Specifically, assessment identifies the needs of a patient; diagnosis involves interpreting and analyzing patient data; outcome identification involves the nurse and patient, when applicable, in stating desired outcomes; plan outlines the best interventions predicted to meet the patient's needs; implementation requires the activation or delegation of the planned care; and evaluation determines if the patient achieved the desired outcomes from the selected nursing interventions. In this framework, nursing may be described as in-

formed caring for the well-being of others (Swanson, 1993).

THE NURSING PROCESS: PERIOPERATIVE NURSING

The universal components of the nursing process also serve as the conceptual framework for perioperative nursing. The term "perioperative" describes the experience of the patient before, during, and after surgery. The registered nurse who specializes in perioperative nursing is responsible for assessing, determining, and prioritizing nursing diagnoses, identifying desired patient outcomes, planning, implementing (or delegating), and evaluating patient care outcomes preoperatively, intraoperatively, and postoperatively. Since nursing task activities dictated by institutional policy (for example, "a dispersive pad must be attached to the patient before electrocoagulation of vessels") or by medical regimen (for example, "dress incision with collodion") can be completed without an awareness of a patient's individual needs, the assessment phase of the nursing process may be compromised in the rush of the surgical suite. It is tempting to believe that perioperative nursing has a pattern of knowledge that allows the nurse to make a quick assessment of the patient, to establish a diagnosis, and to plan what is best; this may indeed lead to an efficient type of perioperative nursing practice that is based on empirical and experiential knowledge. However, in order for the perioperative nurse to understand, with empathy, the true meaning of the experience of surgery for a patient, the nurse must be open to the subjective nature of each patient; Munhall (1993) termed this openness "unknowing." The variability and uniqueness of the individual patient, therefore, mandates a nursing assessment before any one of the other five components is carried out.

Standards of Perioperative Nursing Practice

The ultimate goal of nursing is to provide safe, effective, high-quality care. The model used to delineate the quality of care delivered before, during, and after surgery is the *Standards of Perioperative Clinical Practice* (Box 1-1), which is also based on the nursing process. These standards require the following:

- A systematic and continuous *assessment* that can be retrieved and communicated to others
- An analysis of the assessment with conclusions written as a *nursing diagnosis*
- Desired *patient outcomes* that should occur as a result of the plan
- A *plan* of nursing care that is written and prescribes nursing behaviors or actions that will help the patient achieve the identified outcomes
- The deliberate *implementation* of the prescribed plan
- A systematic *evaluation* of the plan to determine if the patient outcomes were achieved

Key words of the nursing process are italicized to emphasize the integration of the concept into the standards of care. An understanding of the nursing process is germane to quality care and to perioperative practice.

Using the Nursing Process

When the nursing process is used in perioperative patient care settings—be it an inpatient operating room, an ambulatory surgery setting, a cardiac catheterization laboratory, an endoscopy suite, an interventional radiology department, or an office-based surgery unit—it demonstrates the thoughts and actions taken by the nurse in the care of the patient undergoing an operative or other invasive procedure. The perioperative nurse assesses the patient preoperatively, uses assessment data to identify relevant nursing diagnoses, sets desired patient outcomes, develops a plan of care, implements the plan intraoperatively, and evaluates the effect of the planned interventions postoperatively. Consider the following example. A patient enters the operating room and reports he cannot fully extend his left knee because of arthritic changes. Visual *assessment* confirms the patient can extend his left knee only 60 degrees and the perioperative nurse diagnoses that the knee will be subject to injury unless precautions are taken. The perioperative nurse makes the *diagnosis, High risk for injury during surgical positioning related to arthritic left knee.* The perioperative nurse and patient then *plan* a comfortable position for the knee before general anesthesia is administered. The *desired outcome* is to prevent physical injury to the compromised knee. The perioperative nurse *implements* the planned intervention to secure and protect the knee and prevent injury before the procedure begins. Postoperatively, in the postanesthesia care unit (PACU), the patient responds negatively to an inquiry about leg pain during the *evaluation* of the outcome to prevent additional injury to the left knee. The nursing intervention was successful and the perioperative nurse demonstrated the application of the nursing process intraoperatively. This example of an independent nursing action also illustrates how the definition of nursing is effected intraoperatively. The patient's potential response to injury (a painful left knee) was diagnosed and treatment to prevent the injury was implemented.

Bottoriff and Morse (1994) have suggested an alternate method of classifying nurse-patient interactions that captures patterns of caring. In their framework, the perioperative nurse engages in four types of "doing." "Doing more" is when the nurse does something that goes beyond what is usually required to complete care, as when the nurse reaches out to a patient or takes more time than is usually required. "Doing for" is responding to a patient request or need that is not treatment related; it is a personalized approach to giving assistance. "Doing with" is when the nurse focuses equally on the task and the patient, engaging the patient by seeking his or her thoughts, opinions, and perceptions. "Doing tasks" is when the nurse focuses on equipment, treatment, and getting the job done. Using the nursing process, the patient in the example was nursed

Box 1-1 *Standards of Perioperative Clinical Practice*

The *Standards of Perioperative Clinical Practice* and *Standards of Perioperative Professional Performance* focus on the process of providing nursing care and performing professional role activities. These standards apply to all nurses in the perioperative setting and were developed by the Association of Operating Room Nurses (AORN) using the American Nurses Association (ANA) *Standards of Clinical Nursing Practice.*

It is the nurse's responsibility to meet these standards, assuming that adequate environmental working conditions and necessary resources are available to support and facilitate the nurse's attainment of these standards. Under certain conditions, nurses may not be able to fully meet the standards. It is important to recognize the link between working conditions and the nurse's ability to deliver care. It is the responsibility of employers or health care facilities to provide an appropriate environment for nursing practice.

Several related themes underlie the *Standards of Perioperative Clinical Practice* and *Standards of Perioperative Professional Performance.* Nursing care must be individualized to meet a particular patient's unique needs and situation. This care should be provided in the context of disease or injury prevention, health promotion, health restoration, health maintenance, or palliative care. The cultural, racial, and ethnic diversity of the patient must always be taken into account in providing nursing services.

The nurse must respect the patient's goals and preferences in developing and implementing a plan of care. One of the nurse's primary responsibilities is patient education; therefore nurses should provide patients with appropriate information to make informed decisions regarding their care and treatment. It is recognized, however, that some state regulations or institutional policies or procedures may prohibit full disclosure of information to patients.

The nurse's partnership with the patient and other health care providers is recognized in the standards. It is assumed that the nurse works with other health care providers in a coordinated manner throughout the process of caring for a surgical patient. The involvement of the patient, family, or significant others is paramount. The appropriate degree of participation expected of the patient, family, or other health care providers is determined by the clinical environment and the patient's unique situation.

Throughout the standards, terms such as "appropriate," "pertinent," and "realistic" are used. It is beyond the scope of documents such as these to account for all possible scenarios that the professional perioperative nurse may encounter in practice. The perioperative nurse will need to exercise judgment, based on education and experience, in determining what is appropriate, pertinent, or realistic. Further direction also may be available from documents such as recommended practices guidelines for care, agency standards, policies, procedures, protocols, and current research findings.

Summary

The *Standards of Perioperative Nursing* provide a mechanism to delineate the responsibilities of registered nurses engaged in practice in the perioperative setting. The standards of perioperative nursing and recommended practices serve as the basis for quality monitoring and evaluation systems; data bases; regulatory systems; the development and evaluation of nursing service delivery systems and organizational structures; certification activities; job descriptions and performance appraisals; agency policies, procedures and protocols; and educational offerings.

Standard I: Assessment

The perioperative nurse collects patient health data.

Interpretive statement

Assessment is the systematic and ongoing collection of data, guided by the application of knowledge of physiologic and psychologic principles and experience, and is used to make judgments and predictions about a patient's response to illness or changes in life processes. Assessment is essential to establishing a nursing diagnosis and predicting outcomes. Assessment may occur in a variety of settings.

Criteria

1. The priority of data collection is determined by the patient's immediate condition or needs and the relationship to the proposed intervention. Pertinent data include, but are not limited to,
   - Current medical diagnoses and therapies
   - Physical status and physiologic responses
   - Psychosocial status of the patient
   - Cultural, spiritual, and life-style information
   - The individual's understanding, perceptions, and expectations of the procedure
   - Previous responses to illness, hospitalizations, and surgical, therapeutic, or diagnostic procedures
   - Results of diagnostic studies
2. Pertinent data are collected using appropriate assessment techniques.
3. Data collection involves the patient, significant others, and health care providers when appropriate. It may be accomplished through diverse means, such as interview, review of records, assessment, and/or consultation.
4. Data collection is systematic and ongoing.
5. Relevant data are documented in retrievable form.

Standard II: Diagnosis

The perioperative nurse analyzes the assessment data in determining diagnoses

Interpretive statement

The outcome of assessment is the potential for one or more nursing diagnoses. Nursing diagnoses are concise statements about actual, or high risk for, health problems/clinical conditions that are amenable to

Continued.

Box 1-1 *Standards of Perioperative Clinical Practice—cont'd*

---

nursing intervention. Diagnoses result from analysis and interpretation of data about the patient's problems, needs, and health status.

Criteria

1. Diagnoses are consistent with the assessment data.
2. Diagnoses are validated with the patient, significant others, and health care providers, when possible.
3. Diagnoses are documented in a manner that facilitates the determination of outcomes and plan of care.

Standard III: Outcome Identification

The perioperative nurse identifies expected outcomes unique to the patient

Interpretive statement

Patient outcomes are derived from nursing diagnoses and direct the interventions to correct, alter, or maintain the nursing diagnoses. Areas for the perioperative nurse to consider when formulating outcomes should include, but are not limited to,

- Absence of infection
- Maintenance of skin integrity
- Absence of adverse effects through proper use of safety measures related to positioning, extraneous objects, and chemical, physical, and electrical hazards
- Maintenance of fluid and electrolyte balance
- Knowledge of the patient and significant others of the physiologic and psychologic responses to surgical intervention
- Participation of the patient and significant others in the rehabilitation process

Criteria

1. Outcomes are derived from the diagnoses and are mutually formulated with the patient, significant others, and health care providers, when possible.
2. The patient's present and potential physical capabilities and behavioral patterns are congruent with the expected outcomes.
3. Outcomes are attainable with consideration to human and material resources available to the patient.
4. Outcome statements include measurable criteria for determining expected outcomes as a result of nursing interventions.
5. Outcomes include a time estimate for attainment.
6. Outcomes are prioritized.
7. Outcomes are communicated to appropriate people.
8. Outcomes are documented in a retrievable form.
9. Outcomes provide direction for continuity of care.

Standard IV: Planning

The perioperative nurse develops a plan of care that prescribes interventions to attain expected outcomes

Interpretive statement

The outcome statements become the guide for nursing interventions necessary to achieve the desired re-

sults. The individualized plan of care reflects the perioperative assessment and a logical sequence to attain outcomes. Priorities for the provision of nursing care are established by the perioperative nurse in collaboration with the patient, significant others, and health care providers. Examples of interventions performed include, but are not limited to,

- Provision of information and supportive perioperative teaching specifically related to the surgical intervention and nursing care
- Identification of the patient
- Verification of the surgical site
- Verification of the operative consent and reports of essential diagnostic procedures
- Positioning according to physiologic principles
- Adherence to principles of asepsis
- Provision of appropriate and properly functioning equipment and supplies for the patient
- Provision for comfort measures and supportive care to the patient
- Environmental monitoring and safety
- Evaluation of outcomes in relation to the identified interventions
- Communication of intraoperative information to significant others and the health care team to provide for continuity of care

Criteria

1. The plan of care reflects current nursing practice.
2. The plan of care provides for continuity of care.
3. The plan of care specifies nursing diagnoses, interventions necessary to achieve the outcomes, and a logical sequence of interventions.
4. Human and material resources are available to implement the plan of care.
5. The plan of care is communicated to appropriate people.
6. Evidence of a plan of care is retrievable through documented intervention and evaluation of progress toward expected outcomes.

Standard V: Implementation

The perioperative nurse implements the interventions identified in the plan of care

Interpretive statement

Interventions are consistent with the established plan of care and provide continuity of nursing care in the perioperative period. Interventions are based on expert opinion, scientific principles, and/or consensus. They reflect the rights and desires of the patient and significant others.

Criteria

1. Interventions are consistent with the established plan of care.
2. Implementation of the plan of care is an ongoing process and is based on the patient's response.
3. Interventions reflect the rights and desires of the patient and significant others.

Continued.

Box 1-1 Standards of Perioperative Clinical Practice—cont'd

4. Interventions are implemented with safety, skill, and efficiency and are adjusted according to patient responses.
5. Interventions may be assigned or delegated as appropriate.
6. Interventions are documented and communicated verbally as appropriate to promote continuity of care.

Standard VI: Evaluation

The perioperative nurse evaluates the patient's progress toward attainment of outcomes

Interpretive statement

Evaluation is systematic and ongoing. It is based on observations and patient responses to nursing interventions; the effectiveness of interventions is evaluated in relation to the outcomes. Ongoing assessment data are used to revise diagnoses, the plan of care, and/or outcomes as needed. The patient, significant others, and health care providers are involved in the evaluation process.

Criteria

1. Evaluation of the effectiveness of interventions is systematic and ongoing.
2. The effectiveness of interventions is evaluated in relation to outcomes.
3. Documentation of the patient's progress toward achievable outcomes is retrievable.
4. Ongoing assessment data are used to revise diagnoses, outcomes, and the plan of care, as needed.
5. Revisions in diagnoses, outcomes, and the plan of care are documented.
6. The patient, significant others, and health care providers are involved in the evaluation process when appropriate.

---

carefully, consciously, intellectually, and systematically by the perioperative nurse who did with, for, and more while simultaneously doing the task of positioning. Box 1-2 shows the component parts of the nursing process.

Assessment

Dividing the nursing process into phases is an artificial separation of actions that in actual practice cannot be separated. Separation, however, encourages a thoughtful analysis of each phase and permits a greater understanding of what nursing practice is. Assessment, the first phase of the process, is divided into two parts, data collection and data organization.

Data collection. Data collection is the primary tool of initial patient assessment and is a continual process of obtaining information necessary to provide nursing care. Information changes as more data are added and as the patient's condition alters. Information about potential or actual problems may come directly from the patient, a family member or friend, the medical record, or other health professionals. Data are considered to be either subjective (what the patient states) or objective (what the nurse sees, hears, smells, or touches). Data can be gathered by interview, by physical examination, or by reading reports (that is, laboratory findings, x-ray examinations, progress notes, or consultations). Many sources are available for data collection.

Generally, a comprehensive nursing admission assessment is completed when a patient first enters

---

Box 1-2 The Nursing Process

Assessment
- Systematic data collection
- Data organization
- Data interpretation

Nursing Diagnosis
- Sorting of data cues to form patterns, relationships
- Identifying nursing diagnoses based on patterns and perioperative nursing knowledge of known risks

Outcome Statement
- Derived from nursing diagnosis
- Includes measurable criteria

Planning
- Prioritization
- Planned nursing interventions communicated/retrievable

Implementation
- Preparation
- Interdependent/independent nursing activities
- Appropriate delegation

Evaluation
- Reassessment
- Comparison to desired outcomes
- Variances used to improve care processes

a health care facility. Nursing histories are a primary means of personalizing nursing care. This in-depth admission assessment documents general information about the patient, psychosocial information that is important in planning care, the history, the reason for the current admission, a description of usual activities of daily living, personal preferences, and a complete head-to-toe examination. Factors that affect the patient's psychosocioeconomic adjustment to illness, as well as the patient's perceptions and expectations, are also added to the comprehensive assessment. Once the comprehensive assessment is recorded on the permanent medical record, ongoing assessments by the registered nurse (RN) are initiated.

Specialty assessments focus on information required to deliver safe, effective, high-quality care before a special procedure or treatment. Thus the assessment by the perioperative nurse is directed toward data needed to provide safe, effective, high-quality perioperative patient care.

A focused interview before surgery to collect subjective information may include the following questions, as suggested by Kleinbeck (1978):

> "What do you expect the surgeon to do today?"
> "Have you ever had surgery before?"
> "What did you do to prepare for your surgery?"
> "When did you last eat?"
> "When did you last take medication?"
> "Do you have any problem areas that we should know about?"
> "Who will be with you after surgery?" (Tell them where to wait.)
> "Is there anything you are especially concerned about now?"

Answers to these questions, with additional probing by the perioperative nurse, elucidate the patient's understanding of the surgical events, the surgical history, whether the patient is properly prepared for surgery, potential problem areas, or any personal areas of concern. Although they may seem like simple questions, they illustrate dimensions of perioperative nurse caring as identified by Wolf and her colleagues (1994): respectful deference (treating the patient as an individual, showing respect, listening), assurance of human presence (allowing patient to express feelings, showing concern), positive connectedness (being empathic), professional knowledge and skill (knowing what needs to be asked), and attentiveness to the other's experience (appreciation of the patient's experience, as perceived by the patient).

Objective data the perioperative nurse needs preoperatively are collected from a variety of sources,

such as physical assessment and review of the patient's record. Data may include the following items about the patient:

- *Physical appearance:* Weight, height, baseline vital signs, activity level
- *Physical impairments:* Hearing, sight, speech, motor ability, neurosensory problems, pain, skeletal position limitation, drainage, bowel or bladder dysfunction
- *Skin condition:* Intact, breaks, scars, dry, moist, rash, pale, reddened, bruises, jaundiced, edematous, ulcers
- *Mental-emotional status:* Level of consciousness, responds to name, crying, tremor, anger, talkative, composed, calm, sad
- *Therapeutic devices and measures in use:* Oxygen, transfusions, drains, catheters, tracheostomy, nasogastric tube, cast, traction, colostomy, previous laryngectomy, pacemaker
- *Laboratory values:* On chart, significant abnormal values noted
- *Legal-ethical:* Consent signed? Blood available? Advance directive executed?

The collection of data before decision making is essential. Once collected, the information must also be validated. Action based on inaccurate information is unsafe and nonprofessional.

Organization of data. Organizing and processing information are critical to assisting efficient decision making. Organizing data allows the perioperative nurse to integrate knowledge about the patient and the patient's condition with nursing knowledge. As data are organized, they are interpreted, analyzed, and examined in relation to ensuring that nursing care corresponds with patient needs. Sifting through and sorting data allow the nurse to determine what information is necessary to make nursing diagnoses relative to nursing responsibility. Such a review reveals cues, patterns, or clusters of information that can be organized into diagnostic statements.

Nursing Diagnosis

To diagnose is to study something carefully and critically to determine its nature. The North American Nursing Diagnosis Association (NANDA) has defined nursing diagnosis as a clinical judgment about individual, family, or community responses to actual or potential health problems/life processes; they provide the basis for selection of nursing interventions to achieve outcomes for which the nurse is accountable (Kim, McFarland, & McLane, 1995). The NANDA list of nursing diagnoses grows biannually as nurses identify patterns or clusters of symptoms and signs that require nursing actions to help a patient resolve or prevent a specific problem. Chapter 7 provides the 1994 NANDA list.

Research (Kleinbeck, 1989) using perioperative nursing students as data collectors indicates that examples of intraoperative nursing diagnoses common among adult patients scheduled for general surgery include the following:

> High risk for infection related to exposure to pathogens
>
> High risk for hypothermia related to cool environment
>
> High risk for fluid and electrolyte deficit or excess related to estimated blood loss and intravenous replacement
>
> High risk for impaired tissue or skin integrity related to surgical positioning
>
> High risk for injury by retained foreign body related to open body cavity
>
> High risk for thermal injury (burn) related to use of electrosurgery, laser, or other electrical equipment
>
> High risk for neuromuscular injury related to surgical positioning
>
> High risk for injury by fall or trauma related to mind-altering anesthetic drugs
>
> Anxiety, fear, or pain related to awake status during local or regional anesthesia

Any one of these diagnostic statements could be generated by the perioperative nurse during surgery. Each one is patient oriented, focused on the patient's response to the impairment, requires nursing knowledge to intervene, and anticipates a positive change or outcome following intervention. Although the NANDA list is incomplete and evolving, it offers the advantage of providing a common language within the profession.

The NANDA list also demonstrates sufficient autonomy to warrant the potential of reimbursement based on the patient's nursing requirements (nursing diagnostic groups) rather than solely on the medical diagnosis. Perioperative nurses are encouraged to test and further define the nursing diagnoses that apply to the surgical setting. Guidelines for submitting a nursing diagnosis to NANDA can be obtained from that organization (Box 1-3).

Writing a nursing diagnosis. A utilitarian nursing diagnosis for clinical use by perioperative nurses is divided into two components: the title or health problem/condition label, which then becomes the basis for identification of desired, projected outcomes, and the primary etiological or related factors, which then become the focus of designing interventions to reduce or eliminate them. The health problem may already be present or the patient may be at high risk for the problem to occur. Perioperative

nurses use both actual and high-risk problems in planning patient-care interventions. Seifert (1994) explains this difference nicely: anxiety is a diagnosis that is often present (actual) in surgical patients; most patients do not have an infection as a presenting problem, but are at high risk for infection due to alteration in normal body defense mechanisms, compromised immune responses, inadequate nutritional status, risk of contamination, etc. Thus "high risk for" diagnoses indicate that, in the perioperative nurse's judgment, the surgical patient population is more vulnerable to developing a specific problem or condition than another patient population. High-quality perioperative nursing care demands that perioperative nurses develop diagnoses based on both individual patient assessment and recognition of the various risks imposed on surgical patients, and that they then develop plans for nursing interventions aimed at reducing this risk.

Learning to write diagnostic statements that clearly define both the problem (actual or high risk) and the contributing factors or etiology can be difficult. The following general guidelines are recommended (Carpenito, 1992):

> Write the health problem first and the etiology or contributing factor second. Both statements are necessary to plan nursing interventions and identify patient outcomes. The phrase "related to" is used as a connection between the two statements, indicating a relationship exists between the problem and its etiology; this enables the perioperative nurse to plan nursing interventions. Many factors may influence the problem, but the nurse identifies the patient-focused etiology or factor which he or she will target for intervention.
>
> Statements are limited to the patient's response to health problems/life processes. Avoid incorporating medical diagnoses or the name of a surgical procedure into a nursing diagnosis. Physicians treat cancer; nurses treat the patient's response to cancer. "High risk for pneumonia related to chronic obstructive pulmonary disease (COPD)" should be restated "Ineffective airway clearance related to poor cough effort." Another incorrect example, "High risk for infection related to cholecystectomy," could be given a nursing focus by writing "High risk for infection related to loss of protective barrier secondary to incision." Nurses do not treat the medical or surgical problems of pneumonia, COPD, or cholecystectomy; they minimize the exposure of the patient to pathogens through aseptic technique or instruct the patient in methods to produce a strong cough effort. Interestingly, a patient with one medical diagnosis often has multiple nursing diagnoses that change over the course of the medical treatment.

Box 1-3 North American Nursing Diagnosis Association Guidelines for Submission of Proposed Diagnoses

I. Proposed diagnoses

The North American Nursing Diagnosis Association (NANDA) solicits proposed nursing diagnoses for review by the Association. Proposed diagnoses undergo a systematic review for inclusion in NANDA's list of approved diagnoses. Approval indicates that NANDA endorses the diagnosis for clinical testing and continuing development by the discipline. Partially developed diagnoses are placed on NANDA's "To Be Developed" (TBD) List.

Classification of diagnoses. Approved diagnoses are forwarded to the Taxonomy Committee for review and classification. A working definition of the term "nursing diagnosis" was developed by the NANDA Board and Taxonomy Committee to use in screening accepted diagnoses for fit with Taxonomy I, Revised.

Working definition. A nursing diagnosis is a clinical judgment about individual, family, or community responses to actual or potential health problems/life processes. Nursing diagnoses provide the basis for selection of nursing interventions to achieve outcomes for which the nurse is accountable (approved as working definition at 9th Conference).

II. Types of diagnostic concepts

Actual nursing diagnoses. Actual nursing diagnoses are diagnostic concepts that describe human responses to health conditions/life processes that exist in an individual, family, or community. Actual nursing diagnoses are supported by defining characteristics (manifestations/signs and symptoms) that cluster in patterns of related cues or inferences. Related factors (etiologies) are factors that contribute to the development or maintenance of an actual diagnosis.

High risk. High-risk nursing diagnoses are diagnostic concepts that describe human responses to health conditions/life processes that may develop in a vulnerable individual, family, or community. High-risk nursing diagnoses are supported by risk factors that contribute to increased vulnerability.

Wellness. Wellness nursing diagnoses are diagnostic concepts that describe human responses to levels of wellness in an individual, family, or community that have a potential for enhancement to a higher state.

III. Components of proposed diagnoses

Label. The label provides a name for a proposed diagnosis. It is a concise term or phrase that represents a pattern of related cues. Diagnostic labels may include qualifiers.

Definition. The definition provides a clear, precise description of the diagnostic concept; delineates its meaning; and helps differentiate it from similar diagnoses.

Defining characteristics. Defining characteristics are observable cues/inferences that cluster as manifestations of a nursing diagnosis. Defining characteristics are listed for actual diagnoses. A defining characteristic is described as a "critical indicator" if it *must be present* to make the diagnosis. A defining characteristic is described as "major" if it is *usually* present when the diagnosis exists. A defining characteristic is de-scribed as "minor" if it provides supporting evidence for the diagnosis but may not be present.

Related factors. Related factors are conditions/circumstances that contribute to the development/maintenance of a nursing diagnosis.

Risk factors. Environmental factors and physiologic, psychologic, genetic, or chemical elements that increase the vulnerability of an individual, family, or community to an unhealthful event.

IV. Literature support

A narrative review of relevant literature (theoretical and data-based) is required to demonstrate the existence of a substantive body of knowledge underlying the proposed diagnostic concept. Literature citations (or current research) for each defining characteristic, related factor, or risk factor must be included. Differentiation of major from minor defining characteristics must be logically defended and supported by clinical data.

V. Validation

The validity of a nursing diagnosis refers to the degree to which a cluster of defining characteristics describes a condition that can be observed or inferred in client-environment interactions. One or more descriptive studies and/or content validity indices (Fehring, 1986) are required for a diagnosis to be designated as validated. Higher forms of validity are desirable.

VI. Diagnostic statement

A diagnostic statement with associated outcome criteria and nurse-prescribed interventions must accompany the submission. A three-part statement (label, related factor[s], clinical cues) is required for actual diagnoses; a two-part statement (label and risk factors) is required for high-risk diagnoses; and a one-part statement (label) is used for wellness diagnoses.

VII. Qualifiers for diagnostic labels (suggested/not limited to)

Acute—Severe but of short duration
Altered—A change from baseline
Chronic—Lasting a long time; recurring; habitual; constant
Decreased—Lessened, lesser in size, amount, or degree
Deficient—Inadequate in amount, quality, or degree; defective; not sufficient; incomplete
Depleted—Emptied wholly or partially; exhausted of
Disturbed—Agitated; interrupted, interfered with
Dysfunctional—Abnormal; incomplete functioning
Excessive—Characterized by an amount or quantity that is greater than is necessary, desirable, or useful
Increased—Greater in size, amount, or degree
Impaired—Made worse, weakened; damaged, reduced; deteriorated
Ineffective—Not producing the desired effect
Intermittent—Stopping and starting again at intervals; periodic; cyclic
Potential for enhanced (for use with wellness diagnoses)—Enhanced is defined as made greater, to increase in quality or more desired

From McFarland GK & McFarlane EA. *Nursing diagnosis and intervention: planning for patient care* (2nd ed) St Louis: Mosby, 1993.

A nursing diagnosis requires nursing intervention. The purpose of identifying health problems and their etiologic factors is to plan nursing actions that will modify or change the patient's response. The statement "restricted mobility related to blindness" is inappropriate because blindness is not subject to change through nursing intervention. The nurse should assess for the response to the visual loss and specifically label it, not the deficit. The statement could be improved by writing "high risk for injury related to vision loss"; with this statement, the nurse can intervene by providing protection, orientation, and assistance in transfer with a clear intended outcome of preventing injury. The diagnosis should also reflect an unhealthy or potentially unhealthy state. It would be incorrect to use "anger" or "grieving" as a health problem because neither are necessarily unhealthful. Rather, identify the patient's unhealthy response, for example, "sleep-pattern disturbance" or "dysfunctional grieving." Nursing diagnoses should be patient centered rather than nurse oriented. Nursing diagnoses do not describe the staff's problem in coping with a patient. "Noncompliance related to postoperative ambulation," for example, could be restated to indicate the patient's response: "Activity intolerance related to postoperative incisional pain." Neither do the statements suggest illegal or unethical activity. "High risk for injury related to inappropriate placement of electrosurgical unit (ESU) dispersive pad" or "Impaired tissue integrity related to improper lithotomy positioning" have implications for blame and are inadvisable.

Avoid including treatments, tests, or equipment within the nursing diagnosis. The terms "Foley catheter," "cardiac monitor," "on heparin," or "wheelchair" do not reflect a patient's response to a health problem/life process and do not belong in a nursing diagnostic statement. Neither would it be appropriate to repeat a medical treatment or order in a nursing diagnostic problem statement.

Once assessment data have been collected and organized into patterns, and nursing diagnoses have been formulated, the perioperative nurse proceeds to the third step of the nursing process: the identification of desired patient outcomes.

Patient Outcome Statements

The interest in outcomes measurement has grown dramatically in the 1990s. Some of this interest has been fueled by perplexing and seemingly unexplainable variations in outcomes of care, resource utilization, and cost of care (Batalden, Nelson, & Roberts, 1994). Patient outcome measures come in many forms; desired patient outcomes as identified during patient care planning are the ones the nurse is accountable for and are identified from the nursing diagnosis. To be effective, outcomes should be observable, measurable, attainable, and focused on the patient's response rather than the nurse's actions. The purpose of specifying outcomes is to designate what the nursing actions and interventions are predicted to accomplish. Some outcome measures apply to a broad class of patients. The *Patient Outcomes: Standards of Perioperative Care* (AORN, 1995) has been published by the professional specialty organization and are recommended as a minimal data set in identifying and measuring the outcomes of perioperative patient care. These *Outcome Standards* are listed in Box 2-1 on p. 17.

Plan

The planning phase involves prioritizing the identified health problems and nursing diagnoses, designating the nursing actions to reach the desired patient outcome, and writing the plan itself.

Prioritizing. The refinement of Maslow's (1970) hierarchy of needs by Kalish (1983) into survival, stimulation, safety, love and belonging, esteem, and self-actualization is a useful framework for prioritizing patient problems or nursing diagnoses. Kalish identified the human needs for food, air, water, manageable temperature, elimination, rest, and pain avoidance as survival needs. When these needs are compared with common perioperative nursing diagnoses, it would appear from the following examples that the majority fit the survival description:

Need	Diagnosis
Food and water	Fluid volume deficit related to npo status; *or* High risk for fluid volume deficit related to estimated blood loss and intravenous replacement
Air	High risk for aspiration during recovery from general anesthesia
Temperature	Hypothermia related to exposure to cool environment
Pain	Pain related to awake status during local or regional anesthesia or related to surgical position

A major emphasis in perioperative nursing is safety for the patient through prevention of injuries related to burns, positioning, foreign body, or hemorrhage. These safety requisites, however, are secondary to the basic survival requisites noted earlier.

The nursing diagnoses prevalent in the preoperative and postoperative phases tend to be higher in the hierarchy and thus may be a lower priority for the perioperative nurse. The development of a plan of care for the patient scheduled for surgery cannot realistically incorporate every actual or potential problem. Priority decisions based on a conceptual or theoretical framework similar to that of Kalish or Maslow are an expectation of the perioperative nurse.

Planned nursing intervention. The etiology component of the nursing diagnosis provides direction for selecting interventions. For example, in the diagnosis "High risk for injury from retained foreign body related to open body cavity," the efforts of the perioperative nurse involve keeping an accurate count of needles, sharps, sponges, and instruments while the body cavity is open. Additional interventions may include when to do the counts or directions needed for incorrect counts.

Once interventions are specified, the plan should be documented in a written format acceptable to the health care facility, with a minimal of three headings such as the following:

Nursing diagnosis	Interventions	Desired outcome
High risk for infection related to invasive procedure	Implement and maintain principles of asepsis Determine wound classification Assess contributing factors Follow institutional protocol for room preparation	The patient is free of signs and symptoms of infection

A copy of the signed care plan is then attached to the patient's permanent record. A written plan clearly demonstrates knowledgeable forethought and analysis of patient needs.

Implementation

Preparing, acting, and documenting are the action words of the implementation phase of the nursing process. The nurse employs education, experience, and complex technical skills to activate a plan of care.

Many interventions in the operating room do not require independent nursing actions; rather they are interdependent. Interdependent nursing actions require the *collaboration* of an additional health care specialist(s) before the act can be completed; thus, they are often referred to as collaborative activities. That is, the physician or surgeon cannot reach the desired end without nursing action and/or the nurse requires a physician order to meet a patient need. Examples of collaborative action include monitoring and reporting diagnostic values outside the acceptable range, administering medications or intravenous replacement fluids, and following institutional protocol, routine, or procedure. Many institutions have begun applying critical path methods to the delivery of patient care. In an effort to coordinate and standardize clinical care, an interdisciplinary effort is used to identify the expectations of care, the events that are critical to a designated length of stay,

and methods that will improve the quality and cost-effectiveness of care delivery (Hofmann, 1993).

Delegation. Perioperative nurses are involved in patient care activities that require a clear understanding of nursing science and the clinical inquiry model of the nursing process. The registered nurse in the perioperative practice setting is accountable for the nursing process; nursing is a process-oriented profession. Nursing activities include tasks, but are not limited to them. The registered nurse is also involved in nonnursing tasks that relate to patient care. These tasks include activities such as environmental sanitation, sterilization, clerical activities, supply and equipment maintenance, stocking supplies, and running errands. During perioperative patient care episodes, nonnursing tasks and some nursing activities may be delegated to nonnursing personnel. Perioperative care partners, such as surgical technologists, have provided and will continue to provide valuable assistance as part of a team effort to achieve safe, effective, and high-quality patient outcomes for patients undergoing operative and other invasive procedures. When the perioperative nurse delegates activities and tasks, the registered nurse remains responsible for delegation, supervision, and evaluation of the delegated activities. Delegation should be based on patient complexity, criticality of the nursing diagnoses, and competence of the person to whom the activity or task is being delegated. State Boards of Nursing have defined the professional practice of nursing and inappropriate delegation of these acts may constitute the practice of nursing without a license. Although each definition may vary, broadly, acts such as initial patient assessment, identifying nursing diagnoses, establishing desired outcomes from these diagnoses, developing the plan of care, and evaluating the patient's progress toward outcome attainment constitute the practice of nursing. These core components of the nursing process require specialized knowledge, skill, and judgment. It is during the implementation of the plan of care that the nurse may decide to delegate. The American Association of Critical-Care Nurses (AACN, 1990) has suggested that the potential for harm, the complexity of the nursing activity, the required problem solving and innovation, and the predictability of the outcome be used as part of the decision grid for delegation. To that must be added the determination that the person to whom the activity or task is being delegated has the necessary qualifications and competencies to perform it.

The implementation phase is concluded when the nursing interventions and the patient's response to the interventions are documented. The *AORN Recommended Practices for Documentation*

(AORN, 1995) suggests the patient's operating room record should (1) reflect assessment and planning as well as identify patient outcomes, (2) depict intraoperative care and the results, and (3) show evaluation of care and its outcomes. Intraoperative documentation includes objective and subjective data about the patient, equipment and supplies provided, counts taken, drugs administered by the nurse and surgeon, fluid intake and output, safety measures implemented, and persons providing care. The written record testifies to the delivery of professional nursing care, provides a legal reference to the sequence of events as they occurred in the operating room, and encourages accountability through comparison with the standards of care. Chapter 4 provides an in-depth discussion of documenting patient care.

Evaluation

Evaluation completes the circle of the nursing process. It involves reassessment of the patient and formulation of judgments about the patient's progress toward the identified outcomes. It is a comparison of the actual outcomes with the desired outcomes. Documentation of the results of care cannot be in vague, ambiguous terms such as "poor," "fairly well," or "good." The meaning of these terms varies with each individual and could cause confusing interpretations of the reassessment. If nurses are to value or measure their success, they must evaluate the patient's response to nursing intervention objectively and regularly. Postoperative evaluation of intraoperative care may begin with the closure of the incision and end with a telephone or mail follow-up in 2 or 3 weeks. The process of evaluating care has a simple and direct relationship to the clarity and comprehensive nature of the nursing plan for care. If that plan is clear, with stated nursing diagnoses, interventions and actions, and outcomes, then it becomes the basis for evaluation. It is very difficult for evaluation to take place, or to be meaningful, when plans for care are not explicit, since such an evaluation attempts to somehow measure success or a positive outcome without knowing the intent of nursing care. The evaluative process should also enable nursing awareness of additional data on which to plan or adapt subsequent nursing care.

Specific guidelines for evaluation are usually devised by the health care facility. Evaluation can be formal or informal; based on observation; determined from data collected retrospectively; objective or subjective, or both. Chapter 2 provides some discussion of issues and directions in measuring and evaluating patient outcomes and quality in nursing care delivery.

SUMMARY

The components of assessment, diagnosis, outcome identification, planning, implementation, and evaluation have been explored to illustrate their essential characteristics. As a model of clinical inquiry, the process is ongoing and nonlinear; steps overlap one another and decisions are made and then remade on the basis of reassessment. One area deserving further research is the study of the ways in which perioperative nurses make decisions related to nursing diagnoses and interventions (Hamers et al., 1994). Studies that focus on factors related to particular perioperative nursing diagnoses would further validate them and provide insight into the decision-making process in sorting clues and deciding on interventions. Even without such studies, however, the perioperative nurse's importance to the patient during a critical life event such as surgery requires a blend of scientific knowledge with the therapeutic use of self in an act of caring, supporting, teaching, and bonding (Mezey et al., 1994). To practice the professional discipline of perioperative nursing requires lifelong learning. The following chapters facilitate the application of such an intersubjective process by perioperative nurses.

References

American Association of Critical-Care Nurses. (1990). *Delegation of nursing and nonnursing activities in critical care.* Aliso Viejo, CA: The Association.

American Nurses Association. (1994). *Nursing: A social policy statement* (2nd draft). Washington, DC: The Association.

Association of Operating Room Nurses. (1995). Patient outcomes: Standards of perioperative care. In *AORN standards and recommended practices for perioperative nursing* (pp. 109-110). Denver: The Association.

Association of Operating Room Nurses. (1995). Recommended practices for documentation of perioperative nursing care. In *AORN standards and recommended practices for perioperative nursing* (pp. 137-140). Denver: The Association.

Association of Operating Room Nurses. (1995). Standards of perioperative clinical practice. In *AORN standards and recommended practices for perioperative nursing* (pp. 91-94). Denver: The Association.

Batalden PB, Nelson EC, & Roberts JS. (1994). Linking outcomes measurement to continual improvement. *Journal on Quality Improvement, 20*(4), 167-177.

Bottoriff JL & Morse JM. (1994). Identifying types of attending: Patterns of nurses' work. *Image—the Journal of Nursing Scholarship, 26*(1), 53-60.

Carpenito LJ. (1992). *Nursing diagnosis: Application to clinical practice.* Philadelphia: JB Lippincott.

Gordon M. (1993). *Manual of nursing diagnoses, 1993-1994.* St. Louis: Mosby.

Hamers JPH, Abu-Saad HH, & Halfens RJG. (1994). Diagnostic process and decision making in nursing: A literature review. *Journal of Professional Nursing, 10*(3), 154-163.

Hofmann P. (1993). Critical path method: An important tool for coordinating clinical care. *Journal on Quality Improvement, 19*(7), 235-246.

Kalish R. (1983). *The psychology of human behavior* (5th ed.). Monterey, CA: Brooks/Cole Publishing.

Kim MJ, McFarland GK, & McLane AM. (1995). *A pocket guide to nursing diagnoses* (6th ed.). St. Louis: Mosby.

Kleinbeck SVM. (1978). Soaping the preoperative interview. *AORN Journal, 28,* 1031-1035.

Kleinbeck SVM. (1989). Prevalent perioperative nursing diagnoses: A classroom research project. *AORN Journal, 49,* 1613-1625.

Koldjeski D. (1993). A restructured nursing process model. *Nurse Educator, 18*(4), 33-38.

Maslow A. (1970). *Motivation and personality.* New York: Harper & Row.

Mezey M, et al. (1994). The patient self-determination act: Sources of concern for nurses. *Nursing Outlook, 42*(1), 30-38.

Munhall PL. (1993). "Unknowing": Toward another pattern of knowing in nursing. *Nursing Outlook, 41*(3), 125-128.

Seifert PC. (1994). *Cardiac surgery.* St. Louis: Mosby.

Swanson KM. (1993). Nursing as informed caring for the well-being of others. *Image—the Journal of Nursing Scholarship, 25*(4), 352-357.

Wolf ZR, et al. (1994). Dimensions of nurse caring. *Image—the Journal of Nursing Scholarship, 26*(2), 107-111.

Chapter 2

The Relationship of Outcomes Management and Performance Assessment to Improvement

Jane C. Rothrock

There is no more silly or universal question scarcely asked than this, "Is he better?" . . . What you want are facts, not opinions—for who can have any opinion of any value as to whether the patient is better or worse, excepting the constant medical attendant, or the really observing nurse?

NIGHTINGALE, 1860

*H*istorically, the nursing profession has provided firm leadership in promoting high-quality patient care in the nation's hospitals. During the past few decades, this effort has intensified. Although nursing's achievements are noteworthy, there is little room for complacency in defining and measuring quality and evaluating its effect on patient outcomes. In today's rapidly changing health care environment, resource limitation, changing reimbursement incentives, issues of liability, and increased competition for patients have made quality of health care a major public-policy issue. There is a perva-

sive demand for greater public accountability of hospitals, nurses, physicians, and other health care providers (Markson & Nash, 1994). This demand comes from patients, accrediting bodies, the government, and third-party payors, as well as from within the institution. Concern about the quality of care focuses not only on improving quality; there is simultaneous concern about maintaining quality while reducing costs. The challenge to provide and monitor quality on behalf of the diverse groups that demand it begins with the following questions: "What is quality?" and "How is quality measured?"

DEFINING AND MEASURING QUALITY

Defining quality and assessing institutional outcomes and performance in relationship to it are not easy tasks. Quality is an elusive concept, the perceptions of which may vary. Definitions of quality are inextricably intertwined with societal, professional, and patient expectations. Society may expect improvements in the overall health of the population or some segment of the population. Improvements in the rate of infant mortality, in cancer detection and treatment, and in long-term care facilities are some common societal expectations. Professional concern with quality may relate to societal concerns or may focus on issues that seem less important to society. For example, the professional may prize shortened lengths of stay as an indicator of improved quality; society, however, may see decreased lengths of stay as a burden and drain on family resources because care that was previously included in the hospital stay must be provided by the family or community. The patient may define improved quality as a successful outcome from a specific health intervention or the absence of complications, or in terms of the promptness with which requests were met, the palatability of meals, and the attractiveness of the environment. Without clear delineation of what is meant by quality, it cannot be definitively assessed. Nonetheless, the urgent need persists for health care professionals and the institutions in which they work to monitor and improve the quality and effectiveness of health care within society (Institute of Medicine, 1994).

Quality of Care Measures

Quality of care measures generally fall into three categories: outcome measures, process measures, and structural measures.

Structure. Structural measures reflect the setting in which care is provided and the nature of the resources assembled to provide care. For perioperative nursing this component may be defined as providing patient care within an environment that is conducive to its effective and efficient administration; the AORN *Standards of Perioperative Administrative Practice* are a useful framework for a structural model standard. From an administrative viewpoint, structural measures are attractive for measuring quality of care. Much of the information they require can be readily gathered from existing data sources or inspection of the perioperative suite. The basic assumption underlying the use of structural measures is if the structure is optimal—that is, all standards are being met—then the appropriate processes will follow and outcomes will be maximized (LoGerfo & Brook, 1988). Although this assumption cannot be accepted unequivocally, some level of

structure must be obtained, maintained, and evaluated. Such structural criteria as peer review, verification and credentialing of nurses' continuing education, protocols for fire safety, and so on, are necessary if adequate processes are to occur. Nonetheless, good structure does not serve as a stand-alone correlate of good care.

Process. Process measures reflect what was conducted. For perioperative nursing, this component may be defined as meeting the needs of the patient in a caring manner and conforming to established standards of nursing practice; the AORN *Standards and Recommended Practices for Perioperative Nursing* are a useful framework for studying some of the processes of perioperative patient care. AORN has elaborated the processes of care to mean more than just what was performed; there is an integration of the notions of content of care, or activities performed, with the sequence of activities as contained in the standard nursing process framework, with the affective and interpersonal aspects of meeting the patient's needs in a caring manner.

In the early 1990s, many quality-improvement activities stressed the study of processes to understand them and simplify them; many models for process simplification, such as plan-do-study-act, were implemented as interdepartmental teams worked together in brainstorming, flow-charting, and using quality tools to improve patient care processes. Process measures have considerable attraction as indicators of quality; they are operationally easier to define, require less time for data collection, and depend less on extensive follow-up studies than what might be required in outcome studies. In a limited view, process studies depend on some agreed-on list of criteria, which are considered elements of good care. Data are subsequently reviewed for evidence of these criteria. A common criticism of such study is that it does not provide a strong enough link between process and outcome, which is important in overall determination of quality. The process improvement models seek to overcome such a limitation. In the mid-1990s, process performance measurement in health care continues to be underdeveloped, due, in part, to its complexity.

Outcome. Outcome measures reflect the results or effect of care processes on the health and well-being of patients and populations (*Health Outcomes Research Primer*, 1993). For perioperative nursing, this component may be defined as "improving the probability of achieving desired patient outcomes and/or reducing the probability of undesired outcomes as perceived by the patient and according to a well-defined and properly implemented practice" (Patterson, 1994); the *AORN Patient Outcomes: Standards for Perioperative Nursing* are useful as the beginning place for identifying such desired patient outcomes. Chapter 7 demonstrates one method of integrating process and outcome standards for generic perioperative care planning. Box 2-1 presents the AORN patient outcome standards.

There are inherent problems with simply accepting the notion that outcomes are the best measure of quality of care. Outcomes depend on many variables (Fig. 2-1). Patients are not discrete disease entities; the outcome of dietary instruction and education after coronary artery bypass grafting (CABG), for example, cannot be solely measured as "good" based on reduction in serum cholesterol levels. Health status is multidimensional; it includes physical, emotional, cultural, spiritual, ethnic, and social aspects. Thus an independent assessment of the effect of dietary instruction on cholesterol levels in CABG patients is not a fair or good measure of the quality or content of the instruction if it does

---

Box 2-1 Patient Outcomes: Standards of Perioperative Care

The *Patient Outcome Standards for Perioperative Care* were developed by the AORN Nursing Practices Committee and approved by the AORN Board of Directors in November 1983.* In November 1991, these standards were renamed *Patient Outcomes: Standards of Perioperative Care* to reflect the philosophy that standards of care describe the desired results that a patient can expect to receive during surgical and other diagnostic or therapeutic intervention.

Patient outcomes are observable or measurable physiologic, psychosocial, and psychologic responses to perioperative nursing intervention. These outcome statements and accompanying criteria provide direction for judging patient responses. Patient outcomes result from care provided by the other members of the health care team as well as from independent nursing activities. The achievement of patient outcomes from care provided by the health care team is of primary concern for the perioperative nurse in planning, implementing, and evaluating care.

The outcome standards focus on high-risk areas for patients undergoing surgical, diagnostic, or therapeutic intervention where the patient's protective reflexes may be compromised. They reflect the nurse's scope of responsibility in all phases of the perioperative period. The individual perioperative nurse may use the standards to establish a data base to support current nursing practice or as a rationale for changes.

Standard I

The patient demonstrates knowledge of the physiologic and psychologic responses to surgical intervention.

Interpretive statement

The patient has a right to information regarding the operative procedure and potential physical and psychologic effects. The information is shared with the patient's family or significant others. The patient has the right to expect the assurance of privacy, confidentiality, and maintenance of personal dignity. This standard is most relevant in the preoperative phase, but may also be used for postoperative evaluation.

Criterion

Dependent upon physical and psychologic status, the patient:
1. Confirms, verbally or in writing, consent for the operative procedures
2. Describes the sequence of events during the perioperative period
3. States outcome expectations in realistic terms
4. Expresses feelings about the surgical experience

Standard II

The patient is free from infection.

Interpretive statement

Prevention of infection requires the application of the principles of microbiology and aseptic practice. Preexisting patient conditions can increase susceptibility to infection. Other factors independent of nursing care can contribute to the development of infections. Examples of these factors are:
- Type of operative procedure
- Systems transected
- Tissue trauma
- Wound classification (that is, clean, clean contaminated, contaminated, dirty)
- Length of procedure
- Implants
- Presence of devices (that is, urinary catheters, IVs, endotracheal tubes)

Criterion

Dependent upon physical and psychologic status, the patient will be free from infection following the operative procedure.

Standard III

The patient's skin integrity is maintained.

Interpretive statement

Skin integrity is assessed preoperatively. Existing conditions such as diabetes and obesity may compromise skin integrity. No anticipated alteration to skin occurs during the intraoperative phase.

Reprinted with permission from *AORN Standards and Recommended Practices.* (1994). Denver: The Association.
*Kneedler J. (1976). A standard—What is it and how to use it. *AORN Journal 23*, 551-554.

Continued.

Box 2-1 Patient Outcomes: Standards of Perioperative Care—cont'd

Criterion

Dependent upon physical and psychologic status, the patient is free from evidence of skin breakdown or altered state.

Standard IV

The patient is free from injury related to positioning; extraneous objects; or chemical, physical, and electrical hazards.

Interpretive statement

Prevention of injury requires application of the principles of positioning, knowledge of instrumentation and equipment, and the proper use of chemical agents.

Criterion

Dependent upon physical and psychologic status, the patient is free from injury during the intraoperative phase and any sequelae during the postoperative phase.

Standard V

The patient's fluid and electrolyte balance is maintained.

Interpretive statement

Continual monitoring of fluid losses and replacement therapy occurs during the intraoperative phase.

Decisions relating to replacement therapy are generally not within the scope of practice of the OR nurse.

Criterion

Dependent upon physical and psychologic status, the patient's:
1. Mental orientation is consistent with the preoperative level
2. Elimination processes correlate with activities related to the operative procedure
3. Fluid and electrolyte balance is consistent with preoperative status

Standard VI

The patient participated in the rehabilitation process.

Interpretive statement

The patient should be able to participate in his or her own care, decision making, and discharge planning, and expect a reasonable continuity of care.

Criterion

Dependent upon physical and psychologic status, the patient:
1. Identifies problem areas related to surgical experience
2. Performs activities related to care

Reprinted with permission from *AORN Standards and Recommended Practices*. (1994). Denver: The Association.

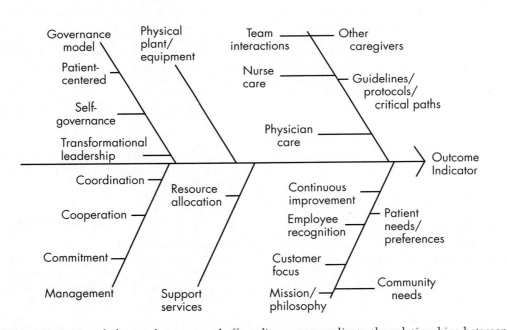

Fig. 2-1. Beginning skeleton of a cause-and-effect diagram to explicate the relationships between the structures and processes that affect the selected indicators of successful outcomes.

not take into account other factors that may influence a patient's dietary patterns and compliance with instructions.

Despite some of the problems with outcome measures, they can be used to identify variations in care, to compare the effectiveness of various treatments and procedures, to develop appropriateness criteria, and to measure health status and consumer preferences (*Health Outcomes Research Primer*, 1993). Adverse outcomes related to nursing interventions or treatment modalities can be monitored, as in electrosurgical burns. Wound infection rates, if they include intrinsic factors present in the patient and classification of the surgical procedure as part of surveillance, can be used as indicators of inadequate aseptic practices. When outcomes are used as indicators of quality of care, it is important that they take into account different levels in the quality of the process or content of care. By relating these two components of quality measurement, determinations can be made about the relationship of change or attempts at improvement. Thus it should be possible to determine if outcomes change when process changes, in what direction the change occurs, and the significance of the change. If a process change is expensive, for example, and produces only a minimal or statistically insignificant change in outcomes, then the process may not be worthy of implementation. Outcomes measurement in health care is in its early stages of development. Innovative projects like the Maryland Hospital Association's Quality Indicator Project (Kazandjian, et al., 1993) suggest that the interpretation of reports of outcomes be done carefully; they should not be used to interpret the quality of the institution's care, but instead as a document that presents various possible interpretations of the data and the necessary next steps in improving performance. O'Leary (1993) recommends that the limitation of using performance outcomes, which describe past performance, should be overcome by evaluating organizations against standards, which he predicts will sharply limit the randomness of certain outcomes.

Efficiency, Outcomes, and Quality

The cost of health care has become a national issue. In 1993, 14.4% of the gross national product was related to health care costs. This expenditure represented a 10% increase from the previous year (Himmelstein & Woolhander, 1994). The Health Care Financing Administration (HCFA) estimates that health care costs will continue to grow 9.2% until the year 2000 unless major reform is enacted.

With concern over the rising costs of health care, increased attention is given to efficient and inefficient use of health care resources. Efficiency of care reflects how much care of a given quality is provided for a specified cost. This measure can be expressed as net outcomes achieved per unit of cost. As efforts to improve quality of care are explored, frameworks relating quality, costs, and outcomes will be needed.

Critical paths. One way in which nursing is addressing the issue of effective use of human and material resources is through the development of critical paths. These are part of an outcomes management process that simultaneously attempts to deliver high-quality service, decrease service fragmentation, improve patient outcomes, and constrain costs. The multidisciplinary, collaboratively designed critical path for a specific patient population is initiated on patient admission. A diagnostic-related group (DRG) classification or a common event, such as the surgical experience, may be used. Moss and O'Connor (1993) describe a perioperative critical path that is used for documentation, identification of variances, cost management, and as a teaching tool. They note that such a tool not only improved patient and financial documentation, but also improved the outcome focus of perioperative nursing practice, reduced operating room time, improved nurse satisfaction with regard to control over care processes, assisted in the orientation of new staff members, and enhanced collaboration among disciplines. Although the critical path is just one example of how specialty nursing professionals can monitor the quality and efficient use of resources during care episodes, it is a frequently used method of outcomes management in the latter part of the 1990s. Leape and his colleagues (1993) further suggest that such protocols for care can prevent adverse events such as failure to employ indicated tests, failure to act on results of monitoring or testing, avoidable delays, and inadequate monitoring or follow-up treatment. Protocols and critical paths minimize oversights and errors, increasing their contribution to outcomes management.

Restructuring work. To achieve cost reductions while maintaining or enhancing quality, many health care institutions turn to the process of work restructuring (Smeltzer, 1993). Restructuring challenges the basic structures that separate care delivery by specialization and fragmentation of work processes. Restructuring and redesigning these processes improve measures of performance such as cost, quality, and service. Processes, not organizations, should be the focus of restructuring. Restructuring requires a strategic examination of what patients need and whether those needs are being met, and then building processes and a surrounding organizational system specifically designed to meet the identified needs. As processes are examined, non–

value-adding activities are eliminated; thus the demands of the care and work processes determine the size and composition of the work force. However, to be done correctly, efforts to restructure and redesign care-delivery processes must focus on mechanisms for developing interventions that meet patient needs as perceived by the patient, not by the provider. This has led to the terms "patient-focused care" and "patient-centered care." An emerging work-force issue, restructuring spurred debates in 1994 on appropriate staffing ratios and skill mixes. The nursing community identified a comprehensive strategic plan linking cost, quality, and staff mix with patient outcomes. As part of the plan, a research agenda was called for that would demonstrate the effectiveness of professional nurses in maintaining and/or improving patient outcomes (Ketter, 1994).

Practice guidelines. Unexplained variance in the style, delivery, and costs of health care coupled with the seemingly uncontrollable rise in health care expenditures have contributed to interest in developing scientifically based practice guidelines. Hastings (1993) defines a guideline as a tool to inform both practitioners and patients, to modify behavior (by improving health care decision making), and to negotiate health care treatment choices and options. Although there are numerous methodologies for developing these guidelines, and criteria by which to evaluate their attributes, the need is explicit for guidelines that are outcome based. Clearly, in such a framework, the guideline is linked to the outcome that needs to be improved (or prevented). Both qualitative (consensus development by experts) and quantitative (direct and indirect scientific evidence) methods are synthesized to predict the effect of an intervention on an outcome (Owens & Nease, 1993). For practice guidelines to be effective, however, they must be acceptable to providers, widely disseminated, and used in the day-to-day practice of care delivery. Then they must be linked with the improvement of that care delivery if they are to have their intended effect (Kibbe, Kaluzny, & McLaughlin, 1994).

Performance improvement and risk management. Early risk-management programs were modeled after those established in industry. They were often poorly implemented, widely misunderstood, and caused frustration and confusion among health care workers. Risk management has as its primary and foremost aim the reduction of unplanned or unexpected financial loss to an institution. In the traditionally nonprofit health care industry, such a mission appeared selfish and incongruent with the broad institutional mission of relieving pain and suffering of patients. In an environment that highly prized improving patient care, the financial considerations of the risk manager appeared unenviable and inconsistent with the altruism that characterized health care delivery.

Risk management, in its broadest sense, is related to and concerned with quality of care. This link is especially evident in the high-tech environment of operating rooms. Risk-management departments work in part to prevent new technology from overpowering the nursing staff's ability to work with and safely use new technologic developments. In ensuring that safety accompanies the introduction of new technologies, both patients and staff are protected, and high quality is attained. As exposure to new risks in facilities occurs, risk managers work to identify, measure, handle, and control risks. This requires a complex articulation and integration of tasks, functions, and decisions. Performance assessment and improvement should not be perceived as a minor component of risk management, but as a full, complementary partner in the facility's excellence-ensuring activities. To do this, Penchansky and Macnee (1993) recommend a reconceptualization of the quality-risk management link that focuses on five attributes of care delivery processes: the appropriateness of care, its proficient delivery, its coordination, amelioration of existing problems, and satisfaction of patients. Managerial responsibilities include defining desired performance by setting standards, measuring the performance, and maintaining or improving it. Activities included within these areas integrate ensuring quality and containing costs. Data collection efforts that measure performance and assess risk include occurrence screening, incident reports, utilization analyses, satisfaction surveys, patient complaints analyses, clinical outcome reviews, malpractice claims analyses, and benchmarking studies. With these essential measurement processes, the interface between management of risks and assessing performance can assist in the identification of areas of future research to further reconceptualize the activities of performance improvement and risk management in ensuring high-quality care while ameliorating the consequences of poor outcomes.

CURRENT INFLUENCES ON QUALITY-OF-CARE MEASUREMENT

It has become increasingly necessary to develop a continuing nursing and health care focus on assessment, monitoring, and improvement of the quality-of-care. Recent developments in health policy have given impetus to the quality of care movement. Development and implementation of financing mechanisms such as prospective payment and capitation have affected the quantity of services, raising questions about the effects of such mechanisms on the quality of services rendered. Information on variation among hospitals or providers in costs, processes, and outcomes of care has raised questions about the clinical appropriateness of such variation. The Joint Commission on Accreditation of Healthcare Organizations requires routine reporting of indicators of quality of care. The health care community is inescapably going to be involved in collecting data to address these issues. Society is beginning to expect such specified data. Both state and federal reform movements rely on the existence of some formal mechanism for reporting standards for clinical quality, service, access, and efficiency (Lansky, 1993). Basic tenets of the measurement mandate include the maintenance of an ever-repeating cycle of improvement with health care professionals who are committed to meeting and exceeding patient expectations for satisfaction with care delivery and improved health status (Davies, et al., 1994). Improvement efforts must then be linked closely with ongoing research on medical outcomes and clinical effectiveness (Cohen, 1994).

The Joint Commission on Accreditation of Hospitals

In 1917 the American College of Surgeons established the Hospital Standardization Program. The following year, a "Standard of Efficiency" was published. Of 692 hospitals surveyed, only 89 met the standard. In December of 1919, five official standards were accepted for hospitals seeking approval under this program. Known as the "Minimum Standard," it defined factors considered integral to proper care and treatment of hospitalized patients. With the establishment of these standards, the accreditation process was begun. The intent was, and continues to be, to focus on issues that protect and promote quality of care. By 1950, 3290 hospitals were approved; this represented over half the hospitals in the United States. It became obvious to the American College of Surgeons that the size and scope of the program would continue to grow and change. In 1951, the Joint Commission on Accreditation of Hospitals (JCAH) was formed as an independent, nonprofit organization.

In 1966 the JCAH undertook a major revision of the standards to reflect optimal, achievable levels of care, rather than essential minimums. These were published in the 1970 *Accreditation Manual for Hospitals*. These standards maintained the early approval focus on review and evaluation of quality of care. However, the process of evaluation within the institution itself was often informal, subjective, and dependent on the individual practitioner's knowledge and experience in evaluating records and observing the performances of others. Thus, in the

1970s, the use of systematic review procedures with objective and valid measurement criteria became common elements for assessing quality of care. Medical audits were promoted by JCAH; as a result, outcome-oriented audits began to be conducted throughout the country. Although the intent of these audits was quality assurance, it appeared that institutions were often preoccupied with the audit requirement rather than quality of care itself (Roberts, Coale, & Redman, 1987).

To reconcile this problem, in 1979 the Joint Commission published a new quality assurance standard for hospitals. The intent of this standard was to invest meaning in quality assurance activities by integrating quality assurance into the management systems of health care facilities. Nonetheless, the structure and function standards by which accreditation was determined only ensured that the health care institution was *capable* of delivering high-quality care; the actual determination of whether that care was effectively or ineffectively provided was not necessarily a part of data collection. In 1985 the JCAH embarked on a broad set of initiatives to address the complex measurement of quality of care. Two important aspects were substantial emphases on clinical performance and management performance. One of the expected results was that the medical and administrative leadership of a health care facility would become aware and responsive to the quality-of-care issues they faced in light of the results of clinical monitoring.

Joint commission definition of quality. In 1989 the Joint Commission on Accreditation of Healthcare Organizations approved an official definition of patient care quality as "the degree to which patient care services increase the probability of desired patient outcomes and reduce the probability of undesired outcomes, given the current state of knowledge," which is still their definition in 1994 (Patterson, 1994). Thus the Joint Commission has directed the attention of health care organizations and health care professionals to the delivery of high-quality care through regular monitoring of clinical performance and patient outcomes. By 1995 the Joint Commission's intent became the formation of a system for more effective and accurate measurement of the health care organization's performance (Box 2-2) through the use of a systematic schema for planning, designing, measuring, assessing, and improving outcomes in all important institutional functions, processes, and activities that are undertaken in support of the institution's patient care mission.

In addition to a focus on performance, the Joint Commission instituted an Indicator Measurement System (IMSystem), in which organizations

Box 2-2 Improving Institutional Performance

The organization has a planned, systematic, organization-wide approach to designing, measuring, assessing, and improving its performance of processes in all patient care and organizational functions.

The process must enable collection of data needed to:

- Design and assess new processes
- Assess the dimensions of performance relevant to functions, processes, and outcomes
- Measure the level of performance and stability of important existing processes
- Identify areas for possible improvement of existing processes
- Determine whether changes improved the processes

Adapted from Patterson CH. (1994). *Joint Commission focus on important functions: The management of human resources. Emerging Issues*, Chicago: National Council of State Boards of Nursing.

Table 2-1 Using clinical indicators to improve performance of laparoscopic cholecystectomy (lap chole)

Process	Application to lap chole
1. Identify area requiring assessment	Laparoscopic cholecystectomy
2. Determine study objective	Appropriate use for symptomatic gallstone patients
3. Identify practice guidelines or standards	Literature review
4. Evaluate practice parameters	Safety, efficacy, efficiency
5. Select and modify practice parameters	Two are selected: qualifications/training of physicians and procedural complications
6. Develop clinical indicators to measure	Did surgeons who perform lap choles assist or receive supervision before performing their first unsupervised procedure? Are their complication variances related to different training?
7. Assess current practice	Mail survey regarding training. Do retrospective review of lap chole patient records for complications and length of stay. Analyze findings.
8. Provide feedback on results	Make recommendations based on findings
9. Assess modified practice and outcomes	Re-review in 6 months
10. Review relevance of clinical indicators and practice parameters	Revise guidelines in 1 year, if indicated

Adapted from Bernstein SJ & Hilborne LH. (1993). *Journal on Quality Improvement*, 19(11), 507-508.

could voluntarily enroll beginning in 1994. Participating institutions submit data to the Joint Commission via electronic networks every quarter. The Joint Commission, in return, provides the institution with comparative reports, reflecting the institution's performance against that of all other participants. These "report cards" are also issued for each indicator used by the institution. Once the value of these data have been demonstrated in the accreditation process, they will become an integral part of that process (Nadzam, et al., 1993).

Clinical indicators, when they are linked to patient outcomes, become powerful tools for assessment of quality and for institutional benchmarking. Some indicators, such as mortality and morbidity data, do not directly depict quality of clinical performance, but instead raise questions about quality of care by acting as screens or flags. Problem investigation and analysis are then required. Indicators are grouped into two broad categories. *Sentinel-event indicators* identify events or phenomena that always require further investigation and analysis. *Aggregate-data indicators* usually measure an event that is expected to occur with some frequency, can express data on either processes or outcomes, provide an early warning of performance areas requiring attention, can be either desirable or undesirable, and guide the organization in improving norms of performance (Nadzam, et al., 1993). When linked to outcomes management, clinical indicators may fo-

cus on a clinical area that requires assessment or potential improvement (Finlan & Zibrat, 1994). Table 2-1 presents an example of a process for integrating clinical indicators and performance improvement in laparoscopic cholecystectomy (Bernstein & Hilborne, 1993).

Benchmarking. Health care institutions and health care providers are working on methods to compare their practices, processes, and outcomes with other organizations to discover "best practices." Many of the basic ideas on which benchmarking is founded have existed for years; the Japanese word "dantotsu," meaning to be the "best of the best," captures its essence (Camp & Tweet, 1994). Two general types of benchmarking are used, depending on the level of analysis desired. *Comparative benchmarking* allows comparison of the organization's performance against that of competing organizations by focusing on key measures and indicators, hence the term "comparative" or "competitive." This type of benchmarking may also be used internally by the institution. In multihospital benchmarking, the group selects the measures to be compared and then each institution collects specific measurement data. Green (1992) suggests data sources for indicators that include patient records, laboratory reports, incident reports, medical logs, financial data, patient satisfaction surveys, autopsy reports, infection control reports, utilization review findings, and direct observation and measurement. Results of comparative data analysis can suggest to the institution ways in which various improvement opportunities can be approached. A compelling comparative benchmarking effort is the Health Plan Employer Data and Information Set, a core set of health plan performance measures covering quality, access, patient satisfaction, membership, and finance to assess health plan performance. Currently in the second version, these performance measures may ultimately be used as "report cards" on the quality of care provided by various competing health plans (Corrigan & Nielson, 1993).

In *process benchmarking*, comparative data analysis begins the process but then involves evaluation of processes (Patrick & Alba, 1994). Core processes are selected that drive critical functions. The numerous steps and procedures involved in each process are referred to as "practices." By the evaluation of processes, the institution begins to identify best practices.

Through such performance assessment and improvement processes, health care organizations should be able to determine patient care quality via outcome determination.

Federal Initiatives

In the mid-1960s the U.S. government wrote its conditions for participation in Medicare. By 2025 one in five Americans will be over 65 years of age. The segment of the population over 85 years old is growing at a faster rate than any other. The rate of surgery for people 90 years old and over has increased almost 5 times in the late 1980s. Clearly, the government's concern will be directed not only toward quality of and access to care, but also toward restraining the escalation of health care costs and improving long-term care for the elderly and infirm.

Research on health services has uncovered wide variations in the types and amounts of care furnished to individuals with apparently similar conditions. This has become front-page news and of great interest to health consumer groups. Questions have been raised as to whether variations in practice represent patient needs, due consideration to alternative treatments, or physician practice styles, and whether the variations are appropriate or inappropriate. These findings have led policy makers, health care providers, insurers, and consumers to believe that improvement may be possible in many currently accepted practice variations through outcomes-based research.

Patient outcomes research. In an amendment to the Omnibus Budget Reconciliation Act of 1986, P.L. 99-509, the National Center for Health Services Research and Health Care Technology Assessment (NCHSR) was authorized to establish a patient outcome assessment research program (POARP). This Center became the Agency for Health Care Policy and Research (AHCPR) in 1989. Within its mission, AHCPR promotes research on patient outcomes of selected medical treatments and surgical procedures for the purpose of assessing their appropriateness, necessity, and effectiveness. The largest AHCPR-funded outcomes studies are the Patient Outcomes Research Team (PORT) projects. These involve 5-year studies with experts from different clinical or scientific fields who conduct multisite research. Each PORT study is designed to identify and analyze outcomes and costs of alternative practice patterns for specific conditions, to determine the best treatment strategy, and to develop the best ways of reducing inappropriate variations. The agency also conducts other outcomes-related studies.

Cost, quality, and access research. Through its program of health services research, the AHCPR continues to be responsible for gathering and analyzing key health data. The 1994 federal budget increased by $8 million funding for research on "cost, quality, and access," the new name for what was previously known as "general health services research." This program funds a broad range of studies, from interactions between cost, quality, and access to the successful characteristics of quality-improvement programs, the effects of medical liability, managed care, state health reform initiatives, and various financing and reimbursement options.

President Clinton's 1994 budget also boosted funding for health services research for the outcomes research program, the Medical Treatment Effectiveness Initiative (MEDTEP) by $12 million. This funding increased projects in effectiveness research, development of clinical practice guidelines, development of data bases for research, and dissemination of guidelines and research findings (MEDTEP Budget Increases, 1993).

Clearly, there is a clarion call on the part of the federal government to balance quality of care, access to care, cost of care, and the federal budget.

NURSING INITIATIVES

Patient outcomes research has the potential to save lives, improve the quality of care, increase and maintain patients' functional abilities, and conserve resources. Nursing has been and continues to be interested in quality-of-care issues and patient outcomes. Perhaps one of the reasons this is so stems from the similarity between the clinical process of nursing and the quality process; important similarities include a scientific combination of theory and fact, systematic analysis of variation, research, the refinement and use of measurement methodologies, and the development of a collaborative professional community (Berwick, 1992).

Nightingale's Contribution to Improving Outcomes

In February of 1855 mortality in the main British hospital in Crimea was staggering. Death resulted from diseases such as cholera, typhus, dysentery, scurvy, and widespread malnutrition. In March of that year, Florence Nightingale initiated sanitary improvements; mortality improved significantly. By the end of the war, mortality among all of the troops in Crimea was two thirds of what it was for the troops at home, which led Nightingale to push for domestic reforms. Using her statistics, which compared mortalities for soldiers at home with those of civilians in the same age groups, she was able to effect formal investigations of military health care (Aiken, 1988). Her recommendations for reform were instituted, and both quality and outcomes of care were improved.

Nursing's Research Agenda

In 1989, a nursing conference to explore nursing resources and patient care delivery came to the general conclusion that the biggest deficit in quality was the inability to link nursing care to patient outcomes. Some of the items and questions resulting from this conference that continue to deserve the attention of nurse scientists are presented in Table 2-2.

Mullinix (1988) proposed a research focus on the effects of nursing care on outcomes such as mortality, complications, infection rates, readmissions to health care facilities, and loss or gain in functional status. Giovanetti (1988) reaffirmed the need for development of valid and reliable measures of the outcomes of nursing care in both acute and long-term facilities. She further advocated studies linking nursing resource (time) and skill mix to costs and quality of nursing care. One of the problems with staffing methods has been their failure to explore measures of the outcomes of nursing care based on staff mix. That has left nursing unable to identify or defend differences in care required and actual care

Table 2-2 Nursing's quality and outcomes research agenda*

Item/question	Proposer
What are the effects of nursing care outcomes: mortality, complications, infection rates, readmissions to hospitals, loss or gain in functional status?	Mullinix
The development of reliable and valid measures of the outcomes of nursing care	Giovannetti
Studies linking nursing resource (time) and skill mix to costs and quality of nursing care	Giovannetti
Studies linking nursing diagnoses with staffing coefficients and diagnosis-related groups per patient and per patient day	Giovannetti
An evaluation of the validity and reliability of outcome screens for the assessment of health care, quality of care, and other intended uses of these measures needs to be undertaken	Hegyvary
The relationship of (1) alternative approaches to resolving the nursing shortage and providing patient care, and (2) the effects on patients and costs of hospital services requires further examination, along with studies regarding the prevalent patterns of nursing care and the alternative structures, processes, and outcomes with altered patterns of care delivery	
What is the impact of nurse education on patient outcomes and health care costs?	Higgerson
What is the impact of various RN, LPN, and nursing assistant staff mixes on patient care outcomes and costs?	Higgerson
What is the effect of a multidisciplinary team approach on patient care outcomes and costs? Can cause and effect be separated?	Higgerson
What is the effect of a generalist versus a specialized nurse on patient care outcomes and costs?	Higgerson

*Research agenda relating to quality care and patient outcomes that were identified at the State-of-the-Science Invitational Conference: Nursing Resources and the Delivery of Patient Care, sponsored by the National Center for Nursing Research, National Institutes of Health, and Health Services Research Association, February 18-19, 1988.

given, beyond a professional consensus of what level of care is needed. Costs of health care personnel range from 60% to 70% of the institutional budget. Therefore studies linking nursing diagnoses with staffing coefficients and diagnosis-related groups per patient and per day of stay become important in providing adequate staff mix in light of cost-containment strategies.

Need for Multiinstitutional Comparisons

Research about quality of care, although growing in its recognized importance, tends to be limited to single institutions. The next step needs to be multiple-site comparisons. Clinical practice and nursing care processes vary from institution to institution. Organizational variables in institutions also vary. Study of variables in the categories of overall hospital characteristics, patient care unit organization, psychosocial variables among staff, characteristics of leadership, and nursing education indicate that every category of variable has been significantly related to the quality of care (Hegyvary, 1988). There is a need for multiinstitutional comparative studies that take into account the simultaneous organizational variables and variations in clinical practice compared to total patient care and clinical outcomes. Generic design of multiinstitutional quality-of-care research will need to include identifying a patient management problem for study, selecting the target population, measuring the processes of care, measuring the outcomes of care, establishing the reliability and validity of the data, developing or selecting criteria and standards for high-quality care, and validating the criteria and standards (Wells, 1988).

Nursing Practice Standards and Guidelines

Specialty practice organizations like AORN and the American Nurses Association often undertake joint projects. Three initiatives underway include the development and improvement of nursing practice standards and guidelines, creation of data bases to support clinical practice, and nursing payment reform. Standards of nursing practice are authoritative statements that describe a level of care or performance that is common to the profession of nursing and by which the quality of nursing practice can be judged. For clinical nursing practice, standards of care describe competent practice through assessment, diagnosis, outcome identification, planning, implementation, and evaluation of outcomes. Standards of professional performance further explicate the nurse's professional role behaviors, including activities that relate to performance appraisal, education, collegiality, ethics, collaboration, research, and resource utilization. Similarly, nursing has a clear understanding of the importance of practice guidelines, which describe care processes and have the potential of improving both the quality of clinical and patient decision making (ANA, 1993). The suggested format for a clinical practice guideline is presented in Box 2-3. Jacox (1993) additionally recommends the adoption by nursing of the AHCPR guidelines that have relevance for the profession. For perioperative nurs-

---

Box 2-3 Recommended Format for Nursing Clinical Practice Guideline

I. Introduction—describe the nursing diagnosis/clinical condition, its scope (prevalence, population affected, settings where nursing treatment occurs), and its significance (variations in outcomes and cost affected by nursing practice)

II. Clinical Practice Guideline—identify the decisions that need to be made based on patient need/preference, assessment criteria that represent the nursing diagnosis/clinical condition, the requisite interventions, expected outcomes, and major exceptions or alternate management strategies and their linkages, and recommend documentation methods

III. Documentation of Guideline Development—identify organizations/associations involved, process used, evidence used (methods by which data were extracted from the literature, expert opinions, consensus agreement)

IV. Plan for Dissemination and Review—assess practice feasibility, identify dissemination methods, discuss implications for health care professionals and consumers, recommend further research, and make recommendations about periodic review of guideline

A glossary, references, and disclaimer/medical-legal statement conclude the format for nursing clinical practice guidelines.

Adapted from *Format for clinical practice guideline development.* (1991, 1992). Second working paper of the ANA Committee on Nursing Practice Standards and Guidelines, April 14, 1993, Washington, DC: the American Nurses Association.

---

ing, one of these guidelines is for acute pain management for patients undergoing operative procedures. Essential information from that guideline may be found in Box 2-4.

EVALUATION OF NURSING CARE

The important planning aspect of the nursing process is a coupling of outcomes with the interventions required to achieve them. Evaluation is the objective measurement of the effectiveness of the designated actions and interventions that have been purposively designed to achieve the desired outcome. The evaluation process is ongoing throughout each step of the nursing process. Each assessment and plan are reevaluated as new data are discovered and results of care reviewed. As new information is discovered or a change in the patient's status is observed, the ongoing assessment is analyzed and the validity of the nursing diagnoses is tested.

Abbreviated Pain Management Flow Chart

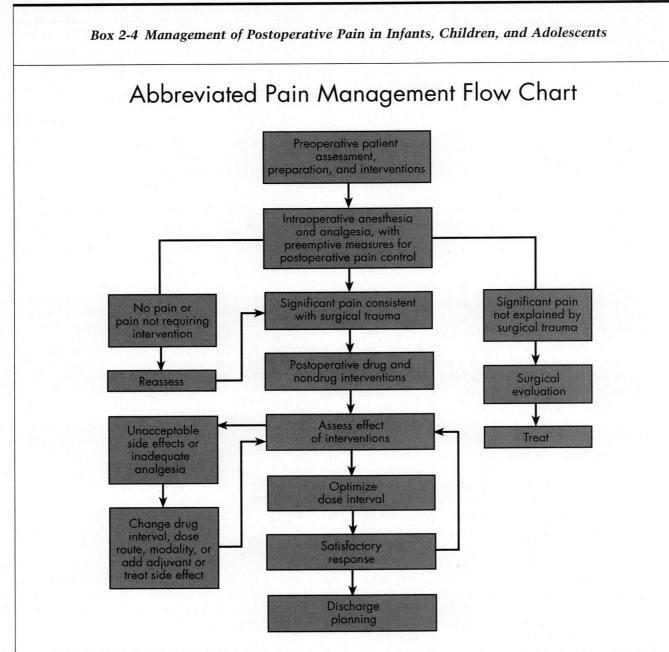

Nonpharmacologic Management of Procedure-Related Pain

Nonpharmacologic strategies can be used alone for less painful procedures, such as venipuncture, or as adjuncts to pharmacologic strategies for more painful procedures. Interventions are tailored to need, preferences, and coping style. The family can encourage and be helpful in facilitating the child's use of these strategies.

- For infants, sensorimotor strategies include pacifiers, swaddling, holding, and rocking.
- Cognitive/behavioral strategies include hypnosis; relaxation; distraction; music, art, and play therapy; preparatory information; and positive reinforcement. Rehearsal before the procedure may be helpful.
- Child participation strategies focus on involving children in age-appropriate decisions about the procedure and in activities related to its conduct.

- Physical strategies include the application of heat or cold, massage, exercise, rest, and immobilization.
- Older children and adolescents who find nonpharmacologic strategies helpful may prefer these strategies over pharmacologic agents for procedures that are not excessively painful.

Pharmacologic Management After Surgery

- Opioid and nonopioid analgesics are the mainstay of postoperative pain management. The approach varies with the child's age, medical condition, type of surgery, and expected postoperative course.
- Pain after minor surgery is usually managed with an oral or rectal nonsteroidal antiinflammatory drug or opioid analgesic (e.g., codeine) singularly or in combination.

Box 2-4 Management of Postoperative Pain in Infants, Children, and Adolescents—cont'd

- Pain after major surgery is managed with parenteral or regional opioids until the child can tolerate oral intake.
- Parent and child instruction in pain control after discharge is important.

Nonsteroidal Antiinflammatory Drugs (NSAIDs)

- Even when insufficient alone to control pain, NSAIDs have significant opioid dose-sparing effects and hence can be useful in reducing opioid side effect.
- NSAIDs must be used with care in patients with thrombocytopenia or coagulopathies and in those patients at risk for bleeding or gastric ulceration. However, acetaminophen does not affect platelet function, and some evidence exists that two salicylates (salsalate and choline magnesium trisalicylate) do not profoundly affect platelet aggregation.

Opioid Analgesics

- Opioid analgesics are the cornerstone for the management of moderate to severe acute pain. Effective use of these agents facilitates postoperative activities, such as coughing, deep-breathing exercises, ambulation, and physical therapy.
- Studies in adults have shown that opioid tolerance and physiologic dependence are unusual in short-term postoperative use in opioid-naive patients, and that psychologic dependence and addiction are extremely unlikely to develop after the use of opioids for acute pain. There is no known aspect of childhood development or physiology that indicates any increased risk of physiologic or psychologic dependence from the brief use of opioids for acute pain management.

Choice of Opioid Agent

- Morphine is the standard for opioid therapy. If morphine cannot be used because of an unusual reaction or allergy, another opioid such as hydromorphone can be substituted.
- Meperidine should be reserved for very brief courses in patients who have demonstrated allergy or intolerance to opioids such as morphine and hydromorphone. It is contraindicated in patients with impaired renal function or those receiving antidepressants of the monoamine oxidase (MAO) inhibitor class. Normeperidine is a toxic metabolite of meperidine and is excreted through the kidney. Normeperidine is a cerebral irritant, and accumulation can cause effects ranging from dysphoria and irritable mood to seizures, even in young, otherwise healthy persons.

Dosage and Schedule

- Titrate the opioid dosage and interval to increase the amount of analgesia and reduce the side effects when necessary. Children vary greatly in their analgesic dosage requirements and responses to opioid analgesics, and the recommended starting dosages may be inadequate.
- Use relative potency estimates to select the appropriate starting dosage, to change the route of administration (for example, from parenteral to oral), or to change from one opioid to another.
- Provide opioids around the clock or by continuous infusion rather than as needed (prn). A prn order is not recommended since it requires the child to communicate the presence of pain and the need for medication. Often children are unable or unwilling to initiate communication about pain. Further, a prn schedule produces delays in administration and intervals of inadequate pain control.
- Start with a dose of 0.02 to 0.04 mg/kg/hr when using a continuous infusion of morphine.
- Offer rescue doses for break-through or poorly controlled pain for children receiving intravenous infusions.
- Consider the use of patient controlled analgesia (PCA) for developmentally normal children 7 years and older.
- Consider writing orders so the child or parent may refuse an analgesic if the child is asleep or not in pain. However, remember that a steady state blood level is required in order for the drug to be continuously effective, and interruption of an around-the-clock dosage schedule (for example, during sleep) may cause a resurgence of pain as blood levels of the analgesic decline.

Route

- Administer opioids through the intravenous catheter (available for postoperative hydration) or orally. The intravenous route is suitable for bolus administration and continuous infusion (including PCA).
- Use intramuscular injections only under exceptional circumstances. They are painful and frightening for children.
- Use oral administration as soon as the patient can tolerate oral intake. It is convenient and inexpensive and is the mainstay of pain management in the ambulatory surgical population.

Other Pharmacologic Approaches

- Regional analgesia, including continuous infusions and intermittent doses of peridural local anesthetics and/or opioids, is used for children and may be particularly applicable for young infants as well as children with problems such as chronic lung disease.
- The administration of regional analgesia is best limited to specially trained and knowledgeable staff, typically under the direction of an acute or postoperative pain treatment service.

Acute Pain Management Guideline Panel. *Acute Pain Management in Infants, Children, and Adolescents: Operative and Medical Procedures. Quick Reference Guide for Clinicians.* AHCPR Pub. No. 92-0020. Rockville, MD: Agency for Health Care Policy and Research, Public Health Service, US Department of Health and Human Services.

Using the Nursing Process

The nursing process has been perceived as the means by which the scientific discipline of nursing practice can develop standards of care and outcomes to measure that care standard. One of the steps of the nursing process is development of nursing diagnoses. Specific and concise outcomes are derived from these diagnoses. If outcomes are specific, they provide a direct statement of the end result the nurse expects the patient to achieve. Nurses have traditionally included goal statements toward which their actions were directed. Often, however, those goals have been vague, nonspecific, and unmeasurable. Outcome statements with specified goals or criteria can serve as parameters for measuring achievement of the patient outcome. According to Guzzetta and Dossey (1992), outcome criteria are accurate statements of something that should (or should not) occur, the level and point in time at which it should occur, or something that is expected to occur as a result of care.

A major difficulty in developing outcome statements and standards is that nursing procedures are not well defined. Systematic use of the nursing process can lend consistency to nursing practice, thereby facilitating evaluation. Standards and outcomes of care provide a sound basis for amending actions and consistently defining nursing procedures. The use of standards and guidelines for evaluating the process of nursing care can become a basis for a unified data base for clinical nursing practice that can be compared among health care institutions across the country.

Because evaluation is an important component of the nursing process, it can assist in developing competencies and thereby affect the results of nursing care. The nursing process can be used as an important first step in identifying nurse competencies. The utilitarian test of nursing performance will be the documented results of nursing care. A major problem in defining outcomes of the care-delivery process is validating patient outcomes based on perioperative nursing care. Eventually, nursing care strategies can be linked to patient outcomes and cost. To evaluate cost-effectiveness, nursing must identify the desired patient outcomes and nursing interventions, determine the cost per unit of service and amount of service rendered, and evaluate the effect or outcome of the interventions on the target group. Clearly, the role of nurse advocacy must extend to the patient's financial welfare as part of outcome design and measurement.

Evaluation, then, is certainly not designed to determine whether nursing actions have been completed as prescribed in the care plan. Its primary goal is to determine whether successful patient outcomes have been achieved and to what degree. Using this framework for evaluation recognizes that it is really involved in all components of the nursing process. Evaluation can determine omissions in the nursing process and its effectiveness. If an outcome is not met, the nursing diagnosis and nursing actions are revised and a new outcome may be established according to a new priority. If an outcome is met, nursing actions used to achieve the outcome may still require evaluation in terms of cost effectiveness. Evaluation of patient care outcomes is a continuous process of refining and improving nursing practice.

Rethinking Care Plans

The nursing shortage of the 1980s precipitated an intensive and overdue discussion and review of the work of nurses and nursing. Much of this debate focused on common practices held sacred by the profession that might infringe on nurses' time for actual care delivery. In light of this desire to explore what might be unnecessary tasks, the time and work of developing the nursing care plan fell under close scrutiny. Sovie (1989) reviewed a study exploring the relationship between three types of nursing care plans and effects on patient outcomes. There was no significant difference in the use of a printed Kardex with physician's orders and a menu of nursing tasks, a standardized nursing care plan with provisions for individualizing the plan, or a Kardex that was a permanent part of the medical record and included nursing diagnoses, nursing orders, and dependent nursing functions (that is, derived from physician orders). Patient outcomes studied were length of stay, number of readmissions within 30 days, patient satisfaction, incidence of nosocomial infections, incident reports related to patient safety, number of analgesics and narcotics administered, and acuity level on discharge.

All of these patient outcomes have been of interest to nursing in the past and have been recommended to continue to be important measurement variables. The questions remain: If there is no significant difference in these outcomes, should nurses take time to develop a care plan systematically for every patient? Is this an essential activity in which every nurse must engage with every patient? Rather, if standardized care plans that allow individualization are deemed as effective as newly, repetitiously created ones, then would the nurse's time be better spent with the work of nursing care delivery? The results of one study cannot answer this question. Nonetheless, it deserves to be answered through replication studies.

Nursing will continue to be interested in patient care outcomes and their relationship to quality-of-care indicators, standards of care, productivity, and cost. Cost should not be viewed in isolation but linked to patient outcome. Patient care outcomes need to be identified and tools developed to measure them. Outcomes then need to be measured. Positive relationships need to be established between nursing interventions and enhanced patient outcomes. Toward this end, nursing leaders at the Invitational Conference for Exploring Nursing Resources and the Delivery of Patient Care recommended identification or development of a generic set of patient outcome indicators that would highlight the role of nursing in the achievement of those outcomes (National Center for Nursing Research, 1988). Using the AORN *Patient Outcomes: Standards for Perioperative Nursing* to begin validation, perioperative nurses have the advantage of starting their research efforts with a generic set of outcome criteria. With identification of nursing's role in achieving these patient outcomes through the development of generic care plans, such as those presented in Chapter 7, perioperative nurses may begin the important business of relating and evaluating clinical nursing practices and patient outcomes.

Summary

Sovie (1990) has challenged nursing to create new and better ways of providing nursing care by critically examining what needs to be done, what difference it makes in patient outcomes, and the best way to produce the desired results. To meet this challenge, information needs to be collected and analyzed to determine the relevance, progress, efficiency, effectiveness, and outcomes of nursing care. This interest is inherent in the profession of nursing and is part of its history; it is supported by influences external to the profession. With this heightened external environment, the questions have intensified. Nursing asks itself whether the nursing care delivered has achieved what it said it would do. The answer to this question lies in serious analysis and self-reflection. We need to determine what evidence there is that current processes of nursing care delivery work well. If these processes do not work, they must be restructured or redesigned. We need to evaluate existing data and collect whatever new data are required to emphasize characteristics of the nursing environment and their effect on enhanced patient outcomes. Outcomes need to be related and connected to stated goals and the requisite nursing care interventions designed to achieve them. It is senseless to measure an outcome if there is no statement of what the nurse expected or planned to occur. Unless our measure of success or lack of success in effecting positive patient outcomes allows us to make changes, there is no sense in doing it. We

would not consider something bought unless it had been sold. The analogy holds for nursing; how can we say something has been achieved if we have no evidence that something was done? Therein may lie the value of the care plan, in whatever form we decide is useful. Its value is not in the fact that it has been written, but rather it is evidence that a process was used to decide on what was to be done. Standardized care plans that collect uniform data on what was done allow us to begin seeing what we do, how well we do it in relation to agreed-on patient outcomes, and then improving it. By operationally defining nursing diagnoses through the process of care planning, the emphasis becomes collecting evidence that patients are meeting the defined outcomes, not writing the care plan. This is one way of understanding differences in patient outcomes and then finding and correcting whatever problems of quality underlie them.

References

Aiken L. (1988). *State-of-the-science invitational conference: nursing resources and the delivery of patient care.* Bethesda, MD: National Institutes of Health.

American Nurses Association. (1993). *Second working paper of the ANA committee on nursing practice standards and guidelines.* Washington, DC: The Association.

AORN Standards and Recommended Practices. (1995). Denver: The Association.

Bernstein SJ & Hilborne LH. (1993). Clinical indicators: the road to quality? *Journal on Quality Improvement, 19*(11), 501-509.

Berwick DM. (1992). The clinical process and the quality process. *Quality Management in Health Care, 1*(1), 1-8.

Camp RC & Tweet AG. (1994). Benchmarking applied to health care. *Journal on Quality Improvement, 20*(5), 229-238.

Cohen AB. (1994). Evaluating new ways of managing quality. *Journal on Quality Improvement, 20*(2), 90-96.

Corrigan JM & Nielson DM. (1993). Toward development of uniform reporting standards for managed care organizations: The health plan employer data and information set (version 2.0). *Journal on Quality Improvement, 19*(12), 566-574.

Davies AR, et al. (1994). Outcomes assessment in clinical settings: a consensus statement on principles and best practices in project management. *Journal on Quality Improvement, 20*(1), 6-16.

Finlan JK & Zibrat FS. (1994). Struggles and successes: Experiences of a Beta test site. *Journal on Quality Improvement, 20*(2), 49-56.

Giovanetti P. (1988). *State-of-the-science invitational conference: Nursing resources and the delivery of patient care.* Bethesda, MD: National Institutes of Health.

Green E. (1992). *Developing indicators, establishing thresholds—letting go of myths.* Annual Conference on Quality Assessment and Quality Improvement, New Orleans.

Guzzetta CE & Dossey BM. (1992). *Cardiovascular nursing: Holistic practice.* St Louis: Mosby.

Hastings K. (1993). A view from the Agency for Health Care Policy and Research: The use of language in clinical practice guidelines. *Journal on Quality Improvement, 19*(8), 335-341.

Health Outcomes Research Primer. (1993). Washington, DC: Foundation for Health Services Research.

Hegyvary S. (1988). *State-of-the-science invitational conference:*

Nursing resources and the delivery of patient care. Bethesda, MD: National Institutes of Health.

Himmelstein D & Woolhander S. (1994). *The national health program book: A source guide for advocates.* Monroe, MI: Common Courage.

Institute of Medicine Special Initiative: America's Health in Transition. (1994). Washington, DC: Institute of Medicine.

Jacox A. (1993). Addressing variations in nursing practice/technology through clinical practice guidelines methods. *Nursing Economics, 11*(3), 170-172.

Kazandjian VA, et al. (1993). Relating outcomes to processes of care: The Maryland Hospital Association's quality indicator project. *Journal on Quality Improvement, 19*(11), 530-538.

Ketter J. (1994). Restructuring spurs debate on staffing ratios, skill mix. *The American Nurse, 26*(7), 26.

Kibbe DC, Kaluzny AD, & McLaughlin CP. (1994). Integrating guidelines with continuous quality improvement: Doing the right thing the right way to achieve the right goals. *Journal on Quality Improvement, 20*(4), 181-190.

Lansky D. (1993). The new responsibility: Measuring and reporting on quality. *Journal on Quality Improvement, 19*(12), 545-551.

Leape LL, (1993). Preventing medical injury. *Quality Review Bulletin, 19*(5), 144-149.

LoGerfo JP & Brook RH. (1988). The quality of health care. In Williams JJ & Torrence PR (Eds.) *Introduction to health services.* New York: John Wiley & Sons.

Markson LE & Nash DB. (1994). Overview: public accountability of hospitals regarding quality. *Journal on Quality Improvement, 20*(7), 359-363.

MEDTEP budget increases $12 million. (1993). *HSR Reports,* 5.

Moss MT & O'Connor S. (1993). Outcomes management in perioperative services. *Nursing Economics, 11*(6), 364-369.

Mullinix C. (1988). *State-of-the-science invitational conference: Nursing resources and the delivery of patient care.* Bethesda, MD: National Institutes of Health.

Nadzam DM, et al. (1993). Data-driven performance in health care: the Joint Commission's indicator measurement system. *Journal on Quality Improvement, 19*(11), 492-500.

National Center for Nursing Research. (1988). *State-of-the-science invitational conference: Nursing resources and the delivery of patient care.* Bethesda, MD: National Institutes of Health.

Nightingale F. (1860). *Notes on nursing.* London: Harrison & Sons.

O'Leary DS. (1993). The measurement mandate: Report card day is coming. *Journal on Quality Improvement, 19*(11), 487-491.

Owens DK & Nease RF. (1993). Development of outcome-based practice guidelines. *Journal on Quality Improvement, 19*(7), 248-263.

Patrick M & Alba T. (1994). Health care benchmarking: A team approach. *Quality Management in Health Care, 2*(2), 38-47.

Patterson CH. (1994). *Re-engineering the environment: TQM beyond the walls.* Paper presented at the National Conference on Restructuring Care, Philadelphia.

Penchansky R & Macnee CL. (1993). Ensuring excellence: Reconceptualizing quality assurance, risk management, and utilization review. *Quality Review Bulletin, 19*(6), 182-189.

Roberts JS, Coale JG, & Redman RR. (1987). A history of the Joint Commission on Accreditation of Hospitals. *Journal of the American Medical Association, 258,* 936-940.

Smeltzer CH. (1993). Lessons learned: Implementing cost reductions and enhancing quality. *Nursing Economics, 11*(6), 373-375.

Sovie MD. (1989). Clinical nursing practice and patient outcomes: Evaluation, evolution, and revolution. *Nursing Economics, 7,* 79-85.

Sovie MD. (1990). Redesigning our future: Whose responsibility is it? *Nursing Economics, 8*(1), 21-26.

Wells KB. (1988). Quality-of-care research in mental health: Policy and personal perspectives. *Focus on Mental Health Services, 3,*1.

Chapter 3

Computerized Patient Care Record

Jeanette X. Polaschek

Hospitals have been purchasing computer-based systems for more than 3 decades, but despite their early adoption within hospital settings, computer-based applications designed for clinical use were not commonplace until the last decade. Around that time personal computers were introduced and the population as a whole gained affordable access to a flexible technology based on microprocessors. More recently, a fundamental shift in managing health care economics has spawned additional interest in providing clinicians with computer-based tools. Hospitals no longer operate independently of outpatient facilities and reimbursement mechanisms are shifting from a fee-for-service system to a capitated payment structure that emphasizes cost-effective utilization of justified services. Services are justified if their delivery is linked to high-quality patient outcomes. It is almost impossible to extract the information needed to compare documented delivery of service to patient outcomes from a system that stores patients' medical records on paper. Clinicians need to enter the information into a computer-based system that later supports the extraction of information for care management decisions.

Government agencies and regulatory bodies recognize that patient medical records need to be automated. The Health Care Financing Administration (HCFA) announced strong incentives to encourage hospitals to submit Medicare claims in a format based on the Electronic Data Interchange (EDI) standard (Work Group for EDI, 1992). The work is sponsored by the Department of Health and Human Services, which also sponsors a work group on the computerization of patient records (Work Group on Computerization of Patient Records, 1993). The Joint Commission on Accreditation of Healthcare Organizations (JCAHO) includes an entire section on information systems standards in the Agenda for Change Project. As of 1996 these standards are being incorporated into the hospital accreditation process, thereby solidifying the need to move to an automated record (JCAHO, 1987). The Computerized Patient Record Institute (CPRI) (Box 3-1) was formed as a result of the recommendations of a committee sponsored by the Institute of Medicine, the National Academy of Sciences, and the National Academy of Engineers (Institute of Medicine, 1991). The institute is involved with several efforts supporting the computer-based medical record. Its members include clinicians, insurance groups, vendors, academic institutions, and government agencies.

OPERATING-ROOM INFORMATION MANAGEMENT SYSTEMS

A computer system designed for use by an operating-room (OR) department is generally referred to as an "operating room information management system" or "OR system." When an OR department fully implements an OR system, much of their dependence on paper forms and manual processing procedures is eliminated. The OR System replaces the forms and procedures with an electronic highway that transmits the information to all individuals who need access. The OR system's software includes a range of applications that automate the following functions:
- Scheduling surgical procedures
- Tracking orders, receipt, and usage of physical inventory

Box 3-1 The Computer-Based Patient Record Institute

Work group products developed:
1. *Codes and structures:* drug coding systems for use in computer-based records
2. *CPR (computer-based patient record) demonstration projects:* compendium of cost/benefit literature
3. *Confidentiality, privacy, and legislation:* compendium of state laws on creation, authentication, and retention of electronic patient records
4. *Professional and public education:* a slide presentation for educating people about cardiopulmonary resuscitation (CPR); available for a one-time purchase or as a subscription for continual updates

The Computer-based Patient Record Institute was founded in January 1992. It is an organization of organizations. Participation in work groups is voluntary and membership in CPRI is not required. Perioperative nurses who are interested in joining one of the work groups may call the CPRI office at 1-800-382-2973.

• Documenting data collected by perioperative nurses
• Storing a permanent record of procedures performed and resources used

Purchase and installation of OR system products continue to increase. A recent survey reported that 61% of all hospital-based OR departments use a computer system (*OR Manager*, 1992). This figure is up 14% from the previous year. Of those reporting using computers, 76% had implemented scheduling applications, and 44% had implemented inventory management applications. There were currently 34 vendors offering an OR system product, with the bulk of the market share divided among three leading vendors (Dorenfest, 1992).

A typical configuration of the OR system's hardware and network structure is shown in Fig. 3-1. Computers are installed in locations that are accessible and convenient to the individuals responsible for data entry and review. They are routinely located in the scheduling office for booking procedures, in the materials coordinator's office for ordering and tracking of physical inventory, in the receiving area for entering receipt of incoming inventory, in the clinical areas for documentation by the nursing staff, and in administrative offices for reviewing historical information and generating summary reports. The cables connecting all the computers form a network, or electronic highway. The network enables users to share devices, such as printers, backup units, and file servers. File servers are computers specifically designed to store large volumes of data. The file server stores the OR system applications and the data bases that support those applications. The data base creates electronic links that allow information to be shared between files. The electronic highway enables users to run the OR system applications from any connected computer. Specialized devices are attached to the network that handle data transmission between computers and monitor the flow of traffic. When transmission problems occur, these specialized devices send warning messages to the OR system's network administrator. The network administrator manages the OR system and is responsible for network security.

Security for an OR system running on a network is achieved by restricted user access. Users gain access to the network by entering a personal password. Once the password is entered, the OR system knows what applications the user is permitted to run, what information the user is permitted to view, and what data fields the user is permitted to modify. Personal network sign-ons not only protect restricted data, they also make the system easier to use. Menu selections are tailored to the type of user. For example, the clerk in the receiving area chooses from a menu of inventory management applications, whereas an OR scheduler works from a selection of scheduling applications.

OR System Applications

OR systems generally include four applications that provide automated tools for managing four key processes of the OR department: scheduling, inventory management, perioperative documentation, and generating summary reports from a historical data base (Fig. 3-2). These four applications work in concert to automate much of the paperwork associated with daily management of an operating-room environment.

OR schedule management. The scheduling application manages the booking of surgical procedures, the associated functions of reserving OR resources, and the tracking of preadmission activities. Automated scheduling eliminates the paper-based appointment book and adds many features only possible using automated tools.

When a surgeon or a surgeon's office staff calls the OR department to schedule a patient, automation assists in several ways. If the physician has booking constraints, such as availability only during certain time intervals or weekdays, the OR scheduler can restrict the search for the next available time slot

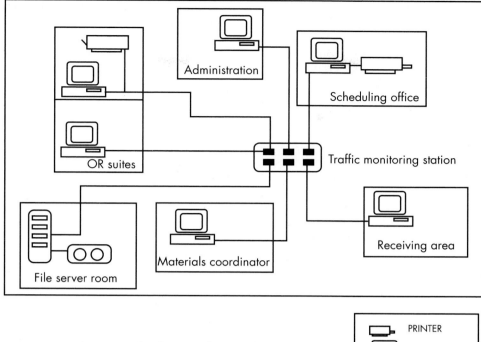

Fig. 3-1. OR system hardware and network configuration.

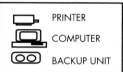

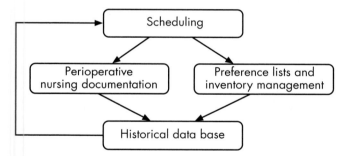

Fig. 3-2. Operating room information management applications.

by entering the specified constraints. Once a potential time slot is selected, the scheduling application checks for a variety of conflicts before confirmation. Conflict checking includes verification that the surgeon and necessary equipment are not already scheduled for another surgery at the same time. For example, the system might discover an equipment conflict when the surgeon requests use of equipment that is in limited supply. If the quantity that the hospital owns is already reserved for other scheduled cases, the system will identify and display the conflict to the OR scheduler. This type of multilevel conflict checking is difficult using manual scheduling procedures.

The patient's electronic record is created when the case is scheduled. The information that the OR scheduler collects and stores in the record varies among different institutions. Most institutions collect patient demographic, insurance, and pertinent medical history information. Some institutions also use the scheduling module for booking preadmission testing and tracking patients' preadmission status. For example, flags can be set in the electronic record indicating whether physician admitting orders have been received and when insurance authorization is obtained. When a case booking is confirmed, the OR system assigns a unique number to the electronic record. If the number is given to the person who schedules the case, the number can be referenced in the future when changes are necessary. The scheduler has immediate access to the record by entering the unique number.

The amount of time it takes to schedule a patient for surgery decreases when the OR scheduler is using a computer. Automated documentation is faster because features such as menu selections and electronic links between files allow users to enter large amounts of data with just a few keystrokes. Menu selections reduce typing errors and standardize the way information about the patient and the surgery is documented. Standardized documentation, unlike free-text data entry, can be stored in a coded format for later use in generating summary reports. Reports are more flexible and accurate if generated from a data base containing coded information.

Links are created between the patient's record and the permanent files stored in the OR system data base. For example, a link to the OR system physician file is established when the patient's surgeon is entered into the record. The physician file contains the surgeon's office number, surgical specialty, and hospital admitting number. The electronic link automatically adds the information to the patient record and the scheduler simply verifies the information. The physician file also contains a list of the procedures that the surgeon is credentialed to perform and will alert the scheduler if the surgeon is on suspension. Once the surgery and procedure are entered into the patient's record, another link to the historical file automatically calculates the estimated case duration. This time is calculated using the actual surgery times from past cases for that particular surgeon and procedure. This calculation replaces the inexact approximations traditionally used by schedulers.

Because OR systems run on a network, the OR schedule and associated patient records are accessible to many individuals simultaneously. Surgeons access the system to check their upcoming case schedules; nurse managers access the system to plan staffing; and admission staff access the system to look up patient demographic and insurance data. In addition, electronic records stored on the network can be updated by individuals spread over a wide geographic area. For example, the anesthesia office adds the anesthesia provider to the scheduled cases, the preadmission office adds the scheduled date for testing, and the admission nurse enters pertinent patient medical history.

Preference lists and inventory management. The purpose of a handwritten preference card is to help the perioperative staff prepare an operating room for a procedure to be performed by one or more surgeons. The card lists supplies and setup procedures that are specific to those surgeons and the procedure to be performed. Another group of one or more surgeons uses a different set of supplies and procedures and therefore has their own set of cards. Unfortunately, the usefulness of a manual card system diminishes over time as product lines are discontinued and procedures are modified. Maintaining the card system becomes increasingly labor intensive and often the best, most accurate information is stored in the minds of the perioperative staff.

The OR system maintains an on-line library of preference cards for each surgeon. The automated version of a preference card is commonly referred to as a "preference list." An example of a preference list for a surgeon performing a coronary artery bypass graft with an internal mammary artery is shown in Fig. 3-3. The top portion contains information on equipment setup and preoperative activities. The middle portion details all required supplies and equipment. Each supply item has an associated description, expected quantity to be used, and a unique code that references the electronic link to a master supply file. The bottom portion includes instructions on postoperative bed preparation and tasks to be completed before patient transfer. Preference lists have critical links to other files within the OR system that broaden their usefulness beyond simply assisting in procedure setup. These links make preference lists the key component to efficiently managing the department's inventory.

A preference list is activated when a procedure is scheduled. Each supply item and piece of equipment contained on the activated preference list is linked to a large master file. The master file stores information on the supplier, the catalogue number, the patient billing amount, and the current stock level. The materials coordinator runs an inventory management application that scans the items on all newly activated preference lists. The current stock level for each item is checked and the application issues a warning for all low-stock items. Using this application, the materials coordinator can quickly take appropriate action for reordering or substituting low-stock items. When the case carts are assembled, another inventory management application is used to generate pick tickets. The electronic pick ticket is generated from the activated preference list. The ticket includes all the items that need to be picked for the procedure. They are viewed online or in printed format and appear in the order that best facilitates case cart picking. For example, items are arranged by location in an order that is consistent with how the bins are physically arranged in the storage area. Any item substitutions made by the materials coordinator are noted on the pick ticket.

The perioperative nurse uses the activated preference list for two activities: preparing the room for surgery and documenting item usage during the procedure. The preference list assists the nurse in room preparation by listing every item that the surgeon expects will be available in the room and by including specific nursing instructions. The instructions include guidelines on operational checks for equipment and procedures for patient preparation. The information provides a valuable learning tool for the novice as well as a handy checklist for the more experienced perioperative nurse. As with accessing pick tickets, the complete preference list is available on-line or in printed format. Instead of viewing the information by how the supply area is arranged, the

Preference list 777   *Coronary artery bypass graft with internal mammary artery*
Surgeon: Dr. X   *Glove size: 7.5, Right-Handed*

Check room for required equipment
Check all equipment for functionality
Check suction for adequacy and setup
Have patient's chest x-rays in room
Confirm availability of blood products

REQUIRED EQUIPMENT			CASE CART ITEMS		
Code #	Qty	Description	Code #	Qty	Description
8213	2	ESU Electrosurgical Unit	7872	1	Cardiovascular Drape
8216	1	Defibrillator	7867	1	Open Heart Basin
8215	1	Light Source	7904	6	Linen Sterile Towel Pack
BASIC SUPPLIES			7905	10	Linen Bath Blanket
4410	1	Pad Cardiac Insulation	2488	1	Tubing Suction 1/4"*12'
5314	1	Aortic Perfusion Cannula	7876	1	Suction Cannister Insert
7826	1	Heart Pump Table Pack	664	3	0.9% NACL 1000 ml Irrigate
3104	2	Gown Extra Large	INSTRUMENTS		
4445	2	ESU Grounding Pad Adult	7828	1	Open Heart Instrument Tray
346	1	Glove UltraDerm 7.5	7829	1	Coronary Art Instrmt Tray
4440	3	Connector 3/8*3/8*3/8	7831	1	Sternal Codman Saw
4364	1	Cell Saver Pack	7834	1	FiberOptic Light Bundle
459	2	Elastic Ace Bandage 4"	SUTURES AND NEEDLES		
678	1	Tape Silk Durapore 2"	5175	1	Silk 2-0 SH CR/8 Suture
6797	1	Surgical Absorbable Hemostat	4934	2	Prolene 4-0 BB DA 36" Sut
8369	2	Physiosol 1000 cc	5625	3	Prolene 3-0 SH-1 DA Sut
5628	1	Dual Drain Venous Return	4203	1	Silk #5 LR DA Suture
4325	1	Aortic Root Cannula	2473	2	Vicryl 3-0 CT 27" Suture
7882	1	Cath Foley Thermister 16FR	4482	3	Vicryl 4-0 PS-1 Suture
845	1	Foam Rubber 1/4*	BANDAGES AND DRESSINGS		
8176	1	Heart Aortic Punch 15.0 mm	4407	4	Steri-strip Antimcrbl 1/2*4
4422	2	Vein Infusion Cannula	8824	4	Betadine Ointment
2480	1	Foley Catheter Tray	8050	2	Liquid Adhesive
CUSTOM PACK SUPPLIES			678	1	Silk Durapore 2" Tape
4173	3	Coverlet Adhesive 4*14	ANESTHESIA SUPPLIES		
4432	1	Polyester Vascular Tape	60	1	Adult Oxygen Mask
926	1	Soft Jaw Insert 61 mm	23	1	Salem Sump Tube 16FR
6635	1	Bone Wax Suture	40	1	Oral Airway Size 5
578	1	Surgical Blade #20	6630	4	Blood Gas Syringe
4576	1	Drape Table Cover Sterile	54	1	ET Cuffed Tube 7.5 mm
7878	1	Drape Ice Saline	234	3	Suction Catheter 14FR
4571	2	Ligaclip Small	2569	1	Esophageal Stethoscope
7884	3	Bulldog Clip	669	1	Suction Cannister 1200 cc

Confirm Intensive Care Unit (ICU) bed availability and send for bed
Prepare bed with oxygen tank, ambu bag, and connection tubing
Notify anesthesia technician to prepare monitoring equipment for bed
Note approximate blood loss after sternal closure
Confirm presence of patient ID band
Notify housekeeping when transferring patient

SIGNATURE: _____   DATE: _____

Fig. 3-3. Preference list for coronary bypass graft with internal mammary artery.

perioperative nurse typically views the information arranged by supply and equipment categories. During the procedure the nurse uses the preference list to track which items are actually used. Because the OR system already knows what quantity of items is expected to be used, the perioperative nurse updates only when those quantities change. If the preference list is well built, changes are the exception, thus reducing nursing documentation time while increasing the accuracy of reported usage.

Two remaining inventory management applications with links to the preference list library are used once the procedure is finished. They are an inventory reconciliation application and a patient billing application. The materials coordinator uses the actual usage information recorded by the perioperative nurse in running the inventory reconciliation application. This application readjusts each item's current stock level and issues reordering notices for items with readjusted levels falling below par. The stock levels are again adjusted when the orders are filled and the items are documented as received. The billing department uses actual usage information to generate patient bills. Patient information, such as demographic and surgery information, is obtained from data entered during case scheduling and surgery. The generated bills include only the items flagged as patient chargeable in the OR system's master supply file.

Perioperative nursing documentation. None of the OR systems available on the market today offers a fully automated system for perioperative nursing documentation. Automated applications for nursing documentation have only in the last few years become available and do not yet demonstrate the rich link functionality that enables a preference list to share data with other applications. The applications in most OR systems today were developed for the intraoperative nurse to record data that is traditionally documented during the course of a patient's stay in a surgical suite. The reason for beginning with intraoperative documentation is related to the kind of computers that run OR systems and to the physical limitation of the network connection. Most OR systems run on standard personal computers and require a physical cable that connects the computer to the network. This setup is easily adapted in the surgical suite, where the perioperative nurse traditionally documents in one designated area. In contrast, preoperative and postoperative nurses move from patient to patient and document where it is convenient. An immobile computer connected to a cable is not as adaptable in this environment. The solution lies with hand-held computers that transmit information to and from the network using wireless communication; these technologies have only recently become available.

Current applications include features that automate the care planning process performed by the perioperative nurse. In fact, the automated care plan becomes the working document the nurse uses to implement patient care and record care activities. The care plan is no longer viewed as a document primarily completed to meet requirements set by institutional policies and JCAHO regulations. Instead, with automated tools, the perioperative nurse uses the care plan as the organizational framework for completing all documentation. Fig. 3-4 illustrates how this process works. The components of the care plan are arranged into corresponding computer modules. Each module contains a set of data-entry screens. From these screens the perioperative nurse creates the care plan by selecting information stored in the permanent files of the OR system data base. The files are electronic references containing information from a variety of sources, some of which are listed in Fig. 3-4. Regulatory requirements, such as Title 22 requirements, JCAHO regulations, and institutional policies, define what is legally required to be stored in the patient record and most often appear on the screen as mandatory data-entry fields. The other sources are used as a format for documentation standards and are most often presented on the screen as menu selections. The Nursing Minimum Data Set (NMDS) was developed in the early 1980s as the first standardized collection of essential nursing data (Delaney, 1992). The NMDS contains 16 elements divided into three categories. These elements have been incorporated into many data bases supporting nursing applications, creating a rich repository for evaluation and outcomes studies.

By the time the patient enters the surgical suite, the electronic record already contains information collected when the procedure was scheduled, as well as any data entered during the preadmission process. The perioperative nurse signs on to the system, selects the patient's name, and enters the *Key Assessment* module to review previously entered information. Basic patient demographic data and procedure information are verified, and the initial nursing assessment is documented. Most OR systems arrange assessment data-entry fields on the screen by physiologic system. Structured data-entry lists dramatically reduce the required typing and once again encourage standardized documentation. The lists are developed by the nursing staff when the perioperative application is implemented. A list of selectable items is created for each appropriate data element and a list-editing tool is included to perform revisions as necessary.

Once the initial assessment is completed, the patient-specific plan of care is created. The perioperative nurse exits the *Key Assessment* module and enters the *Nursing Diagnosis* module. The care plan

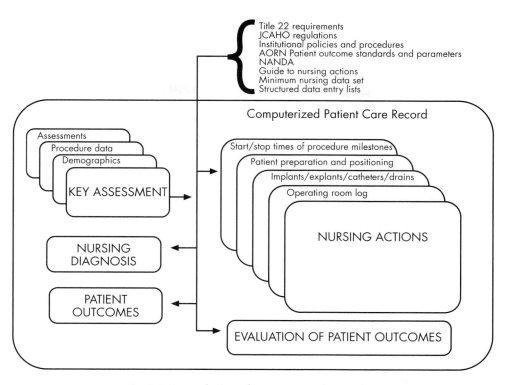

Fig. 3-4. Formulation of an automated care plan.

is created in three steps as the nurse navigates between the modules for *Nursing Diagnosis, Patient Outcomes, Nursing Actions,* and *Outcome Evaluation.* First, the appropriate diagnoses are selected from a menu containing the National Conference Group for Classification of Nursing Diagnoses (NANDA) approved list of nursing diagnoses (NANDA, 1994). Second, the associated patient outcomes, nursing actions, and evaluation parameters for the selected diagnoses are displayed in the corresponding modules. Third, the perioperative nurse adds and deletes items from the plan, depending on what is appropriate for a particular patient. As outcomes are added and deleted from the plan, the associated actions and evaluation parameters are also added and deleted. In this way, the perioperative nurse uses the reference files to quickly develop a plan of care that is both comprehensive and patient specific.

During the surgical procedure most of the documentation is performed from within the *Nursing Action* module. Within this module the perioperative nurse records completed nursing actions and information traditionally documented in the operating room log and associated forms. Fig. 3-5 illustrates an example of a data-entry screen from the *Nursing Action* module. Most of the data elements have an associated data-entry list. A partial list of locations for electrosurgical unit placement is displayed in Fig. 3-5 with "thigh anterior right" as the selected item.

"Start" and "end" times for procedure milestones are recorded as they occur. The system utilizes these data to provide a handy on-line management tool. The tool summarizes recorded time information on one computer screen. Suites are listed down one column, and a time line is listed across the top row. Each case is represented by a color-coded bar. As the perioperative nurse in the suite documents a milestone start or end time, the bar expands and adds a new color. For example, when a patient first enters the room, the perioperative nurse enters the "Patient in Room Time." The tool displays these data as a short bar containing one color. When the time that the patient is intubated and anesthetized is entered, the bar expands and more colors are added. The bar continues to expand and add colors as end times are entered for incision, closure, and final count. Viewing this simple display, a nurse manager receives a quick update on the status of all cases in progress. Without this tool, this same information could be collected only by walking from room to room.

As the procedure is ending, the perioperative nurse finishes documenting within the *Nursing Action* module. Each patient outcome is evaluated in the *Evaluation* module and a brief postoperative assessment is added in the *Key Assessment* module. The perioperative nurse then issues a command to print a copy for the patient's medical record and signs off the network. Whether the perioperative nurse is required to add a handwritten signature and

```
=================================================================
    Patient last name:          Patient first name:        OR suite:
    Surgery date: --|--|--       Surgery time: --:--        Medical record no:
============== |>> Patient preparation <<|================
    Patient in room time: --:--          Delay code:
    Surgeon in room time: --:--          Cancel code:
    ******[PT POSITION]******  ********[Catheter placement]********
        Body position:          Catheter type:     Straight catheter?
           Right arm:           Catheter size:     Cathed amt: ----cc
            Left arm:           *********[PATIENT PREP]*********
        Cooling device:         Prep solution used:
        Warming device:         OP site prepped by:
                                *********[ESU Placement]*********
    ***[Tourniquet placement]***         Site 1   Site 2   Site 3
                Site 1   Site 2  Location:  ==================
        Location:                  No:   ||                    ||
        Settings:                  Mode: ||  Flank left         ||
        Placed by:                 Setting: ||  Flank right      ||
                                   ||  Thigh anterior left   ||
=================================||  Thigh anterior right  || =====
                                 ||  Thigh lateral left    ||
                                 ||  Thigh lateral right   ||
                                 ||  Thigh posterior left  ||
                                  ==================
```

Fig. 3-5. Example of a nursing action data-entry screen.

date to the printed copy is currently under legal review. The OR system tracks when the record is updated and by whom as a by-product of the personal sign-on function. The question is whether the electronic password is considered a legal signature.

Historical data base. The final application to be discussed is the historical data base. The historical data base is the permanent storage unit for all information entered into the OR system. From a management perspective, it is the most powerful component of the system. The information extracted from a well-maintained data base can be used in many areas. Management extracts information to make decisions affecting purchasing activities, block time allocation, and many other daily operational issues. The data base can also be used in tracking quality indicators, screening for risk-management issues, and evaluating patient outcomes. Even staff credentialing can be done because the data base stores a record of the procedures in which each staff member participates.

The historical data base electronically organizes the storage of data in a way that allows users to generate both routine summary reports and ad hoc queries. Routine reports summarize information in a user-specified format and are generated on a regular basis. Examples include:
- Number of procedures by surgical specialty
- Average procedure cost by physician
- High- versus low-volume supply usage
- Wound classification by procedure type
- Surgical delays categorized by reason

The information is extracted by any time frame specified by the user or plotted by time interval to show trending patterns. Ad hoc queries are formulated as necessary in gathering information on a specific issue. The following are examples:
- Number of times Nurse Jones assisted with laser equipment over the past 6 months
- Average turnaround time for liver transplants during the month of May
- Number of times room 6 was used for total knee arthroscopies since renovation
- Patient complications reported when electrosurgical unit 4 was used

It is evident from the content of these queries that the same answers would take many hours of research to extract from a paper-based system. With computers, the data are available for analysis as a by-product of documenting patient care. The OR department spends less time gathering the data and more time analyzing the information.

A well-maintained data base requires effort. If data stored in the historical data base are entered correctly, then summary reports and ad hoc queries generate meaningful information. If data are entered incorrectly, the information is useless. Two mechanisms are used to ensure a well-maintained data base: error-checking routines and structured data entry. Most OR systems include routines that reduce the amount of errors that occur when data are entered. Error-checking routines confirm the validity of entered data. For example, the surgery date field will not accept letters of the alphabet, and the patient gender field will accept only the letters *M* or *F*. Another routine detects missing data. The user

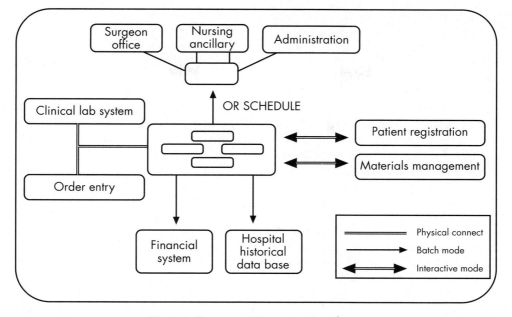

Fig. 3-6. Common OR system interfaces.

is prevented from executing the function until all required fields are completed. For example, an OR scheduler cannot confirm a procedure unless the *Surgery Date, Time, Location,* and *Duration* fields contain data; a materials coordinator cannot place an order without a valid catalog number; and a perioperative nurse cannot print a chart copy of the intraoperative document until all required fields are completed. These error-checking routines ensure that key data needed to generate accurate reports were verified at the time of data entry.

The second mechanism, structured data entry, increases the usefulness of information that is later extracted from the historical data base. Structured data entry standardizes documentation using menu selections that list the valid entries for each field. Menu selections drastically reduce the amount of free-text typing that is required and guarantee that data transferred into the historical data base is in a coded format. Standardized documentation is not a new concept to the nursing profession. This book is dedicated to defining a standard for how the plan of care for the surgical patient is documented. Fig. 3-4 illustrates how the standard's format and content can be accessed in creating an automated care plan. Storing automated care plan documentation in a coded format creates a rich data repository for verifying the content of care plan standards. Goals and patient outcome measurements can be compared to specific nursing actions and patient populations. Studies documenting the validity of care plan standards are easier to conduct when these kinds of data are available.

Interfaces and Additional Applications

Interfaces. No discussion of OR systems is complete without a description of the electronic interfaces typically implemented when an OR system is installed. Although an OR system automates many of the key processes that occur within an OR department, the benefits that automation provides are limited if electronic data sharing is not established with other computer systems installed in the hospital. An interface is defined as an electronic communication link established between two different computer systems that allows those two systems to exchange data. The two systems are different because they run on dissimilar computer models and run applications that support different departments. The simplest interface runs in batch mode, sending data from one system to another system at regular intervals (for example, once a day). The data are transmitted in one direction only. A real-time interactive interface sends data between two systems in both directions whenever there are relevant data to send.

Figure 3-6 summarizes the types of interfaces commonly found in hospitals today. The daily OR schedule can be transmitted to the hospital's main information system, providing access to a broad range of users. Users include physician offices, nursing stations, ancillary departments, and administrative areas. This simple batch-file transfer lowers paper-supply costs, reduces labor associated with photocopying and distribution, and eliminates unnecessary phone calls. A more interactive interface manages the data exchanged between the OR system and the patient registration system. Data are transmitted from the OR system whenever surgical procedures are scheduled, modified, or cancelled. Patient registration data are transmitted back when the patient is admitted.

A real-time, interactive interface is usually employed in developing communication between the OR system and the hospital's materials management system. The ordering, issuing, and replenishing of inventory items is a 24-hour operation in the OR department. The OR system sends order requests as they are entered by OR staff. In response, the materials management system sends order acknowledgments, expected delivery dates, and notifications of delivery. The materials management system may have additional interfaces to automatically route the order information to the appropriate vendor. Complex interfaces such as the two just described greatly reduce documentation redundancy, increase documentation consistency, and improve communication between the two departments.

Patient billing information is sent from the OR system to the hospital financial system. This information is extracted from the documentation of perioperative nurses on preference lists and within the surgical log component. Billing information is usually sent in batch mode on a daily basis. This is because most financial systems generate bills in regular batch mode and cannot process information on a real-time basis. Dynamic data exchange is not required with this type of interface. Summary information from the historical data base can also be extracted and sent to the hospital's information system. The information is incorporated into the hospital's historical database and manipulated on a much larger scale in ways similar to those described earlier.

The final interface shown in Fig. 3-6 is not a true interface in that data exchange does not occur between differing systems. Additional physical cables are connected to the OR system computer to provide access to other systems. The user signs off of the OR system network and signs onto the other system. The primary benefit of these connections is to consolidate the number of computers that are required. Instead of placing three separate computers in each surgical suite, one computer with three cables is installed that provides access to the OR system, the laboratory system, and the order-entry system.

Physician applications. The OR system described in this chapter is used by physicians primarily to review information. Surgeons and anesthesia providers can review the OR schedule for any future time frame or limit the view to just their procedures; they can also review their on-line library of preference lists. Applications for physician documentation do

not exist in most OR systems on the market today (Box 3-2). Surgeons do not document during surgery and rely primarily on dictation services to record the surgery notes. Surgeons do utilize digitized image-management systems intraoperatively to assist with visualization of the surgical field. Systems supporting anesthesia documentation are in abundance but are offered as a separate product line. Some OR systems are beginning to offer applications that allow surgeons or their office staff to submit electronic scheduling requests. Requests can be sent at any time and are processed in the order received. The OR system immediately acknowledges that the request was received, but confirmation of the requested time is not sent until an OR scheduler reviews the information.

Anesthesia documentation systems are designed to process high volumes of data entered at very frequent intervals. Most of the data are automatically downloaded from monitoring equipment and life support systems attached to the patient during a surgical procedure. For example, the ventilator sends all parameter settings and updates as the settings are

---

Box 3-2 Physician Inpatient Order Writing on Microcomputer Workstations

The Agency for Health Care Policy and Research funded a study to examine the effect of personal computers (PCs) on patient and hospital costs. Each participating hospital used a network of three to five PCs to write inpatient physician orders for drugs, diagnostic studies, and nursing care. More than 5000 internal-medicine patients were part of the order-writing on PCs. The study results indicated the following:

- Electronic medical systems helped speed execution of physicians' orders
- The average patient stay was shortened by almost 1 day
- Average admission charges were reduced by nearly 13%

These effects would amount to a cost savings of $3 million for the hospital annually and potentially billions of dollars nationally. In addition to computer-enabled review of the patient's medical history and current status, including medication allergies, the system also facilitates cost-conscious treatment decisions. The computer displays the patient charge for a prescribed item, offers the most cost-effective tests, and suggests other treatments that are less expensive but effective alternatives.

Adapted from Tierney WJ et al. (1993). Physician inpatient order writing on microcomputer workstations. *Journal of the American Medical Association* 269(3), 79-383.

adjusted; the anesthesia gas machine sends similar information. Patient monitoring equipment, such as the cardiac monitor and pulse oximetry unit, transmit hemodynamic measurements every few seconds or minutes, depending on the stability of the patient. The anesthesia provider monitors all of the incoming data from one integrated screen display. Patient intake and output amounts are entered by the anesthesia provider, and running totals and the balance are calculated by the system. A variety of built-in alarms alert the anesthesia provider to early warning signs of patient complications. Numerous studies have been published documenting a decrease in anesthesia-related complications when these systems are used (Gardner, 1990).

SUMMARY

This chapter describes the four applications that comprise an operating room management system and highlights the benefits derived from automating manual processes within an OR department. Electronic scheduling eliminates the traditional appointment book and adds features such as conflict checking and calculated procedure durations. These features increase the overall accuracy in booking procedures, yet decrease the time required to schedule each procedure. Scheduling done using an on-line library of preference lists stimulates a cascade of activities. Activated preference lists are used by materials coordinators to check needed supplies against current stock levels, technicians generate pick tickets that detail the items to be assembled grouped by physical location, and perioperative nurses use preference lists to assist with room preparation and to document actual item usage during the surgical procedure. The actual usage data are used by the materials coordinator to order replacement stock and by the financial office to generate patient bills.

Automated applications for perioperative nursing documentation add new purpose to the process of formulating and documenting patient care plans. Not only are numerous paper forms replaced with one electronic record, the care plan itself becomes the organizational framework that integrates all intraoperative nursing documentation. The perioperative nurse builds the patient-specific plan of care from within the corresponding computer modules and documents intraoperative activities from within the *Nursing Action* module. Once the patient is discharged, the data from the electronic record are transferred to the historical data base. The historical data base is the permanent storage unit for all data entered into the OR system. If data entry functions are supported with mechanisms such as error-checking routines and structured lists, the historical data base serves as a powerful tool for tracking

management issues, quality improvement programs (Box 3-3), and risk management activities.

The OR system of the future will build on the applications that exist in today's products. Current applications will be enhanced, new applications will be added, and interfaces will evolve into seamless communication channels that allow disparate systems to function in an integrated fashion. Three important trends are contributing to the realization of

---

Box 3-3 Using PC Software for Health Care Quality Data Management

Quality teams must manage their own data, which sometimes is overwhelming as they attempt to learn how to produce and use common total quality tools. Microsoft Excel 4.0 is one example of a graphic user interface; it runs on both Windows-based PCs and Apple Macintosh hardware. It is a spreadsheet program, and it can help the quality team with:

- *Process flow and cause-and-effect (fishbone) diagrams.* The process flow diagram is one of the most commonly used first-step tools in process simplification. The cause-and-effect diagram, used in identifying the structures and processes that contribute to a desired outcome (or a problem) can also be easily constructed.
- *Control charts.* These allow plotting of data elements to show variability over time. When a process is studied, it is important to determine if it is in control (a stable process) or has special cause variation.
- *Pareto charts.* These are used to display the frequency of causes of problems. The Pareto principle suggests that the quality team should work on the few causes that lead to the most problems.
- *Histograms.* These are commonly used by quality teams to show the frequency distribution of collected data via a bar chart.
- *Scatter diagrams.* These are a pictorial representation of relationships between two variables, such as the number of medication errors when temporary nursing staff are used. Although it does not "prove" that one thing causes the other, it can indicate the need for further investigation of the problem under study.
- *Statistical analysis.* Statistical procedures are important in validating studies. Sample analyses that can be performed with this software include analysis of variance, correlations, covariance, descriptive statistics, f-test, t-test, z-test, rank and percentile, regression, sampling, and random number generation.

Adapted from Scoville RP & Kibbe DC. (1993). Tutorial: Using Microsoft Excel for health care CQI. *Quality Management in Health Care*, 2(1), 63-71.

these goals. First, computers continue to shrink in size, making them adaptable to any environment. Second, as networking and communications technology continue to evolve, the physical boundaries that create isolated patient documents and separate physician offices from hospitals, clinics, and home health services will be replaced with electronic highways that enable all these facilities to share one medical record. An episode of care will be documented and stored in the same electronic record, whether the episode occurred during a hospital admission for a surgical procedure, a clinic visit, or a visit by a home health nurse. Finally, regional alliances and managed care competition will continue to promote cost-effective delivery of care supported with evidence of quality patient outcomes. In this type of environment it is likely that the organizational tools for coordinating all patient care activities will be based on the concept of care plans. The nursing plan of care will evolve into a multidisciplinary plan formulated and maintained by a variety of clinicians. Multidisciplinary care plans will ensure consistency of care throughout the perioperative stay, as well as throughout the patient's lifetime.

References

Delaney C, et al. (1992). Standardized nursing language for healthcare information systems. *Journal of Medical Systems, 16*(4), 145-159.

Dorenfest SI. (1992). *Hospital information systems: State of the art.* Chicago: Sheldon I. Dorenfest & Associates.

Gardner RM. (1990). Patient-monitoring systems. In E. Shortliffe & L. Perreault (Eds.), *Medical informatics: Computer applications in health care* (pp. 366-399). Reading, MA: Addison-Wesley.

Institute of Medicine. (1991). *The computer-based record: An essential technology for health care.* Washington, DC: National Academy Press.

Joint Commission on Accreditation of Healthcare Organizations. (1987a). *Agenda for change update.* Chicago: The Commission.

More ORs are using computers. (1992). *OR Manager 8*(2), 10.

North American Nursing Diagnosis Association. (1990). Taxonomy I: Revised 1990. *Nursing Diagnosis 1*(50).

Work Group for Electronic Data Interchange (July 1992). *Report to Secretary of US Department of Health and Human Services.* Washington, DC: United States Department of Health and Human Services.

Work Group on Computerization of Patient Records (April 1993). *Toward a national health information infrastructure.* United States Department of Health and Human Services.

Chapter 4

Documenting Patient Care

Jane C. Rothrock

A great point of distinction between the trained and the untrained nurse is, or should be, the ability of the former to observe accurately, and describe intelligently, what comes under her notice. The nurse, who is with the patient constantly, has, if she knows how to make use of it, a much better opportunity of becoming acquainted with his real condition, than the physician. . . . In order to form correct judgments, it is necessary for the physician to know what goes on in his absence . . . and for such information he is forced to rely almost wholly upon the nurse. It is thus of the greatest importance that she cultivate the habit of critical observation, and simple, direct, truthful statement. . . . Do not trust too much to memory, but keep a little memorandum-book in which to note facts [and] take down orders.

WEEKS, 1890

*T*he collection of information about a patient's condition and subsequent "noting" of that information has guided nursing care for more than a century. The importance of the nurse's contribution to patient care has similarly been long-known and respected. Through the years, the process of information collection and notation has become more systematic and scientific. The nursing process has emerged as an accepted clinical inquiry model to describe the nursing actions that support the provision of comprehensive, high-quality care. In order to form the "correct judgments" described by Weeks, the perioperative nurse must demonstrate anticipatory thinking, focus on patient outcomes, strive to individualize care, involve the patient/family/significant others, be committed to continuity, and understand the participative nature of the planning process (Foust, 1994). Inherent in the steps of the nursing process is a means of communicating the sequence of events and important findings that characterize each step or phase.

Documentation of the nursing process, which has as its central core a means of planning and providing patient care, serves a number of purposes: it validates that a thorough plan of care has been formulated for each patient; it serves as a retrievable data base that can be used to evaluate patient care; it provides continuity of care by communicating to other nurses the specific problems/nursing diagnoses, identified patient outcomes, and interventions identified for each particular patient to achieve those outcomes; and it is necessary for legal purposes and for reimbursement. Thus documentation becomes an important tool in ensuring continuity of care and enabling nurses to evaluate care and measure outcomes of care processes.

DOCUMENTING PERIOPERATIVE NURSING CARE

Perioperative documentation is essential in providing outcome-directed care and evaluating the patient's response to care before, during, and after an operative or other invasive procedure. Communication of information about the patient's perioperative care provides an accurate picture of the phases and results of care. This process also provides a permanent record of all care given during the patient's admission to perioperative care units (Spry & Jenkins, 1991).

Using the Nursing Process as a Documentation Framework

The nursing process provides the governing framework for documenting perioperative nursing care (Fig. 4-1).

Assessment. During the *assessment* phase of care, the perioperative nurse collects data about the patient's status. Assessment is an ongoing process; it initiates care planning and continues through each subsequent phase as new problems arise or the patient's status changes. Perioperative nursing assessment is focused inquiry; it is directed toward the individual patient's needs as they relate to and affect perioperative nursing care. The medical and nursing histories, physical examination, and information about the patient's psychosocial, cultural, ethnic, spiritual, and physiologic responses (diagnostic procedures and results) are reviewed in terms of their relevance to perioperative care planning. Subjective and objective data are analyzed and synthesized to guide the perioperative nurse in determining priority needs for perioperative care. The results of relevant assessment data are then documented.

Nursing diagnosis. The *nursing diagnosis* is the critical link in the nursing process. The nursing diagnosis is essential to move on to each subsequent phase of the nursing process. The patient's nursing diagnoses represent the perioperative nurse's judgment of the information derived through the systematic, focused assessment. The nursing diagnoses may be prioritized as affecting the preoperative, intraoperative, or postoperative period. Some nursing diagnoses will characterize the entire perioperative period. In this instance the perioperative nurse plans nursing actions that may continue through each phase of care; the diagnosis remains the same. Perioperative patient care records may then be designed across the continuum of care, with nurses in each phase of care indicating the relevance of the nursing diagnosis and interventional nursing actions taken (Chana, 1992).

Knowledge of perioperative nursing science and biophysical sciences enables the perioperative nurse to move from assessment to the formulation of nursing diagnoses. As a process, nursing diagnosis consists of collecting information, interpreting that information, clustering it, and naming the cluster—that is, the diagnostic statement (McFarland & McFarlane, 1993).

Nursing diagnoses have been characterized as either independent or interdependent/collaborative; in this book, interdependent nursing diagnoses are referred to as "collaborative." Independent nursing diagnoses are those in which the nurse can intervene without supervision or direction by others. Interventions developed for independent nursing diagnoses are those that the nurse can perform within the scope of nursing practice, which is defined in nurse practice acts. *Collaborative nursing diagnoses* require the participation and guidance of other health care professionals. Most perioperative nursing diagnoses are collaborative. The nurse, by virtue of the nurse practice act, might be licensed to intervene in a nursing diagnosis such as *knowledge deficit.* However, the short, intensive time spent in perioperative nursing activities may require that the unit nurse, physician, social worker, dietitian, clinical nurse specialist, nurse practitioner, or others assist in intervening in a patient's knowledge deficit. Working together to achieve common, safe, effective patient outcomes is characteristic of the perioperative patient care team. Few members of the team work independently; perioperative care is mutually interdependent, and the contributions of each team member are recognized and supported. Such a collaborative design for providing care is inherent in the development of care protocols, care maps, clinical pathways, and critical paths.

Outcome identification. Nursing diagnoses lead to the formulation of *desired patient outcomes;* nursing actions are subsequently identified that will facilitate outcome achievement. Outcomes should be concise. Evaluation criteria are developed to measure the predetermined desired outcomes of patient care. Both evaluation criteria and identified outcomes are documented as part of the perioperative nursing care plan. Desired patient outcomes should be stated in patient-behavioral terms, with measurable verbs and specific content. The nursing diagnosis guides the development of the desired outcome, since nursing's intent is to resolve the diagnosis or prevent it, as in the instance of high-risk nursing diagnoses.

Planning. The *planning* phase begins when the perioperative nurse identifies nursing actions that will intervene in the nursing diagnosis. These actions may aim to prevent a high-risk nursing diagnosis (for example, the prevention of injury and infection) or to intervene in an actual nursing diagno-

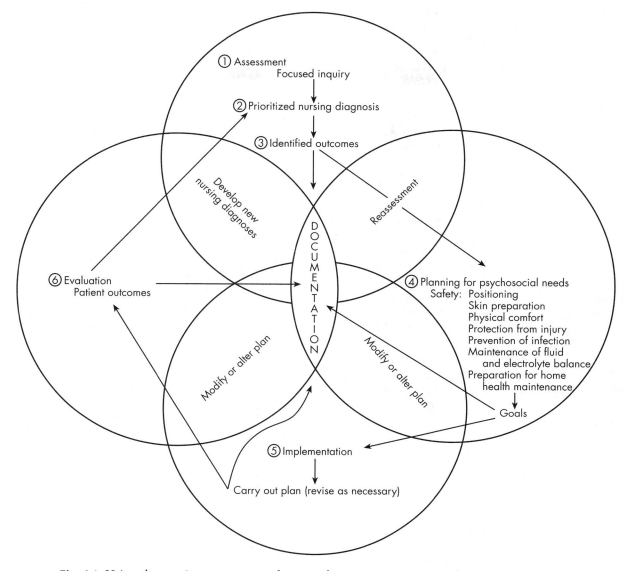

Fig. 4-1. Using the nursing process sets the stage for a systematic approach to perioperative patient care. (Adapted from Manuel BJ. (1980). *Reporting and documenting patient care.* Denver: The Association.)

sis (for example, fluid volume deficit, anxiety, or disturbance in body image). Table 4-1 summarizes the relationships between various nursing diagnoses, expected and desired patient outcomes, and nursing interventions planned.

Implementation. The *implementation* phase depends on assessment, diagnosis, and planning. These activities determine what the nurse does to intervene in patient problems and to prevent high-risk problems from occurring. Implementation requires intellectual, interpersonal, and technical skills; decision making, keen observation, and clear communication are also necessary. During implementation, the perioperative nurse documents the care that is given. Ongoing reassessment during actual care delivery may require that the plan be altered and new

nursing actions be implemented; this requires that the perioperative nurse constantly evaluate new data that become available during the actual process of providing care to the perioperative patient.

Evaluation. The nursing process requires that nurses *evaluate* how well the established patient outcomes were achieved and whether the activities of the perioperative nurse assisted in that achievement. In perioperative nursing, not all desired outcomes are readily apparent at the conclusion of surgery. This problem is not unique to perioperative nursing. At one time, the problems in evaluating care were characteristic of patient care units that provided episodic care (that is, operating rooms, ambulatory surgery units, endoscopy labs, cardiac catheterization labs, interventional radiology depart-

Table 4-1 *The relationships between various nursing diagnoses, expected and desired patient outcomes (as identified in* AORN Patient Outcomes: Standards of Perioperative Care), *and nursing interventions planned*

Diagnoses labels	Interventions	Expected outcomes
Preoperative		
Self-concept, alteration in body image, and role performance	Therapeutic communication Refer to appropriate person Assess for nonverbal cues Include physical or environmental changes in teaching Encourage patient participation (transfer, positioning, and conversation)	The patient demonstrates knowledge of the rehabilitation process.
Activity intolerance or immobility (actual and high risk for)	Assess range of motion, contributing factors (emotional and/or physical) Encourage patient participation Allow for ventilation of feelings (frustration)	The patient demonstrates knowledge of the rehabilitation process.
Intraoperative		
Infection (actual and high risk for)	Implement and maintain principles of aseptic technique Determine wound classification Assess contributing factors Follow hospital policy and procedure for room preparation	The patient is free from signs and symptoms of infection.
Hypothermia (high risk for)	Minimize patient heat loss by conduction (for example, contact with cold surfaces); convection (for example, through air currents); evaporation (for example, via wet solutions); radiation (for example, environmental temperature) Assess determinants (age, weight, dehydration) Compare baseline and intraoperative vital signs	The patient is free from injury related to exposure to heat loss.
Fluid and electrolyte deficit or excess (actual or high risk for)	Assess baseline lab values Note solutions being administered Note changes in monitoring equipment values Document urine/blood loss	The patient's fluid and electrolyte balance is maintained.
Impaired tissue or skin integrity	Assess for contributing factors (allergies, nutrition, disease process, extremes in age or weight) Assess areas at risk during positioning Implement safety measures (pads, safety straps, supports)	The patient's skin integrity is maintained.
Injury, high risk for foreign body	Implement procedures for (correct or incorrect) counts Document results	The patient is free from injury related to extraneous objects and physical hazards.
Injury, high risk for burn	Place ground pad close to incisional site in an area that is dry, free of scars, hair, skin folds, and lesions Select pad appropriate for patient's age and machine Be sure site is not in contact with spilled fluids or other metal objects Follow departmental procedure for assembly and use of electrosurgical unit	The patient is free from injury related to chemical, physical, and electrical hazards.

From Thompson JM, et al. (1993). *Mosby's clinical nursing,* (3rd Ed.) St Louis: Mosby.

Table 4-1 *The relationships between various nursing diagnoses, expected and desired patient outcomes (as identified in* AORN Patient Outcomes: Standards of Perioperative Care*), and nursing interventions planned—cont'd*

Diagnoses labels	Interventions	Expected outcomes
Intraoperative—cont'd		
Injury, high risk for hemorrhage	Assess baseline data of personal history, previous surgeries, and lab values (Hg, Hct, prothrombin time [PT]) Provide sufficient equipment for estimated blood loss (sponges and suction canisters) Monitor patient intake and output status during surgery (blood loss, IV solutions, and irrigations) Coordinate care with staff	The patient's fluid balance is maintained.
Injury, high risk for neuromuscular trauma related to positioning	Assess for contributing factors (allergies, nutrition, disease process, extremes in age or weight) Assess areas at risk during positioning Implement positioning safety measures (pads, safety straps, supports) Position patient for procedure according to hospital policy and procedure	The patient is free from injury related to positioning hazards.
Injury, high risk for fall or trauma	Implement hospital procedures for surgical position Coordinate all patient transfers with sufficient number of personnel Maintain patient alignment during transfer and positioning	The patient is free from injury related to positioning, extraneous objects, or physical hazards.
Injury, high risk for emboli or thrombi formation	Ensure OR bed accommodates patient size and age Assess baseline data for coagulopathy Assess activity level, determinants, and positioning requirements Avoid dependent positioning without cardiovascular supports	The patient is free from injury related to positioning, extraneous objects, or physical hazards.
Anxiety, fear, and alteration in comfort related to local or regional procedure only	Assess baseline emotional and physical status Relate sequence of events intraoperatively and postoperatively Provide emotional support through therapeutic communication Monitor vital signs, oxygen saturation, reported patient pain level; report deviations from baseline	The patient demonstrates knowledge of the physiologic and psychologic responses to surgical intervention.
Postoperative		
Alteration in comfort, pain (actual)	Assess location, duration, and intensity of pain Change position as allowed Therapeutic communication (touch and SOLER) Relate complaints of pain to primary nurse	The patient demonstrates knowledge of the physiologic and psychologic responses to surgical pain.
Infection, high risk for	Maintain aseptic technique and good handwashing practices Assess dressing and incision site for infection Review chart for vital signs and lab results	The patient is free from signs and symptoms of infection.

Continued.

Table 4-1 *The relationships between various nursing diagnoses, expected and desired patient outcomes (as identified in AORN Patient Outcomes: Standards of Perioperative Care), and nursing interventions planned—cont'd*

Diagnoses labels	Interventions	Expected outcomes
Postoperative—cont'd		
Injury, high risk for hemorrhage or emboli	Review chart for recent vital signs and lab results Assess dressing and drainage site where applicable Assess for skin irritation because of prep solutions Check electrosurgical conductive electrode Analyze the effect of surgical position on pressure areas and gross sensory-motor activity Assess patients at risk for circulatory compromise (Homans' sign, respiratory status, consciousness level)	The patient is free from injury related to fluid loss, positioning, extraneous objects, or physical hazards.
Anxiety related to postoperative care	Assess for nonverbal cues (diaphoresis, restlessness) and emotional status Therapeutic communication (SOLER and touch) Identify and include family and significant others Refer to support systems Allow patient to ventilate feelings	The patient participates in the rehabilitation process.
Ineffective airway clearance and breathing (actual or high risk for), aspiration (high risk for)	Assess breathing sounds and respiratory status Have patient demonstrate turn, deep-breathing exercises, and use of incentive spirometer, if applicable Note productive cough Encourage fluids as clinically indicated	The patient is free from respiratory injury related to positioning, extraneous objects, or hypoxia.
Activity intolerance or immobility (actual)	Identify limitations and compare with preoperative baseline Validate knowledge of self-care Assess effects of immobilizing devices applied during surgery (neurovascular checks and pressure areas)	The patient participates in the rehabilitation process.
Grieving, actual related to loss of body part or postoperative surgical diagnosis	Encourage ventilation of feelings Encourage patient participation within limitations Identify and include support systems Refer to other professionals as clinically indicated	The patient participates in the rehabilitation process.

ments, emergency departments, and postanesthesia care units). In episodic care units, the patient's stay is short; access to the patient for outcome evaluation is difficult. Today, changes in hospital reimbursement systems have altered systems of nursing care delivery. All nurses are faced with the problem of patient access, often before and after medical and surgical treatment. Same-day admission, 23-hour stays, and ambulatory surgery require that perioperative nursing develop new ways of initiating nursing data bases and evaluating nursing care. Evaluation of perioperative patient outcomes may need to be collaborative, just as many nursing diagnoses are. Collaborative evaluation may require stronger relationships with the nurse in the discharge unit (postanesthesia care unit, ambulatory recovery, discharge patient care unit), with physicians' offices, with home care providers, and with patients themselves.

Postoperative phone calls and postcare assessment methods will become a routine part of evaluation of nursing care.

Approaches to Documenting Perioperative Patient Care

Every perioperative patient care unit uses a formal system for documenting patient care. Records are different in each setting; the methods selected for documenting perioperative nursing care must fit with the institution's overall philosophy of nursing documentation and its system for record keeping. All documentation forms should contain the patient's name, age, identification number (which in some instances is the social security number), date (day, month, and year), time of documented entry, and the nurse's signature. Whatever documentation system is selected for the perioperative setting, it should have as its goals a legally sound record, reflection of the nursing process and the patient's ongoing status, forms that avoid duplication of information, a plan of care that complements information in the patient record, a mechanism for documenting all nursing interventions, and facilitation of information retrieval (Iyer & Camp, 1992).

Problem-oriented medical records. Once commonly used, problem-oriented medical records (POMR) list the patient's problems and the extent to which the problems are resolved. The POMR system incorporates nursing records, physician records, and documentation by other health care team members. Each problem is defined, labeled, and placed in numeric order. As new problems arise, they are numbered, titled, and added to the problem list. An example of this type of recording is as follows:

1. *Fear/anxiety.* Patient states he is "afraid that the postsurgical pain will be difficult to bear." Patient is perspiring while discussing this problem. Encourage him to discuss the problem, show him splinting techniques to use while coughing, and suggest that when the pain becomes increasingly worse to ask for pain medication.

SOAP and SOAPIE notes. The concept of POMR evolved into SOAP or SOAPIE notes. The six steps in SOAPIE notes are as follows:

1. *Subjective data,* which involves the health status of the patient and what he or she thinks and feels about the health problem.
2. *Objective data,* which includes the physical and laboratory findings as well as observations of the patient.
3. *Assessment,* which includes formulation of a nursing diagnosis/patient problem, the desired patient outcomes, and the evaluation criteria.
4. *Plan,* which identifies the activities necessary to assist the patient to achieve the desired outcomes.
5. *Implementation,* which identifies the nursing activities accomplished.
6. *Evaluation,* which contains the degree to which the patient achieved the specified outcomes.

It is unlikely that many perioperative patient care units use either POMR or SOAP/SOAPIE charting. Even focus charting, which places the symptom, nursing diagnosis, or patient problem in the left column (the focus), followed by the data, action(s), response(s) (DAR) format requires narrative notes. Such documentation systems may still be well suited to in-depth, detailed nursing analyses and interventions, but their practical application to the intensive, focused nature of perioperative care is limited. The dynamic status of the perioperative patient prohibits such detailed nursing data bases. As a consequence, other methods of record keeping have evolved in perioperative care settings.

Preoperative checklists. Preoperative checklists are used in most health care settings. Their major purpose is to document routine procedures that need completion before the patient goes to the surgical suite. The checklist has a dual purpose. The nurse on the patient unit or the presurgical admitting unit uses the form to communicate with the perioperative nurse about care regimens that have been completed before the patient was transferred to the operating room. The perioperative nurse uses the checklist to validate that important preparatory procedures have been completed. Information usually included follows (Fig. 4-2 is an example).

- Time patient left unit or ambulatory holding area
- Vital signs, height and weight
- Allergies
- Pertinent laboratory values and diagnostic procedures
- X-ray films
- Prostheses (dentures, contact lenses, and so on)
- Identification bracelet
- Preoperative medications administered
- Consent and advanced directive
- Blood products available (if prescribed)
- History and physical (completed and in chart)
- NPO status (as applicable)
- Completion of physician orders

Preoperative assessment record. Some institutions use preoperative assessment records to guide the uniform collection of data about patients. Fig. 4-3 presents one such form. The information to be collected is significant for perioperative care planning. Part I, in the upper right-hand corner, provides guidelines for patient education, detailing specific

Mark Appropriate Column with a Check	Yes	No	N/A
Physician consent signed			
Hospital consent signed			
Medical history and physical complete			
Lab results on chart (Department will call OR)			
Blood or blood products available in lab			
Preop studies and results on chart (Department will call OR)			
Addressograph plate attached to chart			
Identification bracelet on patient			
Surgical prep done by: _____			
NPO			
Preop Rxs (enema, Foley, etc.)			
Dentures, cosmetics, nail polish, jewelry, wigs, glasses, underwear, contact lens, etc. removed and placed in S.P.U. closet			
Valuables given to:_____			
Preop medication administered as ordered			
Voided qs			
Comments: _____			
_____			
_____			
Preop vital signs: TPR: _____ BP: _____			

_____   _____
RN Signature   Date

Fig. 4-2. Preoperative checklist. (Courtesy Crozer Chester Medical Center, Chester, PA.)

information that should be conveyed to each perioperative patient and his or her family or significant other, as appropriate. Part II allows the nurse to document in narrative form important assessment data that affect perioperative care. *Social information* might include the patient's ability to communicate; cultural, ethnic, spiritual, and religious practices; support systems; and level of knowledge regarding perioperative routines and events. *Range of motion* information helps the perioperative nurse plan for patient transport, transfer to and from the operating room bed, and patient positioning. Here the perioperative nurse would document any limitations in mobility/motion, musculoskeletal problems, congenital anomalies, or missing extremities.

Respiratory status is of significance to patients undergoing general anesthesia and when planning for transport and positioning if there is respiratory compromise. The perioperative nurse would note the patient's skin color, assess the breath sounds, and review laboratory values (such as arterial blood gases). *Circulation* needs to be assessed for alterations that may affect patient care needs; pulses, skin integrity, and the presence of intravenous or invasive lines would be recorded. *Allergies* and *post-transfusion reactions* relate to information impor-

I. Preoperative Patient Teaching

a. Shave/scrub
b. NPO
c. Anesthesia visit
d. Preoperative medications and effects
e. Transport
f. OR or holding area
g. Never left alone
h. ID check and surgical site checked
i. Sights and sounds of OR
k. Arms tucked and/or stretched out
l. Area may be shaved for grounding pad
m. Sights and sounds of recovery room
n. Vital signs checked
o. When recovered transport to room

II. Patient Assessment

1. Social _____

_____

_____

2. Range of motion _____

_____

_____

3. Respiratory _____

_____

_____

4. Circulation _____

_____

_____

5. Allergies and post blood reactions _____

_____

6. General condition and physical appearance _____

_____

7. Emotional status and level of consciousness _____

_____

8. Medications pertinent to surgery _____

_____

9. Previous medical history _____

_____

_____

10. Preoperative diagnosis _____

Signature RN _____

Date _____

Fig. 4-3. Preoperative assessment record. (Courtesy Delaware County Memorial Hospital, Drexel Hill, PA.)

I. Preoperative Patient Teaching

a. Shave/scrub
b. NPO
c. Anesthesia visit
d. Preoperative medications and effects
e. Transport
f. OR or holding area
g. Never left alone
h. ID check and surgical site checked
i. Sights and sounds of OR
k. Arms tucked and/or stretched out
l. Area may be shaved for grounding pad
m. Sights and sounds of recovery room
n. Vital signs checked
o. When recovered transport to room

II. Patient Assessment

1. Social _Reads, writes understands English No specific religious/cultural needs. Good family support system. Requests report to family when discharged to PACU. Uses hearing aid. R ear Will come to OR with aid, then to PACU for recovery. NDX: sensory perceptual alteration: auditory_

2. Range of motion _Some limitations in daily activity Related to arthritis, both hips affected. No prosthetic devices, muscle weakness. Home maintenance = self. P.E = limited Rom hips   NDX: Impaired physical mobility_

3. Respiratory _No c/o dyspnea.   Resp. 20, regular. No productive cough. Breath sounds equal bilat. Chest x-ray & pulm. functions studies in record - both normal. Does not smoke._

4. Circulation _Skin cool, dry. No rashes, petechiae, lesions. Proposed incision site = unimpaired. Apical rate - 82 BPM. BP (R arm) 136/78. No IV lines. Pedal Pulses +3 bilat. No dependent edema._

5. Allergies and post blood reactions _No previous transfusions. NKA._

6. General condition and physical appearance _Relatively healthy 52 y.o. male. WBC, Diff, HCT, HB = WNL. Well nourished. No Dentures._

7. Emotional status and level of consciousness _Alert, Oriented x 3. Memory intact. No significant problems sleeping. Appropriate behavior. Has realistic questions/perceptions. No recent stress._

8. Medications pertinent to surgery _Uses either aspirin or NSAID for arthritis. Stopped per M.D. recommendation 10 days ago._

9. Previous medical history _Unremarkable. Family Hx of hypertension. Pt. aware of risk factors, practices health-seeking behaviors._

10. Preoperative diagnosis _Basal cell Carcinoma - cheek. For removal 4/1/90_

Signature RN _June H. Johnston RN, CNOR_

Date _3/30/90_

Fig. 4-4. Preoperative assessment record. (Courtesy Delaware County Memorial Hospital, Drexel Hill, PA.)

tant for guiding antimicrobial skin preparation; the administration of antibiotics, local anesthetics, or contrast dye; and planning for anticipated problems with perioperative transfusions. The *general condition* and *physical appearance* of a patient is a useful guide in screening for other problems. *Emotional status,* the patient's perceptions and expectations of the surgery, *verbal ability* (dominant language skills), and *level of consciousness* guide and direct appropriate nursing actions and interventions. Any *medications pertinent to surgery,* such as the use of anticoagulant agents, steroids, antibiotics, diuretics, antihypertensive drugs, and over-the-counter remedies are documented for their possible contribution to intraoperative problems. The *medical history* is reviewed to determine if there are additional system disorders relating to perioperative care; renal, gastrointestinal, endocrine, or genitourinary problems, and so on would be identified here. Information about the *preoperative diagnosis* confirms the planned surgical intervention and suggests needs for the results of selected diagnostic studies or specific supplies and instrumentation needed intraoperatively. Fig. 4-4 depicts a preoperative assessment form with information that leads to nursing diagnoses; these guide the development and subsequent initiation of the perioperative care plan.

Perioperative nursing record. Development of a comprehensive perioperative nursing record should be the goal of each perioperative care unit (Figs. 4-5 and 4-6). The Association of Operating Room Nurses' *Recommended Practices for Documentation of Perioperative Nursing Care* (AORN, 1995) suggests a formalized system of reporting and recording the care administered to each surgical patient. Specific to the perioperative nursing record, the recommended practice suggests that the nursing process be used as the infrastructure for documenting care and include information such as the following:

1. Continual assessment and planning during the intraoperative period of care
2. Identification of all participants providing care and their names, titles, and credentials
3. Initial assessment on arrival in the perioperative care unit (level of consciousness, emotional and physical status)
4. Patient's overall skin integrity on arrival and discharge from the perioperative care unit
5. Presence or absence of communication devices (hearing aids, vocal aids) and prosthetic devices (contact lenses, dentures, wigs, and so on). If these accompany the patient to the operating room, their disposition should be noted.
6. Positioning devices and accessory supports used intraoperatively (such as arm boards, stirrups, safety straps, extremity holder, and gel pads/egg crate mattresses)
7. Area of placement for the electrosurgical dispersive pad, the type of electrosurgical unit, the unit serial numbers, and the settings
8. Wound classification categories so the perioperative nurse can identify patients at high risk for infection and take appropriate preventive measures
9. Placement of electrocardiographic leads, pulse oximeter, or other electronic devices (Doppler, electroencephalograph)
10. Area of placement of thermia units, unit serial numbers, and recording times and temperature
11. Medications administered intraoperatively by the registered nurse (Some institutions require that all medications, including those on the sterile field, be documented and noted as administered per verbal order.)
12. Surgical item counts and outcomes
13. Placement of tourniquet cuffs, identification of the unit, times of inflation and deflation, and pressures of the tourniquet
14. Placement of all drains, packings, dressings, and catheters
15. Prosthetic implants and explants, manufacturer, type and model numbers, size and serial numbers, and application of labels to the patient care record if applicable
16. Local anesthesia administration—agents used, who administered the agents, dosage, route, time, and effects of administration, monitoring devices and equipment used, nursing intervention (for example, oxygen administration), documented results of monitoring by the perioperative nurse, and any untoward reactions
17. Operative site preparation solutions, condition of the skin before and after solution application
18. Diagnostic studies performed intraoperatively
19. Urinary output and estimated blood loss
20. Types of specimens and their disposition
21. Time of completion of surgery and discharge from the operating room suite, along with patient's status and any transfer devices that were used (Patient disposition [postanesthesia care unit, ambulatory recovery, intensive care unit] and who accompanied the patient may also be noted.)

The recommended practice suggests that the patient record should reflect a continual evaluation of the perioperative nursing care and the patient's response to nursing interventions. Documentation of the care and specific outcomes provides a mechanism for evaluating the effects of the perioperative nurse's interventions as well as information that will be useful in the event of a lawsuit.

Operating Room
Perioperative Nursing Record

Patient/ID confirmation by: _____

Date _____   OR _____   Emergency   Yes _____   No _____

Surgeon _____   Surgeon _____   1st Assist _____   2nd Assist _____   Other _____

Scrub _____   Circular _____   Anesthesiologist _____

Relief _____   Relief _____   CRNA _____

Time _____   Time _____   CRNA _____

Relief _____   Relief _____

Time _____   Time _____

Preoperative diagnosis _____   Anesthesia method _____

Procedure _____
_____

Postoperative diagnosis _____   Postoperative condition _____

Complications noted _____   Blood products _____

Specimens: Tissue # _____   Culture # _____   Frozen section # _____   Other # _____

Counts: Sponges _____   Needles and sharps _____   Instruments _____

Drains   Preoperative _____   Postoperative _____

Time   In _____   Procedure start _____   End _____ PACU _____   Other _____

Preoperative Assessment

Patient arrived at: _____   Vai: Litter _____   Bed _____   Crib _____

Permit valid: Yes _____   No _____   Intervention _____

Blood products available _____   Recipient # _____

Shave prep: Yes _____   No _____   N/A _____   Intervention _____

Nursing Assessment and Intervention

Level of consciousness	Musculoskeletal	Skin appearance	Cardiopulmonary	Psychologic	Communications
Alert	No limitations	Cool	Unremarkable	Calm/relaxed	No limitations
Sedated	ROM limited	Warm	Cough	Crying	Language barrier
Drowsy	Traction	Dry	Dyspnea	Withdrawn	Hearing impaired
Asleep	Prosthesis	Flushed	Cyanosis	Restless	Aphasia/ dysphasia
Nonresponsive	Paralysis	Diaphoretic	Shock	Talkative	Blindness
Disoriented	Amputation	Excoriated		Anxious	Retardation
Comatose		Mottled			

Wound classification: 1. Clean _____   2. Clean-contaminated _____   3. Contaminated _____   4. Dirty _____

Interventions _____
_____

Allergies: Denied _____   Yes _____   _____

Prosthesis/support appliances   No _____   Yes _____

Fig. 4-5. Perioperative nursing record. (Courtesy Crozer Chester Medical Center, Chester, PA.)

Intraoperative Asessment

IV: gauge _____   site _____   by _____   N/A _____

A-line: gauge _____   site _____   by _____   N/A _____

PA line: gauge _____   site _____   by _____   N/A _____

CVP line: gauge _____   site _____   by _____   N/A _____

Position for anesthesia/local administration: Supine _____ Prone _____ Lateral _____ Sitting _____ Other _____

Patient positioned for operative procedure (indicate all positions used during procedure) Prone _____ Lithotomy _____

Right Lateral _____   Jacknife _____   Supine _____   Sitting _____   Left Lateral _____   Other _____

Patient positioned by/approved by (Surgeon and Anes) _____

Safety restraints/positioning aids:

Belt _____	R arm/suspended _____	Neuro headrest _____
R arm/board _____	L arm/suspended _____	Vac-Pac _____
L arm/board _____	Foot board _____	Blanket rolls _____
R arm/side _____	Foot rest _____	Traction table _____
L arm/side _____	Laminectomy rest _____	Arthroscopy legholder _____
R arm/chest _____	Foam headrest _____	Wedge _____
L arm/chest _____	Kidney rest _____	Lateral leg post _____
Stirrups _____	Egg crate _____	Other _____

EKG leads: R shoulder _____   L shoulder _____   Other _____

ESU: Unipolar _____   Bipolar _____   N/A _____   Number _____   Settings (cut/coag) _____

Grounding pad location: R thigh _____   L thigh _____   Other _____

Serial # _____   Brand _____   Intervention (shave area) _____

Thermal blanket: No _____   Yes _____   Serial # _____   Temperature _____

Tourniquet   No _____   Yes _____   R arm _____   L arm _____   R thigh _____   L thigh _____

           R ankle _____   L ankle _____   Other _____   mmHg _____

           Time: Up _____   Down _____   Up _____   Down _____

Operative site prepped: Iodophor solution _____   Iodophor scrub _____ (minutes)

                               Alcohol _____   Phisohex scrub _____ (minutes)   Other _____

Local Anesthesia Administration

Agent: _____   Site: _____

Administered by: _____

Time	B/P	P	R	RN Signature	Interventions

Prosthesis implanted   Yes _____   No _____   Implant: _____

Manufacturer: _____   Type/Model # _____

Size/serial # _____   See label on progress note _____

Fig. 4-5. For legend see opposite page.   *Continued.*

Label

Prosthesis removed: Yes _____   No _____

Irrigations solution: No _____   Yes _____   Type _____   Site _____

Drains/packing

        #   Type   Site

_____

_____

_____

X-Ray utilized: Yes _____   No _____   Site _____

C-Arm utilized: Yes _____   No _____   Site _____

Interventions: (document use of aprons/thyroid shields for OR personnel and patient) _____

Postoperative Assessment

Skin condition: N/A (burn patient) _____   Good _____   Other _____

Splint application: No _____   Yes _____   Type/site _____

Cast application: No _____   Yes _____   Type/site _____

Dressings: No _____   Yes _____   Type/site _____

Tape: No _____   Yes _____   Type/site _____

Patient to PACU via: Litter _____   Bed _____   Crib _____

Comments/Evaluations: _____

_____

Circulating Nurse: _____   Verbal report given by: _____
        Signature

Blood: See blood administration record

Medications: See MARPT I/O: See IV I/O record

Counts: See count record

Fig. 4-5. Perioperative nursing record. (Courtesy Crozer Chester Medical Center, Chester, PA.)

Operating room log records. Operating room log records are a permanent copy of all surgical procedures performed in the surgical departments. These records are usually not a part of the patient's permanent record but are for internal departmental use. Types of information in this record are as follows:
- Patient's name and identification number
- Patient's hospital location or outpatient designation
- Operating surgeon, first assistant, second assistant, and scrub and circulating nurses
- Types of anesthesia administered, anesthesia provider, length of anesthesia
- Length of surgical intervention; starting, ending, and PACU disposition times
- Surgical counts done and their results
- Complications during the surgical intervention

In conjunction with the general operating room log, various types of logging systems are kept in the surgical suite. These may include ophthalmologic, orthopedic, or pacemaker implant logs (Fig. 4-7). With the enactment of the Safe Medical Devices Act, forms for reporting complications related to the use of medical devices must be available and understood by perioperative personnel (Fig. 4-8). In addition to the serious adverse events listed, quality, performance, or safety concerns with products should be reported; for example, suspected contamination, questionable sterility, defective components, and poor packaging or labeling (Kessler, 1993).

Date	Consent signed ☐ Yes ☐ No
Id bracelet	Pre-op information obtained
Pre-op Post-op	☐ Pt. room ☐ Holding area

Imprint patient plate

PREOPERATIVE PHASE

Scheduled Preprocedure	**ALLERGIES**

PHYSICAL ASSESSMENT/OBSERVATIONS

Level of consciousness	Musculo/skeletal	Skin appearance	Cardiopulmonary	Psychological	Communications
Pre med	No apparent limitations	Flushed	Cyanosis	Calm/relaxed	Language barrier
No pre med	Traction	Cool	Cough	Crying	Hearing impairment
Alert	Paralysis	Warm	Dyspnea/Orthopnea	Withdrawn	Aphasia/dysphasia
Drowsy	Prosthesis	Dry	Shock	Restless	Diagnosed Retardation
Asleep	ROM limited	Excoriated	Tracheotomy	Talkative	Blindness
Responsive	Amputation	Diaphoretic	Endotracheal Tube	Anxious	No apparent limitation
Disoriented	Other	Mottled	Unremarkable	Other	Other
Comatose		Unusual marks	Other		
Other		Other			

Perioperative communication network		Patient belongings		Supportive systems to operating room	
Time of call	Initials	Item: ☐ N/A		IV	Mechanical ventilator
				Foley	IVAC
				N/G tube	IABP
		Disposition:		Drain	Ostomy
				A-Line	Oxygen
				Swan-Ganz	Other

NURSING INTERVENTIONS

Standard admissions care	Apply non-invasive monitor	Reduce environmental stimuli	Apply soft restraints
Bedpan/urinal/catheterize	Medication	Monitor vital signs	Elevate head of bed
Emotional support/reassurance	Notify surgeon/anesthesiologis	Assist to position of comfort	Ensure proper body alignment
Safety belt	Obtain transfer assistance	Apply padding	Assist with translator
Visual aids	Orientation to environment	Limit unnecessary exposure	Other

INTRAOPERATIVE PHASE

Scrub nurses	Relief/time
Circulating nurses	Relief/time

Positional aids		Prep solutions	Shave	Drip/side towels used:
Bolster/roll	Overhead armboard	Providone solution	Razor	☐ Yes ☐ No ☐ N/A
Egg crate	Traction	Providone scrub	Electric clipper	**POSITION**
Sand bag	Axillary roll	Iodine tincture	Done on pt unit	☐ Supine ☐ Lateral
Pillow	Head support	Soap solution	Depilatory	☐ Prone ☐ Jackknife
Fracture table	Kidney bar	Degreasing agent	None	☐ Lithotomy ☐ Other
Safety belt	Restraint	Other	Other	
Stirrups	Other	None		

SPECIMENS

Pathology				Micro/cytology/other	
Type		Disposition	Signature(s)	Type	Number

Fig. 4-6. Perioperative nursing record. (Courtesy the Hospital of the University of Pennsylvania, Philadelphia, PA.)

Electrosurgery		Grounding Site	Cast/Splint	Tourniquet
Monopolar	Bipolar		☐ Yes ☐ No	Setting:
S/N _____	S/N _____		Type:	Site:
Setting: cut __Coag__	Setting: cut __Coag__		Site:	Time _____ / _____

Medications/Irrigation

X-ray Fluoroscopy

☐ Yes ☐ No

S/N:

Placed by:

Packing–Tubes/Drains

Blood Loss: Blood Loss Estimated ☐ Yes ☐ No

_____ mL _____ mL _____ mL
Sponges   Suction   Total

COUNTS		Correct			Incorrect			N/A	Signatures
		Preliminary	Final	Other	Preliminary	Final	Other		**Preliminary:**
	Sponge								_____
	Cottonoid								Scrub nurse
	Pusher								_____
	Sharps								Circulating nurse
	Instrmts.								**Final:** _____ Scrub nurse _____ Circulating nurse

Discharge from operating room

						Discharge call time
Tubes and drains secure	☐ Yes	☐ No	☐ N/A	Patient checked for cleanliness	☐ Yes ☐ No	
			Transferred to: ☐ Recovery Room ☐ Floor	Transferred by: ☐ O.R. Nurse	☐ Anesthesiologist	
Skin Integrity/Pressure areas	☐ Intact	☐ Other	☐ ICU ☐ Other	☐ Surgeon or Resident	☐ Transporter ☐ Other	

VITAL SIGNS	Time															
	B/P															
	P															
	R															
	O₂ Sat.															

Comments/Nurse's notes

Fig. 4-6. Perioperative nursing record. (Courtesy the Hospital of the University of Pennsylvania, Philadelphia, PA.)

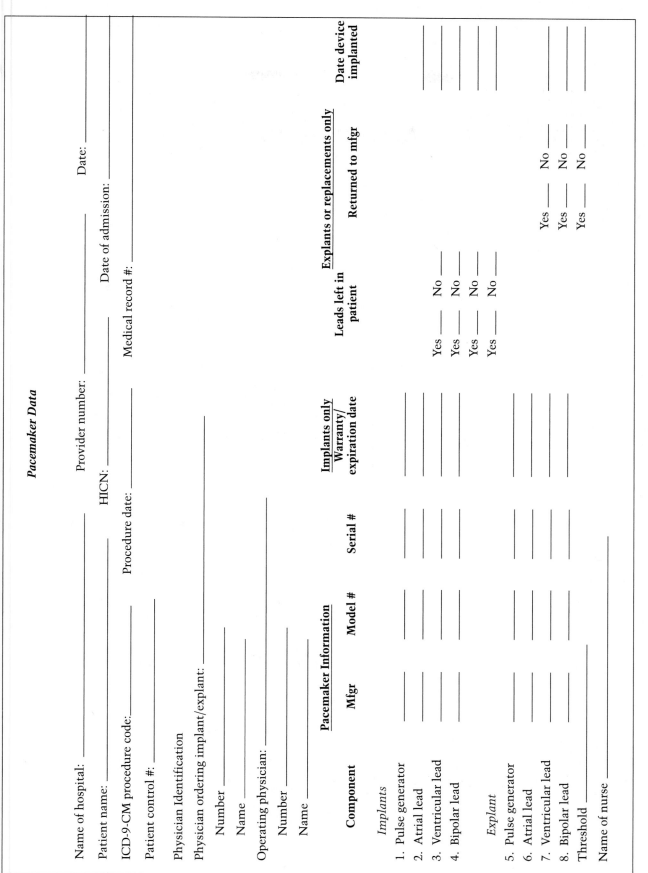

Pacemaker Data

Name of hospital: _____   Provider number: _____   Date: _____

Patient name: _____   HICN: _____   Date of admission: _____

ICD-9-CM procedure code: _____   Procedure date: _____

Patient control #: _____

Physician Identification

Physician ordering implant/explant: _____

   Number _____

   Name _____

Operating physician: _____

   Number _____

   Name _____

Pacemaker Information

| | | | Implants only | Explants or replacements only | | |
Component	Mfgr	Model #	Serial #	Warranty/ expiration date	Leads left in patient	Returned to mfgr	Date device implanted
Implants							
1. Pulse generator	_____	_____	_____	_____			_____
2. Atrial lead	_____	_____	_____	_____			_____
3. Ventricular lead	_____	_____	_____	_____			_____
4. Bipolar lead	_____	_____	_____	_____			_____
Explant							
5. Pulse generator	_____	_____	_____		Yes ___ No ___		
6. Atrial lead	_____	_____	_____		Yes ___ No ___		
7. Ventricular lead	_____	_____	_____		Yes ___ No ___	Yes ___ No ___	
8. Bipolar lead	_____	_____	_____		Yes ___ No ___	Yes ___ No ___	
Threshold	_____					Yes ___ No ___	

Name of nurse _____

Fig. 4-7. Operating room log record.

MEDWATCH
THE FDA MEDICAL PRODUCTS REPORTING PROGRAM

For VOLUNTARY reporting
by health professionals of adverse
events and product problems.

Page ___ of ___

Form Approved: OMB No. 0910-0291 Expires: 12/31/9
See OMB statement on revers

FDA Use Only (MB)

Triage unit
sequence #

A. Patient information

1. Patient identifier

In confidence

2. Age at time of event:
or _____
Date of birth:

3. Sex:
☐ female
☐ male

4. Weight
_____ lbs
or
_____ kgs

B. Adverse event or product problem

1. ☐ **Adverse event** and/or ☐ **Product problem** (e.g., defects/malfunctions)

2. Outcome attributed to adverse event
(check all that apply)

☐ death _____
(mo/day/yr)
☐ life-threating
☐ hospitalization–intial or prolonged

☐ disability
☐ congenital abnormality
☐ required intervention to prevent
permanent impairment/damage
☐ other: _____

3. Date of event:
(mo/day/yr)

4. Date of this report:
(mo/day/yr)

5. Describe event or problem

6. Relevant tests/laboratory data, including dates

7. Other relevant history, including pre-existing medical conditions (e.g., allergies
race, pregnancy, smoking and alcohol use, hepatic/renal dysfunction, etc.)

C. Suspect medication(s)

1. Name (give labeled strength & mfr/labeler, if known)
#1
#2

2. Dose, frequency & route used
#1
#2

3. Therapy dates (if unknown, give duration)
from/to (or best estimate)
#1
#2

4. Diagnosis for use (indication)
#1
#2

4. Event abated after use stopped or dose reduced
#1 ☐ yes ☐ no ☐ doesn't apply
#2 ☐ yes ☐ no ☐ doesn't apply

6. Lot # (if known)
#1
#2

7. Lot # (if known)
#1
#2

8. Event reappeared after reintroduction
#1 ☐ yes ☐ no ☐ doesn't apply
#2 ☐ yes ☐ no ☐ doesn't apply

9. NDC # (for product problems only)
_ - _

10. Concomitant medical products and therapy dates (exclude treatment of event)

D. Suspect medical device

1. Brand name

2. Type of device

3. Manufacture name & address

4. Operator of device
☐ health professional
☐ lay user/patient
☐ other: _____

5. Expiration date
(mo/day/yr)

6.
model # _____
catalog # _____
serial # _____
lot # _____
other #

7. If implanted, give date
(mo/day/yr)

8. If explanted, give date
(mo/day/yr)

9. Device available for evaluation? (Do not send to FDA)
☐ yes ☐ no ☐ returned to manufacturer on _____
(mo/day/yr)

10. Concomitant medical products and therapy dates (exclude treatment of event)

E. Reporter (see confidentiality section on back)

1. Name, address & phone #

2. Health professional?
☐ yes ☐ no

3. Occupation

4. Also reported to
☐ manufacturer
☐ user facility
☐ distributor

**5. If you do NOT want your identity disclosed
to the manufacturer, place an "X" in this box.** ☐

FDA

Mail to: MEDWATCH
5600 Fishers Lane
Rockville, MD 20852-9787

or FAX to:
1-800-FDA-0178

Fig. 4-8. The one-page MEDWatch reporting form.

Do's and don'ts of recording. The do's and don'ts of recording information on patient records for the perioperative nurse are as follows*:

Do's: When recording perioperative patient care, the perioperative nurse should:
- Read the medical record to obtain adequate information about the patient's status before giving care; the nurse is accountable for information contained in that record
- Imprint name, identification number, date, and time on every sheet
- Always use ink for recording data
- Write legibly and spell correctly
- Use appropriate form for charting
- Describe symptoms or patient conditions accurately and completely
- Use patient's own words if possible
- Use institution-approved abbreviations
- Use concise, descriptive terms
- Document factual information (what is seen, heard, or done by the nurse or the source of the nurse's information)
- Use institutional protocol for corrections (usually a line is drawn through the incorrect entry, along with the word "error" and the initials of the individual making the correction, the date, and time)
- Begin each phrase with a capital letter
- Begin each new entry on a separate line
- Document nursing action and patient's response to intervention (designate "A.M." or "P.M." when noting time of actions)
- Document telephone calls that relate to significant events or changes in the patient's condition
- Document communications with the patient's family/significant other when they are important for care and treatment of the patient
- Record all nursing care provided before surgery, in the operative/invasive procedure setting, and afterward
- When recording medications, always designate the dose, site, route, and time of administration (designate "A.M." or "P.M.")
- Record all patient education and discharge instructions
- Note the patient status on discharge from the operative area
- Sign the completed record

Don'ts: When documenting patient care given, the perioperative nurse should not:
- Record without checking name on record
- Record on blank forms
- Use ordinary paper
- Use pencil
- Back-date entry
- Tamper with or add to previous charting
- Skip lines or leave spaces
- Erase
- Chart in advance of nursing actions
- Use broad, nonspecific terms (for example, "good condition," "tolerated well")
- Use medical terminology unless absolutely sure of meaning
- Rely on memory, but should chart immediately
- Discard nurse's notes or records with errors, but should use specific error-correction format
- Repeat in narrative what is recorded in other parts in chart
- Use imprecise terms (for example, "appears to," "seems to," or "apparently")

Even with documentation guidelines, issues related to the collection of irrelevant data, the length of time spent in charting, redundant and repetitive documentation, and inconsistency from nursing unit to nursing unit persist. The nursing community has responded by working on efforts to develop documentation systems that incorporate flow sheets, standardized assessment parameters, and limited narrative charting. Systems similar to charting by exception use formats in which only exceptions to norms or significant findings are charted, eliminating detailed narratives of normal findings. Case management tools, such as clinical pathways, replace progress notes with exception documentation (variances); such tools use written practice guidelines and allow documentation of variations from the guidelines (Zander, 1994). These systems save both time and money (Warne & McWeeny, 1991) while still incorporating medical-legal parameters, the nursing process, and professional standards (Wilhelm-Hass, Rowley, & Robinson, 1991).

Documenting Credentials and Educational Activities

Rapidly changing technology in perioperative care settings mandates that perioperative nurses continue learning to keep current with changes in practice. The Joint Commission on Accreditation of Healthcare Organizations requires that nursing services provide educational programs in which nurses can keep up-to-date with current practice. Documentation of a nurse's participation in an educational program, or that he or she is credentialed to operate a particular piece of equipment, may also be important in legal liability. Credentialing data validate that perioperative nurses who provide patient care services are competent to do so. The *Competency Statements in Perioperative Nursing* (AORN, 1995) can serve as a tool for developing and using a credentialing strategy. The American Nurses Association's *Standards for Nursing Professional Development: Continuing Education and Staff Development* (ANA, 1994) recommend that all aspects of educational activities in the institution be documented; that records be maintained in compliance

*From Manuel BJ. (1980). *Reporting and documenting patient care: OR.* Denver: The Association.

with departmental, institutional, and regulatory requirements; that these data be easily retrievable; and that records be kept confidential.

Computer-Based Documentation

Information management, the assessment of outcomes, performance measurement initiatives, and comparative analysis of performance through benchmarking are all imperative strategies aimed at preserving and improving quality in the delivery of health care services. The need for data that are "good data," as opposed to the view that some data are better than none, is a common thread across federal, state, and regional measurement mandates. The use of computers to support data collection, processing, and use is clearly indicated in health care settings. McCormick (1991) has been developing a taxonomy for measurable outcomes to achieve with verification from automated nursing documentation; these are identified as the essential components for which nursing is responsible in inpatient settings and include data such as nosocomial infection, status of wound, self-care ability, and patient satisfaction. Harris and Conner (1994) suggest that careful consideration be given to the following software options: data manipulation (such as merging files, creating your own variables, converting data from one type of file to another); statistical flexibility (the number of statistical procedures the software is capable of performing); graphics strength (graphic formats for reports); and compatibility with word processors. Automatic data linkages from multiple workstations can make a reporting system very robust and enhance the use of information systems by nursing to support and enhance clinical care. In a study of a bedside computer system for nursing documentation, Dennis and her colleagues (1993) reported a positive impact on efficiency, effectiveness, and satisfaction of the nursing staff with their delivery of patient care; the mechanics of charting as well as documentation of nursing assessments and patient's responses to nursing interventions were improved. As nursing moves to develop a nursing minimum data set (NMDS), computerized records will enable the profession to compare data across patient populations, clinical settings, and geographic areas; to better describe nursing care delivered to patients and their families; to project trends related to nursing care requisites and resource allocation by nursing diagnosis; and to stimulate nursing research through access and linkages to data existing in nursing data sets. In 1994, the Health Industry Manufacturers Association (HIMA), the Center for Health Information Management (CHIM), and the Center for Healthcare Information Management Executives (CHIME) formed an alliance to recommend to Congress the benefits of health information systems. Included in the alliance's recommendations were establishing administrative and clinical data standards, an electronic transmission standard, and security and confidentiality precautions; promoting the use of computer-based patient records; and continuing development and support of financial and clinical implications (Alliance Formed, 1994). Chapter 3 provides a detailed description of some of the possibilities and potentials of an automated system for perioperative patient care.

LEGAL ASPECTS OF DOCUMENTATION

The primary function of documentation is to record pertinent information regarding the patient, the delivery of patient care, and its outcomes. Documentation also helps obtain reimbursement and creates a legal record for the patient. Patient's medical records can and do become evidence in health care litigation (Kemmy, 1993). Standards for documentation come from a variety of sources: professional nursing associations (for example, American Nurses Association, Association of Operating Room Nurses), federal and state statutes or regulations, accrediting bodies such as the Joint Commission on Accreditation of Healthcare Organizations, the nurse practice acts of each state, other health care accreditation groups, and institutional policy and procedure. Failure to document care allows the courts to infer that care was not delivered. In addition, failure to document care may in itself be evidence of negligence (Sensenbrenner, 1993).

Documentation as Evidence in Litigation

Accurate documentation protects both the patient and the nurse; it often plays a critical role in malpractice litigation (Blackwell, 1993). What is or is not documented may be crucial to a strong legal defense. In most cases, the plaintiff (patient) has the burden to prove that the nurse was negligent, or did or did not do what a reasonable and prudent nurse would do (Box 4-1). However, the operating room is an area in which the court may shift the responsibility to the defendant. That is, the court may require the defendants to prove that their activities were not negligent and that their actions were reasonable and prudent. For these reasons, the do's and don'ts of recording patient information ensure patients of quality care and provide nurses with protection in the event of a lawsuit. Murphy (1987) suggested the following five strategies nurses can use to prevent a successful malpractice claim:

- Prevent patient injuries
- Initiate positive patient rapport

Box 4-1 Basis for Professional Liability

Duty—When a perioperative nurse participates in or assumes care of a patient or is charged with a duty to assume potential care of patients, the nurse owes the duty to the patient to possess the degree of learning and skill ordinarily possessed by members of the perioperative nursing profession in good standing, and to exercise the degree of care ordinarily exercised by other perioperative nurses in similar situations.

Breach of duty—A perioperative nurse breaches his or her duty to a patient if there is a failure to act as would a reasonable and prudent perioperative nurse in similar circumstances.

Causation—In order for the perioperative nurse to be held civilly liable to a patient (plaintiff), the perioperative nurse's failure to act in accordance with the standard of care must have resulted in some harm to the patient that the patient would not have otherwise sustained.

Modified from Sensenbrenner EP. (1993, October). *Avoiding liability in the surgical setting: Professional accountability is the key.* Paper presented at Contemporary Forums—Perioperative Nursing, New Orleans.

- Control any damage
- Comply with the standard of care
- Document nursing care

Preventing a successful malpractice claim: an example. One of the goals of perioperative nursing care is the maintenance of skin integrity. Perioperative nurses recognize the high risk for skin injury from electrical hazards, thermal hazards, chemical hazards, surgical positioning, and pressure insults from lengthy surgical procedures. During an admission assessment in the holding area, the perioperative nurse meets the patient. Following introductions, the perioperative nurse checks and verifies the patient's consent, validates information about the patient's condition, determines whether there are risk factors for patient injury or intraoperative complications, and generally determines whether the patient has any specific needs. All of this information helps provide safe, comfortable care. Although the time for patient assessment is brief, the perioperative nurse has established rapport with the patient. The patient feels cared about and cared for.

Based on assessment data and knowledge about the anticipated surgical intervention, the perioperative nurse creates the following care plan:

Nursing diagnosis: High risk for impaired skin integrity

Outcome: The patient's skin integrity will be maintained

Nursing actions: Place electrosurgical dispersive pad on right thigh (the thigh has been assessed as being close to the operative site and has good muscle mass, no scars, excess hair or oil)

Place elbow and heel protectors

Provide sacral and occipital padding

Keep legs uncrossed

The perioperative nurse has designed a plan of care to prevent patient injuries. The plan is not remarkable; it is the kind of plan most perioperative nurses routinely carry out. The perioperative nursing record indicates that these actions were implemented. *Nursing care was documented.* In addition, the *standard of care* was carried out. The care provided was what a reasonable and prudent perioperative nurse would have done under similar circumstances. Nonetheless, hours later, the discharge care unit communicates to the perioperative care unit that a lesion has been found on the patient's buttocks. The lesion is assessed and treated; no further damage occurs (infection), and the skin injury resolves. *Damage to the patient was controlled.* An investigation did not uncover any malfunctioning equipment; the skin injury was unexplained. If a malpractice claim is initiated, the perioperative nurse and the discharge patient care unit staff have acted to control the damage. It would be difficult to establish that the nurse had failed to act in accordance with the standard of care. By complying with the standard of care and documenting the care, the nurse makes it easier for his or her attorney to counter the plaintiff's arguments that the standard of care was not met. The documentation on the perioperative nursing record fortifies the argument that neither the nurse's actions or lack of action contributed to or caused the skin injury.

SUMMARY

The professional challenge to the perioperative nurse is to record the continuity of care accurately and comprehensively. This type of documentation helps nurses position themselves to meet the legal standard of reasonable and prudent nursing care. Each health care facility should have a written policy and procedures for documenting perioperative nursing care. In the perioperative care unit, the nurse should document the continuous monitoring of each patient's nursing diagnosis and the plans and interventions that lead to identified desired patient outcomes. The focus in documentation should be on communicating important data about the patient from one member of the health care team to another. Documentation is an extremely important nursing activity. No matter what form the nursing record takes, its primary focus is the facilitation of patient care through communication, coordination, and evaluation. Accurate and complete perioperative nursing records are important for quality assessment and performance improvement activities and risk management, to accrediting bodies and third-party payors, and in legal proceedings. In the future, an increased emphasis on documentation will be driven by the current economics of the health care system and utilization management, a continued emphasis on quality and its measurement, an emphasis on standardization and standards of care, the identification of nurses' contributions to the care of patients, and the ongoing emphasis on effectiveness and efficiency in delivery systems.

References

Alliance formed to promote health information systems. *AAMI News, 29*(8), 7.

American Nurses Association. (1994). *Standards for nursing professional development: Continuing education and staff development.* Washington, DC: The Association.

Association of Operating Room Nurses. (1995). Competency statements in perioperative nursing. In *AORN standards and recommended practices for perioperative nursing.* Denver: The Association.

Association of Operating Room Nurses. (1995). Recommended practices for documentation of perioperative nursing care. In *AORN standards and recommended practices for perioperative nursing.* Denver: The Association.

Blackwell MK. (1993). Documentation serves as invaluable defense tool. *The American Nurse, 25*(7), 40-41.

Chana CH. (1992). Documenting the nursing process: A perioperative nursing care plan. *AORN Journal, 55*(5), 1231-1235.

Dennis KE, et al. (1993). Point of care technology: Impact on people and paperwork. *Nursing Economics, 11*(4), 229-237, 248.

Foust JB. (1994). Creating a future for nursing through interactive planning at the bedside. *Image—the Journal of Nursing Scholarship, 26*(2), 129-131.

Harris CS & Conner CB. (1994). Building a computer-supported quality improvement system in one year. *Journal on Quality Improvement, 20*(6), 330-342.

Iyer PW & Camp NH. (1992). *Nursing documentation: A nursing process approach.* St. Louis: Mosby.

Kemmy JA. (1993). Legal implications of perioperative documentation. *AORN Journal, 57*(4), 954-958.

Kessler DA. (1993). Introducing MEDWatch. *Journal of the American Medical Association, 269*(21), 2765-2768.

McCormick KA. (1991). Future data needs for quality of care monitoring, DRG considerations, reimbursement, and outcome measurement. *Image—the Journal of Nursing Scholarship, 23*(1), 29-32.

McFarland GK & McFarlane EA. (1993). *Nursing diagnosis and intervention: Planning for patient care.* St. Louis: Mosby.

Murphy EK. (1987). Preventing a successful malpractice claim. *AORN Journal, 46*, 106-110.

Sensenbrenner EP. (1993, October). *Avoiding liability in the surgical setting: Professional accountability is the key.* Paper presented at Contemporary Forums—Perioperative Nursing, New Orleans.

Spry C & Jenkins M. (1991). Intraoperative log: development, revision considerations. *AORN Journal, 53*(3), 740-742.

Warne MA & McWeeny MC. (1991). Managing the cost of documentation: The FACT charting system. *Nursing Economics, 9*(3), 181-187.

Weeks CS. (1890). *Textbook of nursing.* New York: D Appleton.

Wilhelm-Hass E, Rowley S, & Robinson M. (1991). The OR record: Developing a format for documenting care. *AORN Journal, 53*(3), 754-760.

Zander K. (1994). Case management update. *Seminars in Perioperative Nursing, 3*(1), 55-58.

Chapter 5

Joint Commission Recommendations and Requirements

Sheri J. Voss

*T*he need to plan care provided to patients is an accepted fact among nurses. In perioperative patient care settings, planning and organizing are critical to outcome achievement. What is most challenged, both by perioperative nurses and their nursing colleagues, is the need (and time) to document in detail the planning of care. Although nurses have used the nursing process for more than three decades, the planning part of the process has been difficult for perioperative nurses to implement. Chapter 1 describes the nursing process and its application to perioperative patient care. Although few would disagree that perioperative nurses engage in planning care in their everyday practice, the concrete evidence of that planning has most often been absent. The perioperative nurse sets priorities based on assessment data: "This patient has cardiovascular disease and is scheduled to undergo a lengthy surgical intervention. The patient is at high risk for impaired skin integrity." An outcome is identified: "Skin integrity will be maintained. The patient will not experience any skin irritation, reddened areas, or breakdown." Nursing actions are decided on: "Extra padding will be used on dependent pressure areas. Foam booties will be applied to the heels. An anesthesia screen will be placed over the patient's feet to prevent the drapes from weighing on the lower extremities." Mentally, the perioperative nurse engages in these nursing process activities with every patient. Yet the documentation of this process is often missing. Without documentation, it is difficult for other nurses or health caregivers to know what the perioperative nurse planned or did, nor can evaluation of the care or clinical research on its effectiveness be measured. Unless care is documented, neither perioperative nurses nor their professional colleagues can come to any conclusions about the effectiveness of nursing actions. Documentation of nursing care enhances patient care and is professionally and legally expected. It allows for communication about and determination of the effectiveness of the nursing actions performed. The delivery of appropriate, effective, efficient care by nurses and the rest of the health care system is of concern to the profession and the public. Initiatives to monitor the performance of health services have been part of the history and evolution of health care delivery in the United States.

HISTORICAL OVERVIEW

The nursing profession is not unique in its efforts to improve documentation. Initial attempts by the American College of Surgeons to evaluate the results of treatment and to set standards were frustrated by poorly recorded histories and physical findings. When the College was founded in 1913 for the purpose of organizing and standardizing treatment, more than half the potential members were rejected because the records they submitted to validate their competence did not provide enough information (Roberts, Coale, & Redman, 1988). To their credit, these physicians developed standards and surveys to improve the conditions in hospitals, which at that time were deplorable. Improved documentation was inherent in the program. Effective written communication was recognized early as an integral component of organized patient care.

Today, the Joint Commission on Accreditation of Healthcare Organizations is a private voluntary agency that accredits approximately 5300 hospitals and 3000 other types of health care institutions. It was organized in 1951 as an outgrowth of the evaluation process first instituted by the American College of Surgeons in 1917. The earliest Joint Commission standards were structural standards, which attempted to create an environment in which the best possible patient care was provided. The accreditation process focused primarily on medical practice; the standards for nursing were contained on less than one page (Box 5-1). Through the years, the Joint Commission requirements have had a major impact on the provision of high-quality care in hospitals. When the federal government wrote conditions for participation in Medicare in the 1960s, the Joint Commission moved to promote optimal levels of care for hospitalized patients. In addition, other types of health and health-related organizations worked with the Joint Commission to develop new accreditation programs (Roberts, Coale, and Redman, 1988). Today, there are five Joint Commission accreditation programs with established standards and survey procedures. These programs include accreditation of such agencies as long-term care, home care, mental health and ambulatory health care, as well as the accreditation program for hospitals with which perioperative nurses are most familiar.

The Joint Commission has preserved the tradition established by the American College of Surgeons. The accreditation process remains voluntary, and the standards are developed through agreement by health professionals as to their efficacy in providing high-quality care to patients. The accreditation process combines evaluation, education, and consultation.

An important relationship between the Joint Commission and government began in 1965 when the Medicare Act was passed by Congress. A provision was written into that law that allowed for hospitals accredited by the Joint Commission to be "deemed" to meet eligibility requirements for participation in the Medicare program. Government oversight and validation of Joint Commission findings were added in 1972 through amendments to the Social Security Act (Roberts, Coale, and Redman, 1988). Similarly, Joint Commission accreditation requirements were woven into state licensing systems.

Adherence to Joint Commission accreditation requirements represents a commitment to provide a safe, appropriate, and effective standard of care. The standards related to improving organizational performance through continual monitoring and evaluation of important aspects of care are an integral component of a written plan of patient care.

JOINT COMMISSION: PERFORMANCE-FOCUSED STANDARDS

The introduction in 1988 of the chapter on "Surgical and Anesthesia Services" in the *Accreditation Manual for Hospitals* represented the culmination of years of effort by the Association of Operating Room Nurses (AORN) and other organizations. Included in this chapter was an emphasis on the documentation related to perioperative nursing practice. Perioperative nursing practice should be documented in a manner that is easily identified and retrieved during an accreditation visit. This challenge is intensified by the current high demand for perioperative nursing services and the limited time available to document perioperative nursing activities. Nevertheless, the goal must be met.

The 1992 *Accreditation Manual for Hospitals* (AMH) represented the first portion of a multiyear transition to standards that emphasize the application of quality improvement principles and concepts. To accomplish this, major revisions to the manual were made in 1993 that emphasized the organization's role in the continuous improvement of quality (Joint Commission, 1993b). The goal of this reorganization was to change the focus of standards that had been organized around a hospital's departments or services to standards organized around functions most critical to patient care (Box 5-2). Some functions are direct-care activities, such as pa-

---

Box 5-2 An Overview of the Joint Commission and the 1995 Manual

Mission: to improve the quality of care provided to the public. Health Care Functions: Those systems, processes, or jobs that most directly and tangibly affect patient outcomes

Important Functions in the Accreditation Manual for Hospitals

Care of the patient functions
Rights of the patient and organizational ethics
Assessment of patients
Entry to setting or service
Nutritional care
Treatment of patients
Operative and other invasive procedures
Education of patients and family
Coordination of care

Organizational functions
Leadership
Management of human resources
Management of environment of care
Surveillance, prevention, and control of infection
Improving organizational performance

Structures with important functions
Governing body
Management and administration
Nursing

---

tient assessment and discharge planning; others support those care activities, such as information management, competency assessment, and safety management. Thus, in such a framework, "functions" in health care organizations are those that most substantively influence patient outcomes. Patient outcomes may be quantified in terms of many variables; perioperative nurses are particularly interested in physiologic, psychosocial, and qualitative outcomes such as patient satisfaction. The Joint Commission has identified attributes such as accessibility, efficacy, appropriateness, timeliness, safety, continuity, acceptability, and efficiency of care as transcending the eventual determination of the patient's health status, satisfaction with care delivery, and perceptions of the value of that care.

The 1995 AMH represents an underlying premise that, in order for a health care organization to deliver high-quality patient care, its leaders must carefully structure a framework for planning, directing, coordinating, providing, and improving the delivery of health care services that are responsive to patient and community needs and that improve patient outcomes (Patterson, 1994). Performance improvement

requires five processes: plan, design, measure, assess, improve. The Joint Commission sets standards for performance of patient care and organizational *functions*, against which the health care institution is measured (surveyed). The chapter entitled "Surgical and Anesthesia Services" was replaced by the chapter "Operative and Other Invasive Procedures," which contains many of the standards previously found in the surgical and anesthesia section. However, other key standards have been relocated to incorporate this functional approach to the delivery and improvement of patient care. Thus, in the 1995 manual, it is explicit that the health care institution will measure its performance of processes in all patient care and organizational functions identified in the manual.

Before the 1995 *Accreditation Manual for Hospitals,* standards addressing patient assessment and documentation could be found throughout the manual; for example, the "Nursing Care" chapter focused on what nursing staff must document in each patient's medical record relative to the nursing care provided. The "Physical Rehabilitation Services" section focused on documentation requirements for all rehabilitation disciplines. In 1995, functional chapters of standards focused on the nursing process and care performance were transformed into five patient-focused functional chapters of standards: "Patient Rights and Organizational Ethics"; "Assessment of Patients"; "Care of Patients"; "Education of Patient and Family"; and "Continuum of Care." Thus, in the chapter on "Assessment of Patients," aspects of the specific discipline and department or service requirements are presented under one key function. This chapter, which addresses the organization's responsibility to define what must be assessed, by whom, through what processes, and by what criteria, has major implications for perioperative nursing and for planning the care for patients undergoing operative or other invasive procedures. Because perioperative nursing has clear directives from its own professional association and the Joint Commission regarding the importance of planning and documenting care, it is critical for perioperative nurses to identify key components in guiding their efforts.

Key Components

Care planning requirements expected by the Joint Commission are intentionally nonprescriptive. The wide variation among facilities that provide surgery and anesthesia services necessitates widely varying methods of outcome achievement with regard to a standard of care for patients. However, a rationale for focusing on AORN outcome statements and competencies (AORN, 1995) in developing care plans is clearly elucidated in the "Operative and Other Invasive Procedures" chapter if the Joint Commission requirements are to be met. Care plans can be used not only as a guide for delivery of care but as data collection instruments for monitoring and evaluating care given through documentation. Development of care plans should guide nursing activities. A plan of care should direct the activities of the nurse so that care is consistent, coordinated, and outcome directed.

Accreditation surveys have changed throughout their history as they have struggled for the effective measurement of quality of care. As part of the Joint Commission's commitment to patient outcomes, costs, quality, and value, a redesign of the survey process was crucial. By focusing on these four important results, the intent is to measure the effectiveness and efficiency of organizational functions through a "systems-oriented" approach. Current recommendations for nursing require this focus.

Recommendations regarding the nursing process: key components. There are several key components to meeting accreditation recommendations for care planning. One component, use of the nursing process, is addressed as follows in the "Assessment of Patients" chapter of the 1995 *Accreditation Manual for Hospitals* (Joint Commission, 1995):

- A registered nurse assesses the patient's need for nursing care in all settings in which nursing care is to be provided.
  Required Characteristics:
  - Each patient's nursing care is based on identified nursing diagnoses and/or patient care needs and patient care standards and is consistent with the therapies of other disciplines.

The nursing process is also addressed in the "Operative and Other Invasive Procedures" chapter, requiring that:

The plans of care for the patient are formulated and documented in his/her medical record before the procedure(s) is performed and include at least a plan for nursing care.

In breaking down this standard, it is clear that the nursing process is the framework for development of the plan of care. To "provide nursing services to meet the nursing care needs of patients," perioperative nurses must first identify those needs. The *AORN Standards of Perioperative Clinical Practice* (AORN, 1995) guide the nurse in meeting this requirement through specific criteria for assessment and collection of data (Standard I), formulation of appropriate nursing diagnoses (Standard II), outcome identification (Standard III), developing a plan of care (Standard IV), implementing interventions that have been identified (Standard V), and evaluation of outcomes (Standard VI). Because each patient has individual needs, emphasis is placed on identifying not only potential problems/high-risk nursing diagnoses of all patients who undergo surgery, but also on problems unique to the particular patient.

Recommendations for staffing: key components. Ensuring competency of nursing staff members is a key element of staffing as evidenced by standard NC.2 of the AMH (1995), which states:

All nursing staff members are competent to fulfill their assigned responsibilities.

Nursing staff members include registered nurses, licensed practical/vocational nurses, nursing assistants, and other nursing personnel. Additional staffing requirements are noted in the following standards:

NC2.1.2 Nursing care responsibilities are assigned to a nursing staff member in accordance with

NC2.1.2.1 the degree of supervision needed by the individual and its availability; and

NC2.1.2.2 the complexity and dynamics of the condition of each patient to whom the individual is to provide services and the complexity of the assessment required by each patient, including

NC2.1.2.2.1 the factors that must be considered to make appropriate decisions regarding the provision of nursing care; and

NC2.1.2.2.2 the type of technology employed in providing nursing care.

Further information relevant to the appropriateness of staffing is stated as follows:

NC.4.1 The plan for nurse staffing and the provision of nursing care is reviewed in detail on an annual basis and receives periodic attention as warranted by changing patient care needs and outcomes.

Perhaps one of the more important standards related to care planning states:

NC4.1.1 Registered nurses prescribe, delegate and coordinate the nursing care provided throughout the hospital.

NC4.1.2 Consistent standards for the provision of nursing care within the hospital are used to monitor and evaluate the quality of nursing care provided throughout the hospital.

The issue of competency is further elucidated in the chapter, "Management of the Human Resource Function." This chapter clearly posits that the organization's leaders define qualifications and job expectations; provide qualified staff; design processes to ensure that competence of all staff is assessed, maintained, demonstrated, and improved on a continuing basis; and provide ongoing inservice and other education to maintain staff competence. An employee's competence must be assessed at employment and during orientation, and an objective, measurable performance system must be in place. A registered nurse with both clinical and management experience is necessary to determine competence and make subsequent patient care assignments based on that determination. If a nonnurse delegates, instructs, or supervises unlicensed persons in the performance of nursing functions, this constitutes the practice of nursing without a license (Statement on the nursing activities of unlicensed persons, 1994).

In 1988, the standards addressing staffing and the requirement for the registered nurse circulator were found in the chapter, "Surgical and Anesthesia Services." In 1993 the key standards stated:

SA.1.7.1 A registered nurse, qualified by relevant education, training, experience and documented competence is responsible for planning and directing the nursing care of patients who undergo surgery and other invasive procedures when receiving anesthesia.

SA. 1.7.3.1 A qualified registered nurse is assigned to circulating duties for the operating room and obstetric delivery room.

The standards further stated:

SA.1.7.3.1 Other qualified operating room personnel assisting in circulating duties in the operating room and the obstetric delivery room are under the supervision of a qualified registered nurse who is immediately available.

With the reorganization of the 1994 manual, the language from these standards was moved to the scoring guidelines, where the plan of nursing care and a plan for the operative or other invasive procedure are discussed, along with requirements for monitoring patients during anesthesia and the operative procedure. Moving the previous language out of the standards is a concern among perioperative nurses, but is in keeping with the Joint Commission's goal of moving all specific language to the scoring guidelines, which will make the standards more flexible and less prescriptive. These scoring guidelines will be used over time to articulate ongoing expectations in standards compliance. Thus the intent of the scoring guidelines is to assess and determine whether the leaders in the health care organization have carefully planned and exercised due caution when deciding on the type(s) of educational backgrounds and competencies to require in order to have a sufficient number of qualified personnel to deliver high-quality perioperative patient care (Patterson, 1994). The intent of standards on nursing care is clearly that a registered nurse sees the perioperative patient at the time of admission and makes the determination of patient care needs and nursing diagnoses, because these activities require the knowledge, judgment, and skill of a registered nurse. The intent of the Joint Commission relative to the requirement for a registered nurse circulator will be tested as surveys are conducted in 1995 and beyond. Numerous other standards clearly support the registered professional nurse as the individual that must assess, plan, and direct care for patients receiving nursing care throughout the institution. It is inherent in the requirement for patient care planning through the use of the nursing process (Joint Commission, 1994). Thus, in addition to recommendations important from the viewpoint of accreditation, use of the nursing process—with its focus on assessment, planning, implementing, and evaluating—becomes of primary importance in validating the critical reasons why the circulator in perioperative patient care settings should be a nurse, in addition to confirming the need for and skills of the nurse. The nurse must develop the plan of care and accurately identify activities that may be delegated to other personnel "under the supervision" of the nurse. During surveys, the Joint Commission will assess staffing adequacy using indirect measures such as missed treatments, medication errors, incorrect counts, and other risk-management indicators and measures (see Chapter 2 for a more detailed discussion of the relation of risk management and performance improvement).

Recommendations for care planning: key components. The "Nursing Care" chapter of the manual provides additional guidance regarding care planning, as does the chapter, "Management of Information: Patient Specific Data."

Standards related to the documentation of nursing care and the elements of the nursing process may be found in Standard IM.7 (See Chapter 3 for a thorough review of information management [IM] systems and perioperative implications) and more specifically in IM.7.2, which states the following:

The medical record contains sufficient information to identify the patient, support the diagnosis, justify the treatment, document the course and results accurately, and facilitate continuity of care among health care providers. Each medical record contains at least the following:

IM7.2.5 a statement of the conclusions or impressions drawn from the medical history and physical examination;

IM7.2.15 All reassessments, when necessary;

IM7.2.6 The diagnosis or diagnostic impression;

IM7.2.11 Diagnostic and therapeutic orders, if any;

IM7.2.12 All diagnostic and therapeutic procedures and tests performed and the results;

IM7.2.17 The response to the care provided.

Clearly the standards mentioned above have application for and support the use of the nursing process. The reorganization and restructuring of Joint Commission standards have been accomplished to incorporate a cross-functional approach to patient care activities.

The chapter, "Improving Organizational Performance," outlines the Joint Commission's expectations in terms of a focus on performance assessment and improvement, and it represents a significant change from the performance of individuals to the performance of the organization's systems and processes, while continuing to recognize the importance of staff competence in the delivery of patient care. The measurement mandate is a social mandate. With managed competition, key decision making will be driven by performance data. Good measurement systems will demand a focus on delivery processes that are relevant to measure, balancing measures of outcomes and standards with other performance measures. In 1994, the Joint Commission permitted public access to specific information about an organization's performance; the release of accreditation-related data is expected to begin later. Publicly disclosed organization-specific performance information will provide comparative ratings of standards compliance in areas such as nursing care, infection control, patient rights, and life safety (Joint Commission prepares for release of organization specific performance data, 1993).

Essentially, the nurse in perioperative patient care settings is expected to provide perioperative nursing care according to the standards of practice established by the AORN and the American Nurses Association. The process used for documentation should meet the needs of the individual facility. The Joint Commission uses a multidisciplinary team during accreditation surveys consisting of administrator, nurse executive, and physician members. Although all anesthetizing locations in the institution are visited by one or more team members, an accreditation surveyor may obtain only a limited view of actual patient care during a site visit. Therefore, nursing policies and procedures, along with documentation of care in the patient record, are examined to determine if the structure and process used reflect adherence to the standards. The surveyor will look for documented evidence of assessment of each patient undergoing surgery or procedures that require anesthesia. Further, evidence will be required that the individual, ongoing needs of the patient are reflected in the planning and implementation of care. The survey team will also review staffing plans and records.

It should be noted that the accreditation process is a component of an overall mission to improve or maintain a high standard of patient care. This is a goal consistent with institutional or individual nursing goals. The primary purpose of the nursing process and identified standards of care is organized and effective delivery of appropriate, individualized care to patients.

GENERIC CARE PLANS

If the development of a perioperative patient care plan uses the *AORN Standards of Perioperative Clinical Practice*, the *AORN Patient Outcomes: Standards of Perioperative Care*, the *AORN Competency Statements in Perioperative Nursing*, and the *AORN Recommended Practices for Documentation of Perioperative Nursing Care*, the required characteristics as identified in the Joint Commission standards will be met. A generic plan that identifies those nursing diagnoses that apply to all patients who undergo surgery is an acceptable and desirable method. Generic care plans are a viable way of demonstrating that patients with the same health status and condition receive a comparable level of surgical nursing care. This is expected by the Joint Commission. However, the surveyor will want to verify that the plan is dynamic. To make the most effective use of the nurse's time, printed material with space provided for variances is acceptable, but only if the variances are identified and addressed. As generic plans are modified to include nursing diagnoses specific to a particular type of surgery, there must always be space for nursing diagnoses unique to a particular patient's problem or needs. For patients who have a relatively uncomplicated set of nursing diagnoses, the generic plans may include all potential problems and needs. Nurse surveyors for the Joint Commission understand the time constraints placed on nurses, and applaud creative development of care plans that are efficient to use yet guide the nurse in recognizing individual patient needs. Combining a standard that guides patient care planning and implementation with easy-to-document interventions and outcomes provides an effective and valuable tool for perioperative nurses.

Care Plans and Performance-Focused Standards

Improving performance, particularly those processes or systems that have the greatest impact on patient outcomes, is the focus of the 1995 AMH chapter, "Improving Organizational Performance." It is expected that health care institutions will incorporate concepts and methods that include a total quality-management approach to the delivery of care and services within those institutions.

Dynamic care plans can provide a framework for measuring specific "practice guidelines" related to perioperative nursing. The monitoring and evaluation of care may be accomplished through observation and chart review, with a focus on important aspects of care that are high-volume, high-risk, or problem-prone aspects or diagnoses. Findings of monitoring and evaluation activities should not only assist in the identification of problems, but more important, should focus on opportunities to improve care or the delivery of service. Eliminating variances in a process or system, streamlining care activities, and identifying educational needs are important components of the quality-improvement process.

A quality-improvement example. Monitoring and evaluation might be carried out on a selected number of surgery patients. Use of generic care plans that reflect the AORN outcome standards facilitates the efficacy of retrospective surveys in identifying problem areas. Setting a threshold, a point at which opportunities to improve care are identified, guides the corrective action.

For example, a retrospective survey of 50 patient records might focus on information retrieved from the patient care plan and intraoperative record. Assume that the focus on inquiry is on maintaining skin integrity, a perioperative nursing concern common for all patients. The desired patient outcome is, "The patient's skin integrity will be maintained." The measurable goal of nursing care is, "There will be no skin irritation, reddened areas, or breakdown." A threshold might be set at 95% or 100%, with the expectation that this goal would be met for most patients. Of the 50 records reviewed, however, 11 document a reddened area on the patient's heels in the immediate postoperative period. Further review of these records reveals that the reddened area had faded by the time the patient was transferred from the postanesthesia care unit. If the care plan had documented that these 11 patients had folded towels placed under their heels, but did not have foam booties, even more important information would have been collected. The survey does not provide a causal relationship; only clinical research could do that. However, the survey alerts the nursing staff to review positioning devices and accessories in use, to review nursing practice relative to padding and protecting the patient's skin during positioning with all staff, and to schedule a follow-up survey for 3 months later. If patients continue to have reddened areas on their heels, further study would be indicated. If not, the perioperative nursing staff may wish to make the use of foam booties a standard part of their plan of care. Either way, the fact that care plans provided retrievable data is of enormous importance to nursing's quality- and performance-improvement activities.

Use of care plans as data-collection instruments facilitates recognition of potential problems before serious injuries occur, as well as fostering the im-

provement of nursing practice and ultimately the care delivered to patients. Joint Commission requirements for improving organizational performance are designed to promote this type of activity.

CLINICAL INDICATORS

A major developmental project entitled "Agenda for Change" was initiated by the Joint Commission in the fall of 1986. The project goal has centered on development of an outcome-oriented monitoring and evaluation process. Hospitals accredited by the Joint Commission have been participating in the new monitoring, survey, and evaluation process for some time. The clinical emphasis of the accreditation process continues to increase, along with quality-related activities of participating organizations. Performance outcomes continue to be stressed. "Agenda for Change" is a major initiative that is intended to support health care facilities in their attempts to improve quality of care. A major thrust is the formulation of a system for more effective and accurate measurement of a facility's performance through the use of established clinical indicators, which measure patient outcomes and/or the processes that comprise the identified important functions. These indicators involve a more direct review of patient care. A set of 10 indicators was selected by the Joint Commission for voluntary use beginning in 1994. Twenty indicators are available on a voluntary basis in 1995; mandatory use of 30 indicators is anticipated to begin in 1996, requiring health care organizations to demonstrate the effectiveness with which they are using indicator data to monitor and improve their performance. Although clinical indicators may not directly measure quality of clinical performance, they will be useful in raising sound questions about the quality of care. Indicators act as "flags" or "screens" that highlight the need for problem investigation and analysis or may lead to an opportunity to improve. By identifying and selecting acceptable clinical indicators, the Joint Commission intends to direct its attention and monitoring activities to the most important aspects of patient care. Using these indicators, health care facilities should be enabled in asking the important question, "Are we really providing quality care?"

SUMMARY

The Joint Commission requirements reflect important concepts and activities pertaining to perioperative nursing practice. Documentation is inherent in effective communication among professionals through patient care plans. The Joint Commission's documentation requirements reflect nursing's commitment to improve patient care through education and research. Assessment of each patient and subsequent development and modification of a plan of care are in the domain of nursing and underscore the necessity for the registered nurse circulator. The nursing process organizes and guides care planning for effective delivery of appropriate, individualized care to patients. Standards of care imply an expected outcome for each patient. These outcomes are used in monitoring and evaluating care to ensure that a high level of quality is provided. Perioperative nurses are well positioned in the new framework of a patient-focused care environment. They will be increasingly challenged to demonstrate the value they add to perioperative patient care delivery systems and processes and to improving patient outcomes, resource allocation, and cost-effective care. The use of generic care plans, care protocols, and critical pathways will help perioperative nurses develop a unified data base and a research-based practice. Perioperative nurses must be ready to meet these challenges by continuing to refine the "how" and "why" of their care processes so that they may adequately answer questions of "who, when, where, and how much" may be delegated or assigned to their other care partners. When the perioperative nurse delegates selected nursing functions or tasks, the responsibility and accountability to the public for the overall nursing care remains with the nurse (Statement on the nursing activities of unlicensed persons, 1994). Therefore, the processes of caring for and doing for, and their integration with the knowledge, skill, and judgment of perioperative nursing, must be robustly studied and clearly articulated in the interest of appropriate, safe, effective, and efficient perioperative patient care.

References

Association of Operating Room Nurses. (1995). *Standards and Recommended Practices for Perioperative Nursing.* Denver: The Association.

Joint Commission prepares for release of organization specific performance data. (1993a). *Nursing Economics, 11*(5), 314.

Joint Commission on Accreditation of Healthcare Organizations. (1993b). *Agenda for change update: Standards development.* Chicago: The Commission.

Joint Commission on Accreditation of Healthcare Organizations. (1994). *Accreditation Manual for Hospitals, 1995.* Chicago: The Commission.

Patterson CH. (1994). Joint Commission focus on important functions: The management of human resources. *Emerging Issues,* March, 1994, Chicago: National Council of State Boards of Nursing.

Roberts JS, Coale JG, & Redman RR. (1988). A history of the Joint Commission on Accreditation of Hospitals. *Journal of the American Medical Association, 258,* 936.

Statement on the nursing activities of unlicensed persons. (1994). Chicago: National Council of State Boards of Nursing.

Wakefield B. (1994). The evolution of the Joint Commission's nursing standards. *Journal for Health Care Quality, 20*(6), 37-43.

Chapter 6

Delivery of Perioperative Care: Case Management

Nancy J. Girard

*P*erioperative nurses deliver optimal patient care by ensuring the right surgical procedure is performed on the right patient, within the right time frame, using the right skills and resources. The expert perioperative nurse uses problem-solving and critical-thinking skills daily. Decision making, along with competent psychomotor skills, form the core of perioperative nursing. Perioperative nurses must use their extensive cognitive abilities and be able to articulate to others what they contribute to the care of the surgical patient beyond psychomotor skills. This can be done through the planning and delivery of care.

CHANGING HEALTH CARE

The use of a nursing care plan (see Chapter 1) is central to the delivery of high-quality care. In perioperative practice settings, care plans and outcome standards have been incorporated in perioperative nurses' records, computerized care plans (see Chapter 3), or "stand-alone" care plans. However, the carrying out of individualized care plans with identifiable patient outcomes has become more difficult to accomplish in recent years because of the brief time a patient is present with a perioperative nurse. Same-day admission and ambulatory surgery have severely limited the time that a nurse spends with a patient, compromising the amount of time needed and available for professional planning and delivery of care. Rather than facilitating the continuity and integration of care, this may result in pa-

tient dissatisfaction with the confusing, impersonal, and fragmented delivery of care that is frequently costly to the patient and the institution. It also compounds the difficulty of demonstrating quantifiable relationships between perioperative nursing interventions and outcomes such as improved efficacy and efficiency in delivering optimal care to the patient.

These challenges to nursing are also affecting health care institutions. The challenges include technologic advances, shifting patterns of surgical delivery sites, ethical dilemmas, increased competition, higher public expectations, and capped budgets (Petryshen & Petryshen, 1992). Institutions must review the feasibility and viability of their present patient care delivery system and investigate alternatives. Case management is one of the most viable alternatives today.

CASE MANAGEMENT

Case management (CM) was first identified and used by social service providers in the early 1970s. The progressing national economic situation, combined with changing roles for health care personnel and patients' demand for higher quality care, contributed to the development of CM. Today most of the professions and agencies concerned and involved with providing high-quality, effective, and efficient health care have adopted the concept. Because early demonstrations of CM concepts showed favorable results, the federal government began supporting such initiatives; it now provides grants, such as one for the investigation of health care programs that focus on care at the community level (Bower, 1992).

CM can be incorporated within any model because it is not one method of care delivery. CM can be accomplished in any setting, such as ambulatory surgery centers (ASC), inpatient surgery, clinics, and surgeons' offices. There are many variations of CM being developed today in individual institutions. The exact system used depends on the type of institution, the needs and the philosophy of the institution, the knowledge and experience of the staff, and the patient population served.

CM is a very acceptable method of planning, delivering, and evaluating high-quality care because it considers the holistic health care needs of an individual. In an institution that provides tertiary care, such as an acute care hospital, it is called "with-in the walls" (WTW) case management. In primary care settings, such as in the community and outpatient clinics, it is called "beyond the walls" (BTW) case management (Cohen & Cesta, 1993).

Advantages

The American Nurses Association has identified eight advantages of case management (Bower, 1992):

1. Focuses on client and family needs
2. Provides for optimal care outcomes
3. Minimizes fragmentation by coordinating care
4. Promotes cost effectiveness
5. Uses and coordinates multidiscipline health care teams
6. Responds to needs of third-party payors
7. Represents a merger of clinical and financial systems and outcomes
8. Can be a marketing tool for health care institutions

Definitions

One definition of general CM is a multidisciplinary "system of health assessment, planning, service procurement/delivery/coordination, and monitoring to meet the multiple needs of clients" (Zander, 1990). Another definition of CM is "a set of logical steps and a process of interaction with service networks that assures that a patient receives needed services in a supportive, efficient, and cost-effective manner" (McKenzie, Torkelson, & Holt, 1989). The complexity of CM is demonstrated by concurrent descriptions of a "system, a role, a technology, a process, and a service" (Bower, 1992).

As a system, CM has patient outcomes that are cost effective. The major elements are assessment, planning, implementation, and monitoring of the kind of care that is delivered, and proceeds in the delivery of that care within a specific system (such as inpatient surgery or ambulatory surgery centers). CM as a role defines a case manager. This person has the knowledge, authority, and ability to provide and/or plan all aspects of care for a defined patient population. When CM is described as a technology, it considers the new tools and techniques developed to provide timing and sequencing of multiple, complex care activities. Examples are CareMaps, multidisciplinary action plans (MAPs), and critical pathways. The process of CM includes goals, outcomes, plans, interventions, and episode-focused evaluation of care. It is the active accomplishment of the delivery of care and responds to health care needs across the continuum and across multiple settings. Finally, CM as a service provides information, resource identification, and access for personalized care needs (Bower, 1992).

These multiple interpretations of the term "case management" illuminate the reason that understanding and working with the generalized concept are difficult. Before intelligent decisions are made, the CM plan must include precise definitions and terminology that is acceptable to all members of the CM team.

Although there can be many different meanings for CM, there are also many different terms for the concept. These include "case management," "managed care," "care management," "nursing care (or case) management," and "managed competition." Additional new terminology and care descriptions are emerging at an astounding pace as institutions and individuals adapt the concept to their individual needs and label them in an original and innovative way.

Comparison of Case Management and Managed Care

There is a diversity of interpretations of managed care versus case management and many commonly perceived differences.

The focus of managed care is more often geared to control—that is, financial and service—and encompasses a target population. The terminology is usually that of the business world and the most interested parties are the payors of health care. It has also been described as a unit-based, patient-outcome–focused nursing care delivery system (Zander, 1992). Managed care is thus structured to use staff through differentiated practice systems and competency levels of nursing personnel (Zander, 1990). The major change has been the development of new tools and systems to monitor care of a population, such as in a health maintenance organization (HMO).

In comparison, case management is based on the total length of an episode, hospitalization, or health care needs for a specific population of patients

(Etheredge & Lamb, 1989; Zander, 1990; Cohen, & Cesta, 1993). The focus is on individual patients within a defined population and their participation in their own health care. Providers have the major interest and the terminology used is that of the health care provider. Change is evident in the new health care roles.

General Characteristics

The persons or agency providing CM decides its characteristics. The definition and purpose are decided by two factors:

1. Who is paying for patient care delivery? (For example, insurance companies, government, or corporate agencies.)
2. Who is running the program, that is, providing CM? The answer can be nurses, physicians, social service personnel, third-party payors, multidisciplinary health care teams, etc.

The AORN Project 2000 Team to Identify Models of Perioperative Practice (1992) identified characteristics important for a nursing care delivery model. These include using a professional knowledge base, enabling professional autonomy and accountability, providing a framework for standards, having a clear role definition, and contributing to positive patient outcomes. CM exhibits these characteristics.

General characteristics of CM that are consistent in all situations are those that focus on client and institutional needs for quality care that is cost effective (NAMFE Project, 1987). CM includes a patient care plan. It frequently includes a time-specific path called a "critical pathway." Other components that are incorporated into CM are continuous quality improvement (Zander, 1991) and financial analysis. Although formal or informal research has not been historically considered a component of CM, it completes the picture (Fig. 6-1).

Patient Selection

CM is best used for selected patients or populations because not every patient needs such staff-intensive care. Priority determinations for CM are patients who are high in cost, predictably unpredictable, have chronically repeated admissions (or returns to the operating room), significant variances, high-risk socioeconomic factors, or are a high-volume population. Other indications include the institutional strategic mission and when multiple physicians or other disciplines are involved in the patient care (Bower & Falk, 1993). Examples are diabetic patients, HIV positive patients, and multitrauma patients. CM is used with specific populations such as settings, age, diagnostic-related groups (DRGs), or medical diagnoses. CM focuses

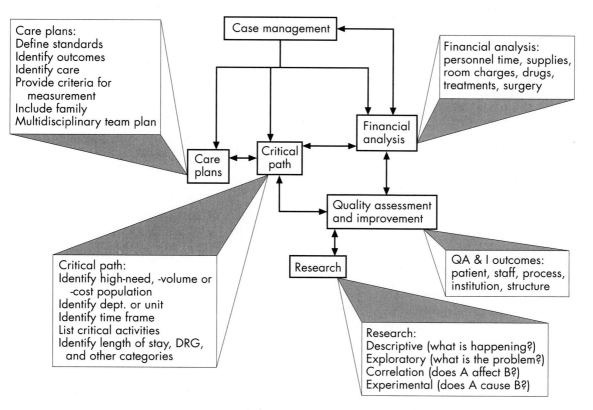

Fig. 6-1. Interaction of components of case management.

on quality-based service and patient participation motivates it.

The CM process starts with the identification of a patient population. Then a complete assessment is accomplished, outcomes are defined with a time frame for accomplishment, the plan is negotiated between the patient and the caregivers, the plan is carried out and monitored, results are analyzed, and needed action is taken. The plan is then reevaluated and adjusted (Zander, 1990).

NURSING CASE MANAGEMENT

The nursing CM concept was developed at the New England Medical Center in Boston in 1980 (Zander, Etheredge & Bower, 1987). CM is considered the second generation of the Primary Care Delivery Model (Zander, 1985) because it is a professional practice model designed to increase nursing involvement in standards of practice. The delivery of nursing care is performed using standards set by the profession (American Nurses Association), the specialty (Association of Operating Room Nurses), and the institution. The delivery of care must also follow regulating bodies such as the Joint Commission on Accreditation of Healthcare Organizations. Nursing CM improves patient care delivery by decreasing fragmentation and increasing collaboration of care, and it integrates patient and provider satisfaction along with cost considerations.

CM is not a new idea in nursing care delivery. Community health nurses and perioperative nurses have used the concepts of CM for their patients for decades. As a model for a care delivery system, it seems especially relevant to ambulatory surgery patients, complex surgical patients, and those in high need, such as the trauma and the elderly patients. The differences between CM today and the delivery of care in the past is the terminology of CM and the use of multidisciplinary teams and new documentation tools.

Perioperative Nursing and Case Management

Perioperative nurses have historically used ideas of nursing CM for complex surgical patients, and they use critical thinking, clinical decision making, and problem-solving abilities in providing this care. For example, perioperative nurses have used care plans with identified outcomes for many years. The plans include the familiar steps of assessment, identifying desired patient outcomes, care planning, implementation, and evaluation. Perioperative nurses have also historically used specific time lines revolving around the preoperative, intraoperative, and postoperative care as a routine practice. Within these time lines, critical activities are identified. In CM, this is called "critical pathways," and the use of this format is the foundation of a CM care plan. Thus perioperative nurses are well qualified to be involved in CM. Furthermore, the clearly defined progression of a surgical patient readily lends itself to a well-defined care plan and critical path in specific units. This is in contrast to patients admitted for medical problems such as renal failure.

Nursing Process and Case Management

Nursing process, the core of professional nursing, is not lost when a CM delivery system is adopted. Rather, the components of the nursing process (that is, assessment, outcomes, plans, implementation, and evaluation) are incorporated into the care, which also includes a time-specific critical path.

The CM care plan incorporates nursing diagnosis or problems identified for a specific population and includes the vital aspects of care. In addition, there is a clearly defined shortened version of care called a "critical path," which defines a specific episode within the patient's hospitalization.

Although there is a generic care plan for an identified population, such as open heart surgery or joint replacement patients, each plan of care is individualized and adapted as needed with the specific patients. The addition of an episodic critical path is usually developed for a determined period within a specific patient care unit, such as the intraoperative or the intensive care episode. Incorporating a critical path into nursing care delivery systems saves time for the patient. Sharing the path with the patient and family enables them to be more knowledgeable of the elements and sequence of care. This can produce satisfaction among patients when they know exactly when and where something will happen, such as when they will be in the postanesthesia care unit (PACU) or discharged from the ambulatory surgical center.

There are identified characteristics for nursing CM that are somewhat different from generalized CM. What makes CM unique as a health care delivery model is the focus on the individual patient in addition to a defined patient population. It is also interdisciplinary or multidisciplinary and works with patients across care settings and areas (Bower & Falk, 1993).

Characteristics of Nursing Case Management

Nursing CM is characterized by the following (McKenzie, et al., 1989):

1. It is collaborative but distinctive from medicine and other health care disciplines
2. It is a cost center and may produce revenue
3. It uses nursing diagnosis and standards of practice
4. It identifies independent nursing decisions and collaborative decisions
5. It is committed to total nursing care for all of the defined patient population

6. It is product-line management
7. It frequently has a clinical nurse specialist (CNS) as manager
8. It considers 20 ongoing patients a manageable case load

DEVELOPING A CASE MANAGEMENT SYSTEM OF DELIVERY

Before developing a CM program, a critical path, CareMap, or MAP, consider the following:

- Why does the institution want CM with critical paths? (Is it to improve quality care/outcomes for patients, decrease fragmented care, improve the efficiency of the product line, save money, make money, etc.?)
- Who will function as case managers and what will their roles be?
- Are CM teams multidisciplinary?
- What is already in place that can be utilized?
- Who in the institution is knowledgeable about CM and can help in development?
- How will the new ideas use past work such as nursing care plans?
- Are standards and theories being used as a basis for development?

Institutional Assessment

An accurate assessment of the institution's individual organizational structure, personnel, and resources will facilitate the planning of CM. It is useful to use a data-gathering form to compile information (Fig. 6-2).

Critical Paths

A main component of CM is the critical path, a tool that is a short version of the care plan. Critical paths are episodic; that is, they are developed for a specific event or episode in a patient's health care experience, such as a surgical intervention. A critical path has clearly defined events within clearly defined areas of service.

Events usually include categories of consultations, tests, treatments, medications, diet or fluid support, safety/activity, and teaching/discharge planning. Areas for the perioperative critical path depend on whether the patient is an ambulatory surgery patient or an inpatient. For example, ambulatory surgery center (ASC) areas could include admission/preoperative, holding, operating room, postanesthesia care unit, and discharge areas. Inpatient surgery critical paths can be incorporated into a complete CM plan for the total hospitalization. Many inpatient CM critical paths are now in existence, but frequently ignore the whole episode of the surgical experience. If mentioned in a critical path, it is listed as "OR day," with none of the intraoperative events identified. It is essential that perioperative nurses join multidisciplinary teams and incorporate the surgical intervention into a care plan in more detail.

Perioperative Critical Paths

The development of a perioperative critical path should follow the format of those used in other areas in the practice setting or health care system. Depending on the needs and structure of the institution, different critical paths may need to be developed for different surgeons doing the same procedure. For example, if five surgeons perform open-heart surgery in a hospital, then the need for development of more than one critical path might be necessary if there is a major difference in protocols for their patients or in speeds of performing the operation. A sample critical path for cataract surgery is shown in Fig. 6-3.

Preplanning for Critical Paths

Before beginning to create a critical pathway, decide the following:

1. Are there any critical paths already developed for the institution? If so:
   - What time frame does the episode encompass?
   - Is it a multidisciplinary plan?
   - What areas are identified?
   - Is the perioperative period defined within the critical path?
2. Is the effort to create critical paths supported?
3. Is there anyone in your department who is knowledgeable about creating critical paths?
4. Who is available for consultation for creating critical paths?
5. How much time will the institution allow for identifying, developing, piloting, and revising critical paths?
6. What support will you have for developing critical paths? (For example, meeting time, secretarial service, library search, computer and photocopying ability)

Steps in Critical Path Development

Once the decision to develop critical paths has been made, the steps to use are to:

1. Assess the position of the critical pathway in the institution's health care delivery method.
2. Identify high-cost, high-need, or high-volume populations.
3. Identify the time frame that the path will encompass.
4. Perform a time-motion study of total critical pathway sequence or episode.
5. Identify specific areas used in the sequence or episode.

1. What kind of hospital is it?
   [ ] Private   [ ] Profit   [ ] Nonprofit   [ ] Community
   [ ] Military   [ ] Other _____

2. What is the personnel mix?
   [ ] RN   [ ] LVN   [ ] Surgical tech   [ ] Administration
   [ ] Advanced practitioner   [ ] Other _____

3. What is the patient mix?
   [ ] Active duty   [ ] Dependent   [ ] Civilian   [ ] Complex
   [ ] Young   [ ] Old   [ ] Acute   [ ] Rehab
   [ ] Emergency/trauma   [ ] Women   [ ] Men
   [ ] Other _____

4. List actual flow/routine the patient goes through for the selected surgery. (Example: physician office, clinic, preadmit visit, telephone, lab, x-ray, diagnosis, pharmacy, admit, preop, holding, OR, PACU, unit, floor, D/C area, other)

5. What disciplines work with the patient during surgical intervention?
   [ ] Physician   [ ] Office personnel   [ ] Radiologist
   [ ] Pharmacist   [ ] Social service   [ ] PT   [ ] OT
   [ ] CRNA   [ ] Anesthesiologist   [ ] RT   [ ] Rehab
   [ ] Dietitian   [ ] Nurses   [ ] Other _____

6. What happens to the patient after leaving the hospital/operating room?

7. What are the discharge planning, community, or home care needs?

8. Who (names, depts) can help you gather data on:
   a. Patient
   b. Procedure
   c. Progression through hospitalization
   d. Care
   e. Cost
   f. Other

9. Who will be of assistance when you implement the project and gather pilot data? Who would (will) you ask to be a member of the development team?

10. What negotiation power/influence or project management skills do you think you will use?

11. What cost figures do you need to gather?
    [ ] Procedure   [ ] Supplies   [ ] Staff   [ ] DRG/other
    [ ] Payment type   [ ] Equipment   [ ] Payor requirements
    [ ] Ratio cost-to-charges   [ ] Private insurance
    [ ] Medicare/Medicaid [ ] Other _____

Fig. 6-2. Organizational assessment form.

6. Follow several patients through the whole time frame.
7. Compute statistical averages of time spent in each area.
8. Obtain input from other members of the case management team if it is a part of a larger critical path.
9. Identify key nursing actions for each activity within each time frame.
10. Identify patient outcomes to be attained.
11. Incorporate professional and institutional standards.
12. Develop a trial critical path.
13. Pilot the critical path on an adequate number of patients.
14. Evaluate the path's ability to do what you want/need it to do (validity).
15. Evaluate the path's ability to determine the same data consistently with every use (reliability).
16. Revise if needed.
17. Have a second trial period of utilization.
18. Evaluate and revise again if needed.
19. Formally adopt critical path.

DRG/ASC # __GRP 9 66884__   LOS __3-4 hours__   Reimbursement_____
Pt. ID _____   Date _____

	Preop (60 min)	Intraop (90 min)	PACU/postop (120 min)
Tests/lab	Preop CBC, EKG	Pulse oximeter - - - - - - - - - - - - ->	D/C oximeter
	Chest X-ray	EKG - - - - - - - - - - - - - - - - ->	D/C EKG
Diet/fluids	NPO ->		as tolerated
	IV Fluids ->		D/C IV fluids
Mobility	Ambulate/ up in chair -> stretcher	Immobile	Ambulate with assistance - - -> ambulate alone
Treatment	Monitor vital signs -> DC	Surgical procedure	
Medication	Eyedrops	Anesthesia	
	Antacid	Analgesia - - - - - - - - - - - - - -> DC	
			Discharge meds
Teaching	Preop activities		
	Surgical info		
	Postop activities		Verbal & written instructions
	Discharge teaching		Clinic appointment instructions
Key nursing actions	Anxiety assessment, History & PE assm't. Create therapeutic environment Assess knowledge level Check permits Eyedrops Vital signs	Position, prep, Monitor physiologic status, Prevent movement during surgery - - - - - - - - - - - - - - - -> Prevent nausea & - - - - - - - - - - - - - - - -> vomiting, Assure safety - - - - - - - - - - - - - - -> Monitor physical status	Assess self-care ability Ensure understanding of discharge instructions
Key patient outcomes	Tolerable anxiety level Knowledgable about procedure and self-care.	Free from injury due to positioning, movement, chemicals, electrical sources	Knows discharge meds Able to care for self, can ambulate safely Able to eat and drink Knows signs & symptoms of complications Can care for eye

Sources: Hampton, 1993; Bower, 1992; Zander, 1991; Guiliano & Poirier, 1991; Cronin & Maklebust, 1989; Etheridge, 1986.

Fig. 6-3. Sample critical path for cataract surgery.

Advantages of such a systematic plan of care include decreased fragmentation of care by anticipating care activities, decreased inadvertent omission of needed care, and increased quality of care by addressing patient outcomes. There is the potential disadvantage of critical paths and care plans of increasing documentation time and initial nursing time (Cohen & Cesta, 1993).

Variations of the Critical Path

A deviation from the defined critical path or a development of a problem is a variance. The constant ability to monitor patient outcomes by the critical path variance trends can form a core component for continuous quality improvement (Petryshen & Petryshen, 1992). All variances are documented and evaluated, with appropriate interventions. Variances can be patient/family focused, caregiver focused, institution focused, or community focused (Hampton, 1993; Zander, 1991). This recorded information can be used for risk management, quality improvement, or research to improve quality of patient care. For example, a patient could deviate from the time frame of the critical path by being delayed in the holding area due to late anesthesia personnel. This minimizes the quality of patient care by increasing apprehension and increases cost time for the institution. Thus by recording the variance for a period, a pattern can be identified, assessed, and improved.

Examples of patient variance might be those caused by absence of required preadmission lab work, preoperative eating or drinking, lack of compliance with preoperative protocols, or unplanned psychosocial conditions. Variances from personnel problems can result from a lack of knowledge, poor technique, presence of students, lack of preparation for all case needs, shortage of staff, or late anesthesia or physician. System-wide variances can result from bumping by cases from the emergency department, from equipment failure, or from unanticipated or unplanned emergencies within the operating suite, such as malignant hyperthermia, cardiac arrest, or unexpected bleeding.

CareMaps

The combination of the critical path and a clearly defined care plan (problem list) with specific outcomes is called a CareMap (Etheredge, 1986; Guiliano & Poirier, 1991).

CareMaps should be multidisciplinary to be the most effective and workable by all health care workers. Physicians are more geared to outcomes than details and are focused on individual activity; they may have difficulty in seeing themselves as participants in a team process (Berwick, 1989). Nevertheless, since society has displayed the desire and need for an effective and efficient patient care delivery system, multidisciplinary CM may be the most viable model. Zander (1992) suggests 30 ways to get physicians involved in CareMaps (Box 6-1).

Perioperative nurses' practice has always been defined by the surgeon and surgical procedure. It makes sense therefore that the surgeon must be involved with any care delivery system. However, nurses have made and are making a significant impact on quality patient care in their own right, and they are not waiting until physicians decide to develop critical paths and care plans (Fig. 6-4).

Exercise caution at this point: if perioperative multidisciplinary plans are substituted for nursing care plans, a decision must be made about whether the plans will be considered standing physician orders and what will happen if the path is not followed.

CASE MANAGEMENT ROLE

Who is a case manager? Case managers have been nurses, administrators, social service agents, insurance companies, health maintenance organizations (HMOs), independent practitioners, physicians, and rehabilitation workers. Each health care profession considers its members to be the most qualified to be the team leader. For example, the medical community has recently discovered critical paths, and many medical publications do not even mention the role nursing has played in developing this process. They recommend MD-directed critical paths because "physicians control the diagnostic and treatment process" (Hart & Musfeldt, 1992).

Qualifications for a case manager include having in-depth knowledge of clinical care, institutional and professional standards, and community resources. To be a successful and contributing members of a multidisciplinary committee, perioperative nurses need knowledge of organizational culture, political dynamics, and change theory. They also need the skills of negotiation, communication, and problem solving.

There are many who support the idea that nurses are uniquely suited to be case managers (Schwartz, Goldman, & Churgin, 1982; Grau, 1984; Bower, 1992). The reasons include nurses' clinical strength and knowledge, the ability to give holistic care, their strong client-focused advocacy, and their knowledge of the services provided by other health care personnel (Mundinger, 1984).

Nurses who lead a multidisciplinary team must also be aware of other members' priorities and needs. For example, many physicians do not want to spend time with anything other than their prime directive: surgery and "their" patients. They have low tolerance for long-winded presentations, rambling and/or unfocused meetings, and typical bureaucratic "work-intensive situations." They prefer a minimum of meetings and a maximum amount of time spent in practice, teaching, and research (Zander, 1992).

Social services personnel may feel an "ownership" of the concept because of their experience with it. Administrators may believe it is their power alone that will affect the delivery of care. The role of the case manager is a challenging and exciting one if there are realistic expectations before commitment of the role.

Preparation for interacting with and providing CM is vital if the program is to succeed. Depending on the education and experience levels of the personnel, it will take from 3 to 12 months to provide proper education (Zander, Etheredge, & Bower, 1987). Each participant's role should be clearly identified and educational sessions should be provided. A self-assessment of educational needs

---

Box 6-1 30 Ways to Involve Physicians in CareMaps

1. Learn what the physicians are worried, angry, excited, or motivated about.
2. Give physicians concrete, case-type related data.
3. Get data if you don't already have it using a 5-20 chart audit if necessary.
4. Relate CareMaps to physicians' goals and desired image.
5. Involve physicians in the initial design: i.e., which case-types, use of variances, measures of success and evaluation.
6. Ask physicians to team the CareMap group about anatomy, physiology, etiology, etc., of the given patient population. Ask them to speak first.
7. Don't get in the middle of an overt or covert interphysician disagreement.
8. Avoid adding layers of people to your system.
9. Avoid adding meetings; use current meeting structures whenever possible.
10. Make time commitments clear.
11. Be honest. No secret data, no secret files.
12. Specify possible physician management changes if any; i.e., documentation, walking rounds.
13. Serve food at meetings.
14. Don't belabor the discussion or meeting process.
15. Cancel CareMap development sessions if physicians can't make it at the last minute. Reschedule immediately.
16. Construct separate CareMaps if interphysician agreement is impossible.
17. Never plan to replace human interaction with a paper information system.
18. Supply your physicians the names of physicians in the same specialty who are currently using CareMaps.
19. If you haven't read "Getting to yes" by Fisher and Ury, do it before you start! It will help you steer clear of territory and personality struggles.
20. Be ready to respond quickly and concretely to valuable physician suggestions.
21. Don't be hesitant to change a term or label if the change encourages cooperation. However, never expect everyone to like the term you finally select.
22. Avoid the word "buy-in." It sounds coercive. Use cooperation, involvement, and commitment in your writing and conversation.
23. Enlist the support of the physician's office manager to confirm appointments as well as for future needs for scheduling, patient education, etc.
24. Develop patient satisfaction questionnaires to include areas physicians want measured.
25. Keep all discussions focused on what is best for the patients and families.
26. Don't be put off by: *"My patients are sicker." "Their hospital is different,"* etc. Approach the CareMap effort as a "feasibility study."
27. Develop CareMaps that don't "box-in" the physicians; this can be done in a variety of ways including actual wording on CareMaps or making some variance analysis "off the record."
28. Have a "neutral" person facilitate CareMap development sessions to keep the process between 1 and 2 hours.
29. Invite hospital administrators to CareMap sessions to reinforce CareMaps as a priority and for administrators to learn about the complex clinical processes they are in a position to support.
30. Realize that when physicians hear of something new that one group of physicians have, they will want it too.

Reprinted with permission Zander K. (1992). Physicians, CareMaps, and collaboration. *Definition,* 7(1) Winter:1-4.

---

can help in program planning and development (Fig. 6-5).

Clinical Nurse Specialist as Case Manager

The American Nurses Association (Bower, 1992) recommends a nurse case manager have a minimum education of a baccalaureate degree. Others believe the complexity of the role is better suited to a masters' prepared clinical nurse specialist (CNS) (Cronin & Maklebust, 1989).

The case manager "should be at the center of think tanks that focus on the what, why, where, and how of health care delivery" (Holt, 1993). This implies an advanced or expanded awareness and knowledge. Job frustration and dissatisfaction can occur among those less qualified than a nurse in an advanced or expanded role, unless they are well prepared before starting.

The CNS role has historically had five basic subroles: caregiver, educator, teacher, researcher, and consultant. The new subrole of case manager may become the predominant one. Some are predicting that this will be the major role of the CNS in the future (Holt, 1993; Cronin & Maklebust, 1989).

A CNS may serve as the actual CM care coordinator. There would be a defined population with whom the CNS team leader interacts to plan the total surgical experience. The CNS must be knowledgeable of surgical health care needs before the surgery and following it, which includes community

Date:_____
Patient:_____   Surgeon:_____
Surgery:_____   DRG:_____

	Preop ( ) min	Holding ( ) min	Or ( ) min	PACU ( ) min	Discharge ( ) min
Assessment /forms	Nurse assm't H & P Informed consent Anes. assm't CareMap -------	--------------	Intraop record, Anes record, Supply record, ----------	PACU record ------------	Discharge record, clinic appointment, pharmacy request ------> D/C
Tests/ monitoring	Routine lab Temperature Vital signs ---------	Psychologic support	Pulse oximeter --- ------------ EKG -------------	------------ ------------	------> D/C ------> D/C ------> D/C
Safety/ activity	Up ad lib BRP Assess allergies	Bed rest Safety rails up	Immobile Safety strap Positioning Aseptic technique ES pad Prep solutions	Bed rest Safety Rails up	Encourage activity with assistance
Fluid support/ diet	Ensure NPO status	Start IV----------	------------	------------	------> D/C Sips of water progressing to discharge diet
Procedures /drugs	Change gown Weigh Preop meds		Prep drape Anesthesia Antibiotics ---- Surgery	PRN pain meds -------	------> D/C ------> D/C Take-home meds
Teaching/ discharge plans	Procedure info, Sensory info Family info	Reinforcement and reassurance		Turn, cough and deep breath Request comfort meds	Wound care Meds Clinic appointment Signs and symptoms of complications Who to call
Other					

Fig. 6-4. Sample of a generic ASC critical path with a care plan.

and home resources. Use of standards, care planning, critical paths, and variance identification and analysis would be among activities for this subrole. Expert clinical and management skills are necessary and are enhanced by the ability to think critically, to make pertinent clinical decisions, and to evaluate resources (Strong, 1992).

CNS case management activities include managing cases across a continuum, establishing the role, identifying how it relates to other roles (especially staff nurses), identifying communication networks, and relating variance analysis to continuous quality improvement (CQI). The advanced practitioner also has skills in management development, including negotiation, change, power/influence, and project development (Bower and Falk, 1993).

Another subrole for the CNS is that of consultant. The case manager must have the communica-

	Preop ( ) min	Holding ( ) min	Or ( ) min	PACU ( ) min	Discharge ( ) min
Patient will not develop an infection related to surgery within 7 days of surgery	Assess potential for wound resistance: nutrition, age, infectious diseases, history, results of CBC	Administer antibiotics as ordered	Maintain aseptic technique, gentle tissue handling, adequate skin prep with appropriate antimicrobial solution	Assess wound, monitor output, assess IV site	Regains ability to eat and drink, voiding sufficient quantities
Patient's surgical intervention will be completed without inadvertent injury	Assistance as needed with procedures, ambulation	Gurney rails in "up" position, restrict ambulation after preop meds, assess allergies	Correct positioning and padding, aware of allergies for solutions, correct placement of ESU pad, lift rather than drag in transfer	Maintain Gurney rails up maintain normothermia, monitor vital signs, assess all skin areas	Assist with producers and ambulation as needed. Return sensory aids (glasses, hearing aid) etc., as soon as possible
Alteration in comfort: physical and mental	Assess anxiety level	Maintain a therapeutic environment, apply warm blankets as needed, administer antianxiety meds as ordered	Monitor and reassure an awake patient, use therapeutic touch and positive words	Assess pain level, give analgesia as needed	Assess comfort level, insure take-home meds as needed
Knowledge deficit	Procedural and sensory information, discharge protocols, critical path activities; begin discharge teaching	Answer questions, provide reassurance, clarify to family or significant others	Maintain awareness if patient is awake so misinterpretation of OR conversation will not occur	Foster orientation × three and accomplishment of deep breathing, active or passive motion	Review discharge teaching verbally and in writing: wound care, ambulation, meds, signs and symptoms of complications, clinic visit, person to notify

Sources: Hampton, 1993; Bower, 1992; Zander, 1991; Guiliano & Poirier, 1991; Cronin & Maklebust, 1989; Etheridge, 1986.

Fig. 6-4, cont'd. For legend see opposite page.

tion, negotiation, and persuasion skills needed to market, develop, implement, and evaluate a program. Consultation is available to health care providers, administrators, industry, and patients and families.

Research is a subrole of CNS practice, and research skills are needed to formally analyze and interpret CM variance data. A CNS has the skills to investigate patient needs and outcomes. In today's complicated health care financial environment, the CNS must be involved in studying financial parameters and data bases. Results can be used for monitoring, evaluation, and payor requirements.

The subrole of CM educator also utilizes the teaching skills of the CNS, teaching CM to new case managers and staff and demonstrating the development of critical paths. A vital function is patient education (content, timing, and sequencing).

Date: _____

Name: _____

Possible case management role: _____

Instructions:

Please review the following topics or concepts in terms of your proposed role in case management. Determine whether you:

    (1) Have no knowledge about the topic
    (2) Are somewhat knowledgeable
    (3) Are competent
    (4) Are an expert in knowledge and application

Please try to be as candid as possible because educational offerings will be planned and given depending on the need.

Thank you.

	Have no knowledge 1	Somewhat knowledgeable 2	Competent 3	Expert in knowledge and application 4
I. Communication Skills				
Written communication				
Verbal communication				
Negotiation				
Conflict management				
Dealing with difficult people				
Confrontation				
II. Manangement Skills				
Budget process				
Supervision				
Counseling				
Delegation				
Effective use of resources				
Priority setting				
Problem identification				
Project management				
Time management				
Management skills, specific				
Disciplinary action				
Performance appraisal				
III. Leadership Skills				
Consultation				
Working with groups				
Running a meeting				
Making agendas				
Mentoring/coaching				
Collaboration				
Organizational dynamics				
Power and influence				
Team building				
Program design & evaluation				
Political awareness				

Fig. 6-5. Case management educational needs self-assessment instrument.

	Have no knowledge 1	Somewhat knowledgeable 2	Competent 3	Expert in knowledge and application 4
IV. Clinical Skills				
Assessment of patient/ family support system	☐	☐	☐	☐
Coordination of care				
Care of complex patient				
Specific knowledge of specialty				
Theory-based care				
Application of empirical findings				
Case presentation				
Product evaluation				
Discharge planning				
Identification of needs				
Resource identification				
Referral ability				
Collaboration with community				
V. Nursing Process/Documentation				
Assessment				
Problem identification				
Goal development				
Developing a plan of care				
Following through on plan				
Evaluation of outcomes				
VI. Patient Education				
Identifying need				
Assessing ability to learn				
Developing content				
Providing content				
Teaching strategies				
Evaluation of learning				
Documentation				

TOTALS:	1	2	3	4
I. Communication skills				
II. Management skills				
III. Leadership skills				
IV. Clinical skills				
V. Nursing process				
VI. Patient education				

Fig. 6-5, *cont'd.* For legend see opposite page.

RN First Assistant and Case Management

RN first assistants (RNFAs) are in an expanded role that may be directly involved with CM. They can provide valuable input for development of critical paths and use of nursing process care plans, and, if available in an institution, should be considered part of the team. Preoperative aspects should include RNFA physical assessment and patient education needs. Intraoperative activity should involve the safety factors used in handling tissue and providing hemostasis. Postoperative care plans included on the CM plan can be the assessment of wound healing and homeostasis, as well as the prevention or early recognition of complications such as shock and systemic infections.

Case Manager Job Description

The institution's job description of a case manager depends on the environment and client needs. However, primary functions include the following (Bower, 1992):

1. Coordinating care and services for identified patient populations
2. Case finding and screening
3. Assessing the biopsychosocial needs of the patient and family
4. Assessing the patient's coping and adaptive abilities, formal and informal support systems, and self-care abilities
5. Gathering all information and synthesizing interdisciplinary problem identification
6. Acting as resource in identifying and linking patients with the most appropriate resource, person, or institution to solve the problems in a timely manner
7. Procuring services, making eligibility decisions, and authorizing hospitalization, rehabilitation, or home care needs
8. Facilitating access to health care
9. Acting as a problem solver and decision maker
10. Providing direct patient care when necessary
11. Acting as a liaison and facilitating communication
12. Educating
13. Documenting
14. Monitoring and evaluating client and program outcomes

RESEARCH AND CASE MANAGEMENT

There is a rapidly growing body of literature describing CM, but accounts most often have been reviews of demonstration projects. However, the components of CM can contribute to the ability to investigate structure, process, and outcome (see Chapter 2) variables more definitively. Structure outcomes refer to how the institution is organized to deliver care (Mitchell, 1993) and include physical and institutional barriers and boundaries to that care system. Process variables are those that define how the system is set up in an organization. This includes how providers deliver and document care. Outcome variables are those that reflect the findings of CM on the quality of patient care (Marschke & Nolan, 1993).

Structure Research

An example of the case study method of research on structure is reported by Johnsson (1991). The study had three goals:

1. To move patients through the hospital cost effectively by removing operational and departmental barriers
2. To develop patient care guidelines by investigating utilization patterns of medical staff and residents
3. To improve hospital financial performance while maintaining good patient outcomes

After implementing CM, the average length of stay decreased 23% and average charges decreased 16%. An additional result was the structural consolidation of three departments (preadmission, concurrent review, and discharge planning) into a single office for managed care.

Another investigation (McKenzie, Torkelson, & Holt, 1989) showed nursing CM contributed to significant cost savings. The investigators developed care plans and critical paths for high-volume DRGs that included coronary artery bypass grafts and cardiac catheterization. There was a decrease in the average length of stay (LOS) of 1.1 days. The result was a savings of an estimated $1 million in one year using the CM system of care.

Process Research

Research of the process of delivering care was reported by Cohen (1991). The effects of nursing CM were investigated with 128 patients undergoing cesarean sections. Analysis included the variances for LOS, hours of nursing care, and resource utilization. The results showed that while more nursing hours were used with CM at the beginning of hospitalization, there were less resources used overall and a 19% decrease in LOS.

The financial effectiveness of CM has been reported in many programs. One such program was developed at Long Regional Hospital in Utah (Bair, Griswold, & Head, 1989). They began a bedside CM model using RNs to plan and control care, evaluate outcomes, and serve as members of a multidisciplinary team. Cost per DRG case type was assessed and compared with the actual cost per case in the average reimbursement for 10 DRGs. They found a decrease of 0.4 days in LOS, an average cost savings of $284 per case, and a total annual savings of $94,572.

The financial aspect has been a driving force in the development of this care delivery model because in instances where the CM model has been carried out, there have been "reduced total costs per patient case, decreased patient length of hospital stay, increased patient turnover, and potential increase in hospital-generated revenues" (Cohen & Cesta, 1993).

Outcome Research

The final component of CM research is that which investigates outcomes. Factors such as LOS, patient satisfaction, rates of nosocomial complications, and improved knowledge for self-care can be studied. One such study by Fleishman, Mor, and Piette (1991) looked at AIDS patients' satisfaction with CM services. Both groups (clinician based and community based) rated case managers as satisfactory. However, the process, especially the access to the case manager, was unsatisfactory.

The analysis of variance from critical path information can identify potential or actual problems and their financial implications. Any areas of care—that is, process, structure, and outcomes—can then be empirically investigated. Thus case management could finally help nurses to support, through empirical findings, what nurses can do, how and where they fit into a multidisciplinary health care team, and their value to perioperative health care.

SUMMARY

The American health care system today has become impersonal, cold, fragmented, expensive, and impractical. Health care workers, government, insurance agencies, and patients themselves are demanding change. One way to effect change is to incorporate case management in the delivery of care.

The main goals of case management are to optimize patient self-care, decrease fragmentation, provide high-quality care across a continuum, enhance the quality of life, decrease the length of stay, increase patient and staff satisfaction, and promote the cost-effective use of resources (Cohen & Cesta, 1993; Bower, 1992; Zander, 1990).

The information obtained with a critical path can help perioperative nurses perform quality-improvement tasks. The analysis will identify whether the "outlier" (deviation from the critical path) is because of patients, personnel, or system. Identification of these variances will provide unique and/or additional data that can add to programs already in place in the institution.

References

American Nurses Association. (1987). Nursing assessment and management of the frail elderly (NAMFE) project. Curriculum of eight models on case management. NAMFE: Project, Kansas City, KS. In Bower K. *Case management by nurses.* Kansas City: The Association. N-32, 25.

Bair N, Griswold J, & Head J. (1989). Clinical RN involvement in bedside-centered case management. *Nursing Economics,* 7(3), 150-154.

Berwick D. (1989). Continuous quality improvement as an ideal in health care. *New England Journal of Medicine,* 320(1), 55.

Bower K. (1992). *Case management by nurses.* Kansas City, KS: The Association.

Bower K. (1993, November). *The managed care environment: Preparation of the advanced practice nurse.* Paper presented at the American Association of Colleges of Nursing Conference, San Antonio, TX.

Cohen (1991).

Cohen E & Cesta T. (1993). *Nursing case management: From concept to evaluation.* St. Louis: Mosby–Year Book. 1993 Mosby.

Cronin C & Maklebust J. (1989). Case-managed care: capitalizing on the CNS. *Nursing Management,* 19, 38.

Etheredge ML. (1986). The maps for managed care. *Definition,* 1(3),1-3.

Etheredge P & Lamb G. (1989). Professional nursing case management improves quality, access, and costs. *Nursing Management,* 20(3), 30-35.

Fleishman JA, Mor V, & Piette J. (1991). AIDS case management: The client's perspective. *Health Services Research,* 26, 447-70.

Guiliano K & Poirier C. (1991). Nursing case management: Critical pathways to desired outcomes. *Nursing Management,* 22(3), 52-55.

Grau L. (1984). Case management and the nurse. *Geriatric Nurse,* 5(6), 372-375.

Hampton D. (1993). Implementing a managed care framework through care maps. *Journal of Nursing Administration,* 23(5), 21-27.

Hart & Musfeldt, 1992.

Holt FM. (1993). The role of the CNS in developing systems of health care delivery. *Clinical Nurse Specialist,* 7(3), 140.

Johnsson J. (1991). Case study: Managed care helps hospitals contain costs. *Hospitals,* 65, 40-44.

Marschke P & Nolan M. (1993). Research related to case management. *Nursing Administration Quarterly,* Spring, 16-21.

McKenzie C, Torkelson N, & Holt M. (1989). Care and cost: Nursing case management improves both. *Nursing Management,* 20(10), 30-34.

Mitchell P. (1993). Perspectives on outcome-oriented care systems. *Nursing Administration Quarterly,* Spring, 1-7.

Mundinger MO. (1984). Community based case: Who will be the case managers? *Nursing Outlook,* 32(6), 294-295.

Petryshen P & Petryshen P. (1992). The case management model: An innovative approach to the delivery of patient care. *Journal of Advanced Nursing,* 17, 1188-1194.

Project team identifies practice model criteria. (1992). *AORN Journal,* 4(56) 630.

Schwartz S, Goldman H, & Churgin S. (1982). Case management for the chronically mentally ill: Models and dimensions. *Hospital and Community Psychiatry,* 33(12), 1006-1009.

Strong S. (1992). Case management and the CNS. *Clinical Nurse Specialist,* 6(1), 64.

Zander K. (1985). Second-generation primary nursing: A new agenda. *Journal of Nursing Administration,* 15(3), 18-24.

Zander K. (1990). Managed care and nursing case management. In Mayer, Madden, & Lawrenz (Eds.), *Patient care delivery models.* Gaithersburg: Aspen.

Zander K. (1991). CareMaps®: The core of cost/quality care. *Definitions,* 6(3), 1-3.

Zander K. (1992a). Differentiating managed care and case management. In K Bower (Ed.), *Case management by nurses* Kansas City, KS: The Association.

Zander K. (1992b). Physicians, CareMaps®, and collaboration. *Definition, 7*(1), 1-4.

Zander K. (1992c). Qualifying, managing, and improving quality: 1. How CareMaps® link CQI to the patient. *The New Definition, 7*(2), 1-3.

Zander K, Etheredge M, & Bower K. (1987). *Nursing case management: Blueprints for transformation.* Boston, Massachusetts: Winslow Printing Systems.

Bibliography

American Hospital Association. (1990). *1990 report of the hospital nursing personnel survey.* Chicago: The Association.

Brown SA & Grimes DE. (1992). *A meta-analysis of process of care, clinical outcomes, and cost-effectiveness of nurses in primary care roles: Nurse practitioners and nurse midwives.* Washington DC: The Association.

Custer ML. (1993). Enhancing case management through computerized patient files. *Clinical Nurse Specialist, 7*(3), 141-147.

Wagner JD & Menke EM. (1992). Case management of homeless families. *Clinical Nurse Specialist, 6*(2), 65-71.

Zander K. (1992). What's new in managed care and case management. *The New Definition, 6*(2), 1-2.

Zander K. (1994). Nurses and case management. In J McClosky & HK Grace (Eds.), *Current issues in nursing* (pp. 254-260). St. Louis: Mosby–Year Book.

Sample Perioperative Care Plans

Chapter 7

Generic Care Planning: AORN Patient Outcome Standards

Jane C. Rothrock

To your patient you owe attention to whatever can affect his health or his comfort. You must be ever on the alert to minister to and even anticipate his many personal wants. These will vary so much in different cases that few directions can be laid down beyond the general ones for constant watchfulness and thoughtfulness.

WEEKS, 1890

*P*lanning for patient care is a nursing strategy designed to ensure that care is outcome directed. Planning often begins as a mental process; however, the plan must be recorded to ensure continuity of care. A complete nursing care plan includes a patient assessment, prioritized nursing diagnoses, identified desired outcomes and criteria by which to measure them, and a plan for achieving the outcomes. Nursing actions must then be identified and implemented to assist the patient in achieving the desired outcomes. Care plans have been described as patient information tools, used as teaching and learning tools in nursing education, developed to ensure individualized care and continuity of care, and referred to as measures of nursing accountability. Most health care institutions require written care plans, in an institutionally specific or approved form, for each patient, as does the Joint Commission

on Accreditation of Healthcare Organizations (see Chapter 5 for a discussion of the Joint Commission requirements). Yet, with all of their attributed benefits and the pressures exerted regarding their development, care plans are not used effectively or consistently in many health care institutions.

Palmer (1988) raised doubt about what she referred to as "nursing's sacred cow—the nursing care plan" when she described some of the findings of a study by Kramer. In interviews with nurses from 16 magnet hospitals, Kramer learned that many of them disliked writing care plans. What the nurses disliked about this part of the nursing process was the repetitive writing of care plans for their own sake, and not as tools in guiding the care planning process. In suggesting that nurses need to use their time to the best advantage of all patients, Palmer concluded that nurses should use standardized, preprinted care plans for the uncomplicated patient whenever possible.

Generation of standardized nursing care plans, based on accepted nursing standards, serves as a conceptual tool for the organization of patient care activities. These plans should be generic enough to apply to all patients in a care setting yet adaptable for individualization. Thus standardized care plans present nursing with the opportunity to plan individualized, outcome-directed nursing care in a timely and efficient manner through the use of the nursing process.

PERIOPERATIVE CARE PLANS

Like other care plans, perioperative care plans depend on the nursing process. After assessment, nursing diagnoses are formulated. They are then ranked or prioritized in relation to their importance and the nurse's ability to intervene during the perioperative period. Outcomes based on actual or high-risk nursing diagnoses are developed, with corresponding evaluative criteria. These criteria become the measures with which the patient's condition is compared to determine if the desired outcomes have been met. Nursing actions are identified for initiation during the perioperative period. The plan is implemented on the day of surgery and is revised and updated as necessary. Evaluation may take place in the operating room, postanesthesia care unit, ambulatory discharge area, patient care unit, physician's office, or in the patient's home; phone or mail surveys may be part of the postdischarge measurement of outcomes. Information accumulated during care plan development and implementation guides further revisions and assists the perioperative care unit in tracking and identifying trends in perioperative nursing care needs. Nonetheless, all who practice this process realize that what is simple in description is not simple in actual practice.

Problems With Planning Perioperative Nursing Care

Planning for patient care needs is a recognized step in the nursing process. Perioperative nurses have consistently and effectively implemented care plans. The myriad nursing activities that accompany safe outcomes in the millions of surgical interventions that take place in the United States attests to the implementation of those plans. In carrying out a plan of nursing care for a patient, the perioperative nurse uses the nursing process quickly and efficiently. Rapid assessment of the skin at the application site of an electrosurgical dispersive pad, proper application of the pad, safety checks during repositioning or requests for higher output settings, and evaluation of the skin at the conclusion of surgery all represent the nursing process in its broad-

est sense. What is often missing, however, is the reason for the care in terms of identifying the desired patient outcome and outcome criteria, the nursing diagnosis, and the actual plan for care. That a plan was carried out is evident from the sequences of the nurse's activity and the patient's outcome. Nonetheless the components of the care plan may be totally absent from the patient record. They exist in the intellect and skill of the nurse delivering the care, but only to those who observe that nurse. That makes the skill very difficult to measure.

Documenting care. In a report of the results of clinical testing of process-oriented criteria to monitor perioperative nursing, it was noted that some criteria that worked well statistically had to be modified because of problems identified by the observers in the research study (Sylvester & Shipley, 1982). The record review criterion "Do records document treatments and procedures performed intraoperatively by the perioperative nurse?" was deleted because observers who reviewed the record postoperatively had no way of knowing what had been done intraoperatively. Patient record reviews that indicate "Patient to OR" and later "Patient received from OR" do little to substantiate the important role played by the perioperative nurse during one of the patient's most vulnerable periods during hospitalization. During the study, several criteria related to the documentation of the preoperative assessment and to the plan of care reflected a high rate of nonapplicability or limited variability (Reeder & Puterbaugh, 1982). Nonapplicability or low rates of variability may indicate that the perioperative nurse subjects had not adopted all aspects of the perioperative role or that those aspects of assessment and care planning were not externally evident. This lack of external evidence may be one of the precipitating factors in "provision of care" debates. If the nursing process functions are not identified and documented by the nurse, can we justify the need for the professional nurse in the operating room? Although nurses may defend the need for their presence by pointing out the routine things they always do for every patient, documentation must more consistently reflect the entire nursing process to validate that standards of nursing practice have been met.

Skill level. Perioperative nurses who function at such a high level have naturalized skills. A naturalized skill evolves from a knowledge and experiential base and is so finely coordinated between the brain, eye, and hand that it occurs naturally. The nurse possesses enormous understanding about the skill actualization, so much so that it becomes routine. Routinization without understanding is secondary ignorance; one knows what to do but not why it is being done. Routinization with knowledge carries the hallmarks of efficiency, quality, and clinical skill. Benner (1984) has described the competency and proficiency that accompany the naturalized care delivery of many perioperative nurses. Competency is developed when nurses see nursing actions in terms of long-range goals or plans of which they are consciously aware. The plan and the outcome-directed nursing behavior guided by the plan dictate to the nurse which aspects in the current situation are most important. The plan, which establishes the nurse's perspective, is based on conscious, abstract, analytic knowledge of the problem or its potential. Roach (1993) has suggested that, for competent nurses, knowledge, judgment, skills, energy, and motivation are required if the nurse is to respond adequately to the demands of professional accountability. Competence, along with compassion, is central to the care process.

Proficient performance is guided by maxims. The word "maxim" arose from the medieval Latin *propositio maxima,* meaning "greatest proposition." In this sense, the maxims that guide the proficient nurse are literally of the greatest importance. As such, they become guiding principles in care delivery. The proficient nurse recognizes the maxim in the total situation, not just in one aspect of it. Thus the nurse's perception of safety, or of the high risk for injury related to the use of the electrosurgical unit in the example cited earlier, and the actions needed to prevent such injury underscore nursing activity. However, the perception of a high risk for injury is not relegated simply to this aspect of the surgical intervention. The guiding principle is prevention of all risks for injuries, not just the high risk presented by the use of the electrosurgical unit.

Putting the plan in writing. Thus by intuition and observation one may logically conclude that, just in the isolated incidence of preparing the patient for electrosurgery, the perioperative nurse is using the nursing process. However, intuition and observation are limited means of documenting care, measuring its quality, or categorizing the nursing diagnoses that led to the nurse's perception of the prevention of injury maxim. In addition, when the plan and most of its directives are in the nurse's mind, the opportunity for exchanging information with nursing colleagues and new nurses is severely limited. The new nurse who enters a clinical setting may be limited to lower levels of performance if the goals and tools of patient care are unfamiliar or inaccessible; steps in perioperative assessment and analysis must be described in great detail for the student nurse or novice nurse (Ryan-Wenger, 1990). Similarly, if those goals and tools are not apparent to the rest of nursing, the notion that perioperative nursing is technical and automatic, rather than intellec-

tual, skilled, and planned, may persist, as may the notion that lesser skilled, lower cost health care workers can replace the perioperative nurse in operative and other invasive procedure settings.

**Relationship of Nursing Standards
to Planning Nursing Care**

All who practice perioperative nursing recognize that it is based on the nursing process and involves standards of care. First published in 1975, the *Standards of Nursing Practice: Operating Room* were revised in 1981 and appear in 1996 as *Standards of Perioperative Clinical Practice* (AORN, 1996). The six standards, presented in Chapter 1, are based on the nursing process. As such, they are process oriented, describing what is to be performed by the nurse.

Process standards. The *Standards of Perioperative Clinical Practice* can be used to monitor nursing care by measuring the presence or absence of the nursing activities deemed relevant to each standard. Although it does not measure outcome per se, process management leads to an understanding of the process and its various steps, which contributes to the outcomes. Thus if it was found that potential injuries from the electrosurgical unit were not being prevented, process management could be an important tool in evaluating why the outcome was poor. For this to be workable, however, there must be a plan for nursing care that prescribes nursing actions to achieve prevention of injury from electrosurgical units. The nursing actions need to be identified, prioritized, sequenced, and specified as to when, where, and by whom they are to be performed. With such specificity of nursing actions, process management can effectively be used to assess and improve many of the outcomes established for individuals undergoing surgery.

Outcome standards. In 1983 the *Outcome Standards for Perioperative Nursing* were approved. The Outcome Standards, which may be found in Chapter 2, provide guidelines for the observable psychologic and physiologic responses of a patient to a surgical intervention. From these six standards, measurable criteria may be elucidated by which to judge patient achievement of each desired outcome. Patient outcomes are another major means, along with process management and improvement, of measuring nursing care. In outcome monitoring, the institution's patient care outcomes can be evaluated by comparing them with established internal or external standards of care (benchmarking or identification of best practices).

As reform of the health care delivery system continues—utilization management, decreasing lengths of stay, same-day surgery, managed care, competition, and capitation plans—it becomes essential to maintain and measure safety, efficiency, and effectiveness of patient care; to understand and improve care processes; and to evaluate the positive nature of patient outcomes. Standards for practice and standards for desired patient outcomes enable the perioperative nurse to deliver care in a patient-centered framework.

GENERIC CARE PLANS FOR PERIOPERATIVE NURSING

The generic care plans presented in this chapter combine the *Standards of Perioperative Clinical Practice,* the *Outcome Standards,* and the *Competency Statements in Perioperative Nursing* (AORN, 1996). Competency, as defined in the statements, is "the knowledge, skills, and abilities necessary to fulfill the professional role functions of a registered nurse in the operating room." Thus the competency statements themselves may be viewed as generic to the whole group of professional perioperative nurses, generalizable to settings and diversified patient populations. The generic care plans are meant to be generalizable. They are based on identified perioperative nursing criteria and competencies. They offer suggestions for nursing interventions and create a mechanism for assessing the quality of the care delivered, as well as the effectiveness of care in meeting patient outcomes. Nonetheless, they are merely suggestions for care. The care plans, in and of themselves, cannot replace or supersede institutional policy and procedure. The nurse who consistently adheres to institutional policy and procedure provides safe patient care. The policies and procedures, in a manner of speaking, become the institution's standard of care (Murphy, 1990). Thus many of the generic care plans indicate that institutional protocol is to be followed when carrying out selected nursing activities. Because this book is not meant to be a nursing textbook, rationales for care have been omitted in most instances. However, each generic care plan is accompanied by an insert with "Guides to Nursing Actions." These guides describe the behaviors identified on the generic care plan, explicating what is meant by a specific nursing action. The generic care plans assist in planning and monitoring care, making public the knowledge, skills, and care that have historically guided perioperative nursing.

Care Plan Design

To help the perioperative nurse in actualizing the nursing process, each generic care plan, as well as the procedure-specific care plans that begin in Chapter 8, has been divided into sections (Fig. 7-1). The following describes the components of the generic care plans.

Key assessment points. This section of the generic care plan provides a summary of the key assessment parameters for the desired outcome or surgical procedure. The perioperative nurse can refer to this section for a quick review of what must be assessed; more detailed information on patient assessment is explicated in the Guides to Nursing Actions that accompany each generic care plan.

Nursing diagnosis. The primary nursing diagnosis is based on the desired patient outcome. In certain instances, secondary nursing diagnoses are offered. North American Nursing Diagnosis Association (NANDA)–approved nursing diagnoses are used except on rare occasions, and these exceptions are clearly identified in a footnote. The NANDA Nursing Diagnosis Taxonomy (Fig. 7-2) is incorporated in the introduction to each generic care plan. Human response patterns to actual or potential health problems are a conceptual framework for the NANDA taxonomy. These nine human-response patterns are not mutually exclusive. As a conceptual framework, they are a loosely organized set of related ideas that provide an overall structure to nursing diagnoses.

Patient outcomes. The patient outcome standard for perioperative nursing is as identified by the AORN. In the procedure-specific care plans that comprise later chapters of the book, the identified outcomes are based on the nursing diagnoses. The outcomes include measurement criteria that are patient centered.

Nursing actions. Nursing actions reflect the specific nursing diagnosis and include nursing behaviors from the AORN Competency Statements. Because perioperative nursing is unique in not always having access to the patient for any period before the surgical intervention, important assessment observations are presented as part of the suggested nursing action. The nursing actions component of the generic care plan becomes, in part, a patient-monitoring guide to prevent complications and provide a positive outcome. Each nursing action is followed by check-off options, indicating that the action was performed or was not applicable to the patient. The nursing action section of the care plan also provides space for additional documentation of nursing actions or assessments. Thus this part of the generic care plan becomes both a guide to patient care delivery and a record of care. It is designed as a double tool to reflect the acuity, rapidity, and intensity with which perioperative nursing care is delivered in an effort to make the most efficient use of the nurse's knowledge, skill, and time.

Additional nursing actions and care plan revisions. The additional nursing actions section of the care plan allows for individualization of the plan for the

FIG. 7-1
GENERIC CARE PLAN

KEY ASSESSMENT POINTS

NURSING DIAGNOSIS

PATIENT OUTCOMES

NURSING ACTIONS   Yes   No   N/A

Document additional nursing actions/care plan revisions here:

_____

_____

_____

EVALUATION OF PATIENT OUTCOMES	Outcome met	Outcome met with additional outcome criteria	Outcome met with revised nursing care plan	Outcome not met	Outcome not applicable to this patient
1.	☐	☐	☐	☐	☐
2.	☐	☐	☐	☐	☐
3.	☐	☐	☐	☐	☐

Signature: _____ Date: _____

I. Health Perception—Health Management Pattern

Altered Health Maintenance
Ineffective Management of Therapeutic Regimen
Noncompliance (Specify)
Altered Protection
High Risk for Infection
High Risk for Injury
High Risk for Trauma
High Risk for Poisoning
High Risk for Suffocation
Health Seeking Behaviors (Specify)

II. Nutritional and Metabolic Pattern

Altered Nutrition: High Risk for More Than Body Requirements
Altered Nutrition: More Than Body Requirements
Altered Nutrition: Less Than Body Requirements
Interrupted Breastfeeding
Ineffective Breastfeeding
Effective Breastfeeding
Ineffective Infant Feeding Pattern
High Risk for Aspiration
Impaired Swallowing
Altered Oral Mucous Membrane
High Risk for Fluid Volume Deficit
Fluid Volume Deficit (1)
Fluid Volume Deficit (2)
Fluid Volume Excess
High Risk for Impaired Skin Integrity
Impaired Skin Integrity
Impaired Tissue Integrity
High Risk for Altered Body Temperature
Ineffective Thermoregulation
Hyperthermia
Hypothermia

III. Elimination Pattern

Constipation
Perceived Constipation
Colonic Constipation
Diarrhea
Bowel Incontinence
Altered Patterns of Urinary Elimination
Functional Incontinence
Reflex Incontinence
Stress Incontinence
Urge Incontinence
Total Incontinence
Urinary Retention

IV. Activity-Exercise Pattern

Altered Growth and Development
Fatigue
Bathing/Hygiene Self-Care Deficit
Dressing/Grooming Self-Care Deficit
Feeding Self-Care Deficit
Toileting Self-Care Deficit
Diversional Activity Deficit
Impaired Home Maintenance Management
High Risk for Activity Intolerance
Activity Intolerance
Impaired Physical Mobility
High Risk for Disuse Syndrome
Dysreflexia
Ineffective Airway Clearance
Ineffective Breathing Pattern
Impaired Gas Exchange
Inability to Sustain Spontaneous Ventilation

Dysfunctional Ventilatory Weaning Response
Decreased Cardiac Output
High Risk for Peripheral Neurovascular Dysfunction
Altered (Specify Type) Tissue Perfusion (Renal, Cerebral, Cardiopulmonary, Gastrointestinal, Peripheral)

V. Sleep-Rest Pattern

Sleep Pattern Disturbance

VI. Cognitive-Perceptual Pattern

Pain
Chronic Pain
Sensory/Perceptual Alterations (Specify) (Visual, Auditory, Kinesthetic, Gustatory, Tactile, Olfactory)
Unilateral Neglect
Altered Thought Processes
Decisional Conflict (Specify)
Knowledge Deficit (Specify)

VII. Self-Perception—Self-Concept Pattern

Fear
Anxiety
Hopelessness
Powerlessness
Body Image Disturbance
Personal Identity Disturbance
Self-Esteem Disturbance
Chronic Low Self-Esteem
Situational Low Self-Esteem
High Risk for Self Mutilation

VIII. Role-Relationship Pattern

Impaired Verbal Communication
Social Isolation
Impaired Social Interaction
Relocation Stress Syndrome
Altered Role Performance
Anticipatory Grieving
Dysfunctional Grieving
High Risk for Violence: Self-directed or Directed at Others
Altered Family Processes
High Risk for Altered Parenting
Altered Parenting
Parental Role Conflict
Caregiver Role Strain
High Risk for Caregiver Role Strain

IX. Sexuality-Reproductive Pattern

Sexual Dysfunction
Altered Sexuality Patterns
Rape-Trauma Syndrome
Rape-Trauma Syndrome: Compound Reaction
Rape-Trauma Syndrome: Silent Reaction

X. Coping—Stress Tolerance Pattern

Ineffective Individual Coping
Defensive Coping
Ineffective Denial
Impaired Adjustment
Post-Trauma Response
Family Coping: Potential for Growth
Ineffective Family Coping: Compromised
Ineffective Family Coping: Disabling

XI. Value-Belief Pattern

Spiritual Distress (Distress of the Human Spirit)

Fig. 7-2. NANDA-accepted nursing diagnosis categorized by Gordon's functional health patterns. (From McFarland GK & McFarlane EA. (1992). *Nursing diagnosis and intervention: Planning for patient care* (2nd Ed.). St Louis: Mosby–Year Book.)

specific patient. Documentation of important aspects of care should be entered.

Evaluation of patient outcomes. The evaluation part of the generic care plan provides summary statements that reflect outcome attainment and provide an indicator of the quality and appropriateness of care. Each outcome has the following five evaluation parameters:

- *Outcome not applicable to this patient.* This category is provided for the patient who did not have a nursing diagnosis related to the generic care plan. If institutions choose to package their own generic care plans as part of a paper or computerized record, this category would be applicable to some patients.
- *Outcome met.* This category would be selected if the evaluation of the outcome statement were true.
- *Outcome met with additional outcome criteria.* This category enables the nurse to individualize the nursing care plan and establish additional or different outcomes for selected patients.
- *Outcome met with revised nursing care plan.* This category allows the nurse to add relevant nursing diagnoses and nursing actions to a generic care plan. It also allows discontinuation of part of the plan that may not be appropriate for a given patient.
- *Outcome not met.* It is possible that a patient outcome may not be achieved. Documentation of care needs to reflect the patient's status, and this category allows monitoring of unmet outcomes.

Signature and date. It is possible that a preprinted, generic care plan will meet the needs of some patients without any changes. Therefore it is important that the care plan be signed and dated. This demonstrates the use of the nursing process and accountability on the part of the professional nurse.

GENERIC CARE PLANS FOR PATIENT OUTCOME STANDARDS

Generic care plans for perioperative patient care enable the nurse to use the nursing process to assess, diagnose, identify relevant patient outcomes and outcome criteria, plan, intervene, and evaluate the patient from admission through discharge from perioperative patient care settings. The generic care plan can be individualized to meet each patient's needs and used simultaneously to document care delivered.

Outcome Standard: The Patient Will Demonstrate Knowledge

Outcome Standard I states, "The patient demonstrates knowledge of the physiological and psychological responses to the surgical intervention" (AORN, 1996). In today's health care climate, patients as consumers/members of health plans expect and often demand that their right to information be respected. The climate of the health care environment, on the other hand, may circumscribe the amount of time the perioperative nurse has to give information, teach, assess learning, and verify and validate the retention and understanding of the teaching. Certainly part of the collection of health data should include the patient's understanding, perceptions, and expectations of the procedure; the individual's experience with and responses to surgery; and the identification of any relevant knowledge deficits that may interfere with the individual's response to surgery. In many practice settings, however, it is not realistic for all information about the patient's knowledge level to be collected or corrected by the perioperative nurse. There is, however, a body of information that the perioperative nurse needs to plan and execute nursing care effectively with the outcome that the patient and his significant others will be knowledgeable about physiologic and psychologic responses to the surgery.

Psychoeducational interventions. Critical in enabling the patient to achieve the goal of being knowledgeable, providing information and supportive preoperative education needs to be carried out. The patient also needs information and supportive communication regarding perioperative care and events surrounding the perioperative period. A wide and varied body of literature supports the positive nature of preoperative psychoeducational interventions (Devine, 1992). The nature of these psychoeducational interventions includes the giving of sensory, temporal, and procedural information to patients, as well as support by answering questions and offering reassurance. The many theoretic perspectives that have guided the giving of information view surgery as a stressful event for which the patient needs to develop coping strategies, alter behaviors, learn new techniques, control emotional responses, and otherwise prepare for the impact of the stress. Implicit in the giving of information and offering of support is the notion that the patient can and will use the information to achieve an optimal response to the stressor of surgery. A large body of research supports the benefits of perioperative patient education. Perhaps the most significant finding is the value of communication in influencing emotional response to and recovery from surgery.

Preoperatively, patients have many concerns, ranging from the operative or invasive procedure itself to its effect on their quality of life. The following is a list of nursing diagnoses that represent common patient concerns. They are discussed in terms of possible cause, assessment factors, suggested interventions, and desired outcomes. These nursing diagnoses may exist in perioperative patients and should be considered when an individualized plan of care is developed to help the patient demonstrate knowledge of the physiologic and psychologic responses to surgery.

Anxiety
Body image disturbance
Communication, impaired verbal
Coping, ineffective individual
Fear
Grieving, anticipatory
Hopelessness
Knowledge deficit (specify)
Noncompliance (specify)
Personal identity disturbance
Powerlessness
Role performance, altered
Self-esteem disturbance
Sensory-perceptual alterations: (specify) (visual, auditory, kinesthetic, gustatory, tactile, olfactory)
Sexuality patterns, altered
Social interaction, impaired
Social isolation
Spiritual distress (distress of human spirit)
Violence, high risk for: self-directed or directed at others

These nursing diagnoses are not exhaustive but represent ones that might cause patients concern and interfere with their response to surgery. They also represent areas in which communication by the perioperative nurse can contribute to the patient's outcome.

Nursing diagnoses related to knowledge or its deficit. The most common nursing diagnosis relative to the desired outcome of a knowledgeable patient is a knowledge deficit. This alteration in knowledge, manifested as a deficit, falls under the human response pattern of knowing, a pattern involving the meaning associated with information. A knowledge deficit indicates a state in which a person experiences a lack of cognitive knowledge or psychomotor skill that alters or may alter disease management or health maintenance (McFarland & McFarlane, 1993). In assessing the patient for alterations in knowledge, the nurse needs to determine whether there is a language barrier or decreased auditory or visual comprehension that requires sensory aids. The nurse must also determine if the patient verbalizes or exhibits a lack of knowledge or skill; is willing, able, and ready to learn (Vidmar, 1994); what the patient's comprehension level is (Dixon & Park, 1990); and what stressors and coping behaviors characterize the patient's experience of surgery. Know-

ing about the patient means, in part, knowing the patient's typical patterns of response (Tanner, et al., 1993); this is central to setting up the possibility of intervening and helping preserve the patient's dignity and integrity. Principles of teaching and learning need to be incorporated into a teaching plan, and outcomes need to be set according to priority, the patient's need, and the patient's readiness to learn (Rega, 1993). The teaching plan may be initiated before hospitalization, during preadmission visits, or on the patient care unit. As more patients are admitted to the health care facility on the same day or within 24 hours of their surgery, the reality of implementing a total teaching plan by the perioperative nurse is greatly diminished. It is most likely that the perioperative nurse becomes a participant in the teaching plan, the expert knowledge broker regarding the immediate events of the perioperative period. Collaboration in patient teaching and in helping the patient overcome a knowledge deficit does not take place only in the clinic, physician's office, preadmitting area, or at the bedside. The imparting of information, explanation of events, and support and reassurance during those events continues when the patient is admitted to the perioperative patient care setting. The importance of the perioperative nurse's contribution to a beneficial outcome for the patient is not circumscribed by the geographic location of the nurse-patient interaction. Instead, the nurse in a perioperative practice setting may continue with a plan that has already been initiated, contributing expertise and support during the perioperative period. The desired outcome in correcting a knowledge deficit is that the patient, significant other, or both will demonstrate understanding of the information or skill needed. In practice, the perioperative nurse contributes to and evaluates this understanding in many ways.

Implicit in determining whether the patient has knowledge of the planned surgical intervention or invasive procedure is the evidence of a signed surgical consent in the patient record. The perioperative nurse often encounters issues and dilemmas regarding informed consent. Murphy (1987) points out that "the operating room nurse's role is confined to assuring that informed consent has been obtained and documented in the health record in accordance with the policy of the institution." It is the surgeon's responsibility to inform the patient of the nature of the procedure and its accompanying risks and benefits and to ascertain that the patient understands the procedure. If the consent for a surgical intervention is not on the patient record, then the perioperative nurse has a duty to call the surgeon's attention to that fact. Institutions should have a policy for instances in which a patient arrives in the operating room with incomplete or absent documentation of consent. There is a section in the generic care plan offered in this chapter to indicate that the patient has additional questions. Although not meant to supersede institutional policy, this section can be used by the perioperative nurse to document the patient's possible lack of understanding of the procedure and its risks and benefits.

In addition to the "knowing" part of knowledge is one's feeling about the knowledge. Feeling is a pattern involving the subjective awareness of information. Patients may have many different feelings about undergoing surgery. They may experience fear about the impending surgery, the perceived threat of pain, disfigurement, or even death. Patients who have had no experience with an operative procedure or have memories of a negative experience may have additional fears. Assessing a patient's level of comprehension, degree of insight concerning the surgical procedure and perioperative events, and identifying erroneous perceptions can be useful in helping a patient overcome fears that might be exaggerated by lack of knowledge. Even without a preoperative visit on a patient care unit, the nurse in the holding area can determine if a patient appears upset, is weeping, or is aggressive or irritable.

Observation of those indicators of feeling can lead the perioperative nurse to initiate interactions to allay fears. The patient should be encouraged to express feelings and concerns; mutual inquiry and interchange are powerfully effective tools in engaging the patient (Berry, 1993). The nurse should listen calmly, attentively, and with acceptance. Warm, friendly, sincere support can be one of the most important gestures the perioperative nurse makes in helping the patient overcome or deal with fear. The desired outcome is that the patient will verbalize or otherwise demonstrate a reduction of fear.

Anxiety is another nursing diagnosis that relates to the feeling pattern. Although anxiety and fear can be present simultaneously in a patient, anxiety differs from fear in that the anxious person cannot identify the threat (Gordon, 1993). With fear, the threat can be identified. The anxious patient experiences feelings of uneasiness or apprehension, which often activate the autonomic nervous system. The heart rate may increase, blood pressure may elevate, and respiratory rate may increase, with voice tremors, hand tremors, palpitations, flushing, and feelings of faintness; the unusually anxious surgical patient may be at greater risk for postoperative psychologic distress, elevated blood pressure, and extended length of stay (Kulik, Moore, & Mahler, 1993). The patient may state feeling nervous, tense, or helpless. Often, anxiety interferes with the patient's ability to concentrate, remember, or recall information. It is these interferences with physiologic, emotional, and cognitive responses in which the perioperative nurse is so highly prepared to intervene. Anxiety that has existed as a nursing diagnosis in the preoperative period may persist when the patient gets to the perioperative patient care setting, despite preoperative medications. The patient may not remember what he or she was told during preoperative teaching. Perioperative nurses play a vital role in explaining what to expect in the operating room environment. They can explain attire, sounds, temperature, and sequence of events, as well as offer sensory information about what the patient can expect to feel, see, and hear; they can plan interventions such as guided imagery (Holden-Lund, 1989; Naparstek, 1993) and music therapy with the patient (Steelman, 1990). The desired outcome is that the patient's anxiety will be reduced or minimized.

Patients also have the right to expect that their privacy, confidentiality, and personal dignity will be maintained during the surgical experience and that any cultural, ethnic, spiritual, or religious factors that may affect their plan of care are noted. The potential for spiritual distress exists when a patient experiences or is at risk of experiencing a disturbance in religious, intellectual, cultural, ethical, or moral beliefs (McFarland & McFarlane, 1993). Spiritual distress occurs in the human-response category of valuing, which is a pattern involving the assignment of relative worth. Spiritual distress can occur as a response to the health problem or treatment or to barriers in the hospital situation that interfere with religious, cultural, ethnic, or spiritual practices. The perioperative nurse can assist with spiritual distress by reinforcing the patient's sense of identity and worth; listening with compassion and sensitivity to the patient's need to express feelings; using touch therapeutically; allowing religious symbols such as rosaries or medals to accompany the patient to the operating room; providing the patient time for or sharing in prayer or meditation when appropriate; and arranging for practices important to the patient's spiritual, cultural, ethnic, and religious beliefs when possible. (See Chapter 23 for a complete discussion of culturally competent care). Baptism at birth, circumcision, amputation, transfusion, dietary restrictions or NPO status, cutting or shaving hair, and special rites or practices associated with death may all affect perioperative patient care. The desired outcome is that the patient's spiritual beliefs and practices will be respected, promoted, and maintained.

A number of potential disturbances in self-concept may accompany surgical interventions and other invasive procedures, therefore influencing the patient's psychologic response to surgery. A disturbance in self-concept occurs when the individual experiences or is at risk of experiencing a negative state of change about the way he or she feels, thinks about, or views himself or herself (Gordon, 1993). Disturbances may be related to body image, self-esteem, role performance, or personal identity. Surgery and its threat of accompanying pain, immobility, loss of a body part, or loss of function certainly may effect a disturbance in body image, self-esteem, role performance, or personal identity. If not resolved, such a disturbance may lead to dysfunctional behaviors such as hopelessness, ineffective individual coping, anticipatory grieving, noncompliance, powerlessness, altered sexuality patterns, impaired social interactions, and social isolation. The perioperative nurse should assess the patient's emotional status, perceptions about physical changes, previous adaptive and maladaptive responses to stressors and illness, and potential for self-destructive behavior. The nurse encourages verbalization of emotions and discussion of perceived physical changes, listening actively for nonverbal as well as verbal cues about the patient's self-perceptions. The desired outcome is that the patient will discuss feelings, both positive and negative; seek knowledge; and use resources for support.

Included in diagnoses related to knowledge is the concept of providing the patient with knowledge and support. Through the perioperative nurse's support, the patient may be better able to face the stressful events of surgery. Support does not always have to be expressed in words. A caring, listening, empathic attitude, accompanied by therapeutic touch and comfort measures, can demonstrate support as effectively as the spoken word. Knowledge is provided to the patient after careful assessment of learning needs and selection of appropriate teaching methods. Communication needs to occur between the nurse and the patient, as well as between the nurse and other members of the health care team.

Communicating knowledge about the patient. Communication is important in any health care setting and involves the sharing of information among the persons providing patient care. In their research project to define criteria for monitoring the quality of perioperative nursing care, Reeder and Puterbaugh (1982) noted that communication of preoperative assessment information between the operating room (OR) and unit nurses was often insufficient. A possible interpretation for this finding was that nursing practice had not changed to reflect the perioperative role. The crux of the issue was that perioperative nurses needed to exchange pertinent information with unit nurses on a regular basis to plan

patient care adequately. Coordination, joint participation, and collaboration between unit staff and perioperative nursing staff hold out perhaps the only possibility for continuity of care in an era of cost containment, dwindling resources, and staffing redesign.

In a study conducted by Abbott, Biala, and Pollock (1983) to determine the effect of preoperative assessment on intraoperative nurse performance, communication was one of the few subsets of nursing activity that was found to be significant. The specific subset "communicates patient information" was measured by reviewing the assessment with team members, documenting a plan of care on the chart, and having all necessary equipment available. The second subset, "communicates intraoperative information," was measured by activities such as reviewing the intraoperative care with the post-anesthesia care unit or intensive care unit nursing staff and documenting intraoperative nursing care in the chart. In this study, preoperative assessment related positively to communication by the perioperative nurse.

Although many research hypotheses have been advanced regarding factors accounting for patients' responses to the stress of surgery, that stress is multidimensional. Nonetheless, changes in clinical practice can be made on the basis of a body of knowledge that indicates repeatedly the value of nursing assessment in planning care and the value of psychoeducational interventions in positively influencing the outcomes of care. Perceived barriers to patient education—such as too many other care-related tasks, short patient stays, disparate beliefs about what should be taught and when, doubts about the efficacy of education on behavior change and compliance, and lack of patient interest (Lipetz, et al., 1990; Yount, et al., 1990)—must be overcome in relation to the significance of research findings. Although changes in nursing practice are sometimes predicated on environmental pressures of the work setting, the ability and potential of the unit nurse and perioperative nurse to collaborate in nursing care delivery needs to be ensured to ensure continuity and high quality of care. Communication between these primary care providers is intuitively sound and holds forth great promise for perioperative nurses who assist the patient to demonstrate knowledge of the physiologic and psychologic responses to surgery.

Generic care plan. Figure 7-3 presents the generic perioperative nursing care plan with its associated Guide to Nursing Actions for helping the patient demonstrate knowledge of the physiologic and psychologic responses to surgery.

FIG. 7-3
GENERIC CARE PLAN   The patient demonstrates knowledge of the physiologic and psychologic responses
to surgery

KEY ASSESSMENT POINTS
Physiologic condition
Presence of anxiety/fear/concern
Level of formal education
Cultural/ethnic/language barriers
Current knowledge and understanding
Psychologic response to current condition
Interest in learning
Motivation/readiness to learn
Experience with surgery

NURSING DIAGNOSIS
Risk for knowledge deficit regarding planned surgical intervention

PATIENT OUTCOMES
The patient will demonstrate knowledge of the physiologic and psychologic responses to the planned surgical intervention as evidenced by:
1. Remaining oriented to person, place, and time
2. Confirming, in writing or verbally, consent for the operative procedure
3. Describing the sequence of events during the perioperative period
4. Stating outcomes in realistic terms
5. Expressing feelings about the surgical experience

NURSING ACTIONS

	Yes	No	N/A
1. Patient identified?	☐	☐	☐
2. Sensory aids/prosthetic devices removed?	☐	☐	☐
3. Sensory impairments?	☐	☐	☐
4. LOC: Alert?	☐	☐	☐
5. Verbal verification of operative site?	☐	☐	☐
6. Consent signed? Advance directive?	☐	☐	☐
7. Language barrier?	☐	☐	☐
8. Special religious/spiritual needs?	☐	☐	☐
9. Special cultural/ethnic needs?	☐	☐	☐
10. Perioperative routine explained?	☐	☐	☐
11. Patient expressed understanding?	☐	☐	☐
12. Patient has additional questions?	☐	☐	☐

Document additional nursing actions/care plan revisions here:

_____

_____

_____

EVALUATION OF PATIENT OUTCOMES

	Outcome met	Outcome met with additional outcome criteria	Outcome met with revised nursing care plan	Outcome not met	Outcome not applicable to this patient
1. The patient remained oriented to person, place, and time.	☐	☐	☐	☐	☐
2. Physical and emotional factors which impacted on the patient's response to the planned surgical intervention were alleviated.	☐	☐	☐	☐	☐
3. The patient was physically and emotionally prepared for the planned surgical intervention.	☐	☐	☐	☐	☐
4. The patient correctly reviewed anticipated perioperative events.	☐	☐	☐	☐	☐
5. The patient signed the operative permit.	☐	☐	☐	☐	☐

Signature: _____ Date: _____

FIG. 7-3 (Continued)
GENERIC CARE PLAN **The patient demonstrates knowledge of the physiologic and psychologic responses to surgery**

GUIDE TO NURSING ACTIONS IN ASSISTING THE PATIENT TO DEMONSTRATE KNOWLEDGE OF THE PHYSIOLOGIC AND PSYCHOLOGIC RESPONSES TO THE PLANNED SURGICAL INTERVENTION

1. Introduce yourself to the patient.
2. Confirm patient identity according to institutional protocol.
3. Note any sensory impairments (hearing, visual, tactile). Document these.
4. Note patient's level of orientation.
5. Check for the presence of any sensory aids or prosthetic devices which accompanied the patient to the OR (e.g., artificial limb, dentures, hearing aid, contact lenses, eyeglasses, wigs, etc.). Document presence and disposition of sensory aids or prosthetic devices.
6. Verify operative procedure with patient statement of planned surgery.
7. Verify that operative consent form is complete and correct. Determine whether advance directive has been executed.
8. Determine the patient's knowledge level. Document lack of relevant information.
9. Determine the patient's ability to understand information.
10. Document language barriers, lack of comprehension.
11. Elicit patient's perceptions of the surgery.
12. Elicit patient's expectations of care.
13. Document additional information given regarding planned surgery.
14. Determine the patient's coping mechanisms and plan with the patient to utilize these. Note alterations in effective coping.
15. Identify patient's religious and spiritual beliefs. Document special needs based on those beliefs.
16. Identify patient's cultural and ethnic practices. Identify special patient needs.
17. Elicit patient's feelings and concerns about the planned surgery. Allow the patient time to verbalize fears and anxieties. Document specific patient concerns.
18. Identify patient teaching needs. Document these.
19. Assess the patient's readiness to learn. Document problems with attention span or anxiety.
20. Provide instruction based on the patient's identified needs. Document that instruction.
21. Document additional nursing actions/care plan revisions related to assisting the patient in demonstrating knowledge about the physiologic and psychologic responses to the planned surgical intervention.

Outcome Standard: The Patient Is Free from Infection

Surgical site infections remain the second most common type of nosocomial infection, accounting for approximately one third of all hospital-acquired infections (Lee & Baker, 1994). A surgical site infection (SSI) is a risk for all perioperative patients and therefore becomes a nursing diagnosis for most patients who undergo surgery. The skin, the body's first line of defense, is violated by a surgical incision. Although the incision is aseptically created and controlled, the risk for infection is increased by the presence of a portal of entry for pathogenic microorganisms. Infection control programs have long been in existence to prevent nosocomial infection and its accompanying morbidity and mortality. Adherence to the principles and practices of aseptic technique are part of the perioperative practice setting's infection-prevention program. The potential for minimizing postoperative infections has grown throughout the history of perioperative nursing and is likely to continue with the impetus for clinical research in the nursing community.

Major advances in surgery and perioperative nursing have often occurred as a result of progress in other disciplines. In the second half of the nineteenth century, advances in bacteriology and anesthesiology led to the introduction of antiseptic and aseptic techniques. Semmelweiss observed that puerperal sepsis was the result of contamination carried from patient to patient on the hands of physicians. He also noted that infections were less frequent when women delivered their babies at home than when they delivered in the hospital. Pasteur recognized that certain diseases were caused by bacteria. Lister applied this knowledge to surgery. He recommended the use of phenol to kill microorganisms in the air, on the surgeon's hands, on the instruments, and on the patient's skin. As a result of his work, aseptic technique was introduced into surgery. The surgeon's hands were scrubbed before the operation, the skin was decontaminated with an antiseptic, and instruments were sterilized by boiling.

Assessing patient risk for infection. Advances in aseptic technique have continued since Lister's time. Today, much is known about the cause, treatment, and management of infection. Nonetheless, the focus of perioperative nursing activity is on preventing infection. A number of endogenous (intrinsic) and exogenous (extrinsic) factors contribute to a patient's risk of infection. Many endogenous factors are not under the control of the perioperative nurse, but are important assessment parameters that guide the plan of care. Nurses use a variety of ways to collect data during systematic nursing assessment. One data collection source involves the review of laboratory data.

Reviewing laboratory data. Laboratory data provide a useful index for assessing a patient's clinical status and potential risk for infection. Although they should never be used without reference to other clinical data, the results of laboratory studies can provide important cues to determining perioperative nursing actions. The patient record is usually the source for laboratory data, and the most recent study results should be reviewed first. After the patient's current status is noted, past laboratory results can be scanned to indicate trends over the course of the preoperative stay. A few significant laboratory studies relating to risk for infection are discussed here.

A *decreased hematocrit* level is often related to a decrease in red blood cells (RBCs). "Anemia" is a nonspecific term often used when a patient has a low RBC count. If the patient has a low hematocrit level, which results from anemia with an accompanying iron deficiency, the immunologic defenses can be lessened. Iron deficiency may cause a reduced bacterial killing by white blood cells, thus leading to the risk for infection. A *low hemoglobin level* would indicate the same nursing diagnosis. A *low platelet count* is also associated with some anemias and should be considered in the risk for infection.

Two measurements of white blood cells are commonly done preoperatively. The *total white blood cell (WBC) count* is an absolute number of cells per cubic millimeter. The *differential* is a determination of the proportion of each of the five types of white blood cells in a sample of 100 WBCs. Differentials are reported in percentages. The *neutrophils* seem to be the body's first defense against bacterial infection; their primary function is phagocytosis. When a patient has an elevated neutrophil count, the perioperative nurse should consider whether the patient has an infection. Although WBCs increase in bacterial infections, the differential finding of an increased neutrophil count or the presence of band or stab cells (early immature forms of neutrophils, referred to as a "shift to the left") encourages assessment for signs of an ongoing, acute bacterial infection. Low platelet counts may accompany neutropenia.

Although most bacterial infections increase neutrophil count, a *low neutrophil count* may accompany bacterial infections and viral diseases, specific drug therapies, and radiation therapy. Because neutrophils play an important role in fighting infection, the patient with neutropenia needs perioperative nursing interventions to protect against infection. Maintenance of scrupulous aseptic technique and environmental control measures are important in the perioperative nursing protocol for such patients.

Lymphocytes are the principal component of the body's immune system. In the differential, T-lymphocytes (thymus derived) and B-lymphocytes (bone marrow derived) are grouped together. At times, it is important to identify these types of lymphocytes individually to help assess immune deficiencies. Lymphocytes are mononuclear leukocytes involved in the production of antibodies and cell-mediated immunity. Lymphocyte counts increase in many viral conditions, chronic bacterial infections, and the lymphocytic leukemias. With a *high lymphocyte count* that is unrelated to malignancy, the presence of infection should be considered.

The patient with a *low lymphocyte count* that is unrelated to other shifts in the differential count—that is, whose lymphocyte count is not low because the neutrophil count is high—is immunodeficient. The perioperative patient who is lymphopenic will need extensive protection from infection. Because postoperative infection in such a patient may exhibit very few of the signs or symptoms that ordinarily characterize the presence of infection, postoperative evaluation must be done very carefully.

Protein requirements may greatly increase as a result of surgery. If protein intake is inadequate, the body begins to break down protein tissue (catabolism) in an effort to generate enough amino acids to synthesize serum albumin. A negative nitrogen balance may result if catabolism is greater than anabolism and the protein deficiency is longstanding. The two serum proteins measured in tests for total protein are serum albumin and globulin. Albumin, produced by the liver, is important in maintaining oncotic pressure in the vascular system and in transport in the bloodstream. Patients who lack protein, evidenced by *low serum albumin levels* in the absence of liver disease, have lowered resistance to infection. Patients with *low gamma globulin levels* or *abnormal gamma globulins* are also at risk for infection because of their increased susceptibility to opportunistic infections. There are five types of globulins, which have complex and diversified compositions. The gamma globulins referred to as "immunoglobulins" are made by B-lymphocytes in response to a stimulus from an antigen. The immunoglobulins are classified as IgG, IgA, IgM, IgD, and IgE, and each may be affected in different types of immunologic responses. They are found in the bloodstream and interact with a cellular response to provide optimal immunologic defense. There is usually more diagnostic significance in gamma globulins than in the other globulins. Thus the patient with low gamma globulin levels has an intense need for protection from infection. Because the main defense against invading organisms is the skin and intact mucous membranes, the perioperative patient in whom this defense is violated is extremely dependent on nursing actions to prevent infection.

There are a host of serologic tests for the diagnosis of bacterial and viral disease that have not been addressed in this section. Humans are constantly being exposed to disease as infective agents enter the body. Usually, healthy people with intact immunity either do not contract the disease or have a brief syndrome. Many prospective surgical patients, however, do not have the ability to fight and contain disease-causing infective agents. They depend on the perioperative nurse's skill and vigilance in confining and containing possible contaminants, in providing an environment that protects against exogenous contamination, and in recognizing the conditions that pose risk. Recognizing and understanding the clinical implications of laboratory tests are two of the many ways the perioperative nurse determines risk status.

Diagnostic tests for infectious diseases. Specific microbiologic serologic tests are used for various types of infectious diseases. Hepatitis may be classified as type A, type B, or type C; hepatitis D and E may represent only two different types of non-A/non-B (NANB) diseases, which are not yet serologically detectable. Numerous tests are now available to test for hepatitis B (HBV) antigens and antibodies. A commonly used test is for hepatitis B surface antigen (HBsAg), which rises before the onset of clinical symptoms, peaks during the first week of symptoms, and returns to normal by the time jaundice subsides (Pagana & Pagana, 1995). Detection of this antigen means either that the patient has active hepatitis or is a carrier. In either case, the patient's blood may be a source of infection. Hepatitis B surface antibody (HBsAb) signifies the end of the phase of acute infection and immunity to subsequent infection; this antibody also denotes immunity after administration of HBV vaccine. Hepatitis C (HCV) accounts for up to 80% of all cases of posttransfusion hepatitis; chronic HCV can be detected by electroimmunoassay, but acute infection cannot be detected because of the long time (referred to as a "window") between infection and seroconversion (Curry, 1993). Hepatitis A is primarily spread through the oral-fecal route.

Serum antibodies against human immunodeficiency virus (HIV), the virus that causes acquired immunodeficiency syndrome (AIDS), can be measured and are the basis of tests for the disease. However, the time between exposure to the virus, appearance of antigens in the serum, and seroconversion with antibody production varies. Thus detection of antibodies through laboratory screening and confirmation is unreliable in finding the patient who is at risk of, has been exposed to, or already has early infection of the virus. Whether or not all patients who have the antibodies will progress to active infection with the disease is not known, but the appearance of antibodies is cause for concern and affects the patient's ultimate ability to resist opportunistic infections. The most widely used serologic test for these antibodies is the enzyme-linked immunosorbent assay (ELISA); following repeatedly reactive ELISA results, the Western blot is used to validate the results. Repeatedly reactive ELISA tests and a positive Western blot is highly predictive of HIV infection. Testing policies for HIV, both for patients and for health care workers, continue to be controversial, yet testing plays an important role in prevention and treatment of HIV infection (Phillips, 1994).

Diagnostic and testing issues aside, it is known that HIV infects CD4 cells, which are one of the cell-mediated activities of the immune system. This, in turn, creates a major immune system defect, allowing the body to become susceptible to opportunistic infections and malignancies. The Centers for Disease Control now integrates the CD4 T-cell level as part of their revised HIV classification system in recognition of its importance as a clinical marker and the severity of immunosuppression (Harwell, 1994). Additionally, HIV-positive patients who are treated with certain drugs may have drastically lowered lymphocyte counts; it is estimated that 20% to 25% of patients with HIV have neutropenia (Muma, et al., 1994). Clearly, HIV-positive patients need perioperative care to protect them from the risk of additional infection.

AIDS, caused by human immunodeficiency virus, continues to be an epidemic of the 1990s. Nonetheless, any consideration of risks to health care workers or other patients through contact with blood or body fluids from individuals who may have HIV must also include the risks of other bloodborne pathogens, especially the hepatitis virus. At present, the evidence indicates that HIV and hepatitis B virus may both pose occupational risks for perioperative nurses and other health care personnel. In 1988, the Centers for Disease Control published clarifications of universal precautions, extending them to all patients. In 1992, the Occupational Health and Safety Administration's (OSHA) standard on bloodborne pathogens became effective, making universal precautions mandatory in all health care settings. Universal precautions apply to blood and other body fluids containing visible blood; semen; vaginal secretions; synovial, pleural, cerebrospinal, pericardial, peritoneal, and amniotic fluid; and human tissue and organs, as well as tissue cultures. The standard also addresses exposure-control plans; engineering and work practice controls; personal protective equipment; and training, education, record-keeping requirements, and HBV vaccine pro-

phylaxis. This vaccine is recommended for health care workers in contact with blood; it is on a two-dose primary schedule (each dose 1 month apart), with a third dose 5 months after the second primary dose (Gardner & Schaffer, 1993).

Reducing the risk of blood and body fluid exposures therefore becomes of primary importance in perioperative patient care settings. The use of needles and sharp instruments poses a risk for exposure. In a study to determine which perioperative personnel received the most exposure to blood contamination, how the exposure occurred, and which personnel tended to be at most risk for exposure, 50% of the surgical procedures involved resulted in at least one blood-contamination event (Dobbing, 1993). The risk for the surgeon and the first assistant was 81%, but the scrub and circulator also had frequent exposure incidents. In an analysis of five studies done between 1990 and 1992, which included 4870 surgical procedures, there were exposures in 17% of the procedures, and 3.5% of these were from punctures (Lynch, 1992). In a 1994 study, 47% of gloves failed (had holes in them) during actual-use testing procedures for a device developed to alert the wearer to microscopic holes (New technology lessens infection risks, 1994). Studies such as these make a compelling argument for the use of methods and principles to prevent exposure. The ongoing collaborative operative blood exposure study (COBEX) led to the development of an assessment kit to assist perioperative practitioners with determining procedures in which exposure occurs and analyzing those procedures for epidemiologic characteristics that would lead to appropriate preventive measures (Lynch, 1993).

The OSHA rule requires perioperative personnel to comply with standards during patient care activities. Adherence to principles of infection prevention, long the province of perioperative excellence, along with initiation and implementation of AORN Recommended Practices, which address these principles, can effectively diminish risk to personnel and prevent contaminating events for other patients. The recommended practices address important principles and updates on the use of barriers, gloves, handling and using sharps and other instruments, asepsis, hand washing, universal precautions, environmental sanitation, and waste management (AORN, 1996).

Assessing intrinsic factors that increase risk for infection. A number of important variables in assessing the patient's potential response to surgery relate specifically to increased risk of infection. Children and the elderly have special risks, which are addressed in Chapters 21 and 22, respectively. With any patient, nutritional status is a significant covariate

Table 7-1 *Classification of surgical procedures*

Category	Definition	Characteristics of surgical intervention
Clean operations (example: herniorrhaphy)	Endogenous contamination is minimal; wound should not become infected.	Nontraumatic, uninfected, no inflammation. Respiratory, alimentary, and genitourinary (GU) tracts not entered. No break in aseptic technique. Primary closure; no drains (some institutions allow use of closed-wound suction for clean operations).
Clean-contaminated operations (example: appendectomy)	Bacterial contamination may have occurred from endogenous sources.	Respiratory, alimentary, or GU tract entered without significant spillage (or infected urine or bile, for GU tract and biliary tree). Vagina or oropharynx entered. Minor break in aseptic technique may have occurred. Wound may be drained.
Contaminated operations (example: repair of open, fresh trauma)	Contamination has occurred.	Gross spillage from gastrointestinal (GI) tract; urine or bile is infected (in GU or biliary tract procedures). Fresh, traumatic open wounds; acute, nonpurulent inflammation present. Major break in aseptic technique may have occurred.
Dirty and infected operations (example: drainage of an abcess)	Infection, devitalized tissue, or microbial contamination is present.	Old traumatic wound (more than 12 hours). Wound is infected; viscera may be perforated.

with positive results and diminished risk of infection. The nursing diagnoses *altered nutrition: less than body requirements* and *altered nutrition: more than body requirements* each carry equal but different risks for the surgical patient. Malnourishment from protein, iron, or vitamin deficiencies interferes with tissue repair and the growth necessary for wound healing. Hypoproteinemia is also associated with decreased gastrointestinal motility, decreased antibody production, infection, and wound dehiscence.

Obesity, often accompanied by other medical problems, decreases the efficiency of respiratory muscles, makes obliteration of dead space in the abdominal wall more difficult, and increases the technical difficulty of surgery. Adipose tissue has a very poor vascular supply, thus contributing to the risk for wound infection and complication. Both of these conditions should be corrected before nonemergency surgery.

Any local or systemic infection can result in wound infection. Elective surgery should be avoided for any patient with acute respiratory infections. It is conjectured that the coughing and sneezing that accompany respiratory infections allow patients to "autoinfect" themselves by aerosolizing microorganisms in the operating room or patient unit postoperatively. An infection far removed from the planned surgical site can also contribute to potential surgical site infection. Remote infections are infections of a body site other than the surgical wound. Studies have shown an 18.4% infection rate in patients with remote infections at the time of surgery (Meakins, 1993). The patient should be queried

regarding lesions, rashes, cuts, scratches, and ulcerated or infected areas; these should be inspected.

A variety of underlying diseases alter defense mechanisms or compromise body systems, contributing to an increased risk of infection. Patients who have chronic debilitating diseases or are receiving chemotherapy have lowered resistance resulting from impairment of their immune system. Assessment of pulmonary function is important because significant pulmonary complications are the most common early infection in surgical patients (Dellinger, 1993). The incidence of pulmonary complications may be related to factors such as smoking; location of surgical site, with increased risk in thoracic, upper abdominal, and lower abdominal surgical sites; and presence of preoperative dyspnea, bronchitis, cough, or other symptoms of chronic obstructive pulmonary disease. Accurate identification of risk and preoperative treatment are the goals in reducing perioperative pulmonary complications. Patients with cardiovascular disease, renal complications, liver disease, and certain endocrine disorders may also be at increased risk of developing surgical infections. Because surgical site infections remain the second most common hospital-acquired infection—increasing morbidity and mortality, prolonging hospital stay, and increasing patient care costs—careful assessment of patient risk promotes perioperative care plans to assist the patient in defending against infection.

Wound classification and surveillance. Classification of wounds is an important perioperative nursing function. Table 7-1 presents a system of classifying wounds according to the degree of operative contamination. Wound classification carries varying risk of surgical wound infection. Clean wounds have infection rates ranging from 1% to 5%. Contamination of these wounds usually results from an exogenous source or from bacterial colonization on the patient's skin. The role of perioperative care planning in controlling environmental sources of contamination is critical. Clean-contaminated wounds carry an infection risk that varies from 3% to 11%. Contaminated wounds have a 10% to 17% risk of postoperative infection, and dirty or infected wounds have a 27% or greater risk of infection. These infections are usually caused by either endogenous sources or local, preexisting trauma. The Centers for Disease Control advocate a composite risk index that includes the four wound-classification types and adds to them a measure of patient risk (often using the American Society of Anesthesiology [ASA] classification, with class 3, 4, or 5 scores to quantify patient susceptibility) and duration of the surgical intervention (Flanagan, 1994). Institutions that use this system can compare their risk-stratified data with other aggregate data bases, such as the National Nosocomial Infection Study (NNIS) program at the Centers for Disease Control; this allows for comparison by wound class and by procedure.

Procedure-specific surgical site surveillance should be the basis for calculation of institutional infection rates; this means that data are collected on every patient in the designated populations (such as all coronary artery bypass graft patients). Although it may be desirable to determine surgeon-specific SSI rates, further study of their value and validation of the risk index are necessary for accurate rate comparisons. The need to quantify SSI rates relates to quality measurement and is an important collaborative function of the perioperative nurse. In the future, perioperative nurses will continue to be challenged to develop standards and methods for postdischarge surveillance.

Antibiotic therapy. Major advances in surgery often accompany wartime experience. During World War I, immunization against tetanus, delayed closure of wounds, and blood transfusion were introduced. The clinical use of sulfonamide in 1935 and penicillin in 1941 marked the beginning of drug efficacy in combating important staphylococcal and streptococcal infections. Since that time, numerous new drugs and second and third generations of old drugs have appeared in clinical practice.

Antibiotics have five major actions. They may inhibit bacterial cell wall synthesis, inhibit protein synthesis, interfere with cell metabolism, interfere with the metabolism of bacteria, or interfere with nucleic acid production. Antibiotics may be bacteriocidal or bacteriostatic. In either case, the immune system and the perioperative nurse do much to place the patient at an advantage in the prevention of infection, with or without the use of antibiotic therapy. Patients who are being considered for antibiotic therapy need careful nursing assessment. The signs of infection (such as fever, purulent drainage, and elevated WBC count), as well as the symptoms of infection (such as redness, swelling, and tenderness), need to be evaluated. Culture results may be important in the asymptomatic patient. Temperature and vital signs need to be monitored. Subjective and objective evaluation of any patient thought to have an infection are extremely important pieces of nursing information to be added to the data base. Results of laboratory tests, any history of exposure to an infecting organism, culture and sensitivity of suspected areas of infection, and preexisting medical conditions should be reviewed.

Once the decision is made to place a patient on antibiotic therapy, additional data should be collected regarding any organ or system that might be consequently affected by the antibiotic regimen. Temperature, vital signs, blood counts, and liver and kidney functions should be monitored for desired and undesired side effects. Adequate nutrition and fluid intake should be maintained according to the patient's status, while objective and subjective review of the signs of the infection are ongoing. Knowledge of the nature of the drug, possible interactions, and side effects allows for the detection of new symptoms. The desired outcome of antibiotic therapy is to help the body eliminate infection without side effects. Surgical antibiotic prophylaxis is usually limited to cases in which there is a high risk of infection. The choice of antibiotic is based on the most likely infecting organism. No perioperative antibiotic should be administered without a review of the patient's drug allergies or sensitivities, and any medication administered by the perioperative nurse should be appropriately documented.

Generic care plan. The generic care plan presented in Fig. 7-4, along with its associated Guide to Nursing Actions, involves nursing assessment and activities that help the patient to remain free of surgical site infection. In an early nursing textbook, the operating room nurse's role was described as follows (Colp & Keller, 1927):

> The surgeon in the operating room . . . has come to rely absolutely on a highly educated and trained nurse. To her he leaves the preparation of supplies, of the operating room and instruments and of the patient; [in addition] most of the aftercare of the patient is left entirely to the nurse. It is a great need that the nurse fulfills . . . she . . . must live up to that high social calling by being well-prepared; she must be so educated

FIG. 7-4
GENERIC CARE PLAN   The patient is free from surgical site infection

KEY ASSESSMENT POINTS

Existing health problems that could decrease resistance to infection
Treatments/medications that increase risk for infection
Nutritional status
Vital signs
General physical condition
Laboratory data
Age-related risks
History of exposure to infectious diseases

NURSING DIAGNOSIS

High risk for surgical site infection

PATIENT OUTCOMES

The patient will be free from surgical site infection as evidenced by:
1. Oral temperature below 100°F
2. Incision site free of erythema, edema, undue tenderness, warmth, induration, foul odor, purulent drainage
3. Absence of dehiscence
4. Approximation of wound edges
5. Vital signs within normal limits
6. Normal laboratory values, especially WBC

NURSING ACTIONS

	Yes	No	N/A
1. Risk factors identified from preoperative assessment?	☐	☐	☐
2. Deviations in lab values reported?	☐	☐	☐
3. Baseline preoperative vital signs noted?	☐	☐	☐
4. Sterile field established and maintained?	☐	☐	☐
5. OR attire appropriate for team/patient?	☐	☐	☐
6. Hand scrub by correct protocol?	☐	☐	☐
7. Effective barriers created?	☐	☐	☐
8. Room inspected before opening supplies?	☐	☐	☐
9. Sterility maintained during opening?	☐	☐	☐
10. Sterile field monitored?	☐	☐	☐
11. Corrective action(s) taken?	☐	☐	☐
12. Surgical wound classified?	☐	☐	☐
13. Traffic patterns adhered to?	☐	☐	☐
14. Equipment properly cleaned and processed?	☐	☐	☐
15. OR sanitation protocols implemented?	☐	☐	☐
16. Used/contaminated items properly disinfected or sterilized?	☐	☐	☐
17. Hands washed?	☐	☐	☐
18. OSHA bloodborne pathogen compliance?	☐	☐	☐

Document additional nursing actions/care plan revisions here:

_____

_____

_____

EVALUATION OF PATIENT OUTCOMES

	Outcome met	Outcome met with additional outcome criteria	Outcome met with revised nursing care plan	Outcome not met	Outcome not applicable to this patient
1. The patient's oral temperature was below 100° F.	☐	☐	☐	☐	☐
2. The incision site was free of signs and symptoms of infection.	☐	☐	☐	☐	☐
3. The wound edges were approximated with no evidence of dehiscence.	☐	☐	☐	☐	☐
4. Vital signs remained within the patient's normal limits.	☐	☐	☐	☐	☐
5. Laboratory values remained normal.	☐	☐	☐	☐	☐

Signature: _____ Date: _____

FIG. 7-4 (Continued)
GENERIC CARE PLAN The patient is free from surgical site infection

GUIDE TO NURSING ACTIONS FOR PREVENTING SURGICAL SITE INFECTION

1. Preoperatively assess the patient for preexisting conditions that place the patient at risk for surgical site infection. Resistance to infection depends on the patient's susceptibility (immune response); use the key assessment factors as the beginning of a focused assessment.
2. Report deviations in laboratory values, especially WBC.
3. Check the patient's baseline preoperative vital signs.
4. Establish and maintain a sterile field according to principles of basic aseptic technique.
5. Adhere to institutional policy and protocol for OR attire.
6. Follow institutional policy and protocol for surgical hand scrubs.
7. Create effective barriers to transmission of microorganisms through proper gowning, gloving, and draping procedures. Follow institutional guidelines for barrier masks for tuberculosis patients.
8. Visually inspect room for total cleanliness before opening the case cart/supplies and instrument sets.
9. Inspect sterile items for contamination before opening. Check package integrity, expiration date, chemical process indicator.
10. Maintain sterility while opening sterile items to preserve the sterility of the item and the integrity of sterile field.
11. Constantly monitor the sterile field.
12. Initiate corrective action when break in technique occurs.
13. Communicate maintenance of a sterile field.
14. Classify surgical wound based on the degree of contamination of the wound and surrounding tissues during the operative procedure (clean, clean-contaminated, contaminated, dirty).
15. Control movement of the patient, personnel, and materials in and out of the OR by adhering to established traffic patterns.
16. Minimize risk of cross-infection by properly cleaning and processing anesthesia equipment and all items that have come into contact with the patient and/or sterile field.
17. Select materials for inhospital packaging that are compatible with the sterilization process, effective barriers, easily presented, and nontoxic.
18. Adhere to OR sanitation policies and protocols.
19. Cleanse skin at the operative site through skin preparation procedures.
20. Utilize methods of sterilization and disinfection to decontaminate needed supplies and equipment.
21. Meticulously wash hands following contact with the patient or any object likely to be contaminated with blood or body fluids.
22. Maintain the OR temperature between 20° C and 24° C (68° to 75° F) except where contraindicated for patient care.
23. Maintain relative humidity at 50% ±10.
24. Keep OR doors closed to maintain pressure gradients.
25. Requisition or administer antibiotics as ordered. Check the patient record for drug allergy/sensitivity. Note drug, dosage, route, and time of administration.
26. Remove soiled linen from around patient before transfer to post-anesthesia care unit.
27. Document additional nursing actions related to prevention of surgical site infection.
28. Comply with the OSHA bloodborne pathogen standard:
    - Be familiar with the exposure control plan
    - Use universal precautions
    - Comply with engineering controls
    - Use work practice controls
    - Wear appropriate personal protective equipment
    - Consider HBV vaccination
    - Follow postexposure protocols
    - Participate in education/training sessions
29. The following AORN recommended practices should be consulted to modify/expand this care plan:
    - Cleaning and processing of anesthesia equipment
    - Aseptic technique
    - Surgical attire
    - Disinfection
    - Use and care of endoscopes
    - Protective barrier materials for gowns and drapes
    - Surgical hand scrubs
    - Care of instruments, scopes, and powered surgical instruments
    - Selection and use of packaging systems
    - Sanitation in the surgical practice setting
    - Skin preparation of patients
    - Steam and ethylene oxide sterilization
    - Traffic patterns in the surgical suite
    - Universal precautions

and trained that she will not be a mere automatic tool, but an intelligent, enthusiastic co-worker, filled with a zeal for science and giving her whole mind and heart to the work that is before her—for only recently in the history of surgery is there scientific surgical nursing.

Today, the scientific basis of perioperative nursing is even more well established. The perioperative nurse, however, no longer views only the surgeon as an important person who depends on her skill and knowledge. It is the patient who depends on the perioperative nurse for assistance. The patient's goal is to undergo surgical intervention without the complication of postoperative surgical site infection.

Outcome Standard: The Patient's Skin Integrity Is Maintained

To maintain the patient's skin integrity, a number of physiologic assessment parameters need to be explored. These are all found in the exchanging category, a human response pattern that involves mutual giving and receiving. The exchanging pattern contains primarily physiologic data and is important in assessing the needs and meeting the requirements of perioperative patient populations. In this section, discussion of the risk for alteration in skin integrity will focus primarily on preoperative considerations. The risk for altered skin integrity that may result from intraoperative skin preparation; positioning; extraneous objects; chemical, physical, or electrical hazards will be discussed in the following section as the alterations relate to the various risks for patient injury.

The risk for impairment of skin integrity exists whenever a patient has or is at risk for an alteration in the skin surface that compromises it as an effective protective barrier (McFarland & McFarlane, 1993). Careful and accurate preoperative assessment of the integrity of the patient's skin is essential in differentiating the source of skin injuries that may appear in the postoperative period. Skin injury that occurs during surgery may be related to electrical, thermal, chemical, or mechanical causes. On the other hand, skin injury may be related to pharmacologic, physiologic, or medical conditions that potentiate skin breakdown. Pressure sores, shear ulcers, reddened areas, bruises, and many other indications of a skin injury may be a complication of the patient's condition rather than a result of an intraoperative injury. A risk assessment tool, such as the Braden Scale or the Norton Scale, is very useful in identifying at-risk patients in need of preventive nursing action and the specific factors placing them at risk (Pressure ulcers in adults, 1992). These tools have utility for perioperative nursing. In their report of a pressure ulcer prevention program, Murray and

Blaylock (1994) describe the incorporation of the Braden Scale on the intraoperative flow sheet as part of nursing activity that highlights the importance of skin assessment and pressure reduction/relief strategies.

Skin assessment. In physical assessment of the skin, both subjective and objective data must be collected. The patient should be asked about any complaints of burning, itching, skin discomfort or pain, dryness, blisters, tenderness, or paresthesias. The skin should be examined, and its color, moisture, texture, temperature, and turgor noted. To assess turgor and mobility, a small section of skin is gently pinched between the thumb and forefinger and then released. The skin should feel resilient, move easily when pinched, and return to place immediately when released. It should be determined whether the patient has any allergies to medications, chemical solutions, or tape that might be exacerbated intraoperatively. Any existing pressure areas, open skin lesions, draining wounds, rashes, abrasions, dry skin areas, infections, or other disruptions in skin layers are sought.

Although not strictly considered a part of the skin, alterations in oral mucous membranes may situationally result from prolonged NPO status, presence of nasogastric or endotracheal tubes, malnutrition, dehydration, fractured mandible, radiation to the head and neck, medication therapy, or mechanical trauma. The oral cavity should be assessed for moisture, integrity, cleanliness, edema, color, bleeding, and odor. Status of the teeth and the presence of dentures should be noted. Findings of the assessment of the oral cavity should be incorporated into plans for mouth and lip care, in both the anesthetized and the awake patient. Application of petroleum jelly to the lips and other interventions should be considered to improve the patient's comfort in the perioperative period.

Differential diagnoses related to skin integrity. Many medical conditions may predispose a patient to compromised skin integrity. Cardiac, circulatory, respiratory, liver, endocrine, hematologic, and other systemic diseases discovered in the patient's history lead to the elucidation of differential nursing diagnoses in the care plan. The following is a list of nursing diagnoses that may be related to the risk for impaired skin integrity. These nursing diagnoses may exist in perioperative patients and should be considered when an individualized plan of care to maintain the patient's skin integrity is developed.

Diarrhea
Hyperthermia
Incontinence, bowel
Incontinence, functional
Incontinence, reflex

Incontinence, stress
Incontinence, total
Infection, risk for
Mobility, impaired physical
Nutrition, altered: less than body requirements
Nutrition, altered: more than body requirements
Oral mucous membrane, altered
Skin integrity, impaired
Skin integrity, impaired, high risk
Tissue integrity, impaired
Tissue perfusion, altered: peripheral

Alterations in bowel elimination, resulting in *diarrhea* or *bowel incontinence,* and *urinary incontinence,* whether functional, reflex, or total, may cause a patient to be admitted to the perioperative patient care setting with actual skin breakdown. The moisture resulting from the incontinence diminishes the skin's resistance, often resulting in skin maceration. The ketones in urine further potentiate skin breakdown. *Infection*—present as an abscess, suppurative ulcer, or gangrene—complicates skin integrity by promoting necrotic and dead cells in the epithelial surface and superficial tissue. The patient with *impaired physical mobility* from paralysis or neuromuscular dysfunction; imposed by an orthopedic appliance or other immobilizing device; or relating to pain, fatigue, motivation, or sedation is predisposed to decreased circulation and circulatory pooling, which contribute to altered skin integrity.

The patient with *altered nutrition* is also at risk for altered skin integrity. Where nutrition is *less than body requirements,* the patient may be emaciated, with little protective cushioning over body prominences. The role of protein, described earlier, remains important in the physiologic maintenance of skin integrity. Lack of protein escalates the risk of skin breakdown because cellular nutrition is inadequate. In a study to determine factors contributing to pressure sores in surgical patients, Kemp, et al. (1989) used serum albumin levels as one of the study variables. Their research indicated that serum albumin levels less than 3 g/dl were significant in determining which perioperative patients developed pressure sores. In addition, patients with serum albumin levels below 2.0 to 2.5 g/dl are at risk for the development of edema, as fluid leaks out into the interstitial spaces, making the skin more vulnerable to injury. This type of edema is not found solely in dependent areas; it may manifest itself in puffy eyelids or hands and in the sacral area. Patients with edema are always at risk of skin breakdown. The patient whose nutritional level is *more than body requirements* has added pressure placed on supporting body surfaces, as well as a layer of adipose tissue that is relatively avascular. These relationships etio-

logically predispose the patient to problems in skin integrity.

Alterations in tissue perfusion impair oxygen and nutrient transport to the skin. The patient with peripheral vascular disease, arteriosclerosis, anemia, or cardiopulmonary disorders is at risk of decreased nutrition and respiration at the cellular level because of a decrease in capillary blood supply (Carpenito, 1993). Elderly patients are especially at risk because they have a high incidence of accompanying maturational vascular disease. Their venous and arterial capillaries are fragile, and their vessels are liable to be hard, brittle, and less elastic as a result of the pathophysiologic changes of aging. Elderly patients also have less body fat, with skin that is dry from reduced glandular secretion and thin. Nutritional status may be compromised if the diet is not rich in protein. All of these risks are patient specific in the elderly and need to be considered in planning care that prevents impairment of skin integrity.

Other factors that may contribute to actual or risk for impaired skin integrity include altered immune states; metabolic and endocrine disorders, such as diabetes mellitus, hepatitis, cirrhosis, renal failure, cancer, jaundice, and edema; medication therapy, especially long-term corticosteroid therapy; radiation therapy; poor hygiene; burns; and the presence of fistulas or stomas. The patient who is *hyperthermic* is also at risk for impaired skin integrity. The increased metabolic rate accompanying fever increases oxygen demand and decreases oxygen tension, thus potentiating the risk of pressure injuries to the skin. Finally, surgery itself violates skin integrity. Perioperative care planning has as its outcome that the patient's skin will remain intact. If the patient has a preexisting break in skin integrity, then the desired outcome is that the patient will be free of further skin breakdown.

Defining actual impairment of skin integrity. When a patient is scheduled for a surgical intervention that is unrelated to an existing impairment in skin integrity, the perioperative nurse needs to consider nursing activities that prevent further skin impairment. The stage of pressure ulcer formation should be identified. The clinical practice guideline for Pressure Ulcers in Adults (1992) defines Stage I as nonblanchable erythema of intact skin; Stage II as ulceration of dermis or epidermis; Stage III as ulceration involving subcutaneous fat; and Stage IV as extensive ulceration penetrating muscle, bone, or supporting structure. Perioperative nurses should develop care protocols and specific nursing interventions for each stage of actual impairment of skin integrity. For Stage I patients, perioperative nursing care plans should involve massage of healthy skin around the affected area, avoiding the reddened area itself. Rubbing the affected area may damage the ischemic skin. Pressure on the area should be minimized, and the patient should always be lifted rather than pulled. For Stage II patients, existing ulcerations should be protected during positioning to prevent deterioration of the ulcer. With Stage III patients, the perioperative nurse should attempt to incorporate any of the healing protocol measures that have been instituted on the patient care unit into the perioperative nursing care plan. This may involve keeping the ulcer surface moist and the sterile covering (e.g., film dressing, hydrocolloid wafer dressing, moist gauze dressing) intact intraoperatively. If a patient with a Stage IV impairment has a clean wound, the perioperative nursing care plan will include a nursing protocol for protecting the granulating wound bed from trauma and bacteria.

Incorporation of these activities into the perioperative nursing care plan for a patient with a skin impairment is one method of providing continuity of care.

Preoperative skin preparation. Part of most routine perioperative nursing assessment is determining if the patient's skin has been prepared before arrival in the operating room. Preoperative skin-preparation routines vary from institution to institution. Intraoperative routines for skin preparation should comply with institutional protocol. The AORN Recommended Practices for Skin Preparation of Patients may be used to expand or modify the generic care plan for prevention of infection through preparation of the skin at the operative site before the incision is made (AORN, 1996).

This section relates to the part of the Recommended Practice stating that "the operative site and surrounding areas should be clean." Opinions differ on how to prepare the patient's skin preoperatively so that it is "clean." Cleansing routines may involve bathing, showering, or site cleansing with an antimicrobial agent, soap, or other cleansing solution. Cleansing is accompanied or unaccompanied by the removal of hair at or varying distances around the operative site. Hair removal, if part of the skin preparation protocol, may be accomplished by shaving, clipping, cutting with scissors, or using a depilatory cream (Rothrock, 1993).

There is little doubt that preoperative skin preparation can influence the infection rate in clean surgical procedures. Cumulative evidence from scientific studies indicates that depilatory hair removal or abstinence from razor shaving is preferable to razor shaving, particularly if shaving is done hours before the operation. Nichols (1987) ranked the importance of factors influencing the development of postoperative infections in clean surgical procedures. A "very important factor," which was operationally defined as doubling the infection rate, was shaving the operative site the day before surgery. This increase results from the growth and multiplication of skin microorganisms in the damaged epithelium after the razor shave. For this reason, it is recommended that shaving be done in the immediate preoperative period if it is necessary. An "important factor," operationally defined as one in which infection rate was significantly increased but less than doubled, was failure to have the patient shower with an antiseptic before surgery. Showering with regular soap has not been observed to reduce infection rates; the value of the shower appears to relate to the use of antiseptics, which decrease populations of skin bacteria. Of "unproven" importance was whether an iodophor or hexachlorophene was used as the antiseptic agent.

The choice of antimicrobial agent and skin preparation technique continues to be studied. Traditional and lengthy scrub and paint with an aqueous iodophor solution have been studied in general surgery (Howard, 1991) and orthopedics (Gilliam & Nelson, 1990). Both of these studies showed that a 2-minute application of water insoluble iodophor in alcohol solution was effective in decreasing skin bacterial counts. An ideal skin preparation agent should be easy and fast to apply; dry quickly; be resistant to removal by perioperative fluids; and deliver antimicrobial protection throughout the duration of the surgical intervention (Patient prepping agents, 1994). The iodophor/alcohol combination appears to provide these characteristics as well as broad-spectrum activity against gram-positive and -negative organisms, tuberculosis, fungi, and viruses.

Generic care plan. Figure 7-5 presents a generic care plan with associated Guide to Nursing Actions for maintaining the patient's skin integrity. Developing a perioperative nursing care plan that has a patient outcome of maintained skin integrity is necessary for providing optimal patient care. Part of all care planning involves the evaluation and reevaluation of nursing practice. The special nursing interventions planned and carried out to maintain skin integrity should ensure physical safety and physiologic integrity. They should also explain, provide privacy, and ensure comfort and maintenance of dignity during any nursing activities that may be emotionally distressing or offensive to the patient.

Outcome Standard: The Patient is Free from Injury

Outcome Standard IV states that "the patient is free from injury related to positioning, extraneous objects, or chemical, physical, and electrical hazards" (AORN, 1996). In their efforts to prevent patient injury, perioperative nurses rapidly assess and act, us-

FIG. 7-5
GENERIC CARE PLAN   The patient's skin integrity is maintained

KEY ASSESSMENT POINTS

Nutritional status
Weight
Age
Circulatory problems
Level of mobility/activity
Sensory deficit
Continence
Examination:
  Skin integrity
  Skin condition
  Skin turgor

NURSING DIAGNOSIS

High risk for impaired skin integrity

PATIENT OUTCOMES

The patient's skin integrity will be maintained.
There will be no alteration in the patient's skin condition during the
  intraoperative period.
There will be no:
  Bruises
  Areas of skin breakdown/pressure ulcer
  Reddened areas
  Discolored skin
  Draining wounds
  Open skin lesions
  Excoriation
  Itching

NURSING ACTIONS

	Yes	No	N/A
1. Skin integrity assessed before surgical intervention?	☐	☐	☐
2. Previous incision site checked?	☐	☐	☐
3. Planned incision site checked?	☐	☐	☐
4. Medical condition(s) that might predispose patient to compromised skin integrity?	☐	☐	☐
5. Patient obese?	☐	☐	☐
6. Adequate tissue padding at bony prominences/pressure sites?	☐	☐	☐
7. Padding/support devices applied?	☐	☐	☐
8. Skin care measures provided?	☐	☐	☐
9. Problems with skin turgor/elasticity?	☐	☐	☐
10. Preoperative skin preparation carried out as prescribed?	☐	☐	☐
11. Any allergies/reactions to skin prep solutions or tape?	☐	☐	☐
12. Skin integrity reassessed following surgical intervention?	☐	☐	☐
13. Dressings appropriately applied?	☐	☐	☐
14. Area around dressing site cleansed?	☐	☐	☐
15. Drains present?	☐	☐	☐

Document additional nursing actions/care plan revisions here:

_____

_____

_____

EVALUATION OF PATIENT OUTCOMES

	Outcome met	Outcome met with additional outcome criteria	Outcome met with revised nursing care plan	Outcome not met	Outcome not applicable to this patient
1. The patient's skin remained intact.	☐	☐	☐	☐	☐
If patient was admitted to OR with an existing skin breakdown, then:					
2. The patient is free from further skin breakdown.	☐	☐	☐	☐	☐

Signature: _____ Date: _____

FIG. 7-5 (Continued)
GENERIC CARE PLAN   **The patient's skin integrity is maintained**

GUIDE TO NURSING ACTIONS FOR MAINTAINING THE PATIENT'S SKIN INTEGRITY

1. Note the condition of the patient's skin. Document any existing rashes, bruises, lesions, reddened areas, lacerations. Use a pressure ulcer assessment tool as applicable.
2. Examine previous incision sites, if any. Document location and condition of previous incisions.
3. Examine the site of the planned surgical incision for the current operative procedure. Document the condition of the site for the planned surgical incision.
4. Assess the patient record for medical conditions that might predispose the patient to compromised skin integrity. Document those.
5. Determine the patient's weight and tissue padding at bony prominences. Note obesity or underweight condition. Document plans for tissue massage, padding of bony prominences, and other skin care measures.
6. Check the patient's skin for turgor, elasticity. Note any problems with turgor, elasticity.
7. Verify with the patient/or patient chart that preoperative skin preparation was carried out according to orders/institutional protocol. Document compliance/deviations from orders/protocol.
8. Document condition of surgical site, dressings applied, drainage devices, and other relevant information relating to wound closure/surgical incision at end of operative procedure.
9. Remove excessive blood, solution, and exudate from the dressing site.
10. Document solutions used and any allergies/reactions to skin preparation solutions or tape.
11. Assess whether the patient has any complaints of paresthesia. Note areas of paresthesia.
12. Document additional nursing actions/care plan revisions related to maintaining the skin integrity.

ing manual and intellectual dexterity in such fast-paced sequences that observers may not even realize the nature of the nursing activities. It has, in fact, been suggested that this is one of the problems with OR student rotations—the perioperative nurse's activities are so quickly prioritized and sequenced that the student is unaware of what is being done. It is important for perioperative nursing educators to describe these activities in terms of patient care so that students can assimilate and synthesize the patient-centered nature of perioperative nursing. The following brief description offers perioperative nurses a philosophic premise for the nursing activities they undertake to prevent patient injuries.

Theoretic perspective. During the past few decades, nurses have endeavored to define nursing and its purpose through theoretic frameworks. Such frameworks are useful in providing direction for nursing practice. Theoretic frameworks for nursing often differ in their views of the patient. They define underlying beliefs about the patient, health, nursing, and the environment in relationship to the view of the patient as a being, not just a recipient of health care. Orem's Self-Care Deficit Theory is one framework that can guide perioperative nursing in describing and classifying patients according to their needs, which allows the design of a system of nursing based on those needs (Orem, 1985).

Nursing systems are described by Orem in relation to when and how nurses use their abilities to prescribe, design, and provide nursing care. There are three basic variations in these nursing systems: (1) wholly compensatory nursing, (2) partly compensatory nursing, and (3) supportive educative nursing. Perioperative nurses, depending on patient acuity, develop nursing systems based on each patient's need for self-care and the provision and management of self-care to sustain life and health. When patients are unable to maintain self-care, a wholly compensatory system of nursing is required. This is the premise for the intensive nursing care of anesthetized patients. Because these patient are incapacitated and unable to care for themselves, the perioperative nurse provides care that has as one of its outcomes the prevention of injury. This is an outcome that patients would set for themselves but, because of a medicated or anesthetized state, are unable to achieve. Therefore a self-care deficit exists, an imbalance between a patient's ability to provide self-care and his or her need for care. The patient requires nursing action for this imbalance, and the perioperative nurse becomes the patient's agent in carrying out care activities. Preventing patient injuries is one of perioperative nursing's most critical advocacy roles.

Legal implications. Although preventing patient injury is a desired outcome not only for the anesthetized or medicated patient, those conditions make the patient more vulnerable to injury. The patient's condition makes self-protection impossible. Medicated and anesthetized patients lack protective responses. If positioning stretched the brachial plexus, an electrical injury took place, or a skin reaction to a chemical skin preparation solution caused itching, a conscious, unsedated patient would complain or withdraw from the source of injury. Because the patient cannot sense the beginning of an injury, take any action to discontinue it, or complain about it, the nurse's advocacy role and exposure to potential liability are increased.

Murphy (1987) identifies the doctrine of *res ipsa loquitor* as a legal concept that is applied to perioperative nursing with greater frequency than other areas of nursing. Meaning "the thing speaks for itself," this legal doctrine alters the ordinary burden of proof, shifting it from the injured party to the defendant, which may be the nurse, surgical team, health care institution, or any combination thereof. For this doctrine to be invoked, the injured party, or plaintiff, must establish that the injury would not ordinarily have occurred in the absence of negligence, that the cause of the injury was within the exclusive control of the defendant(s), and that the plaintiff did not contribute to the injury in any way. In perioperative patient care settings, the anesthetized patient is unlikely to have contributed to an injury. The cause of the injury, be it a positioning device, a chemical, an electrosurgical unit, or any of the other potential causative agents, is usually under the control of the defendant. It is unlikely that paralysis or a burn would occur in the absence of negligence. Because such complication or injury is not an expected result of surgery, the inference is made that someone failed to take reasonable care to prevent the injury. Thus "the thing speaks for itself!"

Prevention of injury: positioning for surgery. Surgical position is selected primarily to gain optimal access to the operative site. Positioning may interfere with the physical and physiologic limits of a patient's tolerance. The absence of pain under anesthesia often permits positioning that would be intolerable if the patient were awake. Therefore it clearly becomes a collaborative team function to select, establish, and evaluate the effects of surgical positioning. The generic care plan and Guide to Nursing Actions for patient positioning presented in Fig. 7-6 does not prescribe techniques for establishing the various positions. The plan will require modification based on position selected, patient assessment, and experience with and availability of various positioning devices and accessories. Only the general

FIG. 7-6
GENERIC CARE PLAN   The patient is free from injury related to positioning

KEY ASSESSMENT POINTS

Age
Weight
Current activity level
Mobility restrictions
Overall health status
Range of motion
Presence of implants
Skin condition at positional pressure points
Respiratory, circulatory, and neuromuscular status
Areas of discomfort that will be affected by selected position
(and factors that alleviate discomfort)

NURSING DIAGNOSIS

High risk for injury related to surgical positioning

PATIENT OUTCOMES

The patient will be free of injury related to the surgical position.
1. The patient will maintain effective breathing patterns throughout the surgical intervention. There will be no mechanical restrictions to ventilation.
2. The patient will not experience significant alterations in cardiac output. There will be no episodes of significant hypotension or hypertension.
3. The patient will be positioned in a manner that facilitates gas exchange. Ventilation: perfusion ratios will be adequate.
4. The patient will not experience any neuromuscular damage. There will be no postoperative pain or discomfort upon abduction, flexion, or extension of positioned extremities that was not present preoperatively.
5. The patient will attain normal preoperative comfort level. There will be no tingling, numbness, cramping, stiffness, weakness, aching, or pain in positioned body parts.
6. The patient will not experience alterations in tissue perfusion. There will be no reddened, discolored, ulcerated, edematous, or excoriated skin areas.

NURSING ACTIONS

	Yes	No	N/A
1. Mobility/ROM checked before positioning?	☐	☐	☐
2. Any physical abnormalities/injury present preoperatively?	☐	☐	☐
3. Any external/internal prostheses present?	☐	☐	☐
4. Privacy provided?	☐	☐	☐
5. Potential problems assessed?	☐	☐	☐
6. Appropriate mode of transportation/transfer procedures selected?	☐	☐	☐
7. OR bed properly functioning/positioned in room?	☐	☐	☐
8. Positioning devices/aids placed?	☐	☐	☐
9. Patient checked during/following each positional change?	☐	☐	☐
10. Restraint strap properly placed?	☐	☐	☐

NURSING ACTIONS—cont'd

	Yes	No	N/A
11. Bony prominences/dependent pressure sites checked at end of surgical intervention?	☐	☐	☐
12. Appropriate transfer to postanesthesia care unit?	☐	☐	☐

Document additional nursing actions/care plan revisions here:

_____

_____

_____

EVALUATION OF PATIENT OUTCOMES

	Outcome met	Outcome met with additional outcome criteria	Outcome met with revised nursing care plan	Outcome not met	Outcome not applicable to this patient
1. The patient maintained effective breathing patterns throughout the surgical intervention.	☐	☐	☐	☐	☐
2. There were no significant alterations in cardiac output during the surgery or positional changes.	☐	☐	☐	☐	☐
3. There was no evidence of neuromuscular damage or injury.	☐	☐	☐	☐	☐
4. The patient maintained adequate gas exchange.	☐	☐	☐	☐	☐
5. The patient demonstrated return to preoperative comfort and mobility levels.	☐	☐	☐	☐	☐
6. There was no evidence of impaired skin integrity related to the surgical position.	☐	☐	☐	☐	☐

Signature: _____ Date: _____

FIG. 7-6 (Continued)
GENERIC CARE PLAN   **The patient is free from injury related to positioning**

GUIDE TO NURSING ACTIONS TO PREVENT INJURY RELATED TO POSITIONING

1. Determine mobility and range of motion of body parts. Document any limitations to mobility.
2. Note any physical abnormalities (congenital anomalies) or injury (loss of extremity or body part). Document those.
3. Identify the presence of any external/internal prostheses or implants. Document those.
4. Provide privacy for the patient during positioning activities and patient examination.
5. Assess the patient/patient record for potential patient problems that make the patient vulnerable to positional injury. Such problems might include the length of the planned surgical intervention, cardiovascular disease, smoking, demineralizing bone conditions, elderly patient, obesity, diabetes, anemia, hypothermia, malnourishment, hypovolemia, edema, arthritis, peripheral nerve dysfunction.
6. Based on assessment data, determine appropriate mode of patient transport and transfer to the OR bed. List special plans. Sheets on OR bed should be dry, wrinkle free.
7. When the patient is on the OR bed, place restraint belt snugly above the knees without compromising circulation or exerting pressure on bony prominences or nerves. Document placement of restraining belt.
8. Check the OR bed for proper functioning and position location for optimum lighting during the surgical intervention. Note any problems/corrective actions regarding bed function.
9. Assemble the required positioning aids (pillows, stirrups, padding, bed parts, etc.).
10. With the team, assist the patient into the designated surgical position. Describe pertinent details of the positioning and placement of positioning devices (including body and safety straps).
11. Note any positional changes (i.e., supine to Trendelenburg's to supine) and position checks for each change.
12. Before patient transfer to postanesthesia care unit, check bony prominences and dependent pressure sites. Document assessment.
13. Document time of discharge, method of transfer, and patient status.
14. Document other nursing actions relevant to prevention of injury during surgical positioning.

considerations of safe positioning for the surgical patient are described.

Surgical positioning requires knowledge of the general principles of positioning and a practical understanding of the operating room bed and the safe use of its accessory positioning devices. In addition, it requires specific knowledge of nursing diagnoses that identify potential positioning problems. Patients may have or be at risk for *decreased cardiac output, pain, fluid volume excess or deficit, impaired gas exchange, altered tissue perfusion, impaired physical mobility, sensory/perceptual alterations: kinesthetic, or impaired skin integrity.* These nursing diagnoses, depending on their etiologic and contributing factors, may influence ventilation and perfusion, positional intolerances and neurovascular compromise, and present numerous other possibilities. Creative teamwork is necessary in collaborating during surgical positioning so that the patient's state is not further compromised. Nursing knowledge is integrated into safe transport of the patient to the operating room; transfer to and from the OR bed; and slow, careful, deliberate, and gentle manipulation of the patient during all positioning and repositioning maneuvers.

Prevention of injury: extraneous objects. "Extraneous" is synonymous with "foreign," and that is the primary focus for the nursing diagnosis *high risk for injury from retained foreign object.* In this context, foreign objects are most likely to be sharps, sponges, or instruments, but can be any object that is introduced inadvertently into the patient during surgery. Perioperative nurses are aware of the importance of sharp, sponge, and instrument counts. Only x-ray detectable sponges are used inside the body, and no counted item should be taken from the room during the procedure. All items and their parts need to be accounted for. Institutions have various protocols for initiating and documenting corrective action when counts are incorrect. Because these are institutional standards, they need to be adhered to strictly. Retained foreign objects can result in postoperative pain, infection, obstruction, or other injury that carries morbidity and may require subsequent surgery.

Murphy (1987) identifies retained foreign bodies as the most prevalent injury resulting in litigation for the perioperative nurse. In malpractice suits, the fact that a sharp, sponge, or instrument was left behind may be accepted as evidence of negligence per se, or the doctrine of *res ipsa loquitor* may be applied. In either case, it is very difficult to show that negligence was not involved; these lawsuits tend to revolve around the extent of damages rather than disproving negligence. Clear and consistent count policies are the most effective strategies for prevent-

ing retained foreign objects. The generic care plan and associated Guide to Nursing Actions for preventing this injury is presented in Fig. 7-7.

Prevention of injury: chemical hazards. A number of chemicals may present the possibility of patient injury. Skin-preparation solutions, improperly aerated ethylene oxide sterilized items, improperly rinsed items chemosterilized in a glutaraldehyde solution, intraoperative medications, methyl methacrylate, depilatory agents, and dyes may cause allergic or tissue reaction. Powder or starch on surgical gloves, if it is not removed, may cause intraperitoneal and tissue granulomas; more recently, starch powder has been implicated in latex allergy (Sussman, Tarlo, & Dolovich, 1991). Allergic proteins found in latex can bind to starch powder. Perioperative personnel need to determine whether they are using a glove that needs to be rinsed or whether the glove is "powder free" and should not be rinsed. Because latex in medical devices can pose a significant risk to those with latex sensitivity, the FDA requires that all medical devices that contain natural rubber latex and come into contact with the body either directly or indirectly are to be labeled accordingly. In preventing patient injury from chemical hazards, patient allergies to latex or other allergens need to be verified, skin assessed, and nursing actions taken to prevent wet areas, flammable hazards, pooling of solutions, and tissue burns. The AORN Recommended Practices for Skin Preparation of Patients and for Sterilization and Disinfection provide additional information that may be used to modify or expand the generic care plan. The Guide to Nursing Actions in Fig. 7-8 gives information for preventing injury related to chemical hazards.

Prevention of injury: physical hazards. The generic care plan and associated Guide to Nursing Actions for preventing injury related to physical hazards (Fig. 7-9) takes into account the multiple and varied sources of environmental stressors. Mechanical injury caused by pressure, shearing forces, friction, or moisture may result in tissue necrosis. Other environmental sources of injury include the stressors of anesthesia; a hard OR bed with a thin mattress; cold rooms, which encourage vasoconstriction; anesthetically or surgically induced hypotension; equipment such as Mayo stands, which may exert external pressure on a body part; members of the operative team, who may lean on the patient; and the use of tourniquets, temperature control devices, lasers, and x-ray equipment.

Gendron (1986) suggests that many unexplained skin injuries discovered postoperatively probably relate to a mechanical injury that results in pressure necrosis. These injuries may be more common after cardiovascular surgery. A procedure that involves

FIG. 7-7
GENERIC CARE PLAN   The patient is free from injury related to retained foreign objects

KEY ASSESSMENT POINTS

Risk increases with the depth of the surgical wound and the body cavities/organs opened.
Risk also increases if the procedure is an emergency.

NURSING DIAGNOSIS

High risk for injury related to retained foreign object

PATIENT OUTCOMES

The patient is free from injury related to retained foreign object.
1. The patient will not have any retained sponge following wound closure unless such sponge placement was deliberate and recorded.
2. The patient will not have any retained sharps following wound closure.
3. The patient will not have any retained instruments or instrument parts unless such placement was deliberate and recorded.
4. The patient will be free of any other retained foreign object unless such placement was deliberate and recorded.

NURSING ACTIONS

	Yes	No	N/A
1. Counts performed according to institutional protocol?	☐	☐	☐
2. Patient care items confined and contained?	☐	☐	☐
3. Broken items accounted for in entirety?	☐	☐	☐
4. Corrective actions taken for incorrect counts?	☐	☐	☐
5. Counts/count results documented?	☐	☐	☐
6. Items deliberately left in patient documented?	☐	☐	☐
7. Only x-ray detectable sponges used in wound?	☐	☐	☐

Document additional nursing actions/care plan revisions here:

_____

_____

_____

EVALUATION OF PATIENT OUTCOMES

The patient's wound was closed with all sharps, sponges, instrument parts, and other foreign objects accounted for.

Outcome met	Outcome met with additional outcome criteria	Outcome met with revised nursing care plan	Outcome not met	Outcome not applicable to this patient
☐	☐	☐	☐	☐

Signature: _____ Date: _____

GENERIC CARE PLAN   Guide to nursing actions to protect the patient from injury related to retained foreign objects

1. Follow established policies and institutional protocols for sponge, sharp, and instrument counts.
2. Confine and contain all discarded sponges, sharps, and instruments. Do not remove counted items from the operating room during a procedure. Dispose of contaminated items per institutional protocol.
3. Account for any sharps or instruments broken or disassembled in their entirety.
4. Initiate corrective actions, following institutional protocol, when counts are incorrect. Document corrective actions, persons notified.
5. Document counts taken and results of counts according to institutional policy.
6. Document any sponges, packing, or other objects deliberately left in the patient.
7. Document names of relief persons.
8. Perform counts during changes of shift. Document change of shift counts.
9. Document any implants (type, size, device identification or lot number, etc.).
10. Document any other nursing action relevant to prevention of retained foreign objects.

FIG. 7-8
GENERIC CARE PLAN The patient is free from injury related to chemical hazards

KEY ASSESSMENT POINTS
Allergies
Skin sensitivities
Skin condition
Effectiveness of hair removal, if applicable

NURSING DIAGNOSIS
High risk for injury related to the use of chemical agents

PATIENT OUTCOMES
The patient will be free of injury related to the use of chemical agents.
1. The patient's skin at the operative site will be prepared so that:
   - Dirt and transient microbes are removed.
   - The rapid rebound growth of microbes during the surgical procedure will be inhibited.
2. The patient will experience minimal or no tissue reaction resulting from skin preparation.
3. The patient will be free of allergic or other untoward reactions from the use of dyes, medications, or other chemical agents.

NURSING ACTIONS

	Yes	No	N/A
1. Any patient allergies?	☐	☐	☐
2. Skin condition assessed before procedure?	☐	☐	☐
3. Patient privacy provided?	☐	☐	☐
4. Institutional protocols followed for skin preparation?	☐	☐	☐
5. Agent(s) allowed to air dry before drapes applied?	☐	☐	☐
6. Pooling of prep solutions prevented?	☐	☐	☐
7. OR bed dry and wrinkle-free following skin prep?	☐	☐	☐
8. Prep solutions/instruments/supplies confined and contained?	☐	☐	☐
9. Other chemical agents used?	☐	☐	☐
10. Medications given by nurse?	☐	☐	☐
11. Ethylene-oxide sterilized items aerated properly?	☐	☐	☐
12. Soaked (chemosterilized) items carefully rinsed?	☐	☐	☐
13. Glove powder removed as recommended?	☐	☐	☐

Document additional nursing actions/care plan revisions here:

_____

_____

_____

EVALUATION OF PATIENT OUTCOMES

	Outcome met	Outcome met with additional outcome criteria	Outcome met with revised nursing care plan	Outcome not met	Outcome not applicable to this patient
1. The operative site showed minimal or no tissue reaction from skin-preparation procedures.	☐	☐	☐	☐	☐
2. The patient experienced no allergic or other untoward reactions to the use of other chemical agents.	☐	☐	☐	☐	☐

Signature: _____ Date: _____

GUIDE TO NURSING ACTIONS TO PROTECT THE PATIENT FROM INJURY RELATED TO CHEMICAL HAZARDS

1. Verify with the patient the presence of any allergies related to chemical agents (skin preparation solutions, depilatory agents, dyes, etc.). Document any patient allergies.
2. Assess the patient for the presence of any rashes, urticaria, reddened areas, complaints of itching, and dry or flaky skin before the application/use of any chemical agents. Document skin condition/patient complaints.
3. Provide patient privacy during skin preparation procedures.
4. Follow institutional protocol for the method of application, selected skin antimicrobial agent, and exposure time of antimicrobial agent. Document methods/agents used to prepare skin at operative site.
5. Document area prepared. Allow skin preparation agents to dry before placement of barrier drapes.
6. Do not allow skin preparation solution to pool at bedside or at site of electrode or dispersive pad placement.
7. Following skin preparation, check that all areas within the immediate patient area are dry and free of wrinkles.
8. Confine and contain instruments, sponges, antimicrobial agents, and accessory items used in skin preparation.
9. List other chemical agents (dyes, glue, etc.), time, and method of application.
10. Document any medications given by the perioperative nurse, time, dose, method of administration, and nurse administering.
11. Verify that ethylene-oxide sterilized items have been properly aerated.
12. Thoroughly rinse items soaked in glutaraldehyde or other chemosterilizing agents. Read and follow instructions for use of chemical agents.
13. Adhere to glove manufacturer's (and institutional) protocol for removal of powder from external surface of sterile gloves.
14. Document other nursing actions relevant to prevention of injury from chemical hazards.

FIG. 7-9
GENERIC CARE PLAN   The patient is free from injury related to physical hazards

KEY ASSESSMENT POINTS

Patient condition/acuity
Patient transport/transfer needs
Patient safety/comfort needs
Complexity of procedure
Complexity of equipment required
Extrinsic factors contributing to temperature alteration

NURSING DIAGNOSIS

High risk for injury related to physical hazards
Related nursing diagnoses:
  High risk for alterations in body temperature
  High risk for alterations in comfort and/or safety*

PATIENT OUTCOMES

The patient will be free of injury related to physical hazards.
The patient will be protected from physical injury by:
  1. Having supplies and equipment made available and in working order by nursing staff
  2. Experiencing no untoward delays or scheduling conflicts
  3. Having patient care needs coordinated with other appropriate departments
  4. Having surgical environment controlled by nursing staff
  5. Having vital signs monitored

NURSING ACTIONS

	Yes	No	N/A
1. Supplies and equipment available?	☐	☐	☐
2. Room temperature controlled?	☐	☐	☐
3. Warm blankets provided?	☐	☐	☐
4. Prep solution warmed?	☐	☐	☐
5. Thermia unit used?	☐	☐	☐
6. Patient temperature monitored by nurse?	☐	☐	☐
7. Vital signs monitored by nurse?	☐	☐	☐
8. Tourniquet used appropriately?	☐	☐	☐
9. Noise level controlled?	☐	☐	☐
10. Traffic patterns maintained?	☐	☐	☐
11. Safe patient transfer procedures used?	☐	☐	☐
12. Additional personnel assigned based on qualifications and patient acuity?	☐	☐	☐
13. Equipment operated per manufacturer's instructions?	☐	☐	☐
14. Equipment malfunctions?	☐	☐	☐
15. Radiation safety precautions used?	☐	☐	☐
16. Intraoperative emergencies occurred?	☐	☐	☐
17. Appropriate patient charges filed?	☐	☐	☐
18. Delays documented/reported?	☐	☐	☐
19. Specimens properly disposed? (include cultures, frozen sections)	☐	☐	☐
20. SMDA compliance?	☐	☐	☐

Document additional nursing actions/care plan revisions here:

_____

_____

_____

EVALUATION OF PATIENT OUTCOMES

	Outcome met	Outcome met with additional outcome criteria	Outcome met with revised nursing care plan	Outcome not met	Outcome not applicable to this patient
1. Supplies and equipment were available for patient care.	☐	☐	☐	☐	☐
2. The patient's body temperature was maintained within normal range.	☐	☐	☐	☐	☐
3. The patient expressed satisfaction with comfort measures.	☐	☐	☐	☐	☐
4. The patient remained injury free.	☐	☐	☐	☐	☐

*This is not a NANDA-approved nursing diagnosis

Signature: _____ Date: _____

FIG. 7-9   (Continued)
GENERIC CARE PLAN   **The patient is free from injury related to physical hazards**

GUIDE TO NURSING ACTIONS PROTECTING THE PATIENT FROM INJURY RELATED TO PHYSICAL HAZARDS

1. Use patient supplies judiciously and in a cost-effective manner.
2. Verify and coordinate use of supplies and equipment for intraoperative care. Document unavailability/problems with supplies and equipment.
3. Before bringing the patient into the OR, check that there are no scheduling conflicts. Document delays/conflicts.
4. Adhere to institutional protocol for safe patient transfer procedures (wheels locked, personnel to assist, etc.). Document transfer method and support measures.
5. Coordinate patient care needs with appropriate departments. Document time and nature of interdepartmental communication (pharmacy, pathology, microbiology, housekeeping, radiology, etc.).
6. Control the room temperature per the need of the patient and surgical team.
7. Offer warm blankets, other comfort measures to patient. Expose only the body surface necessary during skin preparation procedures. Consider covering the patient's head with a cap, stockinette, other head covering to conserve heat loss, or use body warming system. Prep solutions may be warmed, but not heated; follow manufacturer's recommendations. Infusion/irrigation solutions should be warmed (or cooled) appropriate to patient's need.
8. Monitor the patient's temperature as indicated. Document area of placement of temperature control devices, identification of unit, and record of time and temperature.
9. Monitor the patient's vital signs as indicated. Note placement of electrocardiographic or other monitoring devices, time and results of monitoring.
10. Place tourniquet cuff as indicated for surgical procedure. Document placement of tourniquet cuff, pressure, time, and identification of unit.
11. Monitor sensory environment. Control sensory stimuli and noise level in the operating room (to include holding area).

12. Adhere to institutional protocol for traffic patterns in the operating room.
13. Assign activities to other personnel based on their qualifications and the patient's needs.
14. Prepare for potential patient emergencies based on assessment data and intraoperative events. Remain with patient, assist anesthesia as indicated, during induction, extubation, emergency drug reactions, other untoward events. Document intraoperative emergency events (i.e., cardiopulmonary or respiratory arrest, malignant hyperthermia, hemorrhage, etc.).
15. Operate mechanical, electrical, and air-powered equipment according to manufacturer's instructions. Be familiar with institutional equipment management program; each piece of equipment used should have written procedures for testing and training designed to reduce risks.
16. Remove malfunctioning equipment from the OR. Document equipment disposition/person notified. Comply with reporting requirements for medication and device adverse effects and product problems.
17. Follow institutional protocols for radiation safety (ionizing and lasers) to protect the patient and personnel. Document safety precautions taken, type of patient protection, and area(s) protected.
18. Send all blood, body fluid, and tissue specimens in a clean, impervious container for transport to appropriate laboratory. Use universal precautions in handling tissue specimens and cultures. Document specimens and cultures.
19. Comply with the Safe Medical Device Act (SMDA), which requires reporting of implants/explants (use institution-approved device tracking report) and device-related serious injury, illness, or death.
20. Document other nursing actions relevant to prevention of injury from physical hazards.

cross-clamping of the aorta increases the risk of tissue necrosis. A cardiovascular surgical intervention that lasts for more than 2 to 3 hours may result in a deep insult to the tissue in the distal vasculature. Other mechanical pressure from positioning devices, supports, stirrups, or straps that are incorrectly placed for more than 3 hours may produce the same type of injury. The patient with preexisting vascular disease is particularly at risk. All patients need supportive cushioning, padding, careful placement of accessories, and verification by the perioperative nurse that there is no mechanical restriction, pinching, or pressure. Gendron (1986) suggests that a wound with the following characteristics is likely to be a pressure injury caused by mechanical forces:

1. Occurred after a lengthy surgical procedure
2. Occurred below the waist in an area under body weight or pressure
3. Discovered some time after surgery
4. Second- or deep third-degree classification
5. On the sacrum, buttocks, or thigh
6. Extensive
7. Slow to heal

High risk for altered body temperature exists when the patient is at risk of failure to maintain body temperature within the normal range (Carpenito, 1993). The use of hypothermia and hyperthermia temperature control devices in the OR makes this a significant risk for perioperative patients. The already altered temperature of the physical environment may contribute to patient hypothermia, as may anesthetic agents. Patients receiving vasoconstricting or vasodilating drug therapy are already at risk for altered body temperature. Nursing measures such as placement of warm blankets, covering the patient's head, and using warm irrigation and intravenous solutions may assist in controlling some of the shivering that often occurs after administration of general anesthesia. Irrigating solutions and instruments that have been flash sterilized must be checked to verify that their temperature does not cause a thermal injury.

Environmental conditions encountered during operative or other invasive procedures may interfere with the patient's safety or comfort. Patients whose surgery is delayed because of scheduling conflicts or unavailability of equipment may be uncomfortable while waiting for surgery to begin. They need to be reassured that they will be cared for as soon as possible and that their family, significant other, or both will be notified of the delay. Patient transfer procedures carry safety threats unless accomplished with the patient's mobility level in mind. There must be enough support personnel, and wheels must be locked on transport devices and the OR bed. Speci-

mens need to be handled correctly and carefully to ensure that they are not lost, mislabeled, or preserved in a way that interferes with pathologic examination. Noise needs to be controlled, as do traffic patterns and the transport of equipment and items that might be frightening to a patient. The patient's comfort, in terms of personal identity, needs to be considered. Patients should be addressed by their preferred name; perioperative personnel should introduce themselves to the patient.

Intraoperative emergencies such as cardiac arrest, malignant hyperthermia, laryngospasm, hemorrhage, and shock carry enormous threats to safe patient outcomes. A vigilant and caring perioperative nursing team, trained in the use of resuscitative equipment and collaborating closely with the other surgical team members, can make a vital difference in patient safety.

Many perioperative nursing activities that seem routine have as their intended outcome the prevention of patient injury. The following AORN Recommended Practices may be consulted to modify or expand the generic care plan and associated Guide to Nursing Actions (Fig. 7-9) for preventing patient injury related to physical hazards: Use of Pneumatic Tourniquet; Reducing Radiological Exposure; Laser Safety; Traffic Patterns in the Surgical Suite; and Monitoring the Patient Receiving Local Anesthesia and Intravenous Conscious Sedation, and Safe Care Through Identification of Hazards in the Surgical Environment. The number of medical devices used in perioperative care settings require a sound equipment maintenance program. The 1995 Joint Commission chapter, "Management of the Environment," requires written policies for equipment management, documentation of preventive maintenance, and performance assessment and improvement activities. Control of risk to patients is a collaborative perioperative nursing activity.

Prevention of injury: electrical hazards. Electrosurgical burns have dropped off sharply as a cause of accidental skin injury since 1973 (Gendron, 1986). Improvements in technology coupled with vigilant perioperative nursing care have done much to eliminate major electrosurgical injury hazards. Because the electrosurgical unit is widely used for cutting and coagulating tissue, the perioperative nurse must continue efforts directed toward preventing injuries. Injuries from the electrosurgical unit can occur at the dispersive site, at the active electrode, or elsewhere. Injuries that occur at the dispersive site, or patient pad, do so because the pad's conductive surface inadvertently becomes reduced. When a dispersive pad separates from the skin, the electricity flowing from the patient back to the source generator becomes highly concentrated at the remaining conductive site, resulting in a burn. Dispersive pads placed incorrectly, such as over an irregular or bony surface, can also reduce the conductive surface. In selecting a placement site for the dispersive pad, the perioperative nurse should assess the skin and choose a site close to the operative site that has good muscle mass and is clean, dry, and smooth. Bony prominences, hairy surfaces, and oily surfaces can all interfere with pad contact. Adherence of the pad to the site and cable connections should be checked whenever the surgeon requests increased power settings or when the patient's position is changed. Dispersive pads should not be placed over bony projections, on a body pressure point, or on scar tissue; the pad should be placed in such a manner that its longest edge is toward the surgery site, and it should be kept free of surgical solutions (Harrington, 1994).

Alternate current burns occur when the electricity seeks a path other than the dispersive pad to return to the generator. Electrocardiograph electrodes are likely alternate current sources and have been implicated in electrosurgical skin injuries. Because the conductive area of an electrocardiograph electrode is greatly reduced, the current is highly concentrated. Other burn sites may include any area of the patient's skin that is in contact with a metal object, including the OR bed, stirrups, and other positioning accessories; a catheter; or a fluid path from the patient to ground. Insulating the patient from contact with metal is important in preventing both electrical and pressure injuries. Newer electrosurgical units have circuits that monitor the coupling of the dispersive pad to the patient. Recommended Practices for Electrosurgery should be consulted to modify or expand the generic care plan and the associated Guide to Nursing Actions in Fig. 7-10 for prevention of injury related to electrical hazards.

Patient advocacy. Normal sensory perception in the skin is absent in the anesthetized patient. The role of the perioperative nurse as advocate in protecting the patient from injury is a vital one. The potential injurious events are many and often interrelated with the patient's medical condition, the nature of the surgery, the necessity of a selected patient position, the required use of surgical accessories, and environmental hazards. Wholly compensatory nursing systems involve nursing actions that remedy the imbalance between the patient's care needs and capability in delivering self-care. As the perioperative nurse compensates for the patient's inability to provide self-care, he or she implements a plan devised to protect the patient from injury during the perioperative period.

Outcome Standard: The Patient's Fluid and Electrolyte Balance is Maintained

The potential for fluid volume deficit, fluid volume excess, or both are significant nursing diagnoses for the perioperative patient. Intraoperative hemostasis is critical for safe and effective surgical outcomes. However, interference with normal clotting mechanisms, preexisting pathologic conditions, the nature and difficulty of the surgical intervention, and the treatments selected to correct resulting problems can interfere with surgery. Guided by knowledge and skill, the perioperative nurse plans for potential alterations in fluid volume with the goal of maintaining fluid and electrolyte balance. Box 7-1 reviews some common laboratory diagnostic test results that alert the perioperative nurse to actual or potential fluid volume changes.

Achieving hemostasis. Bleeding is usually controlled during surgery through the use of clamps, ligatures, clips, and electrosurgical or argon beam coagulation. Adjunctive to these methods may be the application of pressure or the use of topical hemostatic agents. In normal clotting, four physiologic mechanisms act to control blood loss. The injured vessel initially constricts and retracts in an attempt to decrease the blood flow out of the vessel and exert some pressure to control it. A platelet plug is formed within seconds by thrombocytes produced in the bone marrow. The injured vessel, with its damaged endothelium, has exposed connective tissue that contains collagen. Platelets are attracted to this surface and adhere to it. As the platelets adhere, they release a substance that attracts more platelets, and these platelets attach to other platelets in a process known as aggregation. Thus a fragile plug is formed. This platelet plug is reinforced by fibrin. Through intrinsic and extrinsic pathways involving 12 clotting factors, prothrombin, thrombin, and fibrinogen, fibrin is formed to stabilize the clot and prevent its disintegration. Eventually, dissolution of the clot takes place through a chemical reaction of fibrinolysis. This rather complicated but effective process can be altered or interfered with by a number of patient conditions.

As in all perioperative nursing assessment, the patient's preoperative status can greatly influence intraoperative events. Assessment determines prioritized nursing diagnoses, which guide the development of desired patient outcomes and plans for achieving them. In assessing for potential problems with normal clotting, a history of aspirin or nonsteroidal antiinflammatory drug use should be noted. These drugs inhibit platelet aggregation as a natural consequence of their pharmacologic activity. A history of anticoagulant therapy is also important because these medications usually interfere with

FIG. 7-10
GENERIC CARE PLAN   The patient is free from injury related to electrical hazards

KEY ASSESSMENT POINTS

Skin condition:
   At dispersive pad site
   Under ECG electrodes
   At pressure points
   At temperature probe site
Neuromuscular status
Central nervous system status

NURSING DIAGNOSIS

High risk for injury related to use of electrical equipment

PATIENT OUTCOMES

The patient will be free of any injury related to the use of electrical equipment.
The patient will be free of injury as evidenced by:
   1. Absence of apparent skin lesions
   2. Maintained skin integrity under dispersive pad, ECG electrodes, temperature probe entry sites, and positional pressure points
   3. Absence of neuromuscular damage
   4. Absence of central nervous system complications
   5. No signs or symptoms of shock

NURSING ACTIONS

	Yes	No	N/A
1. Electrical safety policies adhered to?	☐	☐	☐
2. Operational directions reviewed?	☐	☐	☐
3. Identification number on unit?	☐	☐	☐
4. Equipment checked for damage?	☐	☐	☐
5. Unit's safety features checked?	☐	☐	☐
6. Gel on pregelled dispersive pad checked?	☐	☐	☐
7. Dispersive pad placed correctly?	☐	☐	☐
8. Pacemaker/internal defibrillator present?	☐	☐	☐
9. Check for alternate ground points performed?	☐	☐	☐
10. Contact of pad checked?	☐	☐	☐
11. Active electrode protected during surgery?	☐	☐	☐
12. Power settings confirmed orally with operator?	☐	☐	☐
13. Position and contact of pad checked when patient moved/repositioned?	☐	☐	☐
14. Generator ID#, settings, pad and ECG electrode placements, patient's skin condition before and after use, and other electrical equipment documented?	☐	☐	☐
15. Special precautions with argon beam coagulator?	☐	☐	☐
16. Laser safety precautions?	☐	☐	☐
17. Hypo/hyperthermia blanket covered with sheet or other material?	☐	☐	☐
18. With surface hypothermia, respiratory status, cardiac status, and signs of frostbite assessed?	☐	☐	☐

Document additional nursing actions/care plan revisions here:

_____

_____

_____

EVALUATION OF PATIENT OUTCOMES

	Outcome met	Outcome met with additional outcome criteria	Outcome met with revised nursing care plan	Outcome not met	Outcome not applicable to this patient
1. There were no apparent skin lesions that did not exist preoperatively.	☐	☐	☐	☐	☐
2. Skin integrity under dispersive pad, ECG electrodes, temperature probe entry site, and positional pressure points was maintained.	☐	☐	☐	☐	☐
3. There was no evidence of neuromuscular damage.	☐	☐	☐	☐	☐
4. There was no evidence of central nervous system complications.	☐	☐	☐	☐	☐
5. There were no signs or symptoms of shock from electrical sources.	☐	☐	☐	☐	☐

Signature: _____ Date: _____

FIG. 7-10   (Continued)
GENERIC CARE PLAN   The patient is free from injury related to electrical hazards

GUIDE TO NURSING ACTIONS TO PROTECT THE PATIENT FROM INJURY RELATED TO ELECTRICAL HAZARDS

1. Adhere to electrical safety policies and institutional protocols.
2. **Before** the use of any electrical equipment, complete the following activities:
   - Review the operational directions on or attached to the unit
   - Verify that the unit has an identification number
3. With electrosurgical units (ESU), BEFORE USE:
   - Check plug, cord, connections, footswitch, dispersive pad, and active electrode (pencil) for damage. Remove for repair if damaged, following institutional protocol for reporting damaged equipment.
   - Test the unit's safety features (alarm, lights, activation signals) before applying dispersive pad if unit has return cable sentry. Otherwise, test before use.
   - Plan dispersive pad placement after patient is positioned and before draping.
   - If using pregelled pad, check for dry spots. Discard if present.
   - Place dispersive pad on clean, dry convex area of skin over a large muscle mass, as close to the operative site as possible. AVOID bony prominences, scar tissue, excessive adipose tissue, areas with poor circulation, hairy surfaces, areas where fluids may pool, circumferential placements that restrict blood flow.
   - If the patient has a pacemaker or internal defibrillator, place ESU dispersive pad away from generator site. Continuous ECG monitoring should be employed when ESU is used. Check with manufacturer regarding function of pacemaker/internal defibrillator during ESU use. A device programmer may be required. A defibrillator should be in the room.
   - If two ESUs are used, they must be of the same technology (grounding system/isolation system). Each dispersive pad should be close to its respective operative site; the pads should not touch each other.
   - Do not use in the presence of flammable agents (alcohol, tincture-based agents).
   - Check that ECG electrodes are placed away from operative site, and NOT between the operative site and the dispersive pad.
   - Inspect the operative field for additional alternate ground points (i.e., no patient contact with grounded metal parts).
   - Be sure dispersive pad maintains uniform body contact before draping. Check that there is no tenting, gapping, or pooling of liquids.
   - Modify equipment check (i.e., no dispersive pad) for bipolar electrosurgical unit.
4. With ESUs, DURING the procedure:
   - Keep the unit clean and protected from spills.
   - Place active electrode in clean, dry, nonconductive, highly visible area to minimize unintentional activation and untoward results.
   - Do not coil the active electrode cable or allow contact with metal instruments.
   - Keep active electrode free of tissue build-up.
   - Keep power setting as low as possible. Confirm settings orally with operator.
   - If higher settings requested, check dispersive pad contact, cable connections, tissue build-up on active electrode.
   - Anytime the patient is moved or re-positioned, check position and contact of dispersive pad.
   Follow institutional protocol for documenting generator identification number, settings used, dispersive pad and ECG electrode placements, patient skin condition prior to and after procedure, and other electrical equipment used.
   - If an adverse skin reaction or injury occurs, comply with SMDA reporting requirements.
5. The argon beam coagulator: safety issues are similar to monopolar ESU use with dispersive pad placement. Check gas cylinders to be sure they are full. If a foot switch is used, place it for the user. Be familiar with type of unit being used (automatic flow system, control options, line obstruction alarm, pad-sensing system). Also be familiar with recommendations to prevent gas embolism (low-level gas flow settings, air purge from gas line prior to first use).
6. Implement laser safety precautions (eye protection, fire safety, controlled room access, smoke evacuation)
7. With hypo/hyperthermia units
   - Place unit at least 3 feet from anesthesia machine.
   - Avoid direct skin contact by covering the thermia blanket with sheets.
   - Avoid folds or creases in blanket or covering material.
   - Inspect skin integrity before and after unit use.
   - Maintain the correct temperature when the unit is being used.
   - With induced hypothermia, observe the patient closely for respiratory depression, impending cardiac arrest, frostbite. Apply lotion to protect the skin as necessary. Use blankets to slowly rewarm the patient.
8. With nerve stimulators, follow instructions for use and care recommended by the manufacturer.
9. Document other nursing actions relevant to prevention of injury from electrical hazards.

Box 7-1 Laboratory Values Indicating Fluid Volume Changes

Laboratory values must be interpreted in view of the perioperative nurse's total knowledge about the patient's status.

Values that may indicate a nursing diagnosis requiring further action for one patient may be a therapeutic result or normal consequence of surgical stress response in another.

Fluid volume deficit	**Fluid volume overload**
↑ Hematocrit	↓ Hematocrit
↑ Urine specific gravity	↓ Urine specific gravity
↑ Urinary glucose	↓ BUN
↑ Blood urea nitrogen (BUN)	↓ Urine osmolality
↑ Urine osmolality	↓ Serum sodium
↑ Blood sugar	↑ Serum aldosterone
↑ Serum amylase	↑ Urine aldosterone
↑ Prothrombin time	
↑ Partial thromboplastin time	
↑ Platelet count (thrombocytosis)	
↓ Platelet count (thrombocytopenia)	
↓ Fibrinogen level	
↓ Serum aldosterone	

---

thrombin formation. Any disease process that decreases or causes an absence of clotting factor, such as hemophilia or von Willebrand's disease, or any history of disseminated intravascular coagulation should alert the perioperative nurse to potential intraoperative clotting problems.

Recognition of types of surgical intervention in which topical agents may be used is also part of planning patient care. Surgery of the gallbladder, liver, pancreas, spleen, and perianal area may involve diffuse, continuous oozing from capillary beds or tissue that is friable and delicate. Deep, extensive surgical interventions, in which visualization is difficult or which involve large denuded areas, and surgeries with vascular anastomoses may also require plans for adjunctive chemical hemostasis.

A number of topical hemostatic agents may be available in the operating room. Epinephrine solution, thrombin in powder or solution, gelatin sponges or film, oxidized cellulose, or collagen hemostatic agents may be selected to control local bleeding. The perioperative nurse needs to plan appropriate nursing actions depending on the type of hemostatic adjunct. Nursing knowledge is necessary in proper reconstitution of thrombin, in providing enough sponges to keep the site dry for application of powders, in cutting sponges to their desired size, and in recognizing special precautions that must be taken with some of the microfibrillar collagen hemostatic agents.

Fluid volume deficits. When a patient experiences or is at risk of vascular, cellular, or intracellular dehydration, there is the potential for a fluid volume deficit (Carpenito, 1993). Water composes 50% of the weight of an average adult female and 60% of the weight of the average adult male. Fifty-five percent of total body water is extracellular fluid, found in plasma, interstitial spaces, bone and dense connective tissue, and body secretions. The other 45% is intracellular. Water diffuses freely across membranes, and a number of physiologic mechanisms are active in influencing fluid movement.

In healthy people, fluid balance is well controlled by the kidneys, lungs, brain, and hormones. Anesthesia alters these normal physiologic mechanisms. For the surgical patient, the goal is to maintain homeostasis or replace lost fluid. Sometimes, this simply means providing intravenous fluids to replace normal losses through secretion and excretion. Other times, it requires rapid assessment and correlation between blood loss, disturbances in acid base balance, and electrolyte balance.

The perioperative nurse acts with the rest of the surgical team to provide and administer fluids to correct intraoperative losses. Selection of type of fluid replacement is not an independent nursing diagnosis. Maintenance of fluid and electrolyte balance is a collaborative effort that requires collaborative nursing diagnoses. However, only through patient assessment and familiarity with the patient's condition can the perioperative nurse act as a collaborator.

It is important to assess whether the patient had any previous fluid volume deficits caused by dehydration, excessive urinary output, infection, abnormal drainage, excessive use of laxatives, dietary problems, shock, or hemorrhage; hypotension can develop quickly with the induction of anesthesia if a preoperative extracellular fluid volume deficit has not adequately been corrected. It is also important to note if the patient had a preexisting fluid volume excess caused by heart or liver disease, renal failure, hormonal disturbances, or iatrogenic causes. A potential complication of fluid therapy is fluid overload, and baseline information regarding the patient's condition is critical in selecting and administering intraoperative fluids. Unusual losses resulting from fever, sweating, vomiting, or third-space fluid sequestration, as in bowel obstruction, ascites, pleural effusion, or pulmonary edema, should also be noted.

Fluid replacement therapy. The best replacement therapy is chosen from a variety of intravenous fluids. Normal saline solution is often used to replace deficits in extracellular fluid. However, since saline solution contains sodium, it must be used cautiously in the patient who has an elevated serum sodium level or pulmonary edema. One-half or one-quarter normal saline is often selected for the osmolar effect it achieves without providing extra sodium. A 5% solution of dextrose and water has an osmolarity slightly less than plasma and is often used for fluid replacement. The balanced electrolyte solutions mimic the content of body fluid in their sodium, potassium, and calcium electrolyte content. Ringer's lactate solution is frequently used in the operating room to correct third-space fluid losses (shifting of intravascular fluid into the surgical site after extensive tissue dissection; fluid can also sequester into the lumen and wall of the small bowel and accumulate in the peritoneal cavity).

Plasma expanders are used when more than maintenance volume expansion is required. Dextran has a number of potential side effects, including rash, urticaria, allergy, nausea and vomiting, and dyspnea. If a patient needs a type and cross-match for blood replacement, it should be obtained before the administration of dextran. The bottle should be checked for crystals; if they are present, the solution will need to be warmed. Dextran is contraindicated in patients with renal failure; severe bleeding, because it interferes with platelets; severe congestive heart failure; and hypervolemia. The patient's prothrombin time, partial prothromboplastin time, and factor VIII level should be monitored during administration of dextran.

Because dextran has so many side effects, albumin is increasingly being used. Albumin is obtained from whole blood, treated by sterilization, and stored. It is available in 5% and 25% solutions. It has rare side effects, although the patient with heart disease may need simultaneous diuretics with albumin administration. Albumin is primarily used in patients with shock and those with low protein or serum albumin levels. Plasma protein fraction is 83% albumin with some globulins and gamma globulins. It is administered slowly and is indicated in hypovolemic shock and hypoproteinemia (Dole, 1987). Hespan may be used in the early management of shock during surgery or in trauma when fluid replacement and plasma volume expansion are required. Circulatory overload can occur with this product and special care needs to be taken with patients who have impaired renal clearance, since this is the principal way Hespan is eliminated.

A number of blood components may be administered intraoperatively. RBCs usually come in units of approximately 250 ml. They are available as fresh, frozen and then thawed, with leukocytes removed, or saline washed. One unit of RBCs increases the hematocrit by approximately 3%. RBCs can be mixed with normal saline to increase their flow rate. They increase oxygen-carrying capability without the risk of hypervolemia. Platelet transfusions are usually limited to major surgery with excessive bleeding or life-threatening bleeding in idiopathic thrombocytopenia purpura (Practice parameter, 1994). WBCs may be used in the patient with bone marrow depression or sepsis with a low granulocyte count. WBCs carry the risk of allergic reaction. Plasma may be transfused either fresh or frozen and thawed in acute volume loss. Fresh frozen plasma (FFP) is plasma separated from the red cells and platelets of whole blood; it contains all of the blood coagulation factors. It is indicated with active bleeding and may be administered prior to an operative or invasive procedure. It is desirable to check ABO compatibility with the administration of platelets, white cells, and plasma.

Whole blood usually comes in units of approximately 500 ml. In most institutions, at least two people must check the patient's nameband against the unit of blood to be administered. The label of whole blood should be carefully checked to ensure that the following agree with the recipient label: product name, patient's name, donor unit number, RH and ABO blood grouping, and expiration date. Visual inspection should ascertain whether the red cell mass looks purple; if a zone of hemolysis is observed above the cell mass; if there are visible clots; murky, red, brown, or purple plasma; and whether there is blood or plasma at sealing joints in tubing or ports. If so, the product should be returned to the lab (Gonterman, Kiracofe, & Owens, 1994). The phenotype of blood depends on the presence of antigens. Type O is universal donor (no antigens) and Type AB is universal recipient (no antibodies but both A and B antigen). Whole blood is indicated for the patient who has lost 50% of volume through a slow bleed,

20% through an acute bleed, or 80% or more. It is not used as commonly today; the crystalloids, balanced solutions, nonprotein plasma volume expanders, and RBCs are more often indicated for losses of less than 50% (Matthewson, 1987).

Monitoring for possible complications of fluid replacement therapy. Surgical patients commonly have intravenous lines in place for maintenance or replacement therapy. However, there are potential problems and consequent precautions that should be taken with intravenous setups. Proper preparation of insertion site, aseptic technique in handling and adding solution, and protection of the lines during transfer and positioning require perioperative nursing care. The nurse needs to know drug incompatibilities when preparing and administering solutions in the OR. Monitoring is necessary to prevent thrombophlebitis, infection, air embolism, and fluid overload. This is especially important for patients with renal or cardiac disease, who may be unable to physiologically tolerate a fluid challenge.

Monitoring becomes even more intensive with the patient who is receiving blood or blood products. Approximately 1% to 3% of patients who are transfused with blood or blood products may experience a hypersensitivity transfusion reaction to the antibodies in the blood (Matthewson, 1987). These reactions range from mild manifestations of hives and itching to severe manifestations of wheezing, bronchospasm, and anaphylaxis. In any patient who manifests a reaction, the blood should be stopped, the reaction treated, and institutional protocols implemented for transfusion reactions. Usually, the unfinished unit of blood is sent back to the laboratory with a specimen of the patient's blood to determine what caused the reaction.

Hemolytic transfusion reactions are caused by ABO incompatibilities, which result in microclots from the hemolysis of red cells. The patient may exhibit fever, chills, hemoglobinuria and hemaglobinemia, hypotension, flushing, and ventricular tachycardia. After the transfusion is stopped, blood and urine specimens should be collected and sent to the laboratory. Urinary output should be carefully monitored, and diuretics may be prescribed to maintain flow through the kidneys.

Febrile transfusion reactions are caused by sensitization to the WBCs, platelets, or antigens in the blood. These reactions are more common in the patient with multiple transfusions. The patient's temperature may increase to 103° to 104° F with headache, chills, back pain, and tachycardia. After discontinuation of the transfusing fluid, steroid therapy may be prescribed. Circulatory overload becomes a potential problem in the elderly, in patients with renal or cardiovascular disease, and when too much

fluid is given too fast. Overload may be seen more often with plasma expanders and whole blood. Circulatory overload is usually indicated by an elevated central venous pressure, distended neck veins, and dyspnea.

True anaphylaxis is a surgical emergency. It is often precipitated by plasma protein incompatibility. The patient develops a cough, respiratory distress, hypotension, tachycardia, and nausea and vomiting. The perioperative nurse must be familiar and immediately ready with resuscitation equipment.

Generic care plan. The generic care plan and associated Guide to Nursing Actions for maintaining fluid and electrolyte balance (Fig. 7-11) assumes that the perioperative nurse knows why the patient is receiving fluid therapy; what the patient's and/or family's beliefs are about blood or blood product replacement; and what the patient's baseline vital signs, laboratory values, weight, and heart and kidney functions are. The importance of the nurse's knowledge, and thus his or her importance as a collaborator in the management of fluid and electrolyte balance, cannot be overstated.

Outcome Standard: The Patient Participates in Rehabilitation

Outcome Standard VI states that "the patient participates in the rehabilitation process" (AORN, 1996). The accompanying interpretive statement clarifies the intent of the standard in terms of patient participation in self-care, decision making, and discharge planning, as well as the patient's right to expect a reasonable continuity of care. Depending on the individual patient's status, outcome measurement includes the patient's ability to describe his or her responsibilities toward achieving optimal benefits from surgery, identifying problem areas related to surgery, and performing activities related to self-care. For the patient to achieve these goals, there is a need for alliance and interdependence with the nurse and health care team. In perioperative ambulatory surgery settings, this nursing role is crucial and primary to safe patient care. In acute care settings, the perioperative nurse becomes a part of the alliance formed to assist the patient in participating in the rehabilitation process. The perioperative nursing role in ambulatory surgery is described in Chapter 19. This section reviews general considerations for planning care that allow the patient to participate in the rehabilitation process.

Patient should be able to participate in own care. Earlier in this chapter, Orem's Self-Care Deficit Theory was introduced as a theoretic basis for the wholly compensatory nursing care delivered during surgery. Many of the nursing actions undertaken to prevent injury are therapeutic in nature; that is, they

FIG. 7-11
GENERIC CARE PLAN   The patient's fluid and electrolyte balance is maintained

KEY ASSESSMENT POINTS

Vital signs/pulse oximetry
Hemodynamic status (central venous pressure [CVP], mean arterial
    pressure [MAP], pulmonary artery pressure [PAP], pulmonary cap-
    illary wedge pressure [PCWP], if available)
Skin turgor
Fluid balance
Venous filling
Mucous membranes
Mental status
Laboratory results

NURSING DIAGNOSIS

High risk for alteration in fluid and electrolyte balance:
    Fluid volume deficit or fluid volume excess

PATIENT OUTCOMES

The patient will be free of fluid and electrolyte imbalances.
1. The patient's mental orientation will be consistent with preoperative levels
2. Fluid and electrolyte values will be consistent with preoperative
   status.
   • Serum electrolytes WNL
   • Arterial blood gases WNL
   • Absence of signs of imbalances
   • CVP WNL
   • Urinary output 30 ml per hour
3. Vital signs and SaO_2 (pulse oximeter reading) will be consistent
   with preoperative measurement

NURSING ACTIONS

	Yes	No	N/A
1. Patency of IV lines and drainage tubes maintained?	☐	☐	☐
2. Fluid replacement therapy instituted?	☐	☐	☐
3. Blood or blood products administered?	☐	☐	☐
4. Blood warmed?	☐	☐	☐
5. Patient observed for transfusion reaction?	☐	☐	☐
6. Autotransfusion system used?	☐	☐	☐
7. Blood loss estimated?	☐	☐	☐
8. Fluid output monitored?	☐	☐	☐
9. Physiologic parameters indicative of fluid/electrolyte balance monitored?	☐	☐	☐
10. Medications given?	☐	☐	☐

Document additional nursing actions/care plan revisions here:

_____

_____

_____

EVALUATION OF PATIENT OUTCOMES

	Outcome met	Outcome met with additional outcome criteria	Outcome met with revised nursing care plan	Outcome not met	Outcome not applicable to this patient
1. The patient's mental status was consistent with preoperative status.	☐	☐	☐	☐	☐
2. Fluid and electrolyte balance was consistent with the patient's preoperative levels.	☐	☐	☐	☐	☐
3. Vital signs were consistent with preoperative measurements.	☐	☐	☐	☐	☐

Signature: _____ Date: _____

FIG. 7-11   (Continued)

GENERIC CARE PLAN   The patient's fluid and electrolyte balance is maintained

GUIDE TO NURSING ACTIONS TO MAINTAIN THE PATIENT'S FLUID AND ELECTROLYTE BALANCE

1. Protect, maintain, and monitor all intravenous lines, insertion sites, and drainage tubes/sites.
2. Obtain, administer, and regulate all fluid replacement therapy as ordered. Document these.
3. Review patient record for blood order; check availability of blood or blood products. Ensure protocol for proper blood storage.
4. Follow institutional protocol for checking and administering blood or blood products. Document.
5. Request additional blood using appropriate protocols for same.
6. Assist with blood warming procedures.
7. Observe the patient for any indications of transfusion reaction and follow institutional protocol for same. Document.
8. Follow procedure for autotransfusion system in use.
9. Estimate and report/record blood loss according to institutional protocol; note sudden or excessive bleeding.
10. Monitor other fluid output as accurately as possible (urinary, drainage tubes). Document insertion of indwelling urinary catheter.
11. Monitor physiologic parameters indicative of fluid/electrolyte imbalance, as applicable, and report/document.
12. Assess the physical condition of the patient and laboratory values for the following imbalances:
    a. **Overhydration** (water excess, sodium deficit)
       Assess for: weakness, polyuria, twitching, hyperirritability, disorientation, nausea, vomiting, elevated CVP, dyspnea, rales, serum Na^+ less than 20 mEq/L, serum HCT less than 40.
    b. **Dehydration** (water and sodium deficit)
       Assess for: weakness, dry skin, poor skin turgor, vomiting, oliguria, decreased capillary refill, increased specific gravity, drop in systolic blood pressure (BP), elevated HCT, normal or elevated serum Na^+, shock.
    c. **Metabolic Acidosis**
       Assess for: apathy; disorientation; rapid, shallow respirations; increase in serum potassium and chloride; Pco_2 less than 35 to 40, pH less than 7.35, and Hco_3 less than 25, acid urine.
    d. **Metabolic Alkalosis**
       Assess for: increased irritability, disorientation, tingling of fingers, tremors, hypoventilation, irregular pulse, pH greater than 7.45 and Hco_3 greater than 29 in arterial blood gases. Serum chloride, potassium, and calcium may also be decreased.
    e. **Respiratory Acidosis** (CO_2 retention)
       Assess for: tachycardia, dysrhythmias, diaphoresis, restlessness, dyspnea, increased respiratory effort, decreased respiratory rate, pH less than 7.4 with Pco_2 greater than 40 and Hco_3 25 to 35 in arterial blood gases.
    f. **Hypokalemia** (potassium deficit)
       Assess for: weakness, confusion, shallow respirations, hypotension, arrhythmias, serum K^+ less than 3.5 mEq/L, flat or inverted T wave on ECG.
    g. **Hyperkalemia** (potassium excess)
       Assess for: intestinal colic, oliguria, bradycardia, serum K^+ greater than 5 mEq/L, flattened P wave, widened QRS complex, and peaked T wave on ECG.
13. Obtain, prepare, administer corrective medications as ordered. Note drug, dosage, route of administration, and time given.
14. Document additional nursing actions related to maintaining the patient's fluid and electrolyte balance.

are devised to provide and maintain patient care needs to sustain life and health. When the patient no longer needs wholly compensatory nursing, partly compensatory or educative-supportive nursing systems are implemented. Orem (1985) defines self-care as an adult's continuous contribution to his or her own continued existence, health, and well-being. The person's ability to engage in self-care is his or her "self-care agency." The goals to be reached through self-care are the person's "self-care requisites." Self-care actions that will need to be carried out for some time for the person to attain those self-care requisites are "therapeutic self-care demands." When the person is unable to attain therapeutic self-care demands, a "self-care deficit" exists. Nursing plays an important role in helping patients overcome self-care deficits and become able to engage in self-care.

One of the ways in which nurses help patients overcome self-care deficits is through education and support. Risks for self-care deficits need to be identified, the patient's abilities assessed, and appropriate educational interventions designed. Teaching methods should be relevant to the patient's ability to comprehend the information. The knowledge exchanged during the education processes is shared between the nurse and patient. Support may be offered in any number of ways, ranging from positive reinforcement, verbal reassurance, nonverbal communication, agency referrals, and involvement of the family and significant others in the rehabilitation processes.

In a phenomenologic study on healing from surgery, Criddle (1993) identified active participation as one of the integral themes to the healing process. Patients indicated a strong need to regain the control over their lives that surgery disrupted. They believed they had a personal responsibility in their recovery from surgery and wanted to know and understand what to expect, and then begin doing whatever they were supposed to do as active participants. Accurate information was very important to these patients, and they attempted to use that information in developing a positive attitude about their healing. Those patients who had been given no substantive information or little information felt less able to participate in their own recovery and rehabilitation. The need for information was also underscored in the work of Schumacher and Meleis (1994) on conditions that may influence the quality of a transition experience, such as the transition from hospital back to home. They stress that the need for new information and the skill required by the patient influences their successful outcome (participation in rehabilitation) and must be sufficient to meet the demands of the transition.

In discussing nursing practice issues that surfaced during an early research project to define perioperative nursing criteria, one of the monitoring criteria was the question, "Is there a statement written by OR nurses preoperatively about information provided to family members?" (Reeder and Puterbaugh, 1982) Although Outcome Standard VI relates to information that needs to be shared to facilitate participation in rehabilitation, some of that information is shared with the patient preoperatively. A number of research studies on the beneficial effects of psychoeducational interventions with surgical patients have explored the timing of giving such information. The research question is, "Is it most advantageous to present information about surgery and the postoperative course while the patient is at home, in the physician's office when the surgery is scheduled, during preoperative testing, on the afternoon before surgery, or on the evening of surgery?" Research including timing as a variable has not provided clear-cut answers. Although there is some disagreement about the timing of information, research supports the validity of the effects of preoperative information and communication in influencing both emotional responses to and recovery from surgery; positive effects on recovery, pain control, psychologic well-being, satisfaction with care, and lower costs have been documented across a wide range of patient populations, types of care provider, and care setting (Redman, 1993). Some research has included the benefits of involving the family in the educational interventions.

Involving the family. Silva's study (1979) explored the effects of giving information to spouses on the spouses' anxiety and attitude toward hospitalization and surgery. The study assumed that behaviors and attitudes of patients and families are interrelated. The experimental research design controlled for internal and external threats to validity. Of the 48 spouses in the study, the ones receiving information had significantly more positive attitudes toward hospitalization and surgery and reported fewer anxieties than the spouses who did not receive information.

In Abrams' study (1982), the resistance behaviors of children in day surgery were related to preoperative educational strategies. The children in the study were either exposed to a slide-tape program that included sensory and mastery information, procedural information, or no specific educational intervention. The children in the group receiving both sensory and mastery information had fewer major resistant behaviors than either of the other two groups. In addition, the parents of these children had fewer complaints about the services in the health care institution.

In Wong and Wong's study (1984) on preoperative patient education, patients who were to undergo total hip arthroplasty were sent a learning activity packet 4 weeks before admission. The packet had five subpackets, describing the surgery, what happens in the hospital, what the patient had to learn before the operation, what would happen in the first 4 hours postoperatively, and what the patient needed to learn before going home. On the day of surgery, patients viewed a slide-tape program on prescribed postoperative activities. Thirty-one patients participated in this descriptive, exploratory study. Postoperatively, they had an 81% to 100% compliance rate with postoperative activities such as coughing, deep breathing, foot dorsiflexion and plantar flexion, and quadriceps and gluteal setting. Ninety-seven percent were free of postoperative complications such as atelectasis, pneumonia, thrombosis, or hip dislocation. They were highly satisfied with the preoperative teaching program. One of the important side benefits of receiving the information at home, as reported by the patients who participated in the study, was the ability to involve their family in preparation for and understanding of the surgery and perioperative experience. The theory of family nursing supports this side benefit. In such a perspective, the family is viewed as having the ability to problem solve together. The perioperative nurse should search for family strengths and resources that will facilitate the family's creative capacity to solve the problems that surgery of a family member poses (Vosburgh & Simpson, 1993).

Hilbert (1989) developed a tool to measure social support in chronic illness. The need for such a measurement grew out of her belief that, with the increasing numbers of chronically ill patients, there was a need to involve the family, significant others, or both in their care. Study respondents selected the one person who was most helpful to them on a day-by-day basis and rated their satisfaction with that person's behaviors. The significant person was rated on scales that yielded information about specific guidance, general guidance and feedback, positive social interaction, material aid, and intimate interaction. The results indicated that support was a unidimensional concept and that intimate interaction and specific guidance were the most important subscales. Because specific guidance was so important to patients, Hilbert concluded that supportive family, significant others, or both should be included in patient teaching programs. In that way, they would be better able to help patients comply with the health care team's recommendations. Hagerty and her colleagues (1993) have added to this perspective with their development of a theory on human relatedness. These theoreticians suggest that discomfort and a lack of a sense of well-being may result when the patient experiences low levels of a sense of belonging, reciprocity, and mutuality. Social support for the patient recovering from surgery may mediate a response to illness and stress that leaves the patient feeling disconnected from normal relationships with significant others.

Borghi (1989) assessed the relationship of surgical progress reports on family members' anxiety. Anxiety was measured both by heart rate and by a valid and reliable self-evaluation anxiety questionnaire. Measurements were obtained from two groups, one that received an intraoperative progress report and one that did not. Each group completed the questionnaire during and at the end of the intraoperative period. Heart rate was not significantly different for either group. However, the group that received the intraoperative progress report had significantly decreased anxiety as measured by the questionnaire. The researcher concluded that surgical progress reports or supportive communication and information provided to surgical patients' families can help to allay anxiety during a normally stressful period.

These few studies have not been reviewed in depth in this chapter, nor has an extensive review of the literature been undertaken. The important point is that perioperative nurses need to be aware of the family's needs and the family's potential contribution in helping the patient participate in the rehabilitation process. Part of patient assessment should include documentation of family support. The family should be included in orientation to the surgical experience, and nursing care should be given to both the patient and family (Reeder and Puterbaugh, 1982). Families are often in as much need of support as the patient. When support is given to the family, their ability to support the patient can be increased.

Patient participates in decision making and discharge planning. Both the American Hospital Association (AHA) and the National League for Nursing (NLN) have issued statements on patients' rights. The AHA Patient's Bill of Rights (1992) states that "the patient has the right to expect reasonable continuity of care when appropriate and to be informed by physicians and other caregivers of available and realistic patient care options when hospital care is no longer appropriate." The NLN (1977) addressed the right of the patient to expect coordination of health care and to receive appropriate instruction or education from health care personnel so that he or she can achieve an optimal level of wellness and an understanding of his or her basic health care needs. At the same time, the patient has the right to refuse treatment without fear of being discriminated against or punished. Nonetheless, to participate in decision making and come to self-determination regarding any treatment option, the patient and family need information presented in terms they can readily understand and on which they can base a decision.

Discharge planning is a critical process in which patients are provided with a link to services in the community that their health care needs might require. This requires that the nurse know about the quality and quantity of available community agencies, and that this knowledge is shared with patients and their families. Discharge planning also involves discharge instructions. Instructions may include information about medications, activity limitations, dietary restrictions or supplements, wound care, exercise regimens, specific treatments, follow-up physician appointments, and other information that relates to the specific patient, the nursing diagnoses involved in the patient's ability to participate in rehabilitation, and the surgical intervention. Earlier in this chapter, the nurse's role in assessing patient indications for and responses to antibiotic therapy was described. Part of the nursing responsibility with the patient receiving antibiotic therapy is to share knowledge with the patient regarding why the therapy has been prescribed, how the medication is to be taken, how long the medication should be taken, side effects that may occur, side effects to be reported immediately to the physician, symptoms indicating that the antibiotic therapy is not effective, and any dietary or fluid restrictions that accompany the prescribed therapy. Tuazon (1993) described a model for discharge planning with the acronym SMART: *s*pecific treatment instructions (dressing changes, etc.), *m*edications, *a*ctivity (allowed and to be avoided), *r*eferrals, *t*herapeutic diet instructions.

It is apparent that the activity of discharge planning and instruction is an important nursing action. Written discharge instructions assist both the nurse and the patient by presenting information clearly and thoroughly. In some settings, the perioperative nurse may assume full responsibility for such planning and teaching. In others, the perioperative nurse is a collaborator, communicating and documenting pertinent information that guides nursing colleagues who do the final planning and teaching for discharge.

Patient can expect a reasonable continuity of care. The goal of discharge planning is continuity of care; the patient's anticipated care needs must be identified and provisions for meeting those needs coordinated with the patient, family, significant others, and community resources and services. Caring is the central and unifying domain for the body of knowledge and practices in nursing. Nurses use the terms "care," "caring," and "nursing care" interchangeably. Leininger (1981) defines professional nursing care as follows:

> Those cognitively learned humanistic and scientific modes of helping or enabling an individual, family, or community to receive personalized services through specific culturally defined or ascribed modes of caring processes, techniques, and patterns to improve or maintain a favorably healthy life or death.

Thus continuity of care has biophysical, psychologic, cultural, social, and environmental dimensions. The perioperative nurse interacts in these caring dimensions across practice settings, giving both technologic and interpersonal care. Knowing the quality of the patient's support systems and the patient's ability to engage in acts of self-care and recognizing the need to involve community resources are only part of the provision of perioperative nursing care and continuity of care for the surgical patient.

Generic care plan. The generic care plan and associated Guide to Nursing Actions (Fig. 7-12) for helping the patient meet the outcome of participating in the rehabilitation process has as the nursing diagnosis *Risk for altered participation (ineffective) in the rehabilitation process.* This is not a nursing diagnosis approved by NANDA. The following list suggests related or secondary NANDA-approved nursing diagnoses that may contribute to a patient's ineffective participation in the rehabilitation process. These nursing diagnoses may exist in perioperative patients and should be considered when an individualized plan of care is developed to help the patient participate in rehabilitation.

Activity intolerance
Activity intolerance, risk for
Anxiety
Coping, ineffective family: compromised
Coping, ineffective individual
Decisional conflict (specify)
Denial, ineffective
Diversional activity deficit
Family processes, altered
Fatigue
Health maintenance, altered
Home maintenance management, impaired
Pain
Parental role conflict
Parenting, altered, risk for
Self-care deficit (specify)
Self-esteem, chronic low
Self-esteem disturbance
Self-esteem, situational low

Perioperative nurses, using their assessment data base, organize, synthesize, analyze, and summarize

FIG. 7-12
GENERIC CARE PLAN   The patient participates in rehabilitation

KEY ASSESSMENT POINTS

Age
Functional abilities
Learning needs
Health beliefs (helping or hindering)
Ability to learn
Home environment
Support systems

NURSING DIAGNOSIS

High risk for altered participation (ineffective) in rehabilitation*

PATIENT OUTCOMES

The patient will participate in rehabilitation.
The patient/family/significant other will:
1. Participate in planning for discharge
2. Correctly state discharge plans and instructions
3. Be aware of appropriate referral sources
4. Be able to identify potential problems related to the surgical intervention
5. Be able to perform activities related to postoperative care

NURSING ACTIONS	Yes	No	N/A
1. Discharge plans/instructions reviewed?	☐	☐	☐
2. Reportable signs and symptoms reviewed?	☐	☐	☐
3. Follow-up appointment with physician made?	☐	☐	☐
4. Postoperative medications reviewed?	☐	☐	☐
5. Ability to perform required postoperative care demonstrated?	☐	☐	☐
6. Appropriate referrals made?	☐	☐	☐

Document additional nursing actions/care plan revisions here:

_____

_____

_____

EVALUATION OF PATIENT OUTCOMES

	Outcome met	Outcome met with additional outcome criteria	Outcome met with revised nursing care plan	Outcome not met	Outcome not applicable to this patient
1. The patient/family/significant other correctly stated discharge plans and instructions.	☐	☐	☐	☐	☐
2. The patient/family/significant other were aware of appropriate referral sources.	☐	☐	☐	☐	☐
3. The patient/family/significant other identified potential problems related to the surgical intervention.	☐	☐	☐	☐	☐
4. The patient/family/significant other were able to perform activities related to postoperative care.	☐	☐	☐	☐	☐

*This is not a NANDA-approved nursing diagnosis.

Signature: _____   Date: _____

GUIDE TO NURSING ACTIONS ASSISTING THE PATIENT AND FAMILY/ SIGNIFICANT OTHER TO PARTICIPATE IN THE REHABILITATION PROCESS

1. Review with patient and family/significant other discharge plans and instructions. Note plans/instructions reviewed.
2. Verify that the patient and family/significant other know what signs and symptoms should be reported to the physician.
3. Check that the patient has a follow-up appointment with physician or knows correct procedure for making appointment.
4. Verify that the patient knows the name, purpose, dosage and times, and potential side effects of postoperative medications. List the patient's postoperative medications.
5. Verify that the patient and family/significant other are able to perform any required postoperative care.
6. Make appropriate nursing/community service referrals as required for this patient.
   Consider additional nursing diagnoses such as:
   • Altered health maintenance (inability to identify, manage, or seek help to maintain health): plan interventions and referrals to help the patient anticipate the realities of the home environment, identify and utilize strengths, recognize need for assistance

   • Noncompliance (inability to adhere to therapeutic recommendations): identify the factors contributing to noncompliant behavior (personal, interpersonal, or environmental); plan interventions and referrals that will assist in resolving conflicts between contributing factors and therapeutic recommendations, help the patient identify the benefits of recommendations
   • Impaired home maintenance management (patient is unable to independently maintain a safe, growth-producing environment): this nursing diagnosis requires the patient and family to discuss capacity for home maintenance and the involvement of the care team in determining if family is able to adapt their life-styles to include caregiving activities and for how long. The goal is to maintain the patient at home with maximal independence; available resources (or their lack) need to be part of a feasible and realistic plan for the patient's rehabilitation.
7. Document other nursing actions relevant to assisting the patient with participation in rehabilitation.

the data to arrive at pertinent nursing diagnoses and a subsequent plan of care. Communication with other members of the health care team regarding assessment data indicative of health needs that can best be met by other appropriate team members is part of perioperative nurses' responsibility. Accomplishment of all aspects of the perioperative planning process is most likely to be a group effort. The perioperative nurse, collaborating with the patient, family, other members of the health care team, and appropriate resource persons from community agencies, is part of the alliance formed to help the patient participate in rehabilitation.

References

Abbott NK, Biala G, & Pollock W. (1983). The impact of preoperative assessment on intraoperative nurse performance. *AORN Journal, 37*, 43-58.

Abrams L. (1982). Resistance behaviors and teaching media for children in day surgery. *AORN Journal, 35*, 244-258.

American Hospital Association. (1992). *A patient's bill of rights.* Chicago: The Association.

Association of Operating Room Nurses. (1996). *AORN standards and recommended practices for perioperative nursing.* Denver: The Association.

Benner P. (1984). *From novice to expert.* Menlo Park, CA: Addison-Wesley.

Berry RK. (1993). Effective patient education. *Nursing Spectrum, 2*(23), 14-15.

Borghi KM. (1989, February). *Surgical progress reports: The effect on family members' anxiety.* Paper presented at the Thirty-sixth Annual Congress of the Association of Operating Room Nurses, Anaheim, CA.

Carpenito LJ. (1993). *Nursing diagnosis: Application to clinical practice.* Philadelphia: JB Lippincott.

Colp R & Keller MW. (1927). *Textbook of surgical nursing* (p. 13). New York: Macmillan.

Criddle L. (1993). Healing from surgery: A phenomenological study. *Image—the Journal of Nursing Scholarship 25*(3), 208-213.

Curry JL. (1993). Hepatitis C. *Nursing Spectrum, 2*(1), 12-13.

Dellinger EP. (1993). Nosocomial infection. In *Care of the surgical patient.* New York: Scientific American Medicine.

Devine EC. (1992). Effects of psychoeducational care for adult surgical patients. *Patient Education and Counseling, 11*(2), 2-29.

Dixon E & Park R. (1990). Do patients understand written health information? *Nursing Outlook, 38*(6), 278-281.

Dobbing EA. (1993). Preventing transfer of bloodborne pathogens in the workplace. *Point of View, 30*(2), 8-12.

Dole LJ. (1987). IV and irrigating solution management. In *Drugs in perioperative nursing.* Aurora: Meyer Communication.

Flanagan E. (1994). Surveillance for surgical site infection. *Asepsis, 16*(1), 16-21.

Gardner P & Schaffer W. (1993). Immunization of adults. *New England Journal of Medicine, 328*(17), 1252-1258.

Gendron F. (1986). Unexplained skin injuries may be pressure sores. *OR Manager,* pp 2, 1, 6.

Gilliam DL & Nelson CL. (1990). Comparison of a one-step iodophor skin preparation versus traditional preparation in total joint surgery. *Clinical Orthopaedics and Related Research 250*, 258-260.

Gonterman R, Kiracofe S, & Owens P. (1994). Administering, documenting, and tracking blood products and volume expanders. *Medsurg Nursing, 3*(4), 269-276.

Gordon M. (1993). *Manual of nursing diagnoses.* St. Louis: Mosby–Year Book.

Hagerty BMK, et al. (1993). An emerging theory of human relatedness. *Image—the Journal of Nursing Scholarship, 25*(4), 291-296.

Harrington DP. (1994). Electrosurgery fact and fiction. *Biomedical Instrumentation & Technology, 28*(4), 331-333.

Harwell T. (1994). CDC revises the classification system for HIV to include CD4+ T-cell counts. *HIV Digest, 4*(1), 2-3.

Hilbert GA. (1989). *An instrument to measure social support in chronic illness.* Unpublished manuscript, Widener University at Chester, PA.

Holden-Lund C. (1989). Effects of relaxation with guided imagery on surgical stress and wound healing. *Research in Nursing and Health, 11*(4), 235-244.

Howard RJ. (1991). Comparison of a 10-minute aqueous iodophor and 2-minute water insoluble iodophor in alcohol preoperative skin preparation. *Complications in Surgery, 70*, 43-45.

Kemp M, et al. (1989, February). *Factors that contribute to pressure sore formation.* Paper presented at the Thirty-Sixth Annual Congress of the Association of Operating Room Nurses, Anaheim, CA.

Kulik JA, Moore PJ, & Mahler HIM. (1993). Stress and affiliation: Hospital roommate effects on preoperative anxiety and social interaction. *Health Psychology, 12*(2), 118-124.

Lee TB & Baker OG. (1994). Surveillance of surgical site infections. *Asepsis, 16*(1), 7-10.

Leininger M. (1981). The phenomenon of caring: Importance, research questions, and theoretical considerations. In *Caring—an essential human need: Proceedings of the three national caring conferences.* Thorofare, NJ: Charles B Slack.

Lipetz MJ, et al. (1990). What is wrong with patient education programs? *Nursing Outlook, 38*(4), 184-189.

Lynch P. (1992). Operative blood exposures among personnel: How frequent an event? *Infection Control Rounds, 15*(4), 1-3.

Lynch P. (1993). Surveillance for nosocomial infections and occupational blood exposures. *Infection Control Rounds, 16*(2), 1-3.

Matthewson M. (1987). Plasma expanders and blood products. In *Drugs in perioperative nursing.* Aurora, CO: Meyer Communication.

McFarland GK & McFarlane EA. (1993). *Nursing diagnosis and intervention: Planning for patient care.* St. Louis: Mosby–Year Book.

Meakins JL. (1993). Guidelines for prevention of surgical site infection. In *Care of the Surgical Patient.* New York: Scientific American Medicine.

Muma RD, et al. (1994). *HIV manual for health care professionals.* Norwalk, CT: Appleton & Lange.

Murphy EK. (1987). Operating room and perioperative nursing. In CE Northrop & ME Kelly (Eds.), *Legal issues in nursing.* St. Louis: Mosby–Year Book.

Murphy EK. (1990). Liability for noncompliance with hospital policies, national standards. *AORN Journal, 52*(5), 1060-1064.

Murray M & Blaylock B. (1994). Maintaining effective pressure ulcer prevention programs. *Medsurg Nursing, 3*(2), 85-92.

Naparstek B. (1993). *Health journeys for people undergoing surgery.* Los Angeles: Time Warner AudioBooks.

National League for Nursing. (1977). *Nursing's role in patient's rights.* New York: The League.

New technology lessens infection risks for OR patients, nurses & surgeons. (1994). *Nurse Extra, 2*(4), 6.

Nichols RL. (1987). Surgical infections and choice of antibiotics. In DC Sabiston (Ed.), *Essentials of surgery.* Philadelphia: WB Saunders.

Orem DE. (1985). *Nursing concepts of practice.* New York: McGraw-Hill.

Pagana KD & Pagana TJ. (1995). *Mosby's diagnostic and laboratory test reference.* (2nd ed.). St. Louis: Mosby–Year Book.

Palmer P. (1988). Nursing care plans: Are we protecting sacred cows or beating dead horses? *AORN Journal, 47,* 1357-1358.

Patient prepping agents: The fight against antibiotic-resistant microorganisms. (1994). *Infection Control Rounds, 17*(1), 1-4.

Phillips KA. (1994). The relationship of 1988 state HIV testing policies to previous and planned voluntary use of HIV testing. *Journal of Acquired Immune Deficiency Syndrome, 7*(4), 403-409.

Practice parameter for the use of fresh frozen plasma, cryoprecipitate, and platelets. (1994). *Journal of the American Medical Association, 271,* 777-781.

Pressure ulcers in adults. (1992). AHCPR Publication No. 92-0047. Rockville, MD: US Department of Health and Human Services.

Redman BK. (1993). *The process of patient education.* (7th ed.). St. Louis: Mosby–Year Book.

Reeder JM & Puterbaugh S. (1982). Issues in perioperative nursing practice. *AORN Journal, 36,* 827-840.

Rega MD. (1993). A model approach for patient education. *Medsurg Nursing, 2*(6), 477-479, 495.

Roach S. (1993). *The human act of caring.* Ottawa: Canadian Hospital Association Press.

Rothrock JC. (1993). *The RN first assistant: An expanded perioperative nursing role.* Philadelphia: JB Lippincott.

Ryan-Wenger NM. (1990). A nursing process methodology. *Nursing Outlook, 38*(4), 190.

Schumacher KL & Meleis AI. (1994). Transitions: A central concept in nursing. *Image—the Journal of Nursing Scholarship, 26*(2), 119-126.

Silva MC. (1979). Effects of orientation information on spouses' anxieties and attitudes toward hospitalization and surgery. *Research in Nursing and Health, 2,* 127-136.

Steelman VM. (1990). Intraoperative music therapy. *AORN Journal, 52*(5), 1026-1034.

Sussman GL, Tarlo S, & Dolovich O. (1991). The spectrum of IgE-mediated responses to latex. *Journal of the American Medical Association, 285,* 2844-2847.

Sylvester DC & Shipley SB. (1982). Development of process-oriented criteria to monitor perioperative nursing: Results of clinical testing. *AORN Journal, 36,* 802.

Tanner CA, et al. (1993). The phenomenology of knowing the patient. *Image—the Journal of Nursing Scholarship, 25*(4), 273-280.

Tuazon NC. (1993). Designing a SMART discharge plan. *Nursing Spectrum, 2*(8), 16.

Vidmar PM. (1994). How to enhance compliance. *Nursing Spectrum, 3*(4), 14-15.

Vosburgh D & Simpson P. (1993). Linking family theory and practice. *Image—the Journal of Nursing Scholarship, 25*(3), 231-235.

Weeks C. (1980). *Textbook of nursing.* New York: D Appleton.

Wong J & Wong S. (1984). Preoperative patient education. *CONA Journal, 6,* 7-11.

Yount ST, Edgell J, & Jakovec V. (1990). Preoperative teaching: A study of nurses' perceptions. *AORN Journal, 51*(2), 572-579.

Chapter 8

General Surgery

Katie Steuer

TREATMENT OF STRANGULATED HERNIA: CASE VI

The strangulation was formed by the ring, and it was with difficulty that a director could be introduced, which was held by an assistant, whilst the surgeon himself removed the intestine by the aid of two fingers placed behind the directors. . . . The surgeon drew out a large portion of intestine . . . compressed it gently with the palm of his hand . . . then reduced it without difficulty. For the dressing, he inserted into the inguinal ring the middle of a fine piece of linen, pierced with small holes and filled with coarse lint. A pledget of lint, three long compresses, and the double T bandage, composed the rest of the dressing.

BICHAT, 1814

The idea of the surgical repair of hernias, rather than the reduction of a strangulation described above, was unlikely in the early 1800s. Indeed, in the text from which the above case description was taken, the description of the operative procedure was preceded by a detailed discussion on available methods to externally reduce hernias. Morbidity and mortality were high, and controlling hemorrhage, pain, and infection were often insurmountable challenges. Initially more of an art than a science, early surgical procedures were often limited to amputations, draining abscesses, treating deformities, and removing bladder stones. It was not until the latter half of the eighteenth century that a more scientific approach to surgery developed, guided by a more precise knowledge of anatomy and physiology. The importance of surgery and its successful execution also depended on other scientific developments.

HISTORICAL PERSPECTIVE: THE DEVELOPMENT OF SURGERY

The history of general surgery parallels important advances in asepsis, anesthesia, and techniques for controlling bleeding. Although surgery was performed hundreds of years ago, it was done without adequate means of controlling pain, hemorrhage, or infection. In fact, early surgical interventions were not performed by physicians. Surgery was considered a specialty within the trade of barbery. Barbers were the real pioneers of anatomy and the teaching of their trade took place via apprenticeships; the neophyte learned from watching and observing the craft of the barber. Efforts to separate surgery from barbery succeeded in 1774, when England's Parliament approved a petition to that effect. Military surgeons were a major impetus in the development of modern surgery. On the battlefield, the number and severity of sustained injuries forced the military surgeon to innovate, experiment, and attempt new successes. Amputations were common; as there was no anesthesia, speed was essential, a leg could often be removed in less than a minute. Boiling oil was used on the stump for hemostasis while hot irons were applied to the raw flesh of other wounds. Postoperative wound infections were expected, and the thick, creamy pus that appeared in the wound was described as praiseworthy, or "laudable" pus.

Development of Anesthesia

Before the introduction of general anesthesia, alcohol, morphia, laudanum, hypnotism, or mesmerism were all employed in attempts to alleviate the agonies of surgery. Joseph Priestly discovered nitrous oxide in 1772, but had no idea of its anesthetic properties. In 1799, Humphrey Davy described it as "laughing gas," reported its exhilarating and anesthetic effects, and recommended its use in surgery. Cartoonists made much sport of this potential use, but surgeons showed little interest.

Both nitrous oxide and ether were inhaled for "fun." Observing ether's intoxicating effects and its ability to render its users pain free, on October 16, 1846, a young dentist named Morton successfully administered ether to a patient having a cyst removed from his neck. The operating room at Massachusetts General Hospital was crowded by students and surgeons, who watched history being made.

Control of Infection

Pain-free surgery allowed the advancement of surgical techniques; injured extremities could be repaired rather than amputated, but infection remained a major barrier to successful outcomes. Surgeons donned dirty frock coats to operate, with the dirtiest and bloodiest coat often belonging to the senior surgeon. Hands were washed after the procedure, not before. Sponges were used on one patient after another, often without being washed in between. Infection rates were attributed to bad air, or miasma; the surgeons did not realize that this "miasma" was actually the bacteria carried on their own hands.

In 1842, Oliver Wendell Holmes accused physicians of carrying puerperal fever from the autopsy room to the ward. He suggested that washing hands in a calcium chloride solution would prevent the spread of infection, a practice initiated by an Austrian physician named Ignaz Phillip Semmelweis. In Vienna, Semmelweis had observed that mortality was much higher on the ward attended by medical students than on the wards attended by midwives. He further noted that the medical students frequently came from the autopsy room and, without washing their hands, did vaginal examinations and assisted with deliveries. Based on these observations, he required all of his students to wash their hands with calcium chloride solution. Mortality

dropped from 9.92% to 3.8% in 1 year, and the next year it fell to 1.27%. Semmelweis published his findings repeatedly between 1847 and 1861, but was ridiculed by his peers, as was Holmes.

In 1870, Joseph Lister, aware of Pasteur's work in discovering bacteria and their relationship to the spread of disease, insisted that the operating teams' hands, the instruments used in surgical procedures, the patient's skin, the dressings applied to open wounds, and even the room air be disinfected with a carbolic acid solution. Nine months after initiating antisepsis on his ward in a Glasgow hospital, not a single case of pyemia, hospital gangrene, or erysipelas existed (Meade, 1968). Previously, controlling infection rates meant improving antisepsis or doing something about infections already present. The work of Lister, Koch, Pasteur, and others heralded the era of asepsis, or preventing the infection from the beginning.

Advances in Asepsis

In the mid-1880s, surgery was often performed on the ward. Gradually, designated operating rooms became the standard setting for surgery, and these rooms were cleaned for the event. Sterilized gowns and caps were introduced in 1883. Halsted introduced rubber gloves in 1890 to protect the hands of his operating room nurse from the solution used to disinfect the hands. Later, gloves were universally adopted to protect the patient from the surgeon's hands. Gauze masks were introduced in 1897. Methods were developed for sterilizing all items that came in contact with the patient's wound during surgery. Heroic operations, once rare and attended by crowds in the operating room amphitheater, became widespread. Although many surgical techniques had been tried in the eighteenth and nineteenth centuries, patients often died of sepsis or blood loss, making long-term effectiveness of surgical intervention difficult to evaluate. Refinement and perfection of surgical technique came only after the advent of safe anesthesia and aseptic technique.

The Early Twentieth Century

Many common general surgery procedures were developed between the late 1880s and the mid-1900s. Total thyroidectomy, radical mastectomy, hernia repair, common duct exploration, elective appendectomy, Billroth I (gastroduodenostomy), and Billroth II (closure of the duodenal stump and gastroenterostomy), Roux-en-Y anastomosis and pyloroplasty, among other procedures, were attempted and refined. This golden age of surgery continued with advancements in blood transfusions and the discovery of antibiotics.

Endoscopic Surgery

General surgery took its next major step forward with the development of the field of endoscopy. Although reflected light was used in the tenth century to examine the cervix, the problem of tissue damage caused by the light's heat limited its utility for surgical applications. Cystoscopy carried its own cooling system and was developed in the nineteenth century, with bladder pathology recorded on film in 1874. The pioneering days of laparoscopy proved to be of considerable risk to the patient. In 1910, surgeons did not have the buffering protection of pneumoperitoneum as they inserted trocars into the peritoneal cavity. Although an insufflation needle was eventually developed, it was 1964 before a device to automatically monitor gas flow and abdominal pressure was used. Oxygen, room air, and nitrous oxide all were used and abandoned for insufflation; carbon dioxide became the gas of choice. It does not support combustion like room air or oxygen, making it safe when a laser or electrosurgery is used. It can enter the bloodstream in amounts up to 100 ml per minute without serious metabolic effect, unlike the uncontrollable and unpredictable absorption of nitrous oxide (Zucher, Bailey, & Reddick, 1991). Fiberoptic light sources—or "cold" light, since a heat shield separates the light source and cable—and bipolar forceps both were developed in the early 1960s, lessening bowel injuries.

Gynecologists developed many instruments and techniques as the field of surgical endoscopy grew more complex. Hook scissors, the metal endoloop applicator, pretied sutures, clip appliers, endoscopic needle holders, and other endoscopic instrumentation are the result of their innovation. When computer-chip television cameras were attached to a laparoscope in 1986, the resulting images displayed on high-resolution video monitors enabled other surgical team members to see and more adequately assist the operating surgeon.

Liver biopsies were among the first laparoscopic general surgery procedures performed, and staging for pancreatic cancer soon followed. Such minimally invasive surgical approaches contributed to accelerated recovery time and shortened length of stay; in the mid-1990s, many of these procedures are same-day visits. The first laparoscopic cholecystectomy was performed in France in 1987, and general surgeons in the United States quickly followed suit; within 2 years of its introduction, nearly three fourths of all practicing general surgeons had taken training courses and were performing laparoscopic cholecystectomy (Austen, 1992). General surgical laparoscopy now commonly encompasses appendectomy, inguinal and hiatal hernia repair, transanal resection of the rectal wall, and bowel resection while new laparoscopic approaches are being refined for treatment of perforated peptic ulcers, transhiatal esophagectomy, and vagotomy (Debas, 1991). It is clear that the future of minimally invasive surgery will grow with the ability of surgeons and engineers to overcome its limitations to other general surgical procedures; what is not as clear is the extent to which cost-benefit studies will support a minimally invasive approach when it appears to cost more, in both instrumentation and operative time, than traditional open approaches (Hunter, 1993).

HISTORICAL PERSPECTIVE: PERIOPERATIVE NURSING

Before the mid-1840s, nurses were ordinarily excluded from the operating room. Strong, able-bodied men were used as assistants to physically restrain patients during the agonies of surgery. However, the preoperative role of the nurse was documented in the history of Nightingale, who often visited with soldiers who refused to undergo surgery during the Crimean War. She soothed and supported them, and was instrumental in helping them agree to surgery.

Surgery in the Home

Before the hospital was routinely used as the place for surgery, operations took place in the patient's home. There, a nurse was in attendance. Before the operation, the nurse readied a room for surgery, often the kitchen. Furniture was removed, the table was prepared, the room and furniture were scrubbed, and the walls were covered with sheets. Weeks' early textbook (1890) on nursing offered explicit instructions to the nurse attending the operative patient in the home. McCallum (1903) described part of the curriculum at the Training School for Nurses in connection with the New York Post-Graduate Medical School where, in their third year, two members of the graduating class demonstrated their ideas on preparing for an operation in a private home. Original ideas for using practical items such as ironing boards, tables with extension leaves, clothes-boilers, ordinary sheets (to make the surgeon's gown), teakettles, chafing dishes, broom handles, and even walking sticks and window poles were ingeniously used to substitute for all manner of equipment and supplies found in traditional operating rooms.

The Nurse in the Operating Room

In the late 1800s, as Lister's work with carbolic acid as an antiseptic agent gained favor, the important role of the nurse in the operating room took seed. There was much to do to prepare the physical environment for surgery, and nursing students undertook operating room rotations to train in this specialty. The nurse was expected to foresee and supply all wants of the surgeon, being watchful but not officious. A great deal of the nurse's time was spent in indirect patient care activities. Operating room sanitation and the preparation of supplies and equipment were primary nursing responsibilities. The preparation of sponges, which were literally seasponges, took up to 2 days. The sponges had to be rid of sand by soaking and rinsing in prescribed solutions before they were ready for use. It was common for the head nurse to scrub these sponges and hand them to the surgeon, hence the term "sponge nurse." Assistants handed, cared for, and cleaned the surgical instruments. The preparation of surgical catgut took several days of soaking, cutting to prescribed lengths, stretching, resoaking, wrapping, sealing, and baking. Silk, on the other hand, was placed in clean test tubes, subjected to 1 hour of dry sterilizing, then boiled for half an hour (Luce, 1901). Early operating room nurses wore black uniforms to hide the blood and dirt that tarnished them; these were the same uniforms they wore on the wards. Gradually, the OR nurse joined the rest of the operating team in donning a gown, gloves, a mask, and an OR cap.

By the mid-1930s, the OR nurse had become essential to the safe and effective execution of surgery. Environmental control remained the charge of the nurse. The OR was often located on the top floor of the hospital to allow the best light and circulation of the purest air. If the room was too hot, the windows were opened, and wet wool was hung to keep out dust. Nurses washed surgical gloves, hung them to dry, inspected them for holes, and powdered and sterilized them. Silk suture was cut into preferred lengths and waxed for easier tissue pull-through. The nurse also prepared linen packs, folding, double-wrapping, and sterilizing them as well as all other surgical supplies. When sea-sponges were replaced with gauze, the nurse cut, folded, and wrapped these. Vaseline gauze was similarly prepared for dressings. The nurse washed the floors, scrubbed the walls, polished the faucets of the scrub sinks, and collected and readied all supplies. Although these tasks were not the patient-centered nursing interventions performed by perioperative nurses of today, they were important in preventing infection. Historically, these tasks might be described as early nursing efforts to manage risks and ensure quality.

Today, perioperative nursing has both independent and interdependent role dimensions. Perioperative nurses are essential members of the surgical team who continue to advocate, prevent, protect, and collaborate. Nurses review the medical record to validate important information, review critical laboratory data to plan for the patient's physiologic needs, interview and teach patients, conduct research on the effectiveness of nursing interventions, and continuously engage in activities that direct the plan of care, beginning with patient assessment.

ASSESSMENT CONSIDERATIONS

In the perioperative setting, it is frequently impractical or impossible for the perioperative nurse to obtain a comprehensive history and assessment. The perioperative nurse's first contact with the surgery patient is often in the holding area. Given the limited time he or she has to assess the patient, the priority is to focus on the essentials, using physical examination as the basis. The perioperative nurse most often relies on inspection and palpation, with auscultation and percussion as patient need indicates.

Confirming the History and Physical Examination

Because the perioperative nurse is well acquainted with the signs and symptoms pertinent to the medical diagnosis, a history and physical examination pertinent to that diagnosis is a good start toward developing a focused plan of care. The perioperative nurse reviews, confirms, and validates clusters of signs and symptoms that lead to the development of perioperative nursing diagnoses. Assessment is conducted in light of the surgical intervention planned. For example, a patient with a diagnosis of acute appendicitis will have a typical history of anorexia, periumbilical pain that shifts to the right lower quadrant, nausea, and vomiting. This can be confirmed by interviewing the patient. The patient's white cell count and temperature may be elevated; laboratory data and nurse's notes are reviewed. On physical examination, the patient will have point and rebound tenderness in the right lower quadrant. There may even be a palpable mass. In doing this basic assessment, the perioperative nurse will identify nursing diagnoses such as high risk for infection or actual infection, and/or pain, both of which are important in planning care for the patient. Development of a trusting relationship has begun, which allows the perioperative nurse to gain useful information regarding the patient's ability to learn and cope, his or her anxiety level, relationships with significant others, and so on.

Psychosocial assessment. Before the perioperative nurse can determine the patient's understanding of the planned surgical intervention or sequence of perioperative events, it is important to assess the patient's psychologic and emotional status. One of the desired outcomes is to help the patient verbalize anxieties or fears. Assessment of mental status should begin with evaluation of the level of consciousness. If this is altered, all nursing activities that follow must be modified. The patient's facial expressions; manner; affect; body language; relationships to persons and things; and rate, volume, and fluency of speech all give clues to his or her emotional status.

Skin assessment. Assessment of the skin is ongoing from the moment the perioperative nurse meets the patient until the patient is admitted to the postanesthesia care unit (PACU). Skin color may yield clues of an underlying pathologic condition; yellow skin can indicate increased bilirubin levels from an obstructed common bile duct or chronic renal disease. Bluish extremities can indicate hypoxia, failing peripheral circulation, or decreased body temperature. Reddish skin can occur with fever, chronic alcohol intake, or local inflammation, whereas pallor is seen in anemia, shock, or syncope. Addison's disease causes the skin to bronze, whereas pregnancy causes it to become brown. The perioperative nurse should note any areas of broken skin (ulcers, lacerations, erosions), acute inflammation, or those tender to touch. These could indicate acute local infection. Also significant are purpuric lesions such as petechiae or ecchymoses, which can suggest bleeding disorders or result from trauma. The presence of previous surgical incisions can signal the likelihood of adhesions, a common complication of prior pelvic surgery, especially in women who have undergone reproductive pelvic surgery (Saunders, 1993). The perioperative nurse can assess the skin when moving and positioning the patient, padding bony prominences, prepping the skin, applying the dispersive electrode, and securing dressings. During these activities, the nurse can perform additional assessment of dryness, skin turgor, or redness over bony prominences.

Respiratory assessment. The rate and rhythm of respiration is another area of ongoing assessment, easily gathered when interviewing the patient, during preoperative preparation in the surgical suite, and during extubation and transport to the PACU. Normal respiratory rate is 8 to 16 breaths per minute. Tachypnea can indicate restrictive lung disease, pleuritic chest pain, or an elevated diaphragm (seen with a distended abdomen). Hyperventilation can be caused by high levels of anxiety or metabolic acidosis. Bradypnea may be seen with increased intracranial pressure or drug-induced respiratory depression. Cheyne-Stokes breathing is also seen with the latter or in heart failure. Prolonged expirations are common in obstructive lung disease. The perioperative nurse should note any physical deformities, such as thoracic kyphoscoliosis, pectus excavatum, or pectus carinatum, that could impair the patient's breathing. Preoperative blood gas values, pulmonary function tests, and previously documented respiratory assessments should be reviewed. If the patient is a smoker, subnormal values are expected. The patient's skin color, use of accessory muscles for respiration, productive or nonproductive cough, need for pillows, and fatigue level should also be noted.

Cardiac assessment. The perioperative nurse should obtain the patient's radial pulse to note cardiac rate and rhythm and should continue to assess it via monitoring equipment in the OR and PACU. A regular pulse that is over 100 beats per minute is considered tachycardic; under 60 beats per minute is considered bradycardic. Any irregularities in rhythm are assessed. A totally irregular rhythm suggests atrial fibrillation or flutter, whereas a rhythmically irregular rate suggests bigeminal pulse or atrial or ventricular premature contractions. A diminished pulse indicates a decreased cardiac output, as in hypovolemia, or increased peripheral resistance, as seen in congestive heart failure. Baseline vital signs, including blood pressure, should be noted, and the preoperative electrocardiogram should be reviewed.

Abdominal assessment. Since a majority of general surgery procedures involve the abdomen, abdominal assessment is common in perioperative patient care. Initial impressions can be gathered by observing the patient. Is the patient lying calmly on the transport vehicle, or are the knees bent up in an effort to relieve abdominal pain? Is there an intravenous access line, or is there also a nasogastric tube, biliary drainage tube, indwelling urinary catheter? Abdominal assessment is conducted in relationship to the usual four quadrants of right and left upper and right and left lower. By visualizing what organs lie in each quadrant, the perioperative nurse can relate the presenting complaints to an underlying pathologic condition (Table 8-1). For example, the patient with acute cholecystitis often has right upper quadrant pain that radiates to the shoulder blades. As its location suggests, the pain of pancreatic carcinoma is epigastric (Table 8-2). As the perioperative nurse inspects the abdomen, any abnormalities such as distention or ascites, or the concave contour of the cachetic patient, is noted. Umbilical, inguinal, and ventral hernias are often identified by asking the patient to take a deep breath and bear down. Visible peristalsis, seen as a rippling motion across the abdomen, is abnormal, and often accompanies intestinal obstruction. If the patient is in pain, a description of the type and quantity should be determined. Is it the intermittent cramping of a small bowel obstruction, the burning pain of a peptic ulcer, or the occasional dull ache or dragging sensation of an inguinal hernia? Did it begin gradually, like appendicitis, or abruptly, like a perforated ulcer?

The perioperative nurse should auscultate bowel

sounds based on assessment findings, realizing that these are often unreliable indicators. Lack of bowel sounds, established after 5 minutes of auscultation, occurs in paralytic ileus and peritonitis. Gastroenteritis can cause increased bowel sounds, whereas a rushed, high-pitched sound may be heard in early bowel obstruction.

The perioperative nurse should also consider the role of the intestine in fluid balance. The small intestine absorbs fluids, electrolytes, and digestive end products, as does the proximal portion of the large intestine. The colon secretes potassium and bicarbonate and absorbs sodium and chloride. Intestinal obstruction thus has an important relationship to fluid and electrolyte balance; this may be further complicated by vomiting, which poses the risk of hypokalemia, hypochloremia, and hyponatremia. Drainage from nasogastric and other intestinal tubes can affect the patient's electrolyte balance if the loss is not replaced.

Fluid and electrolyte loss may be aggravated by preoperative bowel preps and enemas. As increasing numbers of patients are admitted the morning of surgery, this bowel prep will have taken place at home without intravenous fluid replacement therapy; the patient may be seriously dehydrated on arrival in the perioperative patient care setting. Perioperative fluid loss (from tissue damage, suction, dissection) will complicate fluid and electrolyte balance if not carefully assessed and replaced. The perioperative nurse collaborates with the rest of the surgical team in determining the patient's preoperative status and monitoring fluid loss and replacement during surgery.

Additional assessment considerations. Other assessment considerations include the following:

- Laboratory data—Important values to check are serum potassium, sodium, albumin, bilirubin, complete blood count, and arterial blood gas results.
- Age—The very old and very young are at higher risk for intraoperative complications.
- Weight—Extremes in weight carry high risk.
- Nutritional status—Albumin levels below 3 g impair wound healing. Recent dramatic weight loss implies compromised nutritional status.

Table 8-1 Landmarks for abdominal examination

Anatomic correlates of the four quadrants of the abdomen

Right Upper Quadrant	**Left Upper Quadrant**
Liver and gallbladder	Left lobe of liver
Pylorus	Spleen
Duodenum	Stomach
Head of pancreas	Body of pancreas
Right adrenal gland	Left adrenal gland
Portion of right kidney	Portion of left kidney
Hepatic flexure of colon	Splenic flexure of colon
Portions of ascending and transverse colon	Portions of transverse and descending colon
Right Lower Quadrant	**Left Lower Quadrant**
Lower pole of right kidney	Lower pole of left kidney
Cecum and appendix	Sigmoid colon
Portion of ascending colon	Portion of descending colon
Bladder (if distended)	Bladder (if distended)
Ovary and salpinx	Ovary and salpinx
Uterus (if enlarged)	Uterus (if enlarged)
Right spermatic cord	Left spermatic cord
Right ureter	Left ureter

Seidel HM, Ball JW, Dains JE, & Benedict GW (1995). Mosby's Guide to Physical Examination, ed. 3, p. 484, St. Louis, Mosby.

Table 8-2 Some causes of pain perceived in anatomic regions

RIGHT UPPER QUADRANT		**LEFT UPPER QUADRANT**
Duodenal ulcer		Ruptured spleen
Hepatitis		Gastric ulcer
Hepatomegaly		Aortic aneurysm
Pneumonia		Perforated colon
		Pneumonia
RIGHT LOWER QUADRANT	**PERIUMBILICAL**	**LEFT LOWER QUADRANT**
Appendicitis	Intestinal obstruction	Sigmoid diverticulitis
Salpingitis	Acute pancreatitis	Salpingitis
Ovarian cyst	Early appendicitis	Ovarian cyst
Ruptured ectopic pregnancy	Mesenteric thrombosis	Ruptured ectopic pregnancy
Renal/ureteral stone	Aortic aneurysm	Renal/ureteral stone
Strangulated hernia	Diverticulitis	Strangulated hernia
Meckel diverticulitis		Perforated colon
Regional ileitis		Regional ileitis
Perforated cecum		Ulcerative colitis

Modified from Seidel HM, Ball JW, Dains JE, & Benedict GW (1995). Mosby's Guide to Physical Examination, ed 3, p. 507, St Louis, Mosby.

- Chronic diseases—Diabetes; chronic obstructive pulmonary disease; rheumatoid arthritis; heart, renal, or liver disease
- Previous surgical intervention—Including those in which a device was implanted, such as a pacemaker, hip prosthesis, or vascular prosthesis
- Presence of sensory aids or prosthetic devices—Glasses, contact lenses, hearing aids, dentures, and so on
- Medications—Antibiotics, anticoagulants (check for aspirin use), potassium-depleting diuretics, steroids, and so on
- Patient allergies
- Any physical limitations
- Any significant socioeconomic background factors, including language barriers and cultural, ethnic, sexual, religious, or spiritual practices that have perioperative implications
- Presence of correct, signed consent and advanced directive

Reviewing Symptoms and the Diagnostic Workup

The patient's history and physical examination remain the mainstay for the diagnosis of general surgery problems. The perioperative nurse reviews the patient's medical and nursing histories to gain important information about the history of the present illness, past medical history, social and occupational information, and a general review of major body systems. The results of the physical examination should be reviewed in terms of the planned surgery. Conclusions about the patient's diagnosis, prognosis, and anticipated perioperative problems may be facilitated on the basis of the history and physical examination.

Breast and thyroid gland. Breast lumps are often detected by self-examination or mammography, if unpalpable. Thyroid masses are usually detected on physical examination. An ultrasound may be performed to determine if the breast or thyroid mass is cystic or solid. Advances in breast imaging techniques include the use of ultrasound computed tomography, which produces seven or eight sequential "slices" of the breast and may be useful in detection of breast cancer, and digital mammography, which allows digital adjustment at the time of testing to obtain a clearer picture. Digital mammography improves image processing not only to enhance lesion detection, but to enable facilities to transmit images electronically for radiologic consultation (Full breast digital mammography, 1994). Ultrasound is now recommended as the first-line test for women with a breast implant with a suspected rupture or leak; intraoperative ultrasonography may be used to assist the surgeon in removing the implant and any silicone gel that has leaked from it. Fine-needle aspiration biopsy of the mass immediately determines if it is cystic, can provide cells for cytologic examination (Hughes & Ulmer, 1994), and is less costly than ultrasound. If a needle biopsy of a breast mass is positive, an excisional biopsy is usually done to remove the mass completely. Formerly used incisional biopsies are being supplanted by needle-core breast biopsy. In a study of needle-core biopsy, it was concluded that this technique was an effective option to standard surgical biopsy of the breast in diagnosing cancer, a precancerous condition, as well as nonmalignant lesions (Parker, 1994).

To aid the surgeon in locating an unpalpable breast mass for excision, needle localization mammographically assisted biopsy of the breast may be performed. A needle or combination of a needle and fine-hooked wire is placed into the mass using mammography or stereotactic needle-localization equipment; methylene blue combined with a contrast substance may be injected into the area via the localizing needle (Kifer, 1994). This assures that the surgeon can still identify the lesion if the wire is accidentally removed. After the specimen is excised, it is sent for specimen mammography to be certain that the suspicious area has been completely excised. Needle-localization mammographic biopsy of the breast has been shown to be useful in detecting early carcinoma of the breast (Senofsky, et al., 1990). If breast cancer is diagnosed, physical examination should be directed at possible sites of metastasis (axillary and supraclavicular nodes, liver, brain); a bone scan and chest x-ray will be done, as well as blood analyses for serum alkaline phosphatase, carcinoembryonic antigen (CEA), and lactic dehydrogenase levels to rule out metastasis before definitive treatment is selected. Although only 1% to 2% of patients with stage I or II breast cancer have a positive bone scan, it will be done if the laboratory analyses are elevated, whereas a gastrointestinal workup and lung computed tomography (CT) scan will be done only if the CEA is elevated (Hughes and Ulmer, 1994).

A solitary thyroid nodule is considered malignant until proven benign, whereas multiple nodules are considered benign unless there is some consideration suggesting malignancy, such as rapid growth, laryngeal nerve palsy, and enlarged nodes. The history should also document whether the patient has had head, neck, or upper chest radiation in the past. This treatment was historically performed for tonsillitis, acne, mastoiditis, and mastitis. Survivors of breast cancer and Hodgkin's disease may have received radiation as part of their treatment, with thyroid malignancies occurring years later.

Fine-needle aspiration biopsies have largely replaced scintiscans in determining if a nodule is malignant. Thyroid scintiscans determine if the nodule is "hot" or "cold." The patient is given radioactive iodine and the scintillations, or emissions from the iodine, are recorded, yielding a map of the gland. A normal thyroid shows an even distribution, whereas a hyperfunctioning, or "hot," nodule has a higher concentration of iodine. Cysts and many benign adenomas will test as "cold," but some thyroid carcinomas will show as "hot." The perioperative nurse may use techniques of inspection (normally, no bulging of thyroid tissue is seen in the midline of the neck or the lobes behind the sternocleidomastoid muscles), palpation (for an enlarged gland, its consistency, and any nodules), and auscultation (this should be done if the gland is enlarged; the bell of the stethoscope is used to determine the presence of bruits, or vibrations, that are heard as a soft, rushing sound). Since the thyroid gland has effects that are not limited to its anatomic location, behavior, appearance, condition of the eyes and hair, and cardiovascular status are also important. Screening laboratory tests for thyroid dysfunction should be reviewed.

Gallbladder. The patient with acute cholecystitis classically has right upper quadrant pain that radiates around to the scapula. The pain occurs shortly after eating, and symptoms ease after several hours. There may be right upper quadrant guarding and a positive Murphy's sign (aggravation on inspiration). Repeated attacks cause scarring and shrinking of the gallbladder; patients with chronic cholecystitis have nonspecific abdominal pain, fat intolerance, flatulence, and nausea. Ultrasound has a 90% accuracy rate in identifying gallstones and is the diagnostic test commonly used; intraoperative ultrasonography with sterile probes may be used to determine the need for common duct exploration. Other imaging studies may involve intravenous cholangiography with tomography, endoscopic retrograde cholangiopancreatography (ERCP), and magnetic resonance imaging (MRI) cholangiography. Approximately 1 million cases of cholelithiasis are diagnosed in the United States each year, and approximately 50% of these patients undergo cholecystectomy (Royer, 1994). For patients with asymptomatic gallstones, surgery should be avoided until gallstone symptoms arise or complications develop (Biliary tract disease patient outcomes research team, 1994). Cholelithotripsy is an alternative treatment for patients with functioning gallbladders and small, radiolucent gallstones; other nonsurgical therapies include dissolving gallstones with oral bile acids or dissolving them with a contact solution of methyl-tert-butyl-ether delivered via a catheter (American College of Physi-

cians, 1993). A critical path for open cholecystectomy is shown in Table 8-3; laparoscopic cholecystectomy is discussed in the sample care plan (see Fig. 8-3). A National Institutes of Health (NIH) Consensus Development Conference concluded that most cases of symptomatic gallstones can be treated laparoscopically; excluded are those patients with generalized peritonitis, septic shock, severe acute pancreatitis, end-stage cirrhosis of the liver, gallbladder cancer, and pregnant women in their third trimester (NIH, 1992).

Stomach and colon. Stomach cancer has few specific early symptoms. Patients may note weight loss, anorexia, fatigue or anemia, and a palpable epigastric mass may be felt. X-rays and gastroscopy are used for diagnosis, and CT scans are done to identify metastasis. The colon may be afflicted with colorectal cancer or inflammatory bowel disease. Altered bowel habits, rectal bleeding, and weight loss are signs and symptoms of colon cancer. A complete blood count (CBC) often reveals anemia. A family history is extremely important in determining the risk of colorectal cancer, and may justify regular colonoscopy (Nelson, 1991). Maule (1994) concluded from his case-control studies that nurse endoscopists can perform screening sigmoidoscopy as accurately and as safely as experienced gastroenterologists, and perioperative nurses working in these settings may incorporate this procedure into their professional role responsibilities in the future, as numerous medical organizations recommend that asymptomatic adults older than 50 years of age undergo screening by sigmoidoscopy to detect adenomas and early cancer. In addition to sigmoidoscopy, barium enema and colonoscopy are employed in confirming the diagnosis. Polyps may be biopsied or excised during colonoscopy, allowing for definitive diagnosis or resection. Circumscribed masses of tissue that project above the surface of the bowel mucosa, polyps are classified grossly as pedunculated (attached by a stalk) or sessile (attached by a base). Histologically, they are classified as neoplastic (having malignant potential) or nonneoplastic. Polyps are extremely common in Western countries, and they may ulcerate and cause bleeding. Large polyps can cause symptoms of partial bowel obstruction. A summary of the American College of Gastroenterology recommendations for polyp diagnosis, treatment, and surveillance is presented in Box 8-1.

Intestinal obstruction is usually either mechanical, from blockage of the bowel's lumen, or it is the result of a paralytic ileus. Unrelieved mechanical obstruction can progress to strangulation and perforation of the involved portion of bowel, whereas paralytic ileus can often be treated nonsurgically by bowel decompression and treatment of the paraly-

Table 8-3 A critical pathway for an open cholecystectomy

Case Manager _____   Date: _____
Total Expected LOS _____   Case # _____
DRG: _____   MD: _____

AREA: *EXPECTED LOS:	PREOP/WARD	OR HOLDING (83 MIN)	PREP (39 MIN)	SURGERY (117 MIN)	POSTCARE (16 MIN)	PARR (95 MIN)	POSTOP/WARD
Start/end time:							
Consults	Anesthesia/medicine						
Tests:	CBC, CXR, UA, ECG	Verify lab results		Radiology IOC as required	Pathology Surgical specimen		
Activity:	Up ad lib	BR/stretcher	Transfer	BR/OR table	Transfer	Encourage active range of motion	OOB ASAP with assistance
Treatments/procedures:	VS, I&O, NG, Foley, as ordered preop	Check IV site, verify AES	Position, induction, ES pad, scrub/shave prep, drape	VS, I&O, ECG, surgery O₂ sat. position	Clean & dry skin, dressing, check ES pad site	Check dressing, drains, IV, VS, TCDB at least every 2 hrs	TX as ordered
Medications:	As ordered preop	Verify preop	General anesthesia induction	General anesthesia	General anesthia reversal	Pain medication as ordered	Discharge medical instructions
Diet/fluids:	NPO p̄ MN	NPO - - - - - - - - - - - - - - →				DC NPO	Advance as tolerated
Discharge planning/teaching:	Start IV Evaluation of home environment/support, OR environment, processes, procedures	Monitor IV - - - - - - - - → Review preop teaching				DC IV Report to PARR nurse	Coordinate with needed services, instruct family on home care, wound, mobility, diet, signs and symptoms of complications, clinic appts
Documentation:	Consent, preop H&P	Verify consent, check chart	Sponge/sharp count	Report of operation, pathology report, intraop note	Pathology record	PARR nurse's notes	Postop evaluation
Variance:							
Causes & action:							

KEY: *DRG*, diagnostic-related group; *UA*, urinalysis; *OOB*, out of bed; *I&O*, intake and output; *AES*, antiembolism stockings; *ES*, electrosurgical; *Foley*, urethral catheter; *TCDB*, turn, cough, and deep breathing; *TX*, treatment.
*Minutes are calculated by averaging times found on retrospective chart audit of past year.

Box 8-1 Polyp Guideline: Diagnosis, Treatment, and Surveillance

---

Summary of the American College of Gastroenterology Recommendations

1. Initial management
   a. Most patients with polyps detected by barium enema or flexible sigmoidoscopy should undergo colonoscopy to excise the polyp and search for additional neoplasms.
   b. The decision whether to perform colonoscopy for patients with polyps less than 0.5 cm in diameter must be individualized depending on the patient's age, comorbidity, and history of colonic neoplasia.
   c. Small polyps encountered during colonoscopy are usually examined by biopsy and then destroyed by fulguration. Representative biopsies are obtained when these small lesions are numerous.
   d. When a small polyp is encountered during screening flexible sigmoidoscopy, it should be examined by biopsy to determine if it is an adenoma and thus may be an indication for colonoscopy. The balance of current evidence supports the recommendation that a hyperplastic polyp found during flexible sigmoidoscopy is not, by itself, an indication for subsequent colonoscopy.
   e. A patient who has had successful colonoscopic excision of a large sessile polyp (≥2 cm) should undergo follow-up colonoscopy in 3 to 6 months to determine if resection was complete. If residual polyp is present, it should be removed and the completeness of resection documented within another 3- to 6-month interval. If complete resection is not possible after 2 to 3 examinations, the patient should usually be referred for surgical therapy.
2. The malignant polyp
   a. No further treatment is indicated after colonoscopic resection of a malignant polyp if the following criteria are fulfilled:
      (i) The polyp is considered completely excised by the endoscopist and is submitted in toto for pathologic examination.
      (ii) In the pathology laboratory, the polyp is fixed and sectioned so that it is possible to accurately determine the depth of invasion, grade of differentiation, and the completeness of excision of the carcinoma.
      (iii) The cancer is not poorly differentiated.
      (iv) There is no vascular or lymphatic involvement.
      (v) The margin of excision is not involved.
   b. Patients with malignant polyps with favorable prognostic criteria should have follow-up colonoscopy in 3 months to check for residual abnormal tissue at the polypectomy site, especially if the poly was sessile. After one negative result of follow-up examination, the clinician can revert to standard surveillance as is performed for patients with benign adenomas.
   c. When a patient's malignant polyp has poor prognostic features, the relative risks of surgical resection should be weighed against the risk for death from metastatic cancer. The patient at high risk for morbidity and mortality from surgery should probably not have surgical resection. If a malignant polyp is located in that part of the low rectum that would require an abdominal-perineal resection, local excision rather than a standard cancer resection is usually justified.
3. Postpolypectomy surveillance
   a. Complete colonoscopy should be performed at the time of polypectomy to detect and resect all synchronous adenomas. Additional clearing examinations may be required after resection of a large sessile adenoma or of multiple adenomas to ensure complete resection.
   b. Repeated colonoscopy to check for missed synchronous and for metachronous adenomas is performed in 3 years for most patients with a single adenoma, or only a few adenomas, provided they have had a high-quality initial clearing examination.
   c. Selected patients with multiple adenomas or those who have had a suboptimal clearing examination might require colonoscopy at 1 and 4 years.
   d. After one negative 3-year follow-up examination, subsequent surveillance intervals may be increased to 5 years.
   e. The presence of severe or high-grade dysplasia in a resected polyp does not, per se, modify recommendations A through D.
   f. If complete colonoscopy is not feasible, flexible sigmoidoscopy followed by a double-contrast barium enema is an acceptable alternative.
   g. Because patients undergoing resection of a single, small, tubular adenoma (<1 cm) may not have an increased subsequent risk for cancer, follow-up surveillance may not be indicated according to decision analysis of available data.
   h. Follow-up surveillance should be individualized according to the age and comorbidity of the patient. Surveillance should be discontinued when it appears unlikely that continued follow-up is capable of prolonging life expectancy.

---

sis of the bowel wall. There is a 4:1 ratio in the lengths of the intestines; that is, there is approximately 20 feet of small intestine to 5 feet of large intestine. This ratio parallels obstruction occurrence; 80% of obstructions are in the small intestine, and 20% are in the large. Hernias, adhesions, and tumors are the three main causes of bowel obstruction in adults (Liechty & Soper, 1980). The bowel's attempt to push fluids and gas past the obstruction results in typical intermittent, crampy pain. Obstruction causes distention to varying degrees, and the patient vomits in an effort to relieve the distention. Tinkling bowel sounds may occur in rushes, then disappear as the bowel continues to distend. Abdominal x-rays show large, dilated loops of bowel with air and fluid levels.

Spleen. Massive blood loss from a severed splenic artery results in severe shock; tachycardia, restlessness, left upper quadrant tenderness, and Kehr's sign (irritation of the diaphragm referred to the left shoulder) are seen with slower blood loss. Peritoneal lavage, abdominal x-rays, and CT scans may be performed.

Appendix. Pain that begins periumbilically and then moves to the right lower quadrant is a classic sign of appendicitis. The patient may have vomiting, anorexia, or a low-grade fever (elevated about 1° C). Localized and rebound tenderness are common, and Rovsing's sign (applied pressure to the left lower quadrant intensifies right lower quadrant pain) may be elicited. The white cell count is usually elevated, with a shift of the neutrophils to the left; an abdominal flat plate, barium enema, and/or laparoscopy, especially in female patients, may be performed to confirm the diagnosis. The Alvarado score has been useful in predicting acute appendicitis, which can be a difficult diagnosis (Kalan, Talbot & Cunliffe, 1994). It scores based on the symptoms of migratory right iliac fossa (RIF) pain, anorexia, and nausea/vomiting, the signs of RIF tenderness, rebound RIF tenderness, and elevated temperature, and based on laboratory findings of leukocytosis with a neutrophil shift to the left.

NURSING DIAGNOSIS

Managing the health and well-being of the patient intraoperatively is the primary concern of the perioperative nurse. It is more important to design a plan of care that meets the patient's needs than it is to meet one's own need for completing the required forms. If the care plan or nursing activities described in the generic care plans presented in this chapter do not fit the patient, the plan must be modified or eliminated. The plans are designed to encourage individualization based on patient need and priority as well as institutional protocol. Whether a specific diagnosis is included in a care plan depends on the extent to which each is a problem for the individual patient. Thus analysis of the patient data base is important in determining specific nursing diagnoses. However, several nursing diagnoses could conceivably be applied to the general surgery patient population. The following are common nursing diagnoses for surgical patients:

High risk for knowledge deficit
High risk for infection
High risk for injury
Pain

To care for the nutritional and metabolic needs of the surgical patient, the perioperative nurse may need to include nursing diagnoses such as *high risk for altered body temperature* (hyperthermia or hypothermia), *high risk for fluid volume deficit* (or *actual fluid volume deficit*), *high risk for fluid volume excess, high risk for impaired skin integrity* (or *actual impaired skin integrity*), *high risk for decreased cardiac output*, and the risks for alterations in respiratory function—*impaired gas exchange, ineffective airway clearance,* and/or *ineffective breathing patterns.*

Nursing diagnoses dealing with self-perception should be included as they apply to the individual patient. It is difficult to imagine a patient about to undergo a surgical intervention who was not experiencing some degree of *fear* or *anxiety*. The degree to which it affects the patient can vary from mild to high levels of anxiety, which is why perioperative nurses should attempt to classify the level of anxiety, its source, and then work with the patient to identify personally effective coping strategies. The source of the fear or anxiety will also vary widely, from financial concerns, to stressed family dynamics, to fear of death. With a variety of treatment modalities available, *decisional conflict* is frequently encountered preoperatively as well as postoperatively. Patients may be overwhelmed by the lack of control they have in hospital settings, over their own bodies, or over the disease process. In such cases, a diagnosis of *powerlessness* may be appropriate.

Situational low self-esteem can occur, especially in high achievers whose expectations of themselves are unrealistic in this setting. *Body image disturbance* may also be a pertinent diagnosis for surgical patients. A surgical incision may be enough to adversely affect one's body image. A major change in body function is likely to have a negative impact, to some extent, on anyone.

Nursing diagnoses dealing with an individual's perception of his or her role in life and the relationships he or she maintains could also be included. *Grieving*, either anticipatory or dysfunctional, could be included. People grieve more for what the lost body part meant to them than for the actual loss of tissue. For example, the loss of a breast may be seen as a serious threat to a woman's sexuality, femininity, or both. In addition, people may grieve for loss of life-style associated with a change in function.

CARE PLANS

The perioperative patient care plan guides that follow for general surgery are meant to be guidelines.

The plans are designed to assist the perioperative nurse in identifying patient outcomes, evaluative criteria, and nursing actions that effect safe, economical, high-quality patient care. They contain a section for noting additional nursing actions or generic care plans initiated. They should be modified to plan and promote perioperative nursing care that recognizes and is sensitive to the individual needs and feelings of the recipient of that care.

GUIDES TO NURSING ACTIONS
Modified Radical Mastectomy (Fig. 8-1)

1. Psychosocial assessment of the patient scheduled for mastectomy may lead to a nursing diagnosis of *body image disturbance related to change in appearance* from loss of the breast (Mock, 1993), decisional conflict (Pierce, 1993), and fear of death (Knobf, 1994) all of which compound feelings of anxiety and stress. Patients need preparation that adequately includes information about the treatment options, actual treatment experience, recovery, self-care, and the impact of treatment on daily quality of life. Verbalization of feelings and perceptions should be encouraged. Both verbal and nonverbal responses (facial expressions and body language) should be noted. Clarify misconceptions about limitations on future activities. If appropriate, review with the patient and significant others normal sensations associated with mastectomy (diminished sensation at the incision site, possibility of phantom breast pain, numbness or tingling in the inner aspect of the arm caused by loss of the intercostal brachial nerve, chest wall tightness, arm swelling). With breast conservation followed by radiation, review potential side effects of breast soreness and edema, skin reactions, arm swelling, sensory changes in the arm from surgery and in the breast from radiation therapy, the prolonged treatment, and fatigue. If the patient is undergoing immediate reconstruction, review anticipated discomfort from elevation and stretching of muscles for an implant (and prolonged physician visits with expanders) or the extensiveness of the surgery, the location of the two surgical sites, and the prolonged recovery for flap procedures. Patients undergoing polychemotherapy or tamoxifen therapy need information about the treatment course, side effects, and long-term therapy that might be recommended with tamoxifen (Harris, et al., 1992). Demonstrate acceptance of the patient through the use of therapeutic touch. Provide information regarding community agencies and/or support groups if this has not been done (Reach for Recovery; family, individual, or sexual counseling). Do not omit information on rehabilitation for older patients; Hynes (1994) indicates that women older than age 80 are 2 to 3 times less likely to receive information on postmastectomy rehabilitation. If immediate reconstruction is planned, note whether the flap site has been marked; all potentially constricting bands, even institutional ID bracelets, must be removed from the operative hand and arm. Be sure that teaching breast self-examination (BSE) is part of the plan of care for all patients. Mastectomy with the carbon dioxide laser may be performed on an outpatient basis; review plans for home care (Morris, et al., 1992).

2. Verify the operative procedure with the patient's statement of planned surgery. Be sure which breast is specified (possibly both). Note whether the permit indicates the possible need for a skin graft.

3. Compare the procedure stated on the surgical consent with the patient's statement of the planned surgery. Note that the procedure and side of operation (possibly bilateral) are the same for both.

4. If antibiotics are prescribed, compare the drug to be used with the drug and dosage ordered. Document any medications administered intraoperatively. Check patient allergies.

5. Prepare the OR bed before the patient is moved to it. The "lawn chair position" should be used because it reduces tension on the back. The neck should be slightly flexed and the head should rest on a small pillow. To prevent compression of subclavian arteries, the head should not be turned to either side. Properly align and secure the arm and hand on the nonoperative side. When placing the arm at the patient's side, avoid compression on the ulnar, medial, or radial nerves. When using an arm board, the angle should be less than 90 degrees to prevent brachial plexus injury secondary to hyperabduction of the arm. Recheck if the patient is repositioned for any reason. Place the knee strap correctly. Monitor the position of the Mayo tray over the patient throughout the procedure. With adequate assistance, place a rolled towel or small beanbag posterior to the axilla to provide access to the operative site. Place the armboard at slightly less than 90 degrees on the OR bed. Secure a pillow or folded blanket to the armboard before placing the arm on it. The additional height prevents tension on the brachial plexus. The additional padding helps prevent pressure on the medial and ulnar nerves. Secure the arm to prevent inadvertent changes in positioning during the axillary dissection. Recheck the position of elbow and hand during the procedure. Check the radial pulse.

FIG. 8-1
CARE PLAN FOR MODIFIED RADICAL MASTECTOMY

KEY ASSESSMENT POINTS

Prior surgical experiences
Knowledge of this surgery and perioperative events
Operative side
Family history of breast carcinoma
Nipple discharge, pain, changes in breast
Knowledge of breast self-examination
Fear, anxiety, and coping mechanisms

NURSING DIAGNOSIS

All generic nursing diagnoses apply to this patient, with the addition of:

High risk for body image disturbance

PATIENT OUTCOMES

All generic outcomes apply, with the addition of:
The patient will demonstrate acceptance of any alterations in body image by:
1. Verbalizing feelings of physical change
2. Discussing altered body image
3. Participating in self-care activities

NURSING ACTIONS

	Yes	No	N/A
1. Psychosocial assessment performed?	☐	☐	☐
2. Verbal verification of operative site? (left/right/bilateral—indicate)	☐	☐	☐
3. Consent signed correctly? (left/right/bilateral—indicate)	☐	☐	☐
4. Prescribed antibiotics available/administered?	☐	☐	☐
5. Correctly positioned?	☐	☐	☐
6. Privacy maintained during prep, positioning, draping, undraping	☐	☐	☐
7. Condition of skin at prep site noted?	☐	☐	☐
8. Dispersive pad site checked before and after application?	☐	☐	☐
9. Skin prep per institutional protocol?	☐	☐	☐
10. Irrigation/IV solution warmed/other measures to maintain normothermia?	☐	☐	☐
11. Specimen to lab?	☐	☐	☐
12. Dispersive pad site checked at removal?	☐	☐	☐
13. Counts performed and correct?	☐	☐	☐
14. Presence of drain(s) noted?	☐	☐	☐
15. Dressing applied?	☐	☐	☐
16. Other generic care plans initiated? (specify)	☐	☐	☐

Document additional nursing actions/generic care plans initiated here:

_____

_____

_____

EVALUATION OF PATIENT OUTCOMES

	Outcome met	Outcome met with additional outcome criteria	Outcome met with revised nursing care plan	Outcome not met	Outcome not applicable to this patient
1. The patient demonstrated acceptance of alterations in body image.	☐	☐	☐	☐	☐
2. The patient met outcomes for additional generic care plans as indicated.	☐	☐	☐	☐	☐

Signature: _____ Date: _____

6. Maintaining privacy is important for all patients but of priority for the patient with a potential for body image disturbance.

7. Note the condition of the skin at the skin preparation site before and after preparatory procedures.

8. Document the condition of the patient's skin at the site of the dispersive electrode before placement and after removal.

9. When cleansing the skin at the operative site, prepare laterally to the nipple on the nonoperative breast; to the clavicle and shoulder cephalad; and laterally to the bedside, axilla, and anterior surface of the arm to the elbow. The lower edge of the preparation will vary depending on the patient's size. For a small patient with a short thorax, prepare to the navel. For a patient with a normal or long thorax, prepare to the costal margin.

10. Warm irrigation and intravenous solutions when appropriate to help the patient maintain a stable body temperature. Additional measures to keep the patient normothermic include covering the shoulder and arm on the nonoperative side and lower abdomen to feet with warm blankets. Expose only the body surface necessary to prepare the patient.

11. Ascertain the surgeon's requirements for preserving the specimen obtained. Follow institutional policy for labeling, preserving, and delivering tissue for frozen sections, estrogen/progesterone receptors, and permanent pathologic sections.

12. Check skin condition at the electrosurgical unit (ESU) dispersive pad site before discharge from the OR.

13. Follow institutional protocol for performing and recording sponge, sharp, and instrument counts.

14. Document the presence of drains.

15. Apply dressing to prevent "tape burns." Place tape over dressing in axilla first, then the lower arm, and then secure tape loosely to the chest. Allow for normal postoperative swelling to occur without stretching the skin underneath the tape.

Thyroidectomy (Fig. 8-2)

1. Patients with hyperthyroidism are normally given antithyroid medication, such as methimazole (Tapazole) or propylthiouracil (PTU), to inhibit synthesis of thyroxine. This is especially important before surgery, when manipulation of the thyroid and/or stress can trigger a sudden release of thyroid hormones, or thyroid storm. The resulting tachycardia, hyperpyrexia, diaphoresis, and shock can make thyroid storm fatal. In assessing the hyperthyroid patient, it is important to note whether antithyroid medication has been administered. Although an unexpected outcome, a perioperative plan for intervening in thyroid storm should include anticipation of insertion of arterial lines, administration of beta blockers, treatment of acid-base disturbance, and hyperthermia (Martinelli & Fontana, 1990).

2. An enlargement of the thyroid gland is a goiter. While the use of iodized salt is commonly known as a preventive measure, the thyroid gland may also enlarge in an attempt to make needed thyroid hormones. Goiters may grow large enough to cause shortness of breath, compress or deviate the trachea, or extend so far substernally that a median sternotomy is necessary. The size of the goiter should be noted and chest x-rays reviewed to note any tracheal deviation. Based on respiratory function, the need to elevate the head of the bed should be considered during transport and positioning.

3. During admission to the OR room, comfort measures such as placing a pillow under the thighs close to the knees or flexing the OR bed in the lawn chair position should be considered. Warm blankets may or may not be appropriate; the hyperthyroid patient may prefer a cool environment. A thermia unit may be placed on the OR bed in anticipation of the need to cool the patient during the rare event of thyroid storm.

4. Sequential compression stockings are applied if required before the induction of anesthesia.

5. An awake fiberoptic intubation may be undertaken if a goiter is so large that it interferes with the airway. In this event, the perioperative nurse provides emotional support to the patient and assists the anesthesia provider; an emergency tracheotomy set should be available in the room.

6. The patient's arms are normally padded and tucked at the side, avoiding compression on the ulnar, median, or radial nerves. Plexiglas sleds or arm cradles may be used to allow the team to get close to the patient without leaning on or compressing the arms. Special headrests, beanbags, a horizontally placed shoulder roll, and flexion of the head portion of the OR bed are commonly used to achieve safe, stable exposure of the operative site. Place the knee strap about 2 inches above the knee, securely but not too tightly, avoiding compression of the popliteal space. Monitor the position of the Mayo tray over the patient throughout the procedure so that no body part, such as the toes, is compressed. Monitor the position of the operating

FIG. 8-2
CARE PLAN FOR THYROIDECTOMY

KEY ASSESSMENT POINTS

History of thyroid dysfunction, radiation, surgery
Change in temperature preference
Swelling in neck
Changes in texture of hair, skin, nails
Change in emotional stability
Increased prominence of eyes, visual changes
Cardiorespiratory changes
Change in menstrual pattern
Change in appetite, bowel or urinary patterns, weight loss
Family history of thyroid disorders

NURSING DIAGNOSIS

All generic nursing diagnoses apply to this patient, with the addition of:
High risk for ineffective breathing patterns

PATIENT OUTCOMES

All generic outcomes apply, with the addition of:
The patient will demonstrate effective breathing patterns by:
1. Maintaining satisfactory ventilation and oxygenation status preoperatively and postoperatively
2. Exhibiting no signs of respiratory distress

NURSING ACTIONS

	Yes	No	N/A
1. Preop assessment performed?	☐	☐	☐
2. Respiratory distress noted/alleviated?	☐	☐	☐
3. Comfort measures initiated?	☐	☐	☐
4. Sequential decompression stockings applied?	☐	☐	☐
5. Assistance with intubation required?	☐	☐	☐
6. Positioned correctly?	☐	☐	☐
7. ESU dispersive pad site assessed (on application and removal)?	☐	☐	☐
8. Skin prep per institutional protocol?	☐	☐	☐
9. Specimen to lab?	☐	☐	☐
10. Counts performed and correct?	☐	☐	☐
11. Dressings applied?	☐	☐	☐
12. Instruments kept sterile until patient discharge from OR?	☐	☐	☐
13. Postop report given?	☐	☐	☐
14. Other generic care plans initiated? (specify)	☐	☐	☐

Document additional nursing actions/generic care plans initiated here:

_____

_____

_____

EVALUATION OF PATIENT OUTCOMES

	Outcome met	Outcome met with additional outcome criteria	Outcome met with revised nursing care plan	Outcome not met	Outcome not applicable to this patient
1. The patient maintained effective breathing patterns.	☐	☐	☐	☐	☐
2. The patient met outcomes for additional generic care plans as indicated.	☐	☐	☐	☐	☐

Signature: _____ Date: _____

team during the procedure. No one should lean on the patient's abdomen or chest, which may depress respiration or raise venous pressure. Prevent injury to the patient's eye during positioning and draping. The protective mechanisms of the eye may be compromised; they should be lubricated and taped shut during anesthesia.

7. Document the skin condition of the ESU dispersive electrode site before application and after removal of the pad.

8. The skin prep ordinarily extends from the lower lip to the nipple line; extending the prep to the umbilicus will be required if a median sternotomy is planned. Laterally, the prep extends from bedside to bedside.

9. Ascertain the surgeon's requirements for preserving the specimen(s) obtained. Follow institutional policy for labeling, preserving, and delivering tissue for frozen sections and permanent pathologic sections. Subsequently document the results of the frozen section.

10. Follow institutional protocol for performing and recording sponge, sharp, and instrument counts. Document the presence of any drains.

11. The dressing is secured with two pieces of tape in an X shape, applied loosely after the neck has been returned to normal position.

12. Instruments should remain sterile until the patient is extubated and has adequate respiratory exchange. The risk for ineffective breathing patterns and airway clearance must be kept in mind at the conclusion of the surgical procedure and during transfer to the PACU. A semi- or high-Fowler's position may be used during transport; protection and close monitoring of the airway is carried out through admission to the PACU.

Laparoscopic Cholecystectomy (Fig. 8-3)

1. The widespread acceptance of laparoscopic cholecystectomy is partly because it has reduced morbidity. Selection criteria for this procedure are very broad. The perioperative nurse may be planning care for the "ideal" patient (young, slim, never undergone previous abdominal surgery, has recent or mild symptoms, a normal gallbladder wall), the "average" patient (middle-aged, muscular or obese, recurrent biliary colic, normal gallbladder wall, previous pelvic surgery), or the "difficult" patient (elderly, morbidly obese, acute cholecystitis, thick or contracted gallbladder wall, previous upper abdominal surgery) (Fried, 1994). Thus, considerations of modifying the plan of care depend on the patient selection classification. In verifying operative consent, it is necessary to determine the pa-

tient's understanding of the planned procedure, as well as the possibility of open cholecystectomy. Patients in whom the risk for conversion is high include the elderly, those markedly obese, those with a history of acute cholecystitis, and those with thickened gallbladder walls. Intraoperatively, when complications occur that cannot be laparoscopically rectified, the decision to convert will be made by the surgeon. The effects of retained carbon dioxide, experienced as shoulder pain, should be explained, as well as the fact that this will disappear as the gas is absorbed and that pain medication will be available. Cardiorespiratory status should be assessed, as patients with disease may have difficulty with the effects of pneumoperitoneum on cardiac output, lung inflation pressure, acid-base balance, and the lungs' ability to eliminate CO_2. The abdomen should be examined for scars, stomas, and hernias, which will influence special techniques for trocar insertion. Plans for home care should be reviewed; the procedure may be a 23-hour stay, and postoperative instructions should be reviewed and plans for a follow-up telephone call made. Research by Kleinbeck and Hoffart (1994) indicates that patients need significant reinforcement of teaching, and that teaching must be adapted toward home recovery with strategies specific to that environment.

2. Some surgeons routinely administer prophylactic antibiotics since inadvertent entry into the gallbladder can lead to spillage of bile or stones into the peritoneal cavity. In this case, verify that antibiotics have been administered as prescribed and that the patient has remained NPO.

3. Before admitting the patient to the OR room, check that the necessary video equipment is operating properly. One or two video monitors may be used; these are positioned toward the head on either side of the OR bed. The videocassette recorder should have a tape ready to be recorded and the light source should be plugged in. If more than one type of camera is used, determine that the camera and processor are compatible. The insufflator should be set at zero to start and the flow rate at the surgeon's preference, usually around 8 to 12 L/min. Insufflators should provide digital readouts of the actual gas flow rate, the actual intraabdominal pressure, the total amount of CO_2 used, a control for adjusting maximum flow rate, and an audible alarm when the pressure exceeds a certain preset value. Check that the carbon dioxide tank is full, with a reading above 50 or "in the green"; a second full tank should be ready. If irrigation

FIG. 8-3
CARE PLAN FOR LAPAROSCOPIC CHOLECYSTECTOMY

KEY ASSESSMENT POINTS

History of indigestion after high-fat meal
Pain/tenderness right subcostal or right epigastric region
Anorexia, nausea, vomiting, flatulence
Positive Murphy's sign
Jaundice
Fever, elevated WBC
Steatorrhea
Determination of risk for conversion to open procedure
History of bleeding disorders
Abdominal examination

NURSING DIAGNOSIS

All generic nursing diagnoses apply to this patient, with the addition
  of the following:
  Pain

PATIENT OUTCOMES

All generic outcomes apply, with the addition of:
The patient will:
1. Express effectiveness of preoperative medication
2. Describe expected postop discomfort and ways to alleviate it
3. Describe/utilize additional pain relief measures that are personally effective

NURSING ACTIONS

	Yes	No	N/A
1. Preop assessment performed?	☐	☐	☐
Consent checked?	☐	☐	☐
Possible conversion to open procedure explained?	☐	☐	☐
Postoperative discomfort explained?	☐	☐	☐
Cardiorespiratory assessment done?	☐	☐	☐
Abdomen examined?	☐	☐	☐
Plans for home care reviewed?	☐	☐	☐
2. Antibiotics given as prescribed?	☐	☐	☐
3. All equipment assembled/checked?	☐	☐	☐
Full CO_2 tank?	☐	☐	☐
Videotape in recorder?	☐	☐	☐
Irrigation ready (if planned)?	☐	☐	☐
4. Positioned correctly?	☐	☐	☐
5. Nasogastric tube inserted?	☐	☐	☐
6. Sequential decompression stockings applied?	☐	☐	☐
7. ESU dispersive pad site assessed (on application and removal)?	☐	☐	☐
8. Skin prep per institutional protocol?	☐	☐	☐
9. Intraabdominal pressure monitored?	☐	☐	☐
10. Patient monitored during positional changes for CO_2 emboli/vital signs?	☐	☐	☐
11. Supplies in room in anticipation of need to convert to open procedure?	☐	☐	☐
12. Specimens to lab?	☐	☐	☐
13. Counts performed and correct?	☐	☐	☐
Dressings applied?	☐	☐	☐
14. Postop report given?	☐	☐	☐
15. Other generic care plans initiated? (specify)	☐	☐	☐

Document additional nursing actions/generic care plans initiated
here:

_____

_____

_____

EVALUATION OF PATIENT OUTCOMES

	Outcome met	Outcome met with additional outcome criteria	Outcome met with revised nursing care plan	Outcome not met	Outcome not applicable to this patient
1. The patient expressed minimal discomfort.	☐	☐	☐	☐	☐
2. The patient met outcomes for additional generic care plans as indicated.	☐	☐	☐	☐	☐

Signature: _____ Date: _____

is used, heparin may be added to prevent the formation of clots that interfere with visibility. An x-ray–compatible OR bed is required.

4. Antiembolic stockings to minimize venous pooling in the extremities during the reverse Trendelenburg's position are usually applied. A warm blanket should be offered during preparatory maneuvers before the induction of anesthesia.

5. When the patient is admitted to the OR room, a nasogastric tube may be inserted and urinary catheterization may be performed to decompress the bladder; if catheterization is not performed, verify that the patient voided before leaving the preoperative area.

6. The patient will be positioned to optimize exposure of the gallbladder and to give the operative team easy patient access. The patient is most often supine (although, in Europe, the patient is placed in low stirrups with the surgeon on the left or in between the patient's legs) with the OR bed tilted into reverse Trendelenburg's position and rotated to position the right side up, allowing gravity to pull the duodenum, colon, and omentum away from the gallbladder. The arms are tucked carefully at the sides. The side rails of the OR bed are kept clear of overhanging drawsheets or drape towels; if an open conversion is required, a table-mounted retractor is normally used. If cholangiography is anticipated, the patient's left scapula may be elevated to rotate the patient so the bile duct is not superimposed over the spine (Fried, 1994).

7. The condition of the skin at the ESU dispersive electrode site is examined and noted before applying the pad and upon removal.

8. Barriers and/or towels are placed at the patient's sides to prevent pooling of prep solution. A standard abdominal prep (nipples to pubis, bedside to bedside) is done.

9. After the patient is draped, connect the camera, light cable, gas tubing, suction, and electrosurgical cables. Monitor the intraabdominal pressure reading on the insufflator; it should not be above 12 to 14 mm Hg. After 3 to 4 L of CO_2 are insufflated, adequate pneumoperitoneum is achieved and trocars are placed. At this point in the procedure, the surgeon may request Trendelenburg's position. Most surgeons prefer 10-mm trocars for the laparoscope and clip applier and 5-mm trocars for the graspers and dissecting forceps. Either disposable or reusable trocars may be used; reusables should be checked for sharpness and properly functioning valves and seals. A laser may be used; the Nd:YAG or argon laser may be requested.

10. Once the initial trocar is inserted and accessory ports placed, the surgeon is ready to proceed with the cholecystectomy. The patient is placed in reverse Trendelenburg's position; this can cause a decrease in cardiac output, blood pressure, and venous return. Distention from the carbon dioxide can elevate the patient's diaphragm and cause hypoxemia. If large amounts of CO_2 enter the patient's bloodstream, a CO_2 embolus can form in the right ventricle, seen as a sudden, severe drop in blood pressure, a "mill wheel" heart murmur, and cyanosis; this may lead to death. Vital signs must be closely monitored during this surgery.

11. Necessary instruments and supplies must be in the room if a quick conversion to open laparotomy is required.

12. The specimen is handled per institutional policy. If the surgeon requests that the gallbladder be opened off the field and examined for stones, the perioperative nurse must use universal precautions when handling the specimen.

13. Closing counts are done as the trocars are removed. Minimal dressings are required; adhesive skin strips are usually adequate to dress the port sites.

14. After assisting with extubation and transfer to the transport vehicle, accompany the patient to PACU. The patient can anticipate minimal postoperative pain. Nausea and vomiting are often treated with an antiemetic as a routine order in the PACU and to accompany each dose of a parenteral narcotic. By 24 to 48 hours postoperative, most patients no longer need narcotics, are eating a full diet, and are fully ambulatory.

Inguinal Hernia Repair (Fig. 8-4)

1. Numerous approaches to inguinal hernia repair are available, as are various options for sutures, suturing techniques, prosthetic materials, and open versus laparoscopic repair. Conventional, open repair is described in this sample care plan; reference is made to some modifications for laparoscopic repair. Approximately 500,000 patients undergo one of these approaches to inguinal hernia repair each year in the United States (Wexler, 1994). Although surgical intervention may be considered "common" to the perioperative team, the individual patient may experience decisional conflict regarding the type of repair selected, anxiety about the recovery process and the potential for recurrence, and embarrassment due to the close anatomic location of the genitals. During patient assessment and examination, privacy should be provided. Rely on both

FIG. 8-4
CARE PLAN FOR INGUINAL HERNIA REPAIR

KEY ASSESSMENT POINTS

Operative side/site
Type, severity of hernia
History of recurrent deep vein thrombosis
Knowledge of surgery, anesthesia planned
Understanding of discharge plans
Compliance with preparatory instructions

NURSING DIAGNOSIS

All generic nursing diagnoses apply to this patient, with the addition of:
Anxiety
(Consider knowledge deficit for ambulatory surgery patient)

PATIENT OUTCOMES

All generic patient outcomes apply, with the addition of:
The patient will exhibit a reduced level of anxiety by:
1. Displaying relaxed facial expressions
2. Verbalizing less anxiety (or fear)
3. Accurately describing perioperative events

NURSING ACTIONS

	Yes	No	N/A
1. Preop assessment performed?	☐	☐	☐
Verbal verification of operative side? (Left/right/bilateral—indicate)	☐	☐	☐
Consent signed correctly? (Left/right/bilateral—indicate)	☐	☐	☐
Method of anesthesia explained? (Local/regional/IV consc. sedation/general—indicate)	☐	☐	☐
Patient understands type of anesthesia?	☐	☐	☐
2. Prescribed antibiotics administered? (Document drug, dosage, route of administration.)	☐	☐	☐
3. Comfort measures initiated?	☐	☐	☐
4. Positioned correctly?	☐	☐	☐
5. Patient monitoring documented?	☐	☐	☐
6. Hair clipped at operative site?	☐	☐	☐
7. ESU dispersive pad site assessed (on application and removal)?	☐	☐	☐
8. Skin prep site assessed?	☐	☐	☐
9. Prosthetic mesh used/logged?	☐	☐	☐
10. Bowel resection required?	☐	☐	☐
11. Specimen to lab?	☐	☐	☐
12. Counts performed and correct?	☐	☐	☐
13. Local anesthetics recorded?	☐	☐	☐
14. Dressings applied?	☐	☐	☐
15. Discharge teaching done?	☐	☐	☐
16. Other generic care plans initiated? (specify)	☐	☐	☐

Document additional nursing actions/generic care plans initiated here:

_____

_____

_____

EVALUATION OF PATIENT OUTCOMES

1. The patient's anxiety was reduced.
2. The patient met outcomes for additional generic care plans as indicated.

	Outcome met	Outcome met with additional outcome criteria	Outcome met with revised nursing care plan	Outcome not met	Outcome not applicable to this patient
1.	☐	☐	☐	☐	☐
2.	☐	☐	☐	☐	☐

Signature: _____ Date: _____

verbal and nonverbal cues about the patient's concerns. When the consent is checked, ask the patient to state which side is to be repaired; this may be right, left, or both. Determine the patient's understanding of the surgery planned, the anticipated discharge sequence and home care requirements, and the anesthesia planned. Hernia repair may be completed under local, regional, or intravenous conscious sedation; the patient may fear being "awake" or that the method of anesthesia won't be effective. Answer questions and provide correct information to clarify misperceptions and to lessen fear and anxiety. Confirm NPO status. If laparoscopic inguinal hernia repair (LIH) is planned, antiembolic stockings will be applied; a scopolamine patch may be applied to control postoperative nausea.

2. If the surgeon plans a repair using prosthetic mesh (or using laparoscopic repair), antibiotics may be prescribed; verify if these have been administered.

3. Consider warming the OR room before the patient is admitted. Offer warm blankets to enhance patient comfort. For distraction and relaxation during the procedure, offer the patient music selections. Support the patient in utilizing other effective coping strategies (meditation, guided imagery, relaxation techniques).

4. The supine position is used. Adjust the OR bed or provide positioning devices to increase comfort. Place arms on padded armboards; for LIH, arms are often placed on padded foam and secured at the sides. The LIH patient will be placed in Trendelenburg's position after draping.

5. If local anesthesia or nurse-monitored IV conscious sedation is planned, initiate institutional protocols for risk assessment, monitoring, and anticipation of complications (respiratory, cardiovascular, allergic/anaphylactic). In addition to the indications and contraindications for agents used (Table 8-4), the perioperative nurse must be familiar with specific cautions of each drug, pharmacologic actions, side/adverse effects, and usual dosage for various patient categories.

6. Pubic hair may need to be clipped on the operative side. Provide privacy, clipping hair from the umbilicus to the base of the penis for male patients or the top of the mons in female patients. Note skin condition at the prep site, and document any nicks or abrasions.

7. The ESU dispersive pad should be applied to a site where its removal will cause the least discomfort. Note the condition of the skin at the pad site on application and removal. For LIH, urinary catheterization will be performed.

Table 8-4 Agents commonly used in IV conscious sedation

Drug	Indications	Contraindications
Midazolam (Versed)	Sedation/ amnesia	Known hypersensitivity to benzodiazepines Acute narrow-angle glaucoma Untreated open-angle glaucoma
Diazepam (Valium)	Sedative/ hypnotic	Same as for midazolam
Fentanyl (Sublimaze)	Analgesia/ sedation	Hypersensitivity Bradydysrhythmias Head injury/increased intracranial pressure Hepatic impairment Respiratory impairment
Meperidine (Demerol)/ morphine	Analgesia	Respiratory depression Patient on MAO inhibitor Allergy to opioids History of convulsions Diarrhea caused by toxins
Naloxone (Narcan)	Reverse respiratory depression caused by opioids	Hypersensitivity
Flumazenil (Romazicon)	Antagonize benzodiazepine sedation	Hypersensitivity to benzodiazepines/ flumazenil

Modified from Odom J. (1994, March). *IV conscious sedation in the perioperative period.* Handout from the 1994 AORN Congress Resource Manual.

8. Place towels/barrier drapes to prevent pooling of skin preparation solutions. If manufacturer's recommendations permit, consider warming the prep solution. Prep from umbilicus to mid-thigh on operative side. The scrotum and penis are often included in the prepped area to allow the surgeon to palpate the hernia through the external ring.

9. If prosthetic mesh is used, follow institutional protocol for recording information about implanted material.

10. Although infrequent, the possibility of bowel resection during hernia repair should be anticipated, with bowel instruments, staplers, etc., readily available. The patient with strangulation and accompanying signs of small bowel obstruction usually has nausea, vomiting, abdominal distention, hyperactive bowel sounds, pain, fever, point tenderness and inflammation, absence of flatus or stool, and generalized peritonitis.

11. Surgical specimens should be documented per institutional policy.
12. Institutional policy for sponge, sharp, and instrument counts is followed.
13. Medications administered during the procedure should be documented (dose, route, reaction). Local anesthesia may be injected into the incision or trocar sites to decrease postoperative incisional discomfort.
14. At the conclusion of the procedure, wash off preparation solution with warm water, apply a dressing (skin strips may be used), and assist the patient onto the transport vehicle. Accompany the patient to the recovery area, give report, and assure the patient that discharge instruction will be re-reviewed. These will include information on pain-control measures (such as application of ice, scrotal support and elevation, medication), activity restrictions, care of the incisional site, and signs and symptoms of infection. The importance of voiding, especially for patients who received spinal anesthesia, should be emphasized. For LIH patients, some crepitus may persist in the inguinal area for 2 to 3 days; patients should be advised of this (Gonzalez-Cortes & Procuniar, 1994). Plans for a postoperative follow-up telephone call should be made.

Appendectomy (Fig. 8-5)

1. Appendectomy, when performed to remove an acutely inflamed appendix, may involve a patient who is very ill and perhaps even septic. Assessment will need to be modified depending on the patient's circumstance. Since the time between onset of symptoms and hospitalization is ordinarily brief (12 to 48 hours), the perioperative nurse can expect the patient to be anxious regarding this abrupt change in their condition; anticipated changes in usual life-style, roles, or both; fear of death; presence of acute pain (pain medication may be withheld while the diagnosis is being made; abrupt cessation of pain may indicate that the appendix has ruptured); and concern about postoperative pain. Modify nursing interventions based on assessment results; determine how much learning can realistically take place based on the patient's level of anxiety. Simple, repeated explanations, caring behaviors such as touching the patient on the arm or leg, a calm voice, direct eye contact, and reassurance that the patient will be well cared for can do much to lessen anxiety.
2. Verify that the patient expresses an understanding of the urgent nature of the procedure. Review the consent for accuracy.

3. Preoperative antibiotic therapy may be prescribed. Verify that the drugs have been administered. If already hospitalized, the patient may have been receiving them; note the time of next scheduled dose. Check for patient allergies. Document all perioperative medications. If perforation is likely, the patient may also have a nasogastric tube in place; this will be connected to suction (this will be routine if the patient is undergoing laparoscopic appendectomy).
4. The patient is normally positioned supine with both arms secured on padded armboards at less then 90 degrees. For laparoscopic procedures, Trendelenburg's position will be used for trocar insertion. During admission and positioning, continue to offer comfort measures to lessen anxiety. Consider a brief introduction to other team members and explanations of each event as it is happening.
5. Document the condition of the patient's skin at the site of the ESU dispersive electrode before placement and after removal.
6. Protective barrier towels are placed along the patient's sides. Prepare an area to include the nipples to pubis. Prepare laterally as far as possible. (Note: The area prepared should anticipate the need for a larger incision, which is occasionally necessary. For open procedures, a small incision at McBurney's point is usually all that is required. For laparoscopic procedures, a standard abdominal preparation is performed and the patient draped widely to allow access to the entire abdominal area.) Note the condition of the skin at the preparation site before and after skin preparatory procedures. With laparoscopic appendectomy, plan to assist anesthesia with induction and then insert an indwelling urinary catheter.
7. A culture may be taken of the peritoneum, the appendix, or both. Obtain the correct culture tube. Use universal precautions in handling cultures and document them.
8. Some surgeons isolate instruments used in amputating the appendix and sealing the appendiceal stump; prepare a discard basin (as appropriate).
9. Check with the surgeon to properly classify the wound, based on whether the appendix is intact or ruptured.
10. Ascertain the surgeon's requirements for preserving the specimen obtained. Follow institutional policy for labeling, preserving, and delivering tissue for permanent pathologic sections.
11. Follow institutional protocol for performing and recording sponge, sharp, and instrument counts.

FIG. 8-5
CARE PLAN FOR APPENDECTOMY

KEY ASSESSMENT POINTS

Patient knowledge about current condition, anticipated sequence of events

History of last oral intake, frequency of nausea/vomiting, anorexia

Laboratory results for electrolyte imbalance, leukocytosis (shift to the left of neutrophils)

Pain assessment (right iliac fossa [RIF] tenderness or rebound tenderness in RIF; migratory RIF pain)

Elevated temperature

NURSING DIAGNOSIS

All generic nursing diagnoses apply to this patient, with the addition of:

Anxiety

PATIENT OUTCOMES

All generic patient outcomes apply, with the addition of:

The patient will exhibit a reduced level of anxiety by:

1. Displaying relaxed facial expressions
2. Verbalizing less anxiety (or fear)
3. Accurately describing perioperative events

NURSING ACTIONS

	Yes	No	N/A
1. Preop assessment performed?	☐	☐	☐
Consent checked?	☐	☐	☐
2. Urgent nature of procedure explained/understood?	☐	☐	☐
3. Antibiotics given as prescribed?	☐	☐	☐
4. Positioned correctly?	☐	☐	☐
5. ESU dispersive pad site assessed (on application and removal)?	☐	☐	☐
6. Skin prep per institutional protocol?	☐	☐	☐
7. Cultures to lab?	☐	☐	☐
8. Protocol for clean contaminated/contaminated wound initiated?	☐	☐	☐
9. Wound classified?	☐	☐	☐
10. Specimens to lab?	☐	☐	☐
11. Counts performed and correct?	☐	☐	☐
12. Drains noted?	☐	☐	☐
13. Dressings applied?	☐	☐	☐
14. Postop report given?	☐	☐	☐
15. Other generic care plans initiated? (specify)	☐	☐	☐

Document additional nursing actions/generic care plans initiated here:

_____

_____

_____

EVALUATION OF PATIENT OUTCOMES

1. The patient's anxiety was reduced.
2. The patient met outcomes for additional generic outcomes as indicated.

	Outcome met	Outcome met with additional outcome criteria	Outcome met with revised nursing care plan	Outcome not met	Outcome not applicable to this patient
1.	☐	☐	☐	☐	☐
2.	☐	☐	☐	☐	☐

Signature: _____ Date: _____

12. If the appendix has ruptured, a drain will be placed in the peritoneal cavity. Note the type of drain and devices used to secure it.

13. Clean the skin of preparation solution and apply dressing to prevent "tape burns." Allow for normal postoperative swelling to occur without stretching of the skin underneath the tape. If the appendix has ruptured, the wound may be left open and packed with gauze for wet-to-dry soaks.

Splenectomy (Fig. 8-6)

1. The spleen is located in the left upper quadrant of the abdomen. In adults, its four main functions are to store red blood cells, destroy old red blood cells and platelets, produce antibodies, and filter microorganisms from the blood. It is not ordinarily palpable, being soft and located in the retroperitoneal space. If it is palpable, it is probably enlarged. The spleen may be surgically removed to treat various blood dyscrasias, such as idiopathic thrombocytopenic purpura. It can be injured by retraction during abdominal surgery or ruptured by trauma. A patient with a history of blunt trauma to the left upper quadrant, abdominal pain referred to the left shoulder (Kehr's sign), and hypotension, syncope, or increased dyspnea will have x-ray studies done to verify an enlarged spleen. In completing a nursing assessment, consider the risk for knowledge deficit, anxiety (or fear), infection, or other diagnoses based on the need for splenectomy (for example, thrombocytopenia, or Hodgkin's disease). Modify the care plan accordingly. Since removal of the spleen leaves the patient at increased risk for developing systemic infections (due to the absence of macrophage and lymphocyte activity), discharge teaching should address preventive measures.

2. If the outcome goal established for preventing altered tissue perfusion (hemorrhage, thrombosis) is to be used, then important laboratory values (thrombocyte level, electrolytes, hemoglobin and hematocrit, and bleeding and clotting times) and baseline vital sign determinations need to be reviewed.

3. When assisting with transfer to the OR bed, provide special handling and positioning of other injuries if this is a trauma patient.

4. The patient is positioned supine with both arms secured on padded armboards at less than 90 degrees. The side rails of the OR bed are kept clear to allow the use of a table-mounted retractor.

5. Sequential compression stockings are applied before induction. Emergent patients may undergo rapid sequence induction; assist the anes-

thesia provider and be prepared to apply cricoid pressure if required.

6. Note the skin condition at the dispersive electrode site before and after pad application.

7. Protective barriers are placed at the patient's bedsides before prepping. Prepare an area to include the nipples to pubis, extending laterally as far as possible (usually to bedline). Assess the condition of the skin at the preparation site before and after preparatory procedures; note bruising, petechiae, and ecchymoses.

8. Because the spleen stores blood, dissection may involve oozing surfaces or frank bleeding. Prepare an autologous blood transfuser or reservoir as requested. Have hemostatic agents in the room (such as microcrystalline collagen, hemostatic sponge). Have blood, blood products, and a blood warmer readily available. Some surgeons may attempt to salvage the spleen using various mesh materials to achieve hemostasis; have these in the room as requested. Anticipate the need for additional large sponges for packing.

9. The spleen will be sent to the pathology department. Anticipate the possibility of accessory spleen removal in hypersplenic patients. Follow institutional policy for labeling, preserving, and delivering tissue for permanent pathologic sections.

10. Clean preparation solution from the patient's skin before the dressing is applied. Apply dressing to prevent "tape burns." Allow for normal postoperative swelling to occur without stretching of the skin underneath the tape.

11. Drainage is usually only required if there was excessive bleeding or if clotting abnormalities exist. If a drain is inserted, note its presence and method of fixation.

12. Follow institutional protocol for performing and recording sponge, sharp, and instrument counts. Assist as needed with emergence and extubation, then accompany the patient to PACU.

Gastrectomy (Fig. 8-7)

1. Part or all of the stomach may be removed as treatment for gastric carcinoma or ulcer disease, or as part of another procedure such as pancreatoduodenectomy. Depending on the etiology of the patient's disease, there may be nutritional deficits. Significant weight loss and an albumin level below 3 g can impair wound healing and lead to the risk of infection. The patient may be admitted in advance of surgery to correct nutritional deficiencies via parenteral nutrition. Anxiety related to unfamiliar environment; anticipated changes in usual life-style, roles, or

FIG. 8-6
CARE PLAN FOR SPLENECTOMY

KEY ASSESSMENT POINTS

History of blunt trauma
Signs/symptoms of hemorrhage/shock (hypotension, dyspnea, syncope, tachycardia, pallor, diaphoresis)
Abdominal pain, positive Kehr's sign
Expanding mass in left upper quadrant
Lab values (thrombocytes, electrolytes, bleeding time, H&H)
Results of diagnostic studies (CT scan, spleen scan, ultrasound)
Patient knowledge of planned procedure and response

NURSING DIAGNOSIS

All generic nursing diagnoses apply to this patient, with the addition of:
  High risk for fluid volume deficit

PATIENT OUTCOMES

All generic patient outcomes apply, with the addition of:
There will be no signs of fluid volume deficit from hemorrhage as evidenced by:
1. Vital signs that remain within baseline norms
2. An incision site that is dry on discharge to PACU
3. Laboratory values (H & H/bleeding time) that remain within safe limits during the intraoperative period
4. Skin and mucous membranes have a natural color, and are warm and moist

NURSING ACTIONS

	Yes	No	N/A
1. Preop assessment performed?	☐	☐	☐
Consent checked?	☐	☐	☐
Urgent nature of procedure explained/understood?	☐	☐	☐
2. Lab values reviewed?	☐	☐	☐
3. Protected during transfer to OR bed? (Trauma patient)	☐	☐	☐
4. Positioned correctly?	☐	☐	☐
5. Sequential decompression stockings applied?	☐	☐	☐
6. ESU dispersive pad site assessed (on application and removal)?	☐	☐	☐
7. Skin prep per institutional protocol?	☐	☐	☐
Skin at prep site assessed?	☐	☐	☐
8. Autologous transfusion/blood products, hemostatic devices available?	☐	☐	☐
9. Specimen to lab?	☐	☐	☐
10. Dressings applied?	☐	☐	☐
11. Drains noted?	☐	☐	☐
12. Counts performed and correct?	☐	☐	☐
13. Postop report given?	☐	☐	☐
14. Other generic care plans initiated? (specify)	☐	☐	☐

Document additional nursing actions/generic care plans initiated here:

_____

_____

_____

EVALUATION OF PATIENT OUTCOMES

	Outcome met	Outcome met with additional outcome criteria	Outcome met with revised nursing care plan	Outcome not met	Outcome not applicable to this patient
1. There were no signs of fluid volume deficit/bleeding.	☐	☐	☐	☐	☐
2. The patient met outcomes for additional generic care plans as indicated.	☐	☐	☐	☐	☐

Signature: _____ Date: _____

FIG. 8-7
CARE PLAN FOR GASTRECTOMY

KEY ASSESSMENT POINTS

Nutritional status

Pain: heartburn/dyspepsia; relation of pain to ingestion of food; location of pain; relief of pain; use of ulcerogenic substances (ASA, NSAIDS, alcohol)

Results of diagnostic studies (endoscopy, upper GI, gastric analysis, gastric cytology)

Laboratory results (anemia, gastrin levels, positive guaiac in stool)

Current medications

Patient knowledge of planned procedure/response

NURSING DIAGNOSIS

All generic nursing diagnoses apply to this patient, with the addition of:

Anxiety

PATIENT OUTCOMES

All generic patient outcomes apply, with the addition of:
The patient will exhibit a reduced level of anxiety by:
1. Displaying relaxed facial expressions
2. Verbalizing less anxiety (or fear)
3. Accurately describing perioperative events

NURSING ACTIONS

	Yes	No	N/A
1. Preop assessment performed?	☐	☐	☐
Consent checked?	☐	☐	☐
Nature of procedure explained/understood?	☐	☐	☐
2. Postop nasogastric tube/feeding jejunostomy/ urinary catheter explained?	☐	☐	☐
3. Antibiotics ordered/available?	☐	☐	☐
4. GI prep ordered/performed?	☐	☐	☐
5. Urinary catheter inserted?	☐	☐	☐
Sequential compression stockings applied?	☐	☐	☐
6. Positioned correctly?	☐	☐	☐
7. Measures to maintain normothermia initiated?	☐	☐	☐
8. ESU dispersive pad site assessed (on application and removal)?	☐	☐	☐
9. Skin prep per institutional protocol?	☐	☐	☐
Skin at prep site assessed?	☐	☐	☐
10. Special supplies available?	☐	☐	☐
11. Counts performed and correct?	☐	☐	☐
12. Protocol for clean contaminated/contaminated wound initiated?	☐	☐	☐
13. Wound classified?	☐	☐	☐
14. Output from nasogastric tube/urinary catheter recorded?	☐	☐	☐
15. Specimen to lab?	☐	☐	☐
16. Drains noted?	☐	☐	☐
17. Dressings applied?	☐	☐	☐
18. Postop report given?	☐	☐	☐
19. Other generic care plan initiated? (specify)	☐	☐	☐

Document additional nursing actions/generic care plans initiated here:

_____

_____

_____

EVALUATION OF PATIENT OUTCOMES

	Outcome met	Outcome met with additional outcome criteria	Outcome met with revised nursing care plan	Outcome not met	Outcome not applicable to this patient
1. The patient's anxiety was reduced.	☐	☐	☐	☐	☐
2. The patient met outcomes for additional generic care plans as indicated.	☐	☐	☐	☐	☐

Signature: _____ Date: _____

both; death; diagnosis; prognosis; and postoperative pain may be characteristic for this patient. Assess the patient's ability to cope, anxiety level, perception of diagnosis, and perception of change in body image. Assist the patient with anxiety-relieving techniques.

2. Explain to the patient that a nasogastric tube and urinary catheter will be in place postoperatively. A feeding jejunostomy tube is usually inserted to allow anastomoses to heal while providing nutrition; explain the appearance and function of this tube. Total gastrectomy requires esophagojejunostomy; a thoracotomy may be required since the anastomosis is high in the chest. These patients need to be prepared for two incisions (midline abdominal and thoracotomy) and for postoperative chest tubes.

3. Prophylactic antibiotic therapy and heparin therapy will likely be prescribed. Check that these have been administered. Antiembolism stockings may be in place or will be placed in the OR.

4. Preoperative mechanical preparation of the gastrointestinal tract is usually ordered; verify on the medical record that this has been done.

5. A urinary catheter will be inserted preoperatively or immediately following induction. Use aseptic technique for catheter insertion. Place drainage bag (with urimeter, as appropriate) where it is readily observable. Document catheter insertion.

6. Preoperative assessment will have indicated whether the patient's size affects planning for positioning. Obese patients may require special positioning (and instrumentation) considerations, as may the thin, emaciated patient. Prepare the OR bed before the patient is moved onto it. Assist with patient transfer onto the OR bed and position the patient supine with arms secured on padded armboards at less than 90 degrees. A central venous pressure line may be inserted at this time. Reverse Trendelenburg's position is often used during surgery for better exposure; a padded footboard may be placed at right angles to the OR bed.

7. A thermia blanket, thermal drapes, or forced warm air blanket may be used to maintain normothermia. Warm irrigation and intravenous solutions and blood are used when appropriate to help the patient maintain a stable body temperature.

8. Document the condition of the patient's skin at the site of the ESU dispersive electrode before placement and after removal.

9. Place protective barriers at the patient's side and prepare an area that includes the nipples to upper thighs, including the pubis. Prepare laterally as far as possible (usually to the bedline). Note the condition of the patient's skin before and after skin preparatory procedures. Keep the side rails of the OR bed clear to allow placement of a table-mounted retractor.

10. Special supplies, such as stapling instruments, clips for vagotomy, and an endoscope, should be in the room. In a two-part procedure (that is, an abdominal approach followed by thoracotomy), a vacuum pack (beanbag) preplaced on the OR bed, along with pillows, a lateral arm holder, an axillary roll, and other positioning devices will be required for repositioning. A separate instrument table may be used for the thoracotomy, or chest instruments may be added to the abdominal setup. Warm the room as abdominal closure is done for repositioning and reprepping.

11. Follow institutional protocol for counts of multiple instrument sets, if appropriate.

12. Initiate institutional protocol for clean contaminated/contaminated wound protocol. Instruments coming into contact with the gastrointestinal mucosa are isolated in this protocol.

13. Accurate surgical wound classification assists in infection control surveillance procedures.

14. Record output from the nasogastric tube and indwelling urinary catheter.

15. Ascertain the surgeon's requirements for preserving the specimen obtained. Follow institutional policy for labeling, preserving, and delivering tissue for frozen sections, estrogen/progesterone receptors, and permanent pathologic sections.

16. Document the presence of drains and drainage tubes.

17. Apply dressing to prevent "tape burns." Allow for normal postoperative swelling to occur without stretching of the skin underneath the tape. Remain at the patient's side during emergence and extubation. A bed from the patient care unit may be used to avoid multiple patient transfers; a trapeze added to the bed will assist the patient with positional changes when fully awake.

Emergency Small Bowel Resection (Fig. 8-8)

1. An untreated small bowel obstruction will result in death; thus, this patient is a true emergency. As bowel contents pool, unable to be propelled past the obstruction, the bowel wall distends. Continued contractions cause edema of the bowel wall, adding to the accumulating fluid. The more edematous the wall becomes, the less it can absorb, adding to distention (Fig. 8-9). The increasing pressure causes ischemia of the bowel wall and further edema, leading to

FIG. 8-8
CARE PLAN FOR EMERGENCY SMALL BOWEL RESECTION

KEY ASSESSMENT POINTS

Signs/symptoms of hypovolemia, septic shock
Skin turgor
Vomiting
Pain
Bowel sounds
History of previous bowel disorder, abdominal surgery
Respiratory status
Results of diagnostic studies (endoscopy, barium enema/swallow, flat plate)
Laboratory results (blood urea nitrogen [BUN], electrolytes, H&H, acid-base balance)
Patient knowledge of planned procedure/response

NURSING DIAGNOSIS

All generic nursing diagnoses apply to this patient, with the addition of:
  Anxiety

PATIENT OUTCOMES

All generic patient outcomes apply, with the addition of:
The patient will exhibit a reduced level of anxiety by:
  1. Perceiving threat of emergency surgery realistically
  2. Verbalizing less anxiety (or fear)
  3. Accurately describing immediate perioperative events

NURSING ACTIONS

	Yes	No	N/A
1. Preop assessment performed?	☐	☐	☐
2. Urgent nature of procedure explained/understood?	☐	☐	☐
Caring behaviors initiated?	☐	☐	☐
3. Consent checked?	☐	☐	☐
4. Antibiotics ordered/available?	☐	☐	☐
5. Positioned correctly?	☐	☐	☐
6. Assistance to anesthesia provider given?	☐	☐	☐
7. ESU dispersive pad site assessed (on application and removal)?	☐	☐	☐
8. Urinary catheter inserted?	☐	☐	☐
Sequential compression stockings applied?	☐	☐	☐
9. Blood/blood products available?	☐	☐	☐
10. Skin prep per institutional protocol?	☐	☐	☐
Skin at prep site assessed?	☐	☐	☐
11. Cultures to lab?	☐	☐	☐
12. Priority supplies/accessories immediately available?	☐	☐	☐
13. Specimen to lab?	☐	☐	☐
14. Output recorded?	☐	☐	☐
15. Wound classified?	☐	☐	☐
Protocol for clean contaminated/contaminated wound initiated?	☐	☐	☐
16. Counts performed and correct?	☐	☐	☐
17. Drains noted?	☐	☐	☐
18. Dressings applied?	☐	☐	☐
19. Postop report given?	☐	☐	☐
Monitors, oxygen, etc., available for transport?	☐	☐	☐
20. Other generic care plans initiated? (specify)	☐	☐	☐

Document additional nursing actions/generic care plans initiated here:

_____

_____

_____

EVALUATION OF PATIENT OUTCOMES

	Outcome met	Outcome met with additional outcome criteria	Outcome met with revised nursing care plan	Outcome not met	Outcome not applicable to this patient
1. The patient's anxiety level was reduced.	☐	☐	☐	☐	☐
2. The patient met outcomes for additional generic care plans as indicated.	☐	☐	☐	☐	☐

Signature: _____ Date: _____

Table 8-5 *Comparison of symptoms in intestinal obstruction*

Obstruction	Vomiting	Distention	Oliguria	Pain
High small intestine	Occurs early and is severe; emesis is light green and copious; nonfecal odor	Appears late; limited to epigastric area	Present as a result of loss of fluid	Severe; upper quadrants
Low small intestine	Delayed; dark green color; may have fecal odor	Diffuse across abdomen	Less likely to occur	Severe; periumbilical

From: Principles and Practices of Adult Health Nursing; Beare PG, Myers JL, 2nd Ed. p. 1874, St. Louis, Mosby.

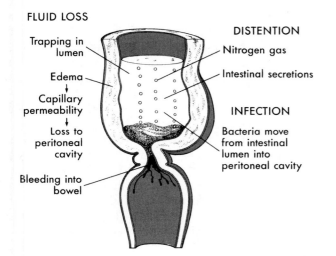

Fig. 8-9. Pathophysiologic events in intestinal obstruction.

bowel wall necrosis and, ultimately, perforation, peritonitis, and septic shock (Table 8-5). The accompanying vomiting, bowel wall edema, and increased bowel secretions lead to dehydration and eventual hypovolemic shock. The nursing diagnosis, *fluid volume deficit*, must be considered; before surgery, fluid losses must be replaced and distention relieved by nasogastric or mercury-tipped intestinal tubes. Passing the latter takes time; the surgeon may opt to decompress the bowel during surgery.

2. The patient who presents for emergency small bowel resection is likely to be very ill, anxious, and frightened. Assess the patient's level of anxiety; anxiety interferes with learning ability, so explanations should be brief and specific (use short, simple sentences; provide factual information relating to immediate events; maintain a calm, unhurried manner). Help the patient to diminish anxious feelings by communicating caring behaviors; call the patient by name, touch the arm or leg, move close and use a soft, gentle voice.

3. Emergency surgery still requires a properly witnessed and signed consent. If the patient is unable to give consent, follow institutional protocol for obtaining consent for emergency surgery.

4. Prophylactic antibiotic therapy may be prescribed. Check to see that these have been given and when the next dose is due. Verify that intraoperative antibiotics are available, correct, and in the right dosage, and that the patient does not have an allergy to the prescribed medication. Document all intraoperative medications given.

5. The patient is admitted to the OR room and positioned supine.

6. Place the ESU pad; document the condition of the patient's skin at the site of the dispersive pad before placement and after removal.

7. Insert an indwelling urinary catheter if one is not already present. Place the bag where it is readily observable. Document the catheter insertion and note any other tubes present on arrival in the OR.

8. Assist the anesthesia provider with induction and intubation, with setting up intravenous lines, and with administering emergency drugs.

9. Verify that blood/blood products are available. Prepare the blood warmer.

10. Perform skin preparation. Cover the patient's upper chest and arms and mid-thighs to feet with warm blankets, or use a warming device, to assist in maintaining normothermia. Prepare an area from the nipples to the upper thighs, including the pubis. Prepare laterally as far as possible. Note the condition of the patient's skin at the preparation site before and after preparation.

11. Peritoneal cultures may be done as soon as the abdomen is opened. Large amounts of peritoneal fluid may be suctioned; monitor fluid loss and anticipate the need to switch suction canisters. Use universal precautions in handling specimens and document their acquisition.

12. Supplies and accessories that need to be immediately available include decompression tubes, staplers, and extra sponges.
13. Ascertain the surgeon's requirements for preserving the specimen obtained. Follow institutional policy for labeling, preserving, and delivering tissue for frozen sections and permanent pathologic sections.
14. Document urine output as well as output from the nasogastric tube. Note output if and when the small bowel is decompressed.
15. Classification of the surgical wound is important for accurate infection control surveillance.
16. Follow institutional protocol for sponge, sharp, and instrument counts.
17. Note the presence of any drains.
18. Apply dressing to prevent "tape burns." Allow for normal postoperative swelling to occur without stretching of the skin underneath the tape. If the patient is going to the intensive care unit (ICU), send for the unit bed and necessary transport equipment. Report is often called to the ICU nurse. Extubation may not be done until the patient is stable. Assist in readying the patient for transport to the ICU; accompany anesthesia providers as required.

Hemicolectomy (Fig. 8-10)

1. Resection of the large intestine may be done for inflammatory diseases (diverticulosis, ulcerative colitis, Crohn's disease), premalignant conditions, or carcinoma; it may be laparoscopically assisted, which is not described in this care plan. The procedure may occur as part of a carcinoembryonic antigen (CEA)-directed "second look" procedure to resect recurrent tumor. If obstruction is present or inflammatory disease is extensive, the surgeon may opt to perform a colostomy if primary anastomosis cannot be done. A colostomy may also be done as a permanent fecal diversion. Assess and classify the patient's level of anxiety (mild, moderate, or severe) and concern over altered body image. Determine if knowledge deficits are contributing to the anxiety. Demonstrate nursing behaviors that indicate caring, such as holding the patient's hand, asking about comfort levels, calling the patient by name, and introducing yourself. If a colostomy is planned, the patient should have been seen by an enterostomal nurse specialist to have an appropriate stoma site marked; note whether this has been done. Collaborate with other members of the patient care team in seeing that available community resources have been discussed with the patient.
2. Explain to the patient that a nasogastric tube, indwelling urinary catheter, and sequential decompression stockings will be in place postoperatively. Verify that the patient understands the functions of these tubes/devices. For the patient who will have an ostomy, explanation regarding peristomal skin care, pouch application, pouch removal, and irrigation should be undertaken.
3. Assess the effectiveness of preoperative bowel preparation. Ineffective preparation raises the risk of postoperative infection.
4. Prophylactic antibiotic therapy will be prescribed; Nelson (1991) suggests that when the parenteral antibiotics are administered 16 to 60 minutes preoperatively, the incidence of wound infection is lower. Antibiotics may also be used in irrigating solution. Check that the drug and dosage available is as ordered. Always check for patient allergies before administering an antibiotic and document all medications given.
5. Prepare the OR bed before the patient is moved onto it. For abdominal incisions, the most common practice is for the OR bed to remain flat. The neck should be slightly flexed and the head resting on a small pillow. To prevent compression of subclavian arteries, the head should not be turned to either side. Align and secure the arms and hands properly. When the arms are placed at the patient's side, avoid compression on the ulnar, median, or radial nerves. When using padded armboards, the angle should be less than 90 degrees to prevent brachial plexus injury secondary to hyperabduction of the arm. Recheck armboard position if the patient is repositioned for any reason. Place the knee strap about 2 inches above the knee. Place the strap securely but not too tightly to avoid compression of the popliteal space. Monitor the position of the Mayo tray over the patient throughout the procedure so that no body part, such as the toes, are compressed.

   If a low anterior resection is planned, the patient is placed in low lithotomy using stirrups; protect vascular and neural structures to prevent positioning injury with stirrups. Apply sequential stockings before induction; remain with the anesthesia provider during intubation, assisting as required.
6. Use aseptic technique for the insertion of indwelling urinary catheters. Document catheter insertion. Place the drainage bag (with urimeter, as appropriate) where it is readily observable.
7. Document the condition of the patient's skin at site of the dispersive electrode before placement and after removal.
8. Place protective barrier towels along the pa-

FIG. 8-10
CARE PLAN FOR HEMICOLECTOMY

KEY ASSESSMENT POINTS

Nutritional status
Knowledge of disease process, possible ostomy
Planned stoma location
Support systems/coping abilities
Pain
Bowel elimination patterns
History of previous bowel disorder, abdominal surgery
Current medications/allergies
Skin integrity
Results of diagnostic studies
Laboratory results (electrolytes, albumin levels)
Patient knowledge of planned procedure/response

NURSING DIAGNOSIS

All generic nursing diagnoses apply to this patient, with the addition of:
  Anxiety

PATIENT OUTCOMES

All generic patient outcomes apply, with the addition of:
The patient will exhibit a reduced level of anxiety by:
  1. Displaying relaxed facial expressions
  2. Verbalizing less anxiety (or fear)
  3. Accurately describing perioperative events

NURSING ACTIONS

	Yes	No	N/A
1. Preop assessment performed?	☐	☐	☐
Consent signed?	☐	☐	☐
Caring behaviors initiated?	☐	☐	☐
Stoma site marked?	☐	☐	☐
2. NG tube/urinary catheter/sequential compression stockings explained?	☐	☐	☐
Stoma care explained?	☐	☐	☐
3. Bowel prep effective?	☐	☐	☐
4. Antibiotics ordered/available?	☐	☐	☐
5. Positioned correctly?	☐	☐	☐
6. Urinary catheter inserted?	☐	☐	☐
7. ESU dispersive pad site assessed (on application and removal)?	☐	☐	☐
8. Skin prep per institutional protocol?	☐	☐	☐
Skin at prep site assessed?	☐	☐	☐
9. Measures to maintain normothermia initiated?	☐	☐	☐
10. Counts performed and correct?	☐	☐	☐
11. Specimens/cultures to lab?	☐	☐	☐
12. Output recorded?	☐	☐	☐
13. Protocol for clean contaminated/contaminated wound initiated?	☐	☐	☐
Wound classified?	☐	☐	☐
14. Dressings applied?	☐	☐	☐
15. Drains noted?	☐	☐	☐
16. Postop report given?	☐	☐	☐
17. Other generic care plans initiated? (specify)	☐	☐	☐

Document additional nursing actions/generic care plans initiated here:

_____

_____

_____

EVALUATION OF PATIENT OUTCOMES

	Outcome met	Outcome met with additional outcome criteria	Outcome met with revised nursing care plan	Outcome not met	Outcome not applicable to this patient
1. The patient's anxiety was reduced.	☐	☐	☐	☐	☐
2. The patient met outcomes for additional generic care plans as indicated.	☐	☐	☐	☐	☐

Signature: _____ Date: _____

tient's sides, then prepare an area that includes the nipples to pubis and laterally as far as possible. Note the condition of the skin (nicks, abrasions, rashes) before and after skin preparation procedures.

9. Warm irrigation and intravenous solutions when appropriate to help the patient maintain a stable body temperature. Use a blood warmer for blood products and document its use. Additional measures to keep the patient normothermic include covering the patient's upper chest and arms and mid-thighs to feet using warm blankets, thermal drapes, or forced warm air blankets. Expose only the body surface necessary to prepare the patient. The room temperature may be increased.

10. Follow institutional procedures for counts if the procedure requires more than a single setup.

11. Ascertain the surgeon's requirements for preserving the specimen; frozen sections may be done to check for metastases. Cultures may be obtained. Use universal precautions when handling cultures/specimens. Follow institutional protocol for documenting and delivering cultures or tissue for frozen sections and permanent pathologic sections.

12. Record all output from nasogastric tube, urinary catheter, and other drainage tubes.

13. Follow institutional policy, if applicable, for closure of a clean/contaminated or contaminated wound (bowel technique).

14. Apply dressing to prevent "tape burns." Allow for normal postoperative swelling to occur without tension on the skin underneath the tape.

15. Note the presence of any drains.

16. Assist the anesthesia provider with extubation, apply warm blankets to the patient, then accompany the patient to the PACU.

Abdominal Perineal Resection (Fig. 8-11)

1. The nursing diagnosis of *anxiety* may be related to an unfamiliar environment; anticipated changes in usual life-style, roles, or both; fear of death; diagnosis of cancer; prognosis; or postoperative pain. The potential for change in body image is very real with this surgical procedure, and it has implications for adversely affecting interpersonal relationships with significant others. Gather data regarding the patient's coping mechanisms. Note alterations in effective coping and lack of adequate support systems. Assess the patient for signs and symptoms of anxiety. Allow additional time with the patient to develop a trusting relationship. Verify the patient's understanding of the following: the planned surgical intervention; fears and misconceptions regarding the diagnosis and/or prognosis; previous experiences with cancer, hospitalizations, and surgery; and feelings of decreased self-worth, powerlessness, or disruptions in relationships with significant others. Based on the nursing assessment, implement a care plan for knowledge deficit. Use nursing measures that communicate caring. Encourage the patient to verbalize feelings. Reinforce positive feelings and accurate perceptions. Clarify misconceptions. Allow the patient as much control as possible by giving choices whenever you can and including the patient and significant others in postoperative planning.

2. Verify the stoma site marked by the enterostomal therapy nurse. Assess and document the condition of the skin at the stoma site. Determine the patient's level of understanding and emotional acceptance of the permanent alteration in bowel function.

3. A nasogastric tube will be inserted intraoperatively if it is not already in place. Verify that the patient knows and understands about the nasogastric tube.

4. Because of the potential for a spill of bowel contents into the peritoneal cavity, antibiotics will likely be ordered. Compare the drug name and dosage with the physician's order. Document medications administered. Check patient allergies.

5. Assess the effectiveness of the preoperative bowel preparation. Ineffective preparation raises the risk of postoperative infection.

6. Prepare the OR bed before the patient is moved onto it; a half-size warming blanket may be used. For abdominal incisions, the most common practice is for the OR bed to remain flat. The neck should be slightly flexed and the head should rest on a small pillow. To prevent compression of subclavian arteries, the head should not be turned to either side. The lithotomy position can result in nerve, fascial, or muscle injury as tissue is stretched or compressed. Hyperflexion of the hip or excess external rotation can damage sciatic and femoral nerves. When positioning the patient in lithotomy, secure enough personnel to raise and lower both legs simultaneously, supporting the foot with one hand and the leg just under the knee with the other. Do not allow the hip to abduct excessively. If metal stirrups are used, prevent them from coming in contact with the skin. To prevent injury to the brachial plexus, shoulder, finger, or elbow joints and nerves, place the arms across the chest when moving the patient. Place the arms on arm boards at a 10- to 15-degree angle from the

FIG. 8-11
CARE PLAN FOR ABDOMINAL PERINEAL RESECTION

KEY ASSESSMENT POINTS

Nutritional status
Level of anxiety
Planned stoma location
Support systems/coping abilities
Limitations in mobility
History of knee/hip prosthesis
Current medications/allergies
Skin integrity
Results of diagnostic studies, laboratory results
Level of home care planning (ostomy care, management of frequently encountered problems, dietary considerations)
Patient knowledge of planned procedure/response

NURSING DIAGNOSIS

All generic nursing diagnoses apply to this patient, with the addition of:
    Anxiety
    (Consider additional nursing diagnoses based on results of nursing psychosocial assessment.)

PATIENT OUTCOMES

All generic patient outcomes apply, with the addition of:
The patient will exhibit a reduced level of anxiety by:
1. Displaying relaxed facial expressions
2. Verbalizing less anxiety (or fear)
3. Accurately describing perioperative events

NURSING ACTIONS

	Yes	No	N/A
1. Preop assessment performed?	☐	☐	☐
Consent signed?	☐	☐	☐
Caring behaviors initiated?	☐	☐	☐
2. Stoma site marked?	☐	☐	☐
3. Nasogastric tube/urinary catheter explained?	☐	☐	☐
4. Antibiotics ordered/available?	☐	☐	☐
5. Bowel prep effective?	☐	☐	☐
6. Positioned correctly?	☐	☐	☐
7. Urinary catheter inserted?	☐	☐	☐
8. Skin prep per institutional protocol?	☐	☐	☐
Skin at prep site assessed?	☐	☐	☐
9. ESU dispersive pad site assessed (on application and removal)?	☐	☐	☐
10. Measures to maintain normothermia initiated?	☐	☐	☐
11. Counts performed and correct?	☐	☐	☐
12. Specimens to lab?	☐	☐	☐
13. Output recorded?	☐	☐	☐
14. Protocol for clean contaminated/contaminated wound initiated?	☐	☐	☐
Wound classified?	☐	☐	☐
15. Drains/tubes noted?	☐	☐	☐
16. Ostomy appliance secure?	☐	☐	☐
17. Dressings applied?	☐	☐	☐
18. Patient returned to supine position safely?	☐	☐	☐
19. Other generic care plans initiated? (specify)	☐	☐	☐

Document additional nursing actions/generic care plans initiated here:

_____

_____

_____

EVALUATION OF PATIENT OUTCOMES

	Outcome met	Outcome met with additional outcome criteria	Outcome met with revised nursing care plan	Outcome not met	Outcome not applicable to this patient
1. The patient's anxiety was reduced.	☐	☐	☐	☐	☐
2. The patient met outcomes for additional generic care plans as indicated.	☐	☐	☐	☐	☐

Signature: _____ Date: _____

OR bed when the move is complete so respiration is not depressed. Sequential support stockings are applied once the patient is on the OR bed. Once the legs are in the stirrups, be sure they are symmetrically positioned. The buttocks should not extend beyond the break of the table. Pad the sacrum. The calves should be parallel to the table. If additional exposure is required, flexion should be done at the hip, not the knee. Awake positioning should be considered for the patient with severe arthritis or hip/knee prostheses (Graling & Colvin, 1992). Monitor the position in which the operating team stands so that no one leans on the inner aspect of the patient's thigh; compression of the knee or calf by leaning on the patient can compress the saphenous nerve against the tibia. Immoderate abduction of the thighs with external rotation of the hips can cause a femoral neuropathy. In the groin, the obturator nerve can also be placed under tension in this way.

7. Use aseptic technique to insert the indwelling urinary catheter. Place the drainage bag so that it is readily observable.

8. A full abdominal preparation should be done, including the nipples and pubis to mid-thighs. Prepare laterally as far as possible. For the perineal resection, preparation should include the pubis, bilateral groins, perineum, lateral and medial aspects of the thighs to mid-thighs, and buttocks. Care should be taken to avoid washing off any marks made preoperatively to designate the stoma site. Note the condition of the skin (nicks, abrasions, rashes) at the preparation site before and after preparatory procedures.

9. The ESU dispersive pad is placed after positioning is completed to avoid tenting of the pad or poor contact. Note skin condition at the placement site before placement and after removal.

10. Warm irrigation solutions and intravenous fluids when appropriate to help the patient maintain a stable body temperature. Use a blood warmer for blood products and document its use. Thermal drapes, forced warm air blankets, and warming the room until draping is completed also assist the patient in maintaining normothermia.

11. Follow institutional procedures for counts when the procedure requires multiple incisions or when more than one setup will be used.

12. Ascertain the surgeon's requirements for preserving the specimen obtained. Follow institutional policy for labeling, preserving, and delivering tissue for frozen sections, estrogen/progesterone receptors, and permanent pathologic sections. Use universal precautions when handling specimens.

13. Record urinary output and output from the nasogastric tube.

14. Follow institutional policy, if applicable, for closure of a clean/contaminated or contaminated wound.

15. Document the presence of tubes and drains.

16. Clean and prepare the skin at the stoma site appropriately before applying the ostomy appliance. The appliance should be securely attached. As little skin as possible should be exposed to colostomy drainage around the stoma. Apply the stomal appliance securely to prevent bacteria-laden colostomy drainage from coming into contact with the incision.

17. Apply dressing to prevent "tape burns." Allow for normal postoperative swelling to occur without tension on the skin underneath the tape.

18. Slowly return the patient to supine position. Assist with extubation. Cover the patient with warm blankets and accompany the patient to PACU.

References

American College of Physicians. (1993). Guidelines for the treatment of gallstones. *Annals of Internal Medicine, 11*(7), 620-622.

Austen WG. (1992). Presidential address. *ACS Bulletin, 77*, 7-22.

Bichat X. (1814). *Desault's surgery* (Vol. 2) (pp. 301-302). Philadelphia: Thomas Dobson.

Biliary tract disease patient outcomes research team. (1993). AHCPR report HS06481.

Debas HT. (1991). What's new in gastrointestinal and biliary operations. *ACS Bulletin, 76*, 19-22.

Fried GM. (1994). Laparoscopic cholecystectomy. *Scientific American* (Scientific American Surgery, Surgical Technique Suppl. 4),

Full-breast digital mammography. (1994). *Biomedical instrumentation and technology, 28*, 171.

Gonzalez-Cortes SB & Procuniar CE. (1994). Laparoscopic inguinal herniorrhaphy. *AORN Journal, 60*(3), 419-430.

Graling PR & Colvin DB. (1992). The lithotomy position in colon surgery. *AORN Journal, 55*(4), 1029-1039.

Harris JR, et al. (1992). Breast cancer. *New England Journal of Medicine, 7*:473-480.

Hughes KS & Ulmer B. (1994, March). *Breast cancer: Current treatment modalities.* Paper presented at the 1994 AORN Congress, New Orleans.

Hunter JG. (1993, October). *Other laparoscopic procedures: What does the future hold?* Paper presented at Contemporary Forums, New Orleans.

Hynes DM. (1994). The quality of breast cancer care in local communities. *Medical Care, 32*:328-340.

Kalan M, Talbot D, & Cunliffe WJ. (1994). Evaluation of the modified Alvarado score in the diagnosis of acute appendicitis: A prospective study. *Annals of the Royal College of Surgeons of England, 76*, 418-419.

Kifer DJ. (1994). Case management of needle-localized breast biopsy patients. *Seminars in Perioperative Nursing, 3*:46-54.

Kleinbeck SVM & Hoffart N. (1994). Outpatient recovery after laparoscopic cholecystectomy. *AORN Journal 60*(3), 394-402.

Knobf MT. (1994). Treatment options for early stage breast cancer. *Medsurg Nursing, 3:*249-257.

Liechty R & Soper T. (1980). *Synopsis of surgery.* St. Louis: Mosby–Year Book.

Luce M. (1901). The duties of an operating room nurse. *American Journal of Nursing, 1:*404-406.

Martinelli AM & Fontana JL. (1990). Thyroid storm: Potential perioperative crisis. *AORN Journal, 52*(2), 305-313.

Maule WF. (1994). Screening for colorectal cancer by nurse endoscopists. *New England Journal of Medicine, 330*(3), 183-187.

McCallum J. (1903). An improved outfit for operation in a private house. *American Journal of Nursing, 3:*619-621.

Meade R. (1968). *An introduction to the history of general surgery.* Philadelphia: WB Saunders.

Mock V. (1993). Body image in women treated for breast cancer. *Nursing Research, 42:*153-157.

Morris PB, et al. (1992). Outpatient carbon dioxide laser mastectomy. *AORN Journal 55*(4), 984-992.

National Institutes of Health. (1992, September). Gallstones and laparoscopic cholecystectomy: NIH Consensus development conference. *Consensus statement 10*(3), 14-16.

Nelson RL. (1991). Colon and rectal surgery. *ACS Bulletin, 76*(1), 12-14.

Parker SH. (1994, April). *Effectiveness of needle core breast biopsy.* Paper presented at the Society of Cardiovascular and Interventional Radiology, Washington DC.

Pierce PF. (1993). Deciding on breast cancer treatment: A description of decision behavior. *Nursing Research, 42:*22-27.

Royer K. (1994). A case management experience with cholecystectomies. *Seminars in Perioperative Nursing, 3*(1), 3-12.

Senofsky GM, et al. (1990). The predictive value of needle localization mammographically assisted biopsy of the breast. *ACS Bulletin Abstract, 75*(12), 63.

Weeks CS. (1890). *Textbook of nursing.* New York: D Appleton.

Wexler MJ. (1994). Laparoscopic inguinal herniorrhaphy. *Scientific American* (Scientific American Surgery, Surgical Technique Suppl. 5)

Zucher KA, Bailey RW, & Reddick EJ. (1991). *Surgical laparoscopy.* St. Louis: Quality Medical Publishing.

Chapter 9

Neurosurgery

Joann Marshall
Diana L. Wadlund

MEMOIR UPON WOUNDS OF THE HEAD

No subject in surgery has given more employment to the pens of authors, than that of wounds of the head. It would be reasonable to suppose, on reviewing the immense collection of their works, that art had nearly reached perfection on this subject. And yet how distant it is still from it! How many doubts are to be removed, how many uncertainties to be cleared up in the diagnosis, prognosis and treatment! The unfavorable influence of these wounds upon the important organ with whose functions those of all other organs are so intimately connected . . . seem [to obstruct] the path of the practitioner.

BICHAT, 1814

*P*eople with nervous system dysfunction constitute one of the largest groups of patients who use the services of health care institutions. The patient undergoing neurosurgical intervention requires intricate, complex nursing care and persistent, long-term rehabilitative care. Despite more than 180 years since Bichat's time, there remains more to know and discover about the complex neurologic system and its control over other systems. Bichat was also correct in identifying that, in 1814, there was already a body of historical knowledge regarding neurosurgery.

PAST AND PRESENT DEVELOPMENTS

Unraveling the mystery of the human brain and its interrelated nervous system controls and functions has been and continues to be of interest to physicians, scientists, perioperative nurses, and the public at large.

History

There is evidence that trephination was performed in widely separate parts of the world from the earliest times of human civilization. Bullard's account (1987) of the history of this intervention suggests that the creation of holes in the skull was accomplished to treat mania (mental illness), melancholy (depression), headache, and trauma. It was believed that the underlying cause of some of these disorders was an evil spirit or noxious humor; the creation of a hole in the skull allowed the offending cause to escape.

Despite the fact that there was interest in and early documentation of treatment of head injuries, descriptions of the brain and cerebrospinal fluid, epilepsy, spinal cord compression, and the anatomy and physiology of the nervous system, it was not until the late nineteenth century that significant advances were made in neurosurgery. As is generally true in the history of surgery, it was the development of asepsis and anesthesia that heralded progress. In 1884, Godlee first localized and operated on an intracranial tumor. In 1887, Horsely removed a neoplasm from the spinal cord; his pioneering work in the field included stereotactic neurosurgery and treatment of trigeminal neuralgia. Cushing went on to develop the science of neurosurgery to a degree perhaps unparalleled; his contributions were many and profound. The field has continuously progressed, with new knowledge about neurologic anatomy and pathophysiology, diagnostic modalities, the work of neurotransmitters, and the ability to surgically intervene with precision and accuracy constantly being added. These advances have led to important trends in the expansion of neurosurgical perioperative nursing roles and patient management.

Current Influences

During the past 20 to 25 years, there has been an explosion of scientific knowledge that has directly influenced the practice of neurology, neurosurgery, and neurosurgical perioperative nursing. These scientific developments, coupled with changing social forces, have affected the health care delivery system and the practice of nursing. Hickey (1992) has characterized these changes as follows:

- Changing trends in life expectancy and morbidity
- Funding patterns and application of research findings addressing neurologic problems
- Development of sophisticated diagnostic and assessment tools
- Establishment of innovative protocols for patient management
- Development of regional trauma centers, neurologic intensive care facilities, and community resources
- Increased emphasis on rehabilitative services
- Attention to legal and ethical considerations of patient care

Trends. Increased life expectancy has allowed people to develop age-related disorders such as cardiovascular disease (stroke and arteriosclerosis) and degenerative conditions (Parkinson's disease). At the same time, more people are showing signs of occupational disease caused by long-term exposure to environmental chemicals. The central nervous system is very susceptible to cell degeneration; as people live longer, the potential for degenerative nervous system disorders increases. Additionally, the incidence of trauma from motor vehicle accidents, violence, and sports has increased. All of these factors require additional nursing knowledge and skills to meet the changing needs and characteristics of the neurosurgery patient population.

Research. Advances in laboratory investigations have led to research focusing on such neurotransmitters as neuromonamines and amino acids. These transmitters regulate excitatory or inhibitory influences on neuronal activity. Research is ongoing on the changes in cellular activity that occur in response to chemical alterations within neurons and spinal fluid. Such research has as its goal the prevention of irreversible cell damage. Other research focuses on the ability and effects of drugs to cross the blood-brain barrier either to maintain sufficient concentrations or to cause therapeutic changes. Advances in computer systems in research centers have made available a large aggregate of data about selection of treatment protocols. Funding for research to collect data on protocols for brain tumors, spinal cord tumors, head injuries, stroke, and other diseases continues to yield hope and promise for improved patient diagnosis, prognosis, and treatment.

Diagnostic and assessment techniques. Computed tomography (CT) has revolutionized neurodiagnosis (Arbit & Krol, 1994). Introduced in 1974, CT uses the same principle as tomography but additionally employs multiple radiation detectors and a computer to digitize and reconstruct the data. By combining intravenous or intrathecal iodinated contrast material, a high degree of resolution can be obtained. By comparing tissue densities on the screen or hard copy, the radiologist can detect anatomic abnormalities (changes in position, shape, and size, such as atrophy or hypertrophy) and attenuate changes. These changes in density can detect abnormalities such as inflammation, edema, hemorrhage, neoplasms, blood clots, calcium deposits, tissue necrosis, cysts, and abscesses. The introduction of CT has made other diagnostic procedures, such as pneumoencephalograms, obsolete. Magnetic resonance imaging (MRI), an even more promising technique, eliminates exposure to radiation. Using magnetic and radio waves to study cranial and spinal structures, MRI offers even better detail of most intracerebral structures. Both CT and MRI provide detailed information on brain anatomy; the configuration and size of ventricular chambers, midline displacements, herniations, and the position of vascular structures may be determined. For patients with suspected cerebral aneurysms, intraarterial cerebral angiography may be performed. Before the development of CT scanning, cerebral angiography was the primary diagnostic tool for providing information about the lumen of cerebral vessels, their size, and any irregularities such as aneurysms, arteriovenous malformation (AVMs), occlusion, or vascular tumors. However, magnetic resonance angiography (MRA) with three-dimensional gradient echo sequence has become increasingly effective in detecting cerebral an-

---

Box 9-1 Glasgow Coma Scale

Best eye opening response	Spontaneously	4
	To verbal command	3
	To pain	2
	No response	1
Best verbal response	Oriented, converses	5
	Disoriented, converses	4
	Inappropriate words	3
	Incomprehensible sounds	2
	No response	1
Best motor response		
To verbal commands	Obeys	6
To painful stimulus	Localized pain	5
	Flexion—withdrawal	4
	Flexion—decorticate	3
	Extension—decerebrate	2
	No response	1

---

eurysms (Rovit, Murali, & Hirschfeld, 1994). As the quality of images obtained through MRA improves, it may become the investigative study of choice for screening cerebral aneurysms. Similarly, the need for myelography, which provides for visualization of the lumbar, thoracic, and/or cervical area for herniated or ruptured discs, tumor or compression, or congenital anomaly, has decreased with the availability of CT and MRI.

Sophisticated intracranial monitoring devices allow definitive action for the prevention of cerebral anoxia, ischemia, and irreversible brain damage. Other assessment techniques, such as Botterell's scale for categorization of patients following intracranial bleeds, have aided the surgeon in selecting the most advantageous time for surgery, thus improving survival rates. The Glasgow coma scale is a standardized method of assessing levels of consciousness. The scale (Box 9-1) grades the best motor, verbal, and eye-opening responses to verbal or painful stimuli, eliminating the use of less objective terms such as "lethargic" or "comatose." Such standardized assessment clearly communicates consistent clinical information to the patient care team.

Surgical advancements. Advances in neurosurgery are directly related to the development of surgical instrumentation and equipment, along with safer anesthetic techniques. The advent of the microscope has allowed better visualization and access to the neurologic system. Surgical tools such as high-speed drills and lasers have increased the precision with which difficult procedures can be performed.

In addition to the laser, profound change in surgical approaches to lesion biopsy, small tumor exci-

sion, and even treatment of hydrocephalus has come about with the introduction of neuroendoscopy. As compatible instrumentation for dealing with central nervous system tissue develops, the role of the neuroendoscope has an expanding place in modern neurosurgery (Williams, Galbraith, & Duncan, 1995). The use of intracranial images as navigational guides during neurosurgery has developed through the use of investigational interactive, image-guided, stereotaxic neurosurgery systems. This "frameless" stereotactic system integrates a computer, optical component (infrared-seeking cameras with infrared-emitting instrumentation), and keyboard to yield precise, accurate preoperative and intraoperative patient information (League, 1995).

In the future the development of closely integrated multidisciplinary groups, such as neurologic science, will continue to result in improved patient care and better timing of surgical treatment.

Specialized facilities. Craniocerebral trauma is one of the most significant areas in American medicine. Each year, approximately a half million Americans require medical attention for head injuries (Barker, 1994). With the development of organized trauma evacuation systems and regional neurotrauma centers, more trauma patients now reach medical care; mortality and complications from neurologic injuries have been, and should continue to be, reduced. (Trauma surgery is fully discussed in Chapter 20.) In the field of nursing, specialization in trauma, neurointensive care, and neurosurgery has evolved in response to the intricate and complex care required by neurosurgery patients. The perioperative nurse is constantly challenged in scrub, circulator, and first-assistant roles. The role of the registered nurse first assistant in neurosurgery has evolved from the former privately employed neurosurgery scrub nurse. Today the registered nurse first assistant may be institutionally or privately employed. Depending on the practice setting and the nurse's expertise, the registered nurse first assistant may make preoperative and postoperative rounds, conduct histories and physicals, perform teaching and discharge planning, and make home visits, as well as assist during surgery.

The extensive needs of neurosurgical patients often require long-term rehabilitation and support services. Physical, speech, recreational, and occupational therapy; occupational and psychologic counseling; and transportation are required and often available in the community. Aggressive rehabilitation therapy, coupled with nursing's community-based focus, have positively changed long-term outcomes for the neurosurgical patient.

Legal and ethical considerations. To offer intelligent and informative support to patients' families and significant others, the nurse must be familiar with criteria to determine brain death and the use of resuscitative measures. Decisions not to resuscitate (DNR) or to discontinue life-support equipment continue to pose legal and ethical dilemmas for health care providers and for patients and their families. Patients may be more likely to discuss with nurses what resuscitation, if any, should be undertaken for them.

In a discussion of withholding, withdrawing, and refusal of treatment, the American Nurses Association (ANA) (1994) has suggested that although there is no ethical or legal distinction between withholding or withdrawing treatments, the latter may create more emotional distress for the perioperative nurse and others involved. Honoring the wish to refuse treatments that the patient does not desire, that are felt by the patient to be disproportionately burdensome, or that will not benefit the patient is ethically and legally permissible. Neurosurgical patients who have made a DNR decision preoperatively have the right to suspend that decision, completely or partially, during the intraoperative period. The Association of Operating Room Nurses (AORN) (1994) recommends that discussion with the patient and family should include the goals of the surgical treatment, the possibility of resuscitative measures, a description of what those measures include, and the possible outcomes with and without resuscitation. If the patient chooses to suspend the DNR order intraoperatively, it must be clearly indicated in the medical record, as it must be when the DNR order is to be reinstated. Ethics committees will continue to assist perioperative nurses as they deal with these and other ethical dilemmas.

Carrying out the patient's wishes places the nurse in a precarious legal stance. It is a philosophic, ethical, and legal dilemma if a neurologic patient has vital functions sustained by technology that forestall death, but that do not improve the basic disease or disease process. In the future, ethics committees will continue to grapple with such difficult decisions.

NEUROLOGIC ASSESSMENT

Perioperative nursing assessment provides critical data needed to plan nursing interventions and effect safe, positive patient outcomes. Assessment establishes the knowledge needed to coordinate a team approach to the management of perioperative patient care, and it allows the perioperative nurse to establish a relationship with the patient and family and to validate findings that will guide the intraoperative care plan. The neurologic problem may limit the patient's participation in self-care or his or her ability to participate in care planning; thus preoperative assessment, teaching, and communication should involve both the patient and family or sig-

nificant other. Preoperative contact allows the nurse to explain perioperative events; this helps to allay fear and anxiety associated with the anticipated surgical intervention.

The components of this assessment should include the patient's physical appearance, health history, mental status, speech and language functions, assessment of cranial nerves, cerebellar functions, sensory functions, and vital signs. The sum of this data base will provide the nurse with the necessary information to formulate nursing diagnoses for the patient's care. This assessment may then be repeated to monitor the patient's progress or to develop a new data base if any surgical or medical intervention has occurred to alter the patient's condition.

Patient History

Before beginning the history, the nurse should spend a few minutes talking with the patient, assisting in his or her comfort, and making sure that he or she can hear and understand what is being said. The neurosurgery patient may have a cognitive or sensory deficit that impedes communication; the family or significant other should be involved in and confirm the exchange of information (Box 9-2).

Patient observation. During the history or perioperative assessment the patient should be closely observed and evaluated. The perioperative nurse should watch the patient's face as questions are asked, noting whether the patient appears alert and attentive, makes eye contact, is drowsy, or has inappropriate facial expressions or affect. Lack of an appropriate affective response may indicate preoccupation, mental illness, drug abuse, subnormal intelligence, or facial paralysis. The perioperative nurse also notes whether the patient is restless or irritable. This may indicate pain, anoxia, or increased intracranial pressure.

The patient's appearance and behavior are important. The patient's face is inspected. Are the features symmetric? Does the eyelid droop? Does the patient twitch, make constant movements, or pill-roll his or her fingers? The nurse generally notes whether the patient can speak appropriately. Are responses logical, clear, and understandable, or are they garbled, unclear, or confused? Does the patient misuse or make up words or lose the train of thought when answering questions? Is there any mood swing, sudden outburst, or inappropriate behavior during the interview?

Assessing Cerebral Function

Another component of neurologic assessment is assessment of the patient's intellectual performance, including memory, orientation, and abstract reasoning. Questions during this part of the assessment

---

Box 9-2 Health History

General Considerations

Demographic data: Age, sex, race, home address, religion

Occupation: Description of typical daily activities

Exposure to occupational and environmental hazards: Solvents, insecticides, pesticides, arsenic, lead, and other chemicals; use of heavy equipment; works with electricity, in or near water, or at heights

Intellectual level: Educational history, general communication pattern

Emotional status: Expression of emotion; feelings about self, family, and health care workers; perceived stresses; usual coping methods

Hand, eye, and foot dominance

Medication history: Current medications (note name, purpose, dosage, frequency, route, and time of last dose); significant past medications; recent changes in medications; use of over-the-counter drugs; drug and food allergies

Use of alcohol, tobacco products, mood-altering drugs

Source of health care: Family physician, nurse practitioner, clinic

Current Problem

Trauma: Sequence of events, elapsed time, extent of known injury, care provided, medications administered, current status

Acute infection: Onset, symptoms, site of infection, source of infection, intervention done, and related response

Seizures/convulsions: Sequence of events, character of symptoms, possible precipitating factors, history of previous seizures, use of anticonvulsants

Pain: Location, quality, intensity, duration (acute or chronic), constancy, related or precipitating activities or symptoms, interventions done and their effectiveness

Gait coordination: Balance, falling, related activities

Vertigo/dizziness: Onset, precipitating activity, sensation, nausea or vomiting, tinnitus, associated symptoms (loss of consciousness, numbness or tingling, cognitive changes, visual changes, chest pain, falling)

Weakness/numbness: Onset, duration, location, characteristics, precipitating activities, associated symptoms (pain, muscle spasms, shortness of breath)

Swallowing difficulties: Onset of drooling, presence of gagging or coughing, problems swallowing liquids or solids

Medical History

Trauma: head, back, spinal cord, birth trauma, nerve injuries

Congenital anomalies, deformities

Cerebrovascular accident

Encephalitis, meningitis

Cardiovascular problems: hypertension, aneurysm, cardiac dysrhythmias or surgery, thrombophlebitis

Neurologic disorders

Psychiatric counseling

Prior surgical procedures

Family History

Epilepsy or seizures

Headaches

Mental retardation

Cerebrovascular accidents

Psychiatric Disorders

Use of alcohol, tobacco products, or mood-altering drugs

Hereditary disorders: Huntington's chorea, muscular dystrophy, neurofibromatosis, Tay-Sachs disease

Neurologic diseases or disorders

From Chipps E, et al. (1992). *Neurologic disorders* (p. 19). St. Louis: Mosby.

---

should be limited to those to which a person with an average education can respond. To test short-term memory, the patient is asked to repeat a short phrase, then to do so again after a short interval. The perioperative nurse asks the patient to repeat a series of numbers, asks about any problems the patient has noticed or that have been called to his or her attention, and asks about changes in his or her ability to remember things. The patient's long-term memory was tested during the history. The patient's level of orientation is determined by asking questions about the time, date, and place. It is important to remember that patients often become confused about time and dates during hospitalization. If this is a problem, ask for the patient's own name, the name of the president, the capital, or something else that the patient would be likely to know. To test abstract reasoning, have the patient explain a simple proverb, such as, "Do unto others as you would have them do unto you."

Recognition. Specific functions of the cerebral cortex may be tested, beginning with the ability to recognize familiar objects by sight, sound, or feel. The inability to recognize common objects through the senses is called *agnosia*. Visual agnosia is the inability to recognize common objects by sight. To test this ability, the perioperative nurse would show a pen or a chair to the patient and ask for the object's name. Auditory agnosia is the inability to identify common environmental signs, such as the ringing of a telephone. The patient cannot attach proper meaning to the sound, despite being able to hear it.

This deficit is often caused by temporal lobe damage. Tactile agnosia is the inability to identify common objects, such as a pencil, by touch. The patient, with eyes closed, is asked to identify an object placed in his or her hand. A parietal lobe lesion may cause tactile agnosia. Autotopagnosia is a special type of agnosia in which the patient has difficulty identifying body parts or their relationship to other parts. A lesion in the posteroinferior parietal lobe may cause autotopagnosia.

Cortical motor integration. Another area of assessment is cortical motor integration. The performance of a skilled motor act requires the performer to understand the act, to remember the directions, and to possess the motor strength to complete the act. For example, if the perioperative nurse asks a patient to brush his or her teeth, the patient must understand what is expected. Inability to comprehend or remember actions is called *ideational apraxia.* The patient must next understand the relationship of his or her body parts. The mental image of the action must be translated to a motor action. A defect in the transmission of an idea into an appropriate image for motor actions is *ideokinetic apraxia.* Finally, the motor execution of the action must take place. Failure of the muscles to carry out the action is *kinetic apraxia.* Performing a skilled act on demand requires integrated function of several areas of the cerebral cortex. A defect in any of the areas is responsible for apraxia.

Communication. Another major area of cerebral function assessment is communication ability. Aphasia, or dysphasia, refers to a disorder of language itself that presents a difficulty in communicating. The cause usually lies in the left cerebral cortex, the outer layer formed by the cellular gray matter (Bates, Bickley, & Hoekelman, 1995). There are several kinds of aphasia. Inability to understand the spoken word is *receptive aphasia.* Inability to express thoughts appropriately is *expressive aphasia.* Careful evaluation of the patient's ability to communicate can help localize the lesion if a specific area of the brain is involved. Hickey (1992) has subdivided four types of aphasia, along with the potential areas of cerebral involvement, as follows:

- Auditory receptive aphasia—lesion at Wernicke's area of the temporal lobe
- Visual receptive aphasia (alexia)—lesion in parietal-occipital area
- Expressive speaking aphasia (agraphia)—lesion at Broca's area of frontal lobe
- Expressive writing aphasia (agraphia)—lesion in posterior frontal lobe

It is important to note the patient's selection of words, the flow, and the fluency of speech. The patient's voice should have inflections, be clear and strong, and be able to increase in volume. Speech should be coherent and relevant; thoughts should be clearly expressed. When the patient has difficulty communicating, more detailed evaluation should be done.

Cranial nerve examination. Assessment of cranial nerves is discussed in Box 9-3.

INTEGRATING ASSESSMENT OF OTHER SYSTEMS

Assessment of the neurosurgery patient cannot be done without correlating neurologic findings with findings from the overall patient assessment. The following list summarizes some of the clinical indications of space-taking lesions:

1. Space-taking lesions above the foramen magnum
   a. Persistent headache, usually unrelieved by analgesic agents and occasionally accompanied by vomiting
   b. Progressive onset of symptoms
   c. History of recent infection, trauma, or neoplasm elsewhere
   d. History of focal or generalized seizures
   e. Personality changes
   f. Slow onset of hemiplegia
   g. Papilledema, increased intracranial pressure, or both
   h. Visual field cuts
   i. Unilateral perceptive deafness
   j. Other unilateral nerve palsies
2. Space-taking lesions below the foramen magnum
   a. Radicular pain
   b. Progressive onset of symptoms
   c. History of recent infection, trauma, or neoplasm
   d. Slow, progressive onset of paraplegia, monoplegia, or hemiplegia
   e. Unilateral or bilateral atrophy of muscles at the level of the lesion
   f. Bladder and rectal sphincter disturbances

Findings from the assessment of skin, vital signs, and other pertinent assessment parameters are part of the complete patient data base.

Cardiovascular Assessment

The triad of increased systolic pressure, widening pulse pressure, and slow pulse are clinical indicators of increased intracranial pressure. They may be observed as signs of rapid neurologic deterioration. In a total evaluation of cardiovascular status, individual vital signs should be correlated with other signs and symptoms.

Pulse. The rate, quality, and rhythm of the pulse should be noted. Abnormalities such as tachycardia,

---

Box 9-3 Assessment of Cranial Nerves (CNs)

CN I (Olfactory)

Test ability to identify familiar aromatic odors, one naris at a time with eyes closed

CN II (Optic)

Test vision with Snellen's chart and Rosenbaum's near vision chart
Perform ophthalmoscopic examination of fundi
Test visual field by confrontation and extinction of vision

CNs III, IV, and VI (Oculomotor, Trochlear, and Abducens)

Inspect eyelids for drooping
Inspect pupils' size for equality and their direct and consensual response to light and accommodation
Assess cardinal fields of gaze

CN V (Trigeminal)

Inspect face for muscle atrophy and tremors
Palpate jaw muscles for tone and strength when patient clenches teeth
Test superficial pain and touch sensation in each branch. (Test temperature sensation if there are unexpected findings to pain or touch)
Test corneal reflex

CN VII (Facial)

Inspect symmetry of facial features with various expressions (smile, frown, puffed cheeks, wrinkled forehead, and so on)
Test ability to identify sweet and salty tastes on each side of tongue

CN VIII (Acoustic)

Test sense of hearing with whisper screening test or by audiometry
Compare bone and air conduction of sound
Test for lateralization of sound

CN IX (Glossopharyngeal)

Test ability to identify sour and bitter tastes
Test gag reflex and ability to swallow

CN X (Vagus)

Inspect palate and uvula for symmetry with speech sounds and gag reflex
Observe for swallowing difficulty
Evaluate quality of guttural speech sounds (presence of nasal or hoarse quality to voice)

CN XI (Spinal Accessory)

Test trapezius muscle strength (shrug shoulders against resistance)
Test sternocleidomastoid muscle strength (turn head to each side against resistance)

CN XII (Hypoglossal)

Inspect tongue in mouth and while protruded for symmetry, tremors, and atrophy
Inspect tongue movement toward nose and chin
Test tongue strength with index finger when tongue is pressed against cheek
Evaluate quality of lingual speech sounds (l, t, d, n)

From Chipps E, et al. (1992). *Neurologic Disorders* (p. 23). St. Louis: Mosby.

---

bradycardia, or cardiac dysrhythmias can relate to neurologic dysfunction. Tachycardia may indicate poor cerebral oxygenation, possible internal bleeding, or a terminal stage of disease. In later stages of increased intracranial pressure, bradycardia may occur; as the major circulation begins to fail, the pulse may become rapid. When the pulse is decreased, it may still be bounding; blood is being pumped under very high pressure. Pulses should be checked bilaterally. It should be determined whether any medications have been given that would alter the pulse rate. The method of checking the pulse (apical, radial, or monitored) should be noted. Cardiac dysrhythmias may be encountered in patients who have had an intracranial bleed or undergone posterior fossa surgery.

Blood pressure. Baroreceptors and chemoreceptors in the carotid artery and aortic arch are responsible for innervating the vasomotor center of the medulla, which regulates blood pressure. When carbon dioxide levels are increased, sympathetic stimulation causes a responsive vasoconstriction with an increase in arterial pressure. Patients need a mean arterial pressure of 60 mm Hg to produce adequate cerebral perfusion pressure, and thus adequate oxygen and glucose for brain metabolism. When vasoconstriction occurs in response to cerebral ischemia with cerebral blood pressure below 50 mm Hg, this is known as the central nervous system ischemic response. Systolic blood pressure may rise above 250 mm Hg. This attempt to supply the brain with oxygen results in an overwhelming peripheral vasoconstriction. Blood pressure should be assessed bilaterally and/or via arterial lines.

Peripheral pulses. Peripheral pulses become important perioperative assessment parameters when there is a threat of thromboembolic events or compromise caused by surgical positioning. Pulses should be assessed and marked as appropriate for the planned surgical intervention. Major arteries may be palpated for pulsating masses and auscultated for bruits. Areas of decreased pulse, pallor, or decreased temperatures, with bruits or masses, should be documented.

Cushing reflex. Increased blood pressure, decreased pulse, and widening pulse pressure (difference between systolic and diastolic measurements) characterize the Cushing reflex. This may be accompanied by an increase in temperature and severely depressed respirations. This reflex may occur with subtentorial (posterior fossa) herniation and subsequent increased intracranial pressure. As cerebrospinal pressure within the ventricles rises to a point where it equals or exceeds arterial pressure, the arteries supplying the brain are compressed. This results in decreased oxygen, blood flow, and ischemia in the brain. The Cushing reflex raises blood pressure to levels higher than systemic pressures, preserving blood flow to the cerebral arterial system.

Hypotension. Normal blood volume, adequate pumping mechanisms, and vascular bed size are necessary to maintain adequate blood supply to all body tissues. In neurogenic shock, blood volume is normal, but the vascular bed size is greatly increased; blood volume cannot fill the blood vessels adequately. Venous pooling, decreased volume return to the heart, and decreased cardiac output ensue. The hypotension is treated with vasopressors.

Temperature. Inability to maintain normal temperature may be caused by damage to the hypothalamus, the heat-regulating center of the body. Subnormal temperatures may be encountered in spinal shock, metabolic or toxic coma, drug overdose, destructive brain stem or hypothalamic lesions, or terminal disease stages. Hypothermia is characterized by decreased metabolic rates; potential dysrhythmias; slowed circulation; reduced oxygen consumption; progressive falling heart rate, blood pressure, and respiratory rate; and reduced cerebral function. Cerebral blood flow is reduced about 6% for every degree centigrade that body temperature is reduced below normal.

Elevated temperature may be encountered with central nervous system infection, subarachnoid hemorrhage, hypothalamic lesions, or brain stem hemorrhage; as a result of cerebral edema; in association with a herniation syndrome; or from traction on the hypothalamus or brain stem, bacterial endocarditis, or other infectious or inflammatory disease. As cell metabolism increases, carbon dioxide byproducts accumulate; this increases intracranial pressure. If oxygen supply to cerebral tissue is compromised, ischemia develops. Intervention is directed at vigorous reduction of the elevated body temperature. Temperature is usually assessed rectally; however, if there are signs of increased intracranial pressure, rectal measurement is contraindicated. Intraoperatively, an esophageal stethoscope with temperature probe or other automatic temperature monitoring device is usually employed.

Respiratory Assessment

The respiratory pattern provides early information of malfunction in a specific area of the brain. Abnormal patterns can be related to damage to respiratory centers as well as to the following conditions:

1. Acidosis
2. Respiratory alkalosis
3. Electrolyte imbalances
4. Congestive heart failure
5. Anxiety
6. Respiratory complications associated with prolonged immobility
7. Primary respiratory dysfunction and disease
8. Infections

Drugs and anesthetics depress respiration. The rate, quality, and patterns of respiration can yield clues to the location of lesions. Patients with underlying neurologic disease are susceptible to abnormal breathing patterns.

Cheyne-Stokes breathing. Cheyne-Stokes breathing is a rhythmic change in rate and depth of respirations, alternating regularly with brief periods of apnea. Causes may include bilateral cerebral infarction, deep cerebral or cerebellar lesions, upper brain stem involvement, hypertensive encephalopathy, and metabolic disorders.

Central neurogenic hyperventilation. With central neurogenic hyperventilation there are sustained, rapid, regular respirations with increased depth; inspiration and expiration are forced. Neurogenic causes may include a lesion or infarction in the middle or low pons, anoxia, ischemia, decreased glucose supply to the midbrain, or tumors.

Apneustic breathing. Apneustic breathing involves a prolonged inspiration with a pause at the point of full inspiration; there may also be expiratory pauses. This breathing pattern may be caused by an extensive brain stem lesion in the middle or low pons or in the upper medulla, or it may be caused by meningitis.

Ataxic breathing. Ataxic respirations are characterized by an irregular and unpredictable pattern. There are random deep and shallow breaths and pauses. Causes may include cerebellar or pontine bleeding, lesions of the medulla, compressing supratentorial tumors, or severe meningitis. *Cluster breathing* differs in that, although the respiratory pattern is irregular, there are longer alternating periods of apnea. A lesion of the low pons or upper medulla may be implicated with cluster breathing.

Genitourinary Assessment

Bladder and/or bowel dysfunction may be related to problems with the autonomic nervous system. Lesions of the nervous system may cause neurogenic bladder, contribute to urinary tract infections, and lead to the formation of stones in the urinary tract.

Neurogenic bladder. "Neurogenic bladder" is a general term for any bladder disturbance caused by a lesion in the central or peripheral nervous system. Loss of bladder control can range from diminished perception of fullness or diminished ability to empty to total loss of control. Neurogenic bladder may be caused by spinal cord injury or tumor, neurologic disease (such as multiple sclerosis), congenital anomalies, and infection. There are a number of types of neurogenic bladder; the two classifications of neurogenic bladder most often referred to are spastic bladder, characterized by automatic, uncontrolled urinary expulsion with incomplete emptying, and flaccid bladder, wherein the sensation of bladder fullness is lost. In this case, the bladder overfills and distends. Neurogenic bladders may also be classified by the level of the lesion in the central nervous system; upper motor neuron dysfunctions produce spastic bladders; lower motor neuron dysfunctions produce flaccid bladders. Major complications of neurogenic bladder include infections, hypertrophy of the bladder wall, eventual reflux, hydronephrosis, and perhaps renal failure.

Urinary tract infection. Urinary infections in the neurosurgery patient can result from urinary stasis or long-term catheter use. Indwelling catheters can erode the integrity of the mucosal lining of the urethra. Static urine is very susceptible to organism growth; therefore urinary stasis greatly contributes to infection.

Urinary stones. Cord-injured and immobile patients are prone to stone formation. Infection, failure to completely empty the bladder, the presence of a foreign body, and urinary tract obstruction all contribute to stone formation. The patient who has bladder stones may be asymptomatic; sometimes cystitis is present. Stones formed in the kidney are accompanied by symptoms of pain, obstruction, and tissue trauma with consequent hemorrhage and infection.

Musculoskeletal Assessment

Neurosurgery patients demonstrate bone, joint, and muscle changes associated with prolonged periods of immobility. These changes include skeletal malalignment, loss of calcium, deformities, joint stiff-

Table 9-1 Segmental spinal cord level and function

Level	Function
C1 to C6	Neck flexors
C1 to T1	Neck extensors
C3 to C5	Supply diaphragm
C5,C6	Shoulder movement; raise arm (deltoid); flexion of elbow (biceps); C6 externally rotates the arm (supinates)
C6 to C8	Extend elbow and wrist (triceps and wrist extensors); pronate wrist
C7,C8,T1	Flex wrist
C8,T1	Supply small muscles of the hand
T1 to T6	Intercostals and trunk above the waist
T7 to L1	Abdominal muscles
L1 to L4	Thigh flexion
L2 to L4	Thigh adduction
L4,L5,S1	Thigh abduction
L5,S1,S2	Extension of leg at hip (gluteus maximus)
L2 to L4	Extension of leg at knee (quadriceps femoris)
L4,L5,S1,S2	Flexion of leg at knee (hamstrings)
L4,L5,S1	Dorsiflexion of foot (tibialis anterior)
L4,L5,S1	Extension of toes
L5,S1,S2	Plantarflexion of foot
L5,S1,S2	Flexion of toes

From Chipps E, et al. (1992). *Neurologic Disorders* (p. 32). St. Louis: Mosby.

ness, ankylosis, muscle weakness, shortening or stretching of muscles, atrophy, and contractures. Patients with disc disease demonstrate muscle spasms, atrophy, and pain. The patient's balance, coordination, strength, muscle mass, and level of discomfort all have important implications for perioperative care planning. Assessment of muscle strength is measured by bilateral comparisons. Muscle tone refers to the amount of firmness or tension of the muscles. It is assessed by determining the resistance to passive stretching of the muscles. The muscle is said to be flaccid if there is no resistance to passive extension or flexion, even with rapid movement. Spasticity is present if there is sustained contraction, most noticeable upon initial movement. Spasticity is unequal in opposing muscle groups. Rigidity refers to continuous, equal tension in opposing muscle groups. The perioperative nurse will note continued resistance to passive motion of both flexion and extension (Table 9-1).

Skin Assessment

Skin changes in the neurosurgery patient are often associated with immobility. The skin should be assessed for abrasions, infections from traumatic wounds, shearing injuries, pressure sores from poor nutritional status, and edema. In addition to assessing skin integrity, color, turgor, and dryness should also be assessed.

Gastrointestinal Assessment

The overwhelming magnitude of their disease places many neurosurgical patients at risk for stress ulcers. Trauma, stroke, cord-injured, and tumor patients are often treated prophylactically to prevent major gastrointestinal bleeds. Patients may be nutritionally supported with intravenous therapy, total parenteral nutrition or hyperalimentation, or enteral tube feedings. Constipation or fecal impactions may result from prolonged immobility and nutritional deficits. Patients with central nervous system disease may also exhibit temporary or permanent bowel incontinence.

DIAGNOSTIC STUDIES

Although the diagnosis for most neurosurgery patients is tentatively derived from a careful history, general examination, and neurologic evaluation, diagnostic studies provide important information in guiding the operative procedure. New neurodiagnostic technology has provided remarkable views and interpretations of the interior of the brain and the structure and function of related components of the nervous system. Understanding which diagnostic studies are used for specific areas of system dysfunction helps the perioperative nurse to incorporate diagnostic results into the plan of care. Box 9-4 presents an overview of common diagnostic studies. The perioperative nurse will need to anticipate the reports of diagnostic studies needed at the time of surgery (Meeker & Rothrock, 1995).

NURSING DIAGNOSES

Using nursing diagnoses in perioperative nursing facilitates the use of common nursing language among practicing nurses. This not only enhances communication for the professional nursing team but also allows for continuity of patient care from nurse to nurse. The selection of nursing diagnoses requires analysis and synthesis of information from the patient data base, critical thinking, and decision making.

Common Nursing Diagnoses (High Risk for or Actual)

The following list of common nursing diagnoses—high risk for or actual—underlines the demanding and complex role of the perioperative nurse caring for neurosurgical patients. It becomes clearly evident that perioperative patient care requires nursing integration and skill in building and maintaining a therapeutic perioperative care team. Continuity and safe care can be provided only through coordination and teamwork. Some of the listed nursing diagnoses

are amenable to independent nursing intervention; most require interdependent collaboration. High skill levels are required for administering and monitoring neurosurgical nursing care if perioperative procedures are to be carried out with minimal patient risk. The perioperative nurse must manage rapidly changing situations, make instantaneous decisions about the nature of problems with equipment and patient care, and use all available coping resources, in addition to the wisdom of experience. Monitoring and ensuring the quality of care delivered by all perioperative team members, along with expert organizational and work role skills, make nursing the neurosurgical patient a challenging area of perioperative practice. Despite the complicated and interrelated physiologic events that affect surgical intervention, the central role of caring, of a committed and patient-centered stance, is evident in the nursing diagnoses. Perioperative care plans must include "care," which is part of nursing's human science.

Altered cerebral tissue perfusion. Cerebral perfusion may be compromised by intracranial pressure changes caused by space-taking lesions, cerebral edema, decreased systemic blood pressure, hypoxia, and direct interruption of cerebral flow by a thrombus or embolus. Patients with marked baseline increases in intracranial pressure are susceptible to further increases with the induction of anesthesia. The *goal* is achievement of cerebral tissue perfusion to maintain cerebral homeostasis.

Ineffective breathing pattern; impaired gas exchange. Compression or injury to respiratory centers alters breathing patterns. This results in fluctuating levels of Pa_{O_2} and Pa_{CO_2}, accompanied either by hypoventilation or by hyperventilation. Disruptions in muscle innervation and tone may jeopardize the airway by relaxation of the tongue or inability to generate an effective cough to clear secretions. Sympathomimetic stimulation causes peripheral vasoconstriction and increased vascular resistance; blood is shunted into the pulmonary vasculature, potentiating the risk of neurogenic pulmonary edema. Intraoperatively, the respiratory system is most vulnerable to compromise from the prone position. This position has the potential to limit diaphragmatic movement, with subsequent hypoventilation if the patient is not properly positioned. The *goal* is to attain and maintain effective respirations.

Impaired swallowing. The patient may have altered sensory reception, transmission, and/or motor integration related to cranial nerve involvement, muscle weakness, or both. To prevent aspiration, a suction line should always be available in the neurosurgery operating room. The *goal* is for the patient

---

Box 9-4 Review of Diagnostic Studies and Their Indications

Radiologic Procedures
Skull series
Fractures, intracranial foreign bodies, bone infections, bone-invading tumors, congenital abnormalities

Orbits
Sphenoid ridge meningioma, optic nerve glioma, orbital tumors

Auditory meati
Cerebellopontine angle tumors

Sinuses and mastoids
Brain abscess, cholesteatoma

Spine (cervical, thoracic, lumbar)
Lesions below foramen magnum, spinal cord trauma, compression fractures, degenerative and congenital diseases

Long bones
Metastasis, lead poisoning

Tomography
Better identification of lesions observed on other studies

Myelogram
Space-taking lesions of cord, extruded disc tumors in posterior fossa of skull, intraspinal soft tissue

Arteriogram
Space-taking lesions of brain, identification of aneurysms, arteriovenous malformations, vascular occlusions

Digital subtraction arteriography (DSA)
Increased visualization of cerebral blood flow and vascular abnormalities; more useful for evaluation of extracranial (as opposed to intracranial) vessels

Computed tomography (CT)
Provides three-dimensional view of intracranial and vertebral structures, which differentiates among tumors, hemorrhage, infarctions, cysts; use of intravenously injected radiopaque contrast agent increases tissue differentiation

Positron emission tomography (PET)
Abnormal isotope concentration identifies areas of tissue damaged by stroke, contusion, or seizure activity

Magnetic resonance imaging (MRI)
Detects structural and biochemical abnormalities by directing magnetic and radio waves at body tissues to determine response to test element; aids in diagnosis of stroke, cerebrovascular disorders, and multiple sclerosis

Other Studies
Electromyography
Detection, recording, and interpretation of electrical activity of muscle at rest or during contraction; used to differentiate muscle disease from lower neuron dysfunction; identifies muscle disease, locates nerve lesions, and quantitates nerve regeneration; may be accompanied by nerve conduction velocity (NCV), which records the rate a stimulated nerve can conduct electrical activity

Evoked potentials (EP)
Recordings of electrical activity from the scalp following specific stimulation of visual, auditory, or somatosensory receptors; valuable in evaluation of multiple sclerosis, optic nerve functioning, and brain stem integrity; used intraoperatively for both posterior fossa and spinal procedures

Electroencephalography (EEG)
Graphic recording and analysis of electrical activity of surface or convexity of cerebral hemispheres; valuable in assessing seizure disorders, brain tumors, abscesses, and cerebral damage

Intracranial pressure monitoring
Measures pressure exerted by brain tissue, blood, and cerebrospinal fluid against skull; three basic types of systems use ventricular catheter, subarachnoid screw, or epidural sensor; indications include head trauma, overproduction or insufficient absorption of cerebrospinal fluid, cerebral hemorrhage, and space-occupying lesions

Brain scan
Detects rays emitted by injected radionuclide and converts them into images; used to detect intracranial masses, vascular lesions, ischemic areas, cerebral infarctions, and intracerebral hemorrhage; especially valuable combined with CT

---

to regain or develop the ability to swallow within the limits imposed by the neurologic dysfunction.

Pain. Head injury, increased intracranial pressure, and brain tumors can cause headache. Spinal cord tumors and disc herniation can result in radicular pain. Patients with progressive paresthesia may have muscle pain. The *goal* is to assist with and achieve relief of pain.

Sensory/perceptual alterations. Cerebral insult may produce altered sensory reception, transmission, and/or integration. Brain dysfunction, physical or chemical alterations, and cranial nerve involvement can result in hearing loss, visual field cuts, cortical blindness, nystagmus, and tactile deficits. The *goal* is protection from injury.

Impaired physical mobility. Altered mobility resulting from decreased consciousness, paralysis, and cognitive impairment potentiates the risk of complications such as skin breakdown, loss of muscle mass and of muscle and joint function, and development of peripheral thrombosis. Damage to motor tracts in the central nervous system can result in various levels of altered motor function. Impaired function impinges on independence, personality, and emotions. It also affects the cardiovascular, musculoskeletal, respiratory, and genitourinary systems. Perioperatively, care needs to be taken in positioning, protecting bony prominences through padding and other support, maintaining body alignment, selecting an appropriate site for the electrosurgical dispersive pad, preventing pressure on joints, and assisting in transfer maneuvers. The *goal* is to maintain mobility within the limits imposed by neurologic dysfunction.

Constipation. Immobility, decreased peristalsis, and altered nutritional status all contribute to problems with bowel elimination. Spinal cord injury disrupts innervation of the bowel and rectum; the patient may be unaware of the need to defecate. The use of narcotics for pain relief further contributes to constipation. There may be fecal impactions. The *goal* is attainment of bowel elimination.

Altered nutrition: less than body requirements. Decreased levels of consciousness, vomiting, or mechanical ventilation disrupt normal food intake. Gastric bleeding (Cushing's ulcers) is a complication that alters gastrointestinal function and nutrient absorption. The patient has increased metabolic needs because of cerebral trauma or tissue injury; these needs may not be met. Muscle weakness with impaired ability to chew and swallow influences nutritional deficits. There may be impaired wound healing and a disturbance in fluid and electrolyte balance. The *goal* is to meet nutritional requirements.

Altered patterns of urinary elimination. Neuromuscular impairment, autonomic dysfunction, and immobility may lead to bladder dysfunction, incontinence, or urinary retention. If the patient does not come to the OR with a urinary catheter in place, one is likely to be inserted. The *goal* is to attain and maintain bladder continence.

Anxiety. Paralysis, pain, and loss of independence, as well as the anticipated surgery, its outcome, and prognosis, are frightening events for patients. Feelings of anxiety may be accompanied by depression, feelings of powerlessness, loss of personal identity, and spiritual distress. Concerns about chronicity, slow recovery, lengthy rehabilitation, or progressive disease compound the situational anxiety of the surgery itself. The *goal* is to reduce or minimize the patient's anxiety.

Body image disturbance; self-esteem disturbance; altered role performance. Drastic changes in physical function and life-style often result from brain and spinal cord deficits. The patient and family or significant other will exhibit a range of emotional responses, including denial, despair, and anger. Loss of hair, bony defects, and loss of function may affect the patient's self-perception. Physical limitations may alter the patient's ability to resume a former role. The *goal* is to help the patient (and family or significant other) to accept altered body function or loss.

Altered thought processes. Cerebral insult and metabolic changes in cerebral tissue may impair memory, judgment, or problem-solving ability; result in inappropriate affect; and change level of consciousness. Depending on the level of alteration, physiologic and emotional support may be required. The *goal* is to maintain orientation within the limits of neurologic dysfunction.

Knowledge deficit. Cerebral disease, unfamiliarity with the disease, prognosis, expectations of surgery, or perioperative activities may result in a patient and family asking many questions, asking few questions, or having misconceptions. Insidious cerebral impairment often handicaps the patient's understanding of the seriousness of the disease. Communication impairments may further contribute to knowledge deficit. The *goal* is to participate in education of the patient and family.

Altered sexuality patterns. Spinal cord injury and severe neurologic deficits may limit sexual function. This affects personal identity. Lack of information about sexual dysfunction, lack of appreciation for alternate methods of expressing sexuality, fear of rejection by partner, or embarrassment that prohibits discussion of fears may lead to depression and social isolation. The *goal* is to participate in education of the patient and significant other.

Self-care deficit. Physical and neurologic limitations may result in various self-care deficits. Patients may have difficulty with feeding, hygiene, toileting, and mobility. The *goal* is to achieve self-care within the limits of neurologic dysfunction.

Fluid volume deficit; fluid volume excess. Neurosurgery patients are at risk for life-threatening fluid and electrolyte imbalances. Injury or disease involving the brain stem and hypothalamus affects mechanisms that regulate water volume. Neurologic disease may interfere with the patient's ability to eat, drink, and recognize thirst sensations. Fever, diarrhea, and hyperventilation increase fluid and electrolyte loss. Drugs such as steroids, diuretics, and hyperosmolar solutions can cause rapid shifts in large volumes of fluids. Osmotic diuretics are often administered intraoperatively; fluid replacement therapy must be carefully monitored and guided by actual and estimated losses. The *goal* is to maintain fluid and electrolyte balance.

Altered body temperature. Neurosurgery patients frequently have temperature alterations because of depressed reflexes, decreased levels of consciousness, and long periods of immobilization. Temperature regulation may be impaired when the hypothalamus is directly involved in the disease or the spinal cord pathways that regulate temperature are injured. Perioperatively, thermia units may be used to cool or warm the patient. The *goal* is to maintain normothermia.

Impaired verbal communication. Damage to the speech center can result in receptive or expressive aphasia or dysarthria. The patient's ability to communicate must be determined during perioperative assessment to plan care effectively. The *goal* is to maintain or attain communication within the limits of the neurologic dysfunction.

Altered family processes. The crisis of critical illness of a family member challenges the normal supportive and effective functioning of the family. Coping skills are compromised by the change in the family member's ability to function and by concerns about the surgery and treatments, the expense of health care, and changes in family roles. The *goal* is for family members to demonstrate ability to cope.

CARE PLANS

If your perioperative nursing staff is interested in developing generic care plans for the neurosurgery patient, as opposed to procedure-specific care plans, the plans presented in Chapter 7 may be adapted or modified. In addition, you may wish to develop care plan protocols for the various surgical positions used in neurosurgery. Because there are so many positioning accessories and modifications of positions, the following care plans are only generally descriptive; they do not specify accessories. You may find it helpful to modify the protocols to reflect what the perioperative nurse in your neurosurgery suite may select.

The care plans that follow are procedure specific, but note that they have been designed to be similar in their flow of information. This has been done deliberately. For risk-management purposes and ease of documentation, standard places to look for and note information decrease opportunities for error. The Guides to Nursing Actions have been tailored for each of the procedure-specific plans. However, in many instances your protocol may vary. It is expected that you will use these guidelines, modifying them to meet individual patient and institutional needs. Neuropsychologic and neurophysiolgic assessments are necessary to develop nursing diagnoses. The following assessments and diagnoses were selected on the basis of their likelihood to occur. However, nursing diagnoses that accurately reflect the individual patient must be identified. The priority for the nursing diagnosis always rests with specific patient considerations. All of the generic patient outcomes identified in Chapter 7 apply to the neurosurgical patient. The outcomes should be so noted on the relevant portion of the care plan.

GUIDES TO NURSING ACTIONS
Cranioplasty (Fig. 9-1)

1. Neurosurgical patients vary significantly in relationship to their underlying disease processes, clusters of signs and symptoms, and adjustment to alterations that result from the disease. The patient undergoing cranioplasty may have a nursing diagnosis of *body image disturbance* because of the cranial defect and the way it influences self-perception. Alteration in body image and situational low self-esteem may result from loss of hair when the head is shaved. There may be knowledge deficits, alterations in thought processes, limitations in mobility, compromised sensory perception, and alterations in levels of consciousness and ability to communicate. Individual nursing diagnoses depend on nursing assessment. Review the medical record to plan for specific patient needs in relation to the planned surgical approach, patient position, special equipment and supply needs, and preliminary maneuvers (lines, catheters, shave, and so on). Check that x-ray films and results of other diagnostic evaluations are available. For the patient undergoing cranioplasty, skull films are usually required. Modify the care plan according to the assessment.

2. Indwelling urinary catheters are usually inserted to monitor urinary output. This procedure may not be long enough for a catheter to be inserted. If it is necessary to catheterize the patient, use aseptic technique for catheter insertion. Place the drainage bag where it is readily observable. Document catheter insertion. Prevent kinking and tension on the tube during position changes.

3. The supine position is usually selected for cranioplasty. Apply elastic bandages or antiembolic stockings to prevent venous stasis if they are not already applied. The head will be elevated. If re-

FIG. 9-1
CARE PLAN FOR CRANIOPLASTY

KEY ASSESSMENT POINTS

Presence/classification of skull fracture
Effects of previously sustained brain injury
History of previous surgery
Headache, vertigo, local tenderness or throbbing
Presence of body image disturbance

NURSING DIAGNOSIS

All generic nursing diagnoses apply to this patient, with the addition of:

Body image disturbance

PATIENT OUTCOMES

All generic outcomes apply, with the addition of:
The patient will demonstrate adaptation to perceived or actual changes in self-image by:
1. Verbalizing feelings about body and image
2. Participating with OR team in plan of care
3. Discussing perceived concerns regarding physical change or function

NURSING ACTIONS

	Yes	No	N/A
1. Assessment performed?	☐	☐	☐
2. Foley catheter inserted?	☐	☐	☐
3. Correctly positioned?	☐	☐	☐
4. Skin prep per institutional protocol?	☐	☐	☐
5. Condition of skin noted at prep site?	☐	☐	☐
6. ESU dispersive pad site checked before application?	☐	☐	☐
7. Aseptic technique monitored during draping?	☐	☐	☐
8. Medications available/administered?	☐	☐	☐
9. Special equipment available?	☐	☐	☐
10. Suction checked?	☐	☐	☐
11. Drills available/checked?	☐	☐	☐
12. Irrigation/IV solutions warmed?	☐	☐	☐
13. Urinary output/blood loss noted?	☐	☐	☐
14. Specimens/cultures to lab?	☐	☐	☐
15. Counts performed and correct?	☐	☐	☐
16. Dispersive pad site rechecked?	☐	☐	☐
17. Drains noted?	☐	☐	☐
18. Dressings applied?	☐	☐	☐
19. Other generic care plans initiated? (specify)	☐	☐	☐

Document additional nursing actions/generic care plans initiated here:

_____

_____

_____

EVALUATION OF PATIENT OUTCOMES

	Outcome met	Outcome met with additional outcome criteria	Outcome met with revised nursing care plan	Outcome not met	Outcome not applicable to this patient
1. The patient demonstrated adaptation to perceived or actual changes in self-image.	☐	☐	☐	☐	☐
2. The patient met outcomes for additional generic care plans as indicated.	☐	☐	☐	☐	☐

Signature: _____ Date: _____

verse Trendelenburg's position is used, apply a padded footboard. Have an appropriate accessory available to stabilize the head. Position the arms to prevent brachial plexus injury by hyperabduction; pad the wrists and elbows to protect vulnerable nerves. Place the safety strap 2 inches above the knees, snugly but not tightly, to prevent compression on the popliteal space. Lumbar and popliteal pads may be used to prevent shearing forces if reverse Trendelenburg's position is used. Always return patients slowly from reverse Trendelenburg's position to prevent volume shifts and changes in vital signs. Monitor the patient closely during positional changes. Pad additional pressure sites.

4. Prepare the skin according to institutional protocol. If hair is removed, explain the procedure and carry it out according to policy, being especially aware of proper disposition of hair. Note the use of skin marking and injections at the incision site.

5. The condition of the skin should be noted before and after skin preparation procedures. Look for and note any nicks, abrasions, and rashes. Because cranioplasty patients may undergo repair of a cranial defect from a previous abscess, note any signs of skin infection or inflammation.

6. The skin should be assessed before and after the placement of electrosurgical dispersive pads.

7. Draping may be complicated for certain neurosurgery procedures. Have special barrier materials available; monitor aseptic technique carefully.

8. Various medications may be used during neurosurgery. These include topical hemostatics, thrombin, bone wax, local anesthetics with or without epinephrine, and antibiotics. All medications on the sterile field must be labeled. Check the patient record for allergies before administering drugs. Document the drug, dosage, route, time administered, and by whom.

9. Special equipment should be readied before patient admission to the OR. Careful review of the medical record, consultation with physician colleagues, and nursing experience should be used to ensure that what will be needed is available and in working order. For cranioplasty, the patient will require craniotomy instrumentation, cranioplasty kit, roller, Carborundum wheel, file, spoon, tongue blade, and mixing bowls (if they are not in the cranioplasty kit). Follow institutional protocol for mixing methyl methacrylate and documenting the use of cranioplasty material.

10. Two suction lines should be available and functioning. Have extra Frazier suction tips, stylets, and tubing ready.

11. Test all drills before use. Follow institutional protocols for the use of electrical and air-powered surgical drills.

12. Warmed irrigation fluid, intravenous solutions, and blood help maintain normothermia. Have a blood warmer available. Have two bulb syringes and adequate irrigating fluid for drilling procedures and bipolar coagulation. Carefully mix and label any antibiotic irrigation fluid.

13. Document urinary output and blood loss.

14. Follow institutional protocol for preserving, labeling, and transporting specimens and cultures; implement universal precautions for handling blood and body tissue. Record specimens and cultures.

15. Perform counts according to institutional protocol. In addition to instrument, sharp, and sponge counts, consider the necessity of counting cottonoids, cotton balls, and electrosurgical tips and cleaning pads. Document the results of counts.

16. Check the electrosurgical dispersive pad site whenever there is a position change and when the pad is removed.

17. Record drains, catheters, silastic tubing, and shunting materials.

18. Assist in the application of dressings. Allow adequate room for postoperative swelling when applying tape to prevent "tape burns."

Craniotomy for Tumor Removal (Box 9-5 and Fig. 9-2)

1. Brain tumors are named according to the tissues from which they arise. Primary intracerebral brain tumors are those in which cells originate from brain substances; these include oligodendrogliomas, ependymomas, astrocytomas, glioblastomas and medulobastomas, acoustic neuromas, and pituitary tumors. Secondary or metastatic tumors arise from metastatic carcinoma or sarcoma (Chipps, Clanin, & Campbell, 1992). The patient undergoing craniotomy for tumor removal may have a nursing diagnosis of *high risk for injury* related to changes in intracranial pressure and sensory-perceptual function. The patient may have additional potential for injury related to seizures. There may be hemiplegia, visual field cuts, hearing loss, and unilateral nerve palsy, all requiring special perioperative nursing care. *Self-esteem disturbance* and *body image disturbance* may result from loss of hair when the head is shaved. There may be knowledge deficits, alterations in thought processes, limitations in mobility, anxiety, and alterations in levels of consciousness

---

Box 9-5 Clinical Manifestations of Brain Tumors Associated with Particular Brain Regions

---

Frontal Lobe

Anterior portion

Disturbance in mental function

Posterior portion

Motor system dysfunction: seizures; aphasia (dominant hemisphere)

Parietal Lobe

Sensory deficits (contralateral)-paresthesia, hyperesthesia; astereognosis, loss of two-point discrimination, finger agnosia; visual field deficits; defects in integrity

Temporal Lobe

Psychomotor seizures; visual field deficits; auditory disturbances; Wernicke's aphasia (dominant hemisphere)

Occipital Lobe

Headache; seizures with visual aura; visual field deficit

Pituitary

Headaches; visual problems; endocrine problems

Cerebellum

Nystagmus; ataxia; unsteady gait; intention tremors; dysmetria; problems with rapid alternating movements.

Brain Stem and Cranial Nerves

Hemiparesis; nystagmus; extraocular nerve palsies; facial paralysis; depressed corneal reflex; hearing loss, tinnitus; difficulty swallowing; drooling; vertigo and dizziness; ataxia; vomiting

From Chipps E, et al. (1992). *Neurologic Disorders* (p. 93). St. Louis: Mosby.

---

and ability to communicate. Individual nursing diagnoses depend on nursing assessment. Review the medical record to plan for specific patient needs in relation to the planned surgical approach, patient position, special equipment and supply needs, and preliminary maneuvers (lines, catheters, shave, and so on). Check that x-ray films and results of other diagnostic evaluations are available. For the patient undergoing craniotomy for tumor removal, CT, MRI, EEG, and brain scans, as well as arteriograms and skull films, are usually required. Modify the care plan according to the assessment and prioritized nursing diagnoses.

2. Indwelling urinary catheters are usually inserted to monitor urinary output. This is especially important in relation to the anticipated length of the procedure and the use of intraoperative diuretics. Use aseptic technique for catheter insertion. Place the drainage bag where it is readily observable. Document catheter insertion. Be sure drainage tubing is not kinked or subject to tension during position changes.

3. Special monitoring equipment that may be used with this patient includes intracranial pressure line, arterial line, Swan-Ganz catheter, epidural catheter, and central venous pressure catheter. Document special monitoring devices and readings as appropriate in the institutional setting.

4. The supine position is usually selected for supratentorial tumors. Refer to positioning for cranioplasty in the previous Guide to Nursing Action. For infratentorial or posterior fossa tumors, the prone position (refer to positioning for laminectomy) or the sitting position is used. Add a padded footboard to the OR bed. Apply antiembolic stockings or sequential decompression hose to prevent venous stasis if they are not already applied. An antigravity suit may be used. The patient is slowly placed in the sitting position, with careful monitoring of vital signs by the anesthesia staff. A head holder, such as the Mayfield or U-frame, is attached to the back or side of the OR bed once the position is achieved. Skull pin attachments are added; the shoulders are stabilized with adhesive tape secured to the U-frame or sitting device. The potential for hypotensive episodes and air emboli must be planned for. A central venous pressure line may be inserted and confirmed by fluoroscopy, with a 50-ml syringe and a three-way stopcock ready to withdraw air. An esophageal stethoscope or Doppler unit will be used. Be prepared to assist the anesthesia staff. Assess pressure areas (occiput, scapulae, elbows, sacrum, heels, and genitals) and pad protectively.

5. Prepare the skin according to institutional protocol. If hair is removed, explain the procedure and carry it out according to policy, being especially aware of proper disposition of hair. Note the use of skin marking and injections at incision site.

6. The condition of the skin should be noted before and after skin preparation procedures. Look for and note any nicks, abrasions, and rashes.

7. The skin should be assessed before and after the placement of electrosurgical dispersive pads.

8. Draping may be complicated for certain neurosurgical procedures. Have special barrier materials available and monitor aseptic technique

FIG. 9-2

CARE PLAN FOR CRANIOTOMY (TUMOR REMOVAL)

KEY ASSESSMENT POINTS

Observe patient for signs/symptoms of increased intracranial pressure (ICP), including restlessness, lethargy, changes in vital signs

Evaluate patient for pain—headache with steady persistent or intractable dull pain or changes in character of headache may indicate intracranial tumor. Sudden severe headache usually beginning as frontal or temporal and then generalizing to the entire head may indicate intracranial aneurysm.

Assess patient's vision. Visual disturbances such as blurring vision, double vision, visual field deficit and unilateral blindness may be present.

Evaluate patient for nuchal rigidity, photophobia, positive Kernig's sign, positive Bruzinski's sign, fever, irritability, or restlessness. All these could be signs of meningeal irritation.

Assess patient's autonomic function. Look for diaphoresis, chills, changes in heart rate and blood pressure, slight temperature elevation.

NURSING DIAGNOSIS

All generic nursing diagnoses apply to this patient, with the addition of:

High risk for injury related to changes in ICP and sensory-perceptual function

PATIENT OUTCOMES

All generic patient outcomes apply, with the addition of:
The patient will remain injury free as evidenced by:
1. Seizure precautions maintained
2. Maintenance of baseline level of consciousness
3. Adequate respiratory function
4. Absence of signs of increased intracranial pressure

NURSING ACTIONS

	Yes	No	N/A
1. Assessment performed?	☐	☐	☐
2. Foley catheter inserted?	☐	☐	☐
3. Special monitoring devices?	☐	☐	☐
4. Correctly positioned?	☐	☐	☐
5. Skin prep per institutional protocol?	☐	☐	☐
6. Condition of skin at prep site noted?	☐	☐	☐
7. ESU dispersive pad site checked before application?	☐	☐	☐
8. Aseptic technique monitored during draping?	☐	☐	☐
9. Medications available/administered?	☐	☐	☐
10. Special equipment available?	☐	☐	☐
11. Laser safety precautions implemented?	☐	☐	☐
12. Suction checked?	☐	☐	☐
13. Drills available/checked?	☐	☐	☐
14. Irrigation/IV solutions/blood warmed?	☐	☐	☐
15. Urinary output/blood loss noted?	☐	☐	☐
16. Specimens/cultures to lab?	☐	☐	☐
17. Counts performed and correct?	☐	☐	☐
18. Dispersive pad site rechecked?	☐	☐	☐
19. Drains/catheters noted?	☐	☐	☐
20. Dressings applied?	☐	☐	☐
21. Other generic care plans initiated? (specify)	☐	☐	☐

Document additional nursing actions/generic care plans initiated here:

_____

_____

_____

EVALUATION OF PATIENT OUTCOMES

	Outcome met	Outcome met with additional outcome criteria	Outcome met with revised nursing care plan	Outcome not met	Outcome not applicable to this patient
1. The patient was injury free.	☐	☐	☐	☐	☐
2. The patient met outcomes for additional generic care plans as indicated.	☐	☐	☐	☐	☐

Signature: _____ Date: _____

carefully. Assist in draping the microscope and other special equipment.

9. Various medications may be used during neurosurgery. These include topical hemostatics, thrombin, bone wax, local anesthetics with or without epinephrine, and antibiotics. All medications on the sterile field must be labeled. Check the patient record for allergies before administering drugs. Document the drug, dosage, route, time administered, and by whom.

10. Special equipment should be readied before patient admission to the OR. Careful review of the medical record, consultation with physician colleagues, and nursing experience should be used to ensure that what will be needed is available and in working order. For craniotomy for tumor, the patient may require craniotomy instrumentation, cottonoids, cotton balls, self-retaining brain retractors, clips and appliers, artificial dura, ventricular needles, Raney clips or other skin hemostatic clips, pituitary forceps, and microinstruments as requested. Headlights, microloops, microscope, bipolar cautery, intraoperative ultrasound and Cavitron aspirator unit may all be necessary adjuncts. Check all equipment before use. Document special safety precautions taken.

11. Laser-assisted tumor excision or laser-assisted neuroendoscopy may be used for select tumors, depending on their size and vascular supply. Tumors that are 2 cm in diameter or smaller, such as colloid cysts, small ependymomas, and pineal region tumors, may be excised via neuroendoscopy (Nurre-Miller, 1994); the endoscopy system is required for this approach. In addition, the laser requires a sterile hand piece, laser director, exhaust hose wand, and arm drape. Nonsterile equipment includes a smoke evacuator, exhaust machines, filter hose, and safety goggles. Follow institutional protocols for laser safety.

12. Two suction lines should be available and functioning. Have extra Frazier suction tips, stylets, and tubing ready.

13. Test all drills before use. Follow institutional protocols for the use of electrical and air-powered surgical drills.

14. Warmed irrigation fluids, intravenous solutions, and blood help maintain normothermia. Have a blood warmer available. Have two bulb syringes and adequate irrigating fluid for drilling procedures and bipolar coagulation. Carefully mix and clearly label antibiotic irrigation fluid.

15. Document urinary output and blood loss.

16. Follow institutional protocol for preserving, labeling, and transporting specimens, frozen sections, and cultures; implement universal precautions when handling blood and body tissue. With tumor removal, it may be necessary to strain suction contents for the specimen. Record specimens and cultures.

17. Perform counts according to institutional protocol. In addition to instrument, sharp, and sponge counts, consider the necessity of counting cottonoids, cotton balls, and electrosurgical tips and cleaning pads. Document the results of counts.

18. Check the electrosurgical dispersive pad site whenever there is a position change and when the pad is removed.

19. Record drains, catheters, Silastic tubing, and shunting materials.

20. Assist in the application of dressings. Allow adequate room for tissue swelling to prevent "tape burns."

Craniotomy for Intracranial Aneurysm (Fig. 9-3)

1. A cerebral aneurysm is a localized dilation that develops secondary to a weakness of the arterial wall (Chipps, Clanin, & Campbell, 1992). Aneurysms are classified according to their characteristics. Saccular aneurysms are thin walled and appear to be berry shaped as they protrude from the artery wall. They are usually found near the Circle of Willis. Fusiform aneurysms are characterized by their occupation of the entire circumference of the artery and appear spindle shaped. These are found on the basilar artery, and when they rupture are usually fatal. Mycotic aneurysms are the result of a septic embolus from another infection that damages the artery. These may be found near the middle and anterior cerebral arteries. Traumatic aneurysms occur from shearing forces to the artery secondary to skull fracture, or they may be the result of surgery to remove tumors, or hematomas. The patient undergoing craniotomy for an intracranial aneurysm may have nursing diagnoses of *altered cerebral tissue perfusion* and *altered peripheral tissue perfusion*. The goals and criteria suggested as evaluation for outcomes may need to be modified according to the patient's mental status. The potential for rupture, followed by hemorrhage and emergency intervention, must be anticipated. The patient's airway and vital signs must be monitored. There may be weakness or paralysis, aphasia, nuchal rigidity, severe headache, or extreme sensitivity to light, all of which require special perioperative nursing care. *Self-esteem disturbance* and *body image disturbance* may result from loss of hair when the head is shaved. There may be knowledge

FIG. 9-3
CARE PLAN FOR INTRACRANIAL ANEURYSM

KEY ASSESSMENT POINTS

Location of aneurysm
Presence/degree of hemorrhage
Headache (acute; generalized; migraine-like)
Visual defects (photophobia, eye deviation, ophthalmoplegia, papilledema)
Neck discomfort
Lethargy
Transient ischemic attacks
Paresis (motor and sensory impairment)
Level of consciousness
Vital signs
Meningeal signs (Brudzinski's and Kernig's)

NURSING DIAGNOSIS

All generic nursing diagnoses apply to this patient, with the addition of:
Altered cerebral/peripheral tissue perfusion

PATIENT OUTCOMES

All generic outcomes apply, with the addition of:
The patient will demonstrate no alteration in cerebral/peripheral tissue perfusion as evidenced by (depending on preoperative status):
1. Remaining alert and oriented
2. Maintaining intact cognitive processes
3. Having normal speech and range of motion

NURSING ACTIONS

	Yes	No	N/A
1. Assessment performed?	☐	☐	☐
2. Foley catheter inserted?	☐	☐	☐
3. Special monitoring devices?	☐	☐	☐
4. Correctly positioned?	☐	☐	☐
5. Skin prep per institutional protocol?	☐	☐	☐
6. Condition of skin at prep site noted?	☐	☐	☐
7. ESU dispersive pad site checked before application?	☐	☐	☐
8. Aseptic technique monitored during draping?	☐	☐	☐
9. Medications available/administered?	☐	☐	☐
10. Special equipment available?	☐	☐	☐
11. Deliberate hypotension safely achieved?	☐	☐	☐
12. Suction checked?	☐	☐	☐
13. Drills available/checked?	☐	☐	☐
14. Irrigation/IV solutions/blood warmed?	☐	☐	☐
15. Urinary output/blood loss monitored?	☐	☐	☐
16. Special measures taken during aneurysm repair?	☐	☐	☐
17. Specimens/cultures to lab?	☐	☐	☐
18. Counts performed/correct?	☐	☐	☐
19. Dispersive pad site rechecked?	☐	☐	☐
20. Drains/catheters noted?	☐	☐	☐
21. Dressings applied?	☐	☐	☐
22. Other generic care plans initiated? (specify)	☐	☐	☐

Document additional nursing actions/generic care plans initiated here:

_____

_____

_____

EVALUATION OF PATIENT OUTCOMES

	Outcome met	Outcome met with additional outcome criteria	Outcome met with revised nursing care plan	Outcome not met	Outcome not applicable to this patient
1. The patient maintained adequate cerebral/peripheral tissue perfusion.	☐	☐	☐	☐	☐
2. The patient met outcomes for additional generic care plans as indicated.	☐	☐	☐	☐	☐

Signature: _____ Date: _____

deficits, alterations in thought processes, limitations in mobility, anxiety, and alterations in levels of consciousness and ability to communicate. Individual nursing diagnoses depend on nursing assessment. Review the medical record to plan for specific patient needs in relation to the planned surgical approach, patient position, special equipment and supply needs, and preliminary maneuvers (lines, catheters, shave, and so on). Check that x-ray films and results of other diagnostic evaluations are available. For the patient undergoing craniotomy for intracranial aneurysm, CT scans and arteriograms are usually required. Modify the care plan according to the assessment.

2. Indwelling urinary catheters are usually inserted to monitor urinary output. This is especially important in relation to the anticipated length of the procedure and the use of intraoperative diuretics. Use aseptic technique for catheter insertion. Place the drainage bag where it is readily observable. Document catheter insertion. Be sure drainage tubing is not kinked or subject to tension during positional changes.

3. Special monitoring equipment that may be used with this patient includes intracranial pressure line, arterial line, Swan-Ganz catheter, epidural catheter, and central venous pressure catheter. Document special monitoring devices and readings as appropriate to the institutional setting.

4. Either the supine or sitting position may be selected. Refer to the two previous Guides to Nursing Actions for positioning for cranioplasty and craniotomy for tumor removal.

5. Prepare the skin according to institutional protocol. If hair is removed, explain the procedure and carry it out according to policy, being especially aware of proper disposition of hair. Note the use of skin marking and injections at incision site.

6. The condition of the skin should be noted before and after skin preparation procedures. Look for and note any nicks, abrasions, and rashes.

7. The skin should be assessed before and after the placement of electrosurgical dispersive pads.

8. Draping may be complicated for certain neurosurgery procedures. Have special barrier materials available and monitor aseptic technique carefully. Assist in draping the microscope and other special equipment.

9. Various medications may be used during neurosurgery. These include topical hemostatics, thrombin, bone wax, local anesthetics with or without epinephrine, and antibiotics. Papaverine HCl may be used for the patient with intracranial aneurysm. All medications on the ster-

ile field must be labeled. Check the patient record for allergies before administering drugs. Document the drug, dosage, route, time administered, and by whom.

10. Special equipment should be readied before patient admission to the OR. Careful review of the medical record, consultation with physician colleagues, and nursing experience should be used to ensure that what will be needed is available and in working order. For aneurysm repair, the patient may require craniotomy instrumentation, cottonoids, cotton balls, self-retaining brain retractors, aneurysm clips and appliers (both temporary and permanent, with two appliers for each type of clip), microinstruments as requested, and an aneuroplasty kit. Headlights, microloops, microscope, bipolar cautery, and laser may all be necessary adjuncts. Check all equipment before use. Document special safety precautions taken.

11. To control the possibility of hemorrhage, deliberate or artificial hypotension may be instituted. Sodium nitroprusside is often the agent of choice to induce hypotension. Collaborate with the anesthesia staff in managing drug therapy and monitoring vital signs. Sometimes, with difficult aneurysm repair involving prolonged periods of hypotension, it becomes necessary to "protect" the brain with the use of barbiturate coma. The loading dose of pentobarbital (Nembutal) is 1 to 2 g; the perioperative nurse should have this available for prompt use should the situation arise.

12. Two suction lines should be available and functioning. Have extra Frazier suction tips, stylets, and tubing ready.

13. Test all drills before use. Follow institutional protocols for the use of electrical and air-powered surgical drills.

14. Warmed irrigation fluids, intravenous solutions, and blood help maintain patient normothermia. Have a blood warmer available. Have two bulb syringes and adequate irrigating fluid for drilling procedures and bipolar coagulation. Carefully mix and clearly label antibiotic irrigation.

15. Document urinary output and blood loss.

16. During the actual repair, special precautions must be taken. The OR team should not lean on the bed; any movements that affect the field can affect the repair. Environmental noise and stimulation should be controlled. Except in urgent cases, perioperative nursing staff should not be relieved during this part of the procedure. Aneurysm clips should not be compressed between the fingers. Once the clip has been compressed, it should be discarded. The aneuro-

plasty kit should be ready to use, as should the bipolar unit. Have suction immediately available.

17. Follow institutional protocol for preserving, labeling, and transporting specimens and cultures; implement universal precautions when handling blood and body tissue. Record specimens and cultures.

18. Perform counts according to institutional protocol. In addition to instrument, sharp, and sponge counts, consider the necessity of counting cottonoids, cotton balls, electrosurgical tips, and cleaning pads. Document the results of counts.

19. Check the electrosurgical dispersive pad site whenever there is a position change and when the pad is removed.

20. Record drains, catheters, Silastic tubing, and shunting materials.

21. Assist in the application of dressings. Allow adequate room for tissue swelling to prevent "tape burns."

Evacuation of Hematoma (Fig 9-4)

1. Neurosurgical patients vary significantly in relationship to their underlying disease processes, clusters of signs and symptoms, and adjustment to alterations that result from the disease. Patient presentation will vary according to the location of the hematoma. Epidural hematomas may be surgical emergencies. This patient may have a rapidly increasing intracranial pressure, demanding careful monitoring. If this is a trauma patient, additional nursing measures will be required. (Refer to Chapter 20 for a discussion of trauma nursing.) If the patient is conscious, anxiety or fear may be present. For the patient with either subdural or epidural hematoma, it may be helpful to classify anxiety levels as low, moderate, or severe. Nursing behaviors that demonstrate caring are helpful in assisting patients to cope with anxiety. A calm voice, short sentences, and a gentle touch all reassure the patient that he or she will be well cared for. If it is not an emergency situation, attempt to determine what anxiety-reducing techniques (imagery, relaxation) have worked for the patient in the past and provide encouragement or assistance in using them. Disturbances in self-esteem and body image may result from loss of hair when the head is shaved. There may be knowledge deficits, alterations in thought processes, limitations in mobility, compromised sensory perception, and varying alterations in levels of consciousness and ability to communicate. Individual nursing diagnoses depend on nursing assessment. Review the medical record to plan for specific patient needs in relation to the planned surgical approach, patient position, special equipment and supply needs, and preliminary maneuvers (lines, catheters, shave, and so on). Check that x-ray films and results of other diagnostic evaluations are available. For evacuation of hematomas, CT scans, angiograms, and skull films are usually required. Modify the care plan according to the assessment.

2. Indwelling urinary catheters are usually inserted to monitor urinary output. This is especially important in relation to the anticipated length of the procedure and the use of intraoperative diuretics. Use aseptic technique for catheter insertion. Place the drainage bag where it is readily observable. Document catheter insertion. Prevent tubing from kinking and tension during any positional changes.

3. Intracranial pressure monitoring and arterial lines may be used. Assist with insertion and set up of equipment. Record monitoring results according to institutional protocol.

4. A modified supine position is usually selected for hematoma evacuation. Apply elastic bandages or antiembolic stockings to prevent venous stasis if they are not already applied. The head will be elevated during this procedure. If reverse Trendelenburg's position is used, apply a padded footboard. Have an appropriate accessory available to stabilize the head. Position the arms to prevent brachial plexus injury by hyperabduction; pad wrists and elbows to protect vulnerable nerves. Place the safety strap 2 inches above the knees, snugly but not tightly, to prevent compression on the popliteal space. Lumbar and popliteal pads may be used to prevent shearing forces if reverse Trendelenburg's position is used. Always return patients slowly from reverse Trendelenburg's position to prevent volume shifts and changes in vital signs. Monitor the patient closely during positional changes. Pad additional pressure sites. The table may be turned to allow for maximal use of room in the OR.

5. Prepare the skin according to institutional protocol. If hair is removed explain the procedure and carry it out according to policy, being especially aware of proper disposition of hair. Note the use of skin marking and injections at incision site.

6. The condition of the skin should be noted before and after skin preparation procedures. Look for and note any nicks, abrasions, and rashes.

7. The skin should be assessed before and after the placement of electrosurgical dispersive pads.

FIG. 9-4
CARE PLAN FOR EVACUATION OF HEMATOMA

KEY ASSESSMENT POINTS

Type of hematoma (epidural, subdural, intracerebral)
Presence of skull fracture
Level of consciousness (and change in)
Signs of increased intracranial pressure
Evidence of penetrating injury
History of past significant injury

NURSING DIAGNOSIS

All generic nursing diagnoses apply to this patient, with the addition
   of:
   Anxiety (Fear)

PATIENT OUTCOMES

All generic patient outcomes apply, with the addition of:
The patient will exhibit a reduced level of anxiety by:
   1. Displaying relaxed facial expressions
   2. Verbalizing less anxiety (or fear)
   3. Accurately describing perioperative events

NURSING ACTIONS

	Yes	No	N/A
1. Assessment performed?	☐	☐	☐
2. Foley catheter inserted?	☐	☐	☐
3. Special monitoring devices?	☐	☐	☐
4. Correctly positioned?	☐	☐	☐
5. Skin prep per institutional protocol?	☐	☐	☐
6. Condition of skin noted at prep site?	☐	☐	☐
7. ESU dispersive pad checked before application?	☐	☐	☐
8. Aseptic technique monitored during draping?	☐	☐	☐
9. Medications available/administered?	☐	☐	☐
10. Special equipment available?	☐	☐	☐
11. Suction checked?	☐	☐	☐
12. Drills available/checked?	☐	☐	☐
13. Irrigation/IV solutions warmed?	☐	☐	☐
14. Urinary output/blood loss monitored?	☐	☐	☐
15. Specimens/cultures to lab?	☐	☐	☐
16. Counts performed/correct?	☐	☐	☐
17. Dispersive pad site rechecked?	☐	☐	☐
18. Drains/catheters noted?	☐	☐	☐
19. Dressings applied?	☐	☐	☐
20. Other generic care plans initiated? (specify)	☐	☐	☐

Document additional nursing actions/generic care plans initiated
here:

_____

_____

_____

EVALUATION OF PATIENT OUTCOMES

1. The patient's anxiety was reduced.
2. The patient met outcomes for additional generic care plans as
   indicated.

	Outcome met	Outcome met with additional outcome criteria	Outcome met with revised nursing care plan	Outcome not met	Outcome not applicable to this patient
1.	☐	☐	☐	☐	☐
2.	☐	☐	☐	☐	☐

Signature: _____ Date: _____

8. Draping may be complicated for certain neurosurgery procedures. Have special barrier materials available; monitor aseptic technique carefully.

9. Various medications may be used during neurosurgery. These include topical hemostatics, thrombin, bone wax, local anesthetics with or without epinephrine, and antibiotics. All medications on the sterile field must be labeled. Check the patient record for allergies before administering drugs. Document the drug, dosage, route, time administered, and by whom.

10. Special equipment should be readied before patient admission to the OR. Careful review of the medical record, consultation with physician colleagues, and nursing experience should be used to ensure that what will be needed is available and in working order. For evacuation of hematomas, the patient will require craniotomy instrumentation, self-retaining retractors, brain retractors, hemostatic skin clips, a bipolar unit, and clips to tag the former bleeding site. A Cavitron surgical aspirator may be used. Headlights with a backup light should also be available.

11. Two suction lines should be available and functioning. Have extra Frazier suction tips, stylets, and tubing ready. Large amounts of irrigation solution will be used until return is clear. Have two bulb syringes or irrigating catheters ready.

12. Test all drills before use. Follow institutional protocols for the use of electrical and air-powered surgical drills.

13. Warmed irrigation fluids, intravenous solutions, and blood help maintain patient normothermia. Have a blood warmer available. Have two bulb syringes and adequate irrigating fluid for drilling procedures and bipolar coagulation. Carefully mix and label any antibiotic irrigation.

14. Document urinary output and blood loss.

15. Follow institutional protocol for preserving, labeling, and transporting specimens and cultures; implement universal precautions when handling blood and body tissue. Record specimens and cultures.

16. Perform counts according to institutional protocol. In addition to instrument, sharp, and sponge counts, consider the necessity of counting cottonoids, cotton balls, and electrosurgical tips and cleaning pads. Document the results of counts.

17. Check the electrosurgical dispersive pad site whenever there is a position change and when the pad is removed.

18. Record drains, catheters, Silastic tubing, and shunting materials.

19. Assist in the application of dressings. Allow adequate room for postoperative swelling when applying tape to prevent "tape burns."

Lumbar Laminectomy (Fig. 9-5)

1. A laminectomy is a surgical procedure performed to relieve compression of the spinal cord or spinal nerve roots or both. Laminectomy is most commonly performed in the lumbar and cervical regions, and this care plan is generally applicable to either site. This care plan does not, however, apply to percutaneous laser disc decompression (PLDD), which requires the Nd:YAG laser lateral recumbent position, an 18-gauge needle for the laser fiber, antibiotic ointment, and a small bandage (Wright, 1995). The traditional surgical treatment for herniated disc is described here. The patient undergoing lumbar laminectomy may have a nursing diagnosis of *pain*. If this nursing diagnosis is used, it is necessary to assess the location, type, and duration of pain. Because laminectomy offers hope of reducing pain, patients may anticipate the surgery with relief. Determine the effectiveness of preoperative medications. Assist the patient to a position of comfort. Encourage the patient to use pain control techniques (imagery, relaxation) that have worked in the past. Consider any neurovascular changes (numbness, decreased mobility) when planning patient transfer and positioning. Individual nursing diagnoses derived for the neurosurgery patient depend on nursing assessment. Review the medical record to plan for specific patient needs in relation to the planned surgical approach, patient position, special equipment and supply needs, and preliminary maneuvers (lines, catheters, shave, and so on). Check that x-ray films (plain spine x-rays) and results of other diagnostic evaluations are available, such as CT or MRI scans or myelograms. Modify the care plan according to the assessment.

2. Indwelling urinary catheters are usually inserted to monitor urinary output. This is especially important in relation to the anticipated length of the procedure if the patient has a spinal cord tumor. Use aseptic technique for catheter insertion. Place the drainage bag where it is readily observable. Document catheter insertion. Prevent kinking and tension on the tube during position changes.

3. The prone position is often selected for laminectomy. There are many options in selecting positioning accessories for the prone position. Whichever accessory is selected, prepare the OR bed before patient transfer. The patient is usually anesthetized on the stretcher. Under careful monitoring by anesthesia personnel, the pa-

FIG. 9-5
CARE PLAN FOR LUMBAR LAMINECTOMY

KEY ASSESSMENT POINTS

Sensory impairment (numbness, tingling, cold in extremity)
Motor impairment (weakness)
Location of pain (that is, in low back/radiates down leg to inner calf, to dorsum of foot and big toe, or to sole of foot and heel)
Muscle spasm
Aggravating factors
Positive Lasegue's test (pain produced before 70° straight leg elevation, dorsiflexion of foot aggravates pain, pain relief occurs with flexion of knee)
Medications taken
Reflexes affected (patellar in L3 and L4; Achilles in L5 and S1)

NURSING DIAGNOSIS

All generic nursing diagnoses apply to this patient, with the addition of:
Pain

PATIENT OUTCOMES

All generic patient outcomes apply, with the addition of:
The patient's pain will be controlled. The patient will:
1. Express effectiveness of preoperative medication
2. Be in a position of comfort in holding area
3. Describe/utilize additional pain control measures that are effective

NURSING ACTIONS

	Yes	No	N/A
1. Assessment performed?	☐	☐	☐
2. Foley catheter inserted?	☐	☐	☐
3. Correctly positioned?	☐	☐	☐
4. Skin prep per institutional protocol?	☐	☐	☐
5. Condition of skin noted at prep site?	☐	☐	☐
6. ESU dispersive pad site checked before application?	☐	☐	☐
7. Aseptic technique monitored during draping?	☐	☐	☐
8. Medications available/administered?	☐	☐	☐
9. Special equipment available?	☐	☐	☐
10. Suction checked?	☐	☐	☐
11. Drills available/checked?	☐	☐	☐
12. Irrigation/IV solutions warmed?	☐	☐	☐
13. Urinary output/blood loss monitored?	☐	☐	☐
14. Specimens/cultures to lab?	☐	☐	☐
15. Counts performed/correct?	☐	☐	☐
16. Dispersive pad site rechecked?	☐	☐	☐
17. Drains/catheters noted?	☐	☐	☐
18. Dressings applied?	☐	☐	☐
19. Other generic care plans initiated? (specify)	☐	☐	☐

Document additional nursing actions/generic care plans initiated here:

_____

_____

_____

EVALUATION OF PATIENT OUTCOMES

1. The patient's pain was controlled.
2. The patient met outcomes for additional generic care plans as indicated.

	Outcome met	Outcome met with additional outcome criteria	Outcome met with revised nursing care plan	Outcome not met	Outcome not applicable to this patient
1.	☐	☐	☐	☐	☐
2.	☐	☐	☐	☐	☐

Signature: _____ Date: _____

tient is log-rolled onto the abdomen. The positioning accessory (beanbag, prone frame, intratrochanteric rolls) should be placed appropriately. Check support for the abdominal wall. Protect wrists, feet, genitals, breasts, eyes, ears, and dependent pressure areas from injury. The head needs to be carefully positioned to prevent injury to the facial nerve. A safety strap should be placed and patient stability verified. Antiembolic stockings may be applied to prevent venous stasis.

4. Prepare the skin according to institutional protocol. Note the use of skin marking and injections at the incision site.

5. The condition of the skin should be noted before and after skin preparation procedures. Observe for and note any nicks, abrasions, and rashes.

6. The skin should be assessed before and after the placement of electrosurgical dispersive pads.

7. Draping may be complicated for certain neurosurgery procedures. Have special barrier materials available; monitor aseptic technique carefully.

8. Various medications may be used during neurosurgery. These include topical hemostatics, thrombin, bone wax, local anesthetics with or without epinephrine, antibiotics, steroids, and diuretics. All medications on the sterile field must be labeled. Check the patient record for allergies before administering drugs. Document the drug, dosage, route, time administered, and by whom.

9. Special equipment should be readied before patient admission to the OR. Careful review of the medical record, consultation with physician colleagues, and nursing experience should be used to ensure that what will be needed is available and in working order. For laminectomy, the patient will require laminectomy instrumentation, self-retaining retractors, laminectomy retractors, root retractors, curettes, and pituitary forceps. Headlights and a bipolar unit may be used. If the patient requires spinal fusion, a bone graft from the iliac crest may be taken or allograft may be used for stabilization. Implants of plates and screws may also be needed for stabilization; documentation of all implantable materials should be made part of the patient's medical record. If there is a cord tumor (Boxes 9-6 and 9-7), the microscope and a laser may be used. Dura film and dura suture should be available in case of a leak or replacement of pathologic dura.

10. Two suction lines should be available and functioning. Have extra Frazier suction tips, stylets, and tubing ready.

Box 9-6 Classification of Spinal Cord Tumors

Intramedullary Tumors
Ependymoma
Astrocytoma
Oligodendroglioma
Hemangioblastoma
Congenital (dermoid, epidermoid)

Extramedullary Tumors
Intradural
Meningioma
Neurofibroma

Extradural
Metastatic carcinomas
Lymphomas
Multiple myeloma

Box 9-7 Characteristics of Spinal Cord Tumors

Intramedullary Tumors
Ependymomas and astrocytomas are most common types
Usually extend over many spinal cord regions
Most have slow, progressive onset
Cord compression occurs on central fiber tracts rather than on nerve roots
Sensory loss of pain and temperature
Tumors in caudal region may cause bowel, bladder, and sexual dysfunction

Extramedullary Tumors
Intradural
Most common spinal cord tumor
Meningiomas and neurofibromas are most common types
Thoracic spine is frequent site
Slow, gradual onset
Local and radicular pain may be present, but isn't always
Symptoms of cord compression may be gradual

Extradural
Mostly malignant
Rapid onset of symptoms
Local pain at area of tumor and along spinal nerve dermatomes
Increased pain with bed rest, movement, and straining
Pain appears before symptoms of spinal cord dysfunction

11. Test all drills before use. Follow institutional protocols for the use of electrical and air-powered surgical drills.
12. Warmed irrigation fluids, intravenous solutions, and blood help maintain patient normothermia. Have a blood warmer available. Have two bulb syringes and adequate irrigating fluid for bipolar coagulation. Carefully mix and label any antibiotic irrigation.
13. Document urinary output and blood loss.
14. Follow institutional protocol for preserving, labeling, and transporting specimens and cultures; implement universal precautions when handling blood and body tissue. Record specimens and cultures.
15. Perform counts according to institutional protocol. In addition to instrument, sharp, and sponge counts, consider the necessity of counting cottonoids, cotton balls, electrosurgical tips, and electrosurgical cleaning pads. Document the results of counts. With laminectomies, attempts are made to secure hemostasis without the use of topical hemostatics. If topical hemostatics are used, be sure to document their removal after hemostasis is secured.
16. Check the electrosurgical dispersive pad site whenever there is a position change and when the pad is removed.
17. Record drains and catheters.
18. Assist in the application of dressings. Allow adequate room for postoperative swelling when applying tape to prevent tape blisters.

Anterior Cervical Fusion (Fig. 9-6)

1. Neurosurgical patients vary significantly in relationship to their underlying disease processes, clusters of signs and symptoms, and adjustment to alterations that result from the disease. The patient undergoing anterior cervical fusion may have a nursing diagnosis of *pain*. If this nursing diagnosis is used, it is necessary to assess the location, type, and duration of pain. It is also important to assess any neurovascular changes that may be present (numbness of shoulder, arm, and fingers). Traumatic injuries may be accompanied by paralysis; the patient may arrive in the OR in traction. Note all preoperative alterations. Determine the effectiveness of preoperative medications. Assist the patient to a position of comfort. Encourage the patient to use pain control techniques (imagery, relaxation) that have been previously effective. Consider any neurovascular changes in planning patient transfer and positioning. Individual nursing diagnoses depend on nursing assessment. Review the medical record to plan for specific patient needs in relation to the planned surgical approach, patient position, special equipment and supply needs, and preliminary maneuvers (lines, catheters, shave, and so on). Check that x-ray films and results of other diagnostic evaluations are available. For the patient undergoing anterior cervical fusion, CT scan, myelograms, and results of other neurologic function tests (electromyography and sensory evoked potentials) are usually required. It is necessary to determine what kind of grafting procedure will be carried out and whether intraoperative fluoroscopy will be required. Modify the care plan according to assessment.
2. An indwelling urinary catheter may be inserted to monitor urinary output. This is especially likely with the anticipated length of the procedure if the patient has a cord tumor. Use aseptic technique for catheter insertion. Place the drainage bag where is it readily observable. Document catheter insertion. Prevent kinking and tension on the tube during position changes.
3. The supine position is used for anterior cervical fusion. Neck rolls may be used for stability and support. If an autograft is to be taken, the donor site (often the iliac crest) may be elevated.
4. Prepare the skin according to institutional protocol for donor and graft sites.
5. The condition of the skin should be noted before and after skin preparatory procedures. Look for and note any nicks, abrasions, and rashes.
6. The skin should be assessed before and after the placement of electrosurgical dispersive pads.
7. Draping will involve two sites if an autograft is used. Monitor aseptic technique carefully. Technique also needs monitoring during team movement from graft to donor sites.
8. Various medications may be used during neurosurgery. These include topical hemostatics, thrombin, bone wax, local anesthetics with or without epinephrine, and antibiotics. All medications on the sterile field must be labeled. Check the patient record for allergies before administering drugs. Document the drug, dosage, route, time administered, and by whom.
9. Special equipment should be readied before patient admission to the OR. Careful review of the medical record, consultation with physician colleagues, and nursing experience should be used to ensure that what will be needed is available and in working order. For anterior cervical fusion, the patient will require laminectomy instruments, self-retaining retractors, Cloward instruments, spinal needles, cassette drape, and drills (hand and power). If allograft is used, determine the size and follow the manufacturer's

FIG. 9-6
CARE PLAN FOR ANTERIOR CERVICAL FUSION

KEY ASSESSMENT POINTS

Sensory impairment (numbness of shoulder, arm, fingers)
Motor impairment (clumsiness, loss of muscle tone)
Location, type, duration of pain
Paralysis
Aggravating factors
Presence of traction
Medications taken
Problems with sphincter control
Respiratory status

NURSING DIAGNOSIS

All generic nursing diagnoses apply to this patient, with the addition of:
  Pain

PATIENT OUTCOMES

All generic patient outcomes apply, with the addition of:
The patient's pain will be controlled. The patient will:
  1. Express effectiveness of preoperative medication
  2. Be in a position of comfort in holding area
  3. Describe/utilize additional pain control measures that are effective

NURSING ACTIONS

	Yes	No	N/A
1. Assessment performed?	☐	☐	☐
2. Foley catheter inserted?	☐	☐	☐
3. Correctly positioned?	☐	☐	☐
4. Skin prep(s) per institutional protocol?	☐	☐	☐
5. Condition of skin noted at prep site?	☐	☐	☐
6. ESU dispersive pad site checked before application?	☐	☐	☐
7. Aseptic technique monitored?	☐	☐	☐
8. Medications available/administered?	☐	☐	☐
9. Special equipment available?	☐	☐	☐
10. Suction checked?	☐	☐	☐
11. Drills available/checked?	☐	☐	☐
12. Irrigation/IV solutions warmed?	☐	☐	☐
13. Urinary output/blood loss monitored?	☐	☐	☐
14. X-ray precautions taken?	☐	☐	☐
15. Specimens/cultures to lab?	☐	☐	☐
16. Counts performed/correct?	☐	☐	☐
17. Dispersive pad site rechecked?	☐	☐	☐
18. Drains/catheters noted?	☐	☐	☐
19. Dressings applied?	☐	☐	☐
20. Other generic care plans initiated? (specify)	☐	☐	☐

Document additional nursing actions/generic care plans initiated here:

_____

_____

_____

EVALUATION OF PATIENT OUTCOMES

	Outcome met	Outcome met with additional outcome criteria	Outcome met with revised nursing care plan	Outcome not met	Outcome not applicable to this patient
1. The patient's pain was controlled.	☐	☐	☐	☐	☐
2. The patient met outcomes for additional generic care plans as indicated.	☐	☐	☐	☐	☐

Signature: _____ Date: _____

instructions. If bone chips and acrylic cement are used for fusion, have the kit available. Plates and screws may be required for the patient with an unstable spine; record all implantable devices used. Headlights and a bipolar unit may be used.

10. Two suction lines should be available and functioning. Have extra Frazier suction tips, stylets, and tubing ready.

11. Test all drills before use. Follow institutional protocols for the use of electrical and air-powered surgical drills.

12. Warmed irrigation fluids, intravenous solutions, and blood help maintain patient normothermia. Have a blood warmer available. Have two bulb syringes and adequate irrigating fluid for bipolar coagulation. Carefully mix and label any antibiotic irrigation.

13. Document urinary output and blood loss.

14. X-ray films may be taken to localize and verify the correct operative interspace. Check that the radiology department has been notified. Have the cassette drape and spinal needles ready; the surgeon may request that the needle be bent so that insertion depth is minimal. Follow institutional protocol for radiation safety.

15. Follow institutional protocol for preserving, labeling, and transporting specimens and cultures; implement universal precautions when handling blood or body tissue. With fusion, the disc material may be weighed before laboratory disposition. Record specimens and cultures.

16. Perform counts according to institutional protocol. In addition to instrument, sharp, and sponge counts, consider the necessity of counting cottonoids, cotton balls, and electrosurgical tips and cleaning pads. Proceed to document the results of counts.

17. Check the electrosurgical dispersive pad site whenever there is a position change and when the pad is removed.

18. Record drains and catheters.

19. Assist in the application of dressings. Allow adequate room for postoperative swelling when applying tape to prevent "tape burns."

Stereotaxic Surgery (Fig. 9-7)

1. The first practical instruments for stereotaxic surgery were developed in 1947. Stereotaxis pertains to the precise localization of a specific target point based on three-dimensional coordinates derived with the use of a stereotaxis frame and instrumentation (Hickey, 1992). Its advantage for deep lesion biopsy, implantation of radioactive seeds, and aspiration of hematomas with little trauma to adjacent tissue has increased its use. The use of a computer and CT scanner and MRI help establish the X,Y,Z coordinates to determine the exact target site. The stereotaxic probe is introduced through the cannula attached to the stereotaxic frame, which has been attached to the patient's head. Endoscopy may be used with stereotaxis for even more precise lesion biopsy. Local anesthesia is recommended to monitor the patient's response to commands. *Anxiety* may be present, related to diagnosis, prognosis, treatment results, being in an awake state, or unfamiliar OR equipment. It is helpful to classify the level of anxiety broadly (mild, moderate, or severe) in planning nursing actions. Assess for signs of increasing anxiety. Provide accurate and factual information to explain perioperative events. Help the patient identify and successfully use coping skills. Individual nursing diagnoses depend on nursing assessment. Review the medical record to plan for specific patient needs in relation to the planned surgical approach, patient position, special equipment and supply needs, and preliminary maneuvers (lines, catheters, shave, and so on). Check that x-ray films and results of other diagnostic evaluations are available. For the patient undergoing stereotaxic endoscopy, CT or MRI scans will be required. Before the surgery the perioperative nurse will need to gather equipment to be sent to the radiology department (stereotaxic apparatus and sterile fixation pins). Consider allowing family members to wait with the patient in the holding area while scan coordinates are processed. Modify the care plan according to assessment and review.

2. The supine position is used with special accessory devices. The awake patient should be assisted to a position of comfort on the OR bed. Positioning is done carefully because the stereotaxic frame is in place. Explain positioning maneuvers.

3. A hyperthermia blanket may be used. Additional warm blankets should be offered for patient comfort. Document the hyperthermia unit's number and temperature setting according to institutional protocol.

4. The incision site may be shaved in the OR after patient positioning. The operative site and stereotaxic frame will then be prepared with an antimicrobial agent that does not corrode the frame. Document agents used.

5. The condition of the skin should be noted before and after skin preparation procedures. Look for and note any nicks, abrasions, and rashes.

6. The skin should be assessed before and after the placement of electrosurgical dispersive pads. The electrosurgical unit may not be used.

FIG. 9-7
CARE PLAN FOR STEREOTAXIC SURGERY

KEY ASSESSMENT POINTS

Verification of surgical site
Normal lab values
Type and cross-match
Signed consent (and investigational permit, if applicable)
Patient understanding of procedure
Medical history
Mobility limitations
Motor or mental deficits (depending on neuroanatomic pathology)

NURSING DIAGNOSIS

All generic nursing diagnoses apply to this patient, with the addition
   of:
   Anxiety

PATIENT OUTCOMES

All generic outcomes apply, with the addition of:
The patient will exhibit a reduced level of anxiety by:
   1. Displaying relaxed facial expressions
   2. Verbalizing less anxiety (or fear)
   3. Accurately describing perioperative events

NURSING ACTIONS

	Yes	No	N/A
1. Assessment performed?	☐	☐	☐
2. Correctly positioned?	☐	☐	☐
3. Thermia unit?	☐	☐	☐
4. Skin prep per institutional protocol?	☐	☐	☐
5. Condition of skin noted at prep site?	☐	☐	☐
6. ESU dispersive pad site checked before application?	☐	☐	☐
7. Aseptic technique monitored?	☐	☐	☐
8. Medications available/given?	☐	☐	☐
9. Special equipment available?	☐	☐	☐
10. Suction checked?	☐	☐	☐
11. Drills available/checked?	☐	☐	☐
12. Irrigation/IV solutions warmed?	☐	☐	☐
13. Urinary output/blood loss monitored?	☐	☐	☐
14. Specimens/cultures to lab?	☐	☐	☐
15. Laser precautions in effect?	☐	☐	☐
16. Counts performed/correct?	☐	☐	☐
17. Dispersive pad site rechecked?	☐	☐	☐
18. Drains/catheters noted?	☐	☐	☐
19. Dressings applied?	☐	☐	☐
20. Other generic care plans initiated? (specify)	☐	☐	☐

Document additional nursing actions/generic care plans initiated
here:

_____

_____

_____

EVALUATION OF PATIENT OUTCOMES

	Outcome met	Outcome met with additional outcome criteria	Outcome met with revised nursing care plan	Outcome not met	Outcome not applicable to this patient
1. The patient's anxiety was reduced.	☐	☐	☐	☐	☐
2. The patient met outcomes for additional generic care plans as indicated.	☐	☐	☐	☐	☐

Signature: _____ Date: _____

7. Monitor aseptic technique carefully during draping procedures.

8. Various medications may be used during neurosurgery. These include topical hemostatics, thrombin, bone wax, local anesthetics with or without epinephrine, and antibiotics. All medications on the sterile field must be labeled. Check the patient record for allergies before administering drugs. Document the drug, dosage, route, time administered, and by whom.

9. Special equipment should be readied before patient admission to the OR. Careful review of the medical record, consultation with physician colleagues, and nursing experience should be used to ensure that what will be needed is available and in working order. For this procedure, stereotaxic instruments, endoscopes (with accessories and light source), laser (with accessories), sterile frame, drill, and bipolar unit may be required.

10. Suction should be checked. Have suction tips, stylets, and tubing ready.

11. Test all drills before use. Follow institutional protocols for the use of electrical and air-powered surgical drills.

12. Warmed irrigation fluids and intravenous solutions help maintain patient normothermia. Have bulb syringes and adequate irrigating fluid for bipolar coagulation. Carefully mix and label any antibiotic irrigation.

13. Document urinary output and blood loss.

14. Follow institutional protocol for preserving, labeling, and transporting specimens and cultures; implement universal precautions when handling blood and body fluids. With this procedure, anticipate frozen sections, cultures, and chemistry and cytology examinations of tissue. Record specimens and cultures.

15. Follow laser safety precautions according to institutional protocol.

16. Perform counts according to institutional protocol.

17. If the electrosurgical unit is used, check the dispersive pad site during any position change and when the pad is removed.

18. Record presence of any drains.

19. Assist in the application of dressings. Allow adequate room for postoperative swelling when applying tape to prevent "tape burns" at the incision site. Apply antimicrobial ointment and bandages to puncture sites.

Decompression of Median Nerve (Fig. 9-8)

1. Neurosurgical patients vary significantly in relationship to their underlying disease processes, clusters of signs and symptoms, and adjustment to alterations that result from the disease. The patient with a compartmental syndrome may have a nursing diagnosis of *pain*, which is related to discomfort or numbness in the thumb, index, middle, and ring fingers. The affected hand may be clumsy or weak. Accurate care planning will depend on nursing assessment. Review the medical record to plan for specific needs in relation to the type of anesthesia planned and special equipment and supply needs. Check that x-ray films and results of other diagnostic evaluations are available. For the patient undergoing median nerve decompression, results of electrodiagnostic studies, wrist films, or MRI scans will be required. Modify the care plan according to the assessment.

2. The supine position is usually selected. Assist the patient to a position of comfort on the OR bed. Place the safety strap and then place the operative arm on the hand table; protect nerves, and pad pressure sites. The OR bed may be turned to accommodate the hand table and sitting stools.

3. Prepare the skin according to institutional protocol. Document agents used.

4. The condition of the skin should be noted before and after skin preparatory procedures. Look for and note any nicks, abrasions, and rashes.

5. Follow institutional protocol for applying and documenting tourniquet use. The unit number, settings, inflation and deflation times, and site of application should be noted.

6. The patient may receive local or regional anesthesia. Follow institutional protocol for monitoring the patient receiving the particular type of anesthesia.

7. Various medications may be used during neurosurgery. Local anesthetics with or without epinephrine may be used. All medications on the sterile field must be labeled. Check the patient record for allergies before administering drugs. Document the drug, dosage, amount, route, time administered, and by whom.

8. When accessories such as a hand table are used, the risk of contamination during draping is increased. Monitor aseptic technique carefully.

9. Special equipment should be readied before patient admission to the OR. Careful review of the medical record, consultation with physician colleagues, and nursing experience should be used to ensure that what will be needed is available and in working order. For this patient, the hand or plastic set along with probes and groove directors will be required.

10. Warmed irrigation fluids and intravenous solu-

FIG. 9-8
CARE PLAN FOR DECOMPRESSION OF MEDIAN NERVE

KEY ASSESSMENT POINTS
Predisposing factors (occupation, obesity, arthritis, diabetes, gout)
Presence of nocturnal paresthesia, other sensory alterations
Pain/discomfort
Relief measures
Symptoms (morning stiffness)
Thenar atrophy
Muscle control loss
Fine motor function
Positive Phalen's test, forced wrist-flexion test, Tinel's sign

NURSING DIAGNOSIS
All generic nursing diagnoses apply to this patient, with the addition
of:
  Pain
  Sensory/perceptual alteration: tactile

PATIENT OUTCOMES
All generic outcomes apply, with the addition of:
The patient will express minimal discomfort. The patient will:
  1. Use pain reduction techniques as appropriate
  2. Be in a position of comfort on the OR bed
  3. Communicate pain sensations intraoperatively (local anesthesia)

NURSING ACTIONS

	Yes	No	N/A
1. Assessment performed?	☐	☐	☐
2. Positioned correctly?	☐	☐	☐
3. Skin prep per institutional protocol?	☐	☐	☐
4. Condition of skin noted at prep site?	☐	☐	☐
5. Tourniquet applied?	☐	☐	☐
6. Special monitoring?	☐	☐	☐
7. Medications available/administered?	☐	☐	☐
8. Aseptic technique monitored?	☐	☐	☐
9. Special equipment available?	☐	☐	☐
10. Irrigation/IV fluids warmed?	☐	☐	☐
11. Specimens/cultures to lab?	☐	☐	☐
12. Counts performed/correct?	☐	☐	☐
13. Dressings/cast/immobilizer applied?	☐	☐	☐
14. Other generic care plans initiated? (specify)	☐	☐	☐

Document additional nursing actions/generic care plans initiated here:

_____

_____

_____

EVALUATION OF PATIENT OUTCOMES

	Outcome met	Outcome met with additional outcome criteria	Outcome met with revised nursing care plan	Outcome not met	Outcome not applicable to this patient
1. The patient expressed minimal discomfort.	☐	☐	☐	☐	☐
2. The patient met outcomes for additional generic care plans as indicated.	☐	☐	☐	☐	☐

Signature: _____ Date: _____

tions help maintain patient normothermia. Consider other nursing measures, such as application of warm blankets, to foster comfort.

11. Follow institutional protocol for preserving, labeling, and transporting specimens and cultures; implement universal precautions when handling blood or body tissue. With this patient, a biopsy specimen of the carpal ligament may be obtained. Record specimens and cultures.

12. Perform counts according to institutional protocol.

13. Assist in the application of dressings. Allow adequate room for postoperative swelling when applying tape to prevent "tape burns." Document the application of a cast or immobilizer.

Insertion of Ventricular Shunt (Fig. 9-9)

1. Neurosurgical patients vary significantly in relationship to their underlying disease processes, clusters of signs and symptoms, and adjustment to alterations that result from the disease. Ventricular shunts may be inserted in either infants or adults. (The pediatric patient is discussed in Chapter 21.) The adult may exhibit signs of progressive dementia, headache, or incontinence. The risk for *sensory/perceptual alterations* relates to possible shunt malfunction. Careful neurologic assessment is necessary for postoperative comparison. Individual nursing diagnoses depend on nursing assessment. Review the medical record to plan for specific patient needs in relation to planned surgical approach, patient position, special equipment and supply needs, and preliminary maneuvers (lines, catheters, shave, and so on). Check that x-ray films and results of other diagnostic evaluations are available. For the shunt patient, results of CT scans, skull series, ventriculogram, and psychometric tests should be available. Modify the care plan based on assessment and review.

2. An indwelling urinary catheter may be inserted if the patient is experiencing urinary incontinence. Use aseptic technique for catheter insertion. Place the drainage bag where it is readily observable. Document catheter insertion. Prevent tubing from kinking and tension during any positional changes.

3. Modified supine position is usually selected for shunt insertions. The head will be slightly elevated during this procedure; an accessory may be used to stabilize the head. Position the arms to prevent brachial plexus injury by hyperabduction; pad wrists and elbows to protect vulnerable nerves. Place the safety strap 2 inches above the knees, snugly but not tightly, to prevent compression on the popliteal space. Pad additional pressure sites.

4. Prepare the skin according to institutional protocols for multiple incision sites. Document agents used.

5. The condition of the skin should be noted before and after skin preparation procedures. Look for and note any nicks, abrasions, and rashes.

6. The skin should be assessed before and after the placement of electrosurgical dispersive pads.

7. Draping may be complicated for certain neurosurgery procedures. Have special barrier materials available; monitor aseptic technique carefully.

8. Various medications may be used during neurosurgery. These include topical hemostatics, thrombin, bone wax, local anesthetics with or without epinephrine, antibiotics, and heparin. All medications on the sterile field must be labeled. Check the patient record for allergies before administering drugs. Document the drug, dosage, route, time administered, and by whom.

9. Special equipment should be readied before patient admission to the OR. Careful review of the medical record, consultation with physician colleagues, and nursing experience should be used to ensure that what will be needed is available and in working order. For ventricular shunt insertion, the following will be required: shunt instrumentation, shunt kit with parts (reservoir, valves if not incorporated into system), packing forceps, and ventricular needles with stylets. Check the valve assembly according to the manufacturer's instructions. Have a sterile basin for the shunt; keep it free from lint or other contaminants. Neuroendoscopy may be used for shunt insertion; this technique enables the surgeon to see and correctly place the shunt away from tissues of high risk for obstruction, bleeding, or neurologic injury (Nurre-Miller, 1994); the endoscopy system is required for this approach.

10. Two suction lines should be available and functioning. Have extra Frazier suction tips, stylets and tubing ready.

11. Test all drills before use. Follow institutional protocol for the use of electrical and air-powered surgical drills.

12. Warmed irrigation fluids and intravenous solutions help maintain patient normothermia. Have available two bulb syringes and adequate irrigating fluids for drilling procedures and bipolar coagulation. Carefully mix and label any antibiotic irrigation.

13. Document urinary output and blood loss.

FIG. 9-9
CARE PLAN FOR INSERTION OF VENTRICULAR SHUNT

KEY ASSESSMENT POINTS

Observe patient for signs of increased intracranial pressure (restlessness, lethargy, change in level of consciousness (LOC), widening pulse pressure, bradycardia, change in respiratory status).

Evaluate patient's mental status (apathy, inattentiveness, declining memory).

Observe pediatric patients for severely enlarged head, irritability, vomiting, seizure, change in LOC, bulging fontanels, visible distended scalp veins, poor feeding behavior.

NURSING DIAGNOSIS

All generic nursing diagnoses apply to this patient, with the addition of:

Potential for sensory/perceptual alterations

PATIENT OUTCOMES

All generic outcomes apply, with the addition of:
Baseline neurologic status will remain unchanged
(Depending on preoperative status). The patient will:
1. Remain oriented
2. Cooperate with the perioperative team by following commands
3. Describe sequence of perioperative events

NURSING ACTIONS

	Yes	No	N/A
1. Assessment performed?	☐	☐	☐
2. Foley catheter inserted?	☐	☐	☐
3. Correctly positioned?	☐	☐	☐
4. Skin prep per institutional protocol?	☐	☐	☐
5. Condition of skin noted at prep site?	☐	☐	☐
6. ESU dispersive pad site checked before application?	☐	☐	☐
7. Aseptic technique monitored during draping?	☐	☐	☐
8. Medications available/administered?	☐	☐	☐
9. Special equipment available?	☐	☐	☐
10. Suction checked?	☐	☐	☐
11. Drills available/checked?	☐	☐	☐
12. Irrigation/IV solutions warmed?	☐	☐	☐
13. Urinary output/blood loss noted?	☐	☐	☐
14. Specimens/cultures to lab?	☐	☐	☐
15. X-ray precautions taken?	☐	☐	☐
16. Counts performed/correct?	☐	☐	☐
17. Implant/drains noted?	☐	☐	☐
18. Dispersive pad site rechecked?	☐	☐	☐
19. Dressings applied?	☐	☐	☐
20. Other generic care plans initiated? (specify)	☐	☐	☐

Document additional nursing actions/generic care plans initiated here:

_____

_____

_____

EVALUATION OF PATIENT OUTCOMES

	Outcome met	Outcome met with additional outcome criteria	Outcome met with revised nursing care plan	Outcome not met	Outcome not applicable to this patient
1. Baseline neurologic status was unchanged.	☐	☐	☐	☐	☐
2. The patient met outcomes for additional generic care plans as indicated.	☐	☐	☐	☐	☐

Signature: _____ Date: _____

14. Follow institutional protocol for preserving, labeling, and transporting specimens and cultures; implement universal precautions when handling blood or body tissue. Record specimens and cultures.
15. X-ray films or image intensification will be used to verify placement of the distal catheter with atrioventricular shunt procedures. Have cassette drape and follow institutional protocol for radiation safety.
16. Perform counts according to institutional protocol. Document the results of counts.
17. Check the electrosurgical dispersive pad site whenever there is a position change and when the pad is removed.
18. Record drains, catheters, and shunting materials. Follow institutional protocol for documenting implants.
19. Assist in the application of dressings. Allow adequate room for postoperative swelling when applying tape to prevent "tape burns."

References

American Nurses Association. (1994). *Position statement on assisted suicide.* Washington, DC: The Association.

Arbit E & Krol G. (1994). Coma, seizures, and brain death. In *Care of the surgical patient* (Vol. 2), Emergency care, New York: Scientific American.

Association of Operating Room Nurses. (1994). Proposed position statement on perioperative care of patients with do-not-resuscitate (DNR) orders. *AORN Journal, 61*(1), 60.

Barker E. (1994). *Neuroscience nursing.* St. Louis: Mosby.

Bates B, Bickley LS, & Heokelman RA. (1995). *A guide to physical examination and history taking* (6th ed.). Philadelphia: JB Lippincott.

Bichat X. (1814). *Desault's surgery.* Philadelphia: Thomas Dobson.

Bullard DE. (1987). Neurosurgery. In DC Sabiston (Ed.). *Essentials of surgery.* Philadelphia: WB Saunders.

Chipps E, Clanin N, & Campbell V. (1992). *Neurologic disorders: Mosby's Clinical Nursing Series.* St. Louis: Mosby.

Hickey J. (1992). *The clinical practice of neurological and neurosurgical nursing science.* Philadelphia: JB Lippincott.

League D. (1995). Interactive, image-guided, stereotactic neurosurgery systems. *AORN Journal, 61*(2), 360-370.

Meeker MH & Rothrock JC. (1995). *Alexander's care of the patient in surgery* (10th Ed.). St. Louis: Mosby.

Nurre-Miller M. (1994). Neuroendoscopy. *Lasers and advanced technology newsletter, 1*(4), 1-2.

Rovit RL, Murali R & Hirschfeld A (1994). What's new in neurosurgery. ACS Bulletin, 7(1)35-40.

Seidel HM, et al. (1995). *Mosby's guide to physical examination* (3rd Ed.). St Louis: Mosby.

Williams EM, Galbraith JG, & Duncan CC. (1995). Neuroendoscopic laser-assisted ventriculostomy of the third ventricle. *AORN Journal, 61*(2), 345-359.

Wright JL. (1995). PLDD offers an alternative to traditional back surgery. *Lasers and advanced technology newsletter, 2*(4), 1.

Chapter 10

Otolaryngologic Surgery

Diana L. Wadlund

The patient being seated upon a high chair, with his head supported against the breast of an assistant, he [Desault] began by separating the cheek of the diseased side from the corresponding gums; then he cut with a scalpel the internal membrane of the mouth, and the other parts which unite the internal parts of the cheek to the maxillary bone. The bone being exposed, he . . . took . . . a sharp perforator . . . whose point penetrated by rotary motions into the sinus. The opening was enlarged by a blunt perforator. . . . a portion [of the fistula] was removed . . . the opening was filled by a plug of lint, supported by others, that were placed between the jaw and the cheek . . . On the twentieth [day] the cure had progressed very sensibly, and was completely finished six weeks after the operation.

BICHAT, 1814

Otolaryngology is the specialty involved with the study and surgical treatment of diseases of the ears, nose, and throat (hence the former designation of ENT, by which the specialty was long known). Today there are many subspecialties within the field, such as otology, facial cosmetic surgery, and head and neck oncology. Physicians who practice in this specialty are certified by the American Board of Otolaryngology. Perioperative nurses are certified through the Association of Operating Room Nurses (AORN) and/or the Society of Otorhinolaryngology and Head and Neck Nurses (SOHN). In 1994, the Society published *Standards and Scope of Practice of Otorhinolaryngology Clinical Nursing Practice* (SOHN, 1994).

HISTORICAL PERSPECTIVE

Records pertaining to abnormal conditions of the ear, nose, and throat date from the Egyptians in 3500 BC. References to tracheostomy, documented as incisions into the "rough artery," can be found in medical records from 1500 BC. In the mid-1800s, the specialty saw a number of significant advances (Farmer, 1987). Tests using a tuning fork were put into use to evaluate hearing. In 1861 Ménière described the relationship between the inner ear labyrinth and vertigo and deafness. Schwartze introduced simple mastoidectomy for the treatment of mastoiditis in 1873. Within 17 years radical mastoidectomy was performed. In 1882 nasal septal surgery was introduced, followed closely by frontal sinus surgery to treat sinus infections. In the early 1900s rhinoplasty was performed, and Caldwell-Luc procedures were developed for maxillary sinusitis. The development of the binocular microscope in 1922 made otolaryngology the first surgical specialty to use the microscope routinely in clinical surgery. By the 1950s stapedectomies were being performed for the management of otosclerosis. With progressive studies on the physiology of the middle and inner ear, the field rapidly developed. Today the use of antibiotics and tympanostomy tubes have effectively reduced the need for formerly common otologic procedures. The laser, advances in endoscopic procedures, pediatric otolaryngology, facial cosmetic surgery, geriatric otolaryngology, and the development of prosthetic devices for head and neck reconstruction have ushered in a host of new surgical procedures.

PERIOPERATIVE NURSING ASSESSMENT

The successful outcome of a perioperative care plan depends largely on accurate preoperative patient assessment and preparation. The extent of a perioperative nursing history and evaluation is determined somewhat by the type of surgical intervention planned; the patient's psychosocial responses to the contemplated surgery; and findings from the nursing and medical history, physical examination, and laboratory test results. The perioperative nurse should review the results of the initial medical and nursing unit histories. This review helps in forming a plan based on the nature of the patient's disease and planned operative management. These "routine" preparatory activities guide and direct the perioperative nurse's effort to focus on essential elements related to the perioperative period.

Patient History

A review of the patient's history will detail the history of the present illness and previous symptoms, treatment, and operations. Specific criteria are age, sex, nature and duration of symptoms, and associated risk factors (Table 10-1). This is important information for developing a plan of care. Knowing whether the episode is acute or chronic assists in hypotheses about nursing diagnoses that may distinguish patients with acute conditions from those who have attempted to cope with chronicity. Clusters of signs and symptoms that are amenable to nursing actions are clearly important for planning care. The patient who has had numerous surgeries may bring an entirely different set of knowledge, fears, or expectations to the operating room (OR) than the patient who has never had surgery. The history, therefore, is important for its contribution to a plan that assists the patient to demonstrate knowledge about the physiologic and psychologic responses to surgery.

Medication history. Anticipating potential perioperative complications affects the achievement of safe and effective patient outcomes. Medication history, especially the use of steroids, nonsteroidal antiinflammatories, aspirin, tranquilizers and seda-

Table 10-1 Diagnostic criteria by history for head and neck masses

Age

Children	80% benign, congenital
Adults	80% malignant, secondary

Sex

Male to female malignancy ratio is 2:1

Symptoms	Average duration	Pain
Congenital	7 years	(−)
Neoplastic	7 months	(±)
Inflammatory	7 days	(+)

Risk factors for malignancy

Previous head and neck cancer
Tobacco/alcohol abuse
Genetic
Other environmental factors

From James EC, Corry RJ, & Perry JP. (1987). *Principles of basic surgical practice.* Philadelphia: Hanley & Belfus.

tives, diuretics, anticoagulants, nose drops or sprays, ototoxic antibiotics, and drug allergies, is useful for predicting possible intraoperative and postoperative problems.

Review of Systems

A review of systems is important for establishing the integrity and functioning of all major organ systems. After these other systems are reviewed, inquiry focuses on the system targeted for surgery.

Ear surgery. When assessing the patient undergoing surgery on *one* or *both ears,* baseline levels of hearing acuity must be known. After reviewing the documented physical findings, the nurse asks the patient about hearing loss. Does it affect one or both ears? Does the patient have difficulty hearing with background noise present? Was the onset gradual or sudden? How closely must one stand by the patient for words to be heard? The perioperative nurse documents this information, as well as information about the use of hearing aids, lip reading, and sign language, and notes subjective data related to ear pain, tinnitus (ringing), vertigo (dizziness), drainage, or feelings of fullness in the ear. If the patient experiences dizziness or vertigo, it is important to identify related symptoms, such as nausea and vomiting, as well as precipitating events. Knowing whether vertigo is related to positional change or movement of the head and neck assists in planning and carrying out patient transfer maneuvers. History of previous ear problems, surgery, and occupational exposure to loud noises should be elicited. The color or any deformities of the auricle are also noted.

Nasal surgery. The nose and nasopharynx, like the oral cavity and oropharynx, are major portals of entry for microorganisms. Inflammation of the nasal mucosa causes local edema, redness, pain, bleeding, mucous production, and sneezing. The patient scheduled for *nasal surgery* should be queried about allergies, frequency of colds, use of decongestants (oral and spray), postnasal drip, and sinus pain. If drainage is a complaint, the nurse should ask about its color and smell or taste. The rate, quality (noisy or congested), and depth of respiratory function should be noted.

Throat surgery. Assessing patients who are undergoing surgery of the *throat* begins with an inspection of the lips. Symmetry, color, texture, edema, or surface abnormalities are recorded. Swelling or lesions may indicate infection; edema may indicate allergies; dry, cracked lips or fissures at the corners of the mouth may indicate the need for perioperative mouth care. The oral mucosa, which should be smooth and moist, is inspected. Small, painful ulcerations can be caused by viral infection, commonly herpes simplex. Immunologic studies have shown altered humoral immunity to herpes simplex in patients with head and neck cancer; they carry an increased risk of squamous cell carcinoma (James, Corry, and Perry, 1987). Local radiation therapy, systemic chemotherapy, or vitamin C deficiency can result in mucositis. The gums should be pink without any apparent lesions, indurations, or ulcers. Gums that are swollen, bleed easily, or contain debris at the tooth margins may be associated wth gingival disease. The perioperative nurse checks for dentures or loose teeth and also examines the tongue to see if it is swollen, ulcerated, or coated. Conditions that present the risk for infection need to be clearly documented and, if possible, treated before surgery of the throat. Inspection of the trachea should reveal that it is in the midline directly above the suprasternal notch. Tracheal deviations can result from respiratory problems, thyroid enlargement, enlarged nodes, or tumors. A history of smoking or excessive alcohol intake is often positively associated with squamous cell (epidermoid) carcinomas. The patient should be questioned about hoarseness, dyspnea, cough, hemoptysis, dysphagia (difficulty swallowing), odynophagia (painful swallowing), the feeling of a lump in the throat (globus), and actual lump in the throat. Deviations from normal are documented.

Head and neck surgery. The patient who is to undergo *head and neck surgery* should be visually examined for head position and facial features. The history is reviewed to see whether any evidence of neurologic impairment or cranial nerve involvement is listed. The neck is observed as the patient

---

Box 10-1 Head and Neck Cancers (by location)	
Tongue/Lips/Floor of mouth Gingiva/ Buccal/Palate	42%
Oropharynx/Hypopharynx/Larynx	40%
Nasopharynx/Nose/Sinuses	8%
Salivary	7%
Other	3.5%

---

swallows. Masses in specific locations have usual causes. A mass filling the base of the neck or one that slides up when the patient swallows may indicate an enlarged thyroid. Neck edema is associated with infection, hyperthyroidism, and abnormal venous or lymphatic drainage (superior vena cava syndrome). The patient should be able to engage in full range of motion without neck pain. If there are enlarged neck nodes, their location, duration, and whether they are tender are determined. The perioperative nurse then asks the patient about associated symptoms of pain, fever, or itching. Nodes that have been present for more than 4 to 6 weeks or are steadily enlarging need further evaluation. Thorough head and neck examination, including endoscopy, may be indicated before biopsy. Fine-needle aspiration biopsy may be replacing open, excisional and incisional biopsy. Despite the fact that lymph node enlargement is often the result of a normal, physiologic response to infection, the patient is likely to be anxious about diagnostic outcomes. If nodes are palpated, a systematic approach, beginning with the head, moving down to the neck, and progressing to the axillae is helpful. Palpation is performed in front of and behind for location, size, consistency, mobility, configuration, and tenderness. The medical and family histories are important considerations when evaluating the significance of enlarged nodes. Head and neck cancers make up approximately 6.29% of all cancers (Box 10-1).

Surgical treatment of head and neck carcinomas requires a highly skilled interdisciplinary team. Staging is based on clinical criteria derived from physical examination and endoscopic evaluation. The results of the staging will dictate the management of the disease process. Twenty to thirty years ago, head and neck surgeons began to use the "TNM" (tumor, node, metastases) method to stage cancers that range from small and localized to advanced and widespread (Box 10-2). Today the goals of surgery are foremost to remove the cancer and secondarily to provide functional and cosmetic re-

Box 10-2 Tumor Classification using the TNM System

T = Size of Primary Tumor.
T_{is} = Carcinoma in situ
T_1 = Invasive cancer 2 cm or less
T_2 = Invasive cancer >2 cm but <4 cm
T_3 = Tumor size >4 cm
T_4 = Massive tumor >4 cm with bone, muscle, skin of neck invasion

N = Spread of Tumor to the Nodes
N_0 = No detectable nodes
N_1 = One node <3 cm, same side as lesion
N_2 = One node >3cm but <6 cm, same side as lesion, *or*
Multiple nodes, same side as lesion with the greatest diameter <6 cm
N_3 = Massive multiple nodes, same side as lesion, *or*
Nodes on both sides of neck, *or*
Nodes on opposite side of neck from the lesion

M = Distant Metastases
M_0 = No metastases found
M_1 = Distant metastases

Staging of Head and Neck Cancer
Stages 1 and 2 T_1, N_0, M_0
Stage 3 T_1, T_2, or T_3, N_1, M_0
T_3, N_0, M_0
Stage 4 T_4, N_0, M_0
Any T, N_2 or N_3, M_0
Any T, Any N

construction. A prime example is tracheoesophageal puncture to provide speech for patients after total laryngectomy. Speech therapists, prosthodontists, social workers, and dietitians are members of the medical and nursing team who care for these patients. With a treatment plan that may include chemotherapy before surgical intervention, patient care becomes increasingly complex, with concomitant complexity in nursing care.

Interdisciplinary Collaboration

The perioperative nurse on the otolaryngology team needs knowledge far beyond what may have been anticipated in the days when tonsillectomy or stapedectomy constituted the bulk of the OR schedule. The perioperative nurse of the 1990s works with a team that constantly seeks better techniques of reconstruction and restoration of funtion after radical surgery. Large defects can now be covered using axial, myocutaneous, or free composite flaps attached to blood vessels. Such reconstruction may begin at the time of the surgery to treat the disease. Flaps, internal and external fixation devices, endoscopic insertion of speech devices, and prostheses for all areas of the head and neck are only a few of the successes of modern surgery underlined by aesthetic and functional considerations (Jones & Wellisz, 1994). Rehabilitation can begin in the immediate postoperative period. Quality, in terms of both aesthetic and treatment outcomes, is constantly improving. Perioperative nursing is similarly concerned with improving the quality of patient care.

NURSING DIAGNOSES

A professional nursing care model constitutes a basic feature of perioperative nursing. Developing a care plan for the patient undergoing otolaryngology procedures maintains a primary focus on the patient throughout the care planning process. It is expected that the nursing care plan will be altered to accommodate the changing conditions and requirements of the patient. Continuous evaluation of patient responses to perioperative nursing interventions is an integral part of planning patient care. Despite the individual nature of this nursing care process, likely nursing diagnoses are correlated to the patient population (Null, Richter-Abt, & Kovac, 1995). The ability to plan care effectively may be positively influenced by the ability to identify successfully the nursing diagnoses that relate to specific patient groups. For the otolaryngology patient, consideration should be given to factors such as airway patency, cranial nerves and sensory perception, communication, swallowing, nutrition, safety, body image, self-care ability, level of comfort or pain, and skin integrity (SOHN, 1994).

Patient Undergoing Surgery for Diagnostic Confirmation

Patients who are being operated on for endoscopy or biopsy may be characterized as being in the diagnostic period. During this time, the patient may experience fears of the outcome; perceptions of threat; and knowledge deficits regarding the meaning and interpretation of diagnostic studies, the reason for the study, and the physical effects of the study. Continuous validation of the patient's understanding is necessary. Correct perceptions should be reinforced, and incorrect perceptions should be identified and explained correctly. The coping methods of the patient, significant others, and family may be stressed and altered. Anxiety, poor communication skills, and worry about disclosing results present difficulties in maintaining open relationships. Apprehension, worry, impatience, inability to sleep or relax, and concentration problems may characterize the patient undergoing diagnostic surgery or waiting for its results.

Intervening in Knowledge Deficits

Once the diagnosis has been confirmed, knowledge deficits regarding the results and the meaning of the diagnostic studies may persist. Confirmation of an illness presents varied threats to individual patients. There may be threats to independence, job and economic security, career goals, and establishment and maintenance of relationships with others, as well as concerns about body functions, intimacy, and sexual attractiveness. Fears related to surgical disfigurement and pain may be paramount. Decision making may be overwhelming when the patient is faced with treatment options. Behavioral responses may be uncharacteristic as the patient works through denial, anger, guilt, or hopelessness. Although defensiveness and denial are considered ineffective coping methods, they may be necessary, transitory strategies until the patient can cope effectively.

The perioperative nurse is an important resource for the patient and family. He or she brings both knowledge and support by providing adequate information regarding all of the following:

- Diet and fluid restrictions
- Diagnostic studies
- Indwelling urinary catheter
- Medications
- Skin preparation protocols
- The surgery and its length
- Waiting areas
- Communication of information during the intraoperative period

These along with simple explanations of what the patient may expect go a long way toward assisting the patient and family to overcome knowledge deficits and cope with their physiologic and psychologic responses to surgery. Nursing research indicates that both factual ("You will be taken to the operating room at 6:30 tomorrow morning. I will meet you in the OR holding area, where there will be other patients waiting for surgery.") and sensory information ("When I ask you to move onto the OR bed, it will *feel* cool and narrow. There will be a lot of special equipment in the room, which may *look* frightening to you. Some of the *sounds* in the operating room may be unfamiliar.") are important in effecting positive patient outcomes. Information regarding postoperative events should also be incorporated into perioperative teaching. Patients are less anxious, have better coping ability, may recover more quickly, and need fewer analgesics postoperatively when they are provided with sensory and factual information (Rothrock, 1989).

Nursing Diagnoses Relating to Specific Areas of Surgical Intervention

In addition to the potential for knowledge deficits, a number of other nursing diagnoses and simple perioperative nursing actions can be incorporated into a plan of care for patients in the otolaryngology OR. Toward that end, the following nursing diagnoses are offered for consideration.

Ear surgery. For the patient having ear surgery, consider the following diagnoses.

- *Fear.* Fear is related to an identifiable source. It may relate to the surgery, diagnosis, prognosis, anesthesia, pain, loss of function, scars, and possibility of greater hearing loss after surgery. As the patient perceives a loss of control associated with the fear-producing source, pulse, respirations, and blood pressure may increase. There may be diaphoresis, voice changes, and increased questioning of the perioperative nurse. Frequent explanations and reassurance are needed.

- *Impaired physical mobility.* In this case, limitations in mobility may be related to vertigo or dizziness. The patient may have limited range of motion of the head and neck and need help in transferring to the OR bed. Transfers should be completed slowly.

- *Body image disturbance.* Surgery on the external ear is visible to others. A scar or reconstructive flap may precipitate a change in body image. The patient may exhibit signs of grieving or withdrawal or appear hostile. Emotional support is necessary whenever there is a potential for disturbance in body image.

- *High risk for injury.* Vertigo and dizziness are often accompanied by falls. Planning for patient assistance during transfer is necessary to prevent injury. Patients with hearing loss may miss danger sounds around them.

- *Pain.* The presence of pain will depend on the underlying disease process. The autonomic response to pain is similar to the one for fear. Assist the patient in assuming a position of comfort and encourage the use of effective pain-control techniques. Offer additional comfort measures such as warm blankets. Use touch when appropriate.

- *Sensory/perceptual alterations.* The patient with partial or total loss of hearing may depend on lip reading to compensate for the deficit. In the OR, lips are not visible. A careful plan for communicating with the patient (such as sign language or symbol board) must be developed to prevent the patient from becoming disoriented or confused about environmental stimuli.

Nasal surgery. For the patient undergoing nasal surgery, the addition of the following nursing diagnoses is considered.

- *Ineffective breathing pattern.* Swollen nasal mucosa, mechanical obstruction from packing for local anesthesia, or anatomic obstructions in nasal passages may alter comfortable respiratory function. As it becomes more difficult to pass air through the respiratory passages, changes may occur in the rate and depth of respirations; nasal flaring, anxiety, or restlessness may be present. When the patient is awake, keep drapes away from the face. Encourage mouth breathing. Perform mouth care as necessary, providing a lip lubricant when the lips become dry. Monitor vital signs and pulse oximeter. Administer oxygen as prescribed.
- *Anxiety.* The patient may experience apprehension unrelated to a specific threat. Situational events that may precipitate anxiety include hospitalization and surgery. A new, unfamiliar environment may be enough for the patient to state that he or she is nervous. Concern about altered body image may be related to anxiety about a changed appearance of the nose and swelling or bruising of the face. There may be sensory changes if the sense of smell is lost. The anxious patient may seem forgetful or unable to concentrate during the perioperative period. A calm manner, short and specific statements, and a quiet environment help to allay anxiety. Explanations and reassurance are necessary. Comfort measures and touch are used when appropriate.

Head and neck surgery. For the patient undergoing head and neck surgery, the following nursing diagnoses are also considered.

- *Activity intolerance.* A preoperative regimen of chemotherapy or radiation therapy may be accompanied by weakness and fatigue. The patient's altered response to activities such as transferring to the OR bed may be manifested by shortness of breath, change in pulse rate, or inability to maintain body alignment. Assistance with transfer as well as the use of accessory positioning devices should be considered.
- *Ineffective individual coping.* The patient may have a number of internal and external stressors with which to cope. When resources for coping become depleted, the patient may or may not be able to verbalize a need for assistance. Protective defense mechanisms may be initiated. A supportive, understanding stance on the part of the nurse is necessary.
- *Impaired verbal communication.* The patient whose speech is hoarse, who is on mandatory voice rest, who is dependent on a ventilator because of trauma, or who already has a tracheostomy or laryngectomy may be unable to communicate verbally with the perioperative team. A writing slate or hand signals should be a part of patient care.
- *Altered nutrition: less than body requirements.* The underlying carcinoma, preoperative chemotherapy or radiation therapy, or preexisting dysphagia may place the patient at risk for inadequate intake of nutrients. The nutritionally debilitated patient is at risk for positioning injuries related to inadequate protective muscle mass. Risk is compounded during lengthy surgical procedures. Careful padding of dependent pressure sites with massage of accessible pressure areas may be required. The potential for impaired wound healing requires careful attention to incisions and aseptic application of dressings.
- *Impaired skin integrity.* Lesions of the mucosa, tongue, gums, or lips may be present. If these are secondary lesions, continuing preoperative care regimens (application of ointments and cool compresses) should be considered when appropriate.
- *High risk for infection.* Although all perioperative patients have this potential, risk is increased with the length of the surgery, exposure of large areas of tissue, surgery involving the nose and mouth, and risk of postoperative serous or hematoma formation. The patient may already be immunosuppressed. Chemotherapy, radiation therapy, presence of invasive lines, and malnutrition can all contribute to the development of infection. Careful attention to aseptic technique and constant and vigilant environmental monitoring are perioperative nursing responsibilities that assist the patient to remain free from infection.

Additional Nursing Diagnostic Considerations

Other nursing diagnoses, such as the following, will depend on the individual patient's emotional and physical status and the length and complexity of the surgery.

- *Ineffective airway clearance* related to bleeding and swelling in head and neck surgery, postoperative packing in nasal surgery, and tracheostomy or laryngectomy
- *Altered body temperature* related to the physical hazards of the OR coupled with the effects of general anesthesia
- *Fluid volume deficit; Fluid volume excess,* which may occur in extensive procedures in

which large tissue areas are denuded and bleeding is encountered
- *Altered growth and development* for pediatric patients
- *Altered oral mucous membrane* with patients who already have lesions
- *Powerlessness* related to feelings of loss of control over surgical events and outcomes, and compounded in patients unable to communicate verbally
- *Impaired swallowing* for patients with tumors or neurologic involvement of the tongue, pharynx, larynx, and esophagus
- *Altered patterns of urinary elimination* related to the presence of an indwelling urinary catheter, depending on the surgical intervention

DIAGNOSTIC STUDIES

Assessment includes collecting, validating, organizing, and identifying patterns in data. The comprehensive nursing assessment is usually conducted in the patient's initial contact with the health care facility. The perioperative nurse engages in additional focused assessment, gathering information about the health problem that has already been identified. Although the patient is the primary source of much data collection, information from the medical record is also an important resource in gathering data during assessment. Laboratory studies, x-ray films, written consultations, and other diagnostic workups should be included in developing a plan of care.

Ear Surgery

Tuning fork tests are useful for determining whether hearing loss is present. Conductive loss (caused by abnormality of the ear canal, tympanic membrane, or middle ear ossicles) versus sensorineural loss (involving the cochlea and vestibulocochlear nerve) should be distinguished. Later, otologic surgical patients should have complete audiometric evaluation of both nerve and bone conduction. The *Weber test* evaluates the presence of conductive hearing loss (the patient perceives the sound as louder in the involved ear) and sensorineural loss (the patient perceives the sound as louder in the uninvolved ear). Postoperatively, the Weber test is used to verify that hearing is intact in the operated ear; sound should lateralize to the side of surgery. The *Rinne test* compares hearing by air conduction and bone conduction. With moderate to severe conductive hearing loss, bone-conducted sound is equal to, or louder and longer lasting, than air-conducted sound. The *Schwabach test* compares the examiner's bone conduction with the patient's. If a tuning fork sound is heard by the examiner but not the patient, an elevated bone conduction threshold for the patient is

suggested. Perioperative nurses may conduct these tests as part of a physical examination, although they are usually performed by otolaryngologists. Formal audiologic evaluation is performed by audiologists with calibrated electronic devices to determine auditory thresholds, speech discrimination, sites of auditory path lesions, and middle ear impedance. Impedance audiometry measures sound reflected from the eardrum to determine tympanic membrane compliance. This information is combined with physical examination findings to determine middle ear effusions, dislocation or fixation of the ossicles, or tympanic perforations and eustachian tube dysfunction. Diagnostic x-ray studies may include plain films (temporal bone and skull), computed tomography (CT) (useful for bony structures and some soft tissue areas), or magnetic resonance imaging (MRI) (particularly valuable for detecting acoustic neuromas). The vestibular system is evaluated by physical examination and electronystagmography. Where indicated, neurologic and ophthalmologic consultations may be requested.

Nasal Surgery

Patients scheduled for nasal surgery may have a sinus series, CT, or MRI as part of the preoperative workup. Sinus films may show obliteration or bony erosion with advanced tumors. The medical record is reviewed for the results of any cultures.

Head and Neck Surgery

Head and neck workups are much more complex. Lateral x-ray films, CT, MRI, and endoscopy are routine preoperative studies. Contrast-enhanced CT, MRI (with or without gadolinium), and angiography provide information about the vascular anatomy of tumors. Baseline chest x-ray studies are routinely done because lesions from the head and neck can metastasize to the mediastinum or lungs. Defects in the palate may be confirmed by speech cinefluoroscopy. Radionuclide bone scans are useful for determining bone invasion, but only in the presence of symptoms. In the absence of symptoms suggesting metastasis and with normal serum alkaline phosphatase levels, bone and liver scans probably will not be performed. Once common, contrast laryngograms and soft tissue films have been replaced by CT and MRI. Direct laryngoscopy, bronchoscopy, and esophagoscopy have remained integral parts of tumor evaluation. Sialography and tomography of the neck are rarely used today. Ultrasonography may be used to differentiate solid from cystic lesions of the thyroid and neck. The use of various diagnostic modalities is constantly changing. Results of diagnostic studies remain an important part of the data review during assessment.

Clinical staging. Clinical staging of head and neck tumors allows accurate description of the primary tumor, its regional spread, and confirmation of any distant metastasis. This information is then used to plan treatment, predict prognosis, and evaluate results of treatment. *Tumor, nodes,* and *metastasis* are indicated by TNM staging; the stage of the disease depends on these three factors (see Box 10-2). The tumor (T) is staged by size and the involvement of additional anatomic areas and is assigned a number of T_1 to T_4. The parameters of nodal (N) staging are increasing size and number of involved lymph nodes and whether the nodes are ipsilateral, contralateral, or bilateral. Nodes are also staged by number, ranging from N_0 (no nodes) through N_3. Metastasis (M) to distant sites is assigned the classification value of either M_0 (no metastasis) or M_1 (metastasis present). The TNM composite determines whether tumors are Stage I, II, III, or IV. Accurate staging influences treatment planning, prognosis, and evaluation of the efficacy of the proposed treatment.

CARE PLANS

Like much of perioperative care planning, collaborative problems are characteristic for the patient presenting for otolaryngology surgery. This is because some of the actual or potential problems relating to the surgical intervention can only be prevented, resolved, or reduced through collaborative nursing interventions. The following eight procedure-specific care plans include both nursing diagnoses that can be treated somewhat independently (for instance, repositioning a patient with ineffective airway clearance) and ones that need collaboration (for instance, administering oxygen therapy). To emphasize the collaborative nature of the perioperative nurse's role, independent and interdependent nursing actions are listed together. Nursing actions are listed in the sequence in which they would likely be carried out. Thus areas of perioperative assessment or preoperative teaching are listed first. As with the other care plans for specific patient populations in this book, it is expected that the perioperative nurse will frequently initiate the generic care plans, because these relate to outcomes that may be achievable for all surgical patients. For the most part, only one additional nursing diagnosis, with a desired outcome and specified measurable criteria, has been identified in each care plan. This diagnosis has been selected on the basis of its likelihood to be present and will need to be confirmed according to the patient's status. The care plan is designed for a simple presentation. Detailed information, along with suggestions for additional nursing diagnoses, is included in the Guides to Nursing Actions. It will be

necessary to modify and adapt these guides according to institutional protocols.

GUIDES TO NURSING ACTIONS
Myringotomy (Fig. 10-1)

1. Otitis media is common in children; in its Guideline for treating otitis media with effusion, the Agency for Health Care Policy and Research (AHCPR) estimated that the condition accounted for an estimated 6.1 million to 8.5 million office visits in 1990. The Agency recommended myringotomy with tympanoplasty tubes if effusion is still present after 4 to 6 months with a bilateral hearing loss of 20 decibels or worse (AHCPR Guidelines, 1994). Preoperative assessment will depend on the child's age and developmental level. (Chapter 21 discusses general nursing considerations for pediatric patients.) Fears about the surgery, separation from parents, and pain are common with these patients. Calm, careful, and comforting nursing behaviors can help reduce the child's resistance behaviors and fear. Verify that the child has been maintained on NPO status. Determine whether there is any problem with hearing acuity (unilateral or bilateral). If the child is old enough, discuss fears and concerns; provide explanations and reassurance.

2. Preoperative teaching through the use of pictures and play is of great value in helping the child overcome fear. Initiate teaching as appropriate for age and developmental status. Allow the child to bring a security object (teddy bear, favorite doll) to the OR as a comfort measure (according to institutional policy). It is also beneficial to have the security object in the child's arms on awakening in the postanesthesia care unit.

3. The microscope and myringotomy (tympanotomy) instruments, suction and suction tips, cotton sponges, and implants (tubes) should be prepared.

4. The supine position, with the affected ear up, is used. The head is gently turned and supported. Protect the eyes and dependent ear. Placement of safety restraints depends on the size of the child (body restraint or knee restraint).

5. The perioperative nurse should remain with the child, providing comfort and reassurance and assisting anesthesia staff as necessary.

6. Depending on institutional philosophy and protocol, parents may be present during induction of anesthesia (parent-present induction). Offer support and explanations to the parents (LaRosa-Nash, et al., 1995).

7. Document the type and size (if appropriate) of tube implanted.

8. At the conclusion of the surgical procedure, wipe

FIG. 10-1
CARE PLAN FOR MYRINGOTOMY

KEY ASSESSMENT POINTS

Otoscopy findings of a slightly infected, dull-gray membrane, obscured landmarks, and a visible fluid level or meniscus behind the eardrum if air is present above the fluid

Mobility of the tympanic membrane may be assessed by pneumatic otoscopy, tympanometry, and acoustic reflectometry

Examination of external auditory canal for presence of purulent discharge (culture required)

Age-specific signs/symptoms of fear

NURSING DIAGNOSIS

All generic nursing diagnoses apply to this patient, with the addition of:

Fear

(Consider also the nursing diagnoses of pain, risk for infection, and altered family processes related to a child undergoing surgery)

PATIENT OUTCOMES

All generic outcomes apply, with the addition of:

The patient's fear will be reduced.

The patient will:

1. Exhibit minimal resistance behaviors
2. Be permitted to bring security object (teddy bear, etc.) to OR (situational)
3. Verbalize fears/concerns (situational)

NURSING ACTIONS

	Yes	No	N/A
1. Preoperative assessment performed?	☐	☐	☐
2. Preoperative teaching performed/reinforced?	☐	☐	☐
3. Equipment/supplies ready?	☐	☐	☐
4. Patient positioned correctly?	☐	☐	☐
5. Assistance provided during induction?	☐	☐	☐
6. Parents present?	☐	☐	☐
7. Implants documented?	☐	☐	☐
8. Discharge teaching performed?	☐	☐	☐
9. Other generic care plans initiated?	☐	☐	☐

Document additional nursing actions/generic care plans initiated here:

_____

_____

_____

EVALUATION OF PATIENT OUTCOMES

	Outcome met	Outcome met with additional outcome criteria	Outcome met with revised nursing care plan	Outcome not met	Outcome not applicable to this patient
1. The patient's fears were reduced.	☐	☐	☐	☐	☐
2. The patient met outcomes for additional generic care plans as indicated.	☐	☐	☐	☐	☐

Signature: _____ Date: _____

the external ear of any preparation solution; assist anesthesia staff with patient transfer and positioning on the postoperative bed (or crib). Accompany the child to the discharge unit as indicated. Explain to the parents, if appropriate, that the child will be unaware of the presence of the tube postoperatively. The tube will fall out naturally in 2 to 8 months, without trauma or pain. Review pain medications (if prescribed), ear drops (when and how to instill), and events to be reported to the physician (early tube extrusion, undue pain, drainage, odor from the ear, fever). Review instructions for keeping ears dry during bathing, showering, and swimming.

9. The generic care plan for the pediatric patient may be initiated (see Chapter 21).

Ear Surgery (Tympanoplasty, Stapedectomy, Mastoidectomy) (Fig. 10-2)

1. Chronic tympanic membrane perforation and conductive hearing loss are surgically repaired by tympanoplasty. Continuity between the ossicles and the reconstructed eardrum is created by using the patient's own ossicle, homograph ossicles, or alloplastic materials. The conduction hearing loss of otosclerosis can be treated surgically by stapes fenestration or by complete stapes removal and insertion of a prosthesis from the incus to a tissue graft (vein or fascia) placed over the oval window. Mastoidectomy is performed for the patient with mastoiditis and middle ear cholesteatoma. With simple or modified radical mastoidectomy, hearing may be preserved; with radical mastoidectomy, it may not. The goals and outcome of this care plan will need to be modified if the patient is not expected to attain or maintain hearing acuity. Preoperative assessment includes determining loss of hearing acuity (unilateral or bilateral and severity). If the patient uses a hearing aid, it should be worn to surgery; it may be properly dispositioned at the time of or after anesthesia induction. If local anesthesia is used, the hearing aid in the unaffected ear should remain in place. Patients with impaired hearing acuity need to be protected from injury. The environment should be controlled; excess stimulation, loud conversations, and use of the intercom interfere with the patient's ability to hear and comply with perioperative instructions and explanations. If hearing loss is uncompensated, a paper and pencil or other means of communicating should be established. This will help to intervene in the patient's anxiety. The facial or abducens nerve may be involved from mastoid abscesses. Assess the patient for nystagmus, inability to look downward, facial asymmetry, and facial paresis. If these are present preoperatively, they should be noted.

2. Preoperative teaching may include the recommendation that hair be shampooed the night before surgery. The sequence of perioperative events should be explained. It is important, at the outset, to explain to the patient that hearing acuity may not return immediately. For the patient receiving a local anesthetic, carefully review the patient's need to remain immobile during the procedure. Explain perioperative monitoring devices and accessories (electrosurgical unit, drills) that may be used if the patient will be awake.

3. Document whether the patient's hearing aid remains in place during surgery or is dispositioned to another area.

4. The patient will be in the supine position, with the head gently turned and supported. The eyes, dependent ear, and other pressure areas should be protected. The arms will be restrained; protect vulnerable nerve sites. Maintain body alignment. Place a safety strap snugly, but not tightly, above the knees. Warm blankets and other comfort measures should be provided.

5. Patient monitoring may be performed by the perioperative nurse. Monitor the patient according to institutional protocol for local anesthesia. Document intravenous solutions (type, rate of flow, location of intravascular catheter) and the results of vital signs, electrocardiogram, and pulse oximetry as applicable.

6. Hair will need to be secured with a cap; shaving may be indicated for postauricular (and sometimes endaural) approaches. Skin preparation should be carried out carefully to protect the eyes and prevent pooling; solution should be placed in the ear canal only per the physician's decision. The preparation solution selected may be a clear one to allow visualization and stimulation of the facial nerve during the procedure.

7. Note and document the condition of the skin (rashes, bruises, abrasions, irritation) at the preparation site.

8. Depending on the surgical procedure, the electrosurgical unit may be needed. The unit should be checked before use.

9. Assess the skin at the electrosurgical dispersive pad site before application.

10. Special equipment and supplies vary depending on the ear procedure. An ear instrument tray, microsurgical ear instruments, suction, microscope, appropriate head and scope drapes, drills, items for local anesthesia, selected prostheses, irrigating accessories, electrosurgical unit, topi-

FIG. 10-2
CARE PLAN FOR EAR SURGERY (TYMPANOPLASTY, STAPEDECTOMY, MASTOIDECTOMY)

KEY ASSESSMENT POINTS

Otoscopy findings (these vary according to etiology)
Culture & sensitivity (ear drainage)
Mastoid films
Presence of hearing loss
Facial palsy
Vertigo

NURSING DIAGNOSIS

All generic nursing diagnoses apply to this patient, with the addition of:
    Sensory/perceptual alteration: auditory
    (Consider also the nursing diagnoses of impaired verbal communication and social isolation related to hearing loss)

PATIENT OUTCOMES

All generic outcomes apply, with the addition of:
    The patient will attain/maintain hearing acuity.
The patient will:
1. Be free from injury related to sensory impairment
2. Wear sensory assistive device (hearing aid) to OR (situational)
3. Have the OR environment controlled to compensate for sensory impairment
4. Be able to communicate needs to perioperative team

NURSING ACTIONS

	Yes	No	N/A
1. Preoperative assessment performed?	☐	☐	☐
2. Preoperative teaching performed/reinforced?	☐	☐	☐
3. Hearing aid to OR?	☐	☐	☐
4. Correctly positioned?	☐	☐	☐
5. Perioperative monitoring by nurse?	☐	☐	☐
6. Skin prep per institutional protocol?	☐	☐	☐
7. Condition of skin noted at prep site?	☐	☐	☐
8. ESU available/operative?	☐	☐	☐
9. Dispersive pad site checked before application?	☐	☐	☐
10. Special equipment/supplies available?	☐	☐	☐
11. Irrigation/IV solution warmed?	☐	☐	☐
12. Medications labeled/documented?	☐	☐	☐
13. Specimen to lab?	☐	☐	☐
14. Implants documented?	☐	☐	☐
15. Counts performed and correct?	☐	☐	☐
16. Dispersive pad site rechecked?	☐	☐	☐
17. Dressings applied?	☐	☐	☐
18. Drains noted?	☐	☐	☐
19. Discharge teaching/planning performed?	☐	☐	☐
20. Other generic care plans initiated? (specify)	☐	☐	☐

Document additional nursing actions/generic care plans initiated here:

_____

_____

_____

EVALUATION OF PATIENT OUTCOMES

	Outcome met	Outcome met with additional outcome criteria	Outcome met with revised nursing care plan	Outcome not met	Outcome not applicable to this patient
1. The patient's hearing acuity was maintained/improved.	☐	☐	☐	☐	☐
2. The patient met outcomes for additional generic care plans as indicated.	☐	☐	☐	☐	☐

Signature: _____ Date: _____

cal hemostatic agents, antibiotic ointment, and local anesthetic agents will be needed. A nerve stimulator may be requested. The argon laser may be used for stapedectomy, in which case the endo-otoprobe will be required. Hydroxyapatite prostheses may be used to rebuild the external auditory canal after canal wall down mastoidectomy (Pillsbury, 1994).

11. Warm intravenous and irrigation solutions assist in maintaining normothermia.

12. All medications on the sterile field should be properly labeled. Check for patient allergies; document all perioperative medications (including intravenous sedation).

13. Follow institutional protocol for the disposition of specimens. Wipe the exterior of any container received from the field with a disinfectant. Document specimens.

14. Note the serial and lot numbers of implants according to institutional protocol.

15. Document the results of sponge, sharp, and instrument counts.

16. Check the dispersive pad site on removal and note the condition of the site.

17. Dressings will vary according to the procedure. Cleanse the site around the dressing of blood, exudate, and preparation solution.

18. Note on the record any drains that have been incorporated into the dressing.

19. Discharge teaching and planning may be initiated by the perioperative nurse. All of the following should be reviwed: precautions and restrictions in ear and dressing care; nutritional, fluid, and activity needs; signs and symptoms to report to the physician (elevated temperature, pain, drainage, loss of hearing acuity, bleeding from operative site, dizziness, facial nerve paralysis [unable to wrinkle eyebrows, nose, close lids, smile, bare teeth symmetrically], nausea, vomiting); and medications (antibiotics, antiemetics, analgesics). Instructions regarding blowing nose, coughing, and sneezing should be provided.

20. The laser may be used. Initiate and document laser safety precautions.

Nasal Surgery (Septoplasty, Rhinoplasty, Nasal Polypectomy) (Fig. 10-3)

1. Nasal septal defects may be congenital anomalies or result from trauma. They often produce nasal obstruction; with sinusitis, the eustachian tube may be obstructed with accompanying middle ear disease. Septal deformities are often associated with external nasal deformities; septoplasty and rhinoplasty may be required for physiologic and cosmetic correction. Nasal pol-

yps may result from acute allergic rhinitis. Respiratory assessment should include the rate, depth, and quality of respirations. The potential for ineffective airway clearance relates to nasal packs placed during and at the conclusion of surgery; patient observation will be required. Because the surgical site involves the face, there is the potential for a disturbance in body image. Anxiety may be related to local anesthesia and being awake during surgery. The patient should be queried regarding allergies, medications taken (including nose drops or sprays), nasal drainage, and any alteration in sense of smell. Inspect the lips and oral mucosa; the awake patient will be mouth breathing during the procedure. Plan mouth and lip care.

2. Preoperative teaching may include suggestions for comfortable breathing during the procedure for the awake patient; explanation or clarification of the procedure and incision site; review of the local anesthesia planned; explanations about postoperative nasal packs and/or splints; restrictions on nose blowing after surgery; and the possibility of postoperative swelling and discoloration. Explain perioperative monitoring devices and accessories that may be used if the patient will be awake.

3. The supine position is usually selected; the head should be supported (accessory headpiece, foam pillow, sandbags, and so on) and the eyes protected. Pressure areas should be padded. The arms will be restrained; protect vulnerable nerve sites. Maintain body alignment. Place a safety strap snugly, but not tightly, above the knees. Warm blankets and other comfort measures should be provided.

4. Patient monitoring may be performed by the perioperative nurse. Monitor the patient according to institutional protocol for local anesthesia. Document intravenous solutions (type, rate of flow, location of intravascular catheter) and the results of vital signs, electrocardiogram, and pulse oximeter as applicable.

5. Follow institutional protocol for anatomic landmarks for preparation. Skin preparation should be carried out carefully to protect the eyes and prevent pooling. A clear preparation solution may be selected for facial surgery.

6. Note and document the condition of the skin (rashes, bruises, abrasions, irritation) at the preparation site.

7. Special equipment and supplies vary depending on the procedure. Nasal and rhinoplasty instrument trays, polyp snares, suction, appropriate head and body drapes, drills, items for local anesthesia, topical hemostatic agents and antibi-

FIG. 10-3
CARE PLAN FOR NASAL SURGERY (SEPTOPLASTY, RHINOPLASTY, SMR, NASAL POLYPECTOMY)

KEY ASSESSMENT POINTS
Patient expectations of surgery
Nasal obstruction, discharge
Distorted speech
Respiratory rate, rhythm, quality
Airway patency (deviated septum, polyps, enlarged turbinates)
Condition of oral mucosa (smooth, pink, moist is normal)
Concerns with altered body image

NURSING DIAGNOSIS
All generic nursing diagnoses apply to this patient, with the addition of:
   Ineffective airway clearance

PATIENT OUTCOMES
All generic outcomes apply, with the addition of:
   The patient will maintain a patent airway
The patient will:
   1. Maintain effective breathing patterns
   2. Maintain respiratory rate and depth within normal baseline values
   3. Be able to swallow, expectorate without difficulty

NURSING ACTIONS

	Yes	No	N/A
1. Preoperative assessment performed?	☐	☐	☐
2. Preoperative teaching performed/reinforced?	☐	☐	☐
3. Correctly positioned?	☐	☐	☐
4. Perioperative monitoring by nurse?	☐	☐	☐
5. Skin prep per institutional protocol?	☐	☐	☐
6. Condition of skin noted at prep site?	☐	☐	☐
7. Special equipment/supplies available?	☐	☐	☐
8. IV solutions warmed?	☐	☐	☐
9. Medications labeled/documented?	☐	☐	☐
10. Specimen to lab?	☐	☐	☐
11. Counts performed and correct?	☐	☐	☐
12. Dressings/splints applied?	☐	☐	☐
13. Drains/packing noted?	☐	☐	☐
14. Discharge teaching/planning performed?	☐	☐	☐
15. Other generic care plans initiated? (specify)	☐	☐	☐

Document additional nursing actions/ generic care plans initiated here:

_____

_____

_____

EVALUATION OF PATIENT OUTCOMES

	Outcome met	Outcome met with additional outcome criteria	Outcome met with revised nursing care plan	Outcome not met	Outcome not applicable to this patient
1. The patient's airway remained patent.	☐	☐	☐	☐	☐
2. The patient met outcomes for additional generic care plans as indicated.	☐	☐	☐	☐	☐

Signature: _____ Date: _____

otic ointment, and local anesthetic agents will be needed. The laser may be used for the treatment of allergic rhinitis; initiate and document laser safety precautions.

8. Warm intravenous solutions assist in maintaining normothermia.

9. All medications on the sterile field should be properly labeled. Check for patient allergies; document all perioperative medications (including intravenous sedation).

10. Follow institutional protocol for the disposition of specimens. Wipe the exterior of any container received from the field with a disinfectant. Document specimens.

11. Document the results of sponge, sharp, and instrument counts. It is critically important to verify that any throat packs placed intraoperatively are removed (that is, if general anesthesia was used).

12. Dressings, nasal drip pad, and/or splints will vary according to the procedure. Cleanse the site around the dressing of blood, exudate, and preparation solution.

13. Note on the record any drains or packing that have been incorporated into the dressing.

14. Discharge teaching and planning may be initiated by the perioperative nurse. Precautions and restrictions regarding the following should be reviewed:
    a. Nose blowing and coughing are to be avoided; sneeze with mouth open
    b. Dressing, splint, or drip pad care
    c. Nutritional, fluid, and activity needs
    d. Mouth breathing until packing is removed
    e. Temporary loss of taste and smell
    f. The temporary nature of nasal and eye edema and discoloration and numbness in the nasal tip and upper lip
    g. Signs and symptoms to report to the physician (nasal bleeding, respiratory difficulty, and vertigo)
    h. Medications (antibiotics and analgesics)
    i. Measures to reduce edema

Sinus Surgeries (Frontal, Ethmoid, and Sphenoid)
(Fig. 10-4)

1. Chronic sinusitis often needs to be corrected by surgery. These patients often experience chronic sinus headache, characterized by dull head pains that are present in the morning, disappear during the day, and reappear the next morning. The patient may have difficulty sleeping, chronic cough, and fatigue. Although the patient may anticipate the surgery as a relief for chronic pain, anxiety may be associated with local anesthesia and concern about disturbance in body image. If the nursing diagnosis of chronic pain is not a priority for this patient, select one that is. The patient should be queried regarding allergies, medications taken (including nose drops or sprays), nasal drainage, and any alteration in sense of smell. Inspect the lips and oral mucosa; the awake patient will be mouth breathing during the procedure. Plan mouth and lip care.

2. Preoperative teaching may include suggestions for comfortable breathing during the procedure for the awake patient, explanation and clarification of the procedure and incision site, review of the local anesthesia planned, explanations about postoperative nasal packs, restrictions on nose blowing and vigorous swallowing after surgery, and the possibility of postoperative swelling and discoloration. If the patient will be awake, explain perioperative monitoring devices and accessories (electrosurgical unit or drills) that may be used.

3. The supine position is usually selected, although a modified sitting position may be used. Pressure areas should be protected. The arms will be restrained; protect vulnerable nerve sites. Maintain body alignment. Place a safety strap snugly, but not tightly, above the knees. Warm blankets and other comfort measures should be provided.

4. Patient monitoring may be performed by the perioperative nurse. Monitor the patient according to institutional protocol for local anesthesia. Document intravenous solutions (type, rate of flow, location of intravascular catheter) and the results of vital signs, electrocardiogram, and pulse oximetry as applicable.

5. The area to be prepared depends on the surgical approach. Skin preparation should be carried out carefully to protect the eyes and prevent pooling. A clear preparation solution may be selected for facial surgery.

6. Note and document the condition of the skin (rashes, bruises, abrasions, and irritation) at the preparation site.

7. Depending on the surgical procedure, the electrosurgical unit may be needed. The unit should be checked before use.

8. Assess the skin at the electrosurgical dispersive pad site before application.

9. Special equipment and supplies vary depending on the sinus procedure. A nasal instrument tray, suction, appropriate head and body drapes, drills, items for local anesthesia, irrigating accessories, the electrosurgical unit, topical hemostatic agents and hemostatic clips, antibiotic ointment, and local anesthetic agents will be needed. The microscope may be used in eth-

FIG. 10-4
CARE PLAN FOR SINUS SURGERY (FRONTAL, ETHMOID, SPHENOID)

KEY ASSESSMENT POINTS
Tenderness, pain over affected sinus
Headache
Chronic cough
Respiratory rate, rhythm, quality
Purulent drainage
Anosmia (absence of sense of smell) or hyposmia (decreased sense of smell)
Sinus films
Condition of oral mucosa (smooth, pink, moist is normal)
Concerns related to surgery, body image, local anesthesia

NURSING DIAGNOSIS
All generic nursing diagnoses apply to this patient, with the addition of:
Chronic pain

PATIENT OUTCOMES
All generic outcomes apply, with the addition of:
The patient will report reasonable comfort during the intraoperative period.
The patient will:
1. Assume a position of comfort on the OR bed
2. Use pain-relief measures that are personally effective
3. Describe the effectiveness of preoperative and intraoperative pain medications/agents

NURSING ACTIONS

	Yes	No	N/A
1. Preoperative assessment performed?	☐	☐	☐
2. Preoperative teaching performed/reinforced?	☐	☐	☐
3. Correctly positioned?	☐	☐	☐
4. Perioperative monitoring by nurse?	☐	☐	☐
5. Skin prep per institutional protocol?	☐	☐	☐
6. Condition of skin noted at prep site?	☐	☐	☐
7. ESU available/operative?	☐	☐	☐
8. Dispersive pad site checked before application?	☐	☐	☐
9. Special equipment/supplies available?	☐	☐	☐
10. Irrigation/IV solution warmed?	☐	☐	☐
11. Medications labeled/documented?	☐	☐	☐
12. Specimen to lab?	☐	☐	☐
13. Counts performed and correct?	☐	☐	☐
14. Dispersive pad site rechecked?	☐	☐	☐
15. Dressings applied?	☐	☐	☐
16. Drains/packing noted?	☐	☐	☐
17. Discharge teaching/planning performed?	☐	☐	☐
18. Other generic care plans initiated? (specify)	☐	☐	☐

Document additional nursing actions/generic care plans initiated here:

_____

_____

_____

EVALUATION OF PATIENT OUTCOMES

	Outcome met	Outcome met with addition outcome criteria	Outcome met with revised nursing care plan	Outcome not met	Outcome not applicable to this patient
1. The patient reported reasonable comfort during the intraoperative period.	☐	☐	☐	☐	☐
2. The patient met outcomes for additional generic care plans as indicated.	☐	☐	☐	☐	☐

Signature: _____ Date: _____

moidectomy. If an endoscopic approach is used, endoscopic sinus surgery instruments, light carriers and cords, pledgets, and so on, will be necessary. The techniques of endoscopic sinus surgery continue to be refined and expanded with the holmium:YAG laser, which has the ability to excise thin bone as well as soft tissue. Institute laser precautions as applicable.

10. Warm intravenous and irrigation solutions assist in maintaining normothermia.

11. All medications on the sterile field should be properly labeled. Check for patient allergies; document all perioperative medications (including intravenous sedation).

12. Follow institutional protocol for the disposition of specimens. Wipe the exterior of any container received from the field with a disinfectant. Document specimens.

13. Document the results of sponge, sharp, and instrument counts.

14. Check the dispersive pad site on removal; note the condition of the site.

15. Dressings vary according to the procedure. Cleanse the site around the dressing of blood, exudate, and preparation solution.

16. Note on the record any drains or packing that have been incorporated into the dressing.

17. Discharge teaching and planning may be initiated by the perioperative nurse. All of the following should be reviewed: precautions and restrictions regarding nose blowing; dressing care; nutritional, fluid, and activity needs; signs and symptoms to report to the physician (elevated temperature, pain, tenderness in the sinus); and medications (antibiotics, analgesics).

18. The laser may be used for treatment of allergic rhinitis. Initiate and document laser safety precautions. Fluoroscopy may be used to guide ethmoidectomy. Initiate radiation safety precautions.

Endoscopic Procedures (Fig. 10-5)

1. Endoscopy may be performed for diagnosis, biopsy, or treatment. Airway procedures, especially if they are performed with the patient under local anesthesia, may cause anxiety. The patient should be provided with an opportunity to discuss fears and concerns. If preoperative medications were not given, intervention in the patient's anxiety becomes an important nursing responsibility. The patient will also have a risk for (or actual) alteration in breathing patterns during and after the procedure. Assess the baseline quality, depth, and rate of respirations for comparison; note any preoperative respiratory difficulty. Consider additional nursing diagnoses of *ineffective airway clearance, impaired swallowing,* and *impaired verbal communication* when individualizing the care plan.

2. Preoperative teaching should be initiated or reinforced. Perioperative events, including the administration of local anesthesia and other medications (intravenous sedation) should be explained. Review breathing techniques that will be used during the procedure. Explain mandatory voice rest after the procedure if applicable; devise an alternate method of communication.

3. Suction and suction catheters for the airway should be available and checked.

4. Teeth, gums, and lips should be inspected before the procedure. Capped or broken teeth or alterations in the oral mucosa should be noted. Remove dentures or partial plates. Permanent teeth may be protected during oral endoscopy with a rubber mouthpiece.

5. Remain with the patient as much as possible. Offer frequent explanations and reassurance. Warm blankets, touch, and a calm and unhurried manner all convey caring.

6. The supine position, with the neck moderately extended and head supported, is used for most endoscopic procedures. Protect the patient's eyes with an ophthalmic ointment, lubricant, or tape (for patients who are not awake). Position the arms on armboards or at the patient's side; prevent hyperabduction and pad vulnerable nerves and pressure points. Provide additional padding and support to prevent injury from positioning. Place the safety strap snugly, but not tightly, above the knees. During laser procedures, the patient's face must be draped with appropriate protection (that is, wet towels).

7. The type of endoscope prepared depends on the procedure (laryngoscope, esophagoscope, or bronchoscope). The operating microscope with laser and microinstruments may be necessary. Supplies and equipment for administration of local anesthetic are required. Suction, light sources and fiberoptic cables, sponge carriers and biopsy forceps, sponges (pledgets), containers for specimens and cultures, and procedure-specific accessories are needed. A standby tracheotomy set should be available for emergency airway management. If laser is used, initiate and document laser safety precautions.

8. Vital signs may be monitored by anesthesia staff or the perioperative nurse. Follow institutional protocol for monitoring and documenting vital signs, electrocardiograph, and pulse oximeter.

9. Note the method, flow rate, and patient response to oxygen administration.

10. All medications on the surgical field should be

FIG. 10-5
CARE PLAN FOR ENDOSCOPIC PROCEDURES

KEY ASSESSMENT POINTS

Verify NPO status, operative permit
Query history of smoking, alcohol intake
Note symptoms of hoarseness, dyspnea, cough, dysphagia, odynophagia
Record respiratory rate, rhythm, quality
Assess neck for tracheal deviation, enlarged thyroid, lymph nodes, tumor
Determine whether the patient has any allergies (local anesthesia, sedation)
Check condition of teeth; verify that dentures, plates are removed
Inspect oral mucosa (smooth, pink, moist is normal)
Concerns related to surgery, diagnosis, local anesthesia

NURSING DIAGNOSIS

All generic nursing diagnoses apply to this patient, with the addition of:
Anxiety (high risk of or actual)
Ineffective breathing patterns (high risk of or actual)

PATIENT OUTCOMES

All generic outcomes apply, with the addition of:
1. The patient will experience minimal anxiety.
2. The patient's breathing patterns will be effective.
The patient will:
3. Discuss anxiety related to procedure/diagnosis
4. Follow intraoperative instructions
5. Describe perioperative sequence
6. Maintain a normal respiratory rate and depth
7. Maintain a patent airway

NURSING ACTIONS

	Yes	No	N/A
1. Perioperative assessment performed?	☐	☐	☐
2. Preoperative teaching performed/reinforced?	☐	☐	☐
3. Suction checked/ready?	☐	☐	☐
4. Dentures/plates removed?	☐	☐	☐
5. Emotional support/comfort measures?	☐	☐	☐
6. Correctly positioned?	☐	☐	☐
7. Special equipment/accessories available?	☐	☐	☐
8. ECG/vital signs monitored?	☐	☐	☐
9. Oxygen administered?	☐	☐	☐
10. Medications labeled/documented?	☐	☐	☐
11. Counts performed?	☐	☐	☐
12. Specimen(s)/culture(s) to lab?	☐	☐	☐
13. Postoperative monitoring?	☐	☐	☐
14. Terminal cleaning/disinfection of scopes?	☐	☐	☐
15. Other generic car plans initiated? (specify)	☐	☐	☐

Document additional nursing actions/generic care plans initiated here:

_____

_____

_____

EVALUATION OF PATIENT OUTCOMES

	Outcome met	Outcome met with additional outcome criteria	Outcome met with revised nursing care plan	Outcome not met	Outcome not applicable to this patient
1. The patient's anxiety was reduced.	☐	☐	☐	☐	☐
2. Respirations were effective.	☐	☐	☐	☐	☐
3. The patient met outcomes for additional generic care plans as indicated.	☐	☐	☐	☐	☐

Signature: _____ Date: _____

properly labeled. Medications administered should be documented; these may include intravenous sedation, local anesthetics (topical or local infiltration), and epinephrine. Check for patient allergies before the administration of any medication. Observe the patient's response to the medication.

11. Perform sponge, sharp, and instrument counts according to institutional protocol.

12. Follow institutional protocol for the disposition of specimens and cultures. Wipe the exterior surface of any container received from the sterile field with a disinfectant.

13. Until discharged from the operating room, the patient should be monitored for signs of respiratory distress, bleeding, and difficulty swallowing. Note whether the gag and swallow reflex have returned. Reinforce the importance of voice rest (if applicable) and initiate alternate means of communication.

14. Follow institutional protocol for the terminal disinfection and sterilization of endoscopic instruments.

Tonsillectomy and Adenoidectomy (Fig. 10-6)

1. Removal of the tonsils and adenoids is usually accomplished during the same surgery. A potential complication of this procedure is airway obstruction caused by accumulation of blood and secretions in the airway during surgery. Bleeding during surgery may be difficult to visualize or reach. During assessment, review the patient's clotting time, platelet count, and hemoglobin and hematocrit levels. Inspect the oral mucous membranes; note any variations in tissue color, missing teeth, and intraoral lesions. The procedure is most often performed on children. Preoperative assessment depends on the child's age and developmental level (Chapter 21 discusses nursing considerations with pediatric patients). Fears about the surgical intervention, separation from parents, and fear of pain are common with these patients. Calm, careful, and comforting nursing behaviors can assist in reducing the child's resistance behaviors and fear. Verify that the child has been maintained on NPO status. Determine whether there is any problem with hearing acuity (unilateral or bilateral); removal of diseased tissue may be performed when ear problems occur related to eustachian tube obstruction. For adults and older children, discuss fears and concerns and provide explanations and reassurance. If the patient is an adult, additionally assess his or her knowledge of the anesthesia planned (often local).

2. Preoperative teaching, through the use of pictures and play, helps the child to overcome fear. Initiate teaching as appropriate for age and developmental status. Allow the child to bring a security object (teddy bear, favorite doll) to the OR as a comfort measure (according to institutional policy). Adult patients benefit from an explanation of perioperative events as well as reassurance and comfort measures.

3. Tonsillectomy and adenoidectomy instruments, suction, sponges, retractors (for mouth, tongue, and operative structures), and grasping and dissecting instruments should be prepared. If the electrosurgery unit is used, initiate the generic care plan for prevention of injury from electrical hazards. Assess and document skin condition at the site of the electrosurgical dispersive pad on application and removal.

4. The supine position is used for children. This may be modified by Trendelenburg's or other maneuver to facilitate removal of secretions. Adult patients are placed in a sitting or modified sitting position. Place safety straps appropriately; protect eyes and dependent body areas per position selected.

5. The perioperative nurse should remain with the child, providing comfort and reassurance and assisting anesthesia staff as necessary. If the patient is an adult, local anesthesia may be used. Check for patient allergies. Reassure the patient and observe for reactions to the anesthetic. Document medications administered. Monitor the patient receiving local anesthesia according to institutional protocol; document monitoring results.

6. Depending on institutional philosophy and protocol, parents may be present during induction of anesthesia if the patient is a child. Offer support and explanations to the parents.

7. Follow institutional protocol for the disposition of specimens. Wipe the exterior surface of any container received from the sterile field with a disinfectant. Record specimens.

8. Record the results of sponge, sharp, and instrument counts.

9. If the patient is a child, assist anesthesia staff during extubation and positioning on the postoperative bed (or crib). The general anesthesia patient is usually placed either prone or sidelying to facilitate drainage from mouth. The adult patient under local anesthesia is positioned with the head elevated 45 degrees to facilitate drainage. The tonsil suction tip should remain attached to suction until the patient is discharged. Observe the patient for signs of respiratory distress or impaired swal-

FIG. 10-6
CARE PLAN FOR TONSILLECTOMY/ADENOIDECTOMY

KEY ASSESSMENT POINTS
Record respiratory rate, rhythm, quality
Examine oropharynx and tonsillar pillars for hypertrophy, infection
Determine whether the patient has any allergies (local anesthesia, sedation in adult patients)
Inspect oral mucosa (smooth, pink, moist is normal)
Identify age-specific concerns related to surgery, postoperative discomfort, local anesthesia, parental separation

NURSING DIAGNOSIS
All generic nursing diagnoses apply to this patient, with the addition of:
Ineffective airway clearance

PATIENT OUTCOMES
All generic outcomes apply, with the addition of:
The patient's airway will remain clear.
The patient will:
1. Maintain a patent airway
2. Have bilateral breath sounds
3. Be free of excess tracheobronchial secretions

NURSING ACTIONS

	Yes	No	N/A
1. Preoperative assessment performed?	☐	☐	☐
2. Preoperative teaching performed/reinforced?	☐	☐	☐
3. Equipment/supplies ready?	☐	☐	☐
4. Patient positioned correctly?	☐	☐	☐
5. Assistance provided during induction?	☐	☐	☐
6. Parents present?	☐	☐	☐
7. Specimen to lab?	☐	☐	☐
8. Counts performed and correct?	☐	☐	☐
9. Postoperative monitoring?	☐	☐	☐
10. Packing documented?	☐	☐	☐
11. Discharge teaching?	☐	☐	☐
12. Other generic care plans initiated? (specify)	☐	☐	☐

Document additional nursing actions/generic care plans initiated here:

_____

_____

_____

EVALUATION OF PATIENT OUTCOMES

	Outcome met	Outcome met with additional outcome criteria	Outcome met with revised nursing care plan	Outcome not met	Outcome not applicable to this patient
1. The patient's airway was clear.	☐	☐	☐	☐	☐
2. The patient met outcomes for additional generic care plans as indicated.	☐	☐	☐	☐	☐

Signature: _____ Date: _____

lowing (swallowing and gag reflex may not have completely returned).

10. Document the presence of any packing left in the oropharynx.

11. Review pain medications (if prescribed), gargling, use of ice collars, fluid intake, dietary restrictions, and oral hygiene measures. Review events to be reported to the physician (persistent temperature elevation, excessive pain, bleeding).

12. The generic care plan for the pediatric patient may be initiated (see Chapter 21).

Radical Neck Dissection (Fig. 10-7)

1. Radical neck dissection is performed to treat metastatic carcinoma to the cervical lymph nodes. With extensive neck dissection, there is a high risk of postoperative edema and airway obstruction; a tracheotomy may be planned for this patient before neck dissection. Respiratory assessment should include the rate, depth, and quality of respirations; note whether there is any dysphagia or hoarseness. Chest x-ray film, arterial blood gas and electrolyte values, and electrocardiogram should be reviewed. These are important criteria for determining whether the goal of maintaining effective breathing patterns is achieved. The patient may additionally have fear and anxiety, disturbance in body image, and alterations in nutrition. Wound healing will be compromised in the patient who has received preoperative irradiation or is anemic, diabetic, malnourished, or otherwise immunodeficient. These patients have a potential for infection. Altered skin integrity may result from pressure on dependent body areas. It will be necessary to initiate multiple generic care plans.

2. Preoperative teaching should include reinforcement of information about the presence of a nasogastric tube, drainage tubes, indwelling urinary catheter, or intravascular lines. If a tracheotomy or laryngectomy is planned, review alternate means of communicating with the patient (magic slate, communication board). Encourage the patient to verbalize fears and concerns, and attempt to answer questions honestly. Help the patient and significant others to cope with the diagnosis of cancer, the change in body image, and possible altered modes of communication. Provide information about changes that will occur as a result of surgery, duration of these changes, changes in the voice and ability to eat, alternate methods of speech, self-help groups and community resources, and anticipated emotional adjustments (Lewis & Collier, 1996).

3. Check whether blood and blood products were ordered and are available. Follow institutional protocol for correctly identifying and requisitioning blood and blood products. Collaborate with anesthesia in the careful estimation of blood and fluid loss.

4. The patient is positioned supinely with the head and neck moderately extended to expose the affected side of the face and neck. The OR bed may be slightly flexed, in the modified "lawn chair" position, to lessen strain on the back. The shoulder on the affected side may be slightly elevated. If the arm on the operative side is placed on an armboard, the locking type should be used to prevent hyperextension from movements of the OR team. Whether the arms are on an armboard or at the patient's side, protect vulnerable nerve sites. Maintain body alignment. Use accessory devices to pad dependent pressure areas. Place a safety strap snugly, but not tightly, above the knees. Warm blankets and other comfort measures should be provided.

5. An indwelling urinary catheter may be inserted. Use aseptic technique for catheter insertion. Place the drainage bag where it is readily observable. Prevent kinks or tension on the catheter and tubing. Document catheter size and insertion.

6. Follow institutional protocol for anatomic landmarks for the skin preparation. Consult with the surgical team regarding the possibility of skin grafting. The skin graft site needs to be incorporated into the preparation and draping. Prevent solutions from pooling, and protect the patient's eyes.

7. Note and document the condition of the skin (rashes, bruises, abrasions, erythema, fragility, and irritation) at the preparation site.

8. The electrosurgical unit will be needed. The unit should be checked before use.

9. Assess the skin at the electrosurgical dispersive pad site before application.

10. A major head and neck tray will be needed. If tracheostomy is planned, instruments and tracheostomy tube will need to be added. The risk for blood and fluid loss is high in this procedure; prepare for adequate suction, sponges, hemostatic clamps, and topical hemostatics. A nerve stimulator may be required (area of dissection involves facial, vagus, hypoglossal, and other nerves). Depending on the extent of the dissection, primary closure may not be possible. Reconstruction of the operative site may be carried out at the time of the primary surgery. Local advancement flaps, free tissue flaps (split-thickness or free composite graft), skin flaps (rotation, forehead flap), and musculocutaneous

FIG. 10-7
CARE PLAN FOR RADICAL NECK DISSECTION

KEY ASSESSMENT POINTS

Nutritional status

History (positive family history; heavy tobacco/alcohol use; exposure to fumes, pollution, radiation; chronic laryngitis; prior radiation therapy)

Throat pain or soreness

Hoarseness, stridor

Referred ear pain

Sensation of lump in throat, cough, hemoptysis, dyspnea, dysphagia

Palpable neck mass, tracheal deviation

Cervical lymphadenopathy

Anxiety related to knowledge deficit, postoperative course, pain management, prevention of complications, impaired verbal communication, body image disturbance

NURSING DIAGNOSIS

All generic nursing diagnoses apply to this patient, with the addition of:

Ineffective breathing patterns

PATIENT OUTCOMES

All generic outcomes apply, with the addition of:

The patient will maintain an effective breathing pattern.

The patient will have:

1. Normal rate, rhythm, and depth of respiration
2. Minimal dyspnea
3. Blood gases within normal range

NURSING ACTIONS

	Yes	No	N/A
1. Preoperative assessment performed?	☐	☐	☐
2. Preoperative teaching performed/reinforced?	☐	☐	☐
3. Blood ordered/available?	☐	☐	☐
4. Correctly positioned?	☐	☐	☐
5. Foley catheter inserted?	☐	☐	☐
6. Skin prep per institutional protocol?	☐	☐	☐
7. Condition of skin noted at prep site?	☐	☐	☐
8. ESU available/operative?	☐	☐	☐
9. Dispersive pad site checked before application?	☐	☐	☐
10. Special equipment/supplies available?	☐	☐	☐
11. Irrigation/IV solution/blood warmed?	☐	☐	☐
12. Specimen(s) to lab?	☐	☐	☐
13. Counts performed and correct?	☐	☐	☐
14. Dispersive pad site rechecked?	☐	☐	☐
15. Output from nasogastric tube/catheter noted?	☐	☐	☐
16. Dressings applied?	☐	☐	☐
17. Drains/catheters/tubes noted?	☐	☐	☐
18. Tracheostomy tube with patient?	☐	☐	☐
19. Postoperative monitoring in OR?	☐	☐	☐
20. Other generic care plans initiated? (specify)	☐	☐	☐

Document additional nursing actions/generic care plans initiated here:

_____

_____

_____

EVALUATION OF PATIENT OUTCOMES

	Outcome met	Outcome met with additional outcome criteria	Outcome met with revised nursing care plan	Outcome not met	Outcome not applicable to this patient
1. The patient maintained an effective breathing pattern.	☐	☐	☐	☐	☐
2. The patient met outcomes for additional generic care plans as indicated.	☐	☐	☐	☐	☐

Signature: _____ Date: _____

flaps may be considered for cosmetic and functional reconstruction. Their selection depends on numerous variables. Consultation with the surgical team is required to plan for graft equipment and supplies.

11. Warm intravenous blood and irrigation solutions help maintain normothermia.
12. Follow institutional protocol for the disposition of specimens. The extent of dissection will be predicated on pathologic analysis of tissue margins. Multiple specimens may be taken for frozen section. Wipe the exterior of any container received from the field with a disinfectant. Document all specimens.
13. Document the results of sponge, sharp, and instrument counts.
14. Check the dispersive pad site on removal; note the condition of the site.
15. Output from the nasogastric tube, urinary catheter, and drains should be noted.
16. A bulky pressure dressing may be applied to the site of the neck dissection. The extent and type of dressings will vary according to the type of reconstruction (grafting). Cleanse the site around the dressing of blood, exudate, and preparation solution.
17. Note on the record any drains that have been incorporated into the dressing and the presence of other tubes and catheters.
18. If a tracheostomy was performed, document the type and size of tube inserted. Send a backup tube with the patient. (See care plan for tracheostomy.)
19. Immediate postoperative monitoring will be initiated by the perioperative team. Observe the patient for restlessness, tachycardia, pallor, or cyanosis. Notify the postanesthesia or intensive care unit if a ventilator will be required. Have a hand-held resuscitation bag with adapter and oxygen available for patient transport. Protect the patient's airway during transfer and positioning on the postoperative transport vehicle or bed.
20. Note on the space provided on the care plan other generic care plans that have been initiated.

Tracheostomy (Fig. 10-8)

1. Patients requiring tracheostomy have some alteration in respiratory patterns. To measure the identified goals, the rate, depth, and pattern of respiration, in addition to the results of blood gas analyses, should be assessed to determine baseline values. The patient may be admitted to the OR already on a ventilator; the airway must be maintained during transfer and positioning. Assistance may be needed by the anesthesia team. This patient may have additional nursing diagnoses; consider *anxiety, impaired verbal communication, fear, ineffective airway clearance, altered mucous membrane, high risk for aspiration,* and *body image disturbance.* Modify the care plan based on assessment findings.
2. The perioperative nurse should teach or reinforce teaching of as much as possible of the following: the purpose of the tracheostomy, methods that will be used for postoperative communication, speech with a tracheostomy tube (Table 10-2), the possibility of suctioning procedures, and the unit to which the patient will be discharged.
3. Any airway compromise is a frightening event. The patient should be given time to verbalize fears and concerns (as time allows). Fears may relate to suffocation, helplessness, body image disturbance, and inability to speak. Reassure the patient and provide emotional support. Remain with the patient as much as possible. Speak calmly and unhurriedly. Use touch as appropriate to communicate caring.
4. Inspect the patient's lips and oral mucous membranes. Lips should be pink, smooth, and free of lesions; mucous membranes should be pinkish red, smooth, and moist. If lips or oral mucosa are dry, provide mouth care.
5. Positioning is a coordinated team effort. Place the patient in the supine position with a roll or other device under the shoulders to extend the neck moderately. Protect the patient's eyes by using an ophthalmic ointment or lubricant or by taping the eyes closed (if the patient is not awake). Position the arms either on armboards or at the patient's side; pad elbows and prevent hyperabduction. Place the safety strap above the knees, snugly but not tightly. Pad other dependent pressure areas and provide protection to joints as indicated.
6. Follow institutional protocol for anatomic landmarks for skin preparation. Do not allow solutions to pool, and protect the patient's eyes.
7. Note the condition of the skin (rashes, abrasions) at the preparation site.
8. A tracheostomy set, tracheostomy tubes, and suction tubing and tips are required.
9. A standby, backup tracheostomy tube of the appropriate size should be available. Other emergency equipment should be available in anticipation of respiratory or cardiac arrest. The patient should be discharged from the OR with a backup tracheostomy tube. The obturator, which had been taped to the patient's bed, is considered contaminated; a tracheostomy tube is preferable. Document the size of tube inserted and discharged with the patient.

FIG. 10-8
CARE PLAN FOR TRACHEOSTOMY

KEY ASSESSMENT POINTS

Determine reason for surgical intervention (upper airway obstruction, removal of respiratory tract secretions, to facilitate weaning from respirator, to permit long-term mechanical ventilations)

Assess/record respiratory function (rate, rhythm, quality)

Observe oral mucosa

Note mucous production, color, odor, consistency

Review blood gas evaluation

For patients unable to be extubated following prolonged (1 to 3 weeks) endotracheal intubation, establish how patient communicates (magic slate, paper/pencil)

Anxiety related to airway obstruction, postoperative course, pain management, prevention of complications, impaired verbal communication, body image disturbance

NURSING DIAGNOSIS

All generic nursing diagnoses apply to this patient, with the addition of:

Impaired gas exchange

Ineffective breathing patterns

PATIENT OUTCOMES

All generic outcomes apply, with the addition of:

The patient will attain effective airway and breathing patterns.

The patient will:

1. Have a patent airway
2. Maintain optimal gas exchange
3. Resume an effective breathing pattern
4. Demonstrate arterial blood gas values within normal limits for the disease process

NURSING ACTIONS

	Yes	No	N/A
1. Preoperative assessment performed?	☐	☐	☐
2. Preoperative teaching performed/reinforced?	☐	☐	☐
3. Opportunity to verbalize fears provided?	☐	☐	☐
4. Mucous membranes intact?	☐	☐	☐
5. Patient positioned correctly?	☐	☐	☐
6. Skin prepped?	☐	☐	☐
7. Condition of skin at prep site noted?	☐	☐	☐
8. Equipment/supplies available?	☐	☐	☐
9. Stand-by tracheostomy tube available?	☐	☐	☐
10. Hand-held resuscitation bag available?	☐	☐	☐
11. Tracheostomy suctioning apparatus prepared?	☐	☐	☐
12. Humidification provided?	☐	☐	☐
13. Aseptic technique used in suctioning?	☐	☐	☐
14. Stoma clean and dry?	☐	☐	☐
15. Head of bed elevated?	☐	☐	☐
16. Breath sounds documented?	☐	☐	☐
17. Respiratory distress noted?	☐	☐	☐
18. Ventilator required in PACU/ICU?	☐	☐	☐
19. Discharge teaching performed/reinforced?	☐	☐	☐
20. Counts performed and correct?	☐	☐	☐
21. Other generic care plans initiated? (specify)	☐	☐	☐

Document additional nursing actions/generic care plans initiated here:

_____

_____

_____

EVALUATION OF PATIENT OUTCOMES

	Outcome met	Outcome met with additional outcome criteria	Outcome met with revised nursing care plan	Outcome not met	Outcome not applicable to this patient
1. The patient attained effective airway and breathing patterns.	☐	☐	☐	☐	☐
2. The patient met outcomes for additional generic care plans as indicated.	☐	☐	☐	☐	☐

Signature: _____ Date: _____

Table 10-2 *Characteristics and nursing management of tracheostomy tubes*

Tube	Characteristics	Nursing management
Fenestrated tracheostomy tube (Shiley, Portex) with cuff, inner cannula, decannulation plug	When inner cannula is removed, cuff deflated, and plug inserted, fenestration in outer cannula allows air to pass over vocal cords. Client can then speak. Low-pressure cuff distributes cuff pressure over large area.	Assess risk of aspiration before removing inner cannula. Deflate cuff. Have client swallow small amount of clear liquid or 30 ml of water colored with methylene blue dye. Note any coughing. Suction trachea to check for the presence of colored secretions. If no aspiration is noted, a fenestrated tube may be used. *Never* insert plug in tracheostomy tube until cuff is deflated and inner cannula is removed. (Prior insertion will prevent client from breathing [no air inflow], which may precipitate cardiac arrest.) Monitor cuff pressure q 8 hr. Clean inner cannula as needed.
Speaking tracheostomy tube (Portex, National) with cuff, two external tubings	This tube has two external tubings, one leading to the cuff and the second to an opening above the cuff. When above-cuff tubing is connected to air source, air flows out this opening and up over the vocal cords, allowing the client to speak when the cuff is inflated. Low-pressure cuff distributes cuff pressure over large area.	Once the tube has been inserted, wait 2 days before instructing the client in its use so that the stoma can close around the tube and prevent leaks. When client desires to speak, connect above-cuff tubing to a source of compressed air (or oxygen). Be certain to identify the correct tubing. (If gas flow enters the cuff, it will rupture, requiring an emergency tube change.) Use lowest flow (typically 4 to 6 L/min) that will result in speech because high flows dehydrate the mucosa. Cover tubing adaptor, which will cause the air to flow upward. Instruct the client to speak in short sentences, since voice will become a whisper with long sentences. To prevent mucosal dehydration, disconnect air inflow system when client does not want to speak. If desired, use system to monitor aspiration risk. Give the client ice chips with 5 or 6 drops of methylene blue with the cuff inflated. Suction via the talk port. (If dye is suctioned, the client has aspirated). Estimate the volume of aspirate by collecting secretions in a sputum trap. Monitor cuff pressure q 8 hr.
Tracheostomy tube (Bivona Fome-Cuf) with foam-filled cuff	This tube has cuff filled with plastic foam. Cuff is deflated *before* insertion and allowed to passively inflate after insertion. Pilot balloon tubing is not capped, and no cuff pressure monitoring is required. Low-pressure cuff distributes cuff pressure over large area.	When inserting tube, withdraw all air with a 20-ml syringe; then cap pilot balloon tubing to prevent air entry. After tube is inserted, remove cap from pilot balloon tubing, allowing cuff to reinflate. Do not inject air into tubing or cap tubing while it is in client because air will flow in and out in response to pressure changes (head turning) and thereby maintain minimal occluding volume.
Tracheostomy button (Olympic) with spacers, outer cannula, plug	This tube maintains stoma patency and ability to talk with plug in place. With plug removed, it allows suctioning and access for emergency ventilation. It can be individualized to client's stoma size with spacers provided with kit.	Do not insert button before assessing aspiration risk. Measure stoma size; add spacers as needed. Insert lubricated button in stoma. Insert plug in button, which causes petals at the back of button to flare and hold button in stoma. After insertion, rotate button 180 degrees to ensure that it is not adhering to tracheal tissue. Instruct client to clean area around stoma daily with hydrogen peroxide and to remove and clean button at least twice a week. Be aware that if button is not removed, tissue may granulate around petals, predisposing to bleeding.

From Lewis SM & Collier IC. (1996). *Medical-surgical nursing* (4th Ed.). St Louis: Mosby.

10. A hand-held resuscitation bag with adapter should be available for patient transport from the OR.

11. A free suction line with attached suction catheters should be prepared and available. The catheter should be of an appropriate size for the tube.

12. Suctioning should be performed using aseptic technique. Suctioning should be swift and gentle. Oxygen is usually administered before and after suctioning; pulse oximetry may be used to assess postsuctioning oxygen saturation (Ackerman, 1993).

13. Following tracheostomy, humidification may be immediately provided by a nebulizer or collar on the tracheostomy tube.

14. Do not allow solutions to pool around the stoma site; suction or wipe the area clean. When the procedure is completed, observe the stoma for erythema and exudate. Ensure that the skin under tracheostomy ties is clean and dry.

15. The patient may be positioned on the transport vehicle with the head of the bed elevated 45 to 60 degrees, unless contraindicated.

16. Breath sounds should be bilateral.

17. Observe for respiratory distress (restlessness, tachycardia, tachypnea, noisy or wheezing respirations, nasal flaring, and use of accessory muscles). Institute and document nursing and team interventions.

18. A ventilator may be required in the postanesthesia or intensive care unit. As part of the nursing report to the discharge unit, type, settings, and special information about ventilatory assistance should be provided.

19. Reinforce discharge teaching. Explain precautions to be taken (Medic-Alert bracelet for permanent stoma) and methods for postoperative communication.

20. Document the results of sponge, sharp, and instrument counts.

21. Specify other generic care plans that have been initiated for this patient (for example, care plan for preventing electrical injury if the electrosurgical unit was used during the procedure).

References

Ackerman M. (1993). The effect of saline lavage prior to suctioning. *American Journal of Critical Care, 2,* 326-330.

Agency for Health Care Policy and Research. (1994). Otitis media with effusion in young children. Silver Spring, MD: The Agency.

Bichat X. (1814). *Desault's surgery.* Philadelphia: Thomas Dobson.

Farmer JC. Otolaryngology. In DC Sabiston (Ed.)., (1987) *Essentials of surgery.* Philadelphia: WB Saunders.

James EC, Corry RJ, & Perry JF. (1987). *Principles of basic surgical practice.* St. Louis: Mosby.

Jones CE & Wellisz T. (1994). External ear reconstruction. *AORN Journal, 59,* 411-422.

LaRosa-Nash PA, et al. (1995). Implementing a parent-present induction program. *AORN Journal, 61,* 526-531.

Lewis SM & Collier IC. (1996). *Medical-surgical nursing* (4th Ed.). St. Louis: Mosby.

Null S, Richter-Abt D, & Kovac J. (1995). Development of a perioperative nursing diagnoses flow sheet. *AORN Journal, 61,* 547-557.

Pillsbury HC. (1994). What's new in otorhinolaryngology. *ACS Bulletin, 79*(1), 55-58.

Rothrock JC. (1989). Perioperative nursing research. Part 1. Psychoeducational interventions. *AORN Journal, 49,* 597-619.

Society of Otorhinolaryngology and Head and Neck Nurses and the American Nurses Association. (1994). *Standards and scope of practice of otorhinolaryngology clinical nursing practice.* Washington, DC: American Nurses Publishing.

Chapter 11

Ophthalmic Surgery

Joanne D. Cimorelli

OPERATION FOR THE FISTULA LACHRYMALIS

1st. Introduce the probe through the superior lachrymal punctum, first from without in, then from above to below, to arrive at the lachrymal sac.

2d. Penetrate into the nasal canal, pass the obstacles to enter the nostrils, and if we cannot reach there, substitute a pointed probe for the blunt one that is commonly employed.

3d. Withdraw the probe with one of the instruments mentioned above, and disengage the thread, which remains thus for twenty-four hours, passing through the lachrymal punctum and the nasal fossae.

4th. Fix to this thread the seton, smeared with digestive ointment, and let it be drawn from below upwards.

5th. Withdraw the seton every day, by means of the thread fixed to its inferior extremity, substitute for it another charged like it, with different medicaments, and continue this treatment until the seton allows no more pus to flow, or until it goes up and down at pleasure.

BICHAT, 1814

Ophthalmic surgical nursing has been transformed over the past few decades. The perioperative nurse has had to adapt to changes resulting from technologic advances as well as changes accompanying the impact of diagnostic related groups (DRGs) and health care reform on the entire health care delivery system. Preoperative and postoperative patient teaching before admission has become critical because most eye procedures are performed as ambulatory surgical procedures. The ophthalmic perioperative nurse must use the nursing process to provide high-quality care to all patients undergoing eye surgery. It is necessary for the nurse to assess patient data, formulate appropriate nursing diagnoses, identify appropriate patient outcomes, develop and implement a plan of nursing care, and effectively evaluate the patient's response to care. The perioperative nurse must also know the proper uses and functions of high-technology ophthalmic surgical equipment to prevent injury to the patient and surgical team.

Ophthalmic surgery is a challenging specialty for perioperative nurses; it allows for role expansion as a registered nurse first assistant (RNFA) and involvement in specialty nursing organizations. In ophthalmic surgery the perioperative nurse demonstrates compassion and understanding, the nursing process, manual dexterity, teaching, assisting, and professional growth.

HISTORICAL ASPECTS

Cataract surgery, the most common surgery performed on Americans 65 years of age or older (AHCPR, 1993), is one of the oldest known ophthalmic procedures. According to Garrison (1929), one illustration in a Renaissance picture book, dated 1583, shows a patient tied in a chair, awaiting cataract removal. An ancient Roman relief sculpture depicts "couching a cataract" (Thorwald, 1960). The earliest printed book on the eye was dated 1475. Most early ophthalmic developments were the work of astronomers and physicists exploring the structures and functions of the eye.

Cataract was not defined as clouding and thickening of the lens until about 1707; before that a cataract was thought to be skin inside the capsule. Jacques Daviel (1696-1762) originated modern treatment for cataracts in 1752. By 1756, only 4 years later, Daviel had performed 434 cataract extractions with only 50 failures.

Three pioneers of ophthalmic surgery in the nineteenth century were Hermann von Helmholtz (1821-1894), Albrecht von Graefe (1824-1870), and Frans Cornelius Donders (1818-1889). von Helmholtz invented the ophthalmoscope and phacoscope. von Graefe was the creator of modern eye surgery and is considered one of the greatest of all eye surgeons. Between 1855 and 1862 he introduced iridectomy for iritis and glaucoma, and in 1857 he performed surgery to treat strabismus. From 1865 to 1868, von Graefe's modified cataract surgery decreased postoperative loss of the eye from 10% to 2.3% (Garrison, 1929). This was a major breakthrough in reducing cataract surgical complications. In Holland, Donders devoted his practice to ophthalmology exclusively; he is given credit for defining aphakia. With the invention of the ophthalmoscope and ophthalmometer, ophthalmology became an exact science.

In 1863 Julius Jacobson used a peripheral incision and chloroform anesthesia. Alexander Pagenstecher performed cataract surgery using a scleral incision in 1866. Henry Willard Williams, an American, developed a method for suturing the flap after cataract extraction in 1866. On September 11, 1884, Carl Koller, an ophthalmologist in Vienna, successfully performed the first cataract surgery using topical cocaine as an anesthetic. This was an important discovery not just for ophthalmic surgery, but for all surgery. A Greek physician, Photinos Panas, operated for congenital and paralytic ptosis in 1886. By 1888, in another major advance, the cataract was extracted within the capsule.

During the early 1900s an officer in India's Medical Service, Lieutenant Colonel Henry Smith, was performing 3000 cataract extractions each year. By 1910 he had performed 24,000 cataract surgeries. Another Indian officer, Major Robert Henry Elliot, developed sclerocorneal trephination for treatment of glaucoma in 1909.

A milestone in ophthalmic surgery occurred on December 7, 1905, in Olmütz, Czechoslovakia, as Edward Zirm successfully operated on a man blinded by lime burns to both corneas. Zirm's patient was sighted for 9 months after the surgery. Corneal transplant surgery was continued by Vlad Petrovich Filatov (1875-1955), who performed more than 1000 corneal transplants in Odessa. After World War II, corneal transplant surgery was refined and good results were obtained.

During the early to middle 1900s advances were also made in cataract surgery, and the intracapsular technique became the standard for cataract extraction. Early attempts at implantation of posterior chamber intraocular lenses during the 1950s were not highly successful. Most of these lenses had to be removed as a result of dislocation (Spaeth, 1994). The next advance was the anterior chamber intraocular lens. Although this did not dislodge as the posterior chamber lens had, it produced some corneal damage. With changes in the design of the modern posterior chamber lens, fewer complications are seen. The development of phacoemulsification (breaking up the lens with ultrasound and removing it with irrigation and suction) has paved the way for smaller incisions. This approach allows for smaller lenses and, in some cases, foldable lenses to be inserted. This technique is now the most frequently used approach in the United States. The posterior chamber lens is most commonly used after phacoemulsification or extracapsular cataract extraction.

Tremendous advances in ophthalmic surgery have occurred during the past few decades. Highly technical equipment has made it possible to improve ophthalmic procedures and expand ophthalmic surgery. Ophthalmology has again taken a leadership role in the field of surgery. Most ophthalmic procedures require a microscope and other sophisticated equipment. Radial keratotomy surgery has been developed and is performed to restore normal vision without the use of corrective lenses in nearsightedness (myopia).

The development of ophthalmic lasers for treating eye disorders has been one of the most important recent breakthroughs in ophthalmology. Laser surgery allows for virtually painless treatment of various types of eye problems. Physicians are using lasers most frequently intraoperatively, as part of the treatment of proliferative diabetic retinopathy (PDR) during vitrectomy and as an adjunct therapy during scleral buckling for retinal detachment. Laser surgery is currently used to treat glaucoma (laser sclerostomy) and myopia (laser photorefractive keratotomy) (Vaughan, Asbury, & Riordan-Eva, 1992). Still in the investigational phase is a new use for lasers: Holmium laser thermokeratoplasty. This involves treating the cornea with a laser to correct hyperopia (Thoman, 1994). Techniques of corrective-vision surgery are rapidly developing, and the topic is controversial in the ophthalmic community. It is important to note here that most ophthalmic laser procedures are performed in the office rather than in the OR.

Today, most surgical ophthalmic procedures are performed as ambulatory surgery in hospitals, free-standing surgery centers, and ophthalmologists' offices. Fewer complications are seen and postoperative restrictions have almost vanished as surgical techniques, instruments, equipment, sutures, and local anesthetics improve (Javitt, Street, & Tielsch, 1994). These advances have contributed to precise treatment of many eye disorders, including the restoration of sight, humans' most treasured sense.

ASSESSMENT CONSIDERATIONS

Assessment of the patient is always the first step in the multistep process of planning care. This involves the systematic collection of data regarding the specific patient for which the plan of care is being developed. This data is then used to make educated judgments and predictions about the patient's response to the illness. The initial assessment of the patient is crucial to establishing a nursing diagnosis and for establishing desired patient outcomes and criteria by which to measure their attainment (AORN, 1996).

Many ophthalmic procedures are elective, and therefore the data on the patient's chart frequently assists the perioperative nurse with completing the initial assessment. It is critical to assess the patient's general status, especially because most of these patients are elderly, and a very large percentage of diabetic patients have retinal pathology. However, the perioperative ophthalmic nurse will also be expected to assess infants, who require unique considerations. Children as well as adults undergo eye surgery, and nursing assessment must address their specific and individual needs.

General Health Status Review

Any patient experiencing health problems needs to obtain medical clearance before surgical intervention regardless of whether the surgical intervention will be performed using general anesthesic or monitored anesthesia care with regional block anesthesic. As with any surgical procedure, routine tests will be completed preoperatively. These should include, but are not limited to, complete blood count (CBC), electrolytes, blood sugar, blood area nitrogen (BUN), and creatinine. Chest x-ray and electrocar-

diogram (ECG) are obtained if the patient is older than a certain age (usually 35 or 40) or if medically indicated. Other tests may be ordered at the discretion of the attending surgeon or practitioner who is ordering testing. During assessment the perioperative nurse reviews data from the chart. This data includes the nurse's admission assessment record, nurse's notes, history and physical examination, laboratory results, chest x-ray, and ECG. The perioperative nurse then incorporates the information to formulate nursing diagnoses for each patient.

Patient Interview

In addition to gathering assessment data from the patient's record, the perioperative nurse conducts a patient interview. The interview can be conducted in a variety of ways, depending on the surgical setting and the policy of the institution. Because most ophthalmic procedures are performed as outpatient surgery, generally the patient is contacted by the perioperative nurse via the telephone on the day before surgery. This is an excellent opportunity to conduct the preoperative interview and gather additional pertinent data. The patient is generally more relaxed at home and may feel less anxious about asking questions regarding the procedure and postoperative routine. Conversing with the patient is an opportunity for the perioperative nurse to establish rapport. This can enable the nurse to obtain the data required for a thorough patient assessment. Telephoning patients the day before surgery may not be possible in all institutions. In some institutions nurses routinely conduct the preoperative patient interview when the patient comes for presurgery testing. The perioperative nurse may also conduct the patient interview in the operating room (OR) holding area.

Patient History

To provide high-quality nursing care, data must be gathered regarding the patient's health history. The nursing history should include, but is not limited to, the following:
- Allergies—Drugs, foods, soap, dyes, tape, environment
- Medications—Ophthalmic and all others (ask patients to bring all medication with them)
- Coexisting health problems
    - Diabetes, endocrine dysfunction (for example, thyroid)
    - Cardiac dysfunction, hypertension, dysrhythmia, congestive heart failure
    - Degenerative joint disease
    - Asthma, chronic obstructive pulmonary disease, coughing attacks, dyspnea while supine

- Previous surgery
    Especially ophthalmic procedures
    Previous anesthesia problems
- Height, weight, and vital signs
- Occupation
- Life-style
    Smoking: How much, how many years?
    Alcohol or substance abuse: Amount? (If significant, there is a risk for symptoms of withdrawal.) When was alcohol last consumed?

As with any surgical patient, it is critical to establish data regarding any history of allergic reaction. The perioperative nurse must also be aware of all medications the patient is currently taking, both prescription and over-the-counter. Because many coexisting health problems can affect the outcome, it is important to assess these problems and plan nursing actions accordingly. Previous surgery can also be a critical element to providing individualized patient care. Also, check for previous anesthesia experiences. The perioperative nurse will want baseline vital signs for comparison with intraoperative measurements. As part of the history, the perioperative nurse needs to inquire about the patient's life-style, self-care ability, and available resources to gather data for the nursing care plan.

Physical Assessment

Ophthalmic surgery presents some unique assessment considerations. Typically the patient has already experienced visual impairment and may fear blindness as a complication of surgery. Emotional assessment is as important as physiologic assessment.

Mental status. Initially the perioperative nurse needs to assess the patient's mental status accurately by establishing the level of consciousness. Most ophthalmic operations are performed with the patient under local anesthesia. Throughout the surgical procedure the patient will be expected to follow the surgical team's instructions. This makes it necessary for the patient to be awake and oriented, while sedated.

Auditory status. The patient's hearing must be assessed. Many elderly patients are hard of hearing and require a hearing device. It is acceptable for patients to wear hearing aids to the operating room so that they can hear the surgical team's instructions; however, hearing aids must be protected from skin prepatory solutions.

Integumentary status. It is also essential to assess the condition of the patient's skin. General condition, temperature, color, and turgor are noted. During the interview the perioperative nurse should ask about any skin problems. As the patient is transferred from the stretcher to the OR bed, the nurse can assess the back, sacral area, and posterior legs.

Ophthalmic Assessment

The perioperative nurse must carry out a complete ophthalmic assessment. This can be performed rapidly and efficiently by establishing guidelines and criteria to follow. A good place to start is the chief complaint as stated by the patient. The patient should also describe any symptoms he or she has experienced. Querying the patient's understanding of the diagnosis will help the perioperative nurse assess for a knowledge deficit.

Ophthalmic history. The perioperative nurse will need to obtain the patient's ophthalmic history, including both personal and family eye problems, and any history of previous eye surgery. If interviewing time is a problem for the perioperative nurse, a questionnaire can be developed for ophthalmic surgical patients and given to them at the time of presurgery testing. The patient can complete the form before the scheduled day of surgery, thus providing the perioperative nurse with important patient data in advance. An ophthalmic history includes all of the following areas:

- Visual symptoms
    Loss of vision
    Blurred vision
    Diplopia (double vision)
    Scotoma (blind spot or area of loss of vision)
    Pain (one or both eyes)
    Dry eyes
    Halos or rainbows around lights
    Floaters, spots, shower of sparks, ascending veil, or light flashes
    Nausea and vomiting
    Tearing
    Discharge
- Personal ophthalmic history
    Corrective lenses
    Previous eye surgery/previous laser surgery
    Glaucoma
    Eye injury
    Occupational exposures or hazards
- Family ophthalmic history
    Strabismus
    Eye tumors
- Eye medications
    Drug name
    Strength of solution
    Dosage
    Times administered
    Length of time taking the medication

While interviewing the patient, the perioperative nurse must inquire about any visual symptoms the patient has experienced. Vision loss can be a symptom of a number of ophthalmic disorders requiring surgical intervention; therefore, it is necessary to assess for all visual symptoms. Floaters, spots, an ascending veil, and light flashes are common symptoms of retinal tear or detachment. Acute angle-closure glaucoma may present with blurred vision, severe pain, halos or rainbows around lights, and nausea and vomiting. These eye conditions must be treated promptly or the patient will suffer permanent vision loss. Because some ophthalmic disorders increase the risk of other eye problems, it is important to obtain a personal ophthalmic history. There is also an increased risk for strabismus, myopia, glaucoma, some eye tumors, and some degenerative eye disorders if the patient has a family history of the disease (Phipps, et al., 1995).

The nurse must also be aware of all eye medications the patient is taking and should request that the patient bring each medication to the surgery setting. Preoperative and intraoperative ophthalmic medications may need to be changed or adjusted for the patient using eye drops to control glaucoma. Glaucoma patients are usually on multiple drops and often systemic diuretics. A thorough ophthalmic history will provide the perioperative nurse with the data necessary to plan and implement individualized nursing care.

Inspection. While the perioperative nurse is interviewing the patient preoperatively, he or she should *observe* the external eye for the following signs and symptoms (always compare both eyes for difference):

- Redness
- Edema
- Abnormal secretions (crusting, scaling, discharge)
- Excessive tearing
- Bulging
- Dilatated pupil(s)
- Constricted pupil(s)
- Squinting
- Strabismus
- Ptosis
- Everted lid
- Inverted lid
- Lesions
- Sagging tissue
- Fasciculations or tremors of the lids
- Inability of eyelid to close completely
- Subconjunctival hemorrhage
- Pterygium (fold of conjunctiva over the cornea)
- Irregularity in the shape of the pupil
- Unequal pupil size (may result from preoperative ophthalmic medications)
- Yellow, green, or dark, rust-colored sclera
- Shallow anterior chamber
- Opacity of the lens

As the perioperative nurse practices the ophthalmic assessment, he or she will develop the skills required to complete a proficient and quick ophthalmic assessment.

Patient's level of understanding. It is also critical to assess the patient's knowledge of the planned procedure, complications, postoperative routine, and follow-up instructions. The approach to preoperative teaching will need to consider the patient's level of comprehension. The perioperative nurse should ask about family members or friends who will be available to assist the patient postoperatively. The patient should be encouraged to have these significant others included during preoperative teaching and instructions for follow-up care. The significant others can be a valuable resource to both the patient and the perioperative nurse. The perioperative nurse should ensure the patient's understanding that it will be necessary for someone to drive him or her home from the hospital following surgery. If there is no other individual in the home, the perioperative nurse may suggest that the patient stay with a friend or relative postoperatively.

After the perioperative nurse has completed a thorough nursing assessment, the actual and high-risk nursing diagnoses can be clearly identified for each patient.

DIAGNOSTIC STUDIES

Technologic advances are evident in the ophthalmic equipment available to assist in the diagnosis of eye disorders requiring surgery. In this section a few of the more commonly used diagnostic studies will be briefly described. Most of these procedures are performed in the ophthalmologist's office by the physician or other qualified professionals.

Visual Acuity Testing

Several different tests can be performed to determine a patient's visual acuity. Generally, patients are routinely screened for visual acuity of the central field by using the familiar Snellen eye chart. This chart is composed of rows of random letters, each becoming progressively smaller. Each eye is tested individually; this test provides a measure of distance vision. A patient may undergo more than one method of testing for visual acuity.

For patients with lens opacities, several techniques are available to help determine visual potential. The most sophisticated instruments in common use project a narrow beam of light containing a pattern of images through any relatively clear portion of the media onto the retina. These techniques are usually able to predict the expected degree of improvement in visual acuity after surgical removal of cataracts.

The laser interferometer uses laser light to generate interference fringes, which the patient sees as a series of parallel lines. These lines are made finer and finer until the patient can no longer distinguish them (Vaughan, Asbury, & Riordan-Eva, 1992). The potential acuity meter projects the Snellen chart onto the retina; the entire chart is carried on a beam of light, 0.15 mm in diameter.

Refractometry

It is essential that all candidates for ocular surgery be examined to determine their best-corrected visual acuity and refractive error. Refractive error is the requirement of corrective lenses needed for the patient to have proper focus for distance. Technology for this examination may involve a computerized automatic refractor, a Phoroptor, or a trial frame with loose lenses.

Perimetry

Both central and peripheral visual fields can be measured by perimetry. Perimetry can be used to detect retinal detachment as well as neural degeneration within the visual pathway. There are many types of perimeters. The current method for assessing visual fields is rapidly shifting to automated perimetry. The Humphrey Field Analyzer, a computerized automated perimeter, provides a much more standardized test than the manual Goldmann perimeter. It can therefore be used to detect the gradual visual field loss seen in the patient with uncontrolled glaucoma, as well as other disorders. However, the Goldmann perimetry is still valuable for patients who are not able to cooperate for the more difficult automated perimetry.

Ophthalmoscopy

One of the first instruments developed to assist in the detection and diagnosis of ophthalmic disorders was the ophthalmoscope. Through this instrument physicians were able to visualize disorders within the inner eye. Today practitioners use the ophthalmoscope for routine screening and diagnostic purposes for patients experiencing altered visual acuity. The different types of ophthalmoscopes will be discussed in more detail.

Direct ophthalmoscopy. Direct ophthalmoscopy is frequently performed as part of a routine physical assessment or examination. It allows monocular examination of the interior of the eye. With use of the direct ophthalmoscope the examiner can directly visualize the fundus (retina, choroid, and sclera) and the transparent media (cornea, aqueous lens, and vitreous). These structures are magnified approximately 15 times their normal size. The examination can be performed without the administration of a mydriatic to dilate the patient's pupils, although in most situations it is necessary to dilatate the pupils. Experienced and skilled nurses can perform direct ophthalmoscopy as part of the physical assessment. The nurse or physician documents the findings on the patient's record.

Indirect ophthalmoscopy. This method is called indirect because the image is formed on a hand-held condensing lens, as opposed to direct ophthalmoscopy where the examiner focuses directly on the retina. To be an effective diagnostic tool, the indirect ophthalmoscope requires acquired skill. The examiner must be experienced to interpret the inverted images correctly. Two advantages, however, are that the procedure provides binocular visualization of the inner eye, and a larger area of the retina is visible than with direct examination. A third advantage is that the brighter light source permits better visualization through cloudy media (Vaughan, Asbury, Riordan-Eva, 1992). In addition to the indirect ophthalmoscope, this examination requires the use of a magnifying lens and, sometimes, a scleral depressor. Because the light of the indirect ophthalmoscope is intense and causes the pupils to constrict, a cycloplegic is administered to dilatate the patient's pupils before the examination. This approach is used preoperatively and also during retinal surgery; the ophthalmologist uses the indirect ophthalmoscope to localize the exact area of retinal detachment.

Tonometry

Tonometry measures intraocular pressure (IOP) and should be a routine part of an ophthalmic examination. With routine screening by tonometry, glaucoma can be detected early and treated before significant damage occurs. This diagnostic test should be performed annually on patients with a family history of glaucoma. Normal IOP is 10.5 to 20.5 mm Hg (Brenner, 1987). The major types of tonometry used are the Schiøtz, the applanation method, and the digital tonopen.

Schiøtz tonometry. Schiøtz tonometry is the older method of tonometry and can be performed by ophthalmologists as well as other health care providers. It also has the advantage of being portable. Topical anesthetic solution is instilled into both eyes first, then the hand-held Schiøtz tonometer is placed directly on the cornea. This is done with the patient in supine position and looking up. As the tonometer indents the cornea, the scale is read and the actual IOP is calculated using a conversion chart. In the OR the Schiøtz tonometer is sterilized to measure IOP during retinal surgery.

Applanation tonometry. Applanation tonometry is more accurate than Schiøtz tonometry. During applanation tonometry the cornea is flattened instead of indented. The most common applanation tonometer is the Goldmann type, which is attached to the slit lamp and is used in an office setting. After the instillation of both anesthetic and fluorescein drops, the cornea is flattened with a small plastic cone, which is (as previously stated) part of the slit lamp, and the IOP is measured.

Slit Lamp Examination

Slit lamp examination, or biomicroscopy, uses a binocular microscope and a special light source to visualize the eye's anterior structures and the small details of the fundus. The patient's head is stabilized in an attached headrest during examination. Mydriatic drops may be administered before the examination; however, iris detail cannot be seen if the eye is dilatated first. Disorders of the lid, cornea, anterior chamber, iris, and lens can easily be detected with the slit lamp. Examination of the retina, vitreous, and optic nerve is performed using a special contact lens.

Fundus Photography and Fluorescein Angiography

Technologic advances have made it possible to photograph the inner structures of the eye. Ophthalmologists can study these photographs to evaluate and record changes in the structures of the fundus. The retinal blood vessels can also be assessed by intravenous injection of fluorescein dye immediately before rapid sequence photographs. The pupil must be well dilatated before the fundus can be photographed. It is important to note that, since this is an invasive procedure, informed consent must be obtained from the patient. Allergic reactions to the fluorescein dye occasionally occur; therefore, the nurse must assess the patient for a history of allergic response to fluorescein dye. Sensitization may develop at any time during routine instillation of topical fluorescein for IOP testing. After the injection the patient must be observed for signs of allergic reaction. It is also important to inspect the intravenous injection site carefully, because any leaking into the subcutaneous tissue can result in intense burning. The patient should be advised that his urine will be orange-green, almost fluorescent, for 1 to 2 days.

Gonioscopy

Gonioscopy enables the ophthalmologist to visualize directly the anterior chamber angle of the eye in patients suspected of having glaucoma. Four types of lenses with mirrors (goniolens) can be used for gonioscopy: Goldmann, Posner/Zeiss, Sussman, and Koepee. The goniolens allows examination of the trabecular region, and the ophthalmologist can distinguish angle-closure from open-angle glaucoma. Topical anesthetic solution is instilled into the eye, and the goniolens is placed directly on it. Depending on the type of lens, the patient is supine or is seated at the slit lamp.

Ultrasonography

High-frequency sound waves are employed to diagnose eye abnormalities and to measure eye structures accurately. Ultrasonography is useful when visualization of the eye is not possible because of opacities. During this examination a transducer probe is gently placed against the eye. Generally, two modes of ultrasound are used in clinical ophthalmology, the A-mode and the B-mode.

A-mode (A-scan). The A-scan provides a one-dimensional tracing of the eye. In the A-mode the sound wave can measure the distance from the cornea to the retina (axial length). This measurement is necessary to calculate the required power for an intraocular lens implant as well as to detect structures within the eye. A-scans can therefore also be used to determine tumor size and monitor any change in size. Most ophthalmologists' offices are equipped to perform A-scan ultrasound.

B-mode (B-scan). The B-scan constructs a two-dimensional image, or cross-section, of the eye. The B-mode is useful in detecting tumors of the orbit or eye. It is also very useful for patients whose posterior segments cannot be visualized because of dense lens opacities or vitreous hemorrhage.

NURSING DIAGNOSES

After reviewing the preoperative assessment data, the perioperative nurse is able to identify high-risk and actual nursing diagnoses accurately for each patient. Individual nursing care plans are critical for high-quality patient care. By developing a list of nursing diagnoses that commonly apply to patients undergoing ophthalmic surgery, the perioperative nurse can incorporate these into a specific, individualized intraoperative plan of care.

All of the generic nursing diagnoses and care plans (Chapter 7) will apply to the ophthalmic patient in surgery. In some instances there may be modifications to the generic care plans, and these will be described under "Guides to Nursing Actions" for the specific surgical procedures. In addition to the generic nursing diagnoses, other nursing diagnoses apply to this specialty. These will be identified and briefly discussed in the following section. It is important to remember that the care plans and Guides to Nursing Actions are provided as samples. As perioperative nurses develop care plans for ophthalmic patients in their institutions, other nursing diagnoses may become applicable. In the OR there is truly a team approach to patient care; interventions for some nursing diagnoses are accomplished through collaborative practice with anesthesia providers and surgeons.

Sensory/Perceptual Alterations: Visual

The nursing diagnosis of visual sensory/perceptual alterations will be appropriate for all patients undergoing eye surgery. This nursing diagnosis is related to (1) opacity of the crystalline lens, (2) increased IOP, (3) damaged cornea, (4) partial or complete detachment of the retina from the choroid, (5) vitreous hemorrhage, (6) deviation of eye muscle alignment, or (7) several different problems involving the eyelids or orbits. Visual sensory/perception alterations may also be related to the covering of both eyes during the perioperative phase. These patients may have experienced either gradual or sudden loss of vision, which may be temporary or permanent. Consequently, the perioperative nurse needs to clearly and verbally communicate to the patient the specifics of the OR environment and routine. The perioperative nurse will also need to introduce the members of the surgical team assigned to provide care to the patient. It is important for the perioperative nurse to identify any noises or sounds heard in the holding area and OR. He or she should also note any difficulty related to the visual disturbance that the patient has when transferring from the stretcher to the OR bed. The degree of visual sensory/perceptual alteration needs to be documented and reported to other nurses caring for the patient. If the patient's unoperative eye has no vision, it is particularly important to communicate this information to other caregivers. This patient should be treated as a blind patient postoperatively, since the operative eye will have a patch on it and the unoperative eye has no vision. Postoperatively, after the eye patch(es) has been applied, the perioperative nurse may identify an increase in the alteration of visual sensory perception.

Pain

The ophthalmic patient may suffer pain related to increased IOP. This is commonly associated with glaucoma; however, it may also result from eye surgery. In addition, the patient undergoing local anesthesia may feel pain as the facial and retrobulbar blocks are injected. In many institutions the anesthesia provider will heavily sedate the patient for a short time while the regional blocks are being given so that the patient has no awareness or memory of the injections. The patient should be instructed to verbalize any pain experienced during the surgery so that a supplemental block may be given. It should not be assumed that nausea in postoperative eye patients is due only to anesthesia; this could be a sign of increased IOP.

Anxiety and Fear

Anxiety and *fear* are closely associated with the patient's emotional status. Anxiety or fear related to visual impairment may vary from patient to patient, depending on the degree of vision loss, the abruptness of onset, and the expected outcome of surgery on the visual impairment. For example, a patient with glaucoma who has had previous surgical interventions that failed to decrease IOP may suffer from increased anxiety and fear. A monocular patient having surgery on his or her seeing eye will most likely have a very high level of anxiety regarding the surgical outcome. If the procedure is being performed with the patient under local anesthesia, the patient may fear pain during the operation. The perioperative nurse plays a vital role in helping ophthalmic patients to reduce or cope with their anxiety and fear.

Ineffective Individual Coping

Ineffective individual coping related to vision loss and change in life-style may be an actual or high-risk nursing diagnosis. Children experiencing eye surgery may have difficulty dealing with the stress of their hospitalization, the perioperative routine, and separation from their parents and familiar surroundings. The hysterical child presents a challenge to even the most experienced perioperative nurse and surgical team. The stress to the child can be minimized by a preoperative visit and patient and family teaching regarding the operation. Some perioperative nurses have been able to incorporate a tour of the surgical suite into the preoperative visit. Familiarity with the surroundings, sounds, odors, equipment, and OR attire can also help reduce the stress the child suffers.

One reaction that adult patients may express is anger. This may be due to the stress of both the change in their life-style and their level of independence. Anger may be directed toward the entire surgical team, especially if the procedure is not well tolerated and does not correct or prevent further visual impairment. In caring for such a patient it is important for the perioperative nurse to be a good listener and provide psychologic support.

PLANNING

The next step in the nursing process is to establish the appropriate plan of perioperative nursing care for ophthalmic patients. Desired patient outcomes guide the nurse in identifying and carrying out the appropriate nursing action.

IMPLEMENTATION AND NURSING ACTIONS

The individual patient assessment and identified desired outcomes will map out the required nursing actions. Specific nursing actions as they relate to different ophthalmic procedures are listed in the care plans in the next section of this chapter. Accompanying each care plan is a Guide to Nursing Actions, which further outlines nursing interventions for the patient having eye surgery. Again, these serve as a model for the perioperative nurse and may require modification to provide individualized, high-quality patient care.

EVALUATION

The final step in the nursing process is evaluation and reassessment of the patient's response to nursing care. During this stage of care the perioperative nurse checks to see if and how the patient outcomes were met. After the evaluation has been completed, the entire nursing process continues, starting with reassessment.

PLANS OF CARE

The remainder of this chapter is devoted to plans of care for specific ophthalmic procedures. The more common and frequently performed procedures are included. Each plan of care is further explained in the Guides to Nursing Actions. The perioperative nurse will need to adapt the plans of care to his or her particular surgical setting, according to institutional policy and procedure.

GUIDES TO NURSING ACTIONS
Muscle Surgery (Fig. 11-1)

1. Preoperatively the perioperative nurse assesses the patient for coexisting health problems that may require modification to nursing actions. It is especially important for the perioperative nurse to assess the extent of the patient's visual impairment. Assessing the level of anxiety and the patient's level of comprehension regarding the planned surgery is also critical. Many of the patients having muscle surgery are children; children should be scheduled early in the morning. The perioperative nurse should keep in mind that patients undergoing strabismus or ptosis surgery are at increased risk for developing malignant hyperthermia during anesthesia.

2. Besides explaining the routine for surgery, the perioperative nurse discusses the specifics for muscle surgery with the patient (and the parents, if the patient is a child). Simple, honest explanations are best with children. If possible the perioperative nurse should include a tour of the OR and show the child the standard OR attire to help familiarize the patient with the surgical surroundings. The child may be encouraged to bring a favorite soft toy to the hospital to alleviate anxiety. Parents will need to know how long they may stay with their child. Preoperative medications are administered, and antibiotic eye medication may be given to prevent infection. Monitoring equipment, such as blood pressure cuff, O_2 saturation monitor clip, and ECG electrodes, will be placed on the patient and used throughout the procedure. Surgical interventions for children are performed with general anesthesia. Postoperatively, eye ointment is applied, which will cause blurred vision tempo-

rarily. The parents and child must be instructed not to rub the eye(s) after surgery. Adult patients will commonly have the operative eye patched postoperatively (if surgery is unilateral).

3. Accurate verification of the operative eye(s) is necessary because the patient often requires surgery on more than one muscle and in both eyes. Verification should be both verbal, obtained from the patient (or parent), and written, obtained through chart review.

4. Compare the operative consent with the patient's verification of the operative eye(s). If the patient is a minor, make sure that the legal guardian is the one who signed the permit; remember that the parent is not always the legal guardian.

5. Check that the ordered preoperative medication was given and evaluate the patient's response and anxiety level.

6. Position the patient in the supine position, using devices for proper head and eye alignment and maximal comfort. The patient's head is stabilized in a headrest. A pillow is placed under the legs superior to the popliteal space and a safety strap is secured over the chest or abdomen. Minor adjustments to the OR bed may be necessary depending on the child's size.

7. The eye is prepared with much care to prevent irritation. In addition to the usual method of prepping the face with Betadine, preparation may also include instillation of Betadine 5% Ophthalmic Prep solution onto the cornea, followed with flushing out with Balanced Salt Solution, after two minutes. Since Betadine is a corneal irritant, its instillation should be preceded with a topical anesthetic, such as tetracaine.

8. Assess and document the condition of the skin and eyes both before and after preparation, and again after the surgery.

9. All medications must be labeled and documented as to date, time, route, and dosage.

10. Special equipment and supplies depend on the physician's preference (disposable cautery or bipolar unit, eye loupes, etc.). Check the physician preference card. Test all equipment according to manufacturers' recommendations and institutional protocol.

11. Ensure that the OR team does not lean on the patient during the procedure.

12. Account for all instruments, ophthalmic sponges, and sharps, including eye needles. Document all counts according to institutional protocol.

13. If a specimen is obtained during muscle resection, follow institutional protocol for preserva-

FIG. 11-1
CARE PLAN FOR MUSCLE SURGERY

KEY ASSESSMENT POINTS

History of previous ocular problems or surgery
Current medications taken/why
Description of visual problems (review behavioral manifestations such as squinting and signs and symptoms such as diplopia, malalignment)
Visual acuity (operative and nonoperative eye)
Physical assessment results (coexisting health problems)
Self-care or parental care ability
Emotional response to eye disorder
Resources available for follow-up care
Operative eye (right eye [OD], left eye [OS], or both eyes [OU])
Allergies

NURSING DIAGNOSIS

All generic nursing diagnoses apply to this patient, with the addition of:
Anxiety related to the stress of hospitalization, surgery

PATIENT OUTCOMES

All generic outcomes apply, with the addition of:
The patient will exhibit a decrease in anxiety by:
1. Pulse, blood pressure, and respirations WNL
2. Displaying relaxed facial expression, unclenched hands
3. Verbalizing less anxiety
4. Accurately describing perioperative events
5. Following instructions

NURSING ACTIONS

	Yes	No	N/A
1. Preoperative assessment performed?	☐	☐	☐
2. Perioperative explanations given?	☐	☐	☐
3. Patient verification/ID bracelet checked?	☐	☐	☐
4. Verbal verification of operative site? (left/right/bilateral)	☐	☐	☐
5. Consent signed correctly?	☐	☐	☐
6. Effect of preoperative medications noted?	☐	☐	☐
7. Positioned correctly?	☐	☐	☐
8. Condition of skin noted at prep site?	☐	☐	☐
9. Prep performed per institutional protocol?	☐	☐	☐
10. Medications labeled/documented?	☐	☐	☐
11. Special equipment/supplies available?	☐	☐	☐
12. Equipment checked/in working condition?	☐	☐	☐
13. Counts performed/correct?	☐	☐	☐
14. Specimens to lab?	☐	☐	☐
15. Ophthalmic ointment applied?	☐	☐	☐
16. Postoperative assessment performed?	☐	☐	☐
17. Other generic care plans initiated? (specify)	☐	☐	☐

Document additional nursing actions generic care plans initiated here:

_____

_____

_____

EVALUATION OF PATIENT OUTCOMES

	Outcome met	Outcome met with additional outcome criteria	Outcome met with revised nursing care plan	Outcome not met	Outcome not applicable to this patient
1. The patient's anxiety was reduced.	☐	☐	☐	☐	☐
2. The patient met outcomes for additional generic care plans as indicated	☐	☐	☐	☐	☐

Signature: _____ Date: _____

tion and disposition of specimens. Document specimens obtained.

14. Apply the eye ointment according to the physician's preference, and dressing if necessary; explain that the ointment will cause blurred vision.

15. Discharge teaching should include verbal and written instructions. These should include when to return to see the physician, and that it is normal to experience light sensitivity, bloody tears, and redness of the eyes. The patient should be instructed to wash his or her hands before touching the eye and to clean the eye using warm water or Dacriose solution while keeping the eye closed. This should be done by wiping gently from nose to ear and by using a new pad for each wipe. It is important to stress to the patient to avoid any pressure on the eye.

Glaucoma Surgery (Fig. 11-2)

1. Preoperatively the perioperative nurse assesses the patient for coexisting health problems (particularly because most glaucoma patients are elderly) that may require modification to nursing actions; for example, diabetic patients should be scheduled early in the morning. It is important for the perioperative nurse to assess the patient's visual impairment. Assessing the level of anxiety and the patient's expectations of the surgical result is also critical. In acute angle-closure glaucoma that does not respond to medical treatment, surgery is performed as an emergency procedure, and the patient may be anxious. In surgery for open-angle chronic glaucoma, check that the patient discontinued the use of certain glaucoma medications according to the physician's instruction. For example, pilocarpine should be discontinued two weeks before surgery if possible because it causes inflammation postoperatively.

2. In addition to explaining the routine for surgery, the perioperative nurse discusses the specifics for glaucoma surgery. Preoperative medications are administered and antibiotic eye medication may also be given to prevent infection. Monitoring equipment, such as blood pressure cuff, O_2 saturation monitor clip, and ECG electrodes, will be placed on the patient and used throughout the procedure. The exact routine varies depending on the specific procedure being performed to increase the outflow of aqueous humor. Often chemotherapeutic agents, mitomycin or fluorouracil, are applied to the trabecular meshwork during surgery (Langseth, 1993; Quigley, 1993). The surgical interventions will be performed with the patient under local anesthesia. Laser procedures usually require only topical anesthetic before the goniolens is placed because this procedure is relatively painless. When laser treatments are performed the perioperative nurse will need to instruct the patient not to move during the treatment. The nurse should also describe the sound of the laser to the patient. Patients undergoing laser treatment are usually discharged a few hours postoperatively, after IOP stabilizes. Those having surgery may need to stay in the hospital to have the IOP monitored. Postoperatively an eye patch and shield are applied. It is important to inform the patient that IOP will be checked frequently in the postoperative period, and that even with a good surgical result it may take several weeks for IOP to stabilize.

3. Accurate verification of the operative eye is necessary because the patient may suffer from glaucoma in both eyes. Verification should be both verbal, obtained from the patient, and written, obtained through chart review.

4. Compare the operative consent with the patient's verification of the operative eye. If the physician intends to implant a valve, make sure that this is delineated on the operative consent.

5. Check that the ordered preoperative medication was given and evaluate the patient's response.

6. Position the patient in the supine position, using devices for proper head and eye alignment and maximal comfort. The head is stabilized in a headrest. A pillow is placed under the legs superior to the popliteal space and a safety strap is secured over the chest or abdomen. During laser procedures the patient sits in a chair, with the head securely positioned in a chin rest.

7. The eye is prepared with much care to prevent irritation. In addition to prepping the operative side of the face with Betadine, preparation may also include instillation of Betadine 5% Ophthalmic Prep Solution followed by flushing with Balanced Salt Solution after 2 minutes. Since Betadine is a corneal irritant, its instillation should be preceded with a topical anesthetic, such as tetracaine. Preparation may not be required for laser procedures.

8. Assess and document the condition of the skin and eye before and after preparation, and again after the surgery.

9. All medications must be labeled and documented as to date, time, route, and dosage. If a chemotherapeutic agent is applied to the trabecular meshwork under the conjunctival flap during the trabeculectomy, vigorous irrigation with Balanced Salt Solution is necessary to prevent corneal epithelial defect (Langseth, 1993).

FIG. 11-2
CARE PLAN FOR GLAUCOMA SURGERY

KEY ASSESSMENT POINTS
Family history of glaucoma
History of previous ocular problems or surgery
Current medications taken/why
Date of last eye exam and IOP measurement
Description of visual problems
Visual acuity (operative and nonoperative eye)
Physical assessment results (coexisting health problems)
Self-care ability
Emotional response to eye disorder
Resources available for follow-up care
Operative eye (OD, OS, or OU)
Allergies

NURSING DIAGNOSIS
All generic nursing diagnoses apply to this patient, with the addition
of:
Sensory/perceptual alterations: visual related to increased intraocular pressure
Anxiety related to stress of hospitalization, surgery, potential loss of vision

PATIENT OUTCOMES:
All generic outcomes apply, with the addition of:
1. The patient will exhibit minimal alteration in sensory perception by:
   a. Recognizing normal sounds and familiar voices
   b. Being oriented to surroundings
2. The patient will exhibit a reduced level of anxiety by:
   a. Pulse, blood pressure, and respirations WNL
   b. Displaying relaxed facial expressions, unclenched hands
   c. Verbalizing less anxiety
   d. Accurately describing perioperative events
   e. Following instructions

NURSING ACTIONS

	Yes	No	N/A
1. Preoperative assessment performed?	☐	☐	☐
2. Perioperative explanations given?	☐	☐	☐
3. Patient verification/ID bracelet checked?	☐	☐	☐
4. Verbal verification of operative site?	☐	☐	☐
5. Consent signed correctly?	☐	☐	☐
6. Effect of preoperative medications noted?	☐	☐	☐
7. Positioned correctly?	☐	☐	☐
8. Condition of skin noted at prep site before and after prep	☐	☐	☐
9. Prep performed per institutional protocol?	☐	☐	☐
10. Medications labeled/documented?	☐	☐	☐
11. Special equipment/supplies available?	☐	☐	☐
12. Equipment checked/in working condition?	☐	☐	☐
13. Laser safety precautions initiated?	☐	☐	☐
14. Counts performed/correct?	☐	☐	☐
15. Postop drops, ointment applied?	☐	☐	☐
16. Dressing/shield applied?	☐	☐	☐
17. Postoperative assessment performed?	☐	☐	☐
18. Other generic care plans initiated? (specify)	☐	☐	☐

Document additional nursing actions generic care plans initiated here:

_____

_____

_____

EVALUATION OF PATIENT OUTCOMES

	Outcome met	Outcome met with additional outcome criteria	Outcome met with revised nursing care plan	Outcome not met	Outcome not applicable to this patient
1. The patient's alteration in visual sensory perception was minimal.	☐	☐	☐	☐	☐
2. The patient's anxiety was reduced.	☐	☐	☐	☐	☐
3. The patient met outcomes for additional generic care plans as indicated.	☐	☐	☐	☐	☐

Signature: _____ Date: _____

10. Special equipment and supplies depend on the type of filtering procedure and the physician's preference (bipolar unit, microscope, laser, goniolens, filtering valve). Check the surgical permit and physician preference card. Test all equipment according to manufacturers' recommendations and institutional protocol.

11. Ensure that the OR team does not lean on the patient during the procedure.

12. Initiate laser safety procedures and document according to institutional protocol.

13. Account for all equipment parts on the sterile field, instruments, ophthalmic sponges, and sharps, including the microsurgery needles. Document all counts according to hospital protocol.

14. Document information regarding implantation of filtering valves according to hospital protocol.

15. Apply (or help apply) any eye ointment and eye dressing according to the physician's preference (moist and/or dry eye patches, plastic eye shield, and tape).

16. Discharge teaching should include instruction to return to see the physician the next day, and that the patch and shield are to be left on until that time. Oral and written instructions are given to the patient regarding time of the follow-up visit, use of medications, and the use of a metal or plastic shield at night. It is important to explain that a scratching, cinderlike feeling in the operated eye is normal, and that there may be crusting or mucous drainage along lid and eyelashes. The patient is instructed to cleanse the eyelids each morning with a cotton ball and warm water. Also the patient should be very careful not to exert any pressure on the eye or upper eyelid to prevent accidentally causing complications. The patient should not sleep on the operated side. Mild pain can be controlled by acetaminophen, but sudden onset of severe pain should be reported immediately to the physician. A general education guide for the patient with glaucoma is presented in Box 11-1.

Retinal Surgery (Fig. 11-3)

1. Preoperatively the perioperative nurse will assess the patient for coexisting health problems that may require modification to nursing actions. Many retina patients are diabetic, especially those undergoing vitrectomy. Diabetic patients should be scheduled early in the morning. It is important for the perioperative nurse to assess the patient's visual impairment and to review the patient's chart for the ophthalmologist's impression and for results of diagnostic studies (indirect ophthalmoscopy, fundus photography, and fluorescein angiography). Assess the level of anxiety related to the vision loss and the patient's expectations of the surgical result. Some retinal detachments are emergencies, and therefore the patient may not be psychologically prepared for hospitalization and surgery.

2. In addition to explaining the routine for surgery, the perioperative nurse discusses specifics for retinal surgery. Retinal surgery is usually performed with the patient under general, but sometimes local, anesthesia and may take many hours. Preoperative medications as well as eye medication to dilatate the pupil of the operative eye are administered. The eyelashes may need to be trimmed; if so, this is usually done before the patient arrives at the OR. Monitoring equipment, such as blood pressure cuff, O_2 saturation monitor clip, and ECG electrodes, will be placed on the patient and used throughout the procedure. During surgery a combination of treatments may be used to repair the detached retina, including vitrectomy, scleral buckle, and intraoperative laser. An eye patch and shield are applied postoperatively, and possibly an antibiotic eye ointment. Inform the patient that light perception will be checked frequently during the postoperative period. Primary retinal detachment requires the patient to remain on bed rest. If a gas bubble (C_3F_8 or SF_6) was injected intraoperatively, the patient will have to remain in a very specific position (for example, face down) depending on where the detachment was located. This should be indicated by the surgeon in the postoperative orders. The patient may remain in the hospital after surgery, but more likely will be discharged following recovery from the anesthesia. Antibiotics and mydriatics for pupillary dilatation will be continued for several weeks postoperatively.

3. Accurate verification of the operative eye is a critical nursing action. Verification should be both verbal, from the patient, and written, obtained through chart review.

4. Compare the operative consent with the patient's verification of the operative eye. If cryotherapy is to be performed intraoperatively on the contralateral eye, make sure that this is delineated on the operative consent.

5. Check that the ordered preoperative medication was given and evaluate the patient's response. Assess pupillary dilatation of the operative eye. If the pathologic condition is present in both eyes, it is possible that dilating drops will be ordered for both eyes so that the unoperative eye may be examined under anesthesia and cryosurgery performed on it if necessary.

Box 11-1 Patient Education Guide for Glaucoma

1. Explain what glaucoma is and the purpose of treatment. Stress that with proper management, blindness can be prevented, but lost vision cannot be restored. Explain the importance of regular, long-term ocular examinations and be sure the patient has the phone number of his or her ophthalmologist.
2. Provide printed material about prescribed medications including the purpose, action, dosage, schedule, any specific instructions (such as refrigeration), and side effects. Evaluate the patient's (and family's) degree of understanding. Advise patient not to use over-the-counter medications before consulting his or her physician.
3. Discuss with patient how to avoid confusing eye medications when several are being used. Discuss methods of storing eye medications for ease of identification and for avoiding double doses or instillation in the wrong eye. Discuss how to improvise a labeling system.
4. Demonstrate and then observe the patient performing correct technique for instillation of eye medications. Observe a family member performing a return demonstration.
5. Demonstrate and observe a return demonstration by patient or family member of any treatments to be done by self or family such as application of dressings, eye shields, eye irrigation, cold or warm compresses, and insertion/removal of contact lens. Give the patient written, step-by-step directions with illustrations. When impaired central vision is a problem, use large print for written instructions. If supplies are to be purchased by the patient, prepare a written list of items needed.
6. Instruct patient to avoid activities that increase IOP. The most important complication of both medical and surgical therapy, including laser trabeculoplasty, is failure to lower IOP far enough to prevent further visual field loss. Some ways to prevent an increase in IOP include the following:
   a. Advise patient to tie shoelaces by bending knee, raising thigh, and bringing foot within hand reach.
   b. Recommend patient move objects weighing 20 pounds or more by pushing the object on the floor using feet or by using a mechanical dolly.
   c. Instruct patient to use poles or rods with hooks on the end to pick up items (avoid bending).
   d. Advise patient to be alert for steroid-type medications prescribed by other physicians for noneye disorders. Steroids tend to increase IOP, especially in patients with glaucoma.
   e. Tell patient about Medic-Alert and other identification worn to alert health care providers in emergency situations about the eye condition and medications used.
   f. Be specific about what activities may be done to ensure patient understanding and obtain compliance.
7. Describe to patient complications to be alert for and measures to avoid them. When a medical term or terms identifying a complication are used, clarify the meaning by describing the signs and symptoms. Tell the patient to seek medical attention for any of the following:
   a. *Upper respiratory infections*—avoid sneezing and coughing, which can increase IOP; avoid crowds of people where respiratory infections can be contracted.
   b. *Retinal detachment*—notify ophthalmologist immediately if sudden painless partial loss of vision (curtain effect) occurs.
   c. *Infection of eye*—seek medical attention for redness, photophobia, lacrimation, and drainage from the eye.
   d. *Blockage of drainage channel*—report to ophthalmologist promptly any eye discomfort, pain, or decreasing visual acuity.
   e. *Cataract formation*—report any change in vision.
8. Review with patient and family a written list of resources available and plan with them how and when to contact selected resources.

From Beare PG & Myers JL. (1994). *Principles and practices of adult health nursing* (2nd Ed.). St Louis: Mosby.

---

6. Before transporting the patient to the OR, verify that the patient has voided.
7. Position the patient in the supine position, using devices for proper head and eye alignment and maximal comfort. The head is stabilized in a headrest. If a wristrest is going to be used during the procedure, make certain that the long plate to secure it to the OR bed is in position before transferring the patient to the operating bed. Armboards are used whenever indicated by the size of the patient, with arms at less than 90° angle to prevent brachial plexus injury. Pad all bony prominences. A pillow is placed under the legs superior to the popliteal space, and a safety strap is secured across the chest or abdomen. Ensure that the feet are uncrossed to prevent peroneal nerve damage. Heel pads are used to prevent pressure breakdown of the skin, as low constant pressure on bony prominences has been shown to cause microscopic changes in even healthy individuals after 2 hours (Kneedler & Dodge, 1994).
8. The eye is prepared with much care to prevent irritation. In addition to prepping the operative side of the face with Betadine, preparation may also include instillation of Betadine 5% Oph-

FIG. 11-3
CARE PLAN FOR RETINAL SURGERY

KEY ASSESSMENT POINTS

History of previous ocular problems or surgery
Current medications taken/why
Visual acuity (operative and nonoperative eye)
Physical assessment results (coexisting health problems; with the diabetic patient, check blood pressure, type, duration and degree of control of diabetes)
Knowledge level (reason for surgical procedure, postoperative care)
Self-care ability
Emotional response and coping style
Resources available for follow-up care
Operative eye (OD, OS, or OU)
Allergies

NURSING DIAGNOSIS

All generic nursing diagnoses apply to this patient, with the addition of:
1. Anxiety related to loss of vision, hospitalization, surgery
2. Sensory/perceptual alterations: visual related to patching of the eye(s)

PATIENT OUTCOMES

All generic outcomes apply, with the addition of:
1. The patient will exhibit a decrease in anxiety by:
   a. Pulse, blood pressure, and respirations WNL
   b. Verbalization of less anxiety
   c. Displaying relaxed facial expression, unclenched hands
   d. Accurately describing perioperative events
   e. Following instructions
2. The patient will exhibit minimal alteration in visual sensory perception by:
   a. Recognizing normal sounds and familiar voices
   b. Being oriented to surroundings

NURSING ACTIONS

	Yes	No	N/A
1. Preoperative assessment performed?	☐	☐	☐
2. Perioperative explanation given?	☐	☐	☐
3. Patient verification/ID checked?	☐	☐	☐
4. Verbal verification of operative site?	☐	☐	☐
5. Consent signed correctly?	☐	☐	☐
6. Effect of preoperative medications/eye drops noted?	☐	☐	☐
7. Positioned correctly?	☐	☐	☐
8. Condition of skin noted at prep site before and after prep?	☐	☐	☐
9. Prep performed per institutional protocol?	☐	☐	☐
10. Medications labeled/documented?	☐	☐	☐
11. Special equipment/supplies available?	☐	☐	☐
12. Equipment checked/in working condition?	☐	☐	☐
13. Counts performed/correct?	☐	☐	☐
14. Implants documented?	☐	☐	☐
15. Postop drops, ointment applied?	☐	☐	☐
16. Dressing applied?	☐	☐	☐
17. Postoperative assessment performed?	☐	☐	☐
18. Other generic care plans initiated? (specify)	☐	☐	☐

Document additional nursing actions generic care plans initiated here:

_____

_____

_____

EVALUATION OF PATIENT OUTCOMES

	Outcome met	Outcome met with additional outcome criteria	Outcome met with revised nursing care plan	Outcome not met	Outcome not applicable to this patient
1. The patient's anxiety was reduced.	☐	☐	☐	☐	☐
2. The patient's alteration in visual sensory perception was minimal.	☐	☐	☐	☐	☐
3. The patient met outcomes for additional generic care plans as indicated.	☐	☐	☐	☐	☐

Signature: _____ Date: _____

thalmic Prep Solution followed by flushing with Balanced Salt Solution after 2 minutes. Since Betadine is a corneal irritant, its instillation should be preceded with a topical anesthetic, such as tetracaine.

9. Assess and document the condition of the skin and eye both before and after preparation, and after the surgery.

10. All medications must be labeled and documented as to date, time, route, and dosage.

11. Special equipment and supplies depend on the type of retinal procedure and the physician's preference. These may include bipolar unit, microscope, diathermy unit, retinal cryoprobe and cryosurgery unit, indirect ophthalmoscope, 20 or 28 diopter lens, tonometer, posterior vitrector unit, endoilluminator, fragmatome, membrane peeler cutter, laser, and assorted Silastic implants. Check the surgical permit and physician preference card. Test all equipment according to manufacturers' recommendations and institutional protocol.

12. Ensure that the OR team does not lean on the patient during the procedure.

13. Account for all equipment parts on the sterile field, instruments, ophthalmic sponges, and sharps, including the microsurgery needles. Document all counts according to hospital protocol.

14. Follow institutional protocol for documenting Silastic retinal implant information.

15. Initiate laser safety procedures and document according to institutional protocol.

16. Apply (or help apply) the eye dressing according to the physician's preference; this may include two dry eye patches, tape, and plastic shield and tape. Make sure that the eye is completely closed before putting the dressing on to prevent corneal abrasion. The dressing should compress the eye.

17. Discharge teaching should include instructions to return to see the physician the next day, and that the patch and shield are to be left on until that time. Oral and written instructions are given to the patient regarding time of the follow-up visit, use of medications, and the use of a metal or plastic shield at night. It is important to explain that a scratching, cinderlike feeling in the operated eye is normal, and that there may be crusting or mucous drainage along the lid and eyelashes. The patient is instructed to cleanse the eyelids each morning with a cotton ball and warm water or Dacriose solution. Also, the patient should be very careful not to exert any pressure on the eye or upper eyelid to prevent accidentally causing complications. The

patient should not sleep on the operated side; however, there may be a very specific position in which the patient will need to remain if gas was injected into the eye. Mild pain should be controlled with acetaminophen, but sudden onset of severe pain should be reported to the physician.

Cataract Surgery (Fig. 11-4)

1. Preoperatively the perioperative nurse assesses the patient for coexisting health problems that may require modification to nursing actions; for example, diabetic patients should be scheduled early in the morning. It is important for the perioperative nurse to assess the patient's mental status and ability to follow simple instructions. Most cataract surgeries are performed with the patient under local block with sedation, and the patient must be able to understand and carry out commands during the procedure. Patients who are not able to follow instructions may need general anesthesia. If the perioperative nurse assesses a hearing impairment the patient is instructed to wear the hearing aid to the OR. Assessing the level of anxiety is also critical.

2. Besides explaining the routine for surgery, the perioperative nurse discusses the specifics for cataract surgery. Preoperatively, eye medications are administered to dilatate the pupil of the operative eye. Vision may become increasingly blurred. Antibiotic eye medication may also be given to prevent infection. The facial and retrobulbar blocks should be described, and the perioperative nurse should emphasize that an anesthesia provider will administer intravenous sedation and/or analgesics to promote comfort. An intermittent pressure device may be applied to the operative eye for 10 minutes after the block is administered; this helps reduce IOP. The intermittent pressure device is not used for patients undergoing cataract surgery who have glaucoma because it may further increase the IOP. The patient should be informed of the draping required: the face will be covered with sterile sheets, but the sheets will be tented off the face to facilitate air circulation. Monitoring equipment, such as blood pressure cuff, O_2 saturation monitor clip, and ECG electrodes, will be placed on the patient and used throughout the procedure. Intraoperatively the patient will be able to hear the sounds of the OR team and the equipment being used. It is critical for the patient to understand that he must not move during the procedure. At the completion of the procedure an eye patch and shield will cover the

FIG. 11-4
CARE PLAN FOR CATARACT SURGERY

KEY ASSESSMENT POINTS

History of previous ocular problems or surgery
Current medications taken/why
Visual acuity (operative and nonoperative eye)
Physical assessment results (coexisting health problems)
Knowledge level (what a cataract is, surgical procedure, postoperative care)
Self-care ability
Emotional response to eye disorder
Resources available for follow-up care
Operative eye (OD, OS, or OU)
Allergies

NURSING DIAGNOSIS

All generic nursing diagnoses apply to this patient, with the addition of:

Anxiety related to local block, surgery
Visual sensory/perceptual alterations related to cataracts

PATIENT OUTCOMES:

All generic outcomes apply, with the addition of:
1. The patient will exhibit a decrease in anxiety by:
   a. Verbalization of less anxiety to perioperative nurse
   b. Pulse, blood pressure, and respirations WNL
   c. Following instructions
   d. Displaying relaxed facial expressions, unclenched hands
   e. Accurately describing perioperative events
2. The patient will exhibit minimal alteration in sensory perception by:
   a. Recognizing familiar sounds and familiar voices
   b. Being oriented to surroundings

NURSING ACTIONS

	Yes	No	N/A
1. Preoperative assessment performed?	☐	☐	☐
2. Perioperative explanations given?	☐	☐	☐
3. Patient verification, ID bracelet checked?	☐	☐	☐
4. Verbal verification of operative site?	☐	☐	☐
5. Consent signed correctly?	☐	☐	☐
6. Effect of preoperative medications/eye drops noted?	☐	☐	☐
7. Positioned correctly?	☐	☐	☐
8. Condition of skin/eye noted at prep site before and after prep?	☐	☐	☐
9. Prep performed per institutional protocol?	☐	☐	☐
10. Medications labeled/ documented?	☐	☐	☐
11. Special equipment/supplies available?	☐	☐	☐
12. Equipment checked/in working condition?	☐	☐	☐
13. Counts performed/correct?	☐	☐	☐
14. Specimens to lab?	☐	☐	☐
15. Implants documented?	☐	☐	☐
16. Postop drops, ointment applied?	☐	☐	☐
17. Dressing/shield applied?	☐	☐	☐
18. Postoperative assessment performed?	☐	☐	☐
19. Other generic care plans initiated? (specify)	☐	☐	☐

Document additional nursing actions generic care plans initiated here:

_____

_____

_____

EVALUATION OF PATIENT OUTCOMES

	Outcome met	Outcome met with additional outcome criteria	Outcome met with revised nursing care plan	Outcome not met	Outcome not applicable to this patient
1. The patient's anxiety was reduced.	☐	☐	☐	☐	☐
2. The patient's alteration in visual sensory/perception was minimal.	☐	☐	☐	☐	☐
3. The patient met outcomes for additional generic care plans as indicated.	☐	☐	☐	☐	☐

Signature: _____ Date: _____

operative eye. Generally the patient will be discharged a few hours after the surgery. Postoperatively the patient will need someone to drive him or her home and to assist with instilling eye drops. The day after surgery the patient will need to be driven to the ophthalmologist's office to be examined.

3. Accurate verification of the operative eye is necessary because the patient may have cataracts in both eyes.
4. Compare the operative consent with the patient's verification of the operative eye. Verification should be both verbal, from the patient, and written, obtained through chart review.
5. Check that the ordered preoperative medication was given and evaluate the patient's response. Also, assess the pupil dilatation of the operative eye.
6. The patient should void immediately before being transported to the OR to promote comfort.
7. Position the patient in the supine position, using devices for proper head and eye alignment and maximal comfort. The head is stabilized in a headrest. Additional padding can be placed on the OR bed and a pillow can be positioned under the legs superior to the popliteal space. Secure the safety strap across the chest or abdomen.
8. The eye is prepared with much care to prevent irritation. Before preparation, topical anesthetic drops are instilled. Preparation may also include instillation of Betadine 5% Ophthalmic Prep solution with subsequent irrigation with Balanced Salt Solution after 2 minutes. Since Betadine is a corneal irritant, its instillation should be preceded with a topical anesthetic, such as tetracaine.
9. Assess and document the condition of the skin and eye both before and after preparation, and again after the surgery.
10. Numerous medications are administered during cataract surgery. All medications must be labeled and documented as to date, time, route, and dosage.
11. Special equipment and supplies depend on the type of cataract extraction and the physician's preference. This may include microscope, phacoemulsification unit and related instruments and supplies, irrigation/aspiration equipment, bipolar unit, and intraocular lens implant. Check the surgical permit and physician preference card. Test all equipment according to the manufacturer's recommendations and institutional protocol. Occasionally the surgeon may wish to convert from a phacoemulsification to an extracapsular cataract extraction (ECCE); have the necessary equipment available in anticipation of this.

Box 11-2 Patient Education Guide After Cataract Removal

1. Assess eye medications, dosage, and schedule for instillation along with patient's ability to correctly administer them. Normally, mydriatics (when intraocular lens not present) and cycloplegics are prescribed. Miotics, corticosteroids, antibiotics, and other medications may be ordered on an individual basis.
2. Explain use of analgesics such as ASA or acetaminophen (Tylenol) for eye discomfort. Also explain that regular daily use of ASA has an anticoagulant effect that could influence postoperative bleeding.
3. Advise patient that when tearing or eye drainage occurs, the eye can be cleansed gently with sterile cotton balls and water (inner canthus outward).
4. Tell patient not to rub or place pressure on eyes.
5. Explain that glasses or shaded lenses should be worn to protect the eye during waking hours after eye dressing is removed. Eye shield should be worn for the prescribed time period.
6. Explain what supplies to purchase and where to buy them for daily eye care at home.
7. Caution against lifting objects over 20 pounds, bending, straining at stool, coughing, or any activities that can increase IOP (for the prescribed period).
8. Explain that showering is usually permissible as long as the eye is shielded and kept dry. Showers are usually advocated because getting in and out of a tub can cause pressure on the eye.
9. Explain that hair can be washed if the head is held backward beauty salon–style under the water with no water getting into the eye.
10. Teach patient to practice safety precautions in daily activities to avoid falling, especially when temporary aphakic lenses are worn.
11. Tell patient to report immediately any decrease in vision, pain, or increased discharge to the ophthalmologist.
12. Explain to patient when sexual activity can be resumed (usually 6 to 8 weeks postoperatively).

From Beare PG & Myers JL. (1994). *Principles and practices of adult health nursing*, (2nd Ed.). St. Louis: Mosby.

12. Ensure that the OR team does not lean on the patient during the procedure.

13. Account for all equipment parts on the sterile field, instruments, ophthalmic sponges, and sharps, including the microsurgery needles. Document all counts according to institutional protocol.

14. According to the type of cataract extraction and hospital policy, the lens may or may not be sent to pathology for gross examination. Document the disposition of the lens, if necessary, according to institutional policy.

15. Follow institutional protocol for documenting intraocular lens implant information.

16. Apply (or help apply) the eye dressing according to the physician's preference (moist and/or dry eye patches, plastic eye shield and tape). Make sure that the eye is completely closed before putting the dressing on to prevent corneal abrasion.

17. Discharge teaching should include instruction to return to see the physician the next day, and that the patch and shield are to be left on until that time. Oral and written instructions are given to the patient regarding time of the follow-up visit, use of medications, and the use of a metal or plastic shield at night. It is important to explain that a scratching, cinderlike feeling in the operated eye is normal, and that there may be crusting or mucous drainage along lid and eyelashes. The patient is instructed to cleanse the eyelids each morning with a cotton ball and warm water or Dacriose solution. Also, the patient should be very careful not to exert any pressure on the eye or upper eyelid to prevent accidentally causing complications. The patient should not sleep on the operated side. Mild pain can be controlled by acetaminophen, but sudden onset of severe pain should be reported to the physician. Box 11-2 summarizes essential patient education that the perioperative nurse should review with patients following cataract surgery.

References

Agency for Health Care Policy and Research. (1993). *Cataract management in adults: Management of functional impairment.* AHCPR Publication No. 93-0542. Rockville, MD: The Agency.

Association of Operating Room Nurses. (1996). *Standards and Recommended Practices for Perioperative Nursing.* Denver: The Association.

Bichat X. (1814). *Desault's surgery.* Philadelphia: Thomas Dobson.

Brenner ZR. (1987). *Diagnostic tests and procedures: Applying the nursing process* (1st Ed.). Norwalk, CT: Appleton & Lange.

Garrison FH. (1929). *An introduction to the history of medicine.* Philadelphia: WB Saunders.

Hykla SC. (1994). Comparative cost analysis of surgical procedures in an ambulatory eye center. *Nursing Economics, 12*(1), 51-55.

Javitt JC, Street DA, & Tielsch JM. (1994). National outcomes of cataract surgery. *Ophthalmology, 101*(1), 100-106.

Kneedler JA & Dodge GH. (1994). *Perioperative nursing care: The nursing perspective* (2nd Ed.). Boston: Jones & Bartlett.

Langseth F. (1993). The use of 5-fluorouracil in glaucoma surgery. *The Journal of the American Society of Ophthalmic Registered Nurses,* 11-13 (vol. 6).

Luckmann J & Sorensen KC. (1987). *Medical-surgical nursing: A psychophysiologic approach* (3rd Ed.). Philadelphia: WB Saunders.

Phipps WJ, et al. (1995). *Medical-surgical nursing: Concepts and clinical practice,* (5th Ed.). St. Louis: Mosby.

Spaeth GL. (1994). What's new in ophthalmology. American College of Surgeons Bulletin, 79(1), 48-50.

Quigley HA. (1993). Open-angle glaucoma. *New England Journal of Medicine, 328*(15), 1097-1106.

Thoman A. (1994). Laser surgery. *Nursing Spectrum, 3*(3), 14-15.

Thorwald J. (1960). *The triumph of surgery.* (1st Ed.). New York: Pantheon.

Vaughan D, Asbury T, & Riordan-Eva P. (1992). *General ophthalmology* (13th Ed.). Norwalk, CT: Appleton & Lange.

Chapter 12

Orthopedic Surgery

Brenda S. Gregory Dawes

Amputation is a last resort, where the ill success that is experienced often effaces the advantages to be obtained; where even these advantages, always gained at an extravagant price, impose upon us the duty of not seeking them, until every other resource has been tried in vain. . . . Such, however, is frequently the progress of accidents, that in a little time amputation is the only obstacle left to oppose them. . . .

The patient was placed almost in a sitting posture upon a bed intended for these kinds of operations, low enough to allow the affected thigh, placed in a horizontal position, to be at a convenient height for the surgeon. An assistant was directed to compress the crural artery, below the fallopian ligament, by means of a cushion. 2d. While other assistants secured the patient, Desault, standing on the right side and grasping firmly with his left hand all the soft parts on the inner side of the thigh above its superior quarter . . . divided these parts with a straight knife, which he entered in front and drew out the point at the inferior part, making it cut down to the bone.

BICHAT, 1814

*T*oday, there are many subspecialties in orthopedic surgery. Patients requiring medical or surgical intervention for an orthopedic or musculoskeletal problem may be referred to a specialist in joint reconstruction, sports medicine, oncologic orthopedics, pediatric orthopedic surgery, hand surgery, spine surgery, foot surgery, orthopedic trauma, or general orthopedics. Many of these subspecialties have their own separate societies that attempt to keep abreast with burgeoning and dramatic advances in the field. Although this was not true of earlier times, the problems of early physicians who treated orthopedic injuries continue to be of interest to the field today.

HISTORICAL ASPECTS

Much of the early history of orthopedic surgery was the treatment of accidents and injuries, many of which eventually required amputation. These surgical procedures, as acknowledged by Bichat, were performed at "an extravagant price" for the patient. Before the development of anesthesia, the "good" surgeon was one who could perform the quickest amputation. Slow, meticulous hemostasis and strict aseptic technique were sacrificed for a quick slash to the bone. Hemorrhage and infection were common complications. The field of orthopedics and successful treatment of injuries to bone became successful with the advent of anesthesia, the development of sutures and other hemostatic techniques, antisepsis, and antibiotics.

Ancient cultures attempted to treat maladies in which today's orthopedist can surgically intervene. Hippocrates discussed the use of traction, counter-traction, bandages, and splints for treatment of long bone fractures. Hippocrates' manipulation involved the surgeon exerting traction on the patient's arm while placing an unshod heel in the axilla to provide countertraction and simultaneously forcing the head of the humerus laterally from beneath the glenoid (Day, et al., 1988). The Irish recognized the benefit of moist heat to treat the "rheumatism" that was so prevalent in their damp climate (Dolan, 1968), including the use of hot compresses, hot water baths, medicated baths, and "sweating houses." The Egyptians developed different types of splints; one was of wood padded with linen (Bullough & Bullough, 1969). The Greeks developed standard types of bandages that were variations of currently used spiral or figure-of-eight bandages; these were used to bind arms or legs or to support limbs. Principles first chronicled in early societies continue to play an important role in the medical treatment of orthopedic problems. Immobilizing a fractured limb is a primary consideration in the emergency and later treatment of fractures. Interestingly, it was Lister's perplexity with differing mortality between cases of simple and compound fractures that led to important theories about the prevention of infection. Applying the theories of Pasteur to open and closed fractures resulted in the conclusion that open fractures communicated with the air, allowing entrance of bacteria. Once prevention of common problems became possible, orthopedic surgery progressed rapidly. By the 1950s, early attempts were being made to replace the hip joint. Today, surgical replacement of joints consumes much of the orthopedic surgery schedule. Orthopedics has become a highly technical environment, including the use of endoscopes, microscopes, specialized power equipment, custom implants, and lasers, resulting in many options for patient care.

ADVANCES IN ORTHOPEDIC SURGERY

Achievements in diagnosis and management of orthopedic injuries have been dramatic in the past decade. Diagnostic studies including computed tomography (CT) and magnetic resonance imaging (MRI) have enabled earlier and more precise diagnosis. Advances in instrumentation, equipment, internal and external fixation devices, and the understanding of physiologic relationships have allowed the restoration of function and relief of pain in diseased bones and joints. Operative arthroscopy has become a valuable procedure for treatment of joints requiring reconstruction with minimal surgi-

cal trauma. Microsurgery has made it possible to attach severed limbs and parts successfully and to transfer vascularized tissue from one body part to another.

Laser application has resulted in trials using carbon dioxide, erbium:YAG, (Er:YAG) and holmium:YAG (Abelow, 1993). Carbon dioxide lasers have been used for removal of polymethylmethacrylate (bone cement) from the medullary canal of the femur during revision hip arthroplasty. The laser vaporizes cement at low temperatures, minimizing bone damage and fracture. The laser is being used to access areas, resulting in less tissue trauma during arthroscopy and microdiscectomy. Safety precautions are a priority during use of the laser. These include understanding the equipment being used, ophthalmic precautions, and fire and plume protection (Michelson, 1990).

Developments in the area of implantable prostheses have improved the restoration of function and have lessened the incidence of complications. Porous ingrowth prostheses are made of titanium alloy with a meshed area to promote bony growth around the implant. These prostheses allow for immediate ambulation with restricted range of motion the day after surgery. The implantation of porous coated prostheses without adjunctive polymethylmethacrylate appears to increase the life and success of the reconstructed joint.

Allograft bone is being used more frequently to restore normal function and mobility. The type most commonly used is the cancellous avascular allograft. The advent of allografts has allowed the reconstruction of limbs affected by bone tumor or trauma. Allograft tissue is also used in sports medicine to replace torn anterior cruciate ligaments (ACLs) in the knee; cadaver ACLs can be placed in the knee joint to replace injured ligaments.

Most diagnoses of orthopedic problems can be made by obtaining a pertinent and complete history and performing a physical examination. Just as this is important for the physician, it is important for the perioperative nurse to review and validate these findings and to link information to the development of nursing diagnoses that will guide perioperative care.

ASSESSMENT CONSIDERATIONS

Assessment by the perioperative nurse is a skill that is usually focused on the area of surgical intervention and must be completed in a very brief time. Knowledge of the anatomy and physiology of the musculoskeletal system is critical for the perioperative nurse's ability to synthesize assessment findings and use them to derive perioperative patient outcomes. The following list presents an overview of a focused history and physical examination for the orthopedic surgery patient:

I. History taking
  A. General
    1. Age
    2. Sex
    3. Occupation
    4. Cultural background
    5. Economic status
  B. Chief complaint (for example, pain, numbness, immobility, deformity)
    1. Location
    2. Quality
    3. Quantity
    4. Onset
    5. Aggravating and relieving factors
    6. Associated manifestations
  C. Specific questions for the orthopedic patient
    1. Ability to carry out activities of daily living?
    2. Change in normal range of motion?
    3. Joint swelling or deformity?
    4. Crepitation or grating sensation?
    5. Change in strength?
    6. Condition of surrounding tissues?
    7. Mechanism of injury (trauma and emergency patients)?
    8. Position of limb during injury (trauma and emergency patients)?
  D. Medical history
  E. Nutritional history
  F. Family history
  G. Social history and life-style
II. Physical examination
  A. General overview
    1. Gait
    2. Posture
    3. Physical activities
    4. General physical appearance
  B. Inspection
    1. Symmetry of parts
    2. Ecchymosis
    3. Lacerations
    4. Obvious deformities
    5. Masses
    6. Skin color
    7. Congenital deformities
  C. Palpation
    1. Crepitus
    2. Temperature
    3. Consistency of muscles
    4. Masses
    5. Tenderness
    6. Deformity
    7. Swelling
  D. Range of motion
  E. Circulation
    1. Pulses
    2. Capillary blanch and refill
    3. Skin color
    4. Skin temperature
  F. Sensory
    1. Touch
    2. Pinprick
    3. Dermatomes
  G. Motor strength

History

A focused history begins with a review of the current problem. Problems requiring surgical intervention are wide and varied; the specific complaints and the patient's condition are important in devising the care plan. Patients may have osteomyelitis for which surgical incision and drainage is planned. There may be a skeletal neoplasm for which intralesional or local resection, or wide local or radical excision, is planned. Fractures may be caused by trauma or pathologic changes such as metastatic carcinoma or lesions of myeloma, requiring implantation of a prosthesis, plates and screws, or intramedullary rodding. When medical treatment fails to relieve pain or a progressive joint deformity produces mechanical disability, surgery may involve synovectomy, arthrodesis, resection arthroplasty, osteotomy, or prosthetic arthroplasty. Thus, the relationship of the patient's current health problem to the perioperative plan of care becomes critical.

Current medications, especially the use of aspirin and steroids, should be determined. A review of other major systems and the medical record should be undertaken to detect heart, lung, kidney, cerebrovascular, or thyroid disease. Gastric or duodenal ulcer should be noted, as should the presence of diabetes. It is helpful to determine if the patient has had previous surgery and to elicit current perceptions and expectations for the planned surgery. The perioperative nurse may be able to correct misperceptions or may need to refer the patient to the physician or discharge unit nurse for additional education about the disease process and realistic expectations regarding the postoperative course and rehabilitation.

Focused Assessment

Reviewing patient information related to specific complaints or conditions provides information for developing the perioperative care plan and outcome criteria. The evaluation and measurement of outcomes is based on assessment information individualized to the patient.

Preoperative education. Assessing the patient's understanding of the surgical procedure and its associated risks or complications is critical for determining educational needs. The patient should be aware of the anticipated length of the hospital stay, operative time, length of incision, and/or need for a second incision. Fixation devices, implants, dressings, and immobilizers such as casts, splints, and orthotics should be explained. The patient's understanding and acceptance of the postoperative activities and projected return to normal activity levels and work should also be discussed.

Risks and complications of the orthopedic surgical procedure should be explained. Blood transfusion or bone grafting are common intraoperative measures requiring explanation. Risks related to the outcome of the surgical procedure, including loss of motor function, paralysis, or those associated with factors that increase operative risk common to each procedure, should be discussed. Assessment of the patient's understanding can be determined by verbalization of the information, compliance measures taken preoperatively, and questions asked during the assessment.

Pain. The evaluation of pain will assist the perioperative nurse with planning a comfortable position for the patient before the induction of anesthesia, as well as with selecting the best positioning accessories for the specific procedure and patient. The evaluation information can be communicated to the nurse caring for the patient postoperatively to assist with pain management. The quality of the pain should be assessed by asking the patient to describe the pain. The pain might be sharp, dull, aching, chronic, or situational (that is, occurs only with a certain activity or position of the body part). By asking the patient to point to the area of pain, the area can be isolated or the areas of pain radiation determined. The patient should be observed for nonverbal indications of pain such as wincing, guarding, massaging, or reluctance to move. Position or external support that assists in alleviating the pain should be determined.

Immobility. It is noted whether the patient has a cast, splint, traction, or brace. The patient's limitations of mobility should be determined, including range of motion, flexion, extension, abduction, adduction, and rotation limitations. These will need to be considered when planning transfer to and from the OR bed, as well as when positioning on the OR bed for surgery. Muscle strength and weakness and movement in the affected body part are determined.

Functional integrity. In addition to mobility limitations, it is important to determine whether there are any functional limitations. Careful neurovascular assessment should determine alterations in sensation including diminished sensory or motor function. The extremity or affected part is observed for color (including paleness, redness) and temperature (coolness or warmth to the touch). Evidence of skin breakdown, ecchymosis, hematoma, or edema should be noted. Pulses should be palpated in an extremity and compared with the presence and quality of pulses in the opposite extremity.

DIAGNOSTIC STUDIES

Useful information about the orthopedic patient may be gained from a variety of diagnostic procedures. Each study is not indicated for all patients. The case study in Box 12-1 demonstrates how the clinical problem guides diagnostic evaluation. In general, however, specific studies may reveal important data about the patient's condition.

CASE STUDY

J.C., a 74-year-old woman, complained of lower back pain radiating to both legs. The pain started 5 days earlier and had been increasing. She also complained of midthoracic pain. Both kinds of pain increased when standing, walking, or lying down. Other problems included fatigue and difficulty climbing stairs.

J.C. had a mastectomy 23 years ago for breast cancer. She also has been diagnosed with non-insulin–dependent diabetes, controlled with oral hypoglycemics.

Routine labwork was completed.

An elderly person with lower back pain may not be easily diagnosed because of the multiplicity of problems that may be encountered. A complete history and physical examination is imperative to diagnose and treat such a patient. Diagnoses to rule out include:

Musculoskeletal disorder or strain
Degenerative disease
Traumatic injury
Osteoporotic collapse
Cancer
Skeletal disorder
Disk herniation

Studies	Results
CBC	Normal
Electrolytes	Normal
Blood chemistry	Normal
Spinal x-ray	Symmetric collapse of vertebral body T4
	Vertebral end plates and disc space normal
	Osteoporosis

Although the first indication of osteoporosis may be x-ray detection of vertebral compression of the spine, bone mineral density can also be measured by dual-energy x-ray absorptiometry (DEXA) and quantitative computed tomography (QCT). Special urine tests include calcium excretion in a 24-hour specimen and a fasting calcium:creatinine ratio (Weigand, 1995).

The patient's history and laboratory values indicate osteoporotic vertebral collapse or spinal metastasis with vertebral collapse. Surgical treatment is not the choice for this patient. Treatment for osteoporosis is started. Bed rest until the pain decreases with a gradual attempt to walk and medication for pain is ordered. If the pain is not eliminated, other studies might include MRI, bone scintigram, or needle biopsy.

Other treatment options for osteoporosis include estrogen or hormone replacement therapy for postmenopausal women, calcitonin, and oral calcium, fluoride, or vitamin D.

Because of the many causes of back pain in the elderly, surgical treatment may or may not be appropriate. In addition to specialized nursing care for the patient undergoing a surgical procedure for a related back problem, psychosocial assessment and interventions are a priority because of the medical assessment regimen these patients may have experienced during diagnostic evaluation. (Brown & Seltzer, 1991).

Noninvasive Diagnostic Studies

X-ray films. X-ray films of bones and joints are the most common noninvasive diagnostic tools available to the orthopedic practitioner. They are used to identify fracture and pathologic conditions such as rheumatoid arthritis, spondylitis, avascular necrosis, and tumor. Joint changes, including joint margin erosion, joint space narrowing, bone spurs, loose bodies, and dislocations may also be detected. Soft tissue injury does not show on x-ray films, but soft tissue swelling can be seen. Evidence of decreased bone mineral content can be visualized when approximately 30% loss has occurred (Evarts, 1992).

Magnetic resonance imaging. The use MRI has increased rapidly. Its advantages are high tissue contrast between normal and abnormal musculoskeletal structures, multiplanar capability, and absence of known complications. MRI uses a magnetic field and radiowaves to depict hydrogen proton density of body tissue. The most common source of these protons is water. It does not require the use of ionizing radiation; contrast medium may be used. MRI can be used to detect tumors, joint disease, avascular necrosis, infection, trauma, or spinal disorders. Cortical bone, in contrast, is not visible with MRI because it contains little or no water. Images may be

produced in three planes: transverse axial (top to bottom), coronal (back to front), and sagittal (left to right) (Watt, 1991).

Computed tomography. CT provides cross-sectional views of the body by passing a narrow x-ray beam from a computerized scanner through the body at different angles. An injected radioiodine contrast agent may or may not be used to highlight blood vessels. A series of x-ray photographs, translated by a computer and displayed on an oscilloscope, produce the CT scan. Images may be in the anterior-posterior, lateral, oblique, coronal, transverse, or sagittal plane. CT is used effectively for assessment of traumatic orthopedic injury. Considerations for use of CT include presence of metal implants, which make imaging difficult, and the patient's medical stability, since bleeding into the equipment causes damage (Evarts, 1992).

Invasive Diagnostic Studies

X-ray using contrast medium

ARTHROGRAM. An arthrogram is an x-ray and fluoroscopic examination of the joint. Following the injection of air, a radiopaque contrast medium is injected into the joint space. The imaging helps to detect injuries of the meniscus, cartilage, and ligaments of the knee and structures of the joint capsule, rotator cuff, and subacromial bursa of the shoulder. CT, MRI, and arthroscopy are replacing arthrography as a diagnostic procedure.

MYELOGRAM. Myelography is the x-ray and fluoroscopic examination of the spinal cord and subarachnoid space following injection of a contrast medium. It is useful in identifying lesions in the intradural and extradural compartments of the spinal canal and in the diagnosis of abnormalities such as herniated disc or tumor. It has been replaced largely by computed tomography (CT) or magnetic resonance imaging (MRI), but continues to be useful for detection of disc lesions.

Radionuclide imaging. Radionuclide imaging (bone scan) permits imaging of the skeleton by use of a scanning camera after the intravenous injection of a radioactive tracer compound, usually technetium (Tc-99m) methylene diphosphate. This compound concentrates at sites of abnormal bone metabolism such as osteoblastic activity. In malignancies, osteoblastic activity occurs at an accelerated rate and appears as "hot spots," which will show in a bone scan 3 to 6 months before x-ray films can reveal any lesion. The procedure also helps to monitor signs of progression in patients with degenerative disease, trauma, and infection or prosthetic loosening. The bone scan is used in conjunction with plain film radiographs.

Arthrocentesis. Joint aspiration is performed to obtain samples of synovial fluid from within the

Table 12-1 Diagnostic studies used in the assessment of the musculoskeletal system

Laboratory study	Orthopedic relevance	Normal values
Alkaline phosphatase (ALP)	Elevated in healing fractures, rheumatoid arthritis	30-85 ImU/ml
Acid phosphatase	Elevated in multiple myeloma, carcinoma of the bone (primary and metastatic to bone)	0.10-0.63 U/ml (Bessey-Lowry) 0.5-2.0 U/ml (Bodansky) 1.0-4.0 U/ml (King-Armstrong) 0.0-0.8 U/6 at 37° C (SI units)
Serum calcium	Elevated (hypercalcemia) in metastatic tumor to the bone	9.0-10.5 mg/dl (total)
Creatinine phosphokinase (CPK)	Elevated in insults to skeletal muscle	5-75 mU/ml
Lactic dehydrogenase (LDH)	Elevated with muscle tissue damage, malignancies	90-200 ImU/ml
Phosphorous (serum)	Elevated in osteoporosis, bone fracture healing Lowered with hypercalcemia, osteomalacia	1.8-2.6 mEq/L or 3-4.5 mg/dl
Serum asparate aminotransferase (AST—formerly SGOT)	Elevated in primary muscle disease, crush injuries	5-40 IU/L
Uric acid (serum)	Elevated (hyperuricemia) in gout, arthritis, soft tissue deposits of uric acid (tophi)	Males: 2.1-8.5 mg/dl Females: 2.0-6.6 mg/dl
C-Reactive protein (CRP) (Rheumatoid factor test)	Elevated in rheumatoid arthritis, malignancies	<60 U/ml
Antinuclear antibody test (ANA)	Elevation (positive titer) in systemic lupus erythematosus (SLE), rheumatoid arthritis	No antinuclear bodies detected at 1:32 titer.
LE cell prep	Elevation in SLE	No LE cells present
Rheumatoid factor test	Elevation (positive titer) in rheumatoid arthritis	No rheumatoid factor present

joint cavity. It aids in determining the presence of aseptic inflammatory processes such as rheumatoid arthritis or septic processes such as bacterial arthritis. The synovial fluid withdrawn is cultured and examined microscopically and chemically. Arthrocentesis with synovial fluid analysis may be performed on any joint to identify the cause of joint effusion.

Biopsy. Biopsy is the removal of tissue for purposes of microscopic examination to confirm a diagnosis, to follow the course of a disease, or to determine the effectiveness of treatment. Muscle biopsy is performed to aid in the diagnosis of myopathic disorders. Synovial biopsy is helpful in differentiating various forms of arthritis. Bone biopsy may diagnose a bone disease or lesion.

Arthroscopy. Arthroscopy is the examination of a joint through a special fiberoptic endoscope called the arthroscope. This procedure is performed in surgery and is being used for joints such as the knee, shoulder, wrist, ankle, and temporomandibular joint.

Electromyography. Electromyography measures electrical activity across muscle membranes by means of needle electrodes. Information regarding the condition of nerve impulses to muscles and the response of muscles to the nerve impulses is obtained. The electrical activity is audible, viewed on an oscilloscope, or printed on a graph. It is helpful in diagnosing lower motor neuron disease, primary muscle disease, and diseases involving defects in the transmission of electrical impulses across neuromuscular junctions.

Routine laboratory studies. Routine blood work, such as complete blood counts, serum electrolyte levels, and clotting studies, are often required for orthopedic patients. Specific laboratory studies will be ordered that are relevant to the patient's overall medical condition and specific diagnosis. Table 12-1 summarizes some of these studies. Indications for elevations (or decreases) have been included only for common orthopedic diagnoses; laboratory studies are altered by many other potential conditions and factors.

NURSING DIAGNOSES
Nursing diagnoses are developed and correlated with patient information and indications for the surgical procedure. Patient assessment includes a physical examination to determine functional ability, presence of pain, deformity, and altered sensory and

motor function resulting from disease process or trauma. The medical history and results of the pre-operative diagnostic tests are reviewed; using the information gathered, patient-specific nursing diagnoses can be developed. Patients undergoing orthopedic procedures may be any age, requiring adaptation of the plan of care to meet age-specific needs. Patient conditions such as traumatic injury or congenital deformity may also require modification of the care plan.

The assessment before any surgical procedure includes affirming NPO status, identifying allergies, ensuring the patient's understanding of the surgical procedure, and confirming the operative consent. Preoperative orders such as antibiotic therapy or skin preparation with an antibiotic scrub should also be confirmed by the patient. Teaching should include exercise/activity regimens and special devices or equipment the patient may expect to use postoperatively.

Common Nursing Diagnoses

Relevant data are collected, then nursing diagnoses are developed and prioritized. Many nursing diagnoses developed for the orthopedic patient are "high risk," indicating that the plan of care is implemented to prevent complications. The generic care plans described in Chapter 7 can be applied to patients undergoing orthopedic procedures. The following nursing diagnoses are not meant to be all inclusive. Each nursing diagnosis must be confirmed or ruled out based on the patient data.

Sensory/perceptual alteration. Pulses, skin color, skin temperature, motor function, and sensory deficits vary among patients and may be a result of injury or may be considered a "normal" response considering the patient's current medical condition. Assessment should occur before induction of anesthesia, and each parameter should be compared with the opposite side or extremity. An anatomic understanding of the neurologic and vascular systems assists with prevention of sensory/perceptual alteration. During the intraoperative period, the neurovascular status can be protected by applying the principles of positioning and by using padding and accessory positioning devices to prevent stretching or compression of nerves. Monitoring may be necessary during the surgical procedure to assess the sensory/perceptual status. Doppler ultrasound may be used to determine vascular status; sensory-evoked potential monitoring may be used to assess spinal integrity.

The desired patient outcome is that the patient will be free from sensory/perceptual alteration(s).

High risk for infection. The potential sequelae of infection following orthopedic procedures can be detrimental to the outcome of the surgical procedure. Factors should be assessed, including determination of high-risk patients, proper use of barriers, and use of routine antibiotics when implants are being used. The patient's medical condition—including presence of diabetes, concurrent infectious processes such as urinary tract infection or dental caries, skin conditions, or other disease processes—may increase the risk of infection. For this reason, surgical procedures that are elective may be delayed until conditions can be controlled or resolved. Other strategies implemented during orthopedic procedures include repetitive skin preparation several days preoperatively, altered airflow systems (laminar airflow or body-exhaust systems), and/or antibiotic therapy delivered intravenously, used as irrigation, or incorporated into bone cement. Implementation of aseptic practices, sterilization practices, and minimizing traffic are a few cost-effective mechanisms for preventing infection (Drez, et al., 1991).

SKIN PREPARATION. Skin preparation is intended to prevent introduction of exogenous microbes into the incision site. Bacteria cannot be totally removed, but can be reduced on the skin surface. Prophylactic skin cleansing may be ordered before surgery and can be completed if the patient is admitted to the hospital preoperatively. Patients arriving for an ambulatory surgical procedure should verify the activity was completed. Patients undergoing a procedure for traumatic injury may require cleansing to eliminate gross debris from the operative site. Hair may or may not be removed before surgery, depending on the amount and area of surgery. If required, shaving is done as close as possible to the time of the procedure. Preferred methods of hair removal include clippers or the use of a depilatory, since there is less disruption of skin integrity (AORN, 1996). Skin cleansing is repeated in the operating room immediately before the procedure using a broad-spectrum antimicrobial agent and aseptic technique.

AIRFLOW. Systems have been promoted as a mechanism of preventing infections when caring for the orthopedic patient. Research using laminar airflow or body-exhaust systems is inconclusive for affirming that the outcome is better than eliminating traffic in the operating room and implementing aseptic practices (McQuarrie, et al., 1990). Body-exhaust systems have the added advantage of protecting the surgical team from fluid contamination (Hester & Nelson, 1991). Body-exhaust systems incorporate a clear plastic face shield with a hood that covers the entire face, head, and shoulders. The face mask is attached to a vacuum system apparatus that exhausts air in the system and replaces air. Isolation drapes may also be used to separate the patient from personnel and equipment.

ANTIBIOTIC THERAPY. Prophylactic antibiotics are recommended when wound exposure will be greater than 2 hours or implants are used (Chapman, 1993). Antibiotics may also be given if the patient has recently undergone surgery, experienced a previous surgical infection, or was exposed to contamination. They may be ordered to be administered 1 hour before the surgical procedure and repeated immediately before the procedure begins. Antibiotics may also be added to the irrigating solutions. Pulsatile irrigation uses force to loosen tissue or bone debris and small pieces of cement. Intravenous antibiotic therapy, given during procedures on an extremity requiring the use of a tourniquet, is delivered before inflation of the tourniquet. Antibiotics may be added to the methyl methacrylate or methyl methacrylate beads impregnated with antibiotic placed in the incision site. Studies have also attributed infection rates to specific surgical procedures (Taylor, 1990), resulting in the need to evaluate activities causing this difference.

DRAPING PROCEDURES. Drapes applied for orthopedic procedures often need to allow for movement of the extremity. They need to be durable, waterproof, and conform easily to the equipment incorporated in the sterile field. Use of fluids for irrigating and use of heavy equipment may compromise the integrity of the drapes. Draping protocols should be followed to accommodate the numerous cords used during endoscopic procedures. Cords and tubes such as those connected to power equipment and polymethyl methacrylate exhaust systems must also be secured during use.

INSTRUMENTATION. Orthopedic procedures require the use of multiple instrument sets and specialty items for implantables. Implant systems may be sterile when provided from the manufacturer for one-time use, purchased for use in the setting, or supplied on consignment for use per procedure. The instrumentation is prepared for use and sterilized following the manufacturer guidelines for the use of the sterilizer and implants (AORN, 1996). Routine monitoring of sterilizers is required. It must be assured that implants are sterile when used. Some instruments may be chemically disinfected for orthopedic procedures.

The desired patient outcome is that the patient will be free from infection.

Impaired tissue integrity. Orthopedic procedures are usually not lengthy, but can result in impaired skin or tissue integrity. Causes of problems can be related to compromised patient condition, the dependent position necessary for the surgical procedure, or forces applied during the procedure causing shearing injury.

The patient's skin integrity must be assessed before the procedure, and bruises, cuts, lacerations, reddened areas, ulcerations, and rashes should be reported and considered when positioning. Traumatic injury may have resulted in exposed bone or a wound contaminated with debris.

Skin and tissue integrity can be maintained by using positioning devices designed to protect the patient. These might include egg-crate foam, gel pads, or a beanbag. Shearing is prevented by ensuring that the patient is secure when force is used that can cause the patient to move during the procedure. In addition, the patient should be protected from solutions that might pool by isolating the boundary of the skin preparation area, electrodispersive pad, or tourniquet with impermeable drapes.

The desired patient outcome is that skin integrity will be maintained.

Impaired physical mobility. The musculoskeletal system is responsible for movement and coordination of the body. Disease or trauma may have caused debilitation of physical mobility. A goal of orthopedic surgery is to restore physical mobility that has been limited by a disease process, injury, or deformity. Perioperative nursing actions should be implemented to ensure that physical mobility is not compromised. Assessing range of motion and limitation will help to determine actions that can be implemented to protect the patient. The plan of care should also include activities to assist the patient with transfer to the OR bed. A smooth transfer requires an adequate number of personnel and adequate time to accommodate the patient's needs.

Patient transfer is as important during the postoperative period, since the patient is usually anesthetized and cannot assist with the transfer. Personnel must support the immobilized body part, as appropriate, and position the patient for transfer to the postanesthesia care unit.

Activities are encouraged postoperatively to restore physical mobility and functional range of motion. The type of surgical procedure will dictate the type of exercise program. Continuous passive motion (CPM) and pain medication using epidural or patient-controlled analgesia (PCA) pumps are used to promote mobility. CPM is commonly used for patients undergoing procedures on the extremity, providing gentle motion at a consistent speed to decrease the effects of immobilization. CPM has proven the ability to inhibit formation of adhesions and stimulate healing of articular cartilage, resulting in decreased postoperative pain, decreased joint stiffness and swelling, and decreased length of hospitalization (Johnson, 1990; Smith 1990). PCA is used to administer a predetermined intravenous dose of narcotic substance to relieve pain (Jones & Brooks, 1990). It has also been reported that patients benefit when using a PCA pump when preoperative teaching has been included in the plan (Timmons & Bower, 1993).

The desired patient outcome is that mobility will be maintained or improved.

Altered peripheral tissue perfusion. The patient's health status, the surgical procedure being performed, or equipment and devices used during the procedure may be criteria used to determine a diagnosis of altered peripheral tissue perfusion. Patient age and activity level are considerations when determining preventive measures for venous stasis. These may include medication therapy, antiembolism stockings, pneumatic stockings, or elastic wrap. Pressure points should be determined preoperatively and padded or protected throughout the procedure. This includes pressure points caused by the body position during the procedure (iliac crest, toes), positioning devices used (breast, genitals), and the patient's body type (bony prominence). Pulse checks preoperatively will help determine the patient's circulatory status. Following positioning, application of a cast or other possible means of occluding the circulation requires that the pulse be checked.

Occluding devices include the tourniquet; this is used to interfere with tissue perfusion, providing a bloodless field. Tourniquets should be applied correctly to prevent tissue damage and inappropriate alteration of perfusion. The tourniquet application, length of time it will remain in place, and the equipment used are important for ensuring patient safety (AORN, 1996).

The desired patient outcome is that tissue perfusion will be maintained.

High risk for injury. Injury may result when caring for the orthopedic patient when activities are not implemented correctly or potential hazards are not recognized. This includes incorrect use of equipment and positioning devices, less than adequate personnel to assist with transfer, or a lack of knowledge related to the surgical procedure. Preventive measures, such as using leaded devices during procedures requiring radiography and thorough rinsing of disinfected instruments, may also eliminate injury. Basic principles of operating room practice guide implementation of activities when caring for the orthopedic patient.

PATIENT TEMPERATURE. Orthopedic procedures may require exposure of body surfaces that may result in rapid loss of body heat. This becomes a critical consideration for the pediatric or geriatric patient. Preventive measures should begin in the preoperative area by using warm blankets. Intraoperative measures include minimizing exposure of the patient before draping and using heating devices. Controlling patient temperature will minimize postoperative complications.

SPECIALTY EQUIPMENT. Use of the electrosurgical unit must be determined; pad placement must be considered for the patient's body type and surgical procedure; and solutions used during the procedure must be compatible with the use of electrosurgery. Saline solution is used during arthroscopic procedures when electrosurgery is not used; water conducts the current and promotes visualization and irrigation when electrosurgery is used.

Laser procedures require implementation of laser-specific safety measures for the patient and personnel. Adequate personnel trained on the operation of laser equipment are assigned to the procedure to ensure that these measures are implemented.

Each type of equipment requires validation of a competent skill level to ensure that the patient is not injured as a result of incorrect use.

Other equipment and special supplies used in orthopedics require that time be planned before moving the patient to the room for checking function. Cameras, endoscopes, microscopes, and power equipment should be connected and checked. Instrument sets should be checked for all parts needed during the procedure. Positioning equipment is needed to maintain supine, lateral, prone, or modifications of these positions. Each type of equipment requires validation of a competent skill level by all personnel to ensure that the patient is not injured as a result of incorrect use.

RADIOGRAPHY. Several procedures requiring confirmation of bone placement or correction caused by trauma require a single x-ray or use of fluoroscopy. This does increase the length of the procedure and possibly the exposure time of an open incision; therefore it must be planned appropriately. The patient is protected during these procedures by use of leaded shields, and sterility is maintained by incorporating draping procedures. Personnel should also be monitored for exposure (AORN, 1996).

STERILIZATION AND DISINFECTION. Instruments can be prepared for procedures using steam, ethylene oxide, or other chemicals. Steam sterilization heats the item during the process; it must be cooled before use to prevent tissue and bone damage. Bone growth may be impeded by exposure to high temperatures. Chemical and ethylene oxide sterilization requires thorough elimination of the chemicals from the surface of the item before use. Practices should be implemented to ensure that the sterilant or disinfectant is in contact with all surfaces of the item and removed before use, and that personnel and the patient are protected.

MEDICATION THERAPY. The common medications used during procedures include antibiotics and local anesthetics. Hemostatics and corticosteroids may also be used. Medications must be labeled, and administration of the medication, route, and dosage must be documented. The route of administration may include topical, intravenous, or irrigation.

The desired patient outcome is that the patient will be free from injury.

High risk for fluid volume deficit. Many orthopedic procedures are completed with minimal fluid and electrolyte changes, resulting in an uneventful intraoperative course. Patients undergoing procedures for primary or revision of total hip replacement, total knee replacement, or spinal fusion may be considered for fluid and electrolyte replacement because of anticipated blood loss. Thorough assessment is important to determine underlying causes of the imbalance. Blood replacement is considered because low hemoglobin and hematocrit levels result in reduced capacity for carrying oxygen to the tissues. A lower Po_2 may precipitate tachycardia, orthostatic hypotension, and decreased exercise tolerance. This affects not only the immediate surgical outcome but the postoperative recovery.

Blood loss is anticipated before the surgical procedure, and blood should be available. If this has not been planned, the blood should be type- and cross-matched. Presurgical autologous blood donation, intraoperative blood salvage, and postoperative autotransfusion/blood collection systems are used to minimize the need for homologous blood donation (Keeling, et al., 1993). Studies have not supported the use of autotransfusion systems when comparing benefit and cost (Arlington, et al., 1992; Mac, et al., 1993).

The desired patient outcome is that fluid and electrolyte balance will be maintained.

Body image disturbance. The type of surgical procedure will influence the patient's concerns about body image. Procedures for correction of deformity may result in this nursing diagnosis because of anticipation of the resulting improved body image. Preoperatively, patients may not recognize the resulting body image change caused by trauma. The ability to cope and understand will influence the postoperative response. Concerns might also be related to the use of assistive devices required during short- and long-term recovery, alterations caused by dressings, immobilizers, and the use of a walker, cane, or other devices. Peer influence often causes adolescents to respond dramatically to anything they perceive as affecting body image.

The desired patient outcome is that the patient will cope with a disturbance in body image.

Pain. Pain is an expected postoperative phenomenon, yet it may be a serious cause of anxiety and worry to the patient. Pain is perceived differently by individuals. Many orthopedic patients live with chronic pain and discomfort, sometimes to the point of debilitation, before the surgical procedure. Disease processes such as osteoporosis and osteomalacia are pain producing. Pain may also be a diagnosis of injury. Pain is assessed in the perioperative environment to determine methods of providing comfort until induction, safety measures used for transfer, and pain levels for postoperative comparison. Pain should be assessed using a pain scale or behavioral measures (Pynsent, et al., 1993); it should be controlled during the preoperative phase by positioning and the use of pain management techniques, including imagery, touch, or medication. A complete assessment can help determine measures to prevent postoperative pain. Careful, deliberate transfer should be planned to minimize pain (Woodin, 1993). Pain management is planned considering expected postoperative pain. This may include use of an epidural, patient-controlled analgesia (PCA) pump (Timmons & Bower, 1993; Johnson, 1990), injection of steroids, or local anesthesia (Woodin, 1993).

The desired patient outcome is that the patient's pain and discomfort will be controlled or minimized.

PLANNING FOR PATIENT CARE

The selection of nursing diagnoses that reflect specific patient conditions and needs allows for a valid and effective plan of care. In orthopedic surgery, planning must also take into consideration the placement of equipment. Video carts, pulsatile lavage pumps, drainage systems, power sources, light sources, electrosurgical units, motorized shavers, holders for positioning the extremity during preparation, the proper OR bed, suspension devices, positioning accessories, and other equipment must not compromise safety or maintenance of the sterile field. Some common concerns in planning for safe patient care are discussed in this section.

Positioning

The variety of operative patient positions in orthopedic surgery, and the inherent risks of each, challenge the planning skills of the perioperative nurse. Discussed here are some of the more common patient positions used in orthopedic surgery and some of the risks involved in each. Basic guidelines appropriate for moving all anesthetized patients include:

1. Provide enough help to move the patient safely, deliberately, and slowly. Maintain alignment and support.
2. Pad all bony prominences and areas sensitive to pressure. Elbows, knees, toes, and axillary regions are some areas susceptible to pressure.
3. Manipulate joints gently, rotating extremities through a "normal" range of motion.

4. Respect the patient's dignity by avoiding unnecessary exposure of the body.
5. Plan the type of positioning accessories needed before induction of anesthesia.
6. Protect intravenous lines, catheters, and airways.
7. Use proper body mechanics to protect personnel.
8. Complete a thorough neurovascular assessment preoperatively, following positioning and, as necessary, to protect the patient.

Supine position. The supine position, also known as the dorsal recumbent position, is used in orthopedic procedures when it provides adequate exposure of an anterior surgical site. Common procedures performed in this position include most knee surgeries, hand surgery using the hand table, and lower leg and foot surgery. The head is in alignment with the body, supported by a headrest. The arms rest on padded armboards with restraints. Each arm is at less than a 90-degree angle to the body, thereby preventing brachial plexus injury. The safety strap is placed snugly 2 inches above the knee. Legs and feet lie on the table uncrossed to prevent peroneal nerve damage.

Prone position. The prone position is modified for procedures involving the spine, requiring the use of a padded laminectomy brace or specially designed bed. This brace lifts the patient's trunk off the OR bed and allows for maximal chest expansion and adequate respiration. An axillary roll is placed to protect the brachial plexus, and the arms are on padded armboards and restrained alongside the patient's head. Elbows are comfortably bent to prevent ulnar nerve injury. The knees and lower legs rest on pillows, keeping the toes and heels free. The safety strap is placed above the knees if appropriate. It is important to remember that anesthesia is usually induced before laminectomy positioning, followed by logroll transfer to the OR bed; in prone position this will require at least six people.

Sitting position. The sitting (Fowler's) position and the lawn chair (semi-Fowler's) position are commonly used for anterior shoulder surgery. The head is on a padded headrest and turned toward the unaffected side. The unaffected arm may either be taped to the abdomen or placed on a padded armboard with the arm restrained at the patient's side. The affected arm and operative shoulder will be draped to expose the surgical site. A 5-pound sandbag may be placed under the operative shoulder or padding placed midline to further expose the surgical site. The OR bed breaks will be at the area of the hips and knees. A pillow should be placed under the knees to prevent stress; a padded footboard should also be used. The safety strap is placed 2 inches above the knees.

Lateral position. The lateral (side-lying) position is used primarily for hip and posterior shoulder proce-

dures. The patient is turned on the side after the induction of anesthesia. The arms are extended on a padded double armboard at less than 90 degrees to the patient's body. An axillary roll is placed dependently to protect the brachial plexus. The dependent arm is rotated to prevent contact of the ulnar nerve with the OR bed. The padded posterior hip positioner is placed at the level of the patient's flank, and the padded anterior hip positioner is placed at the patient's abdomen without causing excessive pressure on the abdomen. The nonoperative leg is flexed in the dependent position, and a pillow is placed between the dependent and operative legs. The safety strap is placed above the knee(s).

Positioning on the fracture table. The orthopedic (fracture) table, used for hip nailings and lower extremity intramedullary roddings, requires a thorough understanding of the anatomic approach and of the accessories needed for positioning. Fracture tables vary widely from manufacturer to manufacturer; it is necessary to be well informed of the operating mechanisms of the table used. The patient may be positioned supine or lateral; in either position, extremity positioning must be carefully planned. With the addition of traction, additional pressure sites at each end of the bone in traction are added. The center perineal post must be well padded, along with the sacral rest. The foot and ankle of the affected leg must be wrapped with protective padding before positioning in the traction boot. The unaffected leg rests on a cushioned leg support, keeping the heel and popliteal space free of excessive pressure.

The numerous potential injuries relating to surgical positioning require that the perioperative orthopedic nurse know the proper use of positioning devices, techniques, and potential complications to ensure optimal patient safety in the OR. Assessment of the patient's skin integrity and neurovascular status preoperatively, intraoperatively, and postoperatively must be documented in the OR record.

Planning for Safe Equipment Use

The Joint Commission on Accreditation of Hospitals, in its *Standards for Management of the Environment of Care*, includes managing equipment and the requirement of a documented plan composed of policies and procedures that support both safe and reliable performance of equipment (Keil, 1995). The plan must be written in language that is understandable, explaining the skills required to operate and service equipment and a mechanism to evaluate the knowledge and skills of the staff using the equipment. Perioperative nurses, physicians, and clinical engineers are expected to have a plan for dealing with failure or loss of function of critical pieces of medical equipment. Performance standards require perioperative staff to be competent in the safe, appropriate, and effective use of equipment. This is a critical area for perioperative nurses in orthopedics as they continue to plan patient care that is underpinned by ensuring high quality.

Pneumatic tourniquet. For most orthopedic surgery procedures involving an extremity, a pneumatic tourniquet will be used to produce a bloodless field. Thus the perioperative nurse must be familiar with the operation and potential risks of the pneumatic tourniquet (AORN, 1996). A tourniquet is used with mechanical or computerized pressure regulation. Persons responsible for application and use of the tourniquet should also be familiar with operating instructions. A cuff size is chosen for the extremity that will allow 3 to 6 inches of overlap. Before putting on the cuff, a smooth layer of cotton Webril padding is applied to the limb on which the cuff will be placed. The skin, cotton padding, and tourniquet cuff should be free of wrinkles. A thorough skin assessment should be performed and documented before tourniquet cuff application. The circulating nurse is responsible for monitoring the tourniquet and documenting the inflation and deflation times. Determination of the amount of pressure at which the tourniquet should be set generally follows these basic guidelines: for the upper extremity add 70 mm Hg to the patient's systolic blood pressure; for the lower extremity multiply the systolic blood pressure by 2. Tourniquet inflation time varies from patient to patient and depends on the extremity and pathologic condition being treated. Generally, tourniquet inflation greater than 2 hours results in postoperative problems, including partial anesthesia, tingling, and hypersensitivity. If it is anticipated that the tourniquet will be used for long periods, it should be deflated for 20 to 30 minutes each hour, after which it may be reinflated (Chapman, 1993). If improperly used, the tourniquet can cause serious nerve and vascular damage, such as mechanical injury, anoxia, ischemic paralysis, posttourniquet syndrome, compartment syndrome, pressure sores, and chemical burns. Postoperatively the perioperative nurse must perform a neurovascular assessment of the extremity and be alert for complications.

Power instruments. In orthopedic surgery, many power-driven instruments such as drills, saws, burrs, and reamers are indicated by the specific procedure. These are powered by compressed nitrogen or a battery. The perioperative nurse must be familiar with the tank, regulator, and power hoses when circulating on a procedure requiring compressed nitrogen as a power source. Guidelines for cleaning, testing, and sterilizing powered instruments must be followed.

Bone cement. Bone cement (polymethyl methacrylate) is often used to hold a metal or synthetic prosthesis in place, such as in total joint replacement. Polymethyl methacrylate is formed by two components, one a liquid and the other a powder. The cement must be mixed properly and continuously for at least 2 to 4 minutes before use. Bone cement may be mixed with antibiotic solution. Manufacturer's recommendations must be followed. Mixing time varies with the humidity and temperature of the room. Most mixing units are equipped with suction that is used to exhaust the toxic polymethyl methacrylate fumes. Changes in blood pressure may occur because of the fusion and subsequent heat generated by the bone cement components. The perioperative nurse should collaborate with anesthesia personnel to monitor vital signs during this time. Polymethyl methacrylate beads impregnated with antibiotic might be placed in a wound to promote healing. The removal time and method will depend on the number of beads implanted.

Immobilizers and orthotics. Temporary immobilization of an extremity may be necessary following open or closed reduction, with or without implants, and with some procedures involving a joint. A cast or splint may be formed and applied using plaster, fiberglass, or thermoplast. Other immobilizers are fit using approximate patient measurements. It is important to measure correctly and pad sufficiently before application of an immobilizer to protect the extremity postoperatively.

A cast or splint of plaster, fiberglass, or thermoplast is applied immediately postoperatively and allowed to dry. Cool water should be used when preparing plaster or fiberglass to prevent an exothermic chemical reaction. Neurovascular status of the extremity should be compared with the status before application of the cast. After the cast or splint is applied, a pillow is placed beneath the extremity to prevent indentations or misshaping of the cast. A plaster cast takes approximately 24 to 48 hours to dry completely. Fingers or toes of the casted limb should be cleaned to allow accurate neurovascular assessments. Removal of a cast from a patient who arrives in the OR suite must take place away from the OR suite so that fine particles of plaster are not released into the air filtering systems of the room. Orthotics required postoperatively will be fitted to meet patient specifications.

Traction. Occasionally a patient may either arrive in the OR with some type of traction already in place or require the application of a traction device for the procedure or postoperatively. An understanding of the classifications, categories, and basic principles of traction maintenance is important.

Traction is the application of a pulling force to a part of the body, and it is an important form of orthopedic immobilization. Traction may be either manual or mechanical. Manual traction is accomplished by an individual exerting a pulling force on an extremity or joint using the hands. Manual traction must be applied firmly, smoothly, and under specific orders and conditions. Mechanical traction uses mechanical devices and is further classified according to the way it attaches and to the nature of the pull. It may be applied to the skin or directly through some part of the skeleton. Skin traction involves the direct application of a pulling force to the patient's skin and soft tissue, thus immobilizing a body part. It may be a continuous or intermittent pull. It may be applied by nursing personnel acting under specific physician orders concerning the amount of weight. Skeletal traction exerts a continuous pull directly on the patient's bones by means of a pin, wire, or tongs.

Mechanical traction is further classified as running (straight) or balanced suspension. Running traction is applied to a body part with a pull in one direction, with countertraction provided by the weight of the patient's body. Balanced suspension traction supports the extremity by means of a splint kept in position by a system of balanced weights attached to an overhead bed frame, thus providing the countertraction.

Traction maintenance is required to prevent complications. Countertraction is maintained by using the patient's body, the position of the bed, or the pull of the weights as dictated by the specific type of traction. Ropes should move freely through the pulleys, and weights hang clear of the bed, floor, footplates, and spreaders. Splints are prevented from resting against the bed, and bed linen is kept from interfering with traction pull. Continuous or intermittent traction is maintained with proper weights as ordered. The traction setup is different for each procedure and varies with equipment.

The perioperative nurse should assess the limb in traction for neurovascular changes (skin color, alterations in sensory or motor ability, peripheral pulses), capillary refill, and pressure areas (Cavendish, 1994).

Drains. Wound drainage systems or blood salvage systems may be used postoperatively to prevent development of hematoma. Hematoma formation can be prevented using other measures, such as obtaining hemostasis or releasing the tourniquet before complete wound closure, but wound drainage may also be the choice of prevention. Blood salvage systems are connected to a drain. These require an understanding of the physiology to assure safe transfusion.

Recognizing and Planning for Potential Complications

All surgical procedures carry inherent risks. Risks during orthopedic procedures relate to the manipulation of tissue and bone, the introduction of foreign bodies during implant surgery, and complications from physiologic alterations related to tissue perfusion in dependently positioned or operative body parts. Knowledge of the pathophysiologic process, the associated risk, and nursing interventions can minimize postoperative complications (Slye, 1991).

Thrombophlebitis. Thromboembolic disease is one of the most common and dangerous of all complications occurring after skeletal trauma (Evarts, 1992). Thrombophlebitis can progress to pulmonary embolism, making preventive measures such as antithrombotic drugs and anticoagulants important considerations (Kaempfee, et al., 1990). The threat is correlated with age, obesity, extent and duration of the procedure, and history and severity of underlying systems. Application of antiembolism devices is commonly performed to increase venous return from the lower extremities. Antiembolism stockings, elastic wraps, or sequential compression stockings may be used. Sequential compression devices are designed to inflate and deflate at regular intervals and at preset pressures to maintain adequate venous return during lengthy procedures.

Fat embolism. Approximately 5000 deaths annually are associated with fat embolism syndrome (Evarts, 1992). This syndrome is a cause of pulmonary insufficiency, commonly associated with long bone fractures and multiple skeletal fractures (crush injury). Fat embolism syndrome is also associated with hypovolemic shock following traumatic injury. Fat globules are released from the marrow and traumatized tissue into the circulation. The globules lodge in the lung and embolize to the local circulation. Resulting pathophysiologic changes cause reduced venous oxygenation and eventual hypoxemia. Early operative fracture stabilization is valuable in prevention of pulmonary complications (Slye, 1991).

Compartment syndrome. Compartment syndrome is caused by edematous tissue compromising circulation and function of tissue. The syndrome begins when a closed space (compartment) that contains muscle becomes edematous, resulting in muscle becoming ischemic. This is followed by cellular swelling that further impairs circulation. The pressure in a compartment may result from trauma to either the lower or upper extremities, circumferential dressing, the patient's skin or muscle, skeletal traction, or ischemia. If left untreated, the entire compartment will be at risk for tissue necrosis. If compartment syndrome is not prevented, fasciotomy will be required to release the distal compartment of the extremity (Mubarak, 1993; Slye, 1991).

Infection. Infection is a serious complication of orthopedic surgery and could result in osteomyelitis. When bone is fractured or surgically disrupted, its local blood supply is damaged. Tissue necrosis occurs to a greater or lesser extent depending on the amount of damage to bone and soft tissue. Associated hematoma and soft tissue damage provide a medium for posttraumatic bone infection. When foreign materials such as prostheses, bone cement, and metallic fracture fixation hardware are inserted in the surgical wound, resistance to bacterial proliferation is further compromised. Strict aseptic technique to prevent contamination, proper tissue handling by the scrub nurse or registered nurse first assistant to prevent unnecessary tissue damage, thorough wound debridement and irrigation, delayed closure of contaminated wounds, and appropriate adjunctive antibiotic therapy are all fundamental principles of orthopedic surgery.

UNIVERSAL PRECAUTIONS IN ORTHOPEDIC SURGERY

Universal precautions are intended to prevent parenteral, mucous membrane, and nonintact skin exposure of health care personnel. In the OR, exposure to bloodborne pathogens is high; contact with blood and other body fluids containing blood, such as synovial fluid, is a routine part of perioperative nursing care. Orthopedic instruments are sharp, and procedures require manipulation of large extremities or equipment, resulting in the potential for violation of the integrity of the surgical glove. Protective barriers that prevent exposure of skin and mucous membranes should be included in the precaution protocols. Protective attire worn during the procedure or when handling instruments and equipment before sterilization reduces the risk of contamination. Protocols for employee handling of fluids, sharps, or other high-risk contaminants should be implemented; all occupational blood exposures must be reported to the individual in the health care facility responsible for postexposure management (Garner, 1995).

CARE PLANS

The ten procedure-specific care plans are representative of the numerous orthopedic procedures for which patients require perioperative nursing care. The nursing diagnoses selected are common for the surgical procedure; identification of nursing diagnoses will follow the individualized patient assessment. Chapter 7 contains generic care plans for meeting general outcome standards. Nursing actions are selected from the generic care plans and added to those specific for the orthopedic procedure. Nursing actions are sequenced in the order they will most likely occur. This will vary with the patient's needs and setting. The Guides to Nursing Actions provide explanation for each activity and will need to be modified to adapt to institutional protocols,

surgeon's preferences, and surgical procedure. Nursing actions to implement the following nursing diagnoses should be included in the care plan:

- High risk for knowledge deficit related to planned surgical interventions and/or rehabilitation process
- High risk for infection (surgical site)
- High risk for impaired skin integrity
- High risk for injury related to surgical positioning
- High risk for injury related to retained foreign object
- High risk for injury related to physical hazards
- High risk for injury related to electrical equipment
- High risk for noncompliance related to rehabilitation

GUIDES TO NURSING ACTIONS
Intramedullary Rodding (Fig. 12-1)

Intramedullary rodding (nailing) is a fixation method effective for the diaphysis of weight-bearing bones that is often required following traumatic injury, including fracture of the femoral shaft, humeral shaft, tibia, or fibula. Rods or nails can be placed using percutaneous closed techniques that minimize soft tissue dissection or as an open procedure. Alignment can be maintained using interlocking nails or fluted nails. The size of the intramedullary canal can be limiting unless extensive reaming is performed. Reaming interferes with the endosteal blood supply and, although revascularization should occur, this is a consideration when determining the method of fixation. Instrumentation and implants may not be owned by the institution, requiring communication with the product representative.

1. Identification is made by asking the patient to state his or her name, operative procedure, and physician. The operative permit should be complete. The hospital identification should correspond with the information stated by the patient.
2. The patient should state the type and verbalize an understanding of the surgical procedure and the anesthesia and confirm the operative site. Assess if the patient has any specific concerns, fears, or anxieties related to the planned anesthesia. General or regional anesthesia may be delivered.
3. Verify any known allergies the patient may have and document them on the OR record.
4. Determine if any preoperative antibiotics are to be administered. Document antibiotic administration.

FIG. 12-1
CARE PLAN FOR INTRAMEDULLARY RODDING

KEY ASSESSMENT POINTS

General physical & mental condition
Type of fracture (stable/unstable)
Type of traction
Presence of chronic health problems (hypertension, diabetes, cardiovascular disease)
Pain, tenderness
Skin integrity (hematoma)
Neurovascular status
Understanding of procedure
Understanding of rehabilitation
Anxiety

NURSING DIAGNOSIS

All generic nursing diagnoses apply to this patient, with the addition of:
Altered tissue perfusion
High risk for peripheral neurovascular dysfunction
Impaired physical mobility
Pain

PATIENT OUTCOMES

All generic outcomes apply, with the addition of:
The patient will maintain peripheral neurovascular function as evidenced by presence of intact sensation and movement of the affected extremity and absence of parasthesia.
The patient will maintain adequate tissue perfusion as evidenced by presence of peripheral pulses, warmth of the extremity, capillary refill in the toes of the affected extremity.
Mobility will be restored as evidenced by movement of the extremity as determined by rehabilitation.
Pain will not be experienced postoperatively as evidenced by vital signs within normal limits, no complaints of pain, responsiveness to directives.

NURSING ACTIONS

	Yes	No	N/A
1. Patient identified and consent verified?	☐	☐	☐
2. Patient verbalized the procedure, operative site, and type of anesthesia?	☐	☐	☐
3. Allergies noted?	☐	☐	☐
4. Preoperative antibiotics administered?	☐	☐	☐
5. Sensory status assessed and documented?	☐	☐	☐
6. Neurovascular status assessed and documented?	☐	☐	☐
7. Skin integrity assessed and cleansed as needed?	☐	☐	☐
8. Medical history verified?	☐	☐	☐
9. Radiologic exams and laboratory values assessed?	☐	☐	☐
10. Blood products available?	☐	☐	☐
11. Equipment prepared for use, including the fracture bed, tourniquet, power equipment?	☐	☐	☐
12. Instrumentation present and function verified?	☐	☐	☐
13. Radiology technician notified and equipment in place?	☐	☐	☐
14. Skeletal traction set prepared?	☐	☐	☐
15. Patient protected during transfer; privacy maintained?	☐	☐	☐
16. Patient positioned and protected with padding?	☐	☐	☐
17. Urinary drainage catheter placed if appropriate and documented?	☐	☐	☐
18. Electrosurgical dispersive pad placed?	☐	☐	☐
19. Patient protected with leaded devices?	☐	☐	☐

NURSING ACTIONS—cont'd

	Yes	No	N/A
20. Temperature maintained?	☐	☐	☐
21. Surgical preparation completed?	☐	☐	☐
22. Patient draped and sterility maintained?	☐	☐	☐
23. Blood loss monitored?	☐	☐	☐
24. Neurovascular status assessed and findings reported?	☐	☐	☐
25. Implant size and sterility ensured?	☐	☐	☐
26. Documentation completed?	☐	☐	☐
27. Dressings and drains secured?	☐	☐	☐
28. Skin integrity assessed?	☐	☐	☐
29. Patient transferred safely?	☐	☐	☐
30. Postoperative evaluation of neurovascular status and skin integrity completed and documented?	☐	☐	☐
31. Patient transferred safely and information communicated?	☐	☐	☐

Document additional nursing actions/generic care plans initiated here:

_____

_____

_____

EVALUATION OF PATIENT OUTCOMES

	Outcome met	Outcome met with additional outcome criteria	Outcome met with revised nursing care plan	Outcome not met	Outcome not applicable to this patient
1. Neurovascular status was intact.	☐	☐	☐	☐	☐
2. Tissue perfusion was maintained.	☐	☐	☐	☐	☐
3. There were no complications related to immobility.	☐	☐	☐	☐	☐
4. Pain was effectively controlled.	☐	☐	☐	☐	☐
5. The patient met outcomes for additional generic care plans as indicated.	☐	☐	☐	☐	☐

Signature: _____ Date: _____

5. The sensory status is assessed as a baseline. Persons may experience postprocedure trauma, resulting in changes in their status.
6. Perform a preoperative neurovascular assessment. Note color, temperature, palpable pulses, capillary refill, sensation, movement, and pain in the affected extremity.
7. Assess the patient's skin integrity and any abnormalities such as hematoma, abrasions, swelling, and/or open fracture sites. Determine the fracture location (midshaft, distal two thirds) and planned approach (open or closed). Perform a skeletal traction assessment if traction is in place; check pin sites, that weights are hanging freely, and alignment of the extremity with the patient's hip and shoulder. Cleanse the skin if needed.
8. Assess the medical status by asking the patient to recollect the incident; evaluate results of diagnostic studies. Injury could have resulted following a change in medical condition (dysrhythmia, cerebrovascular accident).
9. Ensure that all diagnostic studies (for example, x-ray films) are available. Evaluate laboratory values and report abnormal findings, especially decreased hemoglobin or hematocrit levels and an elevated white blood cell count.
10. Ensure that the patient's blood has been typed and cross-matched and that blood products are available for the patient.
11. Prepare the fracture bed for use as appropriate. The room should be arranged to ensure that traffic flow is away from the operative site. Ensure that all pieces are intact and properly functioning before moving the patient into the OR suite. Pad the transfer board and sacral rest and place on the bed. Secure the traction unit with the boot on the abductor bar. Become familiar with the manufacturer's instructions on the recommended use and maintenance of the orthopedic fracture table.
12. Make sure the appropriate intramedullary rodding or nailing system, instrumentation and hardware (such as flexible or solid reamers, intramedullary rods or nails, and locking screws), and power tools (such as a reamer-driver or drill) are available and functioning properly.
   Verify function of equipment including tourniquet and power equipment.
13. Contact the radiology technician and have an image intensifier in the room. Ensure that all personnel and the patient will have adequate lead protection during the procedure.
14. Traction may be applied with free hanging weights if a skeletal traction pin is requested. This reduces the fracture and maintains alignment before the intramedullary rod placement. Prepare basic instrumentation for the skeletal pinning, including a large threaded Steinmann pin, a hand or power drill, and traction bow. Traction weights and rope should be in the room.
15. Ensure that the patient is protected during transfer. OR personnel should be available for safe patient transfer from the bed to the fracture table. Frequently, the patient is anesthetized on the bed before the transfer. During the transfer, maintain support to the fracture site and extremity. Maintain the patient's privacy.
16. Position the patient to ensure that pressure areas are padded. Secure the arm on the affected side across the patient's chest. Secure the arm on the unaffected side on a padded armboard. If the fracture bed is required, insert the perineal post, wrapped with disposable material, into the fracture table. Check that the perineum is in contact with but not pressing against the perineal post. Attach the leg holder to the abductor bar on the unaffected side. Place the unaffected leg securely in a padded leg holder. Keep the knee flexed and the popliteal space free of pressure. Wrap the foot and ankle area of the affected leg with Webril or other protective padding, and secure the foot in the traction boot. The transfer board is removed when limbs are secured.
17. Ascertain if a urinary drainage catheter will be inserted. Use aseptic technique for catheter insertion. Place the drainage bag where it is readily available. Document catheter insertion and urinary output.
18. Place the electrosurgical dispersive pad on the unaffected side. Note the condition of the skin at the placement site.
19. Ensure that the patient's genitals or other sensitive areas are covered with lead protection before the orthopedic surgical skin preparation.
20. Maintain the patient's temperature by placing a thermal blanket on the patient before draping.
21. Complete the surgical prep, including removal of hair if needed, and antimicrobial scrub.
22. Drape the patient. An isolation barrier drape may be placed. The C-arm is placed to prevent contamination of the field and is usually draped.
23. The patient's blood loss is monitored throughout the procedure and the anesthesia staff is informed. If femoral rodding is to be performed as an open procedure, a cell-saver autologous transfusion system may be used.
24. Ongoing assessment of the patient's neurovascular status should be conducted throughout the procedure, and the surgical team should be informed of any abnormal findings.

25. Implant size and sterility are verified before delivery to the sterile field.
26. Follow institutional protocol for documentation of safety and protective precautions, including padding, counts, implanted hardware, tourniquet time, and outcomes.
27. Apply sterile dressings to the incision site, allowing for postoperative swelling. If a drain is placed, ensure that the drain is patent and secured to the patient's skin with tape.
28. Evaluate skin integrity at pressure sites (groin, posterior ankle, and other bony prominences) and beneath the electrosurgical dispersive pad.
29. Replace the transfer board and remove the perineal post from the fracture table. Allow at least six OR personnel for the transfer from the fracture table to the patient's bed. Maintain support of the operative extremity at all times.
30. Perform and document a postoperative neurovascular assessment of the operative extremity. Keep the lower extremities in slight abduction, without rotation. Remove all protective padding, and check all pressure-dependent areas before transfer to the postanesthesia care unit. Note any abnormalities or variances from the preoperative assessment, and alert the surgical team.
31. Maintain the patient in proper position during transfer to the postanesthesia care unit. Communicate the evaluation findings, and communicate other patient information to the PACU staff.

Joint Arthroplasty (Fig. 12-2)

Patients undergoing procedures for joint replacement have often experienced chronic pain and debilitation, resulting in a need for joint replacement to restore mobility caused by arthritis or osteoporosis; as many as one third of elderly men and women have osteoarthritis of the knee (Callahan, Drake, & Heck, 1994). Many joints can be replaced, including the hip, knee, shoulder, elbow, finger, and toe. Partial replacement of anatomic parts may be required following fracture, such as femoral head replacement during hemiarthroplasty. The instrumentation and implants are obtained before the surgical procedure if not owned by the hospital. This may require communication with the product representative and confirmation of the time the procedure is scheduled to ensure availability and sterilization of instruments. Joint replacement may be cemented, noncemented, or hybrid fixation (combination). Joint replacement requiring removal of a nonfunctional joint requires many other considerations and changes in the procedure.

1. Identification is made by asking the patient to state his or her name, operative procedure, and physician. The operative permit should be complete and correct. The hospital identification should correspond with the information stated by the patient.
2. The sensory status is assessed and documented. Older adults undergoing anesthesia sometimes experience postprocedure trauma following delivery of anesthesia. Assessment of sensory status provides a baseline for postoperative comparison.
3. The psychologic and social status of the patient should be assessed. The rehabilitation course requires cooperation and understanding by the patient and family. Reinforcement of the preoperative course of therapy is needed, patient acceptance determined, and social support identified.
4. Identify the patient's understanding of the anticipated outcome. Previous surgical experiences will help identify the patient's understanding of his or her postoperative responsibility. Preoperative teaching should begin at the time the patient determines a surgical procedure is required. Postoperative splints, immobilizers, continuous passive motion, pain management therapy, or other activities should be understood by the patient. (See Box 12-2 for a sample patient education guide to discharge teaching for the patient undergoing total hip replacement.)
5. Assess the range of motion of all extremities. Patients undergoing total joint replacements frequently have arthritis affecting more than one joint.
6. The patient should state the type and verbalize an understanding of the anesthesia. General or regional anesthesia may be delivered.
7. Verify any known drug allergies the patient may have and document them on the OR record.
8. Verify that preoperative orders were completed, including administration of antibiotics, if ordered before surgery, or preparation of the operative site. For example, depilatories or shaving are often employed for hair removal. Verify that these have been completed, if ordered; note the condition of the prepared site.
9. Place compression stockings on the unaffected extremity for patients undergoing joint replacement.
10. Assess and report abnormal laboratory values.
11. Ensure that studies such as x-ray films, MRI scans, or other studies are available. Specific anatomic radiographs, such as long leg x-rays for total knee replacement, should be available.

FIG. 12-2
CARE PLAN FOR JOINT ARTHROPLASTY

KEY ASSESSMENT POINTS

General physical & mental condition
Presence of chronic health problems (hypertension, diabetes, cardio-vascular disease)
Pain, tenderness
Limitations in mobility and protective behaviors
Range of motion
Understanding of procedure
Understanding of rehabilitation
Anxiety

NURSING DIAGNOSIS

All generic nursing diagnoses apply to this patient, with the addition of:
Altered peripheral tissue perfusion
High risk for infection
High risk for peripheral neurovascular function
Pain
High risk for fluid volume deficit

PATIENT OUTCOMES

All generic outcomes apply, with the addition of:
The patient will maintain adequate tissue perfusion as evidenced by the presence of peripheral pulses, warmth of extremity, capillary refill in the toes of the affected extremity.
The patient will maintain peripheral neurovascular function as evidenced by intact movement of the extremity and absence of paras-thesia.
The patient will not experience pain as evidenced by stable vital signs, minimal discomfort, and willingness to move extremity.
Fluid volume will be maintained as evidenced by vital signs within normal limits, blood loss minimal, lab values within normal lim-its.

NURSING ACTIONS

	Yes	No	N/A
1. Patient identified and operative consent veri-fied?	☐	☐	☐
2. Sensory status assessed and documented?	☐	☐	☐
3. Psychologic and social status assessed; preoperative information verified?	☐	☐	☐
4. Verbalized understanding of the procedure and outcomes?	☐	☐	☐
5. Range of motion assessed?	☐	☐	☐
6. Verbalized anesthesia type?	☐	☐	☐
7. Allergies noted?	☐	☐	☐
8. Preoperative orders administered, including medications, skin preparation?	☐	☐	☐
9. Compression stockings placed?	☐	☐	☐
10. Lab values assessed and reported?	☐	☐	☐
11. Diagnostic studies assessed?	☐	☐	☐
12. Blood products available?	☐	☐	☐
13. Equipment function validated, including: Tourniquet as applicable	☐	☐	☐
Positioning equipment (beanbag, foot holder, three point positioner, hand table)	☐	☐	☐
Laminar airflow and/or body exhaust suits	☐	☐	☐
Power equipment	☐	☐	☐
Pulsatile lavage	☐	☐	☐
14. Instrumentation available and sterile?	☐	☐	☐
15. Patient remains covered?	☐	☐	☐
16. Patient protected during transfer and posi-tioning?	☐	☐	☐
17. Output monitored?	☐	☐	☐
18. Patient positioned and padded?	☐	☐	☐

NURSING ACTIONS—cont'd

	Yes	No	N/A
19. Electrosurgical dispersive pad placed?	☐	☐	☐
20. Skin preparation completed?	☐	☐	☐
21. Polymethyl methacrylate (PMMA) mixed correctly and exhaust systems connected?	☐	☐	☐
22. Irrigation system connected?	☐	☐	☐
23. Implant size and sterility verified?	☐	☐	☐
24. Documentation completed?	☐	☐	☐
25. Wound drains protected and secured?	☐	☐	☐
26. Tourniquet removed and skin integrity assessed?	☐	☐	☐
27. Specimens dispensed to pathology?	☐	☐	☐
28. Dressings secured?	☐	☐	☐
29. Electrosurgical dispersive pad removed and skin integrity assessed?	☐	☐	☐
30. Patient protected during transfer?	☐	☐	☐
31. Neurovascular integrity assessed?	☐	☐	☐
32. Position maintained during transfer and patient care information communicated?	☐	☐	☐

Document additional nursing actions/generic care plans initiated here:

_____

_____

_____

EVALUATION OF PATIENT OUTCOMES

	Outcome met	Outcome met with additional outcome criteria	Outcome met with revised nursing care plan	Outcome not met	Outcome not applicable to this patient
1. Tissue perfusion was maintained.	☐	☐	☐	☐	☐
2. There was no evidence of surgical site infection.	☐	☐	☐	☐	☐
3. Neurovascular status was intact.	☐	☐	☐	☐	☐
4. Pain was effectively controlled.	☐	☐	☐	☐	☐
5. Fluid and electrolyte balance was maintained.	☐	☐	☐	☐	☐
6. The patient met outcomes for additional generic care plans as indicated.	☐	☐	☐	☐	☐

Signature: _____ Date: _____

Box 12-2 Discharge Teaching for Total Hip Replacement

Do

Keep legs apart while sitting or lying

Use pillow or blanket between legs as a reminder to keep legs abducted

Sit on a high, firm chair

Use caution when getting in and out of bathtub

Walk with crutches or walker as instructed in physical therapy before discharge

Use elevated toilet seat

Notify physician if operative site becomes reddened or irritated or has any drainage; also if you have pain, swelling, shortening of one leg, or limitation in walking

Advise dentist of prosthesis before dental work so prophylactic antibiotics can be given

Do Not

Sit in low, soft chair

Cross legs

Turn hip or knee inward or outward

Participate in sports activities until advised by physician

Bend forward past 90 degrees to put on shoes or socks or to pick things up

Turn in bed without pillow or blanket between legs

From Beare PG & Meyers JL. (1994). *Principles and Practices of Adult Health Nursing* (2nd Ed.). St Louis: Mosby.

---

12. Verify availability of replacement blood products.
13. Equipment function and availability should be validated as follows:
    a. Tourniquet function for distal joint replacement and correct size of tourniquets obtained
    b. Positioning equipment obtained and assessed for function. Special positioning devices are needed to ensure access of the operative site. The hand table will be used for implantation of prosthesis in the fingers. A beanbag, three-point positioner, sandbag, and pillows may be needed for stabilization of the extremity.
    c. Laminar airflow or body-exhaust apparatus may be employed. Proper functioning must be ensured.
    d. Power equipment (saw, reamer, drill) available and functioning
    e. Supplies for mixing and exhausting polymethyl methacrylate (bone cement) available and functioning.
    f. Pulsatile lavage for removal of bone and other tissue.
14. Verify that the appropriate joint instrumentation system and prostheses are available according to the surgeon's preference and site of the procedure.
15. Protect the patient's privacy and maintain body temperature by ensuring that the patient remains covered during transfer and positioning.
16. The patient is protected during transfer and positioning by ensuring adequate numbers of personnel are available for positioning before and following the procedure. The safety strap may be secured across the thighs and arms secured during induction. This is maintained unless it interferes with the procedure.
17. Output is monitored and documented throughout the procedure by measuring blood loss and urinary output if appropriate. If ordered, a urinary catheter should be inserted before the patient is positioned for surgery using aseptic technique. The drainage bag is placed where it is readily available. Document catheter insertion and urinary output.
18. The patient is positioned for the procedure providing freedom of respiration, maintaining circulatory status, and exposing the surgical site. The principles of positioning are followed. Information obtained during the preoperative assessment regarding range of motion, observation of bony prominences, and areas of sensitivity should be considered when positioning. Patients undergoing the procedure for total joint replacement may have osteoporosis of the affected joint or other anatomic sites, requiring consideration of fragile bone when positioning. Body alignment should be maintained.
19. The electrosurgical dispersive pad should be placed in an area close to the surgical site where there is sufficient healthy tissue without scar tissue, prostheses, or hardware. Note the condition of the skin at the pad placement site.
20. The operative extremity should be suspended with a positioning aid (or with the assistance of personnel) for the surgical skin preparation.
21. If polymethyl methacrylate (PMMA) (bone cement) is used, provide adequate ventilation of fumes; be aware of the room temperature because it is related to the consistency of the cement.
22. A pulsatile irrigation system may be connected to remove loose cement and bone. Antibiotics may be added to irrigation fluids.
23. Implant size and sterility is ensured before delivery of the prostheses to the sterile field.
24. Document safety and protective precautions such as counts and implant type, size, and number.
25. Maintain the patency of wound drains. Ensure that the tubing is not kinked or clotted and that the suction apparatus is properly functioning. Document the presence of drains.

26. The tourniquet is removed following deflation and skin integrity is assessed at the site.
27. The surgical specimen is dispensed following institutional protocol for the preservation and disposition.
28. Apply sterile dressings. An immobilizer appropriate for the surgical site may be applied.
29. Remove the electrosurgical dispersive pad, and evaluate skin integrity. Document findings.
30. Ensure that adequate numbers of personnel are available to provide safe transfer for the patient. Protect the operative area when turning the patient and transferring the patient to the bed. This may require use of special devices to maintain the position.
31. Postoperative neurovascular integrity is compared with the preoperative assessment information, dependent pressure sites are evaluated, and findings are documented.
32. Maintain the patient in the proper position during the transfer to the postanesthesia care unit, and communicate patient care information to the postanesthesia care unit staff.

Open Reduction and Internal Fixation (ORIF) of Fractured Hip (Fig. 12-3)

Open reduction and internal fixation may be performed on any fractured bone. Femoral fractures are each anatomically different, resulting in various modes of treatment. The degree of stability determines the treatment, including implant type, positioning during surgery, and other patient needs.

1. Identification is made by asking the patient to state his or her name, operative procedure, and physician. This should correspond with the name on the patient's identification band and the operative consent form. The operative permit should be complete and correct.
2. The patient should correctly state the type and verbalize an understanding of the anesthesia to be used. Assess if the patient has any specific concerns, fears, or anxieties related to the planned anesthesia.
3. Verify any known allergies the patient may have and document them in the OR record. Determine if any preoperative antibiotics are to be administered.
4. Complete a preoperative neurovascular assessment. Note color, temperature, palpable pulses, capillary refill, sensation, movement, and pain of the affected side, and document accordingly. Also note the patient's skin integrity and any abnormalities such as hematomas and open wounds.
5. Have all diagnostic studies (for example, x-ray films) available.

6. Evaluate laboratory values, and report abnormal findings, especially decreased hemoglobin or hematocrit levels and an elevated white blood cell count.
7. Ensure that the patient's blood has been typed and cross-matched and that blood products are available for the patient.
8. Prepare the orthopedic fracture table. Ensure that all pieces are intact and functioning properly before moving the patient into the OR suite. Become familiar with the manufacturer's instructions on the recommended use and maintenance of the orthopedic fracture table.
9. Ensure the availability and proper functioning of the appropriate internal fixation system; instrumentation and hardware, such as compression screws, plates, and multiple threaded pins; and power tools, such as a reamer, driver, and drill.
10. Contact the x-ray technician and have an image intensifier in the room. Ensure that all personnel and the patient have adequate lead protection for the procedure.
11. Have the orthopedic fracture table set up in the OR suite before the patient's arrival. Make sure that the transfer board and sacral rest are padded and in place on the table. Place a padded armboard on the unaffected side. Have the traction unit with the boot positioned securely on the abductor bar.

    Ensure that personnel are available for safe patient transfer from the bed to the fracture table. Frequently the patient is anesthetized on the bed before the transfer. During the transfer maintain support to the fracture site and extremity. Maintain the patient's privacy.
12. Make sure all pressure areas are padded. Secure the arm on the affected side with a strap or tape to the patient's chest. Secure the arm of the unaffected side on a padded armboard. Insert the perineal post, wrapped with disposable material, into the fracture table. Check that the perineum is in contact with but not pressing against the perineal post. Attach the leg holder to the abductor bar on the unaffected side. Place the unaffected leg securely in a padded leg holder. Keep the knee flexed and the popliteal space free of pressure. Wrap the foot and ankle area of the affected leg with Webril, and secure the foot in the traction boot. When certain that all limbs are secure, remove the transfer board.
13. Ascertain if a urinary drainage catheter will be needed. Use aseptic technique for catheter insertion. Place drainage bag where it is readily observable. Document the presence of the catheter and urinary output.

FIG. 12-3
CARE PLAN FOR ORIF FRACTURED HIP

KEY ASSESSMENT POINTS

General physical and mental condition
Type and location of fracture
Type/weight of traction
Support devices (pillow splint, etc.)
Type of traumatic event
Presence of chronic health problems (hypertension, diabetes, cardio-vascular disease)
Pain (location, severity)
Musculoskeletal condition (spasticity, contractures, range of motion)
Skin integrity
Neurovascular status
Understanding of procedure
Allergies
Availability of blood replacement products

NURSING DIAGNOSIS

All generic nursing diagnoses apply to this patient, with the addition of:
High risk for fluid volume deficit
Pain
High risk for infection
High risk for peripheral neurovascular function

PATIENT OUTCOMES

All generic outcomes apply, with the addition of:
Fluid volume will be maintained as evidenced by vital signs within normal limits, blood loss minimal.
Pain minimal as evidenced by the patient's response to directives, ability to rest.
Infection not experienced postoperatively as evidenced by a clean, dry wound, temperature within normal limits.
Peripheral neurovascular function maintained as evidenced by presence of pulses, presence of intact sensation, movement of extremity, extremity warmth.

NURSING ACTIONS	Yes	No	N/A
1. Patient identified?	☐	☐	☐
2. Patient verbalizes understanding of anesthetic?	☐	☐	☐
3. Allergies noted?	☐	☐	☐
4. Neurovascular assessment completed?	☐	☐	☐
5. Diagnostic studies, including x-rays, available?	☐	☐	☐
6. Laboratory values evaluated and findings reported?	☐	☐	☐
7. Blood replacement available?	☐	☐	☐
8. Fracture table prepared, parts available?	☐	☐	☐
9. Internal fixation instruments and implants available?	☐	☐	☐
10. Radiology technician notified and fluoroscopy prepared?	☐	☐	☐
11. Personnel available for transfer, extremity supported?	☐	☐	☐
12. Pressure areas padded, arm secured, genitals protected?	☐	☐	☐
13. Urinary drainage inserted as appropriate; output documented?	☐	☐	☐
14. Electrosurgical pad placed and skin condition noted?	☐	☐	☐
15. Leaded protection provided for the patient and personnel?	☐	☐	☐
16. Patient draped, isolation barrier placed, and fluoroscopy positioned?	☐	☐	☐

NURSING ACTIONS—cont'd	Yes	No	N/A
17. Blood loss monitored?	☐	☐	☐
18. Neurovascular status assessed throughout the procedure and documented?	☐	☐	☐
19. Safety and precautionary measures documented?	☐	☐	☐
20. Drainage tubes patent and secured?	☐	☐	☐
21. Sterile dressings applied?	☐	☐	☐
22. Skin integrity assessed postoperatively?	☐	☐	☐
23. Patient transferred safely to postoperative bed?	☐	☐	☐
24. Postoperative neurovascular status documented?	☐	☐	☐
25. Patient positioned in postoperative bed; evaluation information communicated?	☐	☐	☐

Document additional nursing actions/generic care plans initiated here:

_____

_____

_____

EVALUATION OF PATIENT OUTCOMES

	Outcome met	Outcome met with additional outcome criteria	Outcome met with revised nursing care plan	Outcome not met	Outcome not applicable to this patient
1. Fluid balance was maintained.	☐	☐	☐	☐	☐
2. An optimal level of comfort was achieved.	☐	☐	☐	☐	☐
3. There was no evidence of surgical site infection.	☐	☐	☐	☐	☐
4. Neurovascular status was intact.	☐	☐	☐	☐	☐
5. The patient met outcomes for additional care plans as indicated.	☐	☐	☐	☐	☐

Signature: _____ Date: _____

14. Place the electrosurgical pad on the unaffected side. Note the condition of the skin at the placement site.
15. Make sure the patient's genitals and other sensitive areas are covered with lead protection before the surgical preparation.
16. The patient is draped. An isolation barrier may be placed. The C-arm of the image intensifier is positioned to prevent contamination of the sterile field. Sterile draping of the C-arm is usually necessary.
17. The patient's blood loss is monitored throughout the procedure, and the anesthesia staff should be informed.
18. The neurovascular status of the patient should be assessed throughout the procedure, and the surgical team informed of any abnormal findings.
19. Document safety and precautionary measures including counts, implanted hardware, and padding.
20. Make sure the drain is patent and secured to the patient's skin with tape.
21. Apply sterile dressings to the incision site allowing for normal postoperative swelling of the skin.
22. Evaluate skin integrity, including pressure sites and beneath the electrosurgical dispersive pad.
23. Replace the transfer board and remove the perineal post from the fracture table. Allow at least six OR personnel for transfer from the fracture table to the patient's bed. Keep the operative extremity supported at all times.
24. Perform and document a postoperative neurovascular assessment of the operative extremity. Note any abnormalities or variances from the preoperative assessment and alert the surgical team. Keep the lower extremities in slight abduction without rotation. Remove all protective padding and check all pressure-dependent areas before transfer to the postanesthesia care unit.
25. Maintain the patient in the proper position during transfer to the postanesthesia care unit. Communicate evaluation information and patient status to the postanesthesia care unit staff.

Bone Grafting for Fusion (Fig. 12-4)

A bone graft is placed in conjunction with a surgical procedure requiring stabilization. Bone may be an autograft from areas other than the iliac crest. In the future, "liquid bone," an artificial bone repair material, may substitute for bone grafts as the agent that stabilizes a fracture site (Fitzgerald, 1995).

1. Identification is made by asking the patient to state his or her name, operative procedure, and physician. The operative permit should be complete, including documentation of bone graft, harvesting, and implantation. The hospital identification should correspond with the information stated by the patient.
2. Verify any known allergies the patient may have and document them on the OR record. Determine if any preoperative antibiotics are to be administered.
3. The bone graft instruments may be prepared as a separate procedure, including a suction tip and electrosurgical pencil. Bone graft is frequently done for nonunion of a fracture site to promote new bone growth. All attempts should be made to prevent cross-contamination between the bone graft and nonunion sites.
4. A 5-pound sandbag is positioned beneath the operative iliac crest to give better exposure of the graft donor site.
5. Before closure of the graft donor site, a preliminary count of sponges, instruments, and sharps should be documented.
6. Ensure patency of the drain. Document insertion, type, and size of the drain.
7. Apply sterile dressings to the incision site and allow for normal postoperative swelling.
8. The scrub nurse should keep the harvested bone graft moistened with a blood-soaked sponge covering the bone in a safe area on the sterile instrument table, away from the recipient site instruments.

Arthroscopy of the Knee (Fig. 12-5)

Arthroscopic surgery is an adjunct to clinical evaluation when used as a diagnostic measure. It can be used to treat loose bodies, meniscus tears, or chondral defect. It is also used in conjunction with an open procedure for anterior cruciate ligament repair or acromioplasty. Arthroscopy can be performed on joints including the shoulder, hip, ankle, or wrist.

1. Identification is made by asking the patient to state his or her name, operative procedure, surgical site (which knee), and physician. The operative permit should be complete. The hospital identification should correspond with the information stated by the patient.
2. Determine the psychologic and social status of the patient. Family support of the patient is important for postoperative recovery. Postoperative activities should be understood, and use of crutches should be reinforced.
3. Verify any known allergies the patient may have and document them on the OR record.
4. Determine if any preoperative antibiotics are to be administered.

FIG. 12-4
CARE PLAN FOR BONE GRAFTING FOR FUSION

KEY ASSESSMENT POINTS

Patient awareness of the procedure
Site of bone graft removal
Physician plan of care (for harvest of bone)

NURSING DIAGNOSIS

All generic nursing diagnoses apply to this patient, with the addition of:
High risk for infection related to cross contamination

PATIENT OUTCOMES

All generic outcomes apply, with the addition of:
Infection is not present as evidenced by temperature within normal limits, absence of redness, warmth, drainage at the incision site.

NURSING ACTIONS

	Yes	No	N/A
1. Patient identified?	☐	☐	☐
2. Allergies verified?	☐	☐	☐
3. Bone graft instruments prepared?	☐	☐	☐
4. Graft site exposed by positioning?	☐	☐	☐
5. Safety measures implemented, including counts?	☐	☐	☐
6. Patency of the drain maintained, documented?	☐	☐	☐
7. Dressings applied correctly?	☐	☐	☐
8. Harvested bone graft secured on the sterile field?	☐	☐	☐

Document additional nursing actions/generic care plans initiated here:

_____

_____

_____

EVALUATION OF PATIENT OUTCOMES

	Outcome met	Outcome met with additional outcome criteria	Outcome met with revised nursing care plan	Outcome not met	Outcome not applicable to this patient
1. Cross-contamination was prevented; there was no wound infection.	☐	☐	☐	☐	☐
2. The patient met outcomes for additional generic care plans as indicated.	☐	☐	☐	☐	☐

Signature: _____ Date: _____

FIG. 12-5
CARE PLAN FOR ARTHROSCOPY OF THE KNEE

KEY ASSESSMENT POINTS

General physical and mental condition
Relevant health problems
History/mechanism of knee injury
Pain (location, severity)
Mobility limitations
Neurovascular status (knee and lower extremity)
Understanding of procedure and its objectives
Understanding of rehabilitation process
Allergies
Psychosocial concerns

NURSING DIAGNOSIS

All generic nursing diagnoses apply to this patient, with the addition
   of:
Impaired physical mobility
Sensory/perceptual alteration (kinesthetic)
High risk for peripheral neurovascular function
Knowledge deficit related to rehabilitation and postoperative course

PATIENT OUTCOMES

All generic outcomes apply, with the addition of:
Patient will experience mobility following rehabilitation.
Sensory/perceptual alteration will not be experienced as evidenced by
   intact movement of the extremities and absence of parasthesia.
Patient will experience peripheral neurovascular function as evidenced by adequate peripheral pulses, warmth of extremity, capillary refill.
Patient will demonstrate an understanding of the procedure and postoperative recovery as evidenced by verbalization of questions, ability to recall information, ability to crutch walk.

NURSING ACTIONS

	Yes	No	N/A
1. Patient identified?	☐	☐	☐
2. Family support, psychosocial status identified?	☐	☐	☐
3. Allergies noted?	☐	☐	☐
4. Preoperative antibiotics given?	☐	☐	☐
5. Patient understands type of anesthesia?	☐	☐	☐
6. Laboratory values evaluated and abnormal findings reported?	☐	☐	☐
7. Radiologic studies, including x-ray and MRI, available?	☐	☐	☐
8. Neurovascular assessment completed?	☐	☐	☐
9. Instrumentation, video equipment, tourniquet and positioning devices available and functional?	☐	☐	☐
10. Patient transferred safely and privacy maintained?	☐	☐	☐
11. Safety strap positioned?	☐	☐	☐
12. Electrosurgical dispersive pad placed and equipment obtained if appropriate?	☐	☐	☐
13. Local anesthetic prepared; medications labeled?	☐	☐	☐
14. Safety and protective measures documented?	☐	☐	☐
15. Specimens handled correctly?	☐	☐	☐
16. Dressings and immobilizer placed if appropriate?	☐	☐	☐
17. Tourniquet cuff placement, identification of equipment, and inflation times documented?	☐	☐	☐
18. Neurovascular assessment completed?	☐	☐	☐
19. Patient transferred safely and postoperative information communicated?	☐	☐	☐
20. Patient teaching completed and patient demonstrated understanding?	☐	☐	☐

Document additional nursing actions/generic care plans initiated
here:

_____

_____

_____

EVALUATION OF PATIENT OUTCOMES

	Outcome met	Outcome met with additional outcome criteria	Outcome met with revised nursing care plan	Outcome not met	Outcome not applicable to this patient
1. Joint motion was regained.	☐	☐	☐	☐	☐
2. Sensation and mobility were normal.	☐	☐	☐	☐	☐
3. Neurovascular status was intact.	☐	☐	☐	☐	☐
4. Rehabilitation program was described by patient and commitment verbalized.	☐	☐	☐	☐	☐
5. The patient met outcomes for additional care plans as indicated.	☐	☐	☐	☐	☐

Signature: _____   Date: _____

5. The patient should correctly state the type and an understanding of the anesthesia to be administered. Assess if the patient has any specific concerns, fears, or anxieties related to the planned anesthesia.

6. Evaluate laboratory values and report abnormal findings.

7. Ensure availability of radiologic studies, including x-ray films and MRI.

8. Perform a preoperative neurovascular assessment of the affected extremity. Note color, temperature, palpable pulses, capillary refill, sensation, movement, and pain. Also note the patient's skin integrity and any abnormalities such as hematomas, swelling, effusion, abrasions, and open areas. Document the findings.

9. Check that all needed instrumentation, video equipment, and positioning devices are available and functioning properly. These may include the following:
   a. Lateral post, which enables the surgeon to position the operative leg fixed and off to the side of the OR bed. This should be attached to the OR bed at or just below the level of the pneumatic tourniquet.
   b. Arthroscopic instruments, including the arthroscope, usually 30-degree angled with sharp and blunt trocars and sheath, fiberoptic light cord, various manual arthroscopic instruments, and motorized intraarticular system.
   c. Video system, including camera and monitor, fiberoptic light source, VCR, printer, and motor for intraarticular system.
   d. Intraarticular irrigation setup, which may or may not involve an arthroscopic pump for infusion. Personnel should be familiar with the operation and manufacturer's recommendations for use of the arthroscopic pump.
   e. Pneumatic tourniquet may be used according to surgeon preference. Follow institutional protocol for preparation, use, and maintenance of the pneumatic tourniquet. Document the unit identification number, site of application, pressure settings, and length of tourniquet time in the OR record.

10. Transfer the patient to the OR bed in supine position. Maintain the patient's privacy at all times. Pad pressure sites. Assist the patient to a position of comfort.

11. Protect the patient by placing the safety strap at the level of the patient's lower abdomen, ensuring the strap does not interfere with respiration.

12. Prepare an electrosurgical unit and a dispersive pad on the unaffected extremity (or have available) in the event that the procedure will be completed with electrosurgery or an arthrotomy needs to be performed. Note the condition of the skin at the site of dispersive pad placement.

13. Prepare a local anesthetic of the surgeon's choice on the sterile field. The operative knee may be injected before the procedure to produce hemostasis. Verify for patient allergies; keep an accurate record of the type and amount of local anesthetic used for the procedure. Label all medications on the sterile field.

14. Document safety and protective measures, including equipment settings and counts.

15. Follow institutional protocol for the preservation and disposition of surgical specimens.

16. After the application of sterile dressings, a knee immobilization device of some type may be requested. This may only be one to two layers of Webril followed by a 6-inch Ace wrap. Ensure that this is applied correctly with all straps secured, and prevent skin folds. Depending on the procedure performed, a knee brace may be required.

17. Document area of tourniquet cuff placement, unit identification, pressure, and inflation and deflation times.

18. Perform postoperative neurovascular assessment including color, warmth, and pulses of the operative leg, and note skin integrity. Document all assessment data in the OR record.

19. Transfer the patient to the postoperative area. Communicate evaluation findings and patient status.

20. Ensure that patient teaching is completed and the patient understands the following:
    a. Symptoms that should be reported including redness and/or alteration in neurovascular status
    b. Dressing and wound care and the need to keep dry and intact
    c. Weight-bearing status of the operative leg and the use of crutches
    d. Length of time the leg must be immobilized
    e. Elevation of the leg
    f. Use of ice packs
    g. Use of analgesics, antiinflammatory agents, and antibiotics
    h. Activities and progression of activity
    i. Scheduling a follow-up appointment

Application of an External Fixator (Fig. 12-6)

An external fixation device may be applied to any extremity. It requires insertion of pins above and below the fracture site, secured to a frame to maintain alignment of the bone. It may be an elective procedure for bone lengthening or

FIG. 12-6
CARE PLAN FOR APPLICATION OF AN EXTERNAL FIXATOR

KEY ASSESSMENT POINTS

General physical and mental condition
Relevant health problems
History/mechanism of injury
Status of injured site (skin integrity, contamination)
Pain (location, severity)
Mobility limitations
Neurovascular status
Understanding of procedure and its objectives
Understanding of rehabilitation process
Allergies
Psychosocial/body image concerns and personally effective coping
  mechanisms

NURSING DIAGNOSIS

All generic nursing diagnoses apply to this patient, with the addition
  of:
Body image disturbance
Sensory/perceptual alteration (kinesthetic)
High risk for infection
Impaired physical mobility

PATIENT OUTCOMES

All generic outcomes apply, with the addition of:
Patient regains a positive body image, copes effectively, and participates in self-care.
Patient maintains sensory/perceptual sensation in the extremity as
  evidenced by adequate pulses, warmth of the extremity, capillary
  refill.
Infection will not be experienced as evidenced by absence of drainage, redness, elevated temperature.
Physical mobility will be restored as evidenced by patient ability to
  resume range of motion and return to routine activities.

NURSING ACTIONS

	Yes	No	N/A
1. Patient identified?	☐	☐	☐
2. Consent signed and accurate for the procedure?	☐	☐	☐
3. Patient understands the surgical procedure and expected outcome?	☐	☐	☐
4. Patient understands anesthesia type?	☐	☐	☐
5. Allergies verified?	☐	☐	☐
6. Preoperative antibiotics given?	☐	☐	☐
7. Neurovascular assessment completed?	☐	☐	☐
8. Laboratory values evaluated and abnormal findings reported?	☐	☐	☐
9. Diagnostic studies available, including x-rays?	☐	☐	☐
10. Instrumentation, fixator devices, and necessary equipment available and function verified?	☐	☐	☐
11. Radiology technician notified, fluoroscopy prepared?	☐	☐	☐
12. Irrigation prepared with antibiotics and irrigation system available?	☐	☐	☐
13. Patient transferred safely?	☐	☐	☐
14. Patient positioned and secured; pressure sites protected?	☐	☐	☐
15. Electrosurgical dispersive pad placed, condition checked?	☐	☐	☐
16. Patient protected with padding and leaded protection?	☐	☐	☐
17. Safety and protective measures documented?	☐	☐	☐
18. Pin edges covered?	☐	☐	☐
19. Pin sites cleaned?	☐	☐	☐
20. Neurovascular assessment completed?	☐	☐	☐
21. Patient transferred safely and evaluation information communicated?	☐	☐	☐

Document additional nursing actions/generic care plans initiated
here:

_____

_____

_____

EVALUATION OF PATIENT OUTCOMES

	Outcome met	Outcome met with additional outcome criteria	Outcome met with revised nursing care plan	Outcome not met	Outcome not applicable to this patient
1. A positive body image will be regained.	☐	☐	☐	☐	☐
2. Neurovascular status was intact.	☐	☐	☐	☐	☐
3. There were no signs of surgical site infection.	☐	☐	☐	☐	☐
4. There were no complications related to immobility.	☐	☐	☐	☐	☐
5. The patient met outcomes for additional care plans as indicated.	☐	☐	☐	☐	☐

Signature: _____ Date: _____

an emergency procedure following traumatic injury.

1. The patient should state his or her name, the operative site, and side. This should correspond with the name on the patient's identification band and the operative consent form.
2. The consent form should be signed by the patient and correspond with the patient information.
3. Explain or reinforce the patient's knowledge of the surgical procedure and expected outcome. The patient should be aware of the appearance and limitations of the external fixator.
4. The patient should correctly state the type of anesthesia to be used as well as display an understanding of it. Assess if the patient has any specific concerns, fears, or anxieties related to the planned anesthesia. The area of fixator application will determine anesthesia type, but regional anesthesia may be used.
5. Verify any known allergies the patient may have and document them in the OR record.
6. Determine if any preoperative antibiotics are to be administered and ensure that this is documented.
7. Perform a preoperative neurovascular assessment of the operative extremity. Note color, temperature, palpable pulses, capillary refill, sensation, movement, and pain. Also note the patient's skin integrity; note such abnormalities as hematomas, swelling, and open wounds. The external fixator may have been selected for fracture reduction if there is extensive soft tissue damage and neurovascular compromise.
8. Evaluate laboratory values and report any abnormal findings, especially an elevated white blood cell count.
9. Have all diagnostic studies available, such as x-ray films.
10. Have all needed instrumentation, external fixation system items (pins, clamps, and connectors), and power drill (reamer driver) available and functioning properly.
11. Notify the radiology technician to plan placement of the image intensifier with the C-arm in the room. Ensure that there is an image OR table in the room. The C-arm will usually require draping.
12. Extensive soft tissue damage may require intraoperative irrigation and debridement before fixation of the fracture. A pulsatile lavage system should be available and will use 9 to 12 L of solution, usually saline, with or without added antibiotics. Document the addition of antibiotics.
13. Transfer the patient to the OR bed, supporting the affected extremity and maintaining the patient's privacy at all times.

14. Position the patient supine on the OR bed. Secure the safety strap. Pad pressure-dependent sites.
15. Place the electrosurgical dispersive pad on the unaffected side. Note the condition of the skin at the site of dispersive pad placement.
16. Protect the patient's genitals and sensitive areas with lead protection before the orthopedic surgical preparation.
17. Document safety and protective measures, including counts, hardware used, and patient needs.
18. Following the procedure, cover all sharp pin edges with plastic caps (usually supplied by the manufacturer of the external fixation system).
19. Clean the pin sites gently of any blood or debris. Pin care protocols remain a debatable issue in orthopedic nursing care; protocols may depend on orders from the surgeon. Basic principles are as follows:
    a. Keep the pin sites clean and open to air, allowing for normal serous drainage.
    b. Use only gentle cleaning techniques to free the sites of crusted material.
    c. Use hydrogen peroxide solution for cleansing pin sites. Povidone-iodine (Betadine) solution corrodes and stains the stainless steel pins. Rinse the sites with saline solution to clean off the peroxide and prevent skin irritation.
20. Perform and document a postoperative neurovascular assessment of the affected extremity. Check skin integrity and note and document any abnormalities (see Table 12-2 for a summary of potential complications and suggested nursing interventions).
21. Maintain the patient in the proper position during transfer to the postanesthesia care unit. Communicate patient care information to the postanesthesia care unit staff.

Rotator Cuff Repair (Fig. 12-7)

Rotator cuff repair is a common procedure for active individuals. It is a soft tissue procedure; bone involvement for the repair will vary with the surgeon's choice of repair type.

1. The patient should state his or her name, operative procedure, and site. This should correspond with the patient's hospital number on the chart and with the patient's nameband.
2. The operative consent should be signed by the patient and include the appropriate shoulder requiring surgery.
3. The patient should state the type of anesthesia to be used and display an understanding of it. Assess the patient for concerns, fears, or anxieties related to the planned anesthesia.

Table 12-2 Nursing intervention summary: external fixation patient

Potential Complications	Nursing Management
Nerve damage	Assess five P's (pain, pallor, paralysis, paresthesia, pulse).
Muscle/vascular damage	Assess five P's and peripheral pulses when assessing vital signs.
Cellulitis and osteomyelitis	Assess skin around pin sites for tenderness, redness, swelling, and serosanguineous or purulent drainage that occurs after pins have been in place 2 to 3 days. Assess for skin tension at pin sites resulting from pressure of pins on skin. Assess for loosening of pins, which may be associated with infection and increased or purulent drainage; loose pins are less effective in immobilizing the fracture site. General pin site care: Clean around entry and exit sites with hydrogen peroxide–soaked sterile applicators. Remove drainage with dry sterile swabs. Leave site uncovered or cover as prescribed by physician. Perform pin site care every 8 hours for first 3 days after insertion of external fixator. After first 3-day period, drainage is minimal to none. Frequency of pin site care is based on presence of drainage. Refer to physician's orders or agency procedure for specific cleaning agents or application of antiseptic ointments.
Hazards of immobility	Determine how restricted patient's activity will be because of external fixator. Patient who is confined to bed in traction will have more limited mobility than patient who can be ambulatory while wearing the device. Promote physical mobility by encouraging patient to put weight on extremity as soon after surgery as physician allows. Patient performs range-of-motion exercises to unaffected extremities. Nurse determines physician's plan for other exercises and assists patient in performing them.
Edema that interferes with healing	Prevent edema by elevating affected extremity above level of heart the first few days after surgery. If a leg is involved, elevation can be achieved by balanced suspension traction or by attaching traction ropes to four different points on the external device and tying the ropes to an overhead bed frame. When swelling has subsided, nurse may elevate leg on pillows or raise foot of bed.
Body image disturbance and knowledge deficit	Assess patient's feelings regarding body image and external fixation device. Acceptance of external fixator may be a problem, because metal frame looks like an "erector set" as it extends outward from extremity. Device is also awkward and heavy, which will make affected leg feel different from the other. This change in appearance and weight may cause concern. Assess patient and family's knowledge of external fixation device and what their concerns are. Prepare patient and family for external fixation by showing them a picture of device. Explain that frame will be visible outside extremity and may be bulky and heavy. Emphasize positive aspects, such as how the device stabilizes the broken bone and that pain usually subsides after early postoperative period. Explain how device works, but caution patient not to tamper with nuts and clamps, which could alter bone alignment and impair healing. Grasp external fixator to lift or move extremity rather than lifting the extremity itself.

From Beare PG & Meyers JL. (1994). *Principles and practices of adult health nursing* (2nd Ed.). St Louis: Mosby.

4. Verify any known allergies the patient may have and document them on the OR record.
5. Verify that preoperative antibiotics have been administered if ordered and document them.
6. Perform the preoperative neurovascular assessment and document it. Note color, temperature, sensory alterations, and capillary refill.
7. Ensure availability of x-ray films, MRI, and CT scans to use for referral during rotator cuff repairs.
8. Review laboratory values and diagnostic studies. Report abnormal values.
9. Obtain instrumentation and equipment for the procedure. A high-speed burr and drill may be required to perform an acromioplasty (if necessary to relieve impingement syndrome). The rotator cuff is usually repaired with nonabsorbable suture.
10. Maintain patient privacy during transfer and positioning procedures.
11. The "lawn chair" position is the most popular for rotator cuff repair. The patient lies supine on the OR bed with the head raised to a semi-Fowler's height and the knees flexed about 40 degrees. If preferred, a 5-pound sandbag is placed under the operative scapula. The operative extremity should then be suspended for surgical preparation.

FIG. 12-7
CARE PLAN FOR ROTATOR CUFF REPAIR

KEY ASSESSMENT POINTS

General physical and mental condition
Presence of chronic health problems
Pain, tenderness, muscle spasm
Limitations in mobility/atrophy
Range of motion
Color, warmth, pulses in affected extremity
Understanding of procedure
Understanding of rehabilitation
Anxiety

NURSING DIAGNOSIS

All generic nursing diagnoses apply to this patient, with the addition of:

High risk for sensory/perceptual alteration (kinesthetic)
Impaired physical mobility
Pain

PATIENT OUTCOMES

All generic outcomes apply, with the addition of:
The patient will maintain kinesthetic sensation/perception and adequate range of motion in affected extremity.
Patient will maintain optimal neurovascular status and mobility in the affected arm as evidenced by:
1. Absence of paresthesias
2. Adequate peripheral pulses
3. Warmth of the extremity
4. Quick capillary refill of the fingers
5. Intact movement and sensation of the upper extremity
6. Minimal edema
Pain will be controlled/minimized as evidenced by:
1. Participation in rehabilitation
2. Satisfactory range of motion
3. Ability to resume normal activities

NURSING ACTIONS

	Yes	No	N/A
1. Patient identified?	☐	☐	☐
2. Consent verified as correct?	☐	☐	☐
3. Patient aware of the type of anesthesia?	☐	☐	☐
4. Allergies verified?	☐	☐	☐
5. Preoperative antibiotics given?	☐	☐	☐
6. Neurovascular assessment completed?	☐	☐	☐
7. Diagnostic studies, including CT, MRI, or x-rays, available?	☐	☐	☐
8. Laboratory studies reviewed and findings reported?	☐	☐	☐
9. Instruments and equipment available and functional?	☐	☐	☐
10. Privacy maintained?	☐	☐	☐
11. Patient positioned safely per physician preference?	☐	☐	☐
12. Electrosurgical dispersive pad placed and skin assessed?	☐	☐	☐
13. Safety strap placed?	☐	☐	☐
14. Local anesthetic delivered to field and medications labeled?	☐	☐	☐
15. Safety and protective measures initiated/documented?	☐	☐	☐
16. Dressings secured?	☐	☐	☐
17. Neurovascular status evaluated and documented?	☐	☐	☐
18. Skin integrity evaluated in pressure areas and beneath the electrosurgical dispersive pad?	☐	☐	☐
19. Patient transferred to the postoperative area safely and patient care information communicated?	☐	☐	☐

Document additional nursing actions/generic care plans initiated here:

_____

_____

_____

EVALUATION OF PATIENT OUTCOMES

	Outcome met	Outcome met with additional outcome criteria	Outcome met with revised nursing care plan	Outcome not met	Outcome not applicable to this patient
1. Kinesthetic sensation/perception and mobility were maintained in the affected extremity.	☐	☐	☐	☐	☐
2. Pain was effectively controlled.	☐	☐	☐	☐	☐
3. The patient met outcomes for additional generic care plans as indicated.	☐	☐	☐	☐	☐

Signature: _____ Date: _____

12. Place the electrosurgical dispersive pad close to the operative site. Note the condition of the skin at the site of pad placement.
13. Place the safety strap 2 inches above the patient's knees.
14. A local anesthetic containing epinephrine may be injected. All medications on the sterile field should be labeled; administration should be documented.
15. Document safety and protective measures including counts, patient needs, and positioning.
16. Apply and secure sterile dressings. A shoulder immobilizer is placed on the operative arm to ensure that the forearm rests across the upper abdomen securely and that motion of the shoulder joint is limited.
17. Evaluate and document changes in neurovascular status.
18. Check skin integrity under pressure points and the electrosurgical dispersive pad.
19. Transfer the patient to the postanesthesia care unit with the operative arm adducted across the upper abdomen. Communicate patient status and information to the postanesthesia care unit staff.

Lumbar Laminectomy (Posterior with or without Implants) (Fig. 12-8)

Laminectomy involves removal of the vertebral lamina for exposure of spinal structures. The procedure may be done via a posterior approach or a combination of anterior/posterior. The procedure is used for correction of herniated nucleus pulposus, spinal cord compression, or fracture.

1. The patient should state his or her name, the operative procedure, and site. This should correspond with the patient's hospital number on the chart and the patient's identification band. The operative permit should be signed for a lumbar laminectomy. The permit should include information related to bone graft or placement of hardware.
2. Verify the level of decompression with the patient to plan the location of the incision site. The patient should state the location of pain radiation; pain will indicate the level of decompression. If this is unclear, clarify the level with the surgeon.
3. Note any drug allergies or sensitivities to topical preparations such as those containing iodine. Verify that preoperative antibiotics have been given if ordered.
4. The patient should have an understanding of anesthesia. The patient may be intubated awake to help move himself or herself into the prone position on the surgical bed.
5. Review laboratory values and diagnostic studies. Report variations from normal as indicated.
6. Obtain diagnostic studies such as x-ray films, CT, and MRI scans, and myelograms for referral during surgery.
7. Blood replacement therapy should be considered in the event blood products are required.
8. An accurate neurovascular assessment should be obtained preoperatively to use as a level of comparison with the postoperative assessment. Note any sensory impairments, numbness, or tingling, as well as the color, temperature, and movement of the legs and feet. Pulses are checked in all areas.
9. Obtain positioning aids needed for the lumbar laminectomy patient, including the laminectomy frame or bed, chest rolls or blocks, and pillows. The patient's size should be assessed to determine correct use of these aids. They should be placed on the OR bed before patient transfer.
10. Ensure that an adequate number of personnel are available to assist with the safe transfer of the patient from the stretcher to the OR bed. A minimum of one person is required to move the head, two on either side, and one at the foot.
11. The Foley catheter may be inserted before patient transfer to the prone position. Use aseptic technique for catheter insertion. Prevent kinks or undue tension on the catheter during transfer and check the patency of the drainage system after positioning. Document urinary output as well as catheter insertion.
12. Logroll the patient slowly from the stretcher to the OR bed. Maintain the patient's privacy. If a laminectomy frame is not being used, place rolls from the shoulders to the iliac crests under the patient to allow for chest expansion and free movement of the diaphragm.
13. Check pressure areas and provide protection. Women's breasts should be free from pressure, and men's genitalia should be positioned freely between the legs. The patient's head is turned to one side and a foam cushion is placed beneath to protect the ear. The integrity of the endotracheal airway is monitored. Protect each knee with padding to reduce patellar pressure. Place a pillow under the ankles to prevent plantar flexion of the feet and to eliminate pressure on the toes. The arms are placed on padded armboards at less than a 90-degree angle and then abducted with the elbows flexed and palms downward. Place the safety strap around the patient's thighs and secure it as appropriate.
14. Place the electrosurgical dispersive pad on the posterior thigh or other muscular area near the

FIG. 12-8
CARE PLAN FOR LUMBAR LAMINECTOMY

KEY ASSESSMENT POINTS
General physical and mental condition
Other relevant health problems/medical diagnoses*
Back pain (location, severity)*
Pain radiation in the leg*
Other pain locations*
Mobility limitations*
Suffering/depression from symptoms*
Reduced work ability*
Type of work/job level*
Social support systems*
Neurovascular status
Understanding of procedure and its objectives
Allergies
Preoperative antibiotic therapy
*Recommended by Junge, Dvorak, & Ahrens. (1995). Predictors of bad and good outcomes of lumbar disc surgery. *Spine, 20*(4), 460-468.

NURSING DIAGNOSIS
All generic nursing diagnoses apply to this patient, with the addition of:
High risk for infection
Impaired physical mobility
High risk for injury
Altered peripheral tissue perfusion
Pain
Ineffective breathing pattern

PATIENT OUTCOMES
All generic outcomes apply, with the addition of:
Patient does not experience infection as evidenced by absence of elevated temperature, redness, drainage.
Physical mobility returns postoperatively as evidenced by return to normal activities.
Patient does not experience injury as demonstrated by postoperative recovery and return of sensation, movement.
Peripheral tissue perfusion maintained as evidenced by presence of pulses, warmth of extremities, capillary refill.
Pain is not experienced postoperatively as evidenced by vital signs within normal limits, return to activities, and minimal discomfort immediately postoperatively.
Patient will be free of respiratory compromise related to ineffective breathing patterns created by positioning as evidenced by vital signs within normal limits, adequate oxygen saturation, and adequate respiratory excursion.

NURSING ACTIONS

	Yes	No	N/A
1. Patient identified?	☐	☐	☐
2. Surgical site and plan of care verified?	☐	☐	☐
3. Allergies verified?	☐	☐	☐
4. Patient verbalizes understanding of anesthetic?	☐	☐	☐
5. Laboratory values and diagnostic studies reviewed; abnormal values reported?	☐	☐	☐
6. Diagnostic studies obtained?	☐	☐	☐
7. Blood replacement products obtained?	☐	☐	☐
8. Neurovascular assessment completed?	☐	☐	☐
9. Positioning aids obtained appropriate for the procedure and the patient?	☐	☐	☐
10. Personnel available for safe transfer?	☐	☐	☐
11. Urinary catheter inserted using aseptic technique, ensuring patency?	☐	☐	☐
12. Patient transferred safely, providing protection?	☐	☐	☐
13. Patient positioned safely; using positioning devices and ensuring physiologic status maintained?	☐	☐	☐
14. Electrosurgical dispersive pad placed?	☐	☐	☐
15. Patient thermoregulation maintained?	☐	☐	☐

NURSING ACTIONS—cont'd

	Yes	No	N/A
16. Skin preparation completed?	☐	☐	☐
17. Blood loss monitored, reported, and documented?	☐	☐	☐
18. Safety and protective measures documented?	☐	☐	☐
19. Specimens handled according to protocol?	☐	☐	☐
20. Patency of drains maintained; drains secured?	☐	☐	☐
21. Dressings secured?	☐	☐	☐
22. Skin integrity and pressure points assessed?	☐	☐	☐
23. Postoperative neurovascular status assessed?	☐	☐	☐
24. Patient transferred safely, with adequate number of personnel?	☐	☐	☐
25. Patient transferred safely; postoperative evaluation communicated?	☐	☐	☐

Document additional nursing actions/generic care plans initiated here:

_____

_____

_____

EVALUATION OF PATIENT OUTCOMES

	Outcome met	Outcome met with additional outcome criteria	Outcome met with revised nursing care plan	Outcome not met	Outcome not applicable to this patient
1. There were no signs of surgical site infection.	☐	☐	☐	☐	☐
2. There were no complications related to immobility.	☐	☐	☐	☐	☐
3. There was satisfactory range of motion with intact motor function and sensation.	☐	☐	☐	☐	☐
4. Peripheral tissue perfusion was adequate.	☐	☐	☐	☐	☐
5. Pain was relieved.	☐	☐	☐	☐	☐
6. Respiratory function was satisfactory.	☐	☐	☐	☐	☐
7. The patient met outcomes for additional care plans as indicated.	☐	☐	☐	☐	☐

Signature: _____ Date: _____

incision site. Note condition of skin at the site of pad placement.

15. Cover the patient with warm blankets; expose only the area to be prepped.
16. Complete the skin prep; the anatomic area of surgical preparation will vary according to the level of planned decompression.
17. The circulating nurse should monitor, report, and record blood loss.
18. Document safety and protective measures including assessment data, counts, positioning needs, and hardware placement.
19. Follow institutional protocol for the preservation and disposition of specimens.
20. Maintain the patency of drains. Ensure suction, and secure the drain and suction apparatus to the patient's dressing. Document the presence of drains.
21. Apply and secure sterile dressings.
22. Skin integrity should be assessed beneath the electrosurgical dispersive pad and at pressure points. Document the results of the evaluation.
23. Assess postoperative neurovascular status and document the findings.
24. Ensure that an adequate number of personnel are available to transfer the patient from the OR bed back to the stretcher. Ensure the drain is secured and not kinked following transfer to the bed.
25. Transfer the patient to the postoperative area. Communicate evaluation information and patient status to the postanesthesia care unit staff.

Anterior Cervical Discectomy (Fig. 12-9)

An anterior cervical fusion will be completed for patients experiencing cervical spondylosis, herniated disc, or cervical lesions. A bone graft may be autograft, allograft, or freeze dried.

1. Identification is made by asking the patient to state his or her name, operative procedure, and physician. The operative permit should be complete, and hospital identification should correspond with the information stated by the patient.
2. The patient's chart is reviewed and symptoms verified. Diagnostic procedures and results of laboratory studies should be obtained.
3. The psychologic and social support systems of the patient should be determined.
4. Because of the nature of the symptoms, patients may express concerns related to the outcome of the procedure. Preoperative teaching should begin at the time the patient determines a surgical procedure is required. The rehabilitation requires cooperation and an understanding by the patient. Immediate postoperative expectations should also be confirmed. The postoperative expectations, including use of a brace postoperatively, responses if there is difficulty breathing, or pain, numbness around the ears or neck, and expected outcomes should be discussed.
5. The physical status should be assessed. Range of motion, pain, and discomfort of the neck and upper extremity is attained to protect the patient during transfer and positioning. Skin integrity, strength of the extremity, and presence or absence of pulses are assessed as a preoperative baseline. The information is documented.
6. Administration of preoperative instructions/orders is verified. Preoperative skin shave and/or scrub instructions may have been given to the patient. Verify that this has been completed. Note the condition of the incision site. Antibiotics may have been ordered to be given before admission to the operating room. Measurements for a cervical collar should have been determined.
7. The patient should verbalize an understanding of the type of anesthesia to be administered and postoperative pain management.
8. Positioning needs are determined and supplies obtained. The goal of positioning is to hyperextend the cervical spine without causing complications. The head may be positioned on a horseshoe headrest and traction placed on the wrists for retraction to expose the area.
9. Equipment function should be validated. Power equipment, microscope, video equipment, and supplies for bone graft placement or plate/screw placement might be used. Use of the image intensifier requires notification of the radiology technician, availability of protective aprons/shields for personnel and the patient, and drapes for the C-arm.
10. The patient is moved to the OR bed maintaining alignment during transfer and positioning. Patient privacy is protected and body temperature is maintained. The safety strap is secured.
11. Output is monitored and documented throughout the procedure by measuring blood loss and urinary output if appropriate. A Foley catheter is inserted preoperatively using aseptic technique per order. The drainage bag is placed in a location where output can be visualized. Blood loss in sponges is monitored as they are counted.
12. The supine position is attained. Cervical traction may be applied or a method of applying traction on the arms may be secured.
13. The patient is protected by placing the electrosurgical dispersive pad in a muscular area, free of abrasions, rash, or breaks in the skin, and

FIG. 12-9
CARE PLAN FOR ANTERIOR CERVICAL DISCECTOMY

KEY ASSESSMENT POINTS

Peripheral pulses
Skin integrity
Limitation of movement, area of radiating pain, sensation
Range of motion
Preoperative antibiotic therapy
Patient understanding of the surgical procedure and outcome
Patient understanding of immediate surgical complications to report

NURSING DIAGNOSIS

All generic nursing diagnoses apply to this patient, with the addition
of:
High risk for infection
Impaired physical mobility
High risk for injury
Altered peripheral tissue perfusion
Pain
Ineffective breathing pattern

PATIENT OUTCOMES

All generic outcomes apply, with the addition of:
Patient does not experience infection as evidenced by absence of elevated temperature, redness, drainage.
Physical mobility returns postoperatively as evidenced by ability to move extremities, return to normal activities.
Patient does not experience injury as demonstrated by postoperative recovery and return of sensation, movement.
Peripheral tissue perfusion maintained as evidenced by presence of pulses, warmth of extremities, capillary refill.
Pain is not experienced postoperatively as evidenced by vital signs within normal limits, return to activities, and minimal discomfort immediately postoperatively.
Patient will be free of respiratory compromise related to ineffective breathing patterns created by edema following surgical procedure as evidenced by vital signs within normal limits, adequate oxygen saturation, and adequate respiratory excursion.

NURSING ACTIONS

	Yes	No	N/A
1. Patient identified?	☐	☐	☐
2. Symptoms, diagnostic studies and plan of care verified?	☐	☐	☐
3. Psychosocial and support system verified?	☐	☐	☐
4. Patient verbalizes understanding of the surgical procedure, postoperative expectations, and rehabilitation?	☐	☐	☐
5. Physical status assessed including range of motion, skin integrity, extremity strength, and presence of pulses?	☐	☐	☐
6. Preoperative orders verified and completed?	☐	☐	☐
7. Patient verbalizes an understanding of the anesthesia?	☐	☐	☐
8. Positioning supplies obtained; functional and appropriate for the procedure and patient?	☐	☐	☐
9. Equipment obtained and verified as functional?	☐	☐	☐
10. Personnel available for safe transfer?	☐	☐	☐
11. Urinary catheter inserted using aseptic technique, ensuring patency?	☐	☐	☐
12. Patient positioned safely; using positioning devices and ensuring physiologic status maintained?	☐	☐	☐

NURSING ACTIONS—cont'd

	Yes	No	N/A
13. Electrosurgical dispersive pad placed?	☐	☐	☐
14. Skin preparation completed?	☐	☐	☐
15. Patient condition monitored throughout the procedure?	☐	☐	☐
16. Dressings and cervical collar applied?	☐	☐	☐
17. Skin integrity assessed?	☐	☐	☐
18. Postoperative neurovascular integrity assessed?	☐	☐	☐
19. Patient transferred safely with adequate number of personnel?	☐	☐	☐
20. Patient observed for airway patency?	☐	☐	☐

Document additional nursing actions/generic care plans initiated here:

_____

_____

_____

EVALUATION OF PATIENT OUTCOMES

	Outcome met	Outcome met with additional outcome criteria	Outcome met with revised nursing care plan	Outcome not met	Outcome not applicable to this patient
1. There were no signs of surgical site infection.	☐	☐	☐	☐	☐
2. There were no complications related to immobility.	☐	☐	☐	☐	☐
3. There was satisfactory ROM with intact motor function and sensation.	☐	☐	☐	☐	☐
4. Peripheral tissue perfusion was adequate.	☐	☐	☐	☐	☐
5. Pain was relieved.	☐	☐	☐	☐	☐
6. Respiratory function was satisfactory.	☐	☐	☐	☐	☐
7. The patient met outcomes for additional care plans as indicated.	☐	☐	☐	☐	☐

Signature: _____ Date: _____

FIG. 12-10
CARE PLAN FOR SURGERY OF THE HAND

KEY ASSESSMENT POINTS
Peripheral pulses
Sensation, warmth, and strength of the extremity
Patient understanding of rehabilitation

NURSING DIAGNOSIS
All generic nursing diagnoses apply to this patient, with the addition of:
Altered tissue perfusion
High risk for impaired peripheral neurovascular function
Impaired physical mobility

PATIENT OUTCOMES
All generic outcomes apply, with the addition of:
The patient will maintain peripheral neurovascular function as evidenced by presence of intact sensation and movement of the affected extremity and absence of parasthesia.
The patient will maintain adequate tissue perfusion as evidenced by presence of peripheral pulses, warmth of extremity, and capillary refill.
The patient will participate in the rehabilitation and therapy.
The patient will experience restored mobility as evidenced by return of function.

NURSING ACTIONS

	Yes	No	N/A
1. Patient identified?	☐	☐	☐
2. Patient verbalizes an understanding of the anesthetic?	☐	☐	☐
3. Patient awareness of rehabilitation?	☐	☐	☐
4. Allergies verified?	☐	☐	☐
5. Neurovascular assessment completed?	☐	☐	☐
6. Instruments and equipment obtained and function verified?	☐	☐	☐
7. Patient transferred and privacy maintained?	☐	☐	☐
8. Patient positioned safely, with access to the surgical site?	☐	☐	☐
9. Tissues protected during the surgical procedure?	☐	☐	☐
10. Safety and protective measures documented?	☐	☐	☐
11. Dressings applied and secured?	☐	☐	☐
12. Postoperative neurovascular assessment completed and compared to preoperative status?	☐	☐	☐
13. Transfer to postoperative area safe and patient evaluation communicated?	☐	☐	☐

Document additional nursing actions/generic care plans initiated here:

_____

_____

_____

EVALUATION OF PATIENT OUTCOMES

	Outcome met	Outcome met with additional outcome criteria	Outcome met with revised nursing care plan	Outcome not met	Outcome not applicable to this patient
1. Neurovascular status was intact.	☐	☐	☐	☐	☐
2. Peripheral tissue perfusion was adequate.	☐	☐	☐	☐	☐
3. Participation in rehabilitation was satisfactory.	☐	☐	☐	☐	☐
4. Mobility and function was restored.	☐	☐	☐	☐	☐
5. The patient met outcomes for additional care plans as indicated.	☐	☐	☐	☐	☐

Signature: _____ Date: _____

close to the surgical site. Prominent bony areas such as elbows and heels are padded. Radial pulses are checked for comparison postoperatively in the event traction is applied intraoperatively.

14. The surgical site is prepped. Pooling of solutions beneath the shoulders should be prevented.

15. Throughout the procedure, attention is paid to the patient's condition. The procedure requires close proximity to the vasculature and spinal cord.

16. Dressings are applied and secured loosely. A drain may be placed before closure of the incision. Ensure the tubing is secured and not kinked. A cervical collar or brace is applied.

17. Skin integrity is assessed, including pressure points, skin beneath the electrosurgical dispersive pad, and around the surgical site. The wrists are assessed if traction is used.

18. Neurovascular integrity is evaluated. Pulses and extremity warmth are evaluated. Mobility is assessed as soon as possible postoperatively to determine possible spinal cord edema or trauma.

19. Adequate numbers of personnel are available for turning, positioning, and transfer to the bed. The patient is moved slowly, maintaining body alignment. The head of bed is elevated, and the patient is transferred to the postoperative area. Patient information is communicated to the postanesthesia care unit staff.

20. The patient is observed closely for 24 hours to ensure that the airway is maintained.

Surgery of the Hand (Fig. 12-10)

Hand procedures may require soft tissue instrumentation or include bone involvement. Numerous procedures are completed on the hand, resulting in application of general orthopedic principles to the extremity. Procedures might be closed or open; may require the use of the microscope or loupes to repair tendons, nerves, or vasculature; or may require implantation of hardware. With improvements in instrumentation and technical refinements, endoscopic methods, currently being evaluated for carpal release, may become state of the art (Murray, 1994).

1. The patient is identified by stating his or her name, surgeon's name, operative procedure, and side. The operative permit should be complete, and hospital identification should correspond with the information stated by the patient.

2. The patient should verbalize an understanding of the type of anesthesia to be used and what to expect during the surgical procedure. A Bier block may be used; the procedure should be explained to the patient.

3. The patient should be assessed for an awareness and understanding of postoperative activities and orthotics. Reinforced teaching is important to promote patient compliance.

4. Note any drug allergies and sensitivities. Verify that preoperative antibiotics have been administered, if ordered, before surgery.

5. Assess and document preoperative neurovascular assessment. Note color, capillary refill, temperature, sensory impairments, and mobility.

6. Prepare instruments and equipment and check their function before surgery. Bipolar electrosurgery equipment, microscope, power equipment, and tourniquet are frequently used. Accessory items should be available before the start of surgery. These include hand table and positioning aids.

7. Patient privacy should be maintained during transfer and positioning procedures.

8. The patient is placed in the supine position with the operative hand resting on the hand table. The opposite hand is placed on a padded armboard at an angle less than 90 degrees. A tourniquet is usually placed high on the operative extremity. The pressure should be set according to the surgeon's specifications. For skin preparation, a positioning device that elevates the operative arm above the hand table (or personnel) will be needed. Document tourniquet cuff placement, pressure settings, inflation and deflation times, and unit identification number. The safety strap should be placed 2 inches above the patient's knees and secured.

9. If possible, the operative hand should be slightly elevated during surgery to decrease edema. The tissues should be kept moist to prevent dryness caused by use of a tourniquet.

10. Document safety and protective measures taken for the patient, including the results of counts.

11. Dressings are applied and secured. Hand surgery often requires postoperative immobilization with a cast or splint. Orthotic devices may be fit at a later time.

12. Compare preoperative and postoperative neurovascular assessments and document any changes.

13. Transfer the patient to the postanesthesia area, ensuring that the patient's hand is elevated during transfer. Communicate patient care information to the postanesthesia care unit staff.

References

Abelow S. (1993). Lasers in orthopaedic surgery: Current concepts. *Orthopaedics, 6*:5, 551-553.

Arlington RG, et al. (1992). Postoperative orthopaedic blood salvage and reinfusion. *Orthopedic Nursing, 11*:3. 30-38.

Association of Operating Room Nurses. (1995). *Standards and recommended practices for perioperative nursing.* Denver: The Association.

Bichat X. (1814). *Desault's surgery.* Philadelphia: Thomas Dobson.

Brown MD & Seltzer DG. (1991). Perioperative care in lumbar spine surgery. *Orthopedic Clinics of North America, 22:2,* 353-358.

Bullough VL & Bullough B. (1969). *The emergence of modern nursing.* London: MacMillan.

Callahan CM, Drake BG, & Heck DA. (1994). Patient outcomes following tricompartmental total knee replacement. *Journal of the American Medical Association, 271*(17), 1349-1357.

Cavendish RC. (1994). Fractures requiring traction. *Nursing Spectrum, 14*(6), 12-14.

Chapman MW. (1993). *Operative orthopaedics.* (2nd Ed., Vol. 1). Philadelphia: J.B. Lippincott.

Day LJ, et al. (1988). Orthopedics. In LW Way (Ed.). *Current surgical diagnosis and treatment.* Norwalk, CT: Appleton & Lange.

Dolan JA. (1968). *History of nursing.* Philadelphia: WB Saunders.

Drez D, et al. (1991). Sepsis in orthopaedic surgery. *Orthopaedics, 14:2.* 157-62.

Evarts CM. (1992). *Surgery of the musculoskeletal system.* New York: Churchill Livingstone.

Fitzgerald S. (1995, March 24). "Liquid bone" could repair breaks faster and less painfully. *The Philadelphia Inquirer,* pp. A1-A2.

Garner BD. (1995). Infection control. In MH Meeker & JC Rothrock (Eds.), *Alexander's care of the patient in surgery* (10th Ed.). St. Louis: Mosby.

Hester RA & Nelson CL. (1991). Current concepts review: Methods to reduce intraoperative transmission of blood-borne disease. *Journal of Bone and Joint Surgery, 73*-A, 7, 1108-1111.

Johnson DP. (1990). The effect of continuous pressure monitor on wound healing and joint mobility after knee arthroplasty. *Journal of Bone and Joint Surgery, 72,* 421-426.

Jones L & Brooks J. (1990). The ABC's of PCA. *RN, 20:5.* 54-63.

Junge A, Dvorak J, & Ahrens S. (1995). Predictors of bad and good outcomes of lumbar disc surgery. *Spine, 20*(4), 460-468.

Kaempfee MD, et al. (1990). Intermittent pneumatic compression versus coumadin: Prevention of deep vein thrombosis in lower-extremity total joint arthroplasty. *Clinical Orthopedics and Related Research, 269,* 89-97.

Keeling MM, et al. (1993). Autotransfusion in the postoperative orthopaedic patient. *Clinical Orthopedics and Related Research, 291,* 251-258.

Keil OR. (1995). Joint Commission Update: Equipment management in the environment of care. *Biomedical Instrumentation and Technology, 29*(2), 108-111.

Mac HL, et al. (1993). Comparison of autoreinfusion and standard drainage systems in total joint arthroplasty patients. *Orthopedic Nursing, 12:3,* 19-25.

McQuarrie DG, et al. (1990). Laminar airflow systems: Issues surrounding their effectiveness. *AORN Journal, 51:4.* 1035-1047.

Michelson SA. (1990). A laser primer for orthopaedic nurses. *Orthopedic Nursing, 9:5.* 57-59.

Mubarak SJ. (1993). Compartment syndromes. In MW Chapman (Ed.), *Operative orthopaedics.* Philadelphia: JB Lippincott.

Murray DG. (1994). What's new in orthopaedic surgery. *ACS Bulletin, 79*(1), 51-52.

Pynsent P, et al. (1993). *Outcome measures in orthopaedics.* London: Butterworth-Heinemann.

Slye DA. (1991). Orthopaedic complications: Compartment syndrome, fat embolism syndrome and venous thromboembolism. *Nursing Clinics of North America, 26:1.* 113-132.

Smith J. (1990). Applying the continuous passive motion device. *Orthopedic Nursing, 9:3* 54.

Taylor CJS. (1990). Perioperative wound infection in elective orthopaedic surgery. *Journal of Hospital Infection Control, 16,* 241-247.

Timmons ME & Bower FL. (1993). The effect of structured preoperative teaching on patients' use of patient-controlled analgesia (PCA) and their management of pain. *Orthopedic Nursing, 12:1,* 23-31.

Watt I. (1991). Magnetic resonance imaging in orthopaedics. *Journal of Bone and Joint Surgery, 73*B, 4, 539-550.

Weigand S. (1995). Osteoporosis. *Nursing Spectrum, 4*(6), 12-13.

Woodin L. (1993). Cutting postoperative pain. *RN, 56:8,* 26-34.

Chapter 13

Gynecologic Surgery

Christine E. Smith

If Levret has justly acquired great reputation by advancing first in a path hitherto unknown, (I mean in passing the ligature round the polypi in the internal surface of the uterus,) he has given us no anatomical details, such as might have been acquired by examining the bodies of women who have died of this disease. Those who have followed have been charged with the same indifference; or more probably, for want of favorable opportunities, their writings represent the same void.

BICHAT, 1814

Although it is not clearly known when gynecology became a part of medicine, descriptions of anatomy by Leonardo Da Vinci, Andreas Vesalius, Gabriel Fallopio, and Julius Arantius in the sixteenth century laid important foundations for the future role of gynecologic surgery. Mystique surrounding the female reproductive system persisted for many years. Victorian notions of propriety hampered efforts to improve the health care of women. Customs of those times prohibited examinations of female patients by male physicians. Even in the middle of the nineteenth century, the vaginal speculum was used only in indicated cases, never in routine examinations. Nurse midwives played a significant role in the early development of knowledge regarding illness of females and influenced provisions of access to health care. The perioperative nurse is challenged to understand current issues that affect women's health care and to translate knowledge of nursing care standards and changing scientific trends to offer holistic, compassionate perioperative nursing care of excellent quality.

GYNECOLOGIC SURGERY: PAST AND PRESENT

The past often yields important direction for the future. Today's gynecologic surgical suite is characterized in part by its heritage from the past. Problems with patients and their care have been identified and overcome, and new problems and risks have been encountered.

Historical Perspective

Information on early gynecologic examinations as far back as Hippocrates' time describe the cervices of pregnant women. The use of the speculum for visualizing the reproductive tract has been described in historical medical writings; specula that might have been used for intravaginal examination have been discovered at the ruins of Pompeii. Egyptian papyri reveal descriptions of abortifacients and contraceptives. Historical descriptions of the irregularities accompanying menstruation and their assumed causes have been well chronicled. Anatomic descriptions of the child in utero, pelvic deformities, and tubes extending from the uterus contributed to the emerging field of obstetrics and gynecology. For many centuries the midwife was society's gynecologist and obstetrician. She was the confidante of women; she, rather than the physician, was consulted on problems with menstruation, abdominal pain, abnormal vaginal discharges, and abnormal child-birthing. As knowledge increased regarding female anatomy and its abnormalities, surgeons began to develop techniques of abdominal and pelvic surgery. According to Sigerist (1960), the gynecologist had two ancestors; the surgeon was his father and the midwife his mother. From the father he inherited techniques, knowledge, and skills; from the mother he received the human touch.

Early records of pelvic surgery describe a cesarean section performed by Jesse Bennett, a physician in Staunton, Virginia, in 1794. His wife was in her first pregnancy and was unable to deliver vaginally because of a contracted pelvis. When a craniotomy was advised, she convinced her husband to attempt a cesarean section. Bennett placed his wife on a crude plank table over two barrels and administered a large dose of opium. He was assisted in surgery by two women. After delivery of the baby and placenta, he removed the ovaries to prevent future pregnancies. He closed the wounds with stout linen thread. Mrs. Bennett survived, and their daughter lived to be 77 years old.

Abdominal surgery is often ascribed as having begun in the backwoods of Kentucky by an intelligent and confident surgeon, Ephram McDowell (Pratt, 1977). He was a pioneer of abdominal surgery whose techniques were rapidly developed after the discovery of anesthetics and the introduction of Lister's theories of antisepsis. At the time of his first successful removal of a large ovarian tumor, he did not know about antisepsis and was without supportive therapy or anesthesia. According to Pratt, McDowell published a report of his first ovariotomy in 1809. From the pelvis of Mrs. Jane Todd Crawford, he removed a 7-pound ovarian tumor. She survived the surgery and lived another 30 years.

Although tubal ligation was originally proposed to prevent the necessity of repeat cesarean sections, efficient and effective surgical approaches to sterilization did not occur until the last years of the nineteenth century, with the refinement of laparoscopy. Early endoscopic efforts actually began in 1805 when Bozzini of Frankfurt visualized the interior of the human urethra with a candle; he was reprimanded for his curiosity. The clinical application of laparoscopy began in the early 1900s by Kelling of Germany and Jacobeus of Sweden. Since these beginnings, techniques and approaches such as culdoscopy, hysteroscopy, and minilaparotomy have become common.

Advances in Gynecologic Surgery

The numerous developments in the progress of operative gynecology expand the options available to women who desire and need surgical intervention for their health maintenance. Certain areas of gynecology, such as oncology, endocrinology, laparoscopy, and infertility, have produced specialists committed to advancement and scientific progress within their specialty. Because of these groups, gynecology has seen a surge of new trends and techniques in each of these areas within the past few years. The perioperative nurse practicing in the gynecologic surgical setting is likewise obliged to increase and expand his or her scientific nursing knowledge base and clinical skill to deliver safe, efficient, and competent patient care and protect the patient from real and perceived risks inherent in all levels of surgery. Critical to the delivery of highly technical procedures with their requisite advanced skills and complex equipment is the nurse's commitment to compassionate and humanistic nursing care attitudes and behaviors.

Infertility. An exciting gynecologic operative trend offers women or couples unable to conceive selected options for retrieval of oocytes from the ovary, fertilization in vitro with sperm, and reimplantation of the fertilized oocytes into the uterus. Gamete intrafallopian transfer (GIFT) technique, an alternative to in vitro fertilization, has successfully been used for women with long-standing infertility who have at least one patent fallopian tube. Oocyte retrieval for GIFT is being performed in the operating room (OR) suite by laparoscopy, minilaparotomy, or vaginal aspiration under ultrasound guidance; ultrasound-directed egg retrieval has made this procedure simpler and more economical (Wilbanks, 1991). Tubal reconstructive surgery corrects defects in tubal patency caused by stenosis from adhesions, pelvic disease, and prior surgical tubal ligation.

Lasers. The role of lasers has and will continue to be a significant factor in improving the cost, morbidity, and efficiency of gynecologic surgery. The advantages of lasers are well known and documented in perioperative nursing literature. They offer precision, instant hemostasis, and have minimal tissue effects. There is decreased mechanical manipulation of anatomic structures and peripheral damage to healthy tissue. Thus surgery is accomplished with less pain, scar formation, and edema. Lasers commonly being used in gynecologic procedures include the carbon dioxide, argon, neodymium:yttrium aluminum garnet (Nd:YAG), and frequency-doubled YAG. Perioperative applications are numerous.

Lasers are being used for infertility surgery for adhesiolysis, anastomosis, and implantation; in neosalpingostomies, ovarian wedge resections, myomectomies, and treatment of endometriosis; and in ectopic pregnancies with segmental excision. Endometrial ablation via the hysteroscope for the treatment of dysfunctional uterine bleeding can now be achieved with laser application (Verrell, 1995). The Nd:YAG laser is used to photocoagulate the endometrium; photocoagulation can control some cases of chronic menorrhagia and possibly prevent the need for hysterectomy. The Nd:YAG may become the gynecologic laser of the future.

Endoscopic advances. Along with culdoscopy, laparoscopy, and culposcopy, hysteroscopy has become a diagnostic tool for evaluation of the intrauterine tissue. The panoramic hysteroscope has been found to be most advantageous, permitting direct visualization of all aspects of the uterine cavity. It has been used for removal of intrauterine devices, removal of polyps, resection of submucous fibroids, lysis of adhesions, and resection of septums as well as for diagnostic intervention in infertility and unexplained bleeding.

Pelviscopy is a fast-growing and safe alternative to abdominal surgery for many procedures. Using a curved, 30-degree angled scope, both endocoagulation and endoligation may be accomplished; ovarian biopsy, ovarian cyst enucleation and resection, oophorectomy, adnexectomy, enucleation of intramural myomas, appendectomy, fimbrioplasty, and removal of tubal pregnancy are procedures that can be performed through a pelviscope. Gynecologic procedures traditionally accomplished through an abdominal approach continue to lend themselves to laparoscopic techniques in total or as an assisted adjunct to a vaginal approach. These techniques offer the patient obvious advantages to open procedures when used prudently and may carry less morbidity (Summit, et al., 1992).

ASSESSMENT CONSIDERATIONS

Comprehensive, individualized perioperative care planning is dependent on patient assessment. The data collected for gynecologic surgery patients will be obtained through review of the nursing and medical history and physical examination results on the medical record. A review of this previously collected information allows the perioperative nurse to analyze, synthesize, prioritize, confirm, and validate information on which to base the perioperative care plan. Gynecologic patient assessment includes a comprehensive history and physical examination; the results of these will be interpreted within the focus area of the planned surgical intervention and related patient care needs. Communication skills will facilitate the nurse/patient exchange of valuable information; it is the responsibility of the nurse to initiate a relationship with the patient in which trust can be developed (Rorden & Taft, 1990). The patient will respond positively to being treated with respect as an individual with demonstration of a concerned and caring attitude by the nurse interviewer. Women generally view well-being as a component of their overall health, are knowledgeable, and articulate about their health status. Hartweg (1993) investigated and described deliberately performed self-care actions that a sample of healthy middle-aged women use to promote well-being. An unexpected finding revealed the importance of diagnostic testing in this group's health construct as improving well-being. The nursing role must acknowledge the personal and complex nature of the individual woman's self-care system, develop trust through tactful honesty, and convey a willingness to share oneself with others.

Key Assessment Points

Key assessment points will guide and focus the perioperative nurse's interview and investigation of the patient to retrieve data pertinent to the formulation of an accurate and individualized plan of care and efficiently utilize the abbreviated time frame that the nurse and patient share before the surgery. These cues both arise from and determine the generic and specific nursing diagnoses particular to gynecologic surgery patients.

> Bleeding history
> Menstrual cycle
> Hormone replacement therapy
> Contraceptive history
> Maternal diethylstilbestrol therapy
> Allergies and/or sensitivities
> Skin integrity
> Positional considerations
> Core body temperature
> Abdominal girth
> Full stomach/last meal
> Vaginal infection
> Sexually transmitted disease (STD) risk/history
> Hemodynamic status
> Anxiety level
> Rh factor status
> Continence status
> Pain/discomfort
> Knowledge of diagnosis/intended intervention

Patient History

The assessment begins with a thorough medical and social history. During this time, important nursing behaviors include providing a supportive and open environment. This is especially important for the perioperative nurse, for whom time is short to establish rapport with the patient. The following should be reviewed for their relationship to the planned surgical intervention: the chief complaint, present problem, relevant medical history, family history (note maternal diethylstilbestrol use, death from gynecologic-related disorders, family history of cancer; three known hereditary syndromes that place a woman at high risk for ovarian cancer are familial site-specific ovarian cancer syndrome, breast-ovarian cancer syndrome, and breast-ovarian-endometrial-colorectal cancer syndrome [NIH, 1994]), social (smoking) and experiential (previous surgery and important life events) history, and review of systems (see Box 13-1 for a review of selected risk factors). A history of previous surgeries is an important assessment consideration; many commonly performed gynecologic procedures result in the formation of pelvic adhesions. Ovarian cystectomy, ectopic pregnancy, abdominal hysterectomy, myomectomy, excision of endometriosis, fim-

---

Box 13-1 Risk Factors

Cervical Cancer

Age—between 40 and 50 years
History—cervical dysplasias, condylomata acuminata lesions, herpes infection
First coitus—early age
Sex partners—multiple or partner with multiple partners
Pregnancies—multiple
History—exposure to diethylstilbestrol, smoking

Endometrial Cancer

Age—postmenopausal
Menarche—early
Menopause—late
Parity—low or infertility
Body weight—obese
History—hypertension, diabetes, endometrial hyperplasia, liver disease
Estrogen—history of replacement
Family history—endometrial, breast, or colon cancer

Ovarian Cancer

Age—between 40 and 60
History—ovarian dysfunction, spontaneous abortions, cancer of breast or endometrium, irradiation of pelvic organs, endometriosis
Family history—ovarian or breast cancer
Environment—exposure to talc or asbestos

From Barkauskas VH, et al. (1994). *Health & Physical Assessment*. St. Louis: Mosby.

---

brioplasty, and cesarean birth have all been implicated in adhesion formation (Saunders, 1993). During abdominal gynecologic surgery, the surgeon may use adjunctive therapy—such as irrigating solutions (for example, saline or Ringer's lactate, with or without heparin) or mechanical barriers such as a biodegradable oxidized cellulose or expanded polytetrafluoroethylene (PTFE)—to separate wound surfaces until healing occurs in an attempt to prevent the formation of adhesions.

The patient's birthplace, nationality, and religion may provide clues to important cultural, spiritual, or religious beliefs that the perioperative nurse will incorporate into the care plan. The history should also include a chronologic listing of each pregnancy, with length of gestation, problems during pregnancy, type of delivery, length of labor, and fetal weight. Note whether the patient has had previous gynecologic surgery or other major abdominal surgery. A medication history should be obtained; note the use of oral contraceptives, estrogen therapy, diuretics, antihypertensive agents, and cardiac drugs.

A brief description of the menstrual cycle is needed and should include length of cycle, duration of bleeding, pain or discomfort associated with menses, date of last menstrual period, and amount of flow. Amount of flow may be assessed in terms of numbers of sanitary napkins or tampons used. A normal interval of menses may vary from 26 to 32 days. The average duration is 3 to 4 days, with average blood loss varying from 10 to 200 ml. While gathering information related to menses, the perioperative nurse should ask the patient about the possibility of current pregnancy. Information about vaginal discharge should include odor, color, consistency, presence of blood, and duration of discharge. The patient should be asked about recent vaginal douching and use of vaginal creams and medications or contraceptives. Risk for sexually transmitted diseases may be raised at this time. If the patient is menopausal, note when menopause occurred and any related symptoms. Gynecologic patients may be instructed to use a povidone-iodine (Betadine) douche before their operative procedure; check to see if this was prescribed and verify with the patient that it was carried out.

Symptoms that may indicate urinary tract problems should be reviewed because these are often associated with gynecologic problems. Stress incontinence or loss of urine while coughing, sneezing, or laughing should be differentiated from urge incontinence. Note whether urination is painful or accompanied by burning sensations. The operative gynecologic patient often has undergone urologic examination before surgery, especially if hysterectomy for uterine prolapse is indicated.

Physical Examination

A complete physical examination will be documented in the patient record. The perioperative nurse should note baseline vital signs, weight, and results of examination of the thyroid (hyperthyroidism, hypothyroidism), chest, heart, breasts, abdomen, pelvis, rectum, and the findings of all laboratory and radiologic studies.

Breasts. The patient's breasts should be inspected for size, symmetry, nipple characteristics, skin condition, venous distribution, presence of prior surgical scars and prosthetic implants. Both breasts are palpated for nodules and tenderness. The nipples should be examined for evidence of discharge. As the perioperative nurse reviews and confirms findings, there may be an opportunity for the nurse to review self–breast examination technique and American Cancer Society guidelines on mammography with the patient. As part of their clinical practice guidelines on quality determinants of mammography, the Agency for Health Care Policy and Research has published a woman's guide about mammograms (AHCPR, 1994). These are well-written consumer versions of important patient education materials.

Abdomen. The results of examination of the abdomen will include findings from inspection, percussion, palpation, and auscultation. Note whether the patient has complaints of pain or abdominal cramping. After review of the medical record, the perioperative nurse confirms significant findings. In general, the perioperative nurse looks for contour, lesions, scars from previous surgeries, stretch marks, visible pulsations, and the presence of bowel sounds. When inspecting the abdomen of the gynecologic patient, protrusion of the abdomen should be noted; this may be related to adipose tissue, ascites, pregnancy, or a protruding large mass or tumor. Palpate the abdomen for fluid, tautness, firmness, areas of tenderness, and tumor outlining. Abdominal girth will guide the perioperative nurse in the selection of appropriately sized instruments and accessories. Percussion of the abdomen for sounds of flatness or tympany may help differentiate fluid, intestines, and tumor. Auscultation to note bowel sounds and rule out pregnancy are also important.

Pelvic and rectal examination. If pelvic and/or rectal examination is performed to confirm findings, patient privacy must be ensured. An appropriate examination area may not always be available; therefore this section of the gynecologic assessment may be confirmed by reviewing the data obtained by the admitting nurse or physician. On the other hand, a patient may be examined by the surgical team once she is admitted to the OR and positioned on the OR bed. If the patient is awake, the perioperative nurse will assist with the examination and collaborate in the confirmation of findings. Before the pelvic examination begins, the patient should be allowed to empty her bladder; if the patient is being examined under anesthesia, straight catheterization will probably be required.

The vulva should be inspected for lesions, cysts on the Bartholin or Skene's gland, and exudate. The perineal body should be inspected for previous episiotomies, edema, excoriation, or scarring that represents vaginal trauma. Relaxation of the anterior and posterior vaginal wall should be noted when the vaginal outlet is inspected; relaxation may represent a rectocele, cystocele, or urethrocele. Uterine prolapse may also be evident on inspection of the vaginal outlet. The vaginal mucosa should be inspected for color, lubrication, or lesions related to herpes, papilloma, or syphilis. The vaginal rugae are prominent in adolescents and young adults but disappear with age. Further vaginal evaluation should include notations of congenital anomalies such as vaginal septa, double vaginas, double cervices, or Gartner duct cysts. These are small, round, or fusiform swellings in the mucosa of the anterolateral wall of the vagina. They usually are asymptomatic and require no surgical treatment unless they are large.

Cervical examination will probably not be conducted by the perioperative nurse. The nurse reviews the medical record for evidence of cervical eversion; ulceration; lesions such as papilloma; polyps; cancer; date and results of most recent Papanicolaou smear; and discharge as found with moniliasis, *Trichomonas* infection, and other vaginal infections.

The uterus is palpated and examined bimanually for size, position, and tenderness. Adnexal areas are palpated for ovarian size, tenderness, and broad ligaments. Often the perioperative nurse assists in a pelvic examination that is repeated with the patient under anesthesia. This allows better pelvic relaxation and therefore better examination. Rectal examination provides information regarding the culde-sac and uterosacral ligaments and allows for further evaluation of rectosigmoid masses, external hemorrhoids, rectal fissures, and other rectal lesions.

Every effort should be directed toward providing the patient with privacy and exposing minimal skin to prevent hypothermia and patient discomfort.

DIAGNOSTIC STUDIES

Numerous diagnostic studies may be found in the data base for the gynecologic patient. Studies will vary from patient to patient; there are many possible indications for any one procedure. For instance, laparoscopy may be either diagnostic or therapeutic. Indications for laparoscopy may include infertility, pelvic pain of uncertain origin, pelvic inflammatory disease, ova collection for in vitro fertilization, lysis of adhesions, evaluation of pelvic mass, or tubal sterilization. With each of these conditions, the indicated diagnostic studies will vary. Boxes 13-2 and 13-3 group diagnostic studies under two common gynecologic procedures. All other procedures will

---

Box 13-2 Preoperative Workup for Diagnostic Laparoscopy/Laparoscopic Bilateral Tubal Ligation*

Complete blood count
Urinalysis
Serum human chorionic gonadotropin
Papanicolaou smear
Hysterosalpingogram
Dehydroepiandrosterone
Serum testosterone
Serum progesterone
Postcoital test
Basal body temperatures
Ultrasound pelvic examination
Intravenous pyelogram
Barium enema

*Diagnostic workups vary according to patient presentation, physician preference, and institutional requirements. The studies indicated here are common but not prescriptive.

Box 13-3 Preoperative Workup for Total Abdominal or Vaginal Hysterectomy/ Exploratory Laparotomy*

Complete blood count, blood chemistry
Urinalysis
Electrocardiogram (if patient >40 years)
Chest x-ray film (if patient >40 years)
Papanicolaou smear
Blood type and Rh factor
Cervical biopsy
Endometrial biopsy
Colposcopy
Previous D/C
Cervical conization
CT/MRI/ultrasound
Intravenous pyelogram
Barium enema
Bowel preparation

*Diagnostic workups vary according to patient presentation, physician preference, and institutional requirements. The studies indicated here are common but not prescriptive.

---

have some of these studies as part of the diagnostic workup.

In addition to studies considered routine for gynecology patients, additional studies may be related to the differential diagnosis. Because the uterus and adnexa are so close to the kidneys, ureter, and bladder, urologic examination via intravenous pyelogram and/or barium enema is often indicated to rule out other existing problems. In the case of a pelvic mass, urologic examination is done to note obstructions or alterations in anatomy.

Ultrasound

The gynecologic patient scheduled for a diagnostic laparoscopy or laparotomy has probably undergone pelvic ultrasound for diagnostic purposes before surgery. Ultrasound is a noninvasive tool used to aid in the diagnosis of ectopic pregnancies and of adnexal and uterine disease. Ultrasound can often allow evaluation of the endometrial cavity by measuring and visualizing its length and thickness. Uterine fibroids can be located and estimates made of size. Adnexal disease such as ovarian cysts or mass, paraovarian cyst, and hydrosalpinx can usually be detected by ultrasound. Abdominal accumulations of blood or fluid may also be evident with ultrasound review, as may evidence of endometriosis.

Computed Tomography

Computed tomography (CT) has advantages over ultrasonography, especially with obese patients and when bowel or stomach distention interferes with interpretation of pulsed ultrasound waves. In a patient with suspected malignancy, CT or magnetic resonance imaging (MRI) is useful for detecting involvement of retroperitoneal lymph nodes or bone.

Hysterosalpingography

Hysterosalpingography is usually the initial diagnostic study for uterine and tubal causes of infertility and provides important information earlier than does laparoscopy. It is a simple procedure that enables assessment of the uterine cavity and detection of anomalies, endometrial polyps, submucous fibroids, and synechiae. In addition, the site of occlusion within the tubal folds can be identified.

Colposcopy

Colposcopy, with colpomicroscopy, is usually performed in the physician's or nurse practitioner's office. It yields cytologic information about cellular irregularity that may involve the vulva, vagina, or cervix; it may define areas of dysplasia and carcinoma in situ. Human papilloma virus (HPV) and cervical condylomata are also frequently diagnosed with colposcopic examination–directed biopsy. Cervical carcinoma is the second most common invasive cancer of the female reproductive tract. It is important to determine the location and extent of a preinvasive cervical neoplasm; this guides the selection of treatment. Preinvasive lesions are classified according to grades of cervical intraepithelial neoplasia (CIN). Mild dysplasia is classified as CIN I, moderate dysplasia as CIN II, and severe dysplasia and carcinoma in situ as CIN III. Colposcopy may be accompanied by punch biopsy or knife cone biopsy and curettage. Colposcopic examination is indicated for the patient with an abnormal Papanicolaou smear suggesting dysplasia or CIN III cytology (see Box 13-4 for information about Papanicolaou smears). Endocervical curettage may also be performed at the time of the colposcopy to rule out invasive carcinoma or to detect early adenocarcinoma. Endocervical curettage is also indicated when a patient has had previous therapy such as multiple biopsies, cryosurgery, conization, or cautery.

CA-125 Tumor Marker

CA-125 is an accurate tumor marker for epithelial tumors of the ovary. It is helpful in making a diagnosis of ovarian carcinoma, may predict whether a repeat (second-look) laparoscopy will be positive, and can be used as posttreatment surveillance for patients with ovarian carcinoma (Pagana & Pagana, 1995). This test on venous blood will be read as positive if the value is above 35 U/ml. Results are usually available in 3 to 7 days. Benign peritoneal disease, pregnancy, or normal menstruation may cause mild elevations.

NURSING DIAGNOSES

Patient assessment is the primary determinant for relevant nursing diagnoses. The gynecology patient may have multiple nursing diagnoses amenable to nursing intervention. The following selected nursing diagnoses will be examined for their specific applicability to the gynecologic surgical patient and are considered concomitant to the universal or generic nursing diagnoses recognized for all surgical patients (see Chapter 7). The utility of these diagnoses will be determined by the defining characteristics of each individual patient. Based on the nursing diagnosis, the perioperative care plan will then identify desired patient outcomes and appropriate nursing actions designed to assist the patient in achieving those outcomes.

Anxiety

The risk for anxiety is a significant nursing diagnosis for the gynecologic patient. Feelings of uneasiness or apprehension may be based on a lack of information; specific fears may be related to the reason for surgery, medical diagnosis, lack of diagnosis, fear of surgery and anesthesia, fear of violation or exposure, fear of prognosis, and/or fear of not being in control. The infertility patient admitted for diagnostic laparoscopy or laparotomy may be anxious about her reproductive potential or the chances for a successful correction of reproductive disorders. The patient admitted for an ovarian mass or second-look laparotomy after chemotherapy for pelvic cancer may be extremely anxious about the diagnostic outcome of her surgery. The patient admitted for "pain of unknown origin" may become anxious when trying to describe her symptoms to the nurse. She may feel inadequate or embarrassed in describing her anatomy. Patients may not know the correct name for a part of their anatomy or may be uncomfortable discussing symptoms in areas of their body they consider "private." Diagnostic workups for the pa-

---

Box 13-4 About Papanicolaou Smears

Client Preparation

No douching, use of vaginal medications or other topical inserts, or tub baths for 24 hours before the procedure

Defer if menstrual flow or infection

Do not use lubricating jelly on the speculum

Findings

Results are reported in classes or in cervical intraepithelial neoplasia (CIN) levels:

Class 1: Benign: absence of atypical or abnormal cells (normal finding).

Class 2: Benign with inflammation: atypical cells, but no evidence of malignancy.

Class 3: Mild dysplasia: cytologic findings suggestive of but not conclusive of malignancy (must receive prompt follow-up).

Class 4: Carcinoma in situ: cytologic findings strongly suggestive of malignancy.

Class 5: Invasive cancer: cytologic changes conclusive of malignancy.

CIN 1: mild and mild-to-moderate dysplasia (similar to classes 2 and 3)

CIN 2: moderate and moderate-to-severe dysplasia (similar to class 3)

CIN 3: severe dysplasia and carcinoma in situ (similar to classes 3 and 4)

Important

Secretions must be fixed before they dry. Drying will distort the cells and make interpretation difficult.

From Barkauskas VH et al. (1994). *Health & Physical Assessment.* St. Louis: Mosby.

tient with pain of unknown origin have often included multiple studies that yielded negative results. The patient may become insecure, doubting her pain and questioning whether her symptoms are psychosomatic. The financial and life-style changes and burdens imposed on patients often go unrecognized by health care providers and fall low on the priority scale when ranking patient concerns to be addressed. When patients have several reasons to be anxious (the outcome of the surgery, its effect on role, relationships, and expectations of self), it is helpful to classify the anxiety as mild, moderate, or severe. This can help the perioperative nurse design interventions appropriate for varying levels of anxiety.

When observing for symptoms that may indicate anxiety, the nurse may note such behavior as fatigue, insomnia, urinary frequency, crying easily, heavy smoking, repetitive gestures with the hands, clearing the throat, or laughing inappropriately. The patient may appear to be antagonistic or uncooperative. Nursing intervention for the gynecologic patient experiencing anxiety would include providing adequate and reliable information in answer to questions she may have about the surgery, anatomy, or body functions. Encourage feedback from the patient after explaining a procedure or answering a question. Allow the patient to express all of her feelings. During this time it is important for the nurse to be a good listener. The patient will evaluate the nurse's nonverbal communication. Maintain good eye contact, apply touch if appropriate, and maintain a private and secure environment. The desired patient outcome is that the patient will experience reduced anxiety and effectively use her coping measures.

Grieving

Grieving is a state in which an individual or family experiences an actual, perceived, or potential loss; this may be the loss of a person, object, function, status, or relationship. These potentials exist for many gynecology patients. The loss of the uterus and/or ovaries alters reproductive function, and may be perceived as having consequences for her status of childbearer, her relationship with a significant other, and her feelings of sexuality and self-esteem. The perioperative nurse may care for a patient admitted for a missed abortion or fetal death. The loss of a pregnancy may initiate grieving in the patient and family. The grief process varies from patient to patient and may include feelings of anger, guilt, denial, and sorrow. The patient may be crying or withdrawn and uncommunicative. Nursing support, through allowing expression of feelings and offering comfort, will be necessary. Touch can be used purposively to provide nurturing and comfort and to convey caring and empathy in perioperative patient care settings. The patient's response to touch should be assessed. Note the patient's nonverbal response to touch; if the patient exhibits a more relaxed posture, touch is an appropriate nursing intervention. The nurse can provide a private, quiet environment, alleviate misconceptions, identify and encourage coping skills, and provide for open and sensitive discussion of the issues.

Body Image Disturbance

Another significant nursing diagnosis is the risk for a disturbance in body image. The gynecologic patient may begin to have feelings of inadequacy before her surgery, which may intensify after the operation. The patient scheduled for hysterectomy may feel a threat to her self-esteem because her body will not allow her to have more children. She may similarly feel a loss of female identity. The infertile patient may perceive her body and self as altered because she is unable to conceive; she may have feelings of inadequacy related to femininity and her role as woman and procreator. Both of these patients may have low self-esteem, which may be chronic or situational, and may express feelings of emptiness and fearfulness. They may feel unneeded and fear rejection from their spouse, significant other, or family. Research on men's views about hysterectomy and women who undergo this procedure indicates that men had concerns about the hysterectomy patient feeling inadequate, being moody, being sexually diminished, and having less sex appeal (Berhhard, 1992). When possible, the perioperative nurse should include male partners in discussions about body image concerns related to gynecologic surgery and correct misperceptions about its effects.

When assessing the patient for disturbances in body image, the perioperative nurse may note behavior suggesting grief, sadness, irritability, depression, anxiety, sensitivity, and withdrawal. It is unreasonable to expect that, during the brief perioperative nursing encounter, disturbances in body image will be completely resolved. Nonetheless, the perioperative nurse can implement nursing interventions that assist the patient in dealing with a negative feeling or view of herself. Expressing understanding, reassuring the patient that her feelings are normal, and allowing the patient to talk about her feelings are important. The nurse can clarify misconceptions, offer feedback, and provide information relevant to the source of the body image disturbance. The desired outcome is that the patient will be able to accept herself and to acquire knowledge and understanding regarding body image. Education can be valuable for the gynecologic patient who is concerned about changes in sexual response because of surgical removal of her uterus and ovaries. Also, many women are concerned with long-term health after removal of their ovaries. The patient may have questions about hormone replacement therapy and the effect of surgery on sexual responses. The perioperative nurse may need to refer these concerns (knowledge deficits) to the patient care unit nurse, nurse practitioner, or the physician.

Pain

The gynecologic patient may be admitted to the OR with acute pain. The patient with an ectopic pregnancy, ovarian cyst, or incomplete abortion may be in pain. The level of pain may vary from tenderness when pressure is applied to the lower abdomen to a throbbing pain associated with an unruptured ectopic pregnancy or ovarian cyst. The abdominal pain may be unilateral or generalized. The patient who is aborting may experience contractions. Pain with a ruptured ectopic pregnancy often is severe; it may be sudden and stabbing, with referred supraclavicular pain. Pain is created by stimuli from the damaged tissues to the nerves that travel to the spinal cord and to the brain. Postoperatively, all gynecologic patients have the potential for some degree of pain. This may range from mild discomfort, as with dilatation and curettage, to moderate to severe pain after hysterectomy.

Patients who are experiencing pain may be irritable or restless, or may cry or breathe irregularly. If the patient is admitted to the OR for cesarean section, she may be hyperventilating in response to hypoxemia. As the fetus presses against the diaphragm, breathing is restricted; compensatory hyperventilation is initiated. Assisting her into a left side-lying position will help this. The patient may have compensated respiratory alkalosis; during contractions, rapid breathing will cause further carbon dioxide loss. Help the patient breathe slowly and deeply between contractions. Additional measures for the patient in pain include assisting her to a position of comfort and encouraging the use of pain control techniques that have been effective for her in the past. Acknowledge the existence of the patient's pain with sincere and empathic responses. Relaxation techniques, guided imagery, or music may be therapeutic.

Urinary Retention

Urinary retention can occur in any postoperative patient. If retention occurs, the bladder overdistends, blood supply is compromised, bacteria proliferate, and infection may result. In abdominal gynecology, or perineal surgery that may result in reflex spasm of the sphincters, an indwelling urinary catheter is often inserted while in the OR. The catheter may remain in place for 24 hours or more. An indwelling catheter allows measurement of urinary output and promotes comfort by relieving bladder pressure. If the patient has had bladder suspension or repair, the catheter will remain for a longer time postoperatively. These patients are also at greater risk for urinary retention after removal of the catheter. Prolonged bed rest and inadequate fluid intake can also interfere with return of the postoperative micturition reflex.

To initiate voiding, the bladder progressively fills until the tension on its walls rises above a threshold value. At that time a nervous reflex, the micturition reflex, either causes urination or a conscious desire to urinate. The micturition reflex is a single complete cycle of progressive and rapid increase in pressure, a period of sustained pressure, and return of the pressure back to the basal tonic pressure of the bladder. The micturition reflex is a completely automatic spinal cord reflex, but it can be inhibited or facilitated by centers in the brain. Therefore urinary retention can be related to a patient's mental and emotional processes. When the time to urinate arrives, the cortical centers can facilitate the sacral nerve centers to initiate a micturition reflex and inhibit the external urinary sphincter so that urination can occur. The muscle of the external sphincter is a voluntary skeletal muscle, in contrast to the muscle of the bladder, which is entirely smooth muscle. Operative trauma, anesthesia, and analgesics cause decreased nerve stimulation to the bladder and sphincter. Prolonged bed rest may interfere with maintenance of normal bladder tone by causing decreased nerve stimulation and inadequate output.

Patients may have questions and misconceptions about an indwelling urinary catheter, how and when it will be removed, and if it will have any effect on resumption of regular patterns of urinary elimination. The perioperative nurse should emphasize the importance of postoperative oral intake and compliance with ambulation. The patient is allowed to express her anxiety about being unable to void. She may fear pain or dysfunction if bladder repair was performed as part of her operation.

Knowledge Deficit

It is quite common for patients to be admitted for surgery, even radical surgery, 1 day before or on the day of their scheduled surgery. The need for a collaborative nursing effort to prepare the patient for surgery, physiologically and psychologically, has never been greater. Some teaching and preparation activities may have occurred in the physician's office, in the surgical admission unit, or through the use of pamphlets, written educational materials, or video instruction. Nonetheless, anticipatory anxiety may interfere with the patient's cognitive functions. The ability to comprehend and remember important information may be impaired; there is a need to repeat and clarify instructions, to reinforce teaching, and to begin preparing the patient for discharge and home care management. The perioperative nurse plays a vital role as a nursing partner in the effort to educate and prepare patients adequately in a short time. Explanations about perioperative events should be a part of all care plans for the patient in surgery. The patient should know what to expect; information about procedures such as insertion of intravenous lines, intravascular monitoring lines, indwelling urinary catheters, nasogastric tubes, drainage devices, and other invasive devices should be communicated to the patient. Information is needed about dressings, the postoperative discharge unit (postanesthesia care unit, intensive care unit, day surgery recovery), postoperative pain management, and the rehabilitation plan. The patient should know where family or significant others will wait and how they will receive communication.

Impaired Skin Integrity

The potential for impaired skin integrity exists when the patient is at risk for an alteration in the skin surface that compromises its effectiveness as a barrier. Gynecology patients vary in their age, state of health, and manifestations of risk factors for impaired skin integrity. Certainly the creation of a surgical incision and stab wounds for drain exits, despite their deliberate and controlled nature, compromises skin integrity. The desired outcome for surgical incisions and drain sites is that they will remain free of infection and in apposition, uncomplicated by dehiscence, drainage, or untoward inflammation. For other skin areas, the desired outcome is that the skin will remain intact. This requires assessment of the skin at dependent pressure sites as well as sites of electrosurgical dispersive pads and electrocardiograph leads. Gynecology patients may be at risk for impaired skin integrity if they have altered nutritional status. Patients whose nutrition is inadequate are at risk, as are patients whose nutritional level is more than body requirements. Additionally, the patient should be assessed for impaired circulation, history of immobility, radiation therapy or chemotherapy, incontinence, or medications (such as long-term corticosteroid therapy). Knowledge regarding factors relating to the risk for impaired skin integrity will be incorporated into the perioperative care plan.

Hypothermia

All surgical patients are at risk for alterations in thermal regulation status due to the environmental conditions, interventions, manipulations, and anesthetic changes inherent in surgery. Considerations specific to gynecologic surgery influence thermal loss. Patient skin exposure during anesthesia induction, positioning, prepreparation pelvic examination, skin preparation, and draping may allow significant cooling of core body temperature. Ambient OR room temperatures below 23° C (72° F) have been identified as a source of body heat loss (Ott, 1991; Seitzinger & Dudgeon, 1993). Cold or room-temperature solutions applied, infused, and irrigated throughout the procedure contribute to thermal loss. Seitzinger and Dudgeon (1993) cite a correlation between length of procedure and hypothermia, and they note the recent surge in advanced laparoscopic procedures, some with significantly prolonged operating times, as contributing to thermal loss. Investigations by Ott (1991) revealed a core body temperature decrease of 0.3° C for each 50 L of room-temperature carbon dioxide delivered to attain pneumoperitoneum during laparoscopic surgery. He describes the surface area of the exposed peritoneal cavity as equal to that of external body surface and an interface for heat exchange, contributing to thermal loss.

Seitzinger and Dudgeon (1993) suggest that this loss may be greater than 0.5° C. Total hypothermic risk for the laparoscopic and open surgical patient is influenced by cumulative factors related to selected anesthetic and operative conditions amenable to nursing intervention.

Measures should be directed toward warming preparation and irrigation solutions, IV fluids, insufflation gas, ambient room temperature, and the patient with thermal devices, coupled with prevention of heat loss by minimizing unnecessary skin exposure.

Aspiration

Although all surgical patients may be at risk for aspiration of secretions or stomach contents, specific circumstances may render the gynecologic surgery patient at risk. The possibility of a full stomach exists with any patient. With the increase in ambulatory and same-day surgery, preoperative preparation may affect compliance with NPO orders; emergency procedures such as ruptured ectopic pregnancies and cesarean births may result in patients with full stomachs. Positional manipulations of lithotomy and Trendelenburg's presentation may mechanically facilitate regurgitation in the presence of relaxation of the pyloric and gastrointestinal sphincters, often seen in pregnancy.

The most serious complication of aspiration of gastric contents into the lungs results from the relative acidity of gastric secretions. Inhalation of material with a pH less than 2.5 will cause an immediate bronchoconstriction and concomitant destruction of the tracheal mucosa. Adult respiratory distress syndrome will follow.

Patients with full stomachs, delayed gastric emptying, and those at risk must be identified, and precautions must be taken to wait when possible to assist gastric emptying and/or to administer prophylactic nonparticulate antacids (sodium citrate) or antagonists to hydrochloric acid (cimetidine or ranitidine). Assistance during anesthesia induction may warrant cricoid pressure during tracheal intubation.

PLANNING FOR PATIENT CARE

The traditional components of nursing care—especially those relating to coordinated, comprehensive care delivered throughout the course of an illness or health dysfunction; inclusion of health promotion; and emphasis on patient education—are integral to the nursing role irrespective of practice setting. The following care plans, with their associated Guides to Nursing Actions, have as their intent the provision of complete, safe, and effective perioperative nursing care. It is expected that many gynecologic patients will meet all of the outcomes for generic care planning identified in Chapter 7. Thus there is a section of the care plan in which the initiation of those generic care plans can be noted. Because perioperative patient care must be individualized, there is also a section in which additional nursing actions for the individual patient may be documented. The nursing actions themselves are listed in the approximate order in which they might be executed. The order and the content will vary in different practice settings. Content that does not apply to the individual patient or the particular setting may be so indicated by checking the appropriate box. It is quite possible that additional outcomes will need to be identified for individual patients, which may be accommodated by selecting the outcome category *Outcome met with additional outcome criteria.* Because so many gynecologic procedures now take place in ambulatory surgical settings, a number of the care plans have information and actions that extend throughout the perioperative period.

Gynecologic surgery frequently is accomplished with the patient in the lithotomy position or some modification thereof. Surgical lasers and endoscopic instruments, accessories, and video systems have created highly technical challenges for the perioperative nurse. Thermal regulation has been identified as a critical consideration in providing optimum patient care. The following protocols will outline nursing care requirements that may be generalized across the perioperative nursing care plans.

Lithotomy Position Protocols

Complications associated with lithotomy position may fall into three categories: muscle and fascia injuries, circulatory complications, and nerve injuries. The anesthetized patient may be at risk for excessive abduction and/or hyperextension. These undesirable outcomes may be attributed to the anatomic posture of the lithotomy position or to the effects of stretching or pressure caused by positioning devices. Positioning devices must be selected to meet the individual needs of each patient (Paschal & Strzelecki, 1992).

Circulatory changes relative to lithotomy position include venous pooling in the lumbar region and vascular compression in the lower extremities and the groin. Blood volume is reduced in the legs during positioning by as much as 500 to 600 ml. Hypotension may result if the legs are not lowered into the supine position slowly and carefully, because the blood volume drains back into the legs from the torso (Rothrock & Sculthorpe, 1993). To prevent patient injury related to the lithotomy position, the perioperative nurse should initiate the following activities:

1. Assess the patient and review the chart for the presence of vascular grafts, orthopedic prostheses, or other mobility limitations.
2. When possible, place the patient in the desired position before anesthesia induction to adjust for comfort and support.
3. Position the patient's arms on armboards abducted 10 to 15 degrees from the OR bed. If arms must be tucked at sides, avoid hyperextension or rotation of arms and compression of the ulnar nerve against the OR bed. Liberate the fingers before raising the foot of the OR bed.
4. First choice for stirrups should be a total leg support system.
5. Place protective padding under dependent pressure sites.
6. Avoid excessive hip abduction and external rotation.
7. If using ankle strap stirrups, use a wide foot strap, and pad the feet and ankles before placement.
8. Apply antithromboembolic stockings and/or devices when appropriate.
9. Elevate both legs into position simultaneously with the leg in the flexed position, supported under the knee and foot. Use two persons to accomplish leg raise.
10. Evaluate for anatomic alignment; the body should be symmetric with the pelvis level and presented at the break of the OR bed.
11. Tuck protective padding under sacrum and buttocks to prevent wetting of sheet and mattress.

12. Maintain and preserve patient privacy and dignity.
13. Avoid placing heavy instruments or accessory items on the groin after draping.
14. Prevent team members from leaning on the groin or legs during the procedure.
15. Return the legs to the supine position in the same manner as they were elevated. Lower legs slowly and with respect to normal range of motion.

LASER PROTOCOLS

The introduction and evolution of surgical lasers has had a tremendous effect on advances in gynecologic surgery and perioperative nursing care in this specialty. This transition to highly technical approaches to surgical care challenges the perioperative nurse to improve organizational skills, mechanical aptitude, and navigation among and between OR room-consuming equipment while providing for the care, comfort, and safety of the patient (Ball, 1995). It is incumbent upon the perioperative nurse to know the responsibilities associated with laser application. Formal programs in laser education, demonstration, hands-on practice, and supervision during the learning process, followed by ongoing continuing education, are recommended. The protocol guidelines listed below suggest nursing actions and considerations for the patient receiving laser intervention in gynecologic surgery. Safety precautions may vary according to the specific wavelength or type of laser. Laser delivery systems vary in their precautions and preoperative preparation considerations.

The nurse should be informed and competent in procuring all necessary laser equipment for the procedure; in sterilization, handling, and testing of laser delivery systems; in specific institutional policies; in trouble-shooting of machinery; in safety precautions of each specific laser unit; and in documentation expectations. A second circulator or laser nurse should be present to manage the laser during the procedure.

1. Follow manufacturer's directions for the use of the laser.
2. Post removable LASER warning signs at the door of the designated OR room.
3. Provide appropriate protective eye wear outside of room.
4. Cover windows of OR room for specific laser wavelength to be used. Carbon dioxide laser does not require covered windows.
5. Procure laser key from authorized person. Do not store in the laser machine.
6. If possible, test-fire laser before the patient is in the room.
7. Have a halon fire extinguisher available in the room.
8. Place the laser in the *standby* mode when not in use.
9. Identify the laser footpedal for the laser operator/surgeon and position for his or her use only. The operator should have only one pedal.
10. Keep fluids and supplies from the laser console. Do not use as a desk.
11. Use only nonreflective instruments and accessories in or near the laser impact site. Cover large instruments (retractors) with sponges or towels to prevent reflection of the beam.
12. Use nonflammable skin preparation solutions.
13. A wet sponge inserted or taped over the rectum will prevent methane gas from escaping into the operative site.
14. Drape with nonflammable drapes, and surround the incision site with frequently moistened towels.
15. Provide sterile back table with container of water or saline.
16. Use the appropriate smoke evacuation system designed for the amount of plume generated. Position smoke evacuation intake tip as close as possible to the laser impact site.
17. Each team member should wear a high-filtration mask.
18. Change the smoke evacuator filters as often as is recommended by the manufacturer. Treat as hazardous waste.
19. Use designated lens cover/filter for the eyepiece of endoscopes.
20. Microscopic procedures require an automatic lens shutter on the microscope head.
21. Cover the anesthetized patient's eyes with moistened gauze sponges. The awake patient may wear protective goggles in place of moistened gauze.
22. Move laser machinery with care to avoid misalignment of critical mirrors or other parts.
23. Handle and store protective eye wear with care to prevent scratches to the surface.

ENDOSCOPY AND INSUFFLATION PROTOCOLS

Advances in endoscopic approaches have expanded the dimension of gynecologic surgery. This technology brings alterations in operating times, issues of instrument sterilization, cost to the facility and patient, changes in postoperative outcome, morbidity, and return to activity for the patient, demands for education and practical experience for health care providers, and controversy among some practitioners. Although it is believed that laparoscopically assisted vaginal hysterectomy (LAVH) may convert some total abdominal hysterectomies to safe vaginal procedures (Tadir & Fisch, 1993) and is less morbid than abdominal hysterectomy, it should be applied cautiously and prudently by trained practitioners. LAVH has been associated with longer operating times, increased cost to the patient and hospital, increased postoperative pain, and increased complications related to the technical aspects of laparoscopy (Summit, et al., 1992).

Hysteroscopic procedures offer an approach to the treatment of dysfunctional bleeding by endometrial ablation using the laser or, more commonly, electrosurgical ablation with the rollerball electrode as an alternative to hysterectomy. Polypectomy and myomectomy may also be accomplished via this approach (Jackson, 1991).

Sterilization of endoscopic instruments and their accessories helps to ensure patient safety and to minimize the risk of infection as outlined in the *AORN Recommended Practices for Care of Instruments, Scopes, and Powered Surgical Instruments* (AORN, 1995). The demand to be able to process these items quickly for immediate reuse and to provide accountability for their sterility and safety of function challenges the perioperative nurse. The perioperative nurse must balance recommendations of avoiding flash sterilization, safety issues with glutaraldehyde and ethylene oxide (ETO), care requirements for heat-sensitive and delicate instruments, cost of disposables versus reusables, turnover time in the OR, universal precautions, and the ethical dimensions of providing the best and equal quality of patient care for all patients (Crow, 1993).

Current developments in sterilization systems offer options for low-temperature sterilization. Peracetic acid systems provide the criteria necessary to address all the issues (Crow, 1993); plasma sterilization provides nontoxic, dry, low-temperature sterilization in about 1 hour (Garner, 1995). Critical attention and choices will have to be made to provide each patient with a sterile scope and accessories.

Manufacturer's recommendations will direct the disassembly, cleaning, and sterilization options while individual institutional policies will guide how these processes will be accomplished and by whom.

The use of automatic surgical stapling devices in gynecologic surgery increased with the development of endoscopic applications and absorbable staples. Staples have been credited with decreasing operating time, decreasing blood loss, less vaginal vault granulation, and a quicker return to work and activity for the patient. Although the use of metal staples formerly caused vaginal migration and dyspareunia, absorbable counterparts have minimized this complication (Beresford & Moher, 1993).

Endoscopic exploration and intervention depend on some means of distention with a medium such as carbon dioxide, dextran 70, or low-viscosity fluids. Low-viscosity fluids such as glycine, sorbitol, dextrose, and saline may support fluid overload and dilutional hyponatremia. Dextran 70 may crystalize with temperature variations or long storage and must be immediately rinsed from instruments with hot water at the end of the procedure. It dries and adheres to surfaces, valves, and opticals, and may cause instrument damage (Jackson, 1991).

Carbon dioxide has evolved as the distention media of choice because of its solubility in blood and tissue; it produces a normal metabolic end product that is easily inhaled through the pulmonary alveoli. It is inexpensive, widely available, and does not present an occupational hazard. It is important to note that the carbon dioxide delivered by the cylinder is not sterile and has, in fact, been found to contain organic and inorganic contaminants. Investigations by Ott (1989; 1991) found particulate matter in the form of iron, chromium, molybdenum, copper, rust particles, metal filings, and Teflon. Organic contaminates were identified to show the presence of *Klebsiella, Serratia, Pseudomonas, Staphylococcus aureus, S. epidermis,* and *Candida*. Ott attributes the presence of these contaminates to the refilling process of tanks and contamination of the inside of the insufflation equipment, possibly due to backflow from the patient. The amount of contamination was directly proportional to the total flow exposure and the amount of remaining gas in the tank. The lower the residual container volume, the greater the contamination. Investigation of the inner lumen of the insufflator tubing revealed similar contamination.

Filtration of the gas can be accomplished with the use of a single-use in-line 0.1 μm filter between the insufflator's patient connector and the patient.

As discussed earlier, room-temperature carbon dioxide will lower core body temperature 0.3° to 0.5° C for every 50 L of gas used to establish and maintain pneumoperitoneum and poses a critical hypothermic risk to laparoscopic patients (Ott, 1991; Seitzinger & Dudgeon, 1993). Attempts to warm the tank and the gas line to the patient have been marginally successful, yet it is not clear what property effect this may have on the gas or the delivery system. Safe recommendations include storing the tank in a warm environment, allowing for passive heat transfer such as in an OR room with a room temperature above 23° C (72° F).

Smoke and plume produced from the thermal tissue interaction of electrosurgical and laser devices creates a toxic aerosol byproduct that can be inhaled via the respiratory tract during open surgical procedures and absorbed in a closed system environment via the peritoneal cavity. Ott (1993) describes a significantly positive correlation between the smoke production in a sample of laparoscopic patients and abnormally elevated methemoglobin levels. The intraabdominal absorption of these toxic products of protein and lipid combustion diminishes the oxygen-carrying capacity of the hemoglobin and will impose a "smoke inhalation syndrome" similar to that of respiratory smoke exposure. Laser smoke and plume may also contain viral contaminants. Thus setting laser and electrosurgical device parameters to desired thermal effect will reduce the risk to the patient; minimal production of smoke coupled with prompt evacuation of the smoke at the point of tissue impact will help protect the surgical team.

The complexity of the video system equipment, cameras, cables, carts, and printers challenges the perioperative nurse to explore creative methods of OR room organization and planning while developing a keen aptitude for electronics. The challenge of providing a sterile camera is best accomplished by the use of a sterile, disposable sleeve.

Although the application of endoscopy as an approach to diagnostic and therapeutic intervention presents identified risks to the patient, awareness of those risks, employment of safe, functional, sterile equipment, and compliance with a structured protocol as suggested below will guide the nurse in maintaining a high standard of care.

1. Follow manufacturer's directions for the assembly, cleaning, sterilization, and operation of equipment and accessories.
2. Formalized instruction and practice should precede using this equipment in patient care situations by each care provider.
3. All removable parts should be disassembled and cleaned at the end of each procedure. Reassembly should be done after sterilization. Rinse glutaraldehyde-soaked instruments with at least two changes of sterile water.
4. Have a second carbon dioxide tank available. Use only the first 75% of the volume in the tank. More accurate volume measure may be accomplished by weighing the tank before and during use.
5. Use tanks that have been stored in environments with temperatures close to or above 23° C (72° F).
6. Use an approved 0.1 μm filter between the insufflator and the patient. Discard after one use.
7. Position the insufflator machine at a higher level than the abdomen.
8. After the procedure, disconnect the insufflation hose from the trocar cannula before deactivating the insufflator to prevent backflow into the insufflator.
9. Flush the insufflator and hose before connecting to the patient to remove any residue and nongas air.
10. Maintain abdominal pressure below the insufflator set pressure throughout the procedure.
11. Position the insufflation machine in view of the surgeon.
12. Initial insufflation should not exceed 1 L/min. After pneumoperitoneum is established, the rate may be increased to a higher rate of 4 to 6 L/min.
13. Before insufflation the intraabdominal pressure monitor should be set at 12 to 16 mm Hg as an upper limit.
14. Wait to turn on fiberoptic light source until the cord is connected to the scope to prevent drape burn.
15. Reduce lens fogging with antifog solution and/or warming the scope before insertion.
16. Calibrate laser and electrosurgical unit settings to get the best effect from the least energy; this reduces smoke production and unnecessary tissue damage.
17. Position smoke evacuation tip as close as possible to the tissue impact site.
18. Handle all instruments and accessories with care.
19. Close tank and flush insufflator at end of procedure.
20. For hysteroscopy with low-viscosity fluid distention media, closely monitor patient intake and output.

THERMAL REGULATION PROTOCOLS

Although intentional physiologic cooling may be a desired effect during selected procedures in other surgical disciplines, it has no place in gynecologic surgery, and efforts will be directed to maintain the patient's core body temperature despite the multiple cooling effects of surgical manipulations. Conservative practice combines the collaborative efforts of anesthesia, surgical, and nursing staff to provide for the thermal regulation needs of the patient. Preventive and corrective measures taken during surgery will decrease the time postoperatively that it takes for the patient to return to normal temperature with the desired level at normal on admission to the recovery unit (Seitzinger & Dudgeon, 1993).

1. Assess patient's core body temperature before admission to the OR room via tympanic membrane thermometer, skin sensor, chart documentation of last value, or patient verbalization of thermal comfort.
2. Set OR room ambient temperature above 23° C (72° F).
3. Provide warmed blankets.
4. Minimize unnecessary skin exposure.
5. Use warmed preparation solutions if manufacturer's recommendations permit.
6. Use warmed irrigation solutions and IV fluids.

7. Place a sheet-covered thermia pad on the OR bed when appropriate.
8. Cover patient's upper torso and arms during surgery with a forced-air thermal warmer if appropriate.
9. Use carbon dioxide tanks that have been stored in the warmed OR room.
10. Cover the patient's head, arms, and legs with occlusive coverings such as insulated hats and leggings or wrap snugly in plastic.
11. Evaluate patient core body temperature before discharge to recovery unit.

GUIDES TO NURSING ACTIONS

These selected guides may be modified and used as institutional protocols. Using the following care plans as suggested guides, the perioperative nurse can develop care plans that assist the patient with attaining the desired outcomes for their perioperative period.

Dilatation and Curettage, Conization of Cervix
(Fig. 13-1)

1. Patient assessment allows for individualization of the nursing care plan. The nursing diagnoses identified in this care plan require patient assessment for positional limitations for lithotomy, as well as any preoperative deficits in range of motion or comfort level or alterations in sensation. The perioperative nurse should verify with the patient that she is not pregnant. The risk for disturbance in body image relates to the exposure of and surgery on the female genitalia. The patient may need reassurance; privacy should be maintained. Expose only those body parts necessary for surgical preparation. Anxiety related to the surgery, its outcome, being in an awake state, and anesthesia may be present. If the patient will be receiving local anesthesia with IV sedation, the perioperative nurse may be responsible for intraoperative monitoring. Follow institutional protocol for monitoring the patient receiving local anesthesia. Record all medications administered. Help the patient use coping strategies that have been effective for her in the past. Assessment includes determining the patient's size and body weight in planning for appropriate instrumentation. A dilatation and curettage set with accessories for conization are required. Conization may be accomplished with a scalpel, cutting electrosurgery electrode (the loop electrosurgical excision procedure [LEEP] may be performed rather than conization), or laser. Confirm, through a review of the operative schedule and the operative consent, the planned conization technique.

2. Refer to the suggested protocol for lithotomy position. Minimize the patient's skin exposure; consider using a warming device/warm blankets, and keep room temperature above 23° C.
3. Perform the vaginal preparation according to institutional protocol. Consider warming preparation solutions.
4. A urinary catheter should be available. If the patient is catheterized, use aseptic technique. Record the amount of urine obtained.
5. Lugol's solution may be used to distinguish normal from abnormal cells. The iodine stains the glycogen of normal cells; abnormal cells contain less glycogen. Consequently, there is little or no staining.
6. The laser may be used. Refer to laser protocol as indicated.
7. The electrosurgical unit should be available for conization.
8. The application site of the electrosurgical dispersive pad should be inspected before and after pad application. Record the condition of the skin and the application site.
9. It is important for the conization specimen to be labeled accurately for pathologic examination.
10. Additional specimens may be obtained. Endocervical and endometrial curettings may need to be separated for fractional specimen analysis. Use universal precautions with all specimen containers received from the sterile field. Record all routine and frozen sections.
11. Follow institutional protocol for sponge, sharp, and instrument counts.
12. Refer to protocol for thermal regulation.
13. Have agents such as Monsel's, Avitene, or gelfoam available for hemostasis. A vaginal pack may be inserted. Record packing.
14. Remove excess preparation solution at the completion of the surgical procedure to prevent skin irritation.
15. The patient may fear damage to or loss of reproductive capacity and reproductive organs. Emotional support is an important perioperative nursing intervention.
16. Postoperative instructions include the following:
    a. Do not wear tampons or douche.
    b. Notify the surgeon if there is excessive pain, nausea, vomiting, significant soiling of three or four pads a day with bright red blood, or a temperature elevation above 100° F.
    c. Review any postoperative medications.
    d. Verify that the patient knows when and with whom to make a follow-up appointment.

FIG. 13-1
CARE PLAN FOR D&C, CONIZATION OF CERVIX WITH FROZEN SECTION

KEY ASSESSMENT POINTS

Anxiety level/psychosocial concerns
Skin integrity
Limitations in mobility, range of motion
Core body temperature
Bleeding history
Hormone replacement therapy
Vaginal infection
Possibility of pregnancy
Allergies/sensitivities

NURSING DIAGNOSIS

All generic nursing diagnoses apply to this patient, with the addition of:

High risk for injury, lithotomy position
Body image disturbance
Anxiety related to diagnostic outcomes
High risk for hypothermia

PATIENT OUTCOMES

All generic outcomes apply, with the addition of:
There will be no injury related to lithotomy position.
The patient will not experience a disturbance in body image.
The patient will effectively cope with anxiety.
The patient's core body temperature will remain unchanged.

1. The patient will be free from injury related to lithotomy position as evidenced by:
   a. Absence of nerve damage
   b. Freedom from skin breakdown
   c. Minimal or no postural hypotension experienced
2. The patient's body image will be sustained through:
   a. Maintaining privacy
   b. Avoiding undue body exposure
   c. Providing emotional support
3. The patient will cope with anxiety by discussing fears/concerns with perioperative nurse.
4. The patient will remain normothermic.

NURSING ACTIONS

	Yes	No	N/A
1. Assessment performed?	☐	☐	☐
2. Patient correctly placed in lithotomy?	☐	☐	☐
3. Vaginal prep performed?	☐	☐	☐
4. Straight or indwelling catheter available?	☐	☐	☐
5. Lugol's solution available?	☐	☐	☐
6. Laser available? Safety protocols initiated?	☐	☐	☐
7. Electrosurgical unit available? (ESU)	☐	☐	☐
8. ESU safety protocols followed?	☐	☐	☐
9. Specimen marked and labeled for orientation for the pathologist? (suture at 1200)	☐	☐	☐
10. Specimen/frozen section to lab?	☐	☐	☐
11. Counts performed/correct?	☐	☐	☐
12. Body temperature monitored?	☐	☐	☐
13. Vaginal pack available?	☐	☐	☐
14. Remove prep solution?	☐	☐	☐
15. Emotional support given?	☐	☐	☐
16. Postoperative instructions given?	☐	☐	☐
17. Other generic care plans initiated? (specify)	☐	☐	☐

Document additional nursing actions/generic care plans initiated here:

_____

_____

_____

EVALUATION OF PATIENT OUTCOMES

	Outcome met	Outcome met with additional outcome criteria	Outcome met with revised nursing care plan	Outcome not met	Outcome not applicable to this patient
1. There was no positional injury.	☐	☐	☐	☐	☐
2. The patient's privacy was maintained.	☐	☐	☐	☐	☐
3. The patient effectively coped with her anxiety.	☐	☐	☐	☐	☐
4. Core body temperature was unchanged.	☐	☐	☐	☐	☐
5. The patient met outcomes for additional generic care plans as indicated.	☐	☐	☐	☐	☐

Signature: _____ Date: _____

e. Discuss resumption of normal sexual activities.

f. If vaginal packing is left in place, be sure the patient is instructed on when and where packing will be removed.

Suction Curettage (Fig. 13-2)

1. Patient assessment allows for individualization of the nursing care plan. The nursing diagnoses identified in this care plan require patient assessment for positional limitations for lithotomy, as well as noting whether there are any preoperative deficits in range of motion or comfort level or any alterations in sensation. The potential for disturbance in body image relates to exposure of and surgery on the female genitalia. The patient may need reassurance; privacy should be maintained. Expose only those body parts necessary for surgical preparation. Anxiety and grief are likely whether the procedure is for a spontaneous, incomplete abortion or a therapeutic abortion. Assist the patient with using coping strategies that have been effective for her in the past. Determine whether there are any cultural or religious beliefs that need to be added to the patient's care plan (for example, the fetus may need to be baptized). Assessment includes determining the patient's size and body weight in planning for appropriate instrumentation. A dilatation and curettage set with accessories for the evacuation of uterine contents are required (cannulas, aspirator tubing, vacuum aspirating unit, and oxytocic drugs). Check the patient's Rh status, because Rhogam may need to be administered.

2. Refer to the suggested protocol for lithotomy position.

3. Refer to protocol for thermal regulation.

4. Perform the vaginal preparation according to institutional protocol. Consider warming preparation solutions.

5. A urinary catheter should be available. If the patient is catheterized, use aseptic technique. Record the amount of urine obtained.

6. In addition to the aspirating unit or suction machine, verify that there is a wide range of cannula sizes.

7. Use universal precautions when handling all specimen containers received from the sterile field. Record all surgical specimens.

8. Follow institutional protocol for sponge, sharp, and instrument counts.

9. Remove excess skin preparation solution at the end of the procedure to prevent skin irritation.

10. The patient may have a great deal of anxiety and grieving regarding the deliberate or unplanned termination of pregnancy. The perioperative nurse needs to be sensitive to how the patient perceives this loss. Encourage her to verbalize her feelings and use coping mechanisms that have worked for her in the past, such as relaxation therapy, imagery, meditation, or prayer. Emotional support is an important perioperative nursing intervention.

11. Document all medications (oxytocic drugs) administered during the surgery.

12. Postoperative instructions include the following:

    a. Do not wear tampons or douche.

    b. Notify the surgeon of excessive pain, nausea, vomiting, significant soiling of three or four pads a day with bright red blood, or temperature elevation above 100° F.

    c. Review any postoperative medications.

    d. Verify that the patient knows when and with whom to make a follow-up appointment.

    e. Discuss the resumption of normal sexual activity (the patient may be advised to wait until a normal menses has occurred) and contraception.

    f. Hormonal changes should be discussed. There may be transitory depression; breasts may be tender and sore (and perhaps leak). A support bra is helpful.

Laparoscopy (Fig. 13-3)

1. Patient assessment allows for individualization of the nursing care plan. The nursing diagnoses identified in this care plan require patient assessment for positional limitations for lithotomy, as well as any preoperative deficits in range of motion or comfort level or any alterations in sensation. The potential for disturbance in body image relates to the exposure of and surgery on the female genitalia. The patient may need reassurance; privacy should be maintained. Expose only those body parts necessary for surgical preparation. Anxiety related to the surgery, its outcome, and anesthesia may be present. Help the patient use coping strategies that have been effective for her in the past. Assessment includes determining the patient's size and body weight in planning for appropriate instrumentation. In addition to laparoscopic instruments and accessories (CO_2 insufflator, light source, television monitor, video cassette recorder, printer, pressurized irrigation), a dilatation and curettage set should be available, as should an abdominal instrument set.

2. Refer to the protocol for lithotomy position; institute additional precautions for placing the patient in Trendelenburg's position.

FIG. 13-2
CARE PLAN FOR SUCTION CURETTAGE

KEY ASSESSMENT POINTS

Anxiety level/psychosocial concerns
Skin integrity
Limitations in mobility, range of motion
Core body temperature
Rh factor status
Hormone replacement therapy
Vaginal infection
Allergies/sensitivities

NURSING DIAGNOSIS

All generic nursing diagnoses apply to this patient, with the addition of:
Body image disturbance
High risk for injury, lithotomy position
Anxiety

PATIENT OUTCOMES

All generic outcomes apply, with the addition of:
The patient will not experience a disturbance in body image.
There will be no injury related to lithotomy position.
The patient will effectively cope with anxiety.
1. The patient's body image will be sustained through:
   a. Maintaining privacy
   b. Avoiding undue body exposure
   c. Providing emotional support
2. The patient will be free from injury related to lithotomy position as evidenced by:
   a. Absence of nerve injury
   b. Freedom from skin breakdown
   c. Minimal or no postural hypotension
3. The patient will cope with anxiety by discussing fears/concerns with perioperative nurse.

NURSING ACTIONS

	Yes	No	N/A
1. Assessment performed?	☐	☐	☐
2. Patient correctly placed in lithotomy position?	☐	☐	☐
3. Vaginal prep performed?	☐	☐	☐
4. Catheterization performed?	☐	☐	☐
5. Suction machine available/working?	☐	☐	☐
6. Specimen to lab?	☐	☐	☐
7. Counts performed/correct?	☐	☐	☐
8. Remove prep solution at end of procedure?	☐	☐	☐
9. Coping mechanisms assessed?	☐	☐	☐
10. Medications documented?	☐	☐	☐
11. Postoperative instructions given?	☐	☐	☐
12. Other generic care plans initiated? (specify)	☐	☐	☐

Document additional nursing actions/generic care plans initiated here:

_____

_____

_____

EVALUATION OF PATIENT OUTCOMES

	Outcome met	Outcome met with additional outcome criteria	Outcome met with revised nursing care plan	Outcome not met	Outcome not applicable to this patient
1. The patient's privacy was maintained.	☐	☐	☐	☐	☐
2. There was no positional injury.	☐	☐	☐	☐	☐
3. The patient effectively coped with her anxiety.	☐	☐	☐	☐	☐
4. The patient met outcomes for additional generic care plans as indicated.	☐	☐	☐	☐	☐

Signature: _____ Date: _____

FIG. 13-3
CARE PLAN FOR LAPAROSCOPY

KEY ASSESSMENT POINTS

Understanding of surgical procedure/possibility of laparotomy
Anxiety level/emotional needs
Skin integrity
Limitations in mobility, range of motion
Core body temperature
Allergies/sensitivities
Relevant health problems

NURSING DIAGNOSIS

All generic nursing diagnoses apply to this patient, with the addition of:
Body image disturbance
High risk for injury, lithotomy position
High risk for hypothermia

PATIENT OUTCOMES

All generic outcomes apply, with the addition of:
The patient will not experience a disturbance in body image.
There will be no injury related to lithotomy position.
1. The patient's body image will be sustained through:
   a. Maintaining privacy
   b. Avoiding undue body exposure
2. The patient will be free from injury related to lithotomy position as evidenced by:
   a. Absence of nerve damage
   b. Free from skin breakdown
   c. Minimal or no postural hypotension experienced
3. The patient's core body temperature will remain unchanged.

NURSING ACTIONS

	Yes	No	N/A
1. Assessment performed?	☐	☐	☐
2. Patient correctly placed in lithotomy/ Trendelenburg's position?	☐	☐	☐
3. Insufflation protocol followed?	☐	☐	☐
4. Thermal regulation measures implemented?	☐	☐	☐
5. Prep per institutional protocol?	☐	☐	☐
6. Patient catheterized? (straight or indwelling? indicate)	☐	☐	☐
7. Counts performed/correct?	☐	☐	☐
8. Medications documented?	☐	☐	☐
9. Prep solution removed at end of procedure?	☐	☐	☐
10. Postoperative pain around diaphragm or shoulder?	☐	☐	☐
11. Postoperative instructions given?	☐	☐	☐
12. Other care plans initiated? (specify)	☐	☐	☐

Document additional nursing actions/generic care plans initiated here:

_____

_____

_____

EVALUATION OF PATIENT OUTCOMES

1. The patient's privacy was maintained.
2. There was no positional injury.
3. Core body temperature was unchanged.
4. The patient met outcomes for additional generic care plans as indicated.

	Outcome met	Outcome met with additional outcome criteria	Outcome met with revised nursing care plan	Outcome not met	Outcome not applicable to this patient
1.	☐	☐	☐	☐	☐
2.	☐	☐	☐	☐	☐
3.	☐	☐	☐	☐	☐
4.	☐	☐	☐	☐	☐

Signature: _____ Date: _____

3. Refer to the protocol for endoscopy and insufflation.

4. Refer to the protocol for thermal regulation.

5. The anatomic skin preparation usually includes the abdomen, perineum, and vagina; it may extend to midthigh. Note the condition of the skin at the preparation site for rashes, bruises, lacerations, and so on.

6. A urinary catheter is usually required. Use aseptic technique. Record the amount of urine obtained. The catheter may remain indwelling for the duration of the procedure to avoid bladder injury during trocar placement.

7. Follow institutional protocol for sponge, sharp, and instrument counts.

8. A long-acting local anesthetic, such as bupivacaine 0.5%, may be injected at the incision site to decrease postoperative discomfort. Antiinflammatory analgesics may also be administered intramuscularly 1 hour before the procedure completion (if patient is free of renal disease and coagulopathy). Document all medications administered, the dose, and the route according to institutional protocol.

9. Remove excess preparation solution at the end of the surgical procedure to prevent skin irritation.

10. Explain to the patient that she may experience referred pain around the diaphragm or shoulder. This is caused by the reabsorption of CO_2. The pain usually lasts only 24 to 36 hours.

11. Postoperative instructions include the following:
    a. Do not wear tampons or douche.
    b. Notify the surgeon of excessive pain, nausea, vomiting, significant soiling of three or four pads a day with bright red blood, or temperature elevation above 100° F.
    c. Review any postoperative medications.
    d. Verify that the patient knows when and with whom to make a follow-up appointment.
    e. Discuss resumption of sexual activity and any other concerns the patient may have.

Laparoscopy with Laser (Fig. 13-4)

1. Patient assessment allows for individualization of the nursing care plan. The nursing diagnoses identified in this care plan require patient assessment for positional limitations for lithotomy, as well as noting whether there are any preoperative deficits in range of motion or comfort level or any alterations in sensation. The potential for disturbance in body image relates to exposure of and surgery on the female genitalia. The patient may need reassurance; privacy should be maintained. Expose only those body parts necessary for surgical preparation. Anxiety related to the surgery, its outcome, and anesthesia may be present. There are multiple indications for diagnostic laparoscopy; the patient may have suspected malignancy, infertility problems, or a tubal pregnancy. Help the patient use coping strategies that have been effective for her in the past. Assessment includes determining the patient's size and body weight in planning for appropriate instrumentation. In addition to laparoscopic instruments and accessories, a dilatation and curettage set should be available, as should an abdominal instrument set. If chromotubation for infertility is being performed, an intrauterine cannula and appropriate dye will be required.

2. Refer to the protocol for lithotomy position. Additional care should be taken when moving patients from lithotomy to Trendelenburg's position. Movement should be slow and deliberate to maintain circulatory stability and prevent shearing forces.

3. Refer to the protocol for insufflation and endoscopy.

4. The laser may be used. Refer to laser protocol.

5. The anatomic skin preparation usually includes the abdomen, perineum, and vagina; it may extend to midthigh. Note the condition of the skin at the preparation site for rashes, bruises, lacerations, and so on.

6. A urinary catheter is usually required. Use aseptic technique. Record the amount of urine obtained. The catheter may be left indwelling during the surgical procedure to prevent bladder injury during trocar placement.

7. Agents such as promethazine, dexamethasone, Hyskon's (dextran 40), and/or heparinized saline may be used to reduce adhesions. Warm irrigating fluids. Label all medications in the sterile field. Record medications administered intraoperatively.

8. Diluted methylene blue or indigo carmine solution may be used to test tube patency in chromotubation. If the tubes are patent, dye will be observed at the fimbriated ends of the fallopian tubes.

9. Follow institutional protocol for sponge, sharp, and instrument counts.

10. Refer to protocol for thermal regulation.

11. Remove excess preparation solution at the end of the surgical procedure to prevent skin irritation.

12. Explain to the patient that she may experience referred pain around the diaphragm or shoulder. This is caused by the reabsorption of CO_2. The pain usually lasts only 24 to 36 hours. Provide

FIG. 13-4
CARE PLAN FOR DIAGNOSTIC LAPAROSCOPY WITH POSSIBLE LASER APPLICATION; CHROMOTUBATION; D&C

KEY ASSESSMENT POINTS

Understanding of surgical procedure/possibility of laparotomy
Anxiety level/emotional needs
Skin integrity
Limitations in mobility, range of motion
Hemodynamic status
Core body temperature
Menstrual history
Allergies/sensitivities
Relevant health problems

NURSING DIAGNOSIS

All generic nursing diagnoses apply to this patient, with the addition of:
Body image disturbance
High risk for injury related to lithotomy position
Anxiety related to diagnostic outcomes
High risk for hypothermia

PATIENT OUTCOMES

All generic outcomes apply, with the addition of:
There will be no injury related to lithotomy position.
The patient will not experience disturbances in body image.
The patient will effectively cope with anxiety.
1. The patient will be free from injury related to lithotomy position as evidenced by:
   a. Absence of nerve damage
   b. Freedom from skin breakdown
   c. Minimal or no postural hypotension experienced
2. The patient's body image will be sustained through:
   a. Maintaining privacy
   b. Avoiding undue body exposure
   c. Providing emotional support
3. The patient will cope with anxiety by discussing fears/concerns with perioperative nurse.
4. The patient's core body temperature will remain unchanged.

NURSING ACTIONS

	Yes	No	N/A
1. Assessment performed?	☐	☐	☐
2. Patient correctly placed in lithotomy?	☐	☐	☐
3. Insufflation protocol followed?	☐	☐	☐
4. Laser available? Safety protocols initiated?	☐	☐	☐
5. Prep per institutional protocol?	☐	☐	☐
6. Patient catheterized?	☐	☐	☐
7. Hyskon or heparinized saline available?	☐	☐	☐
8. Dye available?	☐	☐	☐
9. Counts performed and correct?	☐	☐	☐
10. Thermal regulation measures implemented?	☐	☐	☐
11. Prep solution removed at end of procedure?	☐	☐	☐
12. Emotional support given?	☐	☐	☐
13. Coping mechanisms assessed?	☐	☐	☐
14. Postoperative instructions given?	☐	☐	☐
15. Other generic care plans initiated? (specify)	☐	☐	☐

Document additional nursing actions/generic care plans initiated here:

_____

_____

_____

EVALUATION OF PATIENT OUTCOMES

	Outcome met	Outcome met with additional outcome criteria	Outcome met with revised nursing care plan	Outcome not met	Outcome not applicable to this patient
1. The patient's privacy was maintained.	☐	☐	☐	☐	☐
2. There was no positional injury.	☐	☐	☐	☐	☐
3. The patient effectively coped with her anxiety.	☐	☐	☐	☐	☐
4. Core body temperature was unchanged.	☐	☐	☐	☐	☐
5. The patient met outcomes for additional generic care plans as indicated.	☐	☐	☐	☐	☐

Signature: _____ Date: _____

additional emotional support to the patient as necessary. Ectopic pregnancy, infertility, and diagnostic results have individual meaning to patients. Support and reassurance are important perioperative nursing interventions.

13. Help patients use coping mechanisms that have been effective for them in the past.

14. Postoperative instructions include the following:
    a. Do not wear tampons or douche.
    b. Notify the surgeon of excessive pain, nausea, vomiting, significant soiling of three or four pads a day with bright red blood, or temperature elevation above 100° F.
    c. Review any postoperative medications.
    d. Verify that the patient knows when and with whom to make a follow-up appointment.
    e. Discuss resumption of sexual activity and any other concerns the patient may have.

Total Abdominal Hysterectomy (Fig. 13-5)

1. Patient assessment allows for individualization of the nursing care plan. The potential for disturbance in body image relates to exposure of and surgery on the female genitalia. The patient may need reassurance; privacy should be maintained. Expose only those body parts necessary for surgical preparation. Anxiety related to the surgery, its outcome, and anesthesia may be present. Help the patient use coping strategies that have been effective for her in the past. Pain relates to the surgical intervention and the patient's postoperative status, as does the potential for urinary retention. Assessment includes determining the patient's size and body weight in planning for appropriate instrumentation. An abdominal gynecologic instrument set is required. A dilatation and curettage set should be available. Preparation sets for the abdomen and vagina are necessary.

2. The supine position is used. Assess the patient's skin and muscle mass; pad bony prominences. Place the safety strap snugly, but not tightly, above the knees. Prevent compression of nerves against the OR bed or armboards; prevent hyperabduction of arms on armboards. Apply antiembolism hose/sequential compression stockings as indicated. Care must be taken when moving the patient from supine to Trendelenburg's position. Movement should be slow and deliberate to maintain circulatory stability and prevent shearing. Check the toes for compression against Mayo stands.

3. Perform an external and internal vaginal preparation before prepping the abdomen. Note the condition of the skin at the preparation site (for example, rashes, lacerations, or bruises).

4. An indwelling urinary catheter will be inserted. Use aseptic technique. Keep the drainage bag off the floor, and put it where it is readily observable. Check that tubing is not stretched or kinked, especially during positional changes. Record urinary output.

5. The electrosurgical unit should be available and checked before use. Assess the patient's skin before and after application of the electrosurgical dispersive pad. Document site, condition.

6. Refer to protocol for thermal regulation.

7. If carcinoma is suspected, solution for peritoneal washing should be available. Irrigation fluid should be warmed; heparin may be added. Note the amount of irrigation fluid used; keep this separate from estimated blood loss accounts. Document medications used perioperatively; label all medications on the sterile field.

8. Autosuturing devices may be used according to the physician's preference.

9. Follow institutional protocol for the preservation and disposition of specimens. Use universal precautions when handling all specimens received from the sterile field. Record all routine and frozen sections.

10. Follow institutional protocol for sponge, sharp, and instrument counts.

11. Isolate instruments used in separating the cervix from the vagina.

12. Remove excess preparation solution at the end of the surgical procedure to prevent skin irritation.

13. Apply dressings aseptically. Do not place tape tightly when securing dressings because this may cause "tape burn" or skin breakdown when normal postoperative swelling occurs.

14. Pain is a subjective experience. When assessing pain, ask the patient to rate the pain on a scale of one to ten. Help the patient with pain-reducing strategies such as repositioning herself and splinting her incision. Encourage and explain the role of early ambulation in preventing postoperative complications.

15. If pain medication is administered, record the dosage, drug, and route. Always check for patient allergies before the administration of any medication. Assess the patient's response to and the effectiveness of pain medication. If pain is accompanied by flatulence, a suppository or laxative may be prescribed.

16. You may assist patients with coping by listening and providing explanations. Anxiety may be related to the belief that loss of the uterus also means loss of sexual functioning. If the patient's ovaries remain, they will continue to produce

FIG. 13-5
CARE PLAN FOR TOTAL ABDOMINAL HYSTERECTOMY

KEY ASSESSMENT POINTS

Understanding of surgical procedure/intended outcomes
Anxiety level/emotional needs
Skin integrity
Limitations in mobility, range of motion
Hemodynamic status
Core body temperature
Menstrual history/presence of vaginal infection
Allergies/sensitivities
Relevant health problems

NURSING DIAGNOSIS

All generic nursing diagnoses apply to this patient, with the addition of:

Body image disturbance
Anxiety related to diagnostic outcomes
Pain
High risk for urinary retention
High risk for hypothermia

PATIENT OUTCOMES

All generic outcomes apply, with the addition of:
The patient will adapt to disturbances in body image.
The patient will effectively cope with anxiety.
The patient's pain will be controlled.
The patient will not experience urinary retention.
The patient will remain normothermic.

1. The patient's body image will be sustained through:
   a. Maintaining privacy
   b. Avoiding undue body exposure
   c. Providing emotional support
2. The patient will cope with anxiety by discussing fears/concerns with perioperative nurse.
3. The patient's pain will be controlled as evidenced by:
   a. Vital signs within normal limits
   b. Pain medication is controlling pain
4. The patient will not experience urinary retention as evidenced by:
   a. Patient voids sufficient quantity
   b. Patient experiences no bladder distention
5. The patient's core body temperature will remain unchanged.

NURSING ACTIONS

	Yes	No	N/A
1. Assessment performed?	☐	☐	☐
2. Correctly positioned?	☐	☐	☐
3. Prep per institutional protocol?	☐	☐	☐
4. Indwelling catheter inserted?	☐	☐	☐
5. ESU safety protocols followed?	☐	☐	☐
6. Thermal regulation measures implemented?	☐	☐	☐
7. Supplies available for pertioneal washing if applicable?	☐	☐	☐
8. Stapling devices available?	☐	☐	☐
9. Specimen to lab?	☐	☐	☐
10. Counts performed and correct?	☐	☐	☐
11. Aseptic precautions taken?	☐	☐	☐
12. Prep solution removed at end of case?	☐	☐	☐
13. Dressing applied carefully?	☐	☐	☐
14. Pain assessed?	☐	☐	☐
15. Analgesic administered?	☐	☐	☐
16. Coping mechanisms assessed?	☐	☐	☐
17. Voided 150-200 cc after catheter removed?	☐	☐	☐
18. Postoperative instructions given?	☐	☐	☐
19. RX for:			
a. Antibiotic?	☐	☐	☐
b. Analgesic?	☐	☐	☐
c. Hormones?	☐	☐	☐
d. Iron?	☐	☐	☐
20. Other generic care plans initiated? (specify)	☐	☐	☐

Document additional nursing actions/generic care plans initiated here:

_____

_____

_____

EVALUATION OF PATIENT OUTCOMES

	Outcome met	Outcome met with additional outcome criteria	Outcome met with revised nursing care plan	Outcome not met	Outcome not applicable to this patient
1. The patient's privacy was maintained.	☐	☐	☐	☐	☐
2. The patient effectively coped with her anxiety.	☐	☐	☐	☐	☐
3. The patient's pain was controlled.	☐	☐	☐	☐	☐
4. The patient experienced no urinary retention.	☐	☐	☐	☐	☐
5. Core body temperature was unchanged.	☐	☐	☐	☐	☐
6. The patient met outcomes for additional generic care plans as indicated.	☐	☐	☐	☐	☐

Signature: _____ Date: _____

hormones until normal menopause. If the ovaries have been removed, hormonal therapy will be required. Remind the patient that she will still need gynecologic examinations if her ovaries are intact; some patients think that removal of the uterus indicates cessation of gynecologic examinations. Encourage the patient to ask questions and use coping mechanisms that have worked for her in the past.

17. Measure voidings after removing the indwelling urinary catheter. If the patient is voiding less than 150 ml at a time, she may need to be recatheterized. Provide privacy during voiding; running water or warm perineal rinsing may assist the patient with voiding.

18. Postoperative instructions include the following:
    a. Do not wear tampons or douche until approved by physician.
    b. Notify the surgeon of excessive pain, nausea, vomiting, odorous vaginal discharge, significant soiling of three or four pads a day with bright red blood, any urinary problems (burning, difficulty urinating, frequent urination, passing small amounts of urine), temperature elevation above 100° F, or if the incision appears more swollen or red than it appeared on discharge.
    c. Avoid heavy lifting, activities that increase pelvic congestion (dancing, jogging, aerobics), and resumption of sexual activities until the physician gives clearance.
    d. Begin prescribed abdominal strengthening exercises.
    e. Avoid constrictive clothing.
    f. Verify that the patient knows when and with whom to make a follow-up appointment.

19. Indicate on the care plan whether the patient received prescriptions for any of these medications. Review the medication's purpose, the dosage and times to be taken, and side effects to be expected or reported. It is helpful to involve a family member or significant other in discharge planning.

Laparoscopically Assisted Vaginal Hysterectomy (LAVH)
(Fig. 13-6)

1. Patient assessment allows for individualization of the nursing care plan. The potential for disturbance in body image relates to exposure of and surgery on the female genitalia. The patient may need reassurance; privacy should be maintained. Expose only those body parts necessary for surgical preparation. Anxiety related to the surgery, its outcome, and anesthesia may be present. Assist the patient with the use of coping strategies that have been effective for her in the past. Pain relates to the surgical intervention and the patient's postoperative status, as does the potential for urinary retention. Assessment includes determining the patient's size and body weight in planning for appropriate instrumentation. A vaginal instrument set, along with the laparoscopic instrument set and accessories, is required. An abdominal set should be available. The vaginal walls may be infiltrated with saline or lidocaine solution, with or without epinephrine, to facilitate dissection and decrease bleeding; syringes and needles will then be necessary. Record any medications administered intraoperatively. Label all medications on the sterile field.

2. Refer to protocol for lithotomy position. Care must be taken when moving the patient from supine to Trendelenburg's position. Movement should be slow and deliberate to maintain circulatory stability and prevent shearing. A pelvic examination may be done at this time to assess uterine size, position, and mobility.

3. Perform vaginal and abdominal skin preparation according to institutional protocol.

4. A urinary catheter will be inserted to empty the bladder. Record urinary output. At the conclusion of the procedure, an indwelling urinary catheter may be inserted.

5. The electrosurgical unit should be available and checked before use; determine whether a unipolar or bipolar system will be used. For unipolar systems, assess the patient's skin before and after application of the electrosurgical dispersive pad. Document the site and skin condition.

6. Mechanical stapling systems may be used; have available laparoscopic clips and a reloading mechanical stapling and cutting instrument.

7. Refer to protocol for laparoscopic insufflation.

8. Follow institutional protocol for the preservation and disposition of specimens. Record all routine and frozen sections.

9. Follow institutional protocol for sponge, sharp, and instrument counts.

10. Remove excess preparation solution at the end of the surgical procedure to prevent skin irritation.

11. Pain is a subjective experience. When assessing pain, ask the patient to rate the pain on a scale of one to ten. Assist the patient with pain-reducing strategies. An ice pack may be prescribed for perineal application. Encourage and explain the role of early ambulation in preventing postoperative complications.

12. If pain medication is administered, record the dosage, drug, and route. Always check for pa-

FIG. 13-6
CARE PLAN FOR LAPAROSCOPICALLY ASSISTED VAGINAL HYSTERECTOMY (LAVH)

KEY ASSESSMENT POINTS
Understanding of surgical procedure/possibility of laparotomy
Anxiety level/emotional needs
Skin integrity
Limitations in mobility, range of motion
Hemodynamic status
Significant cardiovascular/pulmonary disease
Core body temperature
Menstrual history/presence of vaginal infection
Recent Papanicolaou smear results
Relevant health problems

NURSING DIAGNOSIS
All generic nursing diagnoses apply to this patient, with the addition of:
Body image disturbance
Pain
High risk for injury related to lithotomy position

PATIENT OUTCOMES
All generic outcomes apply, with the addition of:
The patient will not experience any disturbance in body image.
The patient's pain will be controlled.
There will be no injury related to lithotomy position.
1. The patient's body image will be sustained through:
   a. Maintaining privacy
   b. Avoiding undue body exposure
   c. Providing emotional support
2. The patient's pain will be controlled as evidenced by:
   a. Vital signs within normal limits
   b. Pain medication is controlling pain
3. The patient will be free from injury related to lithotomy position as evidenced by:
   a. Free from nerve damage
   b. Free from skin breakdown
   c. Minimal or no postural hypotension

NURSING ACTIONS

	Yes	No	N/A
1. Assessment performed?	☐	☐	☐
2. Patient correctly placed in lithotomy position?	☐	☐	☐
3. Vaginal/abdominal prep performed?	☐	☐	☐
4. Catheter available/inserted?	☐	☐	☐
5. ESU safety protocols followed?	☐	☐	☐
6. Stapling devices available?	☐	☐	☐
7. Insufflation protocols followed?	☐	☐	☐
8. Specimen to lab?	☐	☐	☐
9. Counts performed/correct?	☐	☐	☐
10. Prep solution washed off at end of case?	☐	☐	☐
11. Postoperative pain assessed?	☐	☐	☐
12. Analgesics administered?	☐	☐	☐
13. Emotional support given?	☐	☐	☐
14. Postoperative instructions given?	☐	☐	☐
15. Rx for:			
a. Antibiotic	☐	☐	☐
b. Analgesic	☐	☐	☐
c. Iron	☐	☐	☐
16. Other generic care plans initiated? (specify)	☐	☐	☐

Document additional nursing actions/generic care plans initiated here:

_____

_____

_____

EVALUATION OF PATIENT OUTCOMES

	Outcome met	Outcome met with additional outcome criteria	Outcome met with revised nursing care plan	Outcome not met	Outcome not applicable to this patient
1. The patient's privacy was maintained.	☐	☐	☐	☐	☐
2. There was no positional injury.	☐	☐	☐	☐	☐
3. The patient met outcomes for additional generic care plans as indicated.	☐	☐	☐	☐	☐

Signature: _____ Date: _____

tient allergies before the administration of any medication. Assess the patient's response to and effectiveness of pain medication. If pain is accompanied by flatulence, a suppository or laxative may be prescribed.

13. You may assist patients in their coping by listening and providing explanations. Anxiety may be related to the belief that losing the uterus means losing sexual functioning. If the patient has remaining ovaries, they will continue to produce hormones until normal menopause. If the ovaries have been removed, hormonal therapy will be required. Remind the patient that she will still need to have gynecologic examinations if her ovaries are intact; some patients think that removal of the uterus indicates cessation of gynecologic examinations. Encourage the patient to ask questions and to use coping mechanisms that have worked for her in the past.

14. Postoperative instructions include the following:
    a. Do not wear tampons or douche until approved by physician.
    b. Notify the surgeon of excessive pain, nausea, vomiting, significant soiling of three or four pads a day with bright red blood, odorous vaginal discharge, problems with urination, or temperature elevation above 100° F.
    c. Verify that the patient knows when and with whom to make a follow-up appointment.
    d. Avoid heavy lifting and activities that increase pelvic congestion (dancing, aerobics, or jogging) until cleared with the physician.
    e. Sexual activity should not be resumed until clearance by the physician is obtained.

15. Indicate on the care plan whether the patient received prescriptions for any of these medications. Review the medication's purpose, the dosage and times to be taken, and any side effects to be expected or reported. It is helpful to involve a family member or significant other in discharge planning.

Cesarean Section (Fig. 13-7)

1. Patient assessment allows for individualization of the nursing care plan. The patient may be anxious if this is an unplanned cesarean section. Assist the patient with breathing techniques during contractions; encourage her to use coping mechanisms she has learned in childbirth classes (Fawcett, et al., 1993). Assessment includes determining the patient's size and body weight in planning for appropriate instrumentation and positioning. A cesarean section instrument set, suction tubing, and accessories for the baby (if these are in a separate set) are required.

Assess for full stomach; have a nasogastric tube and suction line available. See that the consent form is signed. Determine whether blood has been typed and cross-matched. Review relevant preoperative laboratory/diagnostic studies (complete blood count [CBC] with differential, electrolytes, Hgb/Hct, amniocentesis for fetal lung maturity as indicated, ultrasound). Explain preparatory procedures as they are performed. Determine time of last oral intake. Determine core body temperature.

2. The supine position will be used. Pad bony prominences, and place the patient in good body alignment. It may be necessary to assist the anesthesia staff with regional anesthetic injections before the patient is in supine position. Place the safety strap above the knees, snugly but not tightly.

3. Refer to protocol for thermal regulation.

4. Monitor and record maternal vital signs according to institutional protocol. Evaluate breathing (should be controlled with contractions). Continue to evaluate pain and anxiety.

5. Monitor and record fetal heart tones according to institutional protocol (normal: 120 to 160 beats per minute).

6. Monitor and record contractions according to institutional protocol (frequency, duration, intensity). Note and document whether the patient is receiving oxytocin.

7. An indwelling urinary catheter will be inserted if one is not already present. Use aseptic technique. Place the drainage bag where it is readily observable; keep it off the floor. Prevent stretching and kinking of the tubing. Document catheter insertion. Record urinary output.

8. Follow institutional protocol for anatomic landmarks for abdominal preparation. Note the condition of the skin at the preparation site (rashes or bruises).

9. One of the goals of delivery in any patient care setting is that the birthing experience will be perceived as positive and family oriented. A significant other will usually be permitted to accompany the mother to the OR if they have attended childbirthing classes. The significant other may need the nurse's help in preparing for the delivery by washing hands and donning scrub attire or a protective gown. Reassurance may be needed. Encourage the significant other to coach and lend support.

10. Verify that the isolette or baby warmer and other needed equipment are available and in working order.

11. Suction, cord clamps, and oxygen will be needed immediately after the delivery.

FIG. 13-7
CARE PLAN FOR CESAREAN SECTION

KEY ASSESSMENT POINTS

Understanding of precesarean routine/events
Anxiety level/emotional needs
Skin integrity
Limitations in mobility, range of motion
Hemodynamic status
Rh status
Core body temperature
Full stomach
Relevant health problems

NURSING DIAGNOSIS

All generic nursing diagnoses apply to this patient, with the addition of:
Anxiety related to need for cesarean section
High risk for aspiration
High risk for altered patterns of urinary elimination

PATIENT OUTCOMES

All generic outcomes apply, with the addition of:
The patient will effectively cope with anxiety.
The patient will not aspirate stomach contents.
The patient will regain normal voiding patterns.
1. The patient will cope with anxiety by discussing fears/concerns with perioperative nurse. She will:
   a. Display relaxed body posture in between contractions
   b. Verbalize reduction in anxiety
   c. Accurately describe perioperative events
2. The patient will not aspirate stomach contents. She will:
   a. Have normal vital signs
   b. Have regular breath sounds
3. The patient will regain normal voiding patterns. She will:
   a. Void spontaneously without discomfort

NURSING ACTIONS

	Yes	No	N/A
1. Assessment performed?	☐	☐	☐
2. Correctly positioned?	☐	☐	☐
3. Thermal regulation measures?	☐	☐	☐
4. Maternal vital signs monitored?	☐	☐	☐
5. Fetal heart tone monitored?	☐	☐	☐
6. Contractions monitored?	☐	☐	☐
7. Indwelling catheter available/inserted?	☐	☐	☐
8. Prep per institutional protocol?	☐	☐	☐
9. Significant other present?	☐	☐	☐
10. Baby warmer checked?	☐	☐	☐
11. Suction, O_2, cord clamp available for infant?	☐	☐	☐
12. Equipment available for resuscitation of infant?	☐	☐	☐
13. Nursery personnel/pediatrician available?	☐	☐	☐
14. Bulb syringe on sterile field?	☐	☐	☐
15. Infant and mother identified?	☐	☐	☐
16. Tube available for cord blood?	☐	☐	☐
17. Specimen to lab?	☐	☐	☐
18. Counts performed and correct?	☐	☐	☐
19. Remove prep solution at end of procedure?	☐	☐	☐
20. Encourage bonding with infant by mother and family?	☐	☐	☐
21. Report to PACU?	☐	☐	☐
22. Other generic care plans initiated? (specify)	☐	☐	☐

Document additional nursing actions/generic care plans initiated here:

_____

_____

_____

EVALUATION OF PATIENT OUTCOMES

	Outcome met	Outcome met with additional outcome criteria	Outcome met with revised nursing care plan	Outcome not met	Outcome not applicable to this patient
1. The patient effectively coped with her anxiety.	☐	☐	☐	☐	☐
2. Stomach contents were not aspirated.	☐	☐	☐	☐	☐
3. Normal voiding patterns were resumed.	☐	☐	☐	☐	☐
4. The patient met outcomes for additional generic care plans as indicated.	☐	☐	☐	☐	☐

Signature: _____ Date: _____

12. Emergency resuscitative equipment should be available.
13. Nursery personnel and/or the pediatrician are usually in the OR to care for the infant. If they have not arrived at the time of the delivery, the perioperative nurse will need to be prepared to assist a member of the anesthesia team with the newborn.
14. The bulb syringe will be used to clear the nasopharyngeal airway at birth. As soon as this is accomplished, the cord will be clamped and cut and the infant wrapped in a sterile towel or blanket and passed to the pediatrician or nursery personnel. A gown should be provided to this person before transfer.
15. Follow institutional protocol for identifying the mother and baby.
16. A tube is necessary to collect cord blood.
17. Follow institutional protocol for the preservation and disposition of the placenta.
18. Follow institutional protocol for sponge, sharp, and instrument counts.
19. Remove excess preparation solution at the end of the procedure to prevent skin irritation. Apply dressings aseptically. Do not apply tape tightly; allow for postoperative swelling. This will prevent tape burns.
20. After delivery, allow for the mother, baby, and significant other to have time together. Bonding can be initiated in this way. Indications of bonding in the postpartum phase include talking to and about the infant and touching the infant. Research on the stress of cesarean birth indicates that there are numerous physiologic, psychologic, and life-style concerns for most women (Miovech, Knapp, & Borucki, 1994). During the early recovery period (2 weeks postprocedure), pain, incisional problems, activity intolerance, fatigue, and gastrointestinal disturbances were common. At 8 weeks postpartum, concerns related primarily to body image, family interaction, and work. The patient should be encouraged to discuss concerns that might interfere with bonding and return to a balanced life-style and psychologic outlook.
21. Give the nursing report to the postanesthesia care unit staff.

Ruptured Ectopic Pregnancy (Fig. 13-8)

1. When tubal rupture occurs, the patient is in critical need of surgical intervention. She may arrive at the OR with severe pain, nausea and vomiting, and signs and symptoms of shock. Depending on the amount of blood loss, this patient may need transfusion and treatment for shock. The emergent nature of the surgery requires a collaborative nursing focus on maintaining hemodynamic stability. Assess for full stomach. Determine last oral intake. Determine the patient's Rh status. The extensiveness of surgical correction will be determined at the time of operation. Salpingostomy with tubal anastomosis, salpingectomy, or salpingo-oophorectomy may be indicated. Instruments for an abdominal laparotomy will be needed; instruments for tubal anastomosis and accessories (suture, magnifying loops, and microscope) should be available. A calm, supportive environment should be maintained; reassurance and explanations should be provided.
2. Refer to protocol for thermal regulation.
3. The supine position is used. Assess the patient's skin and muscle mass; pad bony prominences. Place the safety strap snugly, but not tightly, above the knees. Prevent compression of nerves against the OR bed or armboards; prevent hyperabduction of arms on armboards.
4. An indwelling urinary catheter may be inserted (if not already present). Use aseptic technique. Keep the drainage bag off the floor. Prevent tubing from kinking or stretching; place the bag where it is readily observable. Document catheter insertion.
5. Perform surgical preparation according to institutional protocol. Note the condition of the skin at the preparation site (rashes, lacerations, or bruises).
6. Intravenous solutions, blood, or blood products should be warmed to help the patient maintain or regain normothermia.
7. If preoperative antibiotics have been ordered, check to see whether they have been given or are available in the OR.
8. The electrosurgical unit should be available and checked before use.
9. Assess the patient's skin before and after application of the electrosurgical dispersive pad. Document the site and skin condition.
10. Follow institutional protocol for the preservation and disposition of specimens. Use universal precautions when handling all specimens received from the sterile field. Record all routine and frozen sections.
11. Follow institutional protocol for sponge, sharp, and instrument counts.
12. Record all intake and output (intravenous infusions, blood and blood products, urinary output).
13. Document all medications administered by the perioperative nursing team. Medication may be added to irrigation to prevent the formation of adhesions.

FIG. 13-8
CARE PLAN FOR RUPTURED ECTOPIC PREGNANCY

KEY ASSESSMENT POINTS
Understanding of perioperative routine/events
Anxiety level/emotional needs
Skin integrity
Limitations in mobility, range of motion
Hemodynamic status
Rh status
Core body temperature
Presence/location of pain
Full stomach
Relevant health problems

NURSING DIAGNOSIS
All generic nursing diagnoses apply to this patient, with the addition of:
Anxiety
Fluid volume deficit (actual or high risk)
Pain
High risk for aspiration

PATIENT OUTCOMES
All generic outcomes apply, with the addition of:
The patient will effectively cope with anxiety.
The patient's fluid volume will be maintained.
The patient's pain will be minimized/controlled.
The patient will not aspirate stomach contents during endotracheal intubation.
The patient will:
1. Perceive threat of emergency surgery realistically
2. Verbalize less anxiety
3. Maintain hemodynamic stability
4. Express pain relief
5. Be intubated without aspiration of stomach contents

NURSING ACTIONS

	Yes	No	N/A
1. Assist with adequate hemodynamic support if patient is in shock?	☐	☐	☐
2. Thermal regulation measures implemented?	☐	☐	☐
3. Correctly positioned?	☐	☐	☐
4. Patient catheterized?	☐	☐	☐
5. Prep per institutional protocol?	☐	☐	☐
6. Blood warmer available?	☐	☐	☐
7. Preoperative antibiotics ordered/given?	☐	☐	☐
8. ESU available?	☐	☐	☐
9. ESU safety protocols followed?	☐	☐	☐
10. Specimen to lab?	☐	☐	☐
11. Counts performed and correct?	☐	☐	☐
12. Intake/output recorded?	☐	☐	☐
13. Medications administered?	☐	☐	☐
14. Prep solution washed off?	☐	☐	☐
15. Dressing applied carefully?	☐	☐	☐
16. Nursing report to postanesthesia care unit?	☐	☐	☐
17. Other generic care plans initiated? (specify)	☐	☐	☐

Document additional nursing actions/generic care plans initiated here:

_____

_____

_____

EVALUATION OF PATIENT OUTCOMES

	Outcome met	Outcome met with additional outcome criteria	Outcome met with revised nursing care plan	Outcome not met	Outcome not applicable to this patient
1. The patient's anxiety was reduced.	☐	☐	☐	☐	☐
2. The patient's fluid volume was maintained.	☐	☐	☐	☐	☐
3. The patient expressed pain relief.	☐	☐	☐	☐	☐
4. The patient did not aspirate stomach contents.	☐	☐	☐	☐	☐
5. The patient met outcomes for additional generic care plans as indicated.	☐	☐	☐	☐	☐

Signature: _____ Date: _____

14. Remove excess preparation solution at the end of the surgical procedure to prevent skin irritation.

15. Apply dressings aseptically. Do not place tape tightly when securing dressings; this may cause "tape burn" or skin breakdown when normal postoperative swelling occurs. Note whether any drains have been incorporated into the dressing.

16. Nursing report should be provided to the nurse in the postanesthesia care unit. If the perioperative nurse is unable to complete full patient education, the postanesthesia care unit staff should be advised of the desirability of a consult with a perinatal nurse specialist. Patients who experience an ectopic pregnancy endure feelings of loss, grief, anger, frustration, or failure. The patient will need support and time to express her feelings. There may be concerns related to the prognosis of future pregnancies; there is evidence of decreased fertility and greater risk for second extrauterine gestation in women with ectopic pregnancy (McCulloch, 1994). The perioperative nurse or perinatal nurse specialist can direct the patient to reliable sources of information as well as sources of support therapy (Wheeler, 1994).

Repair of Cystocele and Rectocele (Fig. 13-9)

1. Patient assessment allows for individualization of the nursing care plan. The potential for disturbance in body image relates to exposure of and surgery on the female genitalia. The patient may need reassurance; privacy should be maintained. Expose only those body parts necessary for surgical preparation. Anxiety related to the surgery, its outcome, and anesthesia may be present. Help the patient use coping strategies that have been effective for her in the past. Pain relates to the surgical intervention and the patient's postoperative status, as does the risk for urinary retention. Assessment includes determining the patient's size and body weight in planning for appropriate instrumentation. A vaginal instrument set is required. A dilatation and curettage set should also be available. Determine core body temperature. Verify that preoperative douche, cathartic, and cleansing enema have been completed as prescribed.

2. Refer to protocol for lithotomy position. Care must be taken when moving the patient from supine to Trendelenburg's position. Movement should be slow and deliberate to maintain circulatory stability and prevent shearing.

3. Perform vaginal preparation according to institutional protocol.

4. A urinary catheter may be inserted. Use aseptic technique. Record the amount of urine obtained from catheterization.

5. Refer to protocol for thermal regulation.

6. The electrosurgical unit should be available and checked before use. Assess the patient's skin before and after application of the electrosurgical dispersive pad. Document the site and skin condition.

7. Vaginal packing may be inserted. Record packing and antibiotic as applicable.

8. Follow institutional protocol for the preservation and disposition of specimens. Use universal precautions with all specimen containers received from the sterile field. Record all routine and frozen sections.

9. Follow institutional protocol for sponge, sharp, and instrument counts.

10. An indwelling urinary catheter (or suprapubic cystotomy catheter) will be inserted at the end of the procedure if not already in place. Use aseptic technique for catheter insertion. Do not allow the drainage bag to lie on the floor. Record the presence of the catheter.

11. Remove excess preparation solution at the end of the surgical procedure to prevent skin irritation.

12. Pain is a subjective experience. When assessing pain, ask the patient to rate the pain on a scale of one to ten. Assist the patient with pain-reducing strategies such as repositioning herself. An ice pack may be prescribed for perineal application. Encourage and explain the role of early ambulation in preventing postoperative complications.

13. If pain medication is administered, record the dosage, drug, and route. Always check for patient allergies before the administration of any medication. Assess the patient's response to and the effectiveness of pain medication. If pain is accompanied by flatulence, a suppository or laxative may be prescribed; enemas should be avoided.

14. Measure voidings after removing the indwelling urinary catheter. If the patient is voiding less than 150 ml at a time, she may need to be recatheterized. Provide privacy during voiding; running water or warm perineal rinsing may help the patient void.

15. Postoperative instructions include the following:
    a. Do not wear tampons or douche.
    b. Notify the surgeon of excessive pain, nausea, vomiting, difficult or painful urination, significant soiling of three or four pads a day with bright red blood, or temperature elevation above 100° F.

FIG. 13-9
CARE PLAN FOR REPAIR OF CYSTOCELE AND RECTOCELE

KEY ASSESSMENT POINTS

Understanding of perioperative routine/events
Anxiety level/emotional needs
Skin integrity
Limitations in mobility, range of motion
Urinary/bowel symptoms
Bladder or vaginal infection
Core body temperature
Hormone replacement therapy
Relevant health problems

NURSING DIAGNOSIS

All generic nursing diagnoses apply to this patient, with the addition
    of:
Body image disturbance
Pain
High risk for injury related to lithotomy position
High risk for altered patterns of urinary elimination

PATIENT OUTCOMES

All generic outcomes apply, with the addition of:
The patient will not experience a disturbance in body image.
The patient's pain will be controlled.
The patient will not experience urinary retention.
There will be no injury related to lithotomy position.
1. The patient's body image will be sustained through:
   a. Maintaining privacy
   b. Avoiding undue body exposure
   c. Providing emotional support
2. The patient's pain will be controlled as evidenced by:
   a. Vital signs within normal limits
   b. Pain medication is controlling pain
3. The patient will not experience urinary retention as evidenced by:
   a. Patient voids sufficient quantity
   b. Patient experiences no bladder distention
4. The patient will be free from injury related to lithotomy position
   as evidenced by:
   a. Absence of nerve damage
   b. Freedom from skin breakdown
   c. Minimal or no postural hypotension

NURSING ACTIONS

	Yes	No	N/A
1. Assessment performed?	☐	☐	☐
2. Patient correctly placed in lithotomy position?	☐	☐	☐
3. Vaginal prep performed?	☐	☐	☐
4. Catheter available/inserted?	☐	☐	☐
5. Thermal regulation measures?	☐	☐	☐
6. ESU safety protocols followed?	☐	☐	☐
7. Vaginal pack available?	☐	☐	☐
8. Specimen to lab?	☐	☐	☐
9. Counts performed and correct?	☐	☐	☐
10. Indwelling catheter inserted at end of procedure?	☐	☐	☐
11. Prep solution washed off at end of procedure?	☐	☐	☐
12. Postoperative pain assessed?	☐	☐	☐
13. Analgesics administered?	☐	☐	☐
14. Voided 150-220 cc after catheter removed?	☐	☐	☐
15. Postoperative instructions given?	☐	☐	☐
16. Other generic care plans initiated? (specify)	☐	☐	☐

Document additional nursing actions/generic care plans initiated
here:

_____

_____

_____

EVALUATION OF PATIENT OUTCOMES

	Outcome met	Outcome met with additional outcome criteria	Outcome met with revised nursing care plan	Outcome not met	Outcome not applicable to this patient
1. The patient's privacy was maintained.	☐	☐	☐	☐	☐
2. The patient's pain was controlled.	☐	☐	☐	☐	☐
3. The patient experienced no urinary retention.	☐	☐	☐	☐	☐
4. There was no positional injury.	☐	☐	☐	☐	☐
5. The patient met outcomes for additional generic care plans as indicated.	☐	☐	☐	☐	☐

Signature: _____ Date: _____

c. Mild laxatives may be prescribed. Straining during bowel movements should be avoided. Fluid intake should be adequate.

d. Heavy lifting and prolonged periods of standing, walking, or sitting should be avoided.

e. Sexual activity should not resume until healing has occurred (consult the physician). Verify that the patient knows there may be a temporary loss of vaginal sensation.

f. Verify that the patient knows when and with whom to make a follow-up appointment.

g. Indicate on the care plan whether the patient received prescriptions for any medications. Review the medication's purpose, the dosage and times to be taken, and any side effects to be expected or reported. It is helpful to involve a family member or significant other in discharge planning.

References

Agency for Health Care Policy and Research. (1994). A woman's guide: Things to know about quality mammograms (AHCPR pub. no. 95-0634). Rockville, MD: The Agency.

Association of Operating Room Nurses. (1993). *Recommended practices for care of instruments, scopes, and powered surgical instruments.* Denver, CO: The Association.

Ball KA. (1995). *Lasers: The perioperative challenge* (2nd Ed.). St. Louis: Mosby.

Beresford JM & Moher MS. (1993). A prospective comparison of abdominal hysterectomy using absorbable staples. *Surgery Gynecology, and Obstetrics, 176*(6), 555-558.

Bernhard L. (1992). Men's views about hysterectomies and women who have them. *Journal of Nursing Scholarship, 24*(3), 177-181.

Bichat X. (1814). *Desault's surgery.* Philadelphia: Thomas Dobson.

Crow S. (1993). Sterilization processes: Meeting the demand of today's health care technology. In V Brinko (Ed.), *Nursing Clinics of North America* (pp. 687-695). Philadelphia: WB Saunders.

Crow S. (1993). Practical innovations. *AORN Journal, 58*(4), 771-774.

Daley J, Espersen C, & Jackson D. (1993). Clinical applications. In JC Rothrock (Ed.), *The RN first assistant: An expanded perioperative nursing role* (pp. 308-336). Philadelphia, PA: JB Lippincott.

Fawcett J, et al. (1993). Effects of information on adaptation to cesarean birth. *Nursing Research, 42*(1), 49-53.

Garner BD. (1995). Infection control. In MH Meeker and JC Rothrock (Eds.), *Alexander's care of the patient in surgery*, (10th Ed.). St. Louis: Mosby.

Hartweg DI. (1993). Self-care actions of healthy middle-aged women to promote well-being. *Nursing Research, 42*(4), 221-227.

Jackson KD. (1991). Endometrial ablation with rollerball electrode. *AORN Journal, 54*(2), 268-282.

Magrina JF. (1994). What's new in gynecology and obstetrics. *ACS Bulletin, 79*(1), 31-34.

McCulloch K. (1994). Ectopic pregnancy. *Nursing Spectrum, 3*(18), 12-14.

Miovech S, Knapp H, & Borucki L. (1994). Major concerns of women after cesarean delivery. *JOGN, 23*(1), 53-59.

National Institutes of Health (1994, June 3). *Consensus statement on ovarian cancer: Screening, treatment, and follow-up.* Washington, DC: The Institutes.

Ott DE. (1989). Contamination via gynecologic endoscopy insufflation. *Journal of Gynecologic Surgery, 5*(2), 205-208.

Ott DE. (1991). Laparoscopic hypothermia. *Journal of Laparoendoscopic Surgery, 1*(3), 127-131.

Ott DE. (1991). Correction of laparoscopic insufflation hypothermia. *Journal of Laproendoscopic Surgery, 1*(4), 183-186.

Ott DE. (1993). Smoke production and smoke reduction in endoscopic surgery: Preliminary report. *Endoscopic Surgery and Allied Technologies, 1*, 1-3.

Pagana KD & Pagana TJ. (1995). *Mosby's diagnostic and laboratory test reference* (2nd Ed.). St. Louis, MO: Mosby.

Paschal CR & Strzelecki LR. (1992). Lithotomy positioning devices, *AORN Journal, 55*(4), 1011-1022.

Pratt JH. (1977). Historical vignette: Ephraim McDowell. *Mayo Clinic Proceedings, 52*, 125.

Rorden JW & Tatt E. (1990). *Discharge planning guide for nurses.* Philadelphia: WB Saunders.

Rothrock JC & Sculthorpe RH. (1993). Anesthesia and patient positioning. In JC Rothrock (Ed.), *The RN first assistant: An expanded perioperative nursing role* (pp. 116-146). Philadelphia: JB Lippincott.

Saunders DB. (1993). Adhesions in pelvic surgery. *Point of View, 30*(1), 10-13.

Seitzinger MR & Dudgeon LS. (1993). Decreasing the degree of hypothermia during prolonged laparoscopic procedures. *Journal of Reproductive Medicine, 38*(7), 511-513.

Sigerist HE. (1960). *The history of medicine.* New York: MD.

Smith CD. (1992). Clinical issues. *AORN Journal, 56*(1), 126-128.

Summitt RL, et al. (1992). Randomized comparison of laparoscopically assisted vaginal hysterectomy with standard vaginal hysterectomy in an outpatient setting. *Obstetrics and Gynecology, 80*(6), 895.

Tadir Y & Fisch B. (1993). Operativew laparoscopy: A challenge for general gynecology? *American Journal of Obstetrics and Gynecology, 69*(1), 7-12.

Verrell C. (1995). Randomized controlled trial of the comparison of two alternative hysteroscopic techniques for the control of dysfunctional uterine bleeding. *British Journal of Theatre Nursing, 4*(10), 7-8.

Wheeler SR. (1994). Psychosocial needs of women during miscarriage or ectopic pregnancy. *AORN Journal, 60*(2), 221-231.

Wilbanks GD. (1991). What's new in gynecology and obstetrics. *ACS Bulletin, 76*(1), 24-26.

BIBLIOGRAPHY

Dripps RD, Eckenhoff JE, & Vandam LD. (1991). *Introduction to anesthesia: The principles of safe practice.* Philadelphia: WB Saunders.

Fishbein EG. (1992). Women at midlife: The transition to menopause. In L Dumas (Ed.), *Nursing Clinics of North America* Philadelphia: WB Saunders.

McMullin M. (1992). Holistic care of the patient with cervical cancer. In L Dumas (Ed.), *Nursing Clinics of North America* Philadelphia: WB Saunders.

Maddox MA. (1992). Women at midlife: Hormone replacement therapy. In L Dumas (Ed.), *Nursing Clinics of North America* Philadelphia: WB Saunders.

Chapter 14

Cardiac Surgery

Patricia C. Seifert

"The road to the heart is only 2 or 3 cm. in a direct line, but it has taken surgery nearly 2,400 years to travel it."

(SHERMAN, 1902)

HISTORY

Because of its mystical attributes, the heart was the last organ to undergo surgical treatment. It was less than 100 years ago in Germany that Ludwig Rehn ushered in the era of cardiac surgery by suturing the right ventricle of a young man hemorrhaging from a stab wound. In the United States, the first cardiac surgery, performed in 1902, was also the closure of a stab wound to the heart. The period surrounding the turn of the century also saw the beginning of efforts to treat valvular heart disease. Early attempts to relieve mitral valve and pulmonary valve stenoses were unsuccessful, and it was not until 1948 that Charles Bailey used a valvulotome to accomplish a closed commissurotomy successfully on a patient with mitral valve stenosis. Techniques for open repair of valvular stenosis or insufficiency would need to await the development of extracorporeal circulation.

Efforts to treat coronary artery disease surgically also began during this early period when sympathectomies were performed for relief of angina pectoris. Epicardial inflammation was then attempted with the hope of developing new blood channels to the ischemic heart. Several modifications of this Beck procedure were made using irritant pastes, talc, magnesium silicate, sand, asbestos, and phenol. Poor results were partly responsible for the development of the Vineberg procedure in 1950, wherein the internal mammary artery was implanted into the myocardium. The procedure was abandoned because it was doubtful how much blood was actually supplied to the heart. It was not until the 1960s that direct surgical revascularization using grafts to bypass coronary obstructions was popularized by Rene Favalaro (Shumacker, 1992).

Perhaps the most significant advancement in cardiac surgery was extracorporeal circulation, which enabled the surgeon to work on a quiescent heart without sacrificing perfusion to the other organs of the body. This achievement by Gibbon in 1953 allowed open heart surgery to flourish in the treatment of congenital and acquired heart disease.

Other technologic improvements in the early twentieth century fostered the growth of heart surgery. Among these were new anastomatic techniques and the development of blood banking, hemodynamic monitoring, and electrocardiography. The discovery of heparin enabled bypass circuits to remain free of blood clots. Diagnostic methods improved with the refinement of chest radiography and the development of angiography, cardiac catheterization, echocardiography, and nuclear imaging techniques. New suture materials were created, and prosthetic grafts and valves enabled surgeons to repair and replace damaged blood vessels, valves, and other cardiac structures. In addition, methods of cardiac resuscitation and refinements in anesthesia, along with improvements in preserving the heart itself, all contributed to the growth of cardiovascular surgery, which numbered over 3.8 million procedures in 1990 (AHA, 1992).

Presently, almost all types of congenital and acquired heart disease are amenable to surgical intervention. Myocardial revascularization with direct coronary artery bypass grafting has shown improved results with antiplatelet therapy and arterial conduits. These conduits, especially the internal mammary artery, show fewer atherosclerotic changes and remain patent longer than the saphenous vein graft, which heretofore was commonly the sole bypass graft used.

New techniques employed for valvular heart disease enable surgeons to repair the native valve or replace it with biologic or mechanical prostheses. Valvular prostheses have been much improved over the years, but bioprostheses can degenerate and fail after 10 years, and mechanical valves require anticoagulation, which creates bleeding risks. When life expectancy is 10 years or more, mechanical valves may be preferable, although within certain populations, such as the elderly or those in whom chronic anticoagulation is contraindicated, biologic valves may be the prosthesis of choice. Whenever possible, valve repair is performed.

Surgery for cardiac dysrhythmias has allowed improved function for patients with abnormal conduction pathways or with ischemic heart disease. Electrophysiologic mapping enables surgeons to locate and then ablate or excise the source of irritable ventricular foci. Pacemakers are now routinely inserted, and the internal cardioverter defibrillator (ICD) can be implanted in patients with intractable lethal dysrhythmias. Current ICDs also have pacing capabilities.

Progress has resulted in decreased mortality from diseases of the aorta. Hypothermic circulatory arrest has decreased the incidence of postoperative complications in patients with aneurysms of the aortic root and of the transverse arch; technical refinements enable early repair of dissecting and atherosclerotic aneurysms.

The majority of congenital lesions have been aggressively attacked, and complex cardiac anomalies, such as single ventricle, truncus arteriosus, and complex transposition of the great arteries, can be palliated or corrected by surgery. Children with the most severe lesions may undergo cardiac transplantation.

Transplantation of the heart itself is no longer considered experimental, largely as a result of improved preservation techniques for donor hearts and advancements in the use of immunosuppressive agents, such as cyclosporine and monoclonal antibodies. A number of mechanical assist devices for the failing heart are available: intraaortic balloon pumps, extracorporeal centrifugal blood pumps, and left and right ventricular assist devices (VADs). Implantable VADs are increasingly employed as a bridge to transplantation. Heart-lung transplantation—a complex, expensive, and resource-intensive procedure—is demonstrating improved 1-year survival rates, although data are still required to establish logical and scientifically sound patient and institutional selection criteria for this procedure (Health Technology Assessment, 1994).

Future trends affecting cardiovascular surgery include disease prevention and a wider array of therapeutic interventions both within and outside the operating room. Efforts to modify risk factors for coronary disease continue to be emphasized. For patients requiring intervention, treatment modalities in the cardiac catheterization laboratory include improved thrombolytic therapy, balloon angioplasty, coronary stents, atherectomy, and the development of laser revascularization. Operative procedures will employ these techniques as well, and new prostheses will be created to bypass stenosed, previously implanted grafts. Finally, experimental research now in progress on heterograft rejection may enable surgeons to implant bovine or porcine hearts in patients with end-stage cardiac disease.

Over the past 100 years progress in surgical interventions for heart disease has been rapid. Until we learn more about the disease process and its progression, we will continue to refine and expand our surgical options and improve our care of patients undergoing these procedures. Nursing research has made important contributions in the study of multiple factors influencing patient care events. Nurse researchers are doing important work in the area of clinical studies. The type of dressing used on central lines and its effect on maintaining line integrity without compromising patient comfort (Dugger, Macklin, & Rand, 1994), rewarming the patient with forced air versus radiant heat (Giuffre, Heidenreich, & Pruitt, 1994), activity patterns and recovery in female bypass surgery patients (Redeker, et al., 1994), gender differences during recovery (Hawthorne, 1994), and coping and emotional response to cardiac surgery (Crumlish, 1994) are just a few examples of this work. The development of clinical paths and benchmarking to describe best processes of care and improve them will be an integral component of future interdisciplinary research (Barnes, Lawton, & Briggs, 1994).

ASSESSMENT CONSIDERATIONS

A patient assessment is performed to develop a plan of care for the cardiac surgical patient. The assessment should reflect a holistic view of the patient, facilitate the use of nursing diagnoses, and incorporate accepted standards of practice (Guzzetta, et al., 1989). Including process and outcome standards developed by the Association of Operating Room Nurses (AORN) for perioperative patients and the standards jointly developed by the American Nurses Association (ANA) and the American Heart Association (AHA) for cardiovascular patients helps the perioperative nurse to document adherence to those standards within the plan of care itself. The *Standards of Cardiovascular Nursing Practice* (ANA, 1981) outline specific data to be collected concerning the health status of the individual within this patient population.

History

The history should include information about the patient's previous health status and his or her perceptions and expectations of the disease and the recommended intervention. The status of the patient, whether emergent, semiemergent, or elective, will affect both the comprehensiveness of the assessment and the extensiveness of the teaching plan. The perioperative nurse should include information about the family (who may also be one of the few sources of information in an emergency).

Symptoms should be identified and described. Patients with ischemic heart disease commonly complain of chest pain (angina pectoris). Patients with valvular heart disease may emphasize shortness of breath, syncope, fatigue, and anginal pain or upper abdominal pain (from hepatomegaly related to right heart failure). The perioperative nurse should note the onset, duration, quality, location, radiation, associated symptoms, precipitating factors, and relieving factors of each symptom.

A detailed list of all recent medications and the patient's response to them should be recorded. Special attention should be given to inotropic, diuretic, and myocardial depressant drugs, such as antiarrhythmics, beta blockers, and calcium channel blockers. Previous antibiotic, antihypertensive, and corticosteroid therapy should be noted as well.

Risk factors. Part of the history should incorporate the risk factor profile. This is important to planning care for hospitalization and discharge because it focuses on areas that may require further patient education. Risk factors include family history of heart disease, hypercholesterolemia or hypertriglyceridemia, smoking, hypertension, obesity, diabetes, alcohol intake, and psychosocial factors such as sedentary living and high stress levels (AHCPR, 1994). Determine if there is a history of rheumatic fever or frequent tonsillitis as a child. The sequelae of rheumatic fever and streptococcal infections can lead to damage of the cardiac valves. The presence of diabetes is notable because diabetes mellitus affects the vascular system and may retard the healing process, predisposing the patient to infection.

Obesity increases the workload of the heart and may also increase the risk for a postoperative infection because adipose tissue is poorly vascularized.

The following personal and social factors should also be assessed:

1. Caffeine intake
2. Nutritional status
3. Sleep patterns
4. Occupational and economic factors
5. Distance from laboratory facilities
6. Activities
7. Living arrangements
8. Family dynamics
9. Education
10. Cultural, ethnic, and spiritual beliefs and values

Physical Assessment

The physical assessment provides the perioperative nurse with baseline data and information about potential problems and risks that may require intervention. Although the cardiovascular system is the focus of the assessment, findings from other assessment parameters guide the perioperative nurse in integrating information into a comprehensive patient care plan. These should be reviewed for their value in planning care for the cardiac surgery patient.

General assessment. Skin appearance offers clues to the patient's cardiovascular status. Dryness, coolness, diaphoresis, paleness, edema, poor capillary refill, bruising, and petechiae can reflect impaired cardiovascular function. Patients with endocarditis may have Osler's nodes in the pads of the fingers or toes. These are painful erythematous skin lesions from infected emboli (Braunwald, 1992).

Visual problems and headaches may alert the perioperative nurse to problems of cerebral perfusion and may be related to inadequate cardiac output or to atherosclerotic disease. However, medications such as digitalis may alter vision and mentation, which can be mistaken for impaired circulation. Sites of chronic infection (tonsils, sinuses, or carious teeth) should be identified and treated to control potential sources of postoperative infection.

Other findings related to the neurologic system include changes in levels of consciousness, memory, comprehension, and emotional status. Confusion, restlessness, slurred speech, numbness, and paralysis can signal impaired cerebral perfusion. Syncope and fainting spells may be associated with reduced cardiac output related to aortic valve stenosis, cerebral emboli originating from an enlarged left atrium in mitral valve stenosis, or cerebral atherosclerotic disease.

Respiratory assessment can indicate the degree of heart failure. What is the respiratory rate, quality, and pattern? Coughing and abnormal breath sounds may point to pulmonary edema and the need for a strict preoperative and postoperative pulmonary toilet. Chest expansion, use of accessory muscles, diaphragmatic excursion, and intercostal retraction or bulging should be assessed. Does the patient suffer from orthopnea or paroxysmal nocturnal dyspnea; does the patient become dyspneic or short of breath after climbing one flight of stairs?

Gastrointestinal problems such as pain, food intolerance, appetite changes, sudden weight gain, heartburn, and difficulty swallowing may signal right ventricular dysfunction. Genitourinary findings such as altered or decreased urinary function or changes in sexual desire or function may indicate compromised cardiac output.

Cardiovascular assessment. Finally, what is the cardiovascular status? Is there discomfort or pain in the chest, arms, shoulders, back, neck, or jaw? Alleviating pain is a prime consideration in the care of the cardiovascular patient because pain is a myocardial stressor. Cold is another stressor because the shivering that accompanies chilling elevates the metabolic rate, making the heart work harder.

Chest wall size, configuration, and movements should be determined. What is the point of maximal intensity? Are there palpable thrills, heaves, or pulsations that may indicate ventricular hypertrophy or aortic stenosis? Heart sounds, murmurs, and friction rubs provide clues to ischemic or valvular heart disease and to pericarditis. Apical, radial, and femoral pulses also reflect cardiac function: what is their rate, rhythm, and quality? An increased heart rate is not well tolerated by cardiac patients because myocardial perfusion is jeopardized during the shortened diastolic filling time that accompanies ventricular tachycardia.

Blood pressure may be high, normal, or low. The hypertensive patient may have left ventricular hypertrophy, and the hypotensive patient may display changes in neurologic, gastrointestinal, and renal function. Blood pressures should be checked bilaterally. Unequal pressures in the arms may be a contraindication for the use of the internal mammary artery on the side of the lower blood pressure, where perfusion may not be optimal. Patients with coarctation of the aorta will demonstrate unequal blood pressures of the upper extremity, and patients with dissecting aneurysms may have unequal carotid, femoral, brachial, or radial artery blood pressures when the dissection occludes one or more of the great vessels.

Because cardiac function affects all the body's organ systems, patient assessment should be comprehensive whenever possible. A thorough assessment will also alert the physician and the perioperative nurse to the need for special diagnostic tests and laboratory procedures.

DIAGNOSTIC STUDIES

Most patients referred for surgery will have had a complete clinical evaluation including both invasive and noninvasive studies. A careful history and physical may bring out pertinent facts not recalled by the patient.

Noninvasive Studies

Electrocardiogram. Initially, most patients seek treatment because of chest pain or other symptoms such as syncope, palpitations, or exertional dyspnea. After the history and physical assessment, a resting electrocardiogram (ECG) is ordered. Even if the resting ECG is normal for a patient suspected of having coronary artery disease (CAD), an exercise ECG (stress test) may be performed because ST segment changes indicating myocardial ischemia are often apparent only during or after exercise. In patients with intractable dysrhythmias, electrophysiologic (EP) studies may be performed to locate the site of irritable ventricular foci, which can be medically treated, surgically removed, or controlled with an implantable defibrillator.

Chest radiography. Chest radiography provides information about the size of the cardiac chambers, thoracic aorta, and pulmonary vasculature, as well as the presence of calcium in valves, pericardium, coronary arteries, and aorta. In patients with coarctation of the aorta, rib notching will be evident on the left side of the thorax due to the tortuous path of hypertrophied intercostal arteries. For patients with suspected thoracic aneurysms, aortography with radiopaque dye is performed to determine the size and location of the lesion and the site of the intimal tear in aortic dissections.

Echocardiography. Echocardiography is a noninvasive test that evaluates both the structure and function of the heart by transmitting sound waves to the heart and measuring those sound waves reflected back to the transducer. These are processed by the transducer, which creates visual images of the structures' movements. Echocardiography is commonly used to assess valvular function and to determine the degree of valvular stenosis or regurgitation. It can also demonstrate a tumor or thrombus in the atrial cavity. Transesophageal echocardiography (TEE) is routinely employed intraoperatively to assess valvular function and reparative techniques, as well as to evaluate ventricular function and the presence of intracardiac air.

Radionuclide imaging. Radionuclide imaging is employed to illustrate wall motion and blood flow through the heart and to quantify cardiac function.

These noninvasive techniques are generally well tolerated by patients, especially when they may be too unstable to withstand a cardiac catheterization. They may also be used as a complement to catheterization. Common radionuclide tests are the multiple-gated acquisition (MUGA) scan (also known as blood pool imaging) and exercise thallium perfusion scintigraphy.

The MUGA scan uses intravenous radioactively tagged red blood cells to provide information regarding cardiac perfusion and function. A computerized camera is programmed to count the distance between R waves on the ECG; the distance is divided into fractions of a second, called gates. The multiple images are viewed to evaluate regional and global wall motion of the heart and to determine the ejection fraction.

Exercise thallium (201 T1) scintigraphy provides additional information about the function of the heart by reflecting deficits in myocardial perfusion at rest and after exercise. The procedure is similar to a MUGA except that there is an exercise portion of the study (often performed on a bicycle).

The integration of computer analysis in imaging techniques has improved quantification of coronary artery disease and produced greater refinements in the diagnostic accuracy of these tests. Computers have also been applied to improve image analysis in techniques such as digital subtraction angiography, computed tomography, and magnetic resonance imaging, all of which are being employed extensively in the diagnosis of heart disease.

Invasive Studies

Cardiac catheterization remains the gold standard in providing the most definitive information about the extent and location of ischemic, valvular, and congenital heart disease, although echocardiography has become a highly reliable tool for valvular and congenital lesions. Coronary angiography demonstrates coronary anatomy, and ventriculography illustrates contractile weaknesses of the ventricles, as well as some congenital intracardiac defects. These studies are used to assess the degree of myocardial dysfunction and to plan interventions, such as coronary artery bypass grafting, mechanical ventricular assistance, or cardiac transplantation, if cardiac function is irreversibly compromised. The cardiologist can compute the orifice of a stenosed valve or determine the degree of regurgitation of an incompetent valve. Ventricular, atrial, and pulmonary pressures are recorded, and cardiac output and ejection fraction estimated. Oxygen saturations of cardiac chambers and the ratio of pulmonary to systemic blood flow (Qp/Qs) are calculated in patients with shunts and congenital or acquired defects. Cinearteriograms provide motion pictures of radiopaque dye flowing through the heart, demonstrating both myocardial contractility and abnormalities of intracardiac flow.

Laboratory Studies

Laboratory tests are used to assess the function of various organ systems. Hematologic tests measure the hemoglobin, hematocrit, and white cell and platelet count, and provide information about the function and oxygen-carrying capacity of the blood. A detailed coagulation profile can uncover hemorrhagic disorders. A low platelet count may alert the perioperative nurse to anticipate prolonged bleeding without replacement of this product. Partial thromboplastin time and prothrombin times are checked to determine deficiencies in the clotting factors of the coagulation system. The patient's blood type is also determined and the appropriate order placed with the blood bank. Precautions are taken to test the blood for viral contamination and for cold antibodies, which could produce agglutination of the patient's blood during surgery when the patient is cooled to hypothermic temperatures.

Liver and kidney function tests may be abnormal for patients with chronic heart failure. This may be due to congestion in the former and reduced blood flow in the latter. Abnormal measurements may be obtained with tests of serum protein, albumin and globulin, serum enzymes, blood urea nitrogen, creatinine, and serum electrolytes. Progressive improvement in hepatic and renal function is anticipated with better perfusion as a result of surgery.

Additional laboratory examinations in the preoperative period may include arterial blood gases and enzyme markers of myocardial damage (such as the creatine-kinase MB isoenzyme, known as MB bands), especially in the presence of persistent angina. Pulmonary function tests are performed to determine baseline data and to plan postoperative care when respiratory function may be impaired due to the use of extracorporeal circulation and stasis of lung secretions that accompany prolonged surgery.

NURSING DIAGNOSES

Because there is often a profound impact on the physical and emotional integrity of the person with cardiovascular disease, many nursing diagnoses are applicable to this patient population. Nursing care plans are developed from more than a pathophysiologic perspective. One method to facilitate the development of nursing diagnoses within a holistic framework is to perform a biopsychosocial assessment and to classify specific diagnoses into the nine human response patterns developed by the North American Nursing Diagnosis Association (NANDA). When assessing the patient, the perioperative nurse can collect the data according to these patterns, cluster the information into signs and symptoms, and determine whether the diagnoses within that pattern are applicable (Box 14-1).

Exchanging

The exchanging pattern includes most of the physiologic diagnoses that are commonly encountered during surgery. It also reflects many of the patient outcomes that pertain to injury, skin integrity, fluid

---

Box 14-1 Nursing Diagnoses for the Cardiac Surgery Patient: Classification by Human Response Patterns

Exchanging: A Human Response Pattern Involving Mutual Giving and Receiving

Airway clearance, ineffective
Aspiration, risk for
Body temperature, altered, risk for
Breathing pattern, ineffective
Cardiac output, decreased
Fluid volume deficit
Fluid volume deficit, risk for
Fluid volume excess
Gas exchange, impaired
Hyperthermia
Hypothermia
Infection, risk for
Injury, risk for (specify) (electrical, physical, chemical hazards, positioning, retained foreign objects)
Nutrition, altered: less than body requirements
Nutrition, altered: less than body requirements
Nutrition, altered: more than body requirements
Nutrition, altered: risk for more than body requirements
Oral mucous membrane, altered
Skin integrity, impaired
Skin integrity, impaired, risk for
Tissue integrity, impaired
Tissue perfusion, altered (specify) (renal, cerebral, cardiopulmonary, gastrointestinal, peripheral)

Communicating: A Human Response Pattern Involving the Sending of Messages

Communication, impaired verbal

Relating: A Human Response Pattern Involving the Establishing of Bonds

Family processes, altered
Parental role conflict
Parenting, altered
Parenting, altered, risk for
Role performance, altered
Sexual dysfunction
Sexuality patterns, altered
Social interaction, impaired
Social isolation

Valuing: A Human Response Pattern Involving the Assigning of Relative Worth

Spiritual distress (distress of the human spirit)

Choosing: A Human Response Pattern Involving the Selection of Alternatives

Adjustment, impaired
Coping, family: potential for growth
Coping, ineffective family: compromised
Coping, ineffective family: disabling
Coping, ineffective individual
Decisional conflict (specify)
Health-seeking behaviors (specify)
Noncompliance (specify)

Moving: A Human Response Pattern Involving Activity

Activity intolerance
Activity intolerance, risk for
Diversional activity deficit
Fatigue
Growth and development, altered
Home maintenance management, impaired
Mobility, impaired physical
Self-care deficit, bathing/hygiene
Self-care deficit, dressing/grooming
Self-care deficit, feeding
Self-care deficit, toileting
Sleep pattern disturbance
Swallowing, impaired

Perceiving: A Human Response Pattern Involving the Reception of Information

Body image disturbance
Hopelessness
Personal identity disturbance
Powerlessness
Self-esteem, chronic low
Self-esteem, disturbance
Self-esteem, situational low
Sensory/perceptual alterations: visual, auditory, kinesthetic, gustatory, tactile, olfactory

Knowing: A Human Response Pattern Involving the Meaning Associated with Information

Knowledge deficit (specify)
Thought processes, altered

Feeling: A Human Response Pattern Involving the Subjective Awareness of Information

Anxiety
Fear
Pain
Pain, chronic

and electrolytes, infection, and the physiologic response to surgery. Grouping diagnoses within this pattern can enable the perioperative nurse to select the appropriate high-risk or actual patient response(s) within a specific body system. Diagnoses related to oxygenation and breathing include *ineffective airway clearance, aspiration, ineffective breathing pattern,* and *impaired gas exchange.* These may all be found in the cardiac patient.

Operative time periods for cardiac surgery are often greater than 2 to 3 hours and may last much longer in complex or difficult cases. The associated immobility and anesthesia time contribute to the retention of secretions that can create a high risk for aspiration and produce impaired gas exchange, as well as ineffective breathing patterns and airway clearance (and lead to altered oral mucous membranes).

Other predisposing factors include a history of smoking and the presence of preoperative pulmonary edema or congestive failure. Pulmonary hypertension also reduces lung compliance and impairs gas exchange. Patients with an altered level of consciousness or who are fatigued, premedicated, in pain, or otherwise unable to breathe deeply may have problems with effective gas exchange and breathing patterns.

Circulatory status. The circulatory status is generally the focal point for patients undergoing cardiac surgery, and the most common nursing diagnoses are *altered cardiac output* and *altered tissue perfusion.* Commonly, patients with cardiac disease either have or are at great risk for a reduction in their cardiac output and subsequently for impaired tissue perfusion. The reasons for this are as varied as the number of diseases related to the heart.

Ischemic heart disease damages the myocardium itself by reducing the supply of nutrients and jeopardizing cellular respiration. Cardiac function is progressively impaired, and less cardiac reserve is available during periods of physical and emotional stress.

Valvular heart disease produces both functional and structural problems. Stenosed valves mechanically obstruct blood flow to the systemic circulation. In the case of aortic valve stenosis, a large pressure gradient between the left ventricular chamber and the ascending aorta can be associated with a sufficiently reduced mean aortic pressure (MAP) that may compromise coronary perfusion and produce anginal symptoms. The compensatory mechanisms that the heart uses to eject blood through a stenosed aortic valve may themselves pose a burden on the heart. Left ventricular hypertrophy eventually reduces ventricular compliance and increases the muscle mass, requiring nutrition from a coronary circulatory system that cannot enlarge to meet increased demands. Systemic changes, such as vasoconstriction, are brought about by the drop in MAP accompanying a decreased cardiac output. Consequently, adequate perfusion of the body's organ systems is impaired. Syncope accompanies reductions in cerebral blood flow or perfusion pressure. Decreased renal perfusion alters kidney function. Incompetent valves produce regurgitation of blood into the originating chamber. The increased volume load produces left ventricular dilatation, which impairs the contractile function of the heart.

Conduction disturbances alter cardiac output by affecting the rate or the rhythm of ejection. Both atrial and ventricular contraction contribute to an adequate output. If there are conduction disturbances, such as atrial fibrillation or premature ventricular contractions, these will impair cardiac output.

Because surgery itself is stressful to the heart, precautions are taken to reduce the possibility of myocardial damage intraoperatively. The possibility of hemorrhage is present intraoperatively and postoperatively. The operative site may contain calcium deposits, fat particles, suture remnants, or other debris that could embolize. Instruments are a source of debris as well, and air bubbles in cardiopulmonary bypass inflow lines can produce air emboli.

Unnecessarily prolonged ischemic times due to lack of preparedness should be prevented. Necessary instruments, supplies, and equipment should be available and in working order. Knowledge of the surgical procedure avoids delays and enhances anticipation of needs.

Although achieving hypothermia during surgery is a method of protecting the heart, hypothermia (and altered body temperature) becomes a problem when it occurs preoperatively or postoperatively. In the preoperative period, the shivering that accompanies chilling should be avoided because of the increased metabolic demands associated with shivering. In the early postoperative period it is not unusual to encounter some residual hypothermia. If rewarming is not gradual, the body has difficulty in rapidly adjusting to the shifting of blood from the core temperature of central organs to the periphery as the patient rewarms and vasodilatation occurs. A precipitous drop in blood pressure can result. It is helpful then to retard heat loss during the period between the end of surgery and admission to the recovering intensive care unit (ICU).

Other diagnoses in the exchanging category applicable to the cardiac patient include injury, impaired skin integrity, and impaired tissue integrity. These diagnoses are related to the same causes of impaired respiratory and circulatory function. In patients with compromised cardiac function who undergo prolonged procedures, special precautions must be taken so that skin and tissue are not damaged. The risk for injury is increased as well due to the use of potentially dangerous equipment, such as defibrillators and electrosurgery devices; chemical hazards, such as the glutaraldehyde storage solution of bioprosthetic valves; and mechanical injury to nerves due to improperly positioned sternal and internal mammary artery (IMA) retractors.

The presence of altered skin and tissue integrity associated with a preexisting metabolic disorder, such as diabetes mellitus, can also increase the risk for infection. Obesity *(altered nutrition, more than body requirements)* and cachexia *(altered nutrition, less then body requirements)* may also impair wound healing and contribute to the development of infection. Obese patients may have retained necrotic tissue at the site of electrosurgical coagulation, and malnourished patients may have insufficient metabolic resources to promote wound healing. A mediastinal infection, or infection of a prosthetic heart valve, is a grave complication that not only prolongs hospitalization and increases costs, but can also lead to generalized sepsis and death. High risk for infection should be routinely included in cardiac care plans.

The last diagnoses to be discussed in the exchanging pattern are *fluid volume excess* and *fluid volume deficit.* These can be related to blood loss, hypertonic or hypotonic infusions, fluid shifts, dehydration, immobility, and an inability to maintain appropriate fluid status due to congestive heart failure or renal failure. Monitoring renal function and hemodynamic status offers clues to the patient's fluid status intraoperatively. Reductions in urine output and low central venous pressures (in the presence of normal or low pulmonary capillary wedge pressures) can indicate fluid volume deficits. A distended heart or elevated central venous and pulmonary pressures may indicate excess volume. Many variables are assessed to confirm either diagnosis.

Communicating

Impaired verbal communication is a diagnosis related to the communicating pattern of human responses. The etiology for this diagnosis is often cardiovascular insufficiency, reduced level of consciousness, sedation, dyspnea, or physical barriers such as endotracheal tubes. The inability to speak or understand the dominant language also impairs communication.

Relating

Establishing and maintaining bonds is frequently affected by heart disease. The heart is perceived by many to be more than just an intricate pump, and the physiologic consequences of heart disease affect the patient's ability to maintain personal, professional, and societal roles. Pain and fatigue, two common symptoms, make social interaction, role performance (such as parenting), and family processes more difficult because the patient is often uncomfortable and tired. Sexual dysfunction may be present as a result of the symptoms described above, and it may also result from poor perfusion.

Valuing

When companionship is denied or compromised by debilitating symptoms, patients may be in *spiritual distress.* They may be unable to engage in religious ceremonies or to benefit from the spiritual support of religious counselors. An awareness of this problem may encourage health care professionals to request visits by ministers, rabbis, or priests. The perception of the heart as the seat of the soul and many patients' fear of death make this a probable nursing diagnosis.

Choosing

When problems with communicating, relating, and valuing exist, it is not unusual to find problems with adjusting and coping. Difficulties are experienced by both patients and families as the disease progresses and its impact is increasingly felt. How does the spouse cope with the disease and its consequences? Who does the housekeeping? Who is responsible for the family's financial welfare? How does the individual respond or adapt to the need for heart surgery? Is the response one of denial, disbelief, anger, regression, lack of cooperation, or acceptance? Do conflicts arise between patient and health care professionals, or patient and significant others?

What about therapeutic regimens prescribed either before or after surgery? Often these regimens necessitate life-style changes that may not be implemented properly unless the patient is in the appropriate frame of mind, adequately educated, and the family supports the changes. Difficulty in following prescribed behaviors may point to a nursing diagnosis of *noncompliance,* but the perioperative nurse should investigate whether failure to adhere to recommendations is purposeful or is the consequence of inadequate knowledge and support (Artinian, 1993).

Patients who demonstrate a willingness to modify life-styles or to follow prescriptive orders may be diagnosed as engaging in *health-seeking behaviors.* This diagnosis is also significant in the rehabilitative period when risk factor modification, laboratory appointments, or awareness of postoperative complications and the appropriate response to them become important.

Moving

Activities of daily living necessitate both a willing mental attitude and the physical ability to perform such activities. Fatigue, pain, and dyspnea can disturb sleep patterns and create self-care deficits in hygiene, grooming, and feeding. *Impaired physical mobility, activity intolerance,* and *impaired home maintenance* would not be uncommon in patients with a cardiac output insufficient to meet exercise-induced demands. These patients would also be likely to have deficits in diversional activity as well. Children with severe congenital lesions would demonstrate altered growth and development.

Perceiving

Activity deficits are likely to influence how individuals perceive themselves. Disturbances in body image and self-concept are related to functional restrictions imposed by disease. Self-esteem and personal identity are affected, and feelings of hopelessness and powerlessness may become apparent with the realization that activities once taken for granted can no longer be accomplished. Sensory and perceptual alterations may become evident as the disease progresses in severity. Both emotional and physical factors may be present in patients who demonstrate changes in vision, hearing, movement, smelling, and tasting.

Knowing

Knowledge deficits are common to patients with heart disease because of the complex nature of the disease and the technical sophistication of its diagnosis and treatment. Moreover, patients employ numerous coping mechanisms to help them adjust to emotional stress. The perioperative nurse must assess the patient within the context of the specific disease and relate that to how the patient perceives the situation. Data from the relating, choosing, and perceiving categories can be used to assess the patient's ability and readiness to learn. Distinctions must be made between what the patient knows, what the patient does not want to know, and what the patient needs to know.

Patient education begins with an assessment of what the patient already knows. Preoperatively, patients are generally unaware of the technical details of a procedure. Many patients do not want vivid descriptions of sternal splitting, saphenous vein excision, or chest wiring. Ignorance of those details should be respected and allowed. Conversely, certain individuals cope through gaining extensive knowledge of a procedure. These patients amaze nurses with their "homework" and inquire about cardiopulmonary bypass, induced arrest, and long-term patency of saphenous vein grafts versus internal mammary artery conduits. Nurses need to meet the patient's needs and answer questions or find someone who can.

Patients need information that facilitates a positive experience. It is easier to have a cooperative patient (and one who will release fewer endogenous catecholamines) if he or she is aware of the sequence of events immediately before surgery. Describe transportation to the OR and explain what the holding area and the OR will look like and feel like (cold? warm?). How many people will be in the room? What do they do? Patients often want to know if they'll be naked and when the urinary catheter goes in and if it hurts. (Read: "Am I awake when these things happen?")

Postoperatively, it is reassuring to know that family members will be able to see, talk, and touch the patient, even though he or she may be heavily sedated. In some cases family members or significant others may not want to go to the ICU. They should be reassured that there is no correct or incorrect ICU protocol about visiting; it is too stressful for some individuals and will only increase their (and the patient's) anxiety.

Patients appreciate being forewarned about being intubated and unable to talk. Recovered patients often mention the frustration of being alert but unable to speak. The perioperative nurse should describe alternative methods of communication available in the ICU.

Feeling

Few patients undergoing surgery are immune to *pain.* Preoperatively, pain may be chronic (for example, angina) or acute (for example, aortic dissection). Postoperatively, pain and altered comfort are related to multiple sources, from the operative procedure itself to the various devices used to monitor postoperative status. Routines such as positioning, and the ICU environment, with its 24-hour illumination and multiple equipment noises, make the achievement of comfort more difficult. Accurate pain assessment and adequate administration of pain medication is imperative for patients experiencing pain and discomfort (Maxam-Moore, Wilkie, & Woods, 1994).

Physical discomfort may be aggravated by *fear* and *anxiety.* By definition, fear has an identifiable source, and the nurse can reduce fear by encouraging the patient to express his or her fear(s), answering questions, and communicating reassurance through body language, caring touch, and tone of voice. Medical questions can be directed to surgeons or attending physicians.

Anxiety is a more unspecified threat and may be the consequence of unformulated fears or some unknown danger. Encouraging the patient to discuss concerns or to verbalize questions facilitates a clearer definition of what is causing the sense of dread. Clarification of these concerns and questions may produce a better sense of control of the situation by the patient. Providing physical comfort measures and reducing noxious stimuli may also foster an increased sense of well-being.

The nursing diagnoses that have been suggested are not all-inclusive. They do, however, represent diagnoses common to cardiac surgical patients. For perioperative nurses who wish to develop a generic care plan for these patients, Box 14-2 presents common nursing actions to help the patient meet outcomes identified by the AORN.

CARE PLANS

Specific cardiac surgery nursing care plans, along with accompanying Guides to Nursing Actions, are presented in the concluding section of this chapter. The nursing diagnoses identified in Box 14-2 may pertain to patients undergoing each of the procedures for which specific care plans have been developed. However, only one or two of the most likely nursing diagnoses for the specific procedure have been incorporated into the care plans. The perioperative nurse needs to modify and adapt these care plans and selected nursing diagnoses, nursing actions, and desired patient outcomes to reflect the individual status of each patient undergoing cardiac surgery.

GUIDES TO NURSING ACTIONS
Coronary Artery Bypass Grafting (CABG) (Fig. 14-1)

1. Fig. 14-1 details key preoperative assessment data for coronary bypass patients. Because of the nursing diagnoses selected for this patient (*decreased cardiac output* and *altered tissue perfusion*), assess parameters that will be used to determine outcome attainment. These may vary but should include a review of baseline vital signs and abnormalities and renal status. Examine the extremities and sacrum for edema. Locate peripheral pulses. In addition to those data, assess legs for varicosities. If present, the surgeon may elect to use an alternative conduit, such as arm veins or the lesser saphenous vein. This will require preparing and draping of arms and draping of legs to expose posteriorly located lesser saphenous vein.

2. Determine both the patient's understanding of the progressive nature of coronary artery disease and readiness to learn about risk factor modification. Assess understanding of the use of internal mammary artery (IMA) (or other arterial conduits) and greater saphenous vein for conduits. Explain possible need for lesser saphenous vein or cephalic vein (or possibly gastroepiploic artery) for conduit if other grafts are unavailable. Determine if additional myocardial revascularization (resection left ventricular aneurysm, intraoperative coronary angioplasty, closure of postmyocardial infarction ventricular septal defect) is to be performed. Determine patient's understanding of these procedures; clarify if necessary. For discharge planning and teaching, assess patient's understanding of warning signs and symptoms of graft closure or occlusion, prescribed medication regimen, nature of disease process, and risk factors and their modification.

3. Thermia unit may be placed on OR bed to reduce heat loss during the closing portion of the procedure. Follow institutional protocol for unit identification, documenting time and temperature, and protecting skin integrity. Note also the placement of additional temperature probes.

4. Urinary drainage catheters are routinely inserted to decompress the bladder, measure output, and monitor renal perfusion and cardiac output. Use aseptic technique for catheter insertion. Check for urine flow. Position drainage bag for easy observation. Prevent kinks or undue pressure on catheter or drainage tubing.

5. Follow institutional protocol for storing, administering, and requisitioning blood or blood products. Document per protocol.

6. Have all IMA table parts and components available and in working order. Place IMA retractor so that injury to the brachial plexus is prevented. Avoid pressure to arms from IMA retractor post. Remove post after IMA dissection, if necessary. For left ventricular aneurysm (LVA) resection, have felt strips or pledgets, suture, and vents available as needed. For intraoperative angioplasty, have coronary balloons, insufflator, syringes, and other items as needed. For coronary endarterectomy, have appropriate dilators, spatulas, and other needed items. For ventricular septal defect (VSD) repair, have felt and suture. If reoperation, have lateral and anteroposterior chest films ready to determine adherence of mediastinal structures to sternum and to identify and count sternal wires; anticipate need for additional blood or blood products. Anticipate need for intraaortic balloon counterpulsation if patient is unable to be weaned from cardiopulmonary bypass (CPB).

7. Prepare legs and feet circumferentially. Use caution if elevating legs to perform circumferential preparation; elevate or lower legs simultaneously; have additional personnel if needed.

Box 14-2 Standard Guide to Nursing Actions for Cardiac Surgery Patient

---

Demonstrates Knowledge of the Physiologic and Psychologic Responses to Surgery

Explain perioperative events

Preoperative

NPO (nothing by mouth, or *non per os*)

Premedication

Time and mode of transportation to OR

Preinduction area events—insertion of peripheral venous and arterial lines

Visit by circulating nurse

Transport to OR and transfer to OR bed

OR environment—cold, numerous staff, light, equipment, apparel

Induction

Central lines, nasogastric tube

Urinary catheter

Skin preparation

Anticipated length of surgery

Intraoperative

Assess patient's desire for knowledge

Respect normal denial

If requested, describe procedure(s) anticipated; use heart model

Answer the patient's and family's questions

Postoperative

Describe surgical intensive care unit (ICU) environment—noises, equipment, protocols

Describe condition of patient on arrival at ICU—tubes, lines, catheters; cool, pale skin; medicated/anesthetized; inability to talk while intubated

Discuss alternative methods of communication

Describe visiting hours, anticipated length of stay

Assess effects of cardiovascular (CV) disease on—functional status, physiologic status, and psychological status

Assess patient's understanding of CV disease

Assess effects of cardiac medications on patient's thought processes

Determine patient's knowledge of current medication regimen

Elicit patient's feelings and understanding of cardiac surgical procedure, possible alternative procedures (e.g., valve repair versus replacement)

Encourage verbalization of fears, "silly questions," concerns

Determine religious beliefs affecting surgical procedure (e.g., Jehovah's Witnesses/attitude toward blood transfusions)

Assess family's fears, concerns, understanding of procedure

Note presence of sternotomy scars; reoperations require longer surgical time and are associated with increased bleeding. Inform patient and family of possible prolonged operative time

Elicit understanding of prior cardiac procedures; if patient has questions or misunderstandings, refer to appropriate health care professional if necessary

Assess the patient's and family's understanding of possible cardiac surgery complications—perioperative myocardial infarction, stroke, hemorrhage, renal failure, atelectasis, mediastinitis, dysrhythmias, death

Ascertain where family will be waiting during surgery

Ascertain wishes related to advance directive

Freedom from Infection

Use depilatories or electric clippers to shave hair; avoid razors if possible

Assess risk factors for postoperative infection—previous cardiac operations, duration of surgery, duration of cardiopulmonary bypass, blood transfusions, postoperative blood loss, length of hospitalization (preoperatively and in ICU)

Dress all intravenous and intraarterial lines

Have prescribed topical antibiotic solution available for irrigation as ordered

Ensure prophylactic antibiotics are given preoperatively

Use closed urinary drainage system; keep drainage bag off floor

Routinely prepare skin from chin to knees (or lower if leg vein needed) in anticipation of inserting femoral artery pressure line, intraaortic balloon, and/or instituting femoral-femoral bypass

Confine and contain instruments and supplies used in groin or leg; change gowns and gloves when moving from lower extremities to chest

If OR bed is elevated, lowered (for some IMA dissection), or turned from side to side (to de-air ventricle), take appropriate measures to retain sterility of field, gowns and gloves; take precautions to maintain sterility of bypass lines.

Keep setup sterile until patient leaves OR (in case incision needs to be reopened for exploration)

Document lot and serial numbers of all implants

Follow institutional guidelines for complying with Safe Medical Devices Act.

Maintenance of Skin Integrity

Pad hands, elbows, and back of head; pad feet when possible

If deep hypothermia is used, protect ears, nose, and other facial prominences; pad hands, arms, and feet. Prevent direct contact of ice and ice chips with skin and tissue

Keep drapes off lower extremities and head; use anesthesia screens or special drape holders and equipment

Prepare ICU bed with mattress padding

Prevent pooling of preparation solutions

Freedom from Injury Related to Positioning

Supine

Maintain proper body alignment; in patients with arthritis or back problems, place in functional position; use extra padding as necessary on arms and under legs

Box 14-2 Standard Guide to Nursing Actions for Cardiac Surgery Patients—cont'd

Supine—cont'd

Maintain accessibility to groin

Have extra personnel to position patient

Lateral

Place patients so that groin is accessible

Use axillary rolls, pillows between legs, padding for arms, elbows, and feet; attach arm boards; use stabilizing pillows, sandbags, or other devices anteriorly and posteriorly; place adhesive tape across buttocks (if it does not interfere with access to the surgical site)

**Freedom from Injury Related to Retained
Foreign Objects**

Account for umbilical tapes, vessel loops, rubbershods, bulldogs, cannulas, pill sponges, connectors for tubing, guidewires, needles, stopcocks, prosthetic obturators and handles, and other items per institutional protocol

Prevent retaining tissue debris on instruments; calcium particles, plaque, thrombus, vegetations, and so forth

Prevent retaining suture particles

Keep instruments clean of blood and particulate matter

Notify surgeon of particulate matter remaining in surgical site

Freedom from Injury Related to Chemical Hazards

Identify fluids, solutions, irrigations, injectates, medications: heparin injectate, heparin solution, topical "slush," cardioplegia, papaverine, calcium chloride, epinephrine, thrombin, antibiotic solution, normal saline, lactated Ringer's solution, and other fluids on field

Test depilatories for allergic reaction

Follow hospital protocol for allergic blood reactions

Inject blood vessels with physiologic solutions or prescribed fluids only

Ensure that temperature of topical solutions is appropriate for use (cold during induced arrest, warm before or after induced arrest)

Remove glove powder from outside of gloves after gloving and before handling tissue

Have cardiac insulating pads, cold lap tapes, and so forth available to retain hypothermic temperature during cardiac repair

Freedom form Injury Related to Physical Hazards

Have additional case carts complete and available in anticipation of emergency procedures

When OR is not in use, keep room prepared for cardiac procedures: sternal saw motor plugged in, light source available, electrosurgery unit(s) in working order (attachments available), OR table attachments on bed, defibrillator and fibrillator available

Test defibrillator (and fibrillator) before use; have alternative defibrillator available

Facilitate moistening of surgeon's and assistant's hands when tying fine suture to prevent snagging

Visualize suture; avoid placing items on free ends of suture; prevent snagging of suture; check suture for knots before handing to surgeon; avoid clamping suture with unprotected metal jaws (use rubbershods or special suture clamps)

Have backup supplies or alternative source of supplies available (grafts, pledgets, valves, special suture, and so forth); list lot and serial numbers of all implants

Prevent overstretching of sternal (or IMA) retractor; remove IMA post after IMA dissection if post is impinging on patient arm

Inspect vascular clamps, forceps, needle holders, and so forth for missing teeth, burrs, and malfunctions

Monitor ECG: during induced arrest, observe for ECG activity and prepare to reinfuse cardioplegia if electrical activity is noted

Maintain extra supply of topical cold solutions ("slush")

Monitor ECG throughout procedure, assess dysrhythmias, ectopic beats for potential cardiac arrest; note bradyarrhythmias, ECG evidence of coronary ischemia (ST changes)

Have epicardial, temporary pacing wires ready for insertion

Monitor cardiac and pulmonary pressures, note drop in blood pressures, increase in pulmonary pressures indicating myocardial dysfunction; if pulmonary artery pressure line has not been inserted, anticipate insertion of line immediately postoperatively; left atrial pressure line may be inserted—have appropriate supplies available

Use sump suction only when patient is fully heparinized; suction with sump suction whenever possible to conserve blood

Use discard suction for irrigating solutions (to reduce amount of irrigation returning to bypass pump and causing a drop in the hematocrit)

Use discard suction to remove topical solutions from pleural cavity (if opened) and pericardial cavity

Use discard suction for antibiotic solutions

Maintain cool temperature in room during period of induced arrest; increase temperature during closing of incision; verify with surgeon; have warming blanket on ICU bed

Monitor patient temperatures (rectal, esophageal, bladder, ventricular, septal, and so forth); verify accuracy of monitoring system; report malfunctions; adjust room temperature as needed

Have chest x-ray films, cardiac catheterization films, arteriograms, angiograms, CAT scans, and so forth available

If reoperation: display lateral and anteroposterior chest x-ray films (to note adherence of mediastinal structures to sternum, to count chest wires, to note presence of prostheses, and so forth); have special supplies and equipment as requested by surgeon (for example, oscillating saw, topical hemostatic agents, and so forth)

Continued.

Box 14-2 Standard Guide to Nursing Actions for Cardiac Surgery Patients—cont'd

Freedom from Injury Related to Electrical Hazards

Ensure appropriate location of ESU dispersive pad site

If more than one ESU is used, place dispersive pads appropriately

Check that defibrillator (and fibrillator) and external pacemaker are in proper working order. Insure regular maintenance checks with biomedical engineering for all equipment

Insulate proximal tip of electrosurgery pencil when using in deep cavities or in retrosternum (for example, during IMA dissection); verify with surgeon

Check epicardial pacing leads and wires for kinks or cracks; if pacing wires are not used postoperatively, place insulating covers over distal tips of each wire; have external pacemaker generator available (unifocal and bifocal)

Verify defibrillator settings with surgeon

Have surgeon verbalize when defibrillator is to be discharged

Have appropriate size internal paddles

For reoperation, have internal and external paddles; verify setting with surgeon before discharging; in adults with extensive pericardial adhesions, consider using pediatric size internal paddle(s) until sufficient space is dissected in pericardial cavity to allow insertion of regular size internal paddle; coordinate changing over to regular paddles with surgeon (use this technique if paddle tips can be changed)

Apply sufficient electrode paste to external paddles before placing paddles on patient's chest

Have appropriate ECG cables for cardioversion

Have appropriate ECG leads for use with intraaortic balloon pump

Maintenance of Fluid and Electrolyte Balance

Maintain adequate blood and blood product supply via communication with blood bank; verify with surgeon and anesthesiologist

Anticipate need for platelets, fresh frozen plasma with reoperations, history of anticoagulation and antiplatelet therapy; have topical hemostatic agents available

Ensure autotransfusion is working properly; have available additional liners and suction tubing

Check bypass lines before instituting cardiopulmonary bypass; note presence of air in arterial lines and notify surgeon or perfusionist, if present; determine whether single or double venous cannulation is to be used (have caval tapes or clamps available for double cannulation, per surgeon's preference); refill venous lines with designated solutions only; prevent air locks in venous lines

If femoral bypass to be instituted, have appropriate supplies and instruments to access femoral artery

Prevent kinks in bypass tubing; avoid pressure on bypass lines; insure that connections in bypass tubing (especially arterial and other high-pressure lines) are secure

Be able to identify inflow lines readily from outflow lines; label if necessary

Verify that suction lines are suctioning (and not infusing); test before using

Prepare antegrade/retrograde cardioplegia infusion lines per protocol

Have correct heparin dosage; have additional heparin available if emergency reinstitution of bypass is required after heparin reversal (with protamine sulfate)

When venting catheters and lines are employed, have appropriate connectors, tubing, and so forth

Verify that urine is draining when catheterizing bladder; notify surgeon if urine is not visualized; if urethral strictures are present, have available dilatators, water-soluble lubricant, large syringe, coudé catheters, and other supplies as requested by surgeon; anticipate possible insertion of suprapubic catheter if other measures fail; have available necessary items

Anticipate need for antiarrhythmic agents if ectopy is noted

Have chest tubes available; if pleural cavity is entered, anticipate placement of a tube in the pleural space (during surgery or immediately postoperatively)

Have available additional chest tubes, Y-connectors, and tubing if extra chest tubes are inserted

Monitor chest tube drainage closely; alert surgeon if drainage exceeds acceptable amount (for example, more than 150 to 200 ml per hour)

Secure tubes and drains (and connections) before leaving OR

In addition to standard postoperative report, include information on cardiac status, dysrhythmias, difficulties with defibrillation, cardiac medications, baseline pulmonary function, location of pressure and infusion lines, electrolyte levels (especially potassium), and any other information that will facilitate nursing care in the ICU

Follow institutional protocol for anatomic landmarks for preparation.

8. Check the condition of the skin before and after preparation procedures. Note rashes, nicks, scratches. Document skin condition.

9. Position according to institutional protocol, taking special care to pad pressure sites. The lower leg may need to be freely mobile so that feet may be wrapped in towels or stockinette.

10. Dispersive pad sites should be checked before application and upon pad removal. Two electrosurgery units (ESUs) may be employed simultaneously. Dispersive pad sites should be appropriate for location of surgical site (that is, legs or

FIG. 14-1

CARE PLAN FOR CORONARY ARTERY BYPASS GRAFTING (CABG)

KEY ASSESSMENT POINTS

Risk factors for heart disease
Functional status
Angina (with/without radiation to neck and arms)
Complaints of tight, crushing, squeezing chest pain
ECG evidence of ischemia (such as ST segment changes) at rest and/or upon exertion
Documented coronary artery lesions (cardiac catheterization report)
Left ventricular status
Previous cardiac surgery
Condition of saphenous veins (variocosities, prior surgery)
Equal, bilateral blood pressure in arms (to assess adequacy of blood flow through IMA)
Psychosocial history (ability to make life-style changes, family support)

NURSING DIAGNOSES

All generic nursing diagnoses apply to this patient, with the addition of:
Risk for decreased cardiac output/altered tissue perfusion

PATIENT OUTCOMES

All generic outcomes apply, with the addition of:
The patient's hemodynamic status will be stable during the perioperative period.
The patient will:
1. Have vital signs that remain within baseline values
2. Have adequate urinary output
3. Be free of peripheral or dependent edema

NURSING ACTIONS

	Yes	No	N/A
1. Preoperative assessment performed?	☐	☐	☐
2. Preoperative teaching performed?	☐	☐	☐
3. Thermia unit?	☐	☐	☐
4. Foley catheter inserted?	☐	☐	☐
5. Blood ordered/available?	☐	☐	☐
6. Special equipment/supplies available?	☐	☐	☐
7. Skin prep per institutional protocol?	☐	☐	☐
8. Condition of skin at prep site noted?	☐	☐	☐
9. Positioned correctly?	☐	☐	☐
10. Dispersive pad site(s) checked before application?	☐	☐	☐
11. Aseptic precautions instituted?	☐	☐	☐
12. Graft properly prepared?	☐	☐	☐
13. Medications labeled/documented?	☐	☐	☐
14. Correct solutions/temperature for irrigation?	☐	☐	☐
15. Autotransfusion prepared?	☐	☐	☐
16. Catheters/tubes/drains documented?	☐	☐	☐
17. Urinary output/other drainage noted?	☐	☐	☐
18. Dispersive pad site rechecked?	☐	☐	☐
19. Counts performed/correct?	☐	☐	☐
20. Specimen to lab?	☐	☐	☐
21. Dressings applied?	☐	☐	☐
22. Other generic care plans initiated? (specify)	☐	☐	☐

Document additional nursing actions/generic care plans initiated here:

_____

_____

_____

EVALUATION OF PATIENT OUTCOMES

	Outcome met	Outcome met with additional outcome criteria	Outcome met with revised nursing care plan	Outcome not met	Outcome not applicable to this patient
1. The patient maintained hemodynamic stability.	☐	☐	☐	☐	☐
2. The patient met outcomes for additional generic care plans as indicated.	☐	☐	☐	☐	☐

Signature: _____ Date: _____

chest); however, both dispersive pads may be placed on the buttocks. Adhere to institutional and manufacturer's recommendations for use of two ESUs. Additional ESU precautions include preventing injury to saphenous vein by inadvertent discharge of ESU active electrode. If using long electrode, insulate all but the tip during IMA use to prevent injury to retrosternal structures.

11. Cross-contamination from the leg to chest should be prevented. Confine and contain instruments and supplies used to excise vein(s). Change gowns and gloves when moving from legs to chest and after retracting heart.

12. Use only physiologically compatible solutions to distend vein.

13. Label syringes containing papaverine and other medications.

14. Solutions on the sterile field should be labeled and maintained at the correct temperature for the correct purpose.

15. Autotransfusion is routine. Fluid is washed, spun, and blood cells collected and infused back into the patient. If antibiotic solution is used, determine whether the irrigant can be washed and reinfused or whether it should be discarded. If discarding is recommended, use discard suction.

16. Peripheral and central lines, urinary drainage catheters, and chest tubes are routinely inserted. Document these.

17. Monitor chest tube drainage for amount, consistency, color. Drainage should not exceed 150 to 200 ml per hour. Some clotting in the tubes is expected; excessive clotting will occlude the tubes, producing cardiac tamponade. Bright red blood indicates arterial bleeding; the chest may need to be reopened. Note amount and color of urinary drainage.

18. Check dispersive pad site(s) at removal. Note any alteration in skin condition.

19. Account for all coronary bulldogs, vein cannulas, coronary dilatators, and epicardial retractors in addition to routine sharp, sponge, and instrument counts.

20. If coronary endarterectomy is performed, ensure that all plaque is removed from the field to prevent embolization. Follow institutional protocol for specimen preservation and disposition. Use universal precautions with material received from the sterile field.

21. Apply dressing to leg, moving from lower to upper leg to prevent venous stasis and seroma formation. Apply sternal dressings and dressings to drain sites and to other sites as applicable.

Aortic Valve Replacement (AVR) (Fig. 14-2)

1. Fig. 14-2 details key preoperative assessment data for aortic valve patients. Because of the nursing diagnoses selected for this patient (*decreased cardiac output, altered cardiopulmonary tissue perfusion,* and *altered cerebral tissue perfusion*), assess parameters that will be used to determine outcome attainment. These may vary but should include review of baseline vital signs and abnormalities, renal status, and neurologic status. Examine the extremities and sacrum for edema. Locate peripheral pulses. Assess patient's ability to comply with postoperative anticoagulant therapy and proximity to laboratory facilities.

2. Determine the patient's understanding of aortic valve disease, possible surgical interventions, and types of valvular prostheses. A demonstration of the prosthesis to be used will facilitate teaching and learning. Clarify misconceptions. In preparing the patient for discharge and rehabilitation, review signs and symptoms of valve failure, of anticoagulant-related hemorrhage, thrombosis, and embolic episodes; determine understanding of postoperative medication regimen (including antibiotic therapy) and the need for follow-up laboratory work.

3. Thermia unit may be placed on OR bed to reduce heat loss during the closing portion of the procedure. Follow institutional protocol for unit identification, documenting time and temperature, and protecting skin integrity. Note also the placement of additional temperature probes.

4. Urinary drainage catheters are routinely inserted to decompress the bladder, measure output, and monitor renal perfusion and cardiac output. Use aseptic technique for catheter insertion. Check urine flow. Position drainage bag for easy observation. Prevent kinks or undue pressure on catheter or drainage tubing.

5. Follow institutional protocol for storing, administering, and requisitioning blood and blood products. Document per protocol.

6. Have available types and ranges of sizes of valvular prostheses. Store in cool, dry location. The following will be needed: sizers (obturators), handles, holders, and other necessary items for sizing and inserting valve; pledgeted and nonpledgeted sutures, with additional pledget material; and AVR instruments. If ball/cage valve with removal poppet is used, ensure that poppet is inserted after valve is sutured to annulus. If alternately colored suture is used, present to surgeon in proper order. Determine whether cardioplegia infusion will take place both retro-

FIG. 14-2
CARE PLAN FOR AORTIC VALVE REPLACEMENT (AVR)

KEY ASSESSMENT POINTS

History of syncope, angina, congestive heart failure, shortness of breath, dyspnea on exertion, fatigue

History of rheumatic fever, bacterial or viral infection

Congenital bicuspid valve, endocarditis, calcific degeneration

Heart murmur/thrill caused by turbulent blood flow through valve

Left ventricular hypertrophy, systolic pressure gradient (aortic stenosis)

Results of cardiac catheterization, echocardiography

Contraindication to anticoagulation

Preexisting or potential site of infection

Psychosocial history (ability to adhere to prescribed postoperative therapeutic regimen, family support)

NURSING DIAGNOSES

All generic nursing diagnoses apply to this patient, with the addition of:

High risk for decreased cardiac output/altered tissue perfusion

High risk for altered cerebral perfusion

PATIENT OUTCOMES

All generic outcomes apply, with the addition of:

The patient's hemodynamic status will be stable during the perioperative period.

The patient will be free of complications from embolic episodes.

The patient will:

1. Have vital signs that remain within baseline values
2. Have adequate urinary output
3. Be free of peripheral or dependent edema
4. Be free of neurologic dysfunction

NURSING ACTIONS

	Yes	No	N/A
1. Preoperative assessment performed?	☐	☐	☐
2. Preoperative teaching performed?	☐	☐	☐
3. Thermia unit?	☐	☐	☐
4. Foley catheter inserted?	☐	☐	☐
5. Blood ordered/available?	☐	☐	☐
6. Special equipment/supplies available?	☐	☐	☐
7. Skin prep per institutional protocol?	☐	☐	☐
8. Condition of skin at prep site noted?	☐	☐	☐
9. Positioned correctly?	☐	☐	☐
10. Dispersive pad site checked before application?	☐	☐	☐
11. Antiembolic precautions instituted?	☐	☐	☐
12. Valve properly prepared?	☐	☐	☐
13. Medications labeled/documented?	☐	☐	☐
14. Correct solutions/temperature for irrigation?	☐	☐	☐
15. Autotransfusion prepared?	☐	☐	☐
16. Catheters/tubes/drains documented?	☐	☐	☐
17. Urinary output/other drainage noted?	☐	☐	☐
18. Dispersive pad site rechecked?	☐	☐	☐
19. Counts performed/correct?	☐	☐	☐
20. Specimen/cultures to lab?	☐	☐	☐
21. Dressings applied?	☐	☐	☐
22. Implants documented?	☐	☐	☐
23. Other generic care plans initiated? (specify)	☐	☐	☐

Document additional nursing actions/generic care plans initiated here:

_____

_____

_____

EVALUATION OF PATIENT OUTCOME

	Outcome met	Outcome met with additional outcome criteria	Outcome met with revised nursing care plan	Outcome not met	Outcome not applicable to this patient
1. The patient maintained hemodynamic stability.	☐	☐	☐	☐	☐
2. The patient's neurologic status remained unchanged.	☐	☐	☐	☐	☐
3. The patient met outcomes for additional generic care plans as indicated.	☐	☐	☐	☐	☐

Signature: _____ Date: _____

grade via coronary sinus and antegrade via aortic root. Have vents ready for aspirating air and fluid during valve replacement; prepare superior pulmonary vein vent catheter. Test vent to be sure it is suctioning. Have venting and aspirating needle and tubing ready for aspirating air during closure of aorta. Switch lines as necessary. If left ventricular hypertrophy is present, anticipate need for additional topical cold solutions and infusion with cardioplegia.

7. Follow institutional protocol for anatomic landmarks for preparation.

8. Check the condition of the skin before and after preparation procedures. Note rashes, nicks, and scratches. Document skin condition.

9. Position according to institutional protocol, taking special care to pad pressure sites. Place anesthesia screen over lower legs and feet to prevent pressure of drapes. Pad feet or place in foam booties.

10. Dispersive pad sites should be checked before application and upon pad removal.

11. Confine and contain specimen(s) from valve containing bacterial vegetations. Keep instruments free of debris (calcium deposits, bacterial vegetation, thrombus, and so forth).

12. Follow protocol for removing glutaraldehyde storage solution from prosthesis. Glutaraldehyde is toxic to tissues; timed, multiple rinsings are recommended to remove all residual storage solution. Label and separate normal saline used to rinse prosthesis; do not use as tissue irrigant. Prevent placing biologic prostheses in antibiotic solution; keep moist with normal saline. Place mechanical prosthesis in antibiotic solution per surgeon request. If aortic homograft is used, prevent contact with valve in frozen condition. Follow manufacturer's instructions for thawing valve. Use insulated gloves when handling cryopreserved valve.

13. Label all medications in syringes and containers. Document medications administered.

14. Solutions on the sterile field should be labeled and maintained at the correct temperature for the correct purpose.

15. Autotransfusion is routine. Fluid is washed and spun, and blood cells are collected and infused back into the patient. If antibiotic solution is used, determine whether the irrigant can be washed and reinfused or whether it should be discarded. If discarding is recommended, use discard suction.

16. Peripheral and central lines, urinary drainage catheters, and chest tubes are routinely inserted. Document these.

17. Monitor chest tube drainage for amount, consistency, and color. Drainage should not exceed 150 to 200 ml per hour. Some clotting in the tubes is expected; excessive clotting will occlude the tubes, producing cardiac tamponade. Bright red blood indicates arterial bleeding; the chest may need to be reopened. Note amount and color of urinary drainage.

18. Check dispersive pad site(s) at removal. Note any alteration in skin condition.

19. Account for all valve obturators, handles, holders, and other items used to size and insert valves in addition to routine sharp, sponge, and instrument counts.

20. Follow institutional protocol for specimen preservation and disposition. Valve sutures, rinse solutions, native valve, and other structures may be cultured. Use universal precautions with material received from the sterile field.

21. Apply sternal dressings and dressings to drain sites and to other sites as applicable.

22. Document lot and serial numbers of implants per institutional protocol.

Mitral Valve Replacement/Repair (MVR) (Fig. 14-3)

1. Fig. 14-3 details key preoperative assessment data for mitral valve patients. Because of the nursing diagnoses selected for this patient (*decreased cardiac output, altered cardiopulmonary tissue perfusion,* and *altered cerebral tissue perfusion*), assess parameters that will be used to determine outcome attainment. These may vary but should include review of baseline vital signs and abnormalities, renal status, and neurologic status. Examine the extremities and sacrum for edema. Locate peripheral pulses. Note presence of chronic atrial fibrillation. Assess patient's ability to comply with postoperative anticoagulant therapy and proximity to laboratory facilities.

2. Determine the patient's understanding of mitral valve disease, possible surgical interventions (replacement, annuloplasty, valvuloplasty, or commissurotomy) and types of valvular prostheses. A demonstration of the prosthesis to be used will facilitate teaching and learning. Clarify misconceptions (that is, repair versus replacement). When preparing the patient for discharge and rehabilitation, review signs and symptoms of valve failure, anticoagulant-related hemorrhage, thrombosis, and embolic episodes; determine understanding of postoperative medication regimen (including antibiotic therapy) and need for follow-up laboratory work.

3. Thermia unit may be placed on OR bed to reduce heat loss during the closing portion of the

FIG. 14-3
CARE PLAN FOR MITRAL VALVE REPLACEMENT/REPAIR (MVR)

KEY ASSESSMENT POINTS

Complaints of fatigue, weakness, shortness of breath, dyspnea

History of thromboembolism, congestive heart failure, atrial fibrillation

History of rheumatic fever, infective endocarditis, ischemic heart disease, connective tissue disorder

Heart murmur caused by turbulent blood flow through diseased valve

Enlarged left atrium or ventricle

Results of cardiac catheterization, echocardiography

Contraindication to anticoagulation

Psychosocial history (ability to adhere to prescribed postoperative therapeutic regimen, family support)

NURSING DIAGNOSES

All generic nursing diagnoses apply to this patient, with the addition of:

High risk for decreased cardiac output/altered tissue perfusion

High risk for altered cerebral perfusion

PATIENT OUTCOMES

All generic outcomes apply, with the addition of:

The patient's hemodynamic status will be stable during the perioperative period

The patient will be free of complications from embolic episodes.

The patient will:

1. Have vital signs that remain within baseline values
2. Have adequate urinary output
3. Be free of peripheral or dependent edema
4. Be free of neurologic dysfunction

NURSING ACTIONS

	Yes	No	N/A
1. Preoperative assessment performed?	☐	☐	☐
2. Preoperative teaching performed?	☐	☐	☐
3. Thermia unit?	☐	☐	☐
4. Foley catheter inserted?	☐	☐	☐
5. Blood ordered/available?	☐	☐	☐
6. Special equipment/supplies available?	☐	☐	☐
7. Skin prep per institutional protocol?	☐	☐	☐
8. Condition of skin at prep site noted?	☐	☐	☐
9. Positioned correctly?	☐	☐	☐
10. Dispersive pad site checked before application?	☐	☐	☐
11. Antiembolic precautions instituted?	☐	☐	☐
12. Valve properly prepared?	☐	☐	☐
13. Medications labeled/documented?	☐	☐	☐
14. Correct solutions/temperature for irrigation?	☐	☐	☐
15. Autotransfusion prepared?	☐	☐	☐
16. Catheters/tubes/drains documented?	☐	☐	☐
17. Urinary output/other drainage noted?	☐	☐	☐
18. Dispersive pad site rechecked?	☐	☐	☐
19. Counts performed/correct?	☐	☐	☐
20. Specimen/cultures to lab?	☐	☐	☐
21. Dressings applied?	☐	☐	☐
22. Implants documented?	☐	☐	☐
23. Other generic care plans initiated? (specify)	☐	☐	☐

Document additional nursing actions/generic care plans initiated here:

_____

_____

_____

EVALUATION OF PATIENT OUTCOMES

	Outcome met	Outcome met with additional outcome criteria	Outcome met with revised nursing care plan	Outcome not met	Outcome not applicable to this patient
1. The patient maintained hemodynamic stability.	☐	☐	☐	☐	☐
2. The patient's neurologic status remained unchanged.	☐	☐	☐	☐	☐
3. The patient met outcomes for additional generic care plans as indicated.	☐	☐	☐	☐	☐

Signature: _____ Date: _____

procedure. Follow institutional protocol for unit identification, documenting time and temperature, and protecting skin integrity. Note also the placement of additional temperature probes.

4. Urinary drainage catheters are routinely inserted to decompress the bladder, measure output, and monitor renal perfusion and cardiac output. Use aseptic technique in catheter insertion. Check urine flow. Position drainage bag for easy observation. Prevent kinks or undue pressure on catheter or drainage tubing.

5. Follow institutional protocol for storing, administering, and requisitioning blood and blood products. Document per protocol.

6. Have available types and range of sizes of valvular prostheses (for example, valves, annuloplasty rings). Store in cool, dry location. The following will be needed: sizers (obturators), handles, holders, and other necessary items for sizing and inserting prosthesis; pledgeted and nonpledgeted sutures with additional pledget material; and MVR instruments. If repair is to be performed with prosthetic annuloplasty ring, have available range of rings and sizers. If valvuloplasty is attempted, have necessary items available. If suture repair (not using a ring) is to be performed, have necessary suture and pledgets. If alternately colored suture is used, present to surgeon in proper order. Have vents ready for aspirating air and fluid during valve replacement (small urinary catheter with 5-cc balloon may be inserted through prosthetic mitral valve to keep it incompetent and thus unable to eject air into the systemic circulation). Prepare superior pulmonary vein vent; test vent to be sure it is suctioning. If used, have aortic root vent ready when left atrial incision is closed. For patients with atrial fibrillation, have cables ready for cardioversion.

7. Follow institutional protocol for anatomic landmarks for preparation.

8. Check the condition of the skin before and after preparation procedures. Note rashes, nicks, and scratches. Document skin condition.

9. Position according to institutional protocol, taking special care to pad pressure sites. Place anesthesia screen over lower legs and feet to prevent pressure of drapes. Pad feet or place in foam booties.

10. Dispersive pad site(s) should be checked before application and upon pad removal.

11. Confine and contain specimen(s) from valve containing bacterial vegetations. Keep instruments free of debris (calcium deposits, bacterial vegetation, thrombus, and so forth).

12. Follow protocol for removing glutaraldehyde storage solution from prosthetic valve. Glutaraldehyde is toxic to tissues; timed, multiple rinsings are recommended to remove all residual storage solution. Label and separate normal saline used to rinse prosthesis; do not use as tissue irrigant. Prevent placing biologic prostheses in antibiotic solutions; keep moist with normal saline. Place mechanical prosthesis in antibiotic solution per surgeon's request. If aortic homograft is used, prevent contact with valve in frozen condition. Follow manufacturer's instructions for thawing valve. Use insulated gloves when handling cryopreserved valve.

13. Label all medications in syringes and containers. Document medications administered.

14. Solutions on the sterile field should be labeled and maintained at the correct temperature for the correct purpose.

15. Autotransfusion is routine. Fluid is washed and spun, and blood cells are collected and infused back into the patient. If antibiotic solution is used, determine whether the irrigant can be washed and reinfused or whether it should be discarded. If discarding is recommended, use discard suction.

16. Peripheral and central lines, urinary drainage catheters, and chest tubes are routinely inserted. Document these.

17. Monitor chest tube drainage for amount, consistency, and color. Drainage should not exceed 150 to 200 ml per hour. Some clotting in the tubes is expected; excessive clotting will occlude the tubes, producing cardiac tamponade. Bright red blood indicates arterial bleeding; the chest may need to be reopened. Note amount and color of urinary drainage.

18. Check dispersive pad site(s) at removal. Note any alteration in skin condition.

19. Account for all valve obturators, handles, holders, and other items used to size and insert valves, in addition to routine sharp, sponge, and instrument counts.

20. Follow institutional protocol for specimen preservation and disposition. Valve sutures, rinse solutions, native valve, and other structures may be cultured. Use universal precautions with material received from the sterile field.

21. Apply sternal dressings and dressings to drain sites and to other sites as applicable.

22. Document lot and serial numbers of implants per institutional protocol.

Tricuspid Valve Repair (Fig. 14-4)

1. Fig. 14-4 details key preoperative assessment data for tricuspid surgery patients. Because of

FIG. 14-4
CARE PLAN FOR TRICUSPID VALVE REPAIR

KEY ASSESSMENT POINTS

Complains of fatigue, abdominal pain (from liver engorgement)

History of associated mitral and/or aortic valve disease, illicit drug use, infective endocarditis, rheumatic fever, cancer metastasis

Edema, ascites, increased systemic venous pressure, pulsatile liver

Right atrial hypertrophy

Results of cardiac catheterization, echocardiography

Contraindication to anticoagulation

Psychosocial history (ability to adhere to prescribed postoperative therapeutic regimen, family support)

NURSING DIAGNOSES

All generic nursing diagnoses apply to this patient, with the addition of:

High risk for decreased cardiac output

PATIENT OUTCOMES

All generic outcomes apply, with the addition of:

The patient's hemodynamic status will be stable during the perioperative period.

The patient will:

1. Have vital signs that remain within baseline values
2. Have adequate urinary output
3. Be free of peripheral or dependent edema
4. Show no signs of conduction arrhythmias

NURSING ACTIONS

	Yes	No	N/A
1. Preoperative assessment performed?	☐	☐	☐
2. Preoperative teaching performed?	☐	☐	☐
3. Thermia unit?	☐	☐	☐
4. Foley catheter inserted?	☐	☐	☐
5. Blood ordered/available?	☐	☐	☐
6. Special equipment/supplies available?	☐	☐	☐
7. Skin prep per institutional protocol?	☐	☐	☐
8. Condition of skin at prep site noted?	☐	☐	☐
9. Positioned correctly?	☐	☐	☐
10. Dispersive pad site checked before application?	☐	☐	☐
11. Antiembolic precautions instituted?	☐	☐	☐
12. Valve properly prepared?	☐	☐	☐
13. Medications labeled/documented?	☐	☐	☐
14. Correct solutions/temperature for irrigation?	☐	☐	☐
15. Autotransfusion prepared?	☐	☐	☐
16. Catheters/tubes/drains documented?	☐	☐	☐
17. Urinary output/other drainage noted?	☐	☐	☐
18. Dispersive pad site rechecked?	☐	☐	☐
19. Counts performed/correct?	☐	☐	☐
20. Specimen/cultures to lab?	☐	☐	☐
21. Dressings applied?	☐	☐	☐
22. Implants documented?	☐	☐	☐
23. Other generic care plans initiated? (specify)	☐	☐	☐

Document additional nursing actions/generic care plans initiated here:

_____

_____

_____

EVALUATION OF PATIENT OUTCOMES

	Outcome met	Outcome met with additional outcome criteria	Outcome met with revised nursing care plan	Outcome not met	Outcome not applicable to this patient
1. The patient maintained hemodynamic stability.	☐	☐	☐	☐	☐
2. There was no evidence of conduction arrhythmias.	☐	☐	☐	☐	☐
3. The patient met outcomes for additional generic care plans as indicated.	☐	☐	☐	☐	☐

Signature: _____ Date: _____

the nursing diagnoses selected for this patient (*decreased cardiac output* and *altered cardiopulmonary tissue perfusion* related to the diseased valve and possible alteration in conduction pathways related to surgical interference with the Bundle of His), assess parameters that will be used to determine outcome attainment. These may vary but should include review of baseline vital signs and abnormalities, renal status, and ECG results. Examine the extremities and sacrum for edema. Locate peripheral pulses. Assess patient's understanding of the disease process and the possibility of valve replacement if repair cannot be achieved. Determine whether the patient realizes that a permanent pacemaker may need to be inserted.

2. Preoperative teaching is the beginning of helping the patient and family to have an increased understanding of the disease process and to start planning for postoperative health management. The perioperative nurse can collaborate with other health care professionals to reinforce information about the nature and type of operation planned and the perioperative events to expect, and to clarify and respond to patient misconceptions and questions.

3. Thermia unit may be placed on OR bed to reduce heat loss during the closing portion of the procedure. Follow institutional protocol for unit identification, documenting time and temperature, and protecting skin integrity. Note also the placement of additional temperature probes.

4. Urinary drainage catheters are routinely inserted to decompress the bladder, measure output, and monitor renal perfusion and cardiac output. Use aseptic technique for catheter insertion. Check urine flow. Position drainage bag for easy observation. Prevent kinks or undue pressure on catheter or drainage tubing.

5. Follow institutional protocol for storing, administering, and requisitioning blood and blood products. Document per protocol.

6. Determine whether suture and annuloplasty, prosthetic ring annuloplasty, or valvuloplasty is planned; have appropriate ring sizers, suture, and annuloplasty rings. Possible need for valve replacement should be considered; atrioventricular prostheses should be available. Right angle superior vena cava venous cannula may be required. Caval snares or clamps may be used to prevent systemic venous return to surgical site. Permanent epicardial leads, generator, and pulse system analyzer (PSA) should be ready. Check leads for kinks or cracks. Pulmonary artery pressure (PAP) line may not be inserted preoperatively (interference in surgical field); plan for line insertion immediately postoperatively. Appropriate supplies will be needed if competency of repair is tested.

7. Follow institutional protocol for anatomic landmarks for preparation.

8. Check the condition of the skin before and after preparation procedures. Note rashes, nicks, and scratches. Document skin condition.

9. Position according to institutional protocol, taking special care to pad pressure sites. Place anesthesia screen over lower legs and feet to prevent pressure of drapes. Pad feet or place in foam booties.

10. Dispersive pad site should be checked before application and upon pad removal.

11. Confine and contain specimen(s) from the valve containing bacterial vegetations. Keep instruments free of debris (calcium deposits, bacterial vegetation, thrombus, and so forth).

12. Follow protocol for removing glutaraldehyde storage solution from prosthesis (consult mitral valve care plan for further discussion).

13. Label all medications in syringes and containers. Document medications administered.

14. Solutions on the sterile field should be labeled and maintained at the correct temperature for the correct purpose.

15. Autotransfusion may be routine. Fluid is washed and spun, and blood cells are collected and infused back into the patient. If antibiotic solution is used, determine whether the irrigant can be washed and reinfused or whether it should be discarded. If discarding is recommended, use discard suction.

16. Peripheral and central lines, urinary drainage catheters, and chest tubes are routinely inserted. Document these.

17. Monitor chest tube drainage for amount, consistency, and color. Drainage should not exceed 150 to 200 ml per hour. Some clotting in the tubes is expected; excessive clotting will occlude the tubes, producing cardiac tamponade. Bright red blood indicates arterial bleeding; the chest may need to be reopened. Note amount and color of urinary drainage.

18. Check dispersive pad site at removal. Note any alteration in skin condition.

19. Account for all items used in valve repair or replacement, in addition to routine sharp, sponge, and instrument counts.

20. Follow institutional protocol for specimen preservation and disposition. Valve sutures, rinse solutions, native valve, and other structures may be cultured. Use universal precautions with material received from the sterile field.

21. Apply sternal dressings, dressings to drain sites, and other sites as applicable.
22. Document lot and serial numbers of implants per institutional protocol, as applicable.

Repair of Atrial Septal Defect (ASD) (Fig. 14-5)

1. Fig. 14-5 details key preoperative assessment data for ASD patients. Because of the nursing diagnosis selected for this patient (*impaired gas exchange* related to the increased pulmonary blood flow associated with ASD), assess parameters that will be used to determine outcome attainment. These may vary but should include review of baseline respiratory function, preoperative catheterization-oxygen saturation studies, and blood gas values. There is also a potential for decreased cardiac output from the right heart failure associated with left-to-right shunting in ASD patients. Modify the care plan to include these assessment parameters (as suggested for the patient undergoing valve replacement). Assess the patient's understanding of types of atrial septal defects and the possible presence of other congenital abnormalities. Determine understanding of patch versus primary closure; refer to physician if appropriate.
2. Teaching may focus on what ASD repair means. Encourage the patient to discuss perceptions about repair, congenital nature of defect, and concerns about progeny. Clarify misconceptions.
3. Thermia unit may be placed on OR bed to reduce heat loss during the closing portion of the procedure. Follow institutional protocol for unit identification, documenting time and temperature, and protecting skin integrity. Note also the placement of additional temperature probes.
4. Urinary drainage catheters are routinely inserted to decompress the bladder, measure output, and monitor renal perfusion and cardiac output. Use aseptic technique for catheter insertion. Check urine flow. Position drainage bag for easy observation. Prevent kinks or undue pressure on catheter or drainage tubing.
5. Follow institutional protocol for storing, administering, and requisitioning blood and blood products. Document per protocol.
6. If sinus venous defect, anticipate need for right angle superior vena cava venous cannula and exploration of right atrium and superior vena cava to determine presence of anomalous pulmonary venous return. Intraoperative oxygen saturation measures may be needed; have appropriate syringes, needles, and so forth. Standard open heart instruments will be used. Patch material should be available (knitted is preferred, since it facilitates more rapid endocardial tissue ingrowth). A permanent pacemaker may be required; have epicardial leads and generator ready. If pulmonary artery pressure catheter was not inserted preoperatively (interference with surgical site), be prepared to insert one immediately postoperatively. Set up sterile field as necessary.
7. Follow institutional protocol for anatomic landmarks for preparation.
8. Check the condition of the skin before and after preparation procedures. Note rashes, nicks, and scratches. Document skin condition.
9. Before induction and intubation, elevate head of bed to facilitate breathing. Position according to institutional protocol, taking special care to pad pressure sites. Place anesthesia screen over lower legs and feet to prevent pressure of drapes. Pad feet or place in foam booties.
10. Dispersive pad site should be checked before application and upon pad removal.
11. Label all medications in syringes and containers. Document medications administered.
12. Solutions on the sterile field should be labeled and maintained at the correct temperature for the correct purpose.
13. Autotransfusion is routine. Fluid is washed and spun, and blood cells are collected and infused back into the patient. If antibiotic solution is used, determine whether the irrigant can be washed and reinfused or whether it should be discarded. If discarding is recommended, use discard suction.
14. Peripheral and central lines, urinary drainage catheters, and chest tubes are routinely inserted. Document these.
15. Monitor chest tube drainage for amount, consistency, and color. Drainage should not exceed 150 to 200 ml per hour. Some clotting in the tubes is expected; excessive clotting will occlude the tubes, producing cardiac tamponade. Bright red blood indicates arterial bleeding; the chest may need to be reopened. Note amount and color of urinary drainage.
16. Check dispersive pad site at removal. Note any alteration in skin condition.
17. Account for all pieces of graft and patch material, instruments and accessories used in ASD repair, in addition to routine sharp, sponge, and instrument counts.
18. Apply sternal dressings and dressings to drain sites and to other sites as applicable.
19. Document lot and serial numbers of prosthetic patch and graft per institutional protocol.

FIG. 14-5
CARE PLAN FOR REPAIR OF ATRIAL SEPTAL DEFECT (ASD)

KEY ASSESSMENT POINTS
Left-to-right shunt at atrial level
Heart murmur from shunted blood
Dyspnea, shortness of breath, pulmonary vascular obstructive disease
Increased pulmonary-to-systemic blood flow ratio of more than 1.5 to 1 (normal: 1 to 1)
Results of cardiac catheterization, echocardiography
Psychosocial history (ability to adhere to prescribed postoperative therapeutic regimen, family support)

NURSING DIAGNOSES
All generic nursing diagnoses apply to this patient, with the addition of:
High risk for impaired gas exchange

PATIENT OUTCOMES
All generic outcomes apply, with the addition of:
The patient will maintain adequate oxygenation and ventilation.
The patient will:
1. Be able to breathe comfortably during transport and positioning on the OR bed.
2. Have P_{O_2} and P_{CO_2} within normal baseline values
3. Maintain a patent airway

NURSING ACTIONS

	Yes	No	N/A
1. Preoperative assessment performed?	☐	☐	☐
2. Preoperative teaching performed?	☐	☐	☐
3. Thermia unit?	☐	☐	☐
4. Foley catheter inserted	☐	☐	☐
5. Blood ordered/available?	☐	☐	☐
6. Special equipment/supplies available?	☐	☐	☐
7. Skin prep per institutional protocol?	☐	☐	☐
8. Condition of skin at prep site noted?	☐	☐	☐
9. Positioned correctly?	☐	☐	☐
10. Dispersive pad site checked before application?	☐	☐	☐
11. Medications labeled/documented?	☐	☐	☐
12. Correct solutions/temperature for irrigation?	☐	☐	☐
13. Autotransfusion prepared?	☐	☐	☐
14. Catheters/tubes/drains documented?	☐	☐	☐
15. Urinary output/other drainage noted?	☐	☐	☐
16. Dispersive pad site re-checked?	☐	☐	☐
17. Counts performed and correct?	☐	☐	☐
18. Dressings applied?	☐	☐	☐
19. Implants documented?	☐	☐	☐
20. Other generic care plans initiated? (specify)	☐	☐	☐

Document additional nursing actions/generic care plans initiated here:

_____

_____

_____

EVALUATION OF PATIENT OUTCOMES

	Outcome met	Outcome met with additional outcome criteria	Outcome met with revised nursing care plan	Outcome not met	Outcome not applicable to this patient
1. The patient maintained adequate oxygenation and ventilation.	☐	☐	☐	☐	☐
2. The patient met outcomes for additional generic care plans as indicated.	☐	☐	☐	☐	☐

Signature: _____ Date: _____

Repair of Ascending Aortic Thoracic Dissection
(Fig. 14-6)

1. Fig. 14-6 details key preoperative assessment data for these patients. Because of the frequently emergent nature of aortic dissections, full patient assessment and teaching will not be possible. Along with life-sustaining measures to support tissue and organ perfusion, the perioperative nurse should consider the patient and the family's *anxiety*. Emotional and physical support should be given. Short, understandable explanations should be offered. Based on the individual nature of the patient situation, modify the care plan accordingly.

2. Thermia unit may be placed on OR bed to reduce heat loss during the closing portion of the procedure. Follow institutional protocol for unit identification, documenting time and temperature, and protecting skin integrity. Note also the placement of additional temperature probes. *If an aortic arch aneurysm or dissection* is present in the patient, deep hypothermia may be instituted. If the head is wrapped in ice, the ears, nose, and other facial prominences must be padded with cotton batting or some other soft material to prevent frostbite. Monitor and assess additional parameters of skin integrity.

3. Urinary drainage catheters are routinely inserted to decompress the bladder, measure output, and monitor renal perfusion and cardiac output. Use aseptic technique in catheter insertion. Check urine flow. Position drainage bag for easy observation. Prevent kinks or undue pressure on catheter or drainage tubing.

4. Follow institutional protocol for storing, administering, and requisitioning blood and blood products. Document per protocol.

5. Ascending aortic dissections are associated with aortic valve insufficiency and may obliterate the entrance to the coronary arteries. Communicate with the physician to determine the nature of the pathology and the type of repair anticipated: Bentall (resection aorta, with AVR and reimplantation of coronary ostia or CABG); resection aorta and AVR (leaving aortic collar); straight resection; insertion intraluminal device. Anticipate institution of femoral bypass. Have eye cautery available (depends on surgeon's technique for heat sealing edges of graft material at site of coronary/bypass graft anastomoses to reduce fraying.) Have grafts ready. If preclotting is required, follow instructions and protocol. If blood components are required for preclotting, order and have ready. Obtain appropriate supplies for graft insertion: suture, tapes for intraluminal device, and so forth. If aortic arch aneu-

rysm is involved, anticipate need for deep hypothermia. Have ice available to cool patient. Have supplies and instruments for arch resection, including additional bypass lines. Monitor blood loss; maintain adequate blood and blood products. Refer to care plans for AVR and CABG for additional equipment and supply needs.

6. Prepare anterior chest with caution (gentle, nonvigorous movements) to prevent traumatizing the enlarged aorta. Prepare entire leg(s) in anticipation of need for saphenous vein grafts.

7. Check the condition of the skin before and after preparation procedures. Note rashes, nicks, and scratches. Document skin condition.

8. Position supinely, allowing access to femoral artery and vein, according to institutional protocol. Take special care to pad pressure sites. Positional modifications will be necessary depending on anticipated repair.

9. Dispersive pad site(s) should be checked before application and upon pad removal.

10. If coronary artery bypass performed, confine and contain instruments and supplies (see care plan for CABG).

11. To reduce the possibility of oozing through graft interstices, the prosthesis may be preclotted with the patient's unheparinized venous blood or with thrombin, albumin, or platelets. Woven grafts are preferred in the thorax. There are grafts manufactured with collagen coating to retard leaking. Follow institutional protocol for type of graft used. If valve is replaced, follow precautions in care plan for AVR.

12. Label all medications in syringes and containers. Document medications administered.

13. Solutions on the sterile field should be labeled and maintained at the correct temperature for the correct purpose.

14. Autotransfusion is routine. Fluid is washed and spun, and blood cells are collected and infused back into the patient. If antibiotic solution is used, determine whether the irrigant can be washed and reinfused or whether it should be discarded. If discarding is recommended, use discard suction.

15. Peripheral and central lines, urinary drainage catheters, and chest tubes are routinely inserted. Document these.

16. Monitor chest tube drainage for amount, consistency, and color. Drainage should not exceed 150 to 200 ml per hour. Some clotting in the tubes is expected; excessive clotting will occlude the tubes, producing cardiac tamponade. Bright red blood indicates arterial bleeding; the chest may need to be reopened. Note amount and color of urinary drainage.

FIG. 14-6
CARE PLAN FOR REPAIR OF ASCENDING AORTIC THORACIC DISSECTION

KEY ASSESSMENT POINTS

Pale, diaphoretic

Unequal bilateral pulses, diminished/absent pulses in extremities

Diminished organ function due to occlusion/malperfusion from dissection (mental changes, gastrointestinal pain, reduced urine output)

Complaints of sudden, severe chest pain (described as ripping or tearing; may radiate to back)

Continued pain (signaling possible impending rupture)

History of hypertension, atherosclerosis, connective tissue disorders, bacterial infection, Marfan's syndrome

Murmur of aortic regurgitation

Results of cardiac catheterization, CAT scan, echocardiography, arteriogram

Psychosocial history (ability to adhere to prescribed postoperative therapeutic regimen, genetic counseling, family support)

NURSING DIAGNOSES

All generic nursing diagnoses apply to this patient, with the addition of:

Altered tissue perfusion

PATIENT OUTCOMES

All generic outcomes apply, with the addition of:

The patient will maintain tissue perfusion and cellular oxygenation

The patient's

1. Vital signs will be maintained
2. Cardiac output will be adequate
3. Intravenous lines will remain patent

NURSING ACTIONS

	Yes	No	N/A
1. Explanations/support given?	☐	☐	☐
2. Thermia unit?	☐	☐	☐
3. Foley catheter inserted?	☐	☐	☐
4. Blood ordered/available?	☐	☐	☐
5. Special equipment/supplies available?	☐	☐	☐
6. Skin prep per institutional protocol?	☐	☐	☐
7. Condition of skin at prep site noted?	☐	☐	☐
8. Positioned correctly?	☐	☐	☐
9. Dispersive pad site checked before application?	☐	☐	☐
10. Aseptic precautions instituted?	☐	☐	☐
11. Graft (and/or valve) properly prepared?	☐	☐	☐
12. Medications labeled/documented?	☐	☐	☐
13. Correct temperature/solutions for irrigation?	☐	☐	☐
14. Autotransfusion prepared?	☐	☐	☐
15. Catheters/tubes/drains documented?	☐	☐	☐
16. Urinary output/other drainage noted?	☐	☐	☐
17. Dispersive pad site rechecked?	☐	☐	☐
18. Counts performed and correct?	☐	☐	☐
19. Specimen/cultures to lab?	☐	☐	☐
20. Dressings applied?	☐	☐	☐
21. Implants documented?	☐	☐	☐
22. Other generic care plans initiated? (specify)	☐	☐	☐

Document additional nursing actions/generic care plans initiated here:

_____

_____

_____

EVALUATION OF PATIENT OUTCOMES

	Outcome met	Outcome met with additional outcome criteria	Outcome met with revised nursing care plan	Outcome not met	Outcome not applicable to this patient
1. The patient maintained tissue perfusion and cellular oxygenation.	☐	☐	☐	☐	☐
2. The patient met outcomes for additional generic care plans as indicated.	☐	☐	☐	☐	☐

Signature: _____ Date: _____

17. Check dispersive pad site(s) at removal. Note any alteration in skin condition.
18. Account for all special instruments and accessories used in repair, for pieces of graft material, and for residual particulate matter if graft has been preclotted, in addition to routine sharp, sponge, and instrument counts.
19. Follow institutional protocol for specimen preservation and disposition. Valve sutures, rinse solutions, native valve, and other structures may be cultured if AVR is performed. Prosthetic grafts and suture may be cultured in aneurysm resection. Use universal precautions with material received from the sterile field.
20. Apply sternal dressings and dressings to drain sites and other sites as applicable.
21. Document lot and serial numbers of implants per institutional protocol.

Repair of Descending Thoracic Aneurysm (Fig. 14-7)

1. Fig. 14-7 details key preoperative assessment data for these patients. Because of the nursing diagnosis selected for this patient (*altered tissue perfusion* related to possible rupture of the aneurysm), assess parameters that will be used to determine outcome attainment. These may vary but should include review of baseline data as suggested for the patient undergoing valve replacement. Assess the patient's understanding of pathophysiology of aneurysms and the potential complications of the repair.
2. Teaching will depend on the results of assessment data. The goal is for the patient to have an understanding of clinical status and to be prepared for home health management.
3. Thermia unit may be placed on OR bed to reduce heat loss during the closing portion of the procedure. Follow institutional protocol for unit identification, documenting time and temperature, and protecting skin integrity. Note also the placement of additional temperature probes.
4. Urinary drainage catheters are routinely inserted to decompress the bladder, measure output, and monitor renal perfusion and cardiac output. Use aseptic technique for catheter insertion. Check urine flow. Position drainage bag for easy observation. Prevent kinks or undue pressure on catheter or drainage tubing.
5. Follow institutional protocol for storing, administering, and requisitioning blood and blood products. Anticipate the need for additional blood and blood products. Document per protocol.
6. Anticipate the need to institute femoral bypass to perfuse kidneys and lower extremities. If shunting will be part of the procedure, have required supplies. Thoracotomy instruments will

need to be added. If *thoracoabdominal aneurysm* is present, have abdominal instruments and supplies. Have low-porosity grafts available; preclot per protocol (see care plan for ascending aortic aneurysm for discussion of preclotting options).

7. Follow institutional protocol for anatomic landmarks for preparation (will vary depending on aneurysm location).
8. Check the condition of the skin before and after preparation procedures. Note rashes, nicks, and scratches. Document skin condition.
9. For *descending thoracic aneurysm*, patient will be in lateral position (left side up). Pad extremities; use axillary roll, pillow between legs, support for feet, arms, and hands so that patient is stabilized anteriorly and posteriorly. Placement of wide tape across buttocks may need to be omitted if access to the groin is necessary. Use anesthesia screen to keep weight of drapes off feet. Pay special attention to preventing nerve injury. For *thoracoabdominal aneurysm*, place patient in supine position with small roll to elevate left side.
10. Dispersive pad site should be checked before application and upon pad removal.
11. Refer to care plan for ascending aortic aneurysm for discussion of graft preparation.
12. Label all medications in syringes and containers. Document medications administered.
13. Solutions on the sterile field should be labeled and maintained at the correct temperature for the correct purpose.
14. Autotransfusion is routine. Fluid is washed and spun, and blood cells are collected and infused back into the patient. If antibiotic solution is used, determine whether the irrigant can be washed and reinfused or whether it should be discarded. If discarding is recommended, use discard suction.
15. Peripheral and central lines, urinary drainage catheters, and chest tubes are routinely inserted. Document these.
16. Monitor chest tube drainage for amount, consistency, and color. Drainage should not exceed 150 to 200 ml per hour. Some clotting in the tubes is expected; excessive clotting will occlude the tubes, producing cardiac tamponade. Bright red blood indicates arterial bleeding; the chest may need to be reopened. Note amount and color of urinary drainage.
17. Check dispersive pad site at removal. Note any alteration in skin condition.
18. Account for all pieces of graft material and particulate matter in addition to routine sharp, sponge, and instrument counts.

FIG. 14-7
CARE PLAN FOR DESCENDING THORACIC ANEURYSM

KEY ASSESSMENT POINTS
(See also ascending aortic thoracic dissection, Fig. 14-6)
Distal thoracic aorta greater than 5 cm
Continued pain (signaling possible impending rupture)
Results of arteriogram, CAT scan, echocardiography
Psychosocial history (ability to adhere to prescribed postoperative therapeutic regimen, risk factor modification, family support)

NURSING DIAGNOSES
All generic nursing diagnoses apply to this patient, with the addition of:
High risk for altered tissue perfusion

PATIENT OUTCOMES
All generic outcomes apply, with the addition of:
The patient's hemodynamic status will be stable during the perioperative period.
The patient will:
1. Have vital signs that remain within baseline values
2. Have adequate urinary output
3. Be free of peripheral or dependent edema

NURSING ACTIONS

	Yes	No	N/A
1. Preoperative assessment performed?	☐	☐	☐
2. Preoperative teaching performed?	☐	☐	☐
3. Thermia unit?	☐	☐	☐
4. Foley catheter inserted?	☐	☐	☐
5. Blood ordered/available?	☐	☐	☐
6. Special equipment/supplies available?	☐	☐	☐
7. Skin prep per institutional protocol?	☐	☐	☐
8. Condition of skin at prep site noted?	☐	☐	☐
9. Positioned correctly?	☐	☐	☐
10. Dispersive pad site checked before application?	☐	☐	☐
11. Graft properly prepared?	☐	☐	☐
12. Medications labeled/documented?	☐	☐	☐
13. Correct solutions/temperature for irrigation?	☐	☐	☐
14. Autotransfusion prepared?	☐	☐	☐
15. Catheters/tubes/drains documented?	☐	☐	☐
16. Urinary output/other drainage noted?	☐	☐	☐
17. Dispersive pad site rechecked?	☐	☐	☐
18. Counts performed and correct?	☐	☐	☐
19. Specimen/cultures to lab?	☐	☐	☐
20. Dressing applied?	☐	☐	☐
21. Implants documented?	☐	☐	☐
22. Other generic care plans initiated? (specify)	☐	☐	☐

Document additional nursing actions/generic care plans initiated here:

_____

_____

_____

EVALUATION OF PATIENT OUTCOMES

1. The patient maintained hemodynamic stability.
2. The patient met outcomes for additional generic care plans as indicated.

	Outcome met	Outcome met with additional outcome criteria	Outcome met with revised nursing care plan	Outcome not met	Outcome not applicable to this patient
1.	☐	☐	☐	☐	☐
2.	☐	☐	☐	☐	☐

Signature: _____ Date: _____

19. Prosthetic grafts and suture may be cultured during resection of aneurysm. Follow institutional protocol for preservation and disposition of specimens and cultures. Document these. Use universal precautions for material from the operative field.
20. Apply sternal dressings and dressings to drain sites and to other sites as applicable.
21. Document lot and serial numbers of prosthetic graft per institutional protocol.

Insertion of Implantable Cardioverter Defibrillator (ICD)
(Fig. 14-8)

1. Fig. 14-8 details key preoperative assessment data for ICD patients. Because of the nursing diagnosis selected for this patient (*decreased cardiac output* related to ventricular dysrhythmia), assess parameters that will be used to determine outcome attainment. These may vary but should include review of baseline vital signs, ECG results, and the signs and symptoms that accompany ventricular tachycardia. These patients have recurrent, sustained, life-threatening episodes of ventricular tachycardia (or ventricular fibrillation). Newer systems incorporate pacing capabilities (for example, pacing cardioverter defibrillator [PCDs]) that allow the device to respond in a pacing mode, a defibrillation mode, or a combination of the two, depending on the underlying rhythm disturbance.

    The patient may be anxious, confused, and cyanotic. The ECG will show a high ventricular rate, with an absent or retrograde P wave, and a wide and bizarre QRS configuration. The patient may arrive with oxygen or a temporary pacing device. Modify the care plan depending on patient acuity. Continuous careful monitoring is necessary for this patient.

2. Urinary drainage catheters are routinely inserted to decompress the bladder, measure output, and monitor renal perfusion and cardiac output. Use aseptic technique for catheter insertion. Check urine flow. Position drainage bag for easy observation. Prevent kinks or undue pressure on catheter or drainage tubing.

3. Follow institutional protocol for storing, administering, and requisitioning blood and blood products. Document per protocol.

4. A sternal, subxyphoid, or thoracotomy (for reoperation) approach will determine instrumentation. Verify that the unit to be used is the one specifically ordered for this patient (this will depend on preoperative workup results and patient capture levels). Have the appropriate leads (there will be two defibrillator patches, one sutured on each side of the heart, and two screw-in epicardial leads). Tunnelers for connecting leads and patches to the generator in the paraumbilical area will be needed. A special analyzer will be used to verify that the leads are capturing and that the device is working. If the device has pacing capabilities, a pacing system analyzer (PSA) is also needed. The patient will be put into induced ventricular tachycardia or fibrillation for repeated tests. Backup leads and devices should be available. If electrophysiologic (endocardial) mapping is to be performed, have appropriate supplies and equipment. Have sterile internal and external defibrillator paddles (and/or external patches); charge paddles when testing.

5. Follow institutional protocol for anatomic landmarks for preparation (this will depend on the surgical approach).

6. Check the condition of the skin before and after preparation procedures. Note rashes, nicks, and scratches. Document skin condition.

7. Supine position will be used for sternotomy or subxyphoid approach; for reoperation, thoracotomy may be used. Position according to institutional protocol, taking special care to pad pressure sites.

8. Dispersive pad site should be checked before application and upon pad removal.

9. Label all medications in syringes and containers. Antiarrhythmic medications should be available in the room. Document medications administered.

10. Special precautions are necessary. Prevent placing defibrillator paddles over generator or leads. The ICD unit must be deactivated if electrosurgery is used to prevent risk of electrical shock to patient. Personnel should not touch the patient while the unit fires (risk of electrical shock to personnel). If a pacemaker is present, it may deactivate the ICD unit; bipolar pacemakers with smaller spikes may be acceptable.

11. Intravascular lines, urinary drainage catheters, and chest tubes (depending on approach) are routinely inserted. Document these.

12. Monitor chest tube drainage for amount, consistency, and color. Drainage should not exceed 150 to 200 ml per hour. Some clotting in the tubes is expected; excessive clotting will occlude the tubes producing cardiac tamponade. Bright red blood indicates arterial bleeding; the chest may need to be reopened. Note amount and color of urinary drainage.

13. Check dispersive pad site(s) at removal. Note any alteration in skin condition.

14. Account for all sharps, sponges, and instruments.

15. Apply sternal dressings and dressings to drain sites and to other sites as applicable.

FIG. 14-8
CARE PLAN FOR IMPLANTABLE CARDIOVERTER DEFIBRILLATOR

KEY ASSESSMENT POINTS
History of ventricular tachycardia/fibrillation, unresponsive to or unable to tolerate pharmacologic therapy

History of coronary artery disease (if yes, refer to key assessment points, Fig. 14-1)

Results of electrophysiologic studies

Surgically unresectable myocardial dysrhythmogenic focus

Psychosocial history (ability to make life-style changes, such as restricting or avoiding driving a car, depending on a "machine"; family support)

NURSING DIAGNOSES
All generic nursing diagnoses apply to this patient, with the addition of:

High risk for decreased cardiac output

PATIENT OUTCOMES
All generic outcomes apply, with the addition of:
1. The patient's hemodynamic state will be stable during the perioperative period.
2. The patient will be free of complications from dysrhythmias.

The patient will:
1. Have vital signs that remain within normal baseline values
2. Have adequate urinary output
3. Be free of peripheral or dependent edema
4. Show no signs of complications from dysrhythmias

NURSING ACTIONS

	Yes	No	N/A
1. Preoperative assessment performed?	☐	☐	☐
2. Foley catheter inserted?	☐	☐	☐
3. Blood ordered/available?	☐	☐	☐
4. Special equipment/supplies available?	☐	☐	☐
5. Skin prep per institutional protocol?	☐	☐	☐
6. Condition of skin noted at prep site?	☐	☐	☐
7. Positioned correctly?	☐	☐	☐
8. Dispersive pad site checked before application?	☐	☐	☐
9. Medications labeled/documented?	☐	☐	☐
10. Electrical safety precautions taken?	☐	☐	☐
11. Catheters/tubes/drains documented?	☐	☐	☐
12. Urinary output/other drainage noted?	☐	☐	☐
13. Dispersive pad site re-checked?	☐	☐	☐
14. Counts performed and correct?	☐	☐	☐
15. Dressings applied?	☐	☐	☐
16. Results of unit test noted?	☐	☐	☐
17. Implants documented?	☐	☐	☐
18. Other generic care plans initiated? (specify)	☐	☐	☐

Document additional nursing actions/generic care plans initiated here:

_____

_____

_____

EVALUATION OF PATIENT OUTCOMES

	Outcome met	Outcome met with additional outcome criteria	Outcome met with revised nursing care plan	Outcome not met	Outcome not applicable to this patient
1. The patient maintained hemodynamic stability.	☐	☐	☐	☐	☐
2. The patient was free of complications from dysrhythmias.	☐	☐	☐	☐	☐
3. The patient met outcomes for additional generic care plans as indicated.	☐	☐	☐	☐	☐

Signature: _____ Date: _____

16. Document results of tests of leads and unit.
17. Document lot and serial numbers of leads, and implantable unit per institutional protocol.

Insertion of Ventricular Assist Device (LVAD, RVAD) (Fig. 14-9)

1. Fig. 14-9 details key preoperative assessment data for VAD patients. Because of the nursing diagnoses selected for this patient (*decreased cardiac output* related to severe myocardial disease, *high risk for infection* related to externalized VAD cables and wires, and *high risk for altered tissue perfusion* related to possible thromboembolic complications), assess parameters that will be used to determine outcome attainment. Because of patient instability, full assessment and teaching may not be possible. Along with life-sustaining measures to support cardiac output, the perioperative nurse should consider the patient's and family's *anxiety*. Emotional and physical comfort should be provided. Offer short, understandable explanations. Keep the family informed of the patient's intraoperative progress. Based on the individual patient situation, modify the care plan accordingly.

2. Thermia unit may be placed on OR bed to reduce heat loss during the closing portion of the procedure. Follow institutional protocol for unit identification, documenting time and temperature, and protecting skin integrity. Note also the placement of additional temperature probes.

3. Urinary drainage catheters are routinely inserted to decompress the bladder, measure output, and monitor renal perfusion and cardiac output. Use aseptic technique for catheter insertion. Check urine flow. Position drainage bag for easy observation. Prevent kinks or undue pressure on catheter or drainage tubing.

4. Follow institutional protocol for storing, administering, and requisitioning blood and blood products. Anticipate the need for additional blood and blood products. Document per protocol.

5. Have available VAD(s), lines, cannulas, connectors, graft material, wrenches, extra vascular clamps, and other implantation supplies, with backups. Handle VAD/VAD components carefully; prevent scratching. Ensure that VAD drive system is functioning. Have defibrillator immediately available. Prepare to cannulate femoral artery for arterial perfusion and right atrium for venous drainage. Ensure that all connections are tight and that there are no kinks in lines. *For LVAD:* Cannula from VAD is placed in ascending aorta, tunnelled through skin to left of abdominal midline; cannula to VAD is placed in left atrial appendage and tunnelled out left abdominal midline (left ventricular apex may be used to preserve atrium for transplantation; have additional suture). *For RVAD:* One cannula is placed in pulmonary artery; other cannula is placed in right atrial appendage; both are tunnelled out of right abdominal midline. *For BiVAD:* Insert LVAD and RVAD; connect pump(s) to cannulas; start drive system. Assist with de-airing measures to lessen risk of embolus. Anticipate insertion of hemodialysis catheter; have necessary supplies. Anticipate heparin reversal; patient may be placed on antiplatelet therapy (dextran) postoperatively. Left atrial and/or femoral pressure lines may be inserted (pulmonary catheters are avoided with VAD); have necessary supplies. Have hemostatic agents ready.

6. Follow institutional protocol for anatomic landmarks for preparation (will vary depending on RVAD/LVAD/BiVAD).

7. Check the condition of the skin before and after preparation procedures. Note rashes, nicks, and scratches. Document skin condition.

8. Patient in supine position; use caution in positioning patient with multiple lines and cables. Patient may come to OR with intraaortic balloon pump. Have femoral artery accessible for cannulation.

9. Dispersive pad site should be checked before application and upon pad removal.

10. Label all medications in syringes and containers. Document medications administered.

11. Solutions on the sterile field should be labeled and maintained at the correct temperature for the correct purpose.

12. Autotransfusion is routine. Fluid is washed and spun, and blood cells are collected and infused back into the patient. If antibiotic solution is used, determine whether the irrigant can be washed and reinfused or whether it should be discarded. If discarding is recommended, use discard suction.

13. Prevent contact between VAD and defibrillator, electrosurgical unit, and pacing wires.

14. Peripheral and central lines, urinary drainage catheters, and chest tubes are routinely inserted. Document these.

15. Monitor chest tube drainage for amount, consistency, and color. Drainage should not exceed 150 to 200 ml per hour. Some clotting in the tubes is expected; excessive clotting will occlude the tubes, producing cardiac tamponade. Bright red blood indicates arterial bleeding; the chest may need to be reopened. Note amount and color of urinary drainage.

FIG. 14-9
CARE PLAN FOR INSERTION OF VENTRICULAR ASSIST DEVICE (LVAD, RVAD)

KEY ASSESSMENT POINTS

End-stage heart disease, reversible or irreversible

Pulmonary artery wedge pressure greater than 25 mm Hg, systolic arterial blood pressure less than 90 mm Hg, cardiac index less than 2 L/min/m^2

Cannot be weaned from cardiopulmonary bypass, cardiomyopathy (candidate for transplant)

Pulmonary function adequate

Results of cardiac catheterization, echocardiography

Failure of maximal medical therapy (volume infusion, pharmacologic support, intraaortic balloon pump)

Psychosocial history (fear of death while awaiting donor organ or recovery of native heart, depending on a "machine"; family support)

NURSING DIAGNOSES

All generic nursing diagnoses apply to this patient, with the addition of:

High risk for decreased cardiac output

High risk for infection

High risk for altered tissue perfusion

PATIENT OUTCOMES

All generic outcomes apply, with the addition of:

The patient's hemodynamic status and tissue perfusion will be stable during the perioperative period.

There will be no signs or symptoms of infection.

The patient will:

1. Have vital signs that remain within baseline values
2. Have adequate urinary output
3. Be free of peripheral or dependent edema
4. Be free of signs/symptoms of infection

NURSING ACTIONS

	Yes	No	N/A
1. Preoperative assessment performed?	☐	☐	☐
2. Thermia unit?	☐	☐	☐
3. Foley catheter inserted?	☐	☐	☐
4. Blood ordered/available?	☐	☐	☐
5. Special equipment/supplies available?	☐	☐	☐
6. Skin prep per institutional protocol?	☐	☐	☐
7. Condition of skin at prep site noted?	☐	☐	☐
8. Positioned correctly?	☐	☐	☐
9. Dispersive pad site checked before application?	☐	☐	☐
10. Medications labeled/documented?	☐	☐	☐
11. Correct solutions/temperature for irrigation?	☐	☐	☐
12. Autotransfusion prepared?	☐	☐	☐
13. Electrical safety precautions taken?	☐	☐	☐
14. Catheters/tubes/drains documented?	☐	☐	☐
15. Urinary output/other drainage noted?	☐	☐	☐
16. Dispersive pad site rechecked?	☐	☐	☐
17. Counts performed and correct?	☐	☐	☐
18. Dressings applied?	☐	☐	☐

Document additional nursing actions/generic care plans initiated here:

_____

_____

_____

EVALUATION OF PATIENT OUTCOMES

	Outcome met	Outcome met with additional outcome criteria	Outcome met with revised nursing care plan	Outcome not met	Outcome not applicable to this patient
1. The patient maintained hemodynamic stability and adequate tissue perfusion.	☐	☐	☐	☐	☐
2. The patient was infection free.	☐	☐	☐	☐	☐
3. The patient met outcomes for additional generic care plans as indicated.	☐	☐	☐	☐	☐

Signature: _____ Date: _____

16. Check dispersive pad site at removal. Note any alteration in skin condition.

17. Account for all items in device insertion in addition to routine sharp, sponge, and instrument counts.

18. The sternum may not be wired closed; only subcutaneous tissue and skin approximated. Apply dressings carefully to sternum, drain, and VAD sites and other sites as applicable. This patient is at increased risk for infection due to the numerous wound sites.

Cardiac Transplantation (Fig. 14-10)

1. Fig. 14-10 details key preoperative assessment data for transplant patients. Because of the nursing diagnosis selected for this patient (*decreased cardiac output, altered tissue perfusion,* and *high risk for infection*), assess parameters that will be used to determine outcome attainment. These may vary but should include review of baseline vital signs and abnormalities, and renal status. Examine the extremities and sacrum for edema. Review the medical record with a focus on cardiopulmonary, neurologic, and psychosocial data.

2. Inpatient preoperative teaching time is often limited for transplant recipients. Transplants are a multidisciplinary effort; the perioperative nurse may collaborate in providing information about incision location, lengthy operative time, and perioperative events. This patient will likely be anxious; in addition to worry about the impending surgery and its success, preoperative narcotics may be withheld due to cardiac decompression. Offer reassurance and focus on necessary information.

3. Thermia unit may be placed on OR bed to reduce heat loss during the closing portion of the procedure. Follow institutional protocol for identification, documenting time and temperature, and protecting skin integrity. Note also the placement of additional temperature probes.

4. Urinary drainage catheters are routinely inserted to decompress the bladder, measure output, and monitor renal perfusion and cardiac output. Use aseptic technique for catheter insertion. Check urine flow. Position drainage bag for easy observation. Prevent kinks or undue pressure on catheter or drainage tubing.

5. Follow institutional protocol for storing, administering, and requisitioning blood and blood products. Ascertain whether there are any special blood requirements (for example, irradiated blood and washed cells). Be alert for hyperacute rejection (antigen/antibody related to improper cross-matching) occurring in OR. Document administration and reactions per protocol.

6. *Procurement:* When team is called, change into fresh OR attire. Assemble needed items: instruments, suture, saw (if requested), medications, plastic bags, IV tubing for cardioplegia administration, crushed ice, and bags of normal saline. At donor facility, prepare sterile work area; assist staff as necessary. Cardioplegia solution, pressure infusers, and myocardial temperature probes may also be required. If multiple procurement, heart will be excised first. Be ready to depart donor facility immediately following excision and preparation of donor heart; no more than 6 hours between excision and implantation is recommended. Notify recipient facility of expected time of arrival. Prevent placing donor heart in direct contact with ice/ice chips/slush during transportation. *Preparation of recipient:* Prepare for central venous line insertion. Have room set up; coordinate with surgeon, anesthesiologist, and procurement team. Following sternotomy, be prepared for double atrial cannulation and ascending aortic cannulation. *Transplantation:* Assess donor heart for residual pieces of tissue (trimmings and so forth) remaining in cardiac cavities. Have long suture, venting catheters, tubing (extensive venting may be performed), and epicardial pacing wires. If heterotopic transplantation (piggyback) is planned, have additional suture and supplies. Notify ICU when new heart is beating.

7. Prepare per institutional protocol for anatomic landmarks.

8. Check the condition of the skin before and after preparation procedures. Note rashes, nicks, and scratches. Document skin condition.

9. Provide comfort measures (warm blanket and pillow) while awaiting verification of viable heart. Patient will be in supine position. Position according to institutional protocol, taking special care to pad pressure sites. This patient has a severely compromised cardiovascular system and will be undergoing a lengthy procedure; impairment of skin integrity is a serious risk.

10. Dispersive pad site should be checked before application and upon pad removal.

11. Sterilize all equipment and supplies; have environmental services clean room before procedure (following institutional protocol). Two circulating nurses are desirable to reduce flow of traffic in and out of room. Use universal precautions with container carrying donor heart before bringing into OR. Procurement team should change OR attire before coming into OR.

FIG. 14-10
CARE PLAN FOR CARDIAC TRANSPLANTATION

KEY ASSESSMENT POINTS

Terminal heart disease, end-stage cardiomyopathy
Presence of VAD or other assist device
Life expectancy less than 12 months
Less than 60 years of age (may vary)
Normal or correctable hepatic, renal, pulmonary, and other major organ function; absence of multiorgan dysfunction
Free of acute infection, cancer
Results of cardiac catheterization, echocardiography
Psychosocial history (emotional stability, coping effectiveness, ability to adhere to prescribed postoperative therapeutic regimen, family support)

NURSING DIAGNOSES

All generic nursing diagnoses apply to this patient, with the addition of:
High risk for decreased cardiac output/altered tissue perfusion
High risk of infection

PATIENT OUTCOMES

All generic outcomes apply, with the addition of:
The patient's hemodynamic status will be stable during the perioperative period.
There will be no signs/symptoms of infection
The patient will:
1. Have vital signs that remain within baseline values
2. Have adequate urinary output
3. Be free of peripheral or dependent edema
4. Be free of signs/symptoms of infection.

NURSING ACTIONS

	Yes	No	N/A
1. Preoperative assessment performed?	☐	☐	☐
2. Preoperative teaching performed?	☐	☐	☐
3. Thermia unit?	☐	☐	☐
4. Foley catheter inserted?	☐	☐	☐
5. Blood ordered/available?	☐	☐	☐
6. Special equipment/supplies available?	☐	☐	☐
7. Skin prep per institutional protocol?	☐	☐	☐
8. Condition of skin at prep site noted?	☐	☐	☐
9. Positioned correctly?	☐	☐	☐
10. Dispersive pad site(s) checked before application?	☐	☐	☐
11. Transplant precautions instituted?	☐	☐	☐
12. Medications labeled/documented?	☐	☐	☐
13. Correct solutions/temperature for irrigation?	☐	☐	☐
14. Autotransfusion prepared?	☐	☐	☐
15. Catheters/tubes/drains documented?	☐	☐	☐
16. Urinary output/other drainage noted?	☐	☐	☐
17. Dispersive pad site re-checked?	☐	☐	☐
18. Counts performed and correct?	☐	☐	☐
19. Specimens/cultures to lab?	☐	☐	☐
20. Dressings applied?	☐	☐	☐
21. Other generic care plans initiated? (specify)	☐	☐	☐

Document additional nursing actions/generic care plans initiated here:

_____

_____

_____

EVALUATION OF PATIENT OUTCOMES

	Outcome met	Outcome met with additional outcome criteria	Outcome met with revised nursing care plan	Outcome not met	Outcome not applicable to this patient
1. The patient maintained hemodynamic stability.	☐	☐	☐	☐	☐
2. The patient was infection free.	☐	☐	☐	☐	☐
3. The patient met outcomes for additional generic care plans as indicated.	☐	☐	☐	☐	☐

Signature: _____ Date: _____

12. Label syringes containing medications. Immunosuppressive drugs may be initiated in OR. Document and report to ICU all medications given.
13. Solutions on the sterile field should be labeled and maintained at the correct temperature for the correct purpose.
14. Autotransfusion is routine. Fluid is washed and spun, and blood cells are collected and infused back into the patient. If antibiotic solution is used, determine whether the irrigant can be washed and reinfused or whether it should be discarded. If discarding is recommended, use discard suction.
15. Peripheral and central lines, urinary drainage catheters, and chest tubes are routinely inserted. Document these.
16. Monitor chest tube drainage for amount, consistency, and color. Be aware that chest tube drainage may not accurately reflect amount of blood in pericardium (related to enlarged pericardial cavity of recipient, with donor heart smaller than excised heart). Note amount and color of urinary drainage.
17. Check dispersive pad site(s) at removal. Note any alteration in skin condition.
18. Account for all items used during transplantation in addition to routine sharp, sponge, and instrument counts.
19. Follow institutional protocol for preservation and disposition of specimens and cultures. Cultures of donor or native heart may be taken. Use universal precautions with material received from the sterile field.
20. Apply dressing to sternotomy incision, to drain sites, and to other sites.

References

Agency for Health Care Policy and Research (AHCPR). (1994). *Heart failure: Evaluation and care of patients with left-ventricular dysfunction.* Rockville, MD: The Agency.

American Heart Association. (1992). *1993 Heart and stroke facts statistics.* Dallas: The Association.

American Nurses Association Division on Medical-Surgical Nursing Practice and the American Heart Association Council on Cardio vascular Nursing. (1981). *Standards of cardiovascular nursing practice.* Kansas City: The Association.

Artinian NT. (1993). Spouses' perceptions of readiness for discharge after cardiac surgery. *Applied Nursing Research, 6*(2), 80-88.

Association of Operating Room Nurses. (1996). *Standards and recommended practices for perioperative nursing.* Denver: The Association.

Barnes RV, Lawton L, & Briggs D. (1994). Clinical bench marking improves clinical paths: Experience with coronary artery bypass grafting. *Journal of Quality Improvement, 20*(5), 267-276.

Braunwald E. (1992). *Heart disease.* Philadelphia: WB Saunders.

Crumlish C. (1994). Coping and emotional response in cardiac surgery patients. *Western Journal of Nursing Research, 16*(1), 57-68.

Dugger B, Macklin D, & Rand B. (1994). Veni-Gard[R] versus standard dressings on hemodynamic catheter sites. *Dimensions in Critical Care Nursing, 13*(2), 84-89.

Giuffre M, Heidenreich T, & Pruitt L. (1994). Rewarming cardiac surgery patients: Radiant heat versus forced warm air. *Nursing Research, 43*(3), 174-178.

Guzzetta CE, et al. (1989). *Clinical assessment tools for use with nursing diagnosis.* St. Louis: Mosby.

Hawthorne MH. (1994). Gender differences in recovery after coronary surgery. *Image—the Journal of Nursing Scholarship, 26*(1), 75-80.

Health Technology Assessment. (1994). Institutional and patient criteria for heart-lung transplantation. Rockville, MD: US Department of Health and Human Services.

Maxam-Moore V, Wilkie D, & Woods S. (1994). Analgesics for cardiac surgery patients in critical care: Describing current practice. *American Journal of Critical Care, 3*(1), 31-39.

Redeker NS, et al. (1994). First postoperative week activity patterns and recovery in women after coronary artery bypass surgery. *Nursing Research, 43*(3), 168-172.

Shumacker HB. (1992). *The evolution of cardiac surgery.* Bloomington, IN: Indiana University Press.

Chapter 15

Thoracic Surgery

Vicki J. Fox

The incision having been made, Desault introduced his fingers into the thorax, and perceived a kind of sac, full of water, which he took for the pericardium. The other consultants, having, like him, examined the parts, were of the same opinion. In consequence, he opened the dilated sac with a blunt knife and gave vent to about a pint of water, which escaped with a hissing at each expiration. The flowing being finished, the finger was again introduced into the orifice and perceived a single substance, pointed and conical, against which it struck. All assistants felt it, and the general opinion was that it was the heart, naked.

BICHAT, 1814

*P*atient care plans have become an accepted part of nursing care that contribute significantly to both the quality and continuity of care. Providing a means of communication among nurses and other health care professionals, care plans are used as planning tools, as measures of patient progress, as resources in determining nursing assignments, and as tools for patient reports among health care providers. Standardized care plans contain nursing diagnoses, expected outcomes, short- and long-term goals, nursing interventions or actions, and statements that describe achievement of desired patient outcomes.

Planning perioperative patient care for the thoracic surgery patient includes physical examination of the chest, nursing assessment of pulmonary status, preparation of the patient for diagnostic procedures, and supporting and educating the patient and family. Patient compliance with postoperative nursing and medical regimens is vastly improved if the patient receives psychoeducational interventions preoperatively (Fox, 1995). Intraoperatively, the perioperative nurse engages in many collaborative activities such as positioning, airway maintenance, and hemodynamic monitoring. During the postoperative period, nursing activities include pulmonary toilet procedures, care of chest tubes, and monitoring of pulmonary efficiency.

HISTORY

Thoracic surgical interventions developed more slowly than general surgery interventions because of the inherent difficulties with entering the chest and the physiologic impact on the lungs. Early thoracic procedures evolved out of a need for an effective treatment of tuberculosis. One of the first successful pulmonary resections was done in 1895. Macewan performed a pneumonectomy on a patient with extensive tuberculosis. The patient survived the procedure, demonstrating that opening the chest and excising a lung was possible. In 1909 Samuel Robinson performed a lobectomy for bronchiectasis. His contributions to managing postoperative pneumothorax included the use of positive pressure. Robinson also treated tuberculosis by purposely creating a pneumothorax (Scannell, 1986); artificial pneumothorax constituted the main treatment for tuberculosis in the United States in the early 1900s. Later, thoracoplasty became widely used to collapse the lungs in the treatment of tuberculosis; through subperiosteal removal of ribs, skeletal support of the chest wall was greatly reduced. The subcostal muscles could no longer lift the chest wall, so a portion of the chest wall fell in toward the mediastinum and the lung collapsed.

In 1910 the Swedish physician, Jacobaeus, introduced thoracoscopy for the diagnosis of tuberculosis and treatment of accompanying pleural effusion. His technique was subsequently employed for cauterizing and lysing intrapleural adhesions. Intrapleural pneumolysis, or the Jacobaeus procedure, was widely used to treat tuberculosis in Europe. In the United States, Bloomberg used intrapleural pneumolysis for approximately 2000 patients between 1936 and 1950. Eventually, thoracoscopy for the treatment of tuberculosis was replaced by antimicrobial agents and effective antituberculosis chemotherapy. Today, health care providers are concerned with both tuberculosis (TB) and multidrug resistant tuberculosis (MDRTB). Altered defense mechanisms place certain groups, including the elderly, IV drug abusers, and the chronically ill who are debilitated by cancer or HIV, at risk for TB (Moody, 1995). Thus, perioperative nurses must once again concern themselves with assessment and diagnostic methods for TB and recognize treatment and follow-up measures for TB and MDRTB. Surgical management of localized resistant mycobacterial infection may involve pulmonary resection, followed by drug therapy (LoCicero, 1993).

As is common in the history of surgery, early thoracic surgeons learned valuable lessons treating battlefield injuries. Surgeons learned the mechanical physiology of respiration from treating penetrating chest wounds. By the 1930s, surgeons had not only mastered techniques that allowed entry into the thoracic cavity, but also had improved resection techniques.

Endoscopy has become common in diagnosing and treating thoracic disease. The first endoscope had a candle as its light source. Since the 1980s, fiberoptic technology has enabled flexible bronchoscopies and video-assisted thoracic procedures to reduce the morbidity associated with diagnosis and treatment of thoracic diseases. Video-assisted thoracoscopy has become the preferred procedure for many clinical situations, including pleural effusions and masses, empyemas, diagnostic lung biopsy, apical blebs, effusive pericarditis, hilar and mediastinal staging of malignant processes, and mediastinal cysts (Coltharp, et al., 1992; Mack, et al., 1992). Clinical situations in which thoracoscopy will find an expanded role in the future are upper extremity sympathetic dystrophies, esopha-

geal achalasia, spine disease, and trauma. Because video-assisted surgery continues to grow so rapidly, a video-assisted thoracic surgical (VATS) study group and registry has been formed to evaluate this new technology in a scientific manner; at the first International Symposium on Thoracoscopic Surgery, over 1800 VATS procedures were reported as part of the first registry (Ginsberg, 1994).

As endoscopic technology has proliferated, so has the equipment used with it. Automatic stapling devices and instruments that enable the use of electrosurgery, laser, and argon beam coagulation in the thoracic cavity also decrease the need for open thoracic procedures. Laser phototherapy for certain types of malignant lesions is under investigation with encouraging results. Double-lumen endotracheal tubes enable the anesthesia provider to deflate or inflate the operative lung as needed, while ventilating the nonoperative lung. This further reduces the risk of intraoperative respiratory and hemodynamic complications. Tube placement may be checked with a fiberoptic bronchoscope. Perioperative nurses who work with patients undergoing thoracic procedures continue to be challenged by these technical advances. Depending on their practice setting, they may be further challenged by single-lung transplantation for patients with chronic obstructive lung disease, restrictive lung disease, or primary pulmonary hypertension or double-lung transplantation for bronchiectasis and the pulmonary complications of cystic fibrosis (DATTA, 1993). Whether caring for a patient undergoing a minimally invasive procedure or a complicated lung transplant, perioperative nurses organize nursing activities and manage collaborative efforts to ensure safe and cost-effective treatments with favorable outcomes for thoracic surgery patients.

PERIOPERATIVE NURSING

In the past, the perioperative nurse cared for patients undergoing thoracic procedures primarily for the treatment of tuberculosis and malignant pulmonary lesions. That is no longer true. Thoracic procedures may be performed for removal of malignant neoplasms or benign cysts arising in the lungs, bronchus, proximal or distal esophagus, or thymus gland; diagnosis of pleural, mediastinal, bronchial, or lung lesions; evacuation of pleural or pericardial effusions and suppurative lesions within lung tissue; lysis of pleural adhesions; obliteration of persistent air leaks from postoperative bronchopleural fistula, cystic fibrosis, or severe chronic pulmonary obstructive disease such as emphysema; decortication of lung, pleura, or heart; pleurodesis; diagnosis and/or repair of ruptured or lacerated diaphragm; removal of thoracic disc; treatment of upper extremity sympathetic dystrophies; treatment of congenital malformations and pathologic conditions of the thoracic aorta; and thoracic injury and trauma of the aorta, lung, and chest wall (McManus & McGuigan, 1994). Planning perioperative patient care for a patient population with such diverse problems requires a broad knowledge base and focused inquiry.

Patient Assessment

The nursing process begins with collecting and organizing assessment data. The perioperative nurse gathers assessment data from a number of sources, reviewing and confirming the medical diagnosis and treatment plan, the patient's presenting complaint and history of the current problem, physical assessment findings, and results of preoperative tests. The perioperative nurse validates, organizes, and interprets data. This assessment is a critical phase of developing a plan of care. Collaboration with other members of the surgical team is essential to achieve a valid and reliable assessment. The perioperative nurse will be especially interested in previous diagnostic tests or treatments the patient has received for the current problem, allergies, nutritional status (particularly the albumin level, because it affects wound healing), current medications, and general skin condition. Vision or hearing impairment; cardiac, urinary, musculoskeletal, or neurologic system dysfunction; results of pulmonary function tests; and arterial blood gas analyses also have implications for perioperative patient care. Since many thoracic procedures are moving to ambulatory settings, the perioperative nurse may very well obtain the initial history. In both inpatient and ambulatory settings, the perioperative nurse should know how to interpret the data and extrapolate the implications for perioperative nursing care from the data.

Assessment of respiratory status. Assessment may begin by taking a patient history specific to respiratory status. Important questions that should be asked about the patient's current respiratory status are presented in Box 15-1. The results of arterial blood gases (ABGs) provide invaluable information for assessing and managing a patient's respiratory and metabolic status preoperatively, intraoperatively, and postoperatively. Box 15-2 presents normal values.

The pH measures alkalinity and acidity. The pH is inversely proportional to the actual concentration of hydrogen ion concentration. In alkalosis, the pH is elevated; in acidosis, the pH is decreased. The P_{CO_2} measures the partial pressure of carbon dioxide in the blood. P_{CO_2} is considered the *respiratory* component of acid-base balance because the CO_2 level is controlled primarily by the lungs (Pagana & Pagana, 1995). If the CO_2 increases, the pH de-

---

Box 15-1 Sample Questions Asked Regarding Respiratory Status

"Are you ever short of breath? For how long?"
"Do you have a cough? Is it a dry or productive cough? When you do cough something up, have you noticed its color? Have you coughed up blood?"
"Do you have chest pain? Show me where it is. How would you describe this pain?"
"Do you ever have a fever? Have you taken your temperature, and if so, what was it?"
"Do you smoke? If so, how many cigarettes do you smoke each day? For how many years have you smoked? If you don't smoke, do you live in the same house as a smoker? For how long?"
"Do you have any allergies or wheezing?"
"Have you ever been exposed to or had tuberculosis?"
"Have you had contact with fumes, chemicals, asbestos, or coal?"

Box 15-2 Normal Arterial Blood Gases

pH	7.35 to 7.45
P_{CO_2}	35 to 45 mm Hg
HCO_3	21 to 28 mEq/L
P_{O_2}	80 to 100 mm Hg
O_2 saturation	95% to 100%

---

creases, and vice versa; the relationship is inversely proportional. The HCO_3 (bicarbonate ion) is a measure of the metabolic or renal component of the acid-base equilibrium. As the HCO_3 level increases, so does the pH; the relationship is directly proportional. An indirect measurement of oxygen content, P_{O_2} is the tension pressure of oxygen dissolved in the plasma. The P_{O_2} level may be decreased in patients who are unable to oxygenate arterial blood. This may be the case with pneumonia, tumor, or mucous plugs of the bronchial tree; in patients who have underventilated pulmonary alveoli as occurs in the anesthetized patient; or when the operative lung is collapsed. Oxygen saturation, O_2, indicates what percentage of hemoglobin is saturated with oxygen. When 95% to 100% of the hemoglobin carries oxygen, the tissues are getting enough oxygen. As P_{O_2} levels decrease, so does the O_2 saturation. As the O_2 saturation level drops below 70%, vital organs are unable to extract enough P_{O_2} to function.

pulmonary function tests

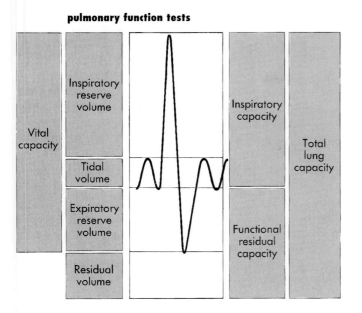

Fig. 15-1. Relationship of lung volumes to capacities. (From Pagana KD & Pagana TJ. (1995). *Mosby's diagnostic and laboratory test reference* (2nd Ed.). St. Louis: Mosby.)

The perioperative nurse must understand the significance of basic pulmonary function studies. These measure the functional ability of the lungs. Pulmonary functions affect preoperative respiratory care, type and duration of anesthesia, methods of postoperative pain control, the type of surgical procedure performed, and the postoperative course. Interpretation of pulmonary functions provides information that differentiates obstructive disease (ventilation is disturbed by an increase in airway resistance and expiration is primarily affected) from restrictive disease (ventilation is disturbed by a limitation in chest expansion and inspiration is primarily affected). Pulmonary function studies are used to evaluate the lungs and pulmonary reserve preoperatively, helping to determine if the patient is even a candidate for a thoracic surgical procedure. There are four basic lung volumes and four derived capacities; these relationships are shown in Fig. 15-1. *Tidal volume* (VT) measures the volume of air inhaled or exhaled during normal breathing. *Inspiratory reserve volume* (IRV) measures the maximal volume of air that can be inhaled following a normal respiration at rest. *Expiratory reserve volume* (ERV) is the maximal volume of air that can be expired following a normal respiration. *Residual volume* (RV) is the volume of air remaining in the lungs after a forced expiration. Four capacities are measured in pulmonary function studies. *Total lung capacity* (TLC) is the volume to which the lungs can be expanded at the end of a maximal inspiration or the sum of vital capacity and residual volume. *Vital capacity* (VC) is

the maximal amount of air that can be expelled from the lungs by a forceful effort after a maximum inspiration. It is the sum of inspiratory capacity and expiratory reserve volume. *Inspiratory capacity* (IC) is the maximal amount of air that can be inhaled from the resting expiratory position after a normal exhalation. It is the sum of the tidal volume and inspiratory reserve volume. *Functional residual capacity* (FRC) is the amount of air contained in the lungs at the end of normal quiet expiration or the sum of expiratory reserve volume and residual volume.

Pulmonary function studies also measure lung function during forced breathing patterns. In the *forced vital capacity* (FVC) maneuver, the patient exhales rapidly and maximally. The amount of air exhaled within 1 and 3 seconds (forced expiratory volumes, FEV_1 and FEV_3) should be within 72% and 92% of FVC at 1 and 3 seconds, respectively. If the FEV_1 is less than 70%, the patient is not a good candidate for resection of lung tissue. Timed vital capacities are reduced in obstructive pulmonary disease and normal or elevated in restrictive disease. Obstructive diseases are those that reduce the elastic properties of the lung tissue, such as emphysema. Restrictive diseases are those that impair the ability of the lung to inflate, such as pleural effusions. Flow-volume loop, obtained both during inspiration and expiration, are widely used pulmonary function tests. During the forced vital capacity maneuver, the airflow is plotted against expired volume.

Physical examination of the chest. Physical examination of the chest involves four common maneuvers reviewed briefly here (Bates, 1995; Stiesmeyer, 1993). *Inspection* begins with observing the size and shape of the chest. Deviations such as barrel chest, as in patients with chronic pulmonary obstructive disease, pectus excavatum, or carinatum; congenital malformations of the chest; and kyphoscoliosis, a structural curvature of the spine, are noted. While inspecting the chest, note breathing patterns and consider the rate and depth of respirations. Restrictive lung disease or pleural pain cause tachypnea, a rapid shallow breathing. Slow respiratory rates can be due to drug-induced respiratory depression or to increased intracranial pressure. Observe for and document dyspnea, use of accessory muscles, forced expiration, and intercostal retraction.

Palpation of the chest is performed with the patient in a sitting position. The hands are placed on the patient's upper chest with the fingertips on the clavicle and the thumbs over the sternum. The patient is asked to take a deep breath. If the hands move apart asymmetrically, atelectasis, pleural thickening, pneumothorax, or bronchial obstruction may be present. Palpate for tenderness and masses, particularly subclavicularly. A crackling feeling under the skin is a sign of subcutaneous emphysema, most often seen in trauma patients with a tension pneumothorax or patients being mechanically ventilated. Also check for tactile fremitus, vibrations that can be felt through the chest wall. When the patient speaks, the examiner's hands should vibrate bilaterally. Higher, unilateral intensity indicates tissue consolidation on that side, as in lobar pneumonia. Diminished intensity or absence of vibration may indicate pleural effusion, pneumothorax, or emphysema.

To palpate for lymph nodes, use the pads of the index and middle fingers. To examine nodes arising from the scalenus anterior muscle, which inserts at the tubercle of the first rib, the patient's neck should be relaxed and flexed slightly forward and toward the side of the examination. Palpate the deep supraclavicular area formed by the clavicle and the sternomastoid muscle. Move the skin over the underlying tissue rather than moving the fingers over the skin. Hard, fixed nodes are ominous and may indicate malignant metastasis. Tender nodes suggest an inflammatory process.

During *percussion,* note sound, pitch, intensity, and quality. Normally, resonance is heard over the entire field with a low pitch, loud intensity, and hollow quality. With pneumothorax and emphysema, percussion notes may be hyperresonant or of louder intensity, lower pitch, and longer duration. With a large pleural effusion, percussion notes may be flat or of soft intensity, high pitch and short duration. With lobar pneumonia, smaller pleural effusions, and atelectasis, percussion notes may be dull or of medium intensity, medium pitch, and medium duration. Resonance normally changes to dullness over an organ, in this case the heart and diaphragm.

Results of *auscultation* vary depending on where the nurse is listening. With the stethoscope placed between the clavicles and midsternum, mainstem bronchial sounds will be heard. These are louder and higher pitched than other sounds. On the anterior chest, low, soft, blowing, vesicular sounds will be heard. Decreased breath sounds may indicate lung consolidation or pleural effusion. If tumor growth obstructs a bronchus, breath sounds may be diminished. Absent breath sounds may indicate pneumothorax. The nurse may also auscultate adventitious sounds, described either as wheezes or crackles. Crackles are discontinuous sounds. Wheezes are heard during either inhalation or exhalation as continuous sounds that are musical or snoring in nature; they are associated with oscillation of the bronchial wall and the opening and closing of the airway (Grap, Glass, & Constantino, 1994). Pleural rub, a grating sound associated with respiratory movements, may indicate pleural effusion. Vocal fremitus may be checked using the stethoscope. Expect results similar to those indicated for palpation.

Diagnostic studies. The perioperative nurse should understand the diagnostic procedures the patient is undergoing or has undergone, incorporating that data into the plan of care. The most common radiologic diagnostic procedures used to evaluate pathologic conditions of the chest are chest x-ray, computed tomography (CT), and magnetic resonance imaging (MRI). The chest x-ray film is ordinarily the first diagnostic step in evaluating the patient. Both the lateral and posterioanterior (PA) views are useful in detecting pulmonary or mediastinal masses, pleural effusion, pneumothorax, cavitating lesions, atelectasis, or pneumonia.

CT is highly accurate in diagnosing and evaluating many pathologic conditions, such as the existence and extent of malignant and benign lesions, pleural effusions, cysts, and abscesses of the lung, pleura, mediastinum, and esophagus. CT is helpful for determining the location and size of pulmonary, mediastinal, and esophageal lesions, as well as in differentiating cystic or cavitating lesions from solid lesions. CT is also useful for determining the stage of malignant pulmonary tumor growth. Tumor invasion to the mediastinum or chest wall or diaphragm rules out thoracic surgery as a curative treatment. However, diagnostic thoracic procedures such as bronchoscopy, mediastinoscopy, or thoracoscopy with lung biopsy may be recommended. When IV contrast is administered to the patient, vascular structures are easily identified. With oral contrast, the esophagus can be evaluated for benign or malignant tumors. CT can also be used to assist the radiologist with locating a pulmonary lesion for needle aspiration.

MRI is a noninvasive diagnostic technique that produces an image based on how hydrogen atoms behave when placed in a magnetic field and then disturbed by radiofrequency waves. It provides better contrast between normal and pathologic tissue than CT, eliminates the bone artifacts that occur in CT, and creates a variety of spatial images (transverse, sagittal, and coronal views). These characteristics make the MRI especially useful for diagnosing the extent of disc disease of the thoracic spinal cord. MRI also can be used to differentiate mediastinal fat from lymph nodes and to detect nodes that were not apparent with CT.

Radioisotope scanning techniques include bone and lung scans. Bone scans are useful for determining if existing tumor has metastasized to distant areas. The degree of uptake of a radionuclide material–injected IV is related to bone metabolism. An increased uptake of the isotope is abnormal and appears as a "hot spot" on the scan. The test is very sensitive, but unfortunately not very specific. It is useful for confirming distant metastasis. A test useful for determining the patient's suitability for pulmonary resection is the ventilation/perfusion scan (VPS). It detects abnormalities in blood perfusion of the lung and in ventilation of the lung fields. It is used to predict what postoperative VC and FEV_1 will be if a certain portion of the lung is removed. If the resection will remove "useful" lung tissue, the resection is less acceptable than if only "nonuseful" lung tissue is to be removed. If the scan shows gross abnormalities throughout the lung fields, a resection is very risky.

Thoracic procedures for diagnosis include thoracentesis (inserting a large bore needle into the pleural space and aspirating fluid; this may also be done for therapeutic reasons to relieve pain, dyspnea, or other signs of pleural pressure); percutaneous transthoracic needle aspiration biopsy (when lesions are located in the periphery of the lung, in the chest wall, or in the superior pulmonary sulcus); and scalene node biopsy, which is one of the simplest, most reliable, and least risky of the diagnostic procedures. If scalene lymph nodes are palpable, biopsy is done in the OR, under either general or local anesthesia with IV sedation. It can also be done on an outpatient basis. Biopsy results positive for malignant cells indicate a malignant lesion has metastasized to a distant location. The patient would not be helped by pulmonary resection. Alternative treatment plans for lung cancer in later stages include radiation or chemotherapy as indicated for cell type (Table 15-1).

Bronchoscopy, mediastinoscopy, or thoracoscopy may also be indicated. Diagnostic bronchoscopies were once done in the OR suite by a general or thoracic surgeon; today, they are commonly done on an outpatient basis in the pulmonary function laboratory by a pulmonologist. If performed in the OR suite, the procedures are likely to be done in combination with a mediastinoscopy or for therapeutic reasons rather than for diagnosis. Diagnostic bronchoscopy is a low-risk procedure, usually performed with the vocal cords and trachea anesthetized with a topical anesthetic agent and using IV sedation. It may be performed under fluoroscopy or may be video-assisted. The flexible bronchoscope is usually used, because it is less traumatic to the trachea and bronchus and offers a better look at the segmental bronchi and lobes of the lung. Diagnostic uses include direct visualization of the tracheobronchial tree for abnormalities, biopsy of suspicious lesions, and aspiration of deep sputum for culture, sensitivity, and cytologic examination. Therapeutic applications of bronchoscopy include aspiration of retained secretions, control of bleeding in the bronchus, removal of foreign bodies, endobronchial radiation using an iridium wire placed with the bronchoscope, and palliative laser obliteration of obstructive bronchial lesions.

Mediastinoscopy, or cervical mediastinal exploration (CME), is indicated when enlarged nodes are

---

Table 15-1 Characteristics of lung cancers

Tumor type	Growth rate	Metastasis	Means of diagnosis	Clinical manifestations and treatment
Squamous cell carcinoma	Slow	Late; mostly to hilar lymph nodes	Biopsy, sputum analysis, bronchoscopy, electron microscopy, immunohistochemistry	Cough, sputum production, airway obstruction; treated surgically
Small cell (oat cell) carcinoma	Very rapid	Very early; to mediastinum or distally in lung	Radiography, sputum analysis, bronchoscopy, electron microscopy, immunohistochemistry, and clinical manifestations (cough, chest pain, dyspnea, hemoptysis, localized wheezing)	Airway obstruction caused by pneumonitis, signs and symptoms of excessive hormone secretion; treated by chemotherapy and ionizing radiation to thorax and central nervous system
Adenocarcinoma	Moderate	Early	Radiography, fiberoptic bronchoscopy, electron microscopy	Pleural effusion; treated surgically
Large cell carcinoma	Rapid	Early and widespread	Sputum analysis, bronchoscopy, electron microscopy (by exclusion of other cell types)	Chest wall pain, pleural effusion, cough, sputum production, hemoptysis, airway obstruction caused by pneumonia (if airways involved); treated surgically

From McCance KL & Huether SE. (1994). *Pathophysiology: The biologic basis for disease in adults and children.* St. Louis: Mosby.

noted on CT. Through a small incision made in the suprasternal notch, a small rigid mediastinal scope allows direct viewing of the superior mediastinum behind the ascending aorta. Peritracheal and mediastinal nodes can be biopsied through the scope. These lymph nodes receive the lymphatic drainage from the lungs. Evaluation of these nodes is useful for diagnosing malignant pulmonary lesions of the lung, granulomatous infections, and sarcoidosis. Biopsy results that are positive for malignant cells indicate the disease has spread to the mediastinum. Thoracotomy for tumor resection is unlikely. Alternative treatments are more appropriate.

Thoracoscopy with pleural or lung biopsy can also be used as a diagnostic procedure. Pulmonary lesions most amiable to thoracoscopic biopsy are located on the peripheral surface of the lung. Deeper lesions may require "hook wire" localization with CT. The hook wire snares the lesion, making it easy to find with thoracoscopy, much like the hook wire procedure used to locate unpalpable breast lesions. Thoracoscopy can be done under either local anesthesia with IV sedation or general anesthesia. If general anesthesia is used, a double-lumen endotracheal tube, which allows the anesthesia provider to deflate the operative lung, while ventilating the nonoperative lung may, be inserted. Deflating the operative lung makes application of endostapling devices easier. Unfortunately, deflating the operative lung makes finding the lesion to be biopsied more difficult. Biopsy of the pleura can be done without deflating one lung. Mediastinotomy, anterior thoracotomy ("minithoracotomy"), or full thoracotomy for diagnosis may be done when all other means of diagnosis have been exhausted.

Cytologic studies. Microscopic classification of cell type is essential to choosing the correct treatment of pulmonary lesions. Some lesion types are not usually treated surgically, except for diagnostic procedures. These cell types grow rapidly, are poorly differentiated, and do not generally respond well to radiation or chemotherapy.

Sputum samples may be cultured for routine, anaerobic, acid-fast, and fungal organisms and examined microscopically for malignant cells. Bronchial washings and brushings can be obtained for cultures, acid-fast bacteria, fungus, and cytologic examination. Pleural or pericardial fluid may be examined for appearance, cell counts, protein and lactic dehydrogenase, cytology, glucose, amylase, and Gram's stain for bacteria. The gross appearance of pleural fluid is checked for color, optical density, and viscosity. Red-tinged fluid is likely to have red blood cells in it, whereas thick fluid with a foul odor may be suppurative. Cell counts may include a differential count, but the most noteworthy is the white blood cell (WBC) count. A WBC count over 1000/ mm^3 suggests an exudate. When more than half of the WBCs are small lymphocytes, the effusion is likely caused by tuberculosis or a malignant process. Protein counts greater than 3 g/dl indicate the presence of an exudate. Exudates are most often found in infectious or malignant diseases. Protein content less than 3 g/dl indicates the presence of transudates. Transudates are most commonly caused by congestive heart failure, cirrhosis, and nephrotic syndromes. A pleural fluid/serum lactic dehydrogenase (LDH) ratio greater than 0.6 is typical of an exudate. An exudate can be identified if the pleural/serum LDH ratio is greater than 0.6 and the pleural/serum protein ratio is greater than 0.5. Pleural glucose levels are similar to serum levels. Values less than 60 mg/dl are occasionally seen in malignant processes. In a malignant effusion, the amylase concentration is slightly elevated.

Staging of malignant pulmonary lesions. The results of tests done on tissue specimens are essential to staging of tumor growth. Physicians use clinical staging and cell type to determine the most appropriate treatment. Options include surgical resection alone, chemotherapy, radiation therapy, or a combination of therapies. The TNM code (primary *tumor*, lymph *node* status, and presence of distant *metastasis*) is used for staging. An international staging system for lung cancer has been developed to enable comparison among treatment modalities. This staging system is presented in Fig. 15-2.

Presenting symptoms and patient history. A wide range of medical problems can require a thoracic surgical intervention. Likewise, patients may have a wide range of presenting symptoms and histories. Patients with Stage I or Stage II malignant pulmonary lesions may be asymptomatic if the tumor has not caused obstructive pneumonitis. These patients are most likely diagnosed with a routine chest x-ray and will probably require further diagnostic thoracic procedures such as needle aspiration, bronchoscopy, mediastinoscopy, or thoracoscopy with lung biopsy to obtain a pathologic diagnosis. Additional treatment of malignant lung lesions depends on the histologic classification of the cell as well as the stage of disease progression. Patients with Stage I lesions have the best prognosis if pulmonary resection is possible via an open thoracotomy or video-assisted thoracoscopy. In later stages, patients may complain of cough with hemoptysis; wheezing; gradually worsening dyspnea; chest wall, shoulder, or back pain; generalized joint pain; and loss of appetite with significant weight loss. The patient may have had intermittent bouts of pneumonia and be febrile, indicating obstructive pneumonitis or atelectasis. Some patients with malignant pulmonary lesions

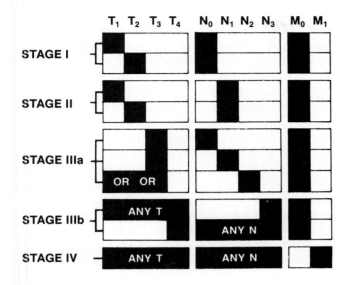

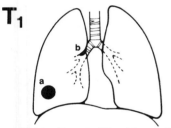

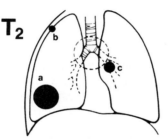

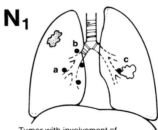

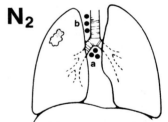

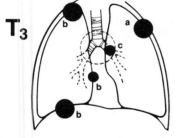

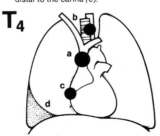

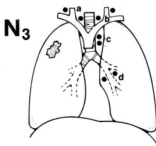

Fig. 15-2. TNM codes for lung cancer Stages I to IV. (From James EC, Corry RJ, & Perry JP: *Principles of basic surgical practice.* Philadelphia: Henley & Belfus).

may have had chemotherapy or radiation to reduce the size of the tumor, making it more amenable to resection. As a result, they may be immunosuppressed or have a radiation pneumonitis.

Patients with lesions in Stage III or later are unlikely to have long-term benefits from pulmonary resection, but may be palliated by thoracoscopic evacuation of pleural or pericardial effusion and pleurodesis. The patient may be hoarse if the tumor invades the laryngeal nerve. These patients may also have palpable, hard scalene nodes. In terminal stages with central nervous system involvement, the patient may experience headaches, seizures, or hemiplegia due to distant metastasis to the brain.

Patients with *spontaneous pneumothorax* may complain of a sudden onset of a sharp, stabbing pain that radiates to the shoulder of the same side (Curry & Casady, 1992). The pain may have been precipitated by coughing, laughing, talking, or simply the movement of breathing. Breath sounds are diminished or absent in the affected area. The patient may have experienced dyspnea and a sputumless cough. The patient will likely have a history of smoking or living with a smoker. The patient may have chronic pulmonary obstructive disease, showing signs of a barrel chest and clubbed fingers. In the case of the young, thin, nonsmoking patient, spontaneous pneumothorax is considered a congenital defect. Obtaining a family history is helpful. Pneumothorax is most frequently diagnosed by chest x-ray. Chest x-rays of patients with pneumothorax caused by mechanical ventilation may show tracheal deviation away from the affected side. These patients may also have subcutaneous emphysema. Pneumothorax for any cause is treated by inserting at least one chest tube. If the air leak does not stop in 24 to 48 hours, the patient may be scheduled for a thoracoscopy with stapling of bleb and possibly for a pleurodesis.

Patients presenting with a *pleural effusion* may have normal to absent breath sounds, depending on the severity of the effusion. A pleural friction rub may also be present. The patient may have a productive cough and complain of sharp pleuritic chest pain and dyspnea if the effusion is severe enough to restrict inflation. The patient may have a fever and pneumonia. The color of the sputum will depend on the pathogen: pink-salmon, *Staphylococcus*; rusty, *Streptococcus*; green, *Pseudomonas*; and currant, *Klebsiella*. Pleural effusions are often the result of an infectious process such as pneumonia or a manifestation of advancing malignant processes such as breast or lung cancer. Obtaining a more comprehensive patient history is relevant.

Patients with *chronic pericardial effusions* will have distant heart sounds, absence of murmurs, and shifting intensity of heart sounds. The chest x-ray will show an enlarged heart shadow. The patient's electrocardiogram (ECG) will show low-voltage S-T segment elevation. The QRS complex is regular in time but shows alteration in height. The patient will relate a history of insidious debilitation and complain of weakness, dyspnea, and easy fatigability. Occasionally, patients have acute cardiac tamponade due to uncompensated chronic pericardial effusions or penetrating trauma. These patients show signs of clinical shock. The patient is cool to the touch; the skin is moist; the heart rate is rapid and heart sounds are dampened. Blood pressure may be normal or low. The S-T segment will be elevated due to compression and consequent myocardial ischemia. The most telling sign is the presence of venous distention at a time when other signs suggest peripheral circulatory failure. The patient may be very apprehensive, if conscious. Acute cardiac tamponade is a life-threatening situation and surgical intervention should be considered an emergency.

Patients with *lesions of the esophagus* will frequently complain of dysphagia, pain, regurgitation, cough, and weight loss. The most common benign lesion requiring a thoracic incisional approach is the leiomyoma in the upper and middle esophagus. Lesions in the lower third can be reached with an abdominal incision. Malignant lesions that require a total esophagectomy may also require a thoracic approach. Diagnosis of either type of lesion is made by barium swallow and CT of the chest. Malignant esophageal lesions may be biopsied through a gastroscope to confirm the diagnosis. There may be no remarkable findings on physical examination.

Patients with *thoracic disc disease* complain of sudden or progressive numbness in the lower extremities. They may show normal coordination on neuroskeletal examination, but are limited by weakness. Range of motion may be limited by pain. Diagnosis is made by history, physical examination, and CT or MRI of the thoracic spine. Many patients can be treated conservatively with an exercise and physical therapy program. However, if conservative, nonoperative treatment does not bring adequate relief of symptoms, thoracic discectomy is recommended. Sudden onset of severe or quickly progressive symptoms often precludes conservative medical treatment.

Nursing Diagnoses, Interventions, and Outcome Determination

Once the assessment data has been collected, organized, and analyzed, the perioperative nurse selects relevant nursing diagnoses, identifies desired patient outcomes with criteria by which to measure them, and plans nursing interventions that will facilitate outcome achievement. The nursing process is cyclic in nature. Evaluation of achievement of outcomes is not only the end, but the beginning of the cycle.

Evaluation leads the perioperative nurse to reassessment, planning, and implementation. Evaluation examines the outcomes of nursing actions according to patient response. The perioperative nurse can then determine the extent to which selected outcomes were met. Did the patient accomplish the outcome statement? To what extent? Do adjustments to the plan need to be made? Was the outcome statement realistic for this patient? How can care be improved? These activities require the perioperative nurse to use his or her professional judgment based on experience and assessment data. Nursing diagnoses for thoracic surgery are derived from relevant assessment data, which are validated with the patient when possible, and identify actual or high-risk respiratory problems, risk factors, symptoms, airway patency, adequate ventilation, adequate oxygen/gas exchange, and respiratory self-care management strategies (Standards of Respiratory Nursing Practice, 1994).

Ineffective airway clearance. If the patient is unable to clear secretions from the bronchotracheal tree to maintain a patent airway, the nursing diagnosis is *ineffective airway clearance.* Depending on the underlying disease, bronchial secretions may be difficult for the patient to clear. As previously discussed, many patients scheduled for thoracic procedures have dyspnea, abnormal breath sounds, changes in respiratory rate and depth, cough, and fever. These are characteristics of ineffective airway clearance. Adequate airway clearance is important to the patient's ability to perform postoperatively (especially for open thoracotomy procedures), to prevent complications, and to speed recovery; nursing interventions include teaching the patient how to cough more effectively. McCloskey & Bulechek (1992) suggest the following nursing interventions:

1. Review results of pulmonary function tests, history of current problem, and planned surgical intervention to determine the underlying cause of ineffective airway clearance. Auscultate lung fields before interventions and document results.
2. Help the patient sit with head slightly flexed with shoulders relaxed and knees flexed (semi-Fowler's to high-Fowler's position), depending on patient's comfort level.
3. Encourage the patient to take three to four deep breaths, holding the last one for 2 to 3 seconds, then coughing three to four times.
4. Instruct the patient to inhale deeply and to exhale with three or four huffs (with vocal cords open).
5. Instruct the patient to inhale deeply, exhale slowly, then cough at the end of the exhalation.
6. Instruct the patient in the use of an incentive spirometer. Document baseline capacity.
7. Promote adequate systemic hydration.
8. Praise the patient for effort.

The desired outcome is that the patient will exhibit improved airway clearance by (a) improved breath sounds in lower or affected lung fields on auscultation, (b) productive cough, an (c) increased capacity on incentive spirometry.

Decisional conflict regarding treatment options. Understanding the rationale for the various treatment options, particularly those for malignant lesions, can be difficult and confusing for the patient and family. With the debilitating nature of pulmonary diseases, the possibility or reality of a malignant diagnosis, and the stress of having to make life-changing decisions about life-threatening situations, the patient's decision-making processes may be impaired. Nursing interventions can include support for the decision-making process, teaching about the disease process, and/or spiritual support. McCloskey and Bulechek (1992) suggest the following:

1. Determine the patient and family's specific learning needs regarding the disease process. Provide information, as appropriate, about the pathophysiology of the disease, the common signs and symptoms, the clinical course of the disease, diagnostic measures, and treatment options.
2. Determine if there are differences in the patient's view of his or her condition and the view of the nurses and physicians providing care. Clarify discrepancies. Help the patient assess his or her condition accurately.
3. Help the patient list the advantages and disadvantages of each treatment option.
4. Facilitate collaborative decision making with other health care team members. Serve as a liaison between patient, family, and other health care providers.
5. Be familiar with institutional policies on informed consent. Obtain informed consent when appropriate.
6. Respect the patient's autonomy: the right to choose any treatment option or none, the right to receive information or not, the right to privacy even from his or her own family.
7. Assess the patient's need for and appropriateness of spiritual support. If relevant, encourage the use of spiritual resource persons, such as clergy. Encourage the use of other spiritual resources, such as meditation, prayer, inspirational reading material, or other religious traditions and rituals. Use values-clarification techniques to clarify spiritual beliefs and values.
8. Help the patient express and relieve anger in appropriate ways.
9. Help the patient explain his or her decision to others.

The desired outcome is that the patient will resolve decisional conflict by (1) seeking appropriate sources of information, support, and consultation, (2) expressing an understanding of treatment options and predicted outcomes of each, (3) determining a course of action regarding treatment, and (4) signing consent for treatment if appropriate.

Ineffective breathing patterns. Reasons for ineffective breathing include impaired lung elasticity, hemothorax or pneumothorax, or intraoperative positioning, such as the lateral position. General anesthesia alters breathing patterns. Nursing interventions for this diagnosis will likely require collaborative efforts. The perioperative nurse will collaborate with the anesthesia provider to insert an artificial airway. For open thoracic and some thoracoscopic procedures, a double lumen endobronchial tube will be inserted. For airway insertion and stabilization, McCloskey and Bulechek (1992) suggest the following nursing interventions:

1. Collaborate with the anesthesia provider to select the correct size and type of endotracheal tube.
2. Assist with insertion by gathering necessary intubation equipment, administering medications as needed, and observing hemodynamic monitors during intubation.
3. Be prepared to assist in difficult intubations by having the 8-mm fiberoptic endobronchial scope, light source, suction, and lubricant ready for use and/or check the position of the tube.
4. Inflate the endotracheal cuff using a minimum amount of pressure.
5. Help to ensure that the double lumen endobronchial tube will function intraoperatively by auscultating the chest laterally on both sides as the cuffs are inflated to occlude bronchus of the operative side and deflated to open the bronchus on the nonoperative side.
6. Stabilize tube with tape.

The desired outcome is that the patient's breathing pattern will provide adequate oxygenation intraoperatively by (1) maintenance of O_2 saturation above 90% on pulse oximetry, (2) maintenance of blood gases within normal limits, and (3) absence of pneumothorax or hemothorax after chest tubes have been inserted and chest wall has been closed.

High risk for fluid volume deficit. Blood loss is the most frequent cause of fluid depletion in the patient undergoing a thoracic surgical procedure. Significant blood loss can occur from the intercostal vessels, the pulmonary arteries and veins during resection, or from other vascular structures in the chest, such as the aorta or azygous vein. Tumor that is adhered to vascular structures can bleed as the tumor is dissected free. There may be blood sequestered in the portion of lung tissue removed. Risk factors that sur-

faced in the assessment data should also be considered. When anticipating planning for electrolyte imbalances, the nurse must consider the chest trauma, the patient who receives massive transfusions (risk for hyperkalemia, hypomagnesemia, hypocalcemia, and infection); the protein depleted, nutritionally deficient patient (risk for hypokalemia and hypocalcemia); the patient receiving total parenteral nutrition (risk for hypokalemia); and the patient with fluid volume depletion (risk for hypokalemia). Nursing interventions focus on fluid management and resuscitation; McCloskey and Bulechek (1992) recommend the following:

1. Insert indwelling urinary catheter.
2. Record accurate intake and output, including blood loss, nasogastric drainage, and urinary output.
3. Monitor hemodynamic status.
4. Monitor vital signs.
5. Ascertain the availability of blood or blood products.
6. Prepare for and administer blood products as appropriate.
7. Obtain and maintain at least one large bore IV site.
8. Collaborate with physicians to ensure administration of both crystalloids (normal saline, lactated ringers) and colloids (volume expanders such as Hespan, etc.).
9. Use blood warming and infusion pumps as appropriate.

The desired outcome is that the patient will maintain adequate fluid volume by (1) maintaining blood pressure within normal limits, and (2) eliminating adequate amounts of urine.

Pain. Postoperative pain is most often associated with the incision site. Trauma to the intercostal nerves during thoracoscopy can cause considerable discomfort. Chest tubes can also cause pleuritic pain. Nursing interventions may include using pain management and splinting; the following are recommended by McCloskey and Bulechek (1992):

1. Conduct a comprehensive assessment of pain to include location, characteristics, intensity, and precipitating factors.
2. Observe nonverbal clues of discomfort, especially for patients with the endotracheal tube still in place.
3. Consider cultural influences on the patient's response to pain.
4. Control environmental factors that may influence the patient's discomfort (room temperature, lighting, noise, etc.).
5. Consider the patient's preoperative preparation to participate in control of postoperative pain.
6. Collaborate with the patient, family, and other

team members to select and implement the appropriate pharmacologic and nonpharmacologic methods of pain control. Pain control should begin in the preoperative phase with appropriate education for the type of pain control method anticipated, and it should continue into the intraoperative phase with injection of intercostal nerve blocks and insertion of intrapleural or epidural catheters for postoperative pain control.

7. Implement the use of a patient-controlled analgesia (PCA) pump or epidural or interpleural analgesia, if appropriate. Because pain in or around the thoracic area can interfere with the patient's ability to breathe effectively and to maintain adequate pulmonary function, the goal of interpleural analgesia is to anesthetize the sensory but not the motor function of the internal intercostal muscles for coughing and the external intercostal muscles used for deep breathing (Polomano, Blumenthal, & Riegler, 1994).

8. Administer analgesics as appropriate.

9. Teach nonpharmacologic techniques to relieve pain (biofeedback, guided imagery, music therapy, distraction, hot/cold application, massage, etc.) preoperatively. Encourage their use during painful activities or before pain occurs or increases.

10. Refer for medical management if pain control measures are inadequate.

11. Incorporate the family in pain control efforts if possible.

The desired outcome is that the patient will select 3 or below on a 0 to 10 numeric pain intensity scale (Fig. 15-3).

Knowledge deficit. A knowledge deficit is most often associated with the preoperative phase. For the thoracic surgery patient, knowledge deficit is particularly meaningful because many thoracic procedures are for diagnostic purposes. The perioperative nurse should plan for individual teaching; McCloskey and Bulechek (1992) recommend the following interventions:

1. Establish rapport and teacher credibility.

2. Determine patient's and family's specific learning needs.

3. Assess the current knowledge level and understanding of the problem.

4. Determine the patient's ability to learn. Assess cognitive, psychomotor, and affective abilities or disabilities. Determine the patient's educational level.

5. Assess the patient's motivation and readiness to learn.

6. Enhance the patient's readiness to learn.

7. Set mutual, realistic goals with the patient.

8. Select teaching style, materials, and content to meet the patient's needs.

9. Instruct the patient when appropriate.

10. Evaluate patient's achievement of learning goals.

11. Refer patient to others team members or agencies when appropriate.

12. Document the content, materials provided, and the patient's understanding of the information or behaviors that indicated learning in the nursing record.

13. Involve the family as appropriate.

For the thoracic surgery patient, the perioperative nurse should plan to add specific information about the type of surgical procedure planned, the presence and purpose of invasive monitoring lines, the location of dressings, the presence and location of the endotracheal tube, ventilator-assisted breathing, the nasogastric tube, chest tubes, interpleural or epidural catheters, and the indwelling urinary catheter. The family should be prepared for the patient's appearance in the intensive care unit (ICU), know the location and visiting hours of the ICU, and understand the perioperative nurse's plan for communicating. The perioperative nurse should consider adding specific information regarding the continuing treatment of the disease that was diagnosed or treated with a thoracic procedure. This should include accurate information regarding the progression of the disease, treatment options, support systems such as cancer support groups, and support resources such as hospice and "I Can Cope." Understanding of home care requirements and follow-up instructions is also important.

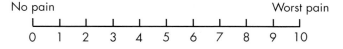

Fig. 15-3. 0-10 Numeric Pain Intensity Scale. To use this scale, explain to the patient that at one end of the line is 0, which means that he or she feels no pain. At the other end is 10, which is the worst pain possible. The numbers 1 to 9 are for very little pain to a great deal of pain. Ask the patient to choose the number that best describes the pain.

The desired outcome is that the patient expresses or demonstrates that learning needs have been met.

PROCEDURE-SPECIFIC CARE PLANS

This section discusses four procedure-specific care plans. The four procedures included are bronchoscopy, mediastinoscopy, thoracoscopy, and open thoracotomy. Each will be discussed with these topics in mind: (1) key assessment points, (2) nursing diagnoses, (3) patient outcomes, (4) nursing actions, and (5) evaluation of patient outcomes.

GUIDES TO NURSING ACTIONS
Bronchoscopy (Fig. 15-4)

1. Preoperative teaching and explanation of the sequence of perioperative events should be done using language the patient can understand. The patient and family should be provided with information about the date, time, and location of procedure; its anticipated length (an uncomplicated bronchoscopy is usually scheduled from 30 to 45 minutes); the sensory effects of preoperative and intraoperative medications (with local anesthesia, the patient will experience an inability to swallow, a very dry mouth, and a swollen tongue and throat; with IV sedation, the patient will feel relaxed, perhaps drowsy, and will not be able to remember the procedure); and location of the surgery waiting room for the family. If the patient is undergoing a diagnostic procedure, the amount of time for specimens to be processed should be reviewed because patients and families are anxious to get these results. Frozen sections are rarely done for bronchoscopies. Pathology reports often take 2 to 4 days. Cultures may take 24 hours to 2 weeks, depending on the type of culture done. Depending on the patient's wish for an explanation of the procedure, bronchoscopy can be described as passing a lighted tube down the windpipe to look at the inside of the tubes to the lungs. For therapeutic reasons, it is done to wash thick secretions loose and remove them with suction. For diagnosis, it is done to collect tissue and cell samples to be looked at under the microscope. The cell samples may be tested for infection. The patient should be instructed to remain NPO 6 hours before the procedure; an empty stomach prevents the patient from inadvertently vomiting while sedated or asleep, thus preventing the stomach contents from getting into the lungs (aspiration pneumonia). The purpose of IV sedation and local anesthetics should be explained; knowing they will be kept relaxed and comfortable is reassuring to patients. A description of how the topical/local anesthetic will be applied (it will be sprayed in the nose and mouth) may also be explained.

2. Document the effect of preoperative and intraoperative sedation as well as the amount given. Frequently used drugs are diazepam (Valium) or midazolam (Versed). Both can be given intravenously, and they should be administered slowly over 2 to 3 minutes and titrated to achieve the desired effect. Both have an amnesic effect.

3. The total amount of IV sedation should be documented. If separate doses were given incrementally, each incremental dose should be documented according to time given, amount given, and who administered it. The usual IV sedation dose for diazepam is 0.1 to 0.2 mg/kg; for midazolam, it is 0.035 mg/kg titrated, with 0.1 to 0.2 mg/kg total dose (Maree, 1993).

4. The cough and gag reflexes should be adequately suppressed. More local anesthetic may be instilled through the bronchoscope for the lower level bronchioles if the patient starts to cough as biopsy forceps, brushes, or irrigation is being used.

5. The total amount of local anesthetic(s) given should be documented. Always check for allergies before the administration of any perioperative medication.

6. If the scope is introduced through the nose, a face mask with an opening cut for the scope allows oxygen to be given to the patient intraoperatively. If the scope is introduced through the mouth, protect the scope with a mouth piece that will hold the teeth apart and prevent the patient from inadvertently biting the scope. A nasal cannula can be used if the scope is passed through the mouth.

7. The pulse oximeter is the easiest way to monitor intraoperative oxygen levels. If the O_2 saturation level drops below 90%, inform the physician. Ask the patient to take deep breaths. The scope may have to be removed if adequate O_2 levels cannot be achieved shortly. Monitor the ECG and vital signs closely for the effects of medications. Epinephrine in some local anesthetic agents can cause the heart rate and blood pressure to increase. IV sedation can decrease respiratory and heart rates. Document monitoring techniques and findings.

8. Reassure the patient that the effects of IV sedation will be carefully monitored during the procedure and that he or she will be kept comfortable. A calm and confident manner, reassurance, and the use of touch by holding the patient's hand are effective for minimizing anxiety.

9. Check the bronchoscope and its accessories to ensure it has been properly disinfected, properly assembled, and is in working order. Apply a de

FIG. 15-4
CARE PLAN FOR BRONCHOSCOPY

KEY ASSESSMENT POINTS

Purpose of procedure (therapeutic/diagnostic)
Medical diagnosis
Type of anesthesia planned
Results of previous treatments/tests
Baseline O_2 saturation
Baseline vital signs
Emotional status
Condition of teeth/oral mucosa

NURSING DIAGNOSIS

All generic nursing diagnoses apply to this patient, with the addition
  of:
High risk for ineffective breathing patterns
High risk for decisional conflict (situational)

PATIENT OUTCOMES

All generic outcomes apply, with the addition of:
1. The patient's breathing patterns will be effective.
2. The patient will begin resolving decisional conflict.
The patient will:
1. Maintain a normal respiratory rate and depth with O_2 saturation
   above 90% on pulse oximetry
2. Seek appropriate sources of information, support, and counseling

NURSING ACTIONS

	Yes	No	N/A
1. Preop teaching done?	☐	☐	☐
2. Effect of sedation assessed?	☐	☐	☐
3. Sedative medication documented?	☐	☐	☐
4. Effect of local anesthesia assessed?	☐	☐	☐
5. Local anesthetic documented?	☐	☐	☐
6. Oxygen administered?	☐	☐	☐
7. Patient monitored?	☐	☐	☐
8. Emotional support/comfort measures?	☐	☐	☐
9. Equipment/supplies prepared?	☐	☐	☐
10. Positioned appropriately?	☐	☐	☐
11. Counts performed/correct?	☐	☐	☐
12. Specimens to lab?	☐	☐	☐
13. Terminal cleaning/disinfection done?	☐	☐	☐

Document additional nursing actions/generic care plans initiated
here:

_____

_____

_____

EVALUATION OF PATIENT OUTCOMES

	Outcome met	Outcome met with additional outcome criteria	Outcome met with revised nursing care plan	Outcome not met	Outcome not applicable to this patient
1. The patient's breathing patterns were effective.	☐	☐	☐	☐	☐
2. The patient began to resolve decisional conflict.	☐	☐	☐	☐	☐
3. The patient met outcomes for additional generic care plans as indicated.	☐	☐	☐	☐	☐

Signature: _____ Date: _____

fogging agent to the lens of the scope. Gather the light source and/or video equipment, biopsy forceps, endoscopic brushes, suction and suction tubing, adaptor for endotracheal tube (for general anesthesia), mouth piece (for local/topical anesthesia, oral insertion of scope), specimen traps, and any special containers or solutions for cultures. Prepare the topical/local anesthetic agent for use.

10. The patient may be positioned in semi-Fowler's. If the patient is in the supine position, elevate the shoulders with a small roll or pillow to allow for extension of the head and neck. Place a safety strap. Secure the arms on armboards or at the patient's side.

11. Counts are performed according to institutional policy.

12. Follow institutional protocol for preserving specimens. Provide the appropriate containers or solutions for the specimen obtained and the tests to be done. Use universal precautions for handling items received from the sterile field. Seal containers to prevent leaking or contamination. Label specimens with appropriate data. Arrange for transport of specimen to laboratory. Document the type of specimens and tests requested. Tissue obtained via bronchoscopy is usually too small for frozen section. A definitive diagnosis must be made by permanent section.

13. Follow institutional protocol for terminally cleaning and disinfecting endoscopic equipment.

Mediastinoscopy (Fig. 15-5)

1. Part of assessment is determining the patient's psychologic response to the planned surgical intervention. Since mediastinoscopy is often performed to detect metastatic lymph node involvement, the patient may have *anxiety* related to the outcome of biopsy, the surgery, and/or the administration of anesthesia. Broad classification of anticipatory anxiety as mild, moderate, or severe, depending on perioperative assessment, may help. Plan for enough time for preoperative medications to become effective; plan other comfort measures. Verify that the patient has maintained NPO status. Reinforce explanations about perioperative events and anesthesia. Using language the patient and family can understand, provide information about the length of time the procedure will take (an uncomplicated mediastinoscopy usually takes about 45 minutes; if it is done following a bronchoscopy, both procedures take 1 hour and 30 minutes), location of incision (just above the breast bone), sensory effects of preoperative and intraopera-

tive medications (the patient will feel relaxed, perhaps drowsy, and may not remember leaving the holding area), and location of surgery waiting room for the family. If the patient and family want a description of the procedure and its purpose, mediastinoscopy can be described as "looking at the lymph nodes that live on the outside of the windpipe and above the heart in the chest." Explain that the surgeon will take a sample or biopsies of tissue from those nodes. Verify that the patient has been NPO for 6 hours.

The nursing diagnosis *high risk for fluid volume deficit* is related to the potential for injury during the surgical intervention. During mediastinoscopy, the peritracheal and mediastinal lymph nodes to be biopsied are situated around the pulmonary vessels and aorta. Therefore, these vascular structures are at risk of being injured with the dissector or biopsy forceps. If the hemorrhage cannot be controlled through the existing small incision, an emergency sternotomy may be necessary. In this case, emergency protocols should be initiated immediately. Consider the addition of the following nursing diagnoses in this emergency situation: (a) *altered cerebral and cardiac tissue perfusion*, (b) *fluid volume deficit*, and (c) *impaired gas exchange.*

2. Mediastinoscopy frequently follows a bronchoscopy. The wound classification for a bronchoscopy and mediastinoscopy are different. A bronchoscopy need not be done as a sterile procedure; a mediastinoscopy should be treated as a sterile procedure. The perioperative nurse should have a sterile field, back table, Mayo stand, and drapes, separate from the bronchoscopy setup. The surgeon and scrub nurse should change gowns and gloves when beginning the mediastinoscopy.

3. Collaborate with the physician and the anesthesia provider to select the correct size and type of endotracheal tube. Check for dentures and loose or capped teeth. Assist with tube insertion by gathering necessary intubation equipment, administering medications as needed, and observing hemodynamic monitors during intubation. Apply tracheal pressure, if needed. Inflate the endotracheal cuff using minimum pressure. Stabilize tube with tape. Ensure that airway stays in place during positioning.

4. Note the condition of the skin at the preparation site. Check for rashes and nicks. Document skin condition. Assess skin at the site of the electrosurgical dispersive pad and document.

5. Positioning for mediastinoscopy will include placing the patient in a reverse Trendelenburg's

FIG. 15-5
CARE PLAN FOR MEDIASTINOSCOPY

KEY ASSESSMENT POINTS

Patient understanding of procedure and anesthesia
Medical diagnosis
Results of previous treatments/tests
Baseline O_2 saturation
Baseline vital signs
Emotional status
General physical condition

NURSING DIAGNOSIS

All generic nursing diagnoses apply to this patient, with the addition
   of:
Anxiety
High risk for fluid volume deficit (vascular injury)

PATIENT OUTCOMES

All generic outcomes apply, with the addition of:
1. The patient's anxiety level will be reduced.
2. Intraoperative bleeding, if it occurs, will be controlled.
The patient will exhibit a reduced level of anxiety by:
1. Displaying relaxed facial expressions
2. Verbalizing less anxiety
3. Accurately describing perioperative events
The patient will maintain adequate fluid volume.

NURSING ACTIONS

	Yes	No	N/A
1. Preop teaching done?	☐	☐	☐
2. Sterile field maintained?	☐	☐	☐
3. Assist with induction?	☐	☐	☐
4. Skin condition assessed?	☐	☐	☐
5. Positioned correctly?	☐	☐	☐
6. Skin prep done?	☐	☐	☐
7. Counts performed/correct?	☐	☐	☐
8. ESU precautions?	☐	☐	☐
9. Blood/blood products given?	☐	☐	☐
10. Equipment/supplies prepared?	☐	☐	☐
11. Specimens to lab?	☐	☐	☐
12. Emergency equipment available?	☐	☐	☐
13. Report to postanesthesia care unit given?	☐	☐	☐

Document additional nursing actions/generic care plans initiated
here:

_____

_____

_____

EVALUATION OF PATIENT OUTCOMES

	Outcome met	Outcome met with additional outcome criteria	Outcome met with revised nursing care plan	Outcome not met	Outcome not applicable to this patient
1. The patient's anxiety was reduced.	☐	☐	☐	☐	☐
2. The patient's fluid/volume status was adequate.	☐	☐	☐	☐	☐
3. The patient met outcomes for additional generic care plans as indicated.	☐	☐	☐	☐	☐

Signature: _____ Date: _____

position to reduce venous pressure in the vessels of the chest, therefore reducing venous bleeding. Extend the neck either by placing a roll under the patient's shoulders or by lowering the headrest on the OR bed. Too much hyperextension can compress the space between the sternum and trachea.

6. Prep the skin from the chin superiorly, to the breast inferiorly, and to the shoulders laterally.

7. Gauze dissectors (kittners, pushers, pill sponges), cottonoids, and sponges are among the items that should be counted. Follow institutional policy for instrument counts.

8. Follow institutional protocol for testing and documenting use of the electrosurgical unit.

9. Determine if blood was ordered and verify availability. Have blood warming and infusion pump readily available. Have volume replacement fluid readily available.

10. Check the mediastinoscope and accessories to ensure they have been properly disinfected, properly assembled, and are in working order. Gather the light source, biopsy forceps, dissecting instruments, aspirating needle, suction tips and suction tubing, electrosurgery tips and cords, and special containers or solutions for cultures and specimens. Have chemical hemostatic agents such as oxidized cellulose (Gelfoam) available.

11. Follow institutional protocol for preserving specimens. Use universal precautions for all material received from the sterile field. Frozen sections may be done to determine if there is enough tissue to make a diagnosis. Definitive diagnosis usually must wait for permanent section. Place tissue for frozen section in saline; place tissue for permanent section in a preservative.

12. In the unlikely event that uncontrolled hemorrhage occurs and a mediastinotomy must be performed, have a sternal saw, chest instruments, and resuscitation cart immediately available.

13. Report the intraoperative events to the postanesthsia care unit nurse. Include the results of the postoperative assessment and pathology reports, if available. Auscultate for appropriate breath sounds. Pneumothorax can occur intraoperatively. Assess for tachycardia and hypotension.

Thoracoscopy (Fig. 15-6)

1. Preoperative teaching should include a general explanation of the sequence of perioperative events, the type of anesthesia planned, and general postoperative care. The depth of teaching depends on the patient's desire for information and his or her specific learning needs. The perioperative nurse should determine what the patient knows or wants to know about events such as postoperative pain control, the use of the incentive spirometer, coughing and deep breathing, the presence of chest tubes, and the purpose of the procedure. The length of time for thoracoscopy is difficult to predict. Knowing what the scheduled procedure entails will help. A thoracoscopy may be therapeutic or diagnostic. Therapeutic thoracoscopies include the following:

   a. Removal of malignant neoplasms or benign cysts arising in the lungs, bronchus, proximal or distal esophagus, or thymus gland
   b. Evacuation of pleural or pericardial effusions and suppurative lesions within lung tissue
   c. Lysis of pleural adhesions
   d. Obliteration of persistent air leaks from postoperative bronchopleural fistula, cystic fibrosis, or severe chronic pulmonary obstructive disease, such as emphysema
   e. Decortication of lung, pleura, or heart
   f. Pleurodesis
   g. Removal of thoracic disc
   h. Treatment of upper extremity sympathetic dystrophies
   i. Repair of ruptured diaphragm
   j. Treatment of congenital malformations and pathologic conditions of the thoracic aorta

   Diagnostic thoracoscopies include diagnosis of pleural, mediastinal, bronchial, or lung lesions and diagnosis of ruptured or lacerated diaphragm. An uncomplicated pleural biopsy can take about 1 hour, including the time necessary to intubate and position the patient. A double lumen endobronchial tube may not be required on pleural biopsies, thus reducing the amount of time required for intubation. Stapling multiple pulmonary blebs and pulmonary resection can take up to 2 hours and 30 minutes. A double lumen tube is almost always required, therefore intubation time may be longer. Operating time will also be longer because of the time required to locate lesions. Although the exact locations of incisions are not predictable, it can be anticipated that there will be one to four incisions on the chest wall. Verify that the patient has maintained NPO status. Provide other information as required by the patient/family/significant other.

2. Thoracoscopy offers special challenges to maintaining a sterile field because of the many lines and tubes leading to and from the field.

3. Thoracoscopy is easier, with the possible exception of pleural biopsy, if the lung on the operative side is deflated by insertion of a double lumen endobronchial tube. Collaborate with the

FIG. 15-6
CARE PLAN FOR THORACOSCOPY

KEY ASSESSMENT POINTS

Patient understanding of procedure and anesthesia
Type of anesthesia planned
Medical diagnosis
Results of previous treatments/tests
Respiratory status
Baseline O_2 saturation
Baseline vital signs
Emotional status
Learning needs
Positional limitations
General physical condition

NURSING DIAGNOSIS

All generic nursing diagnoses apply to this patient, with the addition
  of:
High risk for ineffective breathing patterns

PATIENT OUTCOMES

All generic outcomes apply, with the addition of:
The patient will maintain adequate breathing patterns.
The patient will:
1. Maintain O_2 saturation above 90% on pulse oximetry
2. Be free of pneumothorax or hemothorax following chest tube insertion and wound closure
3. Have improved lung sounds in the lower or affected lung
4. Demonstrate increasing capacity on incentive spirometry
5. Use effective airway clearance techniques

NURSING ACTIONS

	Yes	No	N/A
1. Preop teaching done?	☐	☐	☐
2. Sterile field maintained?	☐	☐	☐
3. Assist with induction?	☐	☐	☐
4. Position of double lumen tube checked?	☐	☐	☐
5. Skin condition assessed?	☐	☐	☐
6. Positioned correctly?	☐	☐	☐
7. Skin prep done?	☐	☐	☐
8. Counts performed/correct?	☐	☐	☐
9. ESU/laser/argon beam coagulator precautions?	☐	☐	☐
10. Blood/blood products given?	☐	☐	☐
11. Equipment/supplies prepared?	☐	☐	☐
12. Specimens to lab?	☐	☐	☐
13. Thoracotomy equipment/supplies available?	☐	☐	☐
14. Chest tubes secured?	☐	☐	☐
15. Report to postanesthesia care unit given?	☐	☐	☐
16. Output(s) recorded?	☐	☐	☐
17. Ventilator-assistance required?	☐	☐	☐
18. Nerve block/epidural catheter?	☐	☐	☐
19. Medications documented?	☐	☐	☐
20. Other generic care plans initiated? (specify)	☐	☐	☐

Document additional nursing actions/generic care plans initiated
here:

_____

_____

_____

EVALUATION OF PATIENT OUTCOMES

	Outcome met	Outcome met with additional outcome criteria	Outcome met with revised nursing care plan	Outcome not met	Outcome not applicable to this patient
1. The patient maintained effective breathing patterns.	☐	☐	☐	☐	☐
2. The patient met outcomes for additional generic care plans as indicated.	☐	☐	☐	☐	☐

Signature: _____ Date: _____

physician and anesthesia provider to select the correct size and type of endotracheal tube. Right or left double lumen tubes go into the right or left mainstem bronchus, depending on which lung is to be ventilated. This most often requires the perioperative nurse to collaborate with and assist the anesthesia provider. Assist with insertion by gathering necessary intubation equipment, administering medications as needed, and observing hemodynamic monitors during intubation. Be prepared to assist in the difficult intubation by having the 8-mm fiberoptic endobronchial scope, light source, suction, and lubricant ready. Stabilize the tube with tape when it is correctly inserted. Arterial lines may be inserted depending on the extent of the planned procedure and the patient's baseline medical condition.

4. The 8-mm scope may be used as a guide when inserting the tube or to check the position of the tube once it is in place. The tubing is clearly marked according to the left or right mainstem. Assist with making certain the double lumen endobronchial tube will function intraoperatively by auscultating the chest laterally on both sides as the cuffs are inflated to occlude the bronchus of the operative side and deflated to open the bronchus on the nonoperative side.

5. The skin is assessed at dependent pressure sites and at the site of intended placement of the electrosurgical dispersive pad. Note any reddened or bruised areas.

6. Most patients will be positioned in the lateral position (lateral decubitis) (Rothrock & Sculthorpe, 1993). Place a beanbag mattress on the bed before the patient arrives in the room. If needed, have suction tubing and a five-in-one adaptor readily available. Positioning is a collaborative effort: the anesthesia provider is at the head of the bed controlling the head, neck, and endotracheal tube; the surgeon is on one side of the patient; and two other team members, one across from the surgeon and the other at the patient's feet, are required. On cue, the team will lift and roll the patient on to his or her side. The lower knee and hip is flexed at nearly a right angle to the bed, a pillow is placed between the thighs, and the upper leg is left straight. A second pillow is placed between the knees lengthwise to pad and support the knee, calf, and ankle. Two team members lift the patient's upper body while the third places a roll near the axilla to allow adequate expansion of the nonoperative lung and to relieve pressure on the head of the humerus, axillary nerve, and ax-

illary vessels. If the patient is obese, a blanket roll or sandbag under the abdomen helps support and stabilize the position. The upper arm is extended forward; a padded Mayo stand may be used for this. Place the lower arm on an armboard and position forward. Press the beanbag next to the patient, aligning the heel and spine. Attach the suction to the beanbag, making it a stable cradle in which the patient lies. Place wide adhesive tape from one side of the bed across the patient's hip to the other side of the bed to prevent the patient from gradually slipping forward or backward. If the patient is undergoing thoracoscopy under regional or local anesthesia and has respiratory insufficiency that makes the lateral position unsafe, the patient may be positioned sitting upright on the OR bed with the arms and torso resting on a padded Mayo stand (Rusch, 1993).

7. Skin should be prepped from the nape of the neck, shoulder, and axilla superiorly; to the iliac crest inferiorly; and to the bedsides laterally. Note the condition of the skin at the preparation site.

8. Follow institutional policy on instrument, sharp, and sponge counts.

9. A traditional electrosurgery unit, an argon beam coagulator, or a laser may be used for a thoracoscopy. Follow institutional protocol for testing and documenting use of the unit, as necessary, and initiate appropriate safety measures.

10. Determine whether blood and blood products have been ordered and are available. Have warmers, infusion pumps, etc., ready. Report estimated blood loss and urine output to the anesthesia provider. A central venous or Swan-Ganz catheter is inserted in patients whose cardiac status demands precise hemodynamic monitoring.

11. Check the scope, video equipment, and its accessories to ensure they have been properly disinfected, properly assembled, and are in working order. Have video monitors and camera, biopsy forceps, dissecting instruments, suction tips and suction tubing, electrosurgery tips and cords, stapling devices, retractors, lung clamps, forceps, and needle holders ready. Any special containers or solutions for cultures or tissue should also be available.

12. Follow institutional protocol for preserving specimens. Use universal precautions for all material received from the sterile field. Document each specimen and its disposition.

13. Occasionally intraoperative events may require conversion to an open procedure. For example, if the lesion for biopsy cannot be located with

the scope, the surgeon may choose to open the chest and palpate the lung to locate it. The perioperative nurse should always have a thoracotmoy setup immediately available for these circumstances.

14. Secure all chest tube connections with tape. Monitor and record the presence of an air leak and the amount, color, and consistency of chest drainage. For thoracoscopy, there may be not an apparent sign of an air leak after the air in the tubing is evacuated. If an air leak is present, suction is applied and continued until the leak ceases. Note if the surgeon used irrigation in the chest; what was not suctioned out will be evacuated by the chest tube. Apply appropriate dressings, securing tube to skin. Postoperatively, inspect areas around tube insertion for skin breakdown.

15. The intraoperative events, the exact nature of the procedure, how the patient tolerated it, and whether an intercostal block was administered to control postoperative pain should be reported to the postanesthesia care unit nurse. Report the presence of a chest tube(s) and the color and amount of drainage. Assist with connecting chest suction devices and monitoring equipment if appropriate. Report results of the postoperative assessment. A chest x-ray may be ordered postoperatively to check for residual air or fluid.

Thoracotomy (Fig. 15-7)

1. Preoperative teaching should include information about time and location of the procedure and the length of time the procedure is expected to take. The length of time for thoracotomy varies according to procedure. A simple wedge resection can take as long as 2 hours, whereas a segmental resection can take up to 4 hours. A double lumen endobronchial tube is used often, but is not required. Occasionally, a preoperative and/or postoperative bronchoscopy may be done; add the time required for these. (See Guide to Nursing Actions for Bronchoscopy.) In addition to explaining the sequence of perioperative events and where the family/significant others will wait, assess the patient's desire for information and specific learning needs. As appropriate, point out the location of the incision (the posterior lateral incision begins near the spine, comes under the scapula, to the anterior chest wall under the breast; an anterior thoracotomy incision may be made just inferior to the nipple). Use language the patient can understand; for example, a thoracotomy can be described as "opening the chest wall to remove lung tissue"

(or whatever is the purpose of the procedure). Verify that the patient has maintained NPO status 6 hours before procedure. Because the patient my be anxious about postoperative pain, techniques and methods may be discussed. Provide further information based on the patient's questions.

2. Procedures that require entry into the respiratory or alimentary tract are considered clean-contaminated.

3. Although deflation of the operative lung is not an absolute requirement, thoracotomy is easier if the lung on the operative side is deflated. Collaboration with the anesthesia provider for insertion of a double lumen endobronchial tube has been discussed (see Guides to Nursing Action for thoracoscopy). Occasionally the operating surgeon will do a diagnostic bronchoscopy preoperatively and a therapeutic one postoperatively. Many bronchoscopes are too large to fit through the lumen of the double lumen tube; therefore, a single lumen tube with a larger lumen may need to be inserted initially. After the bronchoscopy, the single lumen tube is then pulled and the double lumen tube inserted. Postoperatively, if a therapeutic bronchoscopy is performed to remove secretions collected in the operative lung, the double lumen tube may have to be removed and a single lumen reinserted. If the patient is to stay on the ventilator beyond the time spent in postanesthsia care unit, a single lumen tube should be inserted.

4. The 8-mm scope may be used as a guide to inserting the tube or to check the position of the tube once it is in place. The tube is clearly marked according to the left or right mainstem. Assist with making certain the double lumen endobronchial tube will function intraoperatively by auscultating the chest laterally on both sides as the cuffs are inflated to occlude bronchus of the operative side and deflated to open the bronchus on the nonoperative side.

5. Assess the condition of the patient's skin at all dependent pressure sites, the area to be prepared, and at the application site for the electrosurgical dispersive pad. Document skin condition.

6. Patients will be positioned in the lateral position (lateral decubitis) for a posterior approach or in the supine position for an anterior approach. Lateral positioning has been discussed in the Guide to Nursing Actions for Thoracoscopy; the positioning requirements are the same for open thoracotomy in the lateral position. To position for an anterior thoracotomy, place the

FIG. 15-7
CARE PLAN FOR THORACOTOMY

KEY ASSESSMENT POINTS

Patient understanding of procedure and anesthesia
Type of anesthesia planned
Medical diagnosis
Results of previous treatments/tests
Respiratory status
Baseline O_2 saturation
Baseline vital signs
Nutritional status
Emotional status
Learning needs
Positional limitations
General physical condition

NURSING DIAGNOSIS

All generic nursing diagnoses apply to the patient, with the addition of:
High risk for ineffective breathing patterns

PATIENT OUTCOMES

All generic outcomes apply, with the addition of:
The patient will maintain adequate breathing patterns.
The patient will:
1. Maintain O_2 saturation above 90% on pulse oximetry
2. Be free of pneumothorax or hemothorax following chest tube insertion and wound closure
3. Maintain blood gases within normal limits

NURSING ACTIONS

	Yes	No	N/A
1. Preop teaching done?	☐	☐	☐
2. Wound correctly classified?	☐	☐	☐
3. Assist with induction?	☐	☐	☐
4. Position of double lumen tube checked?	☐	☐	☐
5. Skin condition assessed?	☐	☐	☐
6. Positioned correctly?	☐	☐	☐
7. Skin prep done?	☐	☐	☐
8. Counts performed/correct?	☐	☐	☐
9. ESU used?	☐	☐	☐
10. Blood/blood products given?	☐	☐	☐
11. Specimens to lab?	☐	☐	☐
12. Chest tubes secured?	☐	☐	☐
13. Interpleural/epidural catheter inserted?	☐	☐	☐
14. Intercostal block done?	☐	☐	☐
15. Report to postanesthesia care unit?	☐	☐	☐

Document additional nursing actions/generic care plans initiated here:

_____

_____

_____

EVALUATION OF PATIENT OUTCOMES

1. The patient maintained effective breathing patterns.
2. The patient met outcomes for additional generic care plans as indicated.

	Outcome met	Outcome met with additional outcome criteria	Outcome met with revised nursing care plan	Outcome not met	Outcome not applicable to this patient
1.	☐	☐	☐	☐	☐
2.	☐	☐	☐	☐	☐

Signature: _____ Date: _____

patient in the supine position on the OR bed with the operative side elevated slightly by rolls under the shoulder and hip. Place the arm on an armboard with additional padding to support the upper arm. The arm on the nonoperative side may be tucked to the side. Protect invasive monitoring lines when positioning the patient. Pad dependent pressure areas as required. Add the safety strap above the knees, snugly but not tightly. It is preferable to execute these maneuvers before the induction of anesthesia; in this way, you can ascertain with the patient the level of comfort and make adjustments as required.

7. Prepare the skin from the nape of the neck, shoulder, and axilla superiorly; to the iliac crest inferiorly; and to the bedsides laterally.

8. Follow institutional policy for sponge, sharp, and instrument counts.

9. A traditional electrosurgery unit, an argon beam coagulator, or a laser may be used for a thoracotomy. Follow institutional protocol for testing and documenting use of the unit(s) used. Initiate appropriate safety measures.

10. When preparing for the procedure, verify if blood was ordered, whether autologous blood is available, and the location of the blood (in the laboratory or the OR suite). Verify that blood products match the patient's; follow institutional protocol for checking blood products. Use universal precautions in handling blood containers. Document blood administration.

11. Follow institutional protocol for preserving specimens. Frozen sections may be done to check if tissue margins are free of tumor. Use universal precautions when handling all material received from the sterile field. Document specimens obtained and their dispositions.

12. Chest tubes should be secured; in some institutions, the perioperative nurse marks which is anterior and which is posterior. An air leak is expected after a pulmonary resection. For other procedures performed during thoracotomy, there may be not an apparent sign of an air leak. Note the amount, color, and consistency of drainage from chest tubes.

13. An interpleural line is generally inserted by the surgeon intraoperatively. The perioperative nurse may assist the anesthesia provider with inserting an epidural line either preoperatively or postoperatively. Gather and prepare the appropriate epidural catheter. Assist with positioning the patient either in a sitting position with chin dropped to chest or in a lateral position with the knees pulled up to the stomach and the chin dropped to the chest. Securely tape

either type of catheter. Label the line to avoid confusion by postanesthesia care unit and ICU nurses.

14. The surgeon may block the intercostal nerves around the incision with a long-acting local anesthetic such as bupivacaine (Marcaine). Document the agent and amount injected.

15. The intraoperative events, the exact nature of the procedure, blood replacement therapy, urine output, and the patient's tolerance of the surgery should be reported to the postanesthesia care unit nurse. Review the presence of a chest tube(s) and amount, color, and consistency of drainage. Note whether an interpleural catheter, epidural catheter, or intercostal block has been placed for postoperative pain control. Include the results of the postoperative assessment done in the OR (skin condition at dependent pressure sites, electrosurgical unit pad site, prepared areas, etc.). A chest x-ray may be ordered postoperatively to detect residual fluid or air.

References

Bates B. (1995). *A guide to physical examination and history taking.* Philadelphia: JB Lippincott.

Bichat X. (1814). *Desault's surgery.* Philadelphia: Thomas Dobson.

Coltharpe WH, et al. (1992). Videothoracoscopy: Improved technique and expanded indications. *Annals of Thoracic Surgery, 53*(5), 776-779.

Curry K & Casady L. (1992). Managing spontaneous pneumothorax. *The Nursing Spectrum, 7*(1), 12-13.

Diagnostic and Therapeutic Technology Assessment (DATTA): Lung transplantation. (1993). *Journal of the American Medical Association 269*(7), 931-936.

Fox VJ. (1995). Patient teaching and discharge planning: The short stay challenge. *Capsules & Comments in Perioperative Nursing, 1*(2), 99-111.

Ginsberg RJ. (1994). What's new in general thoracic surgery. *ACS Bulletin, 79*(1), 70-72.

Grap MJ, Glass C, & Constantino S. (1994). Accurate assessment of ventilation and oxygenation. *Med-Surg Nursing, 3*(6), 435-442.

LoCicero J. (1993). What's new in general thoracic surgery. *ACS Bulletin, 78*(3), 23-26.

Mack MJ, et al. (1992). Present role of thoracoscopy in the diagnosis and treatment of diseases of the chest. *Annals of Thoracic Surgery, 54*(3), 403-409.

Maree SM. (1993). Benzodiazepines and their reversal. *Current Reviews for Nurse Anesthetists, 15*(7), 54-59.

McCloskey JC & Bulechek GM. (1992). *Nursing intervention classification.* St. Louis: Mosby.

McManus K & McGuigan J. (1994). Minimally invasive therapy in thoracic injury. *Injury, 25,* 609-614.

Moody LE. (1995). Challenges: TB or not TB. *The Nursing Spectrum, 4*(1), 12-13.

Pagana KD & Pagana TJ. (1995). *Diagnostic and laboratory test reference.* St. Louis: Mosby.

Polomano RC, Blumenthal NP, & Riegler FX. (1994). Interpleural analgesia for the management of postoperative pain. *Med-Surg Nursing, 2*(3), 185-190.

Respiratory Nursing Society and the American Nurses Association. (1994). *Standards and scope of respiratory nursing practice.* Washington, DC: The Society.

Rothrock JC & Sculthorpe RH. (1993). Anesthesia and patient positioning. In JC Rothrock (Ed.), *The RN first assistant: An expanded perioperative role* (2nd ed., pp 116-146). Philadelphia: JB Lippincott.

Rusch VM. (1993). Thoracoscopy. In care of the surgical patient, surgical technique, Scientific American Medicine, (Suppl. 2).

Scannell JG. (1986). Samuel Robinson: Pioneer thoracic surgeon. *Annals of Thoracic Surgery, 42,* 692-699.

Stiesmeyer JK. (1993). A four-step approach to pulmonary assessment. *American Journal of Nursing, 93,* 22-31.

Chapter 16

Vascular Surgery

Christy R. Johnson

The noose of thread being passed below the artery, we must make the constriction of it. The surgeon's knot, usually employed with this view, has, in deep seated arteries, the inconvenience of being very difficult to be suitably tightened at the moment of the operation, more difficult still to tighten it anew, when the shrunken artery, at the end of a few days, permits the blood to escape. The reason of these difficulties is, that we must, 1st. Plunge the fingers and forceps deeply upon the artery, in order to tie it. 2d. That the motion impressed upon the threads for their constriction being obliged to be horizontal, the very elevated edges of the wound are necessarily opposed to it. We must, therefore, have a method by which we may, on the one hand, tighten the artery without acting immediately upon it; and on the other hand, draw the threads particular direction. . . . [Desault has used] a small canula of silver wide above, narrower below, into which he passed the two ends of the noose, which, being drawn upward, whilst the canula was pressed against the artery, made the constriction of it; then being separated from each other, they were reversed upon each of the sides; between them he engaged a small wedge of wood, which was exactly fitted to the canula, fixed them invariably, and thus made the constriction sure. To increase it at pleasure, whenever a hemorrhage supervened, it was sufficient to take away the wedge, to draw the thread to himself, and then to replace it between them.

BICHAT, 1814

*M*edical technologic advancements, improved vascular radiology, and progressive surgical techniques have had a marked effect on the progress of vascular surgery. Efforts to devise instruments appropriate to the anatomic structure of the vascular system, as well as sutures, needles, ligature devices, and effective methods of hemostasis, were of primary interest to innovative surgeons. The ligature carrier and hemostatic device described by Bichat is only one example of the strides made by early vascular surgeons in attempting to correct vascular anomalies surgically.

DEVELOPMENTS IN VASCULAR SURGERY

In 1759 the first successful attempt at suturing an artery was reported. Since that time, the aim of surgery has been to repair rather than ligate vessels. As suture materials and technology became more advanced, surgeons became interested in other methods of repair of diseased vessels. Arterial reconstruction, either by enlarging or reestablishing the vessel lumen or by bypassing the stenosis of occlusion, became a surgical goal. Fogarty made a major contribution to improving morbidity and mortality in the management of arterial embolism (Schwartz, Shires,

& Spencer, 1989). With the development of the balloon-tipped Fogarty catheter, it became possible to extract emboli by inflating the balloon at the distal end of the catheter. Later, balloon-tipped catheters were applied to the treatment of stenotic intraarterial lesions. In 1974 Gruentzig developed a balloon that expanded to a constant size and shape. This proved to be the breakthrough in transluminal angioplasty (Porter, 1991). Four years later, Fogarty and Chinn developed the linear extrusion balloon angioplasty catheter; this has been of great utility intraoperatively. Surgical laser-assisted balloon angioplasty has been used in the treatment of patients with involvement of the smaller arteries and those with hard, calcified lesions, which cannot be successfully treated with peripheral balloon angioplasty. This procedure is still considered an investigative procedure; research is currently underway to compare long-term patency rates of the laser-assisted angioplasty to the already accepted surgical modalities (Polk, Gardner, & Stone, 1993).

When correction of atherosclerotic vascular disease is not possible through intraluminal techniques, bypass techniques can be used. Bypass surgery has been performed using the autogenous saphenous vein, umbilical vein allografts, and nonautogenous grafting materials. Nonautogenous grafting materials include monofilament and multifilaments, woven or knitted, with or without velour surface. Expanded polytetrafluoroethylene (PTFE) grafts are also used; these have achieved long-term patency. Infection is a serious complication of any prosthetic graft, which acts as a foreign body.

Bypass surgery using the autogenous saphenous vein graft gives the best result and represents the first choice of arterial substitute for lower extremity bypass (Mannick, 1993). The saphenous vein may be completely excised and reversed as an arterial conduit or it may be used in situ. With in situ artery bypass for limb salvage, the valves in the vein are deliberately rendered incompetent through excision or division of the valve cusps. This procedure, first reported by Hall in 1964, is preferable to reversed graft in the lower extremity because it causes less damage to the intimal surface of the vein, less trauma when preparing the vein, and permits the use of smaller saphenous veins (Veith, 1989). Alternatives to the saphenous vein are being researched. Favorable results have been reported with the lesser saphenous vein, the brachial and cephalic veins, the long saphenous vein, and the superficial femoral-popliteal veins.

Recent developments in endoscopic vascular instrumentation has increased the popularity of peripheral vascular angioscopy (Borgini & Almgren, 1990; Fogarty, 1991). The angioscope, allowing direct visualization of vessel or previous arterial graft bypass lumens, enables the surgeon to assess and correct intraluminal pathologic conditions. This helps to prevent early graft failure and the need for further surgery (Bergan, 1991).

Despite advances in bypassing or improving luminal diameter for occluded vessels, the pathophysiology of the disease process often leads to reocclusion of vascular grafts. Recent laboratory work has focused on recanalizing obstructed segments of PTFE grafts through laser thrombectomy. Unlike balloon catheter or thrombolytic therapy, hot-tip laser thromboablation provides for adjunctive treatment of anastomotic and distal occlusive disease in PTFE grafts, further increasing the potential for limb salvage (Porter, 1991). Thrombolytic therapy is also being used for vein and prosthetic graft thrombosis. Research in graft development is ongoing; the use of bioresorbable polymers shows promise in graft flexibility, but problems with dilatation and aneurysm development remain to be resolved.

Before advancements in arterial reconstruction, amputation was the inevitable treatment for chronic, uncorrectable atherosclerotic disease of the lower limbs. Today, the choice of amputation in the management of a patient with advanced limb ischemia is difficult. Revascularization should be the first option considered in patients with critical limb ischemia. Improvements in vascular surgery and vascular radiology have provided long-term limb salvage for patients who in the past would have required amputation (Martin, et al., 1994).

Developments are also ongoing in the treatment of atherosclerotic stenosis of the infraaortic arterial system. Self-expanding and balloon-expandable stents are currently being evaluated. The Palmaz stent, which can be used in straight, short segments of large vessels, has been approved for use in the iliac system. Early data are encouraging, but further clinical trials are needed to determine the safety, indications, and efficacy of these recent developments to treat large-vessel atherosclerotic stenosis (Johnson, 1994).

Today's vascular surgery operating room (OR) is equipped with fine microvascular instruments, microscopes, headlights and magnifiers, fluoroscopy, and lasers. Laser-assisted balloon angioplasty, using a hot-tipped laser that goes through the obstructed vessel, followed by balloon angioplasty, will be more common. Atherectomy catheters and devices are being used to whittle channels through the stenoses that occur after angioplasty. Minimally invasive techniques to bypass diseased vessels will continue to be clinically tested (Naslund, 1994); the Chuter bifurcated graft is currently being investigated as an alternative to traditional aortic aneurysm repair (Mathias, 1994).

Angioscopy is considered the method of choice for arterial examination of the lower extremity and will likely replace intraoperative arteriography. Intraoperative ultrasound will guide surgical intervention. The aging of the U.S. population will continue to require advances in vascular surgery. ORs will need to be bigger to accommodate all of the devices for surgery and patient monitoring. Sophisticated vascular surgical interventions may increase operating time and necessitate additional personnel to manage the technology. Risks associated with the increased use of equipment and the increased numbers of persons in the OR will need to be investigated and managed. The challenge of balancing technologic advancements with cost and of developing effective outcomes management systems will continue to be a priority for this surgical specialty (Moss, 1993).

ASSESSMENT

Like other health care team members, the perioperative nurse is challenged to plan complicated care regimens for vascular surgery patients, who often have multisystem diseases. As the age of patients who are candidates for vascular surgery increases, so does the complexity of their pathophysiologic alterations. Diabetes, chronic obstructive pulmonary disease, and neurologic deficits may be present. Surgical interventions may be accompanied by anticoagulant therapy, thrombolytic therapy, arterial and other invasive monitoring lines, thermia equipment, monopolar and bipolar electrosurgery, devices for cell saving, prosthetic conduits, lasers, fluoroscopy, and ultrasonography. The perioperative nurse needs assessment skills for functional review of the system or systems involved, the ability to prioritize and synthesize vast amounts of patient data, and planning and coordinating strategies to promote safe, effective patient outcomes.

Circulatory System

Assessment of patients with vascular disease involves a history, physical examination, and review of related history and physical findings. The perioperative nurse will most often be involved in assessing the primary system involved in the disease process; other assessments will be reviewed and integrated into the care plan as they relate to the individual patient's needs and problems. Boxes 16-1 and 16-2 include Key Assessment Points for the circulatory system and patients undergoing surgery for vascular disorders.

History. The type and severity of symptoms present in patients with vascular disease depend on the stage and extent of the disease process. It is important for the nursing history to include onset and characteristics of initial signs and symptoms, course since onset, and related and alleviating factors.

Patients with vascular disease may be asymptomatic, have intermittent pain with exercise, persistent pain at rest, or tissue necrosis with ulceration or gangrene. It is important for the nursing history to coordinate signs and symptoms with resultant functional ability or disability. The patient's exercise ability should be determined. It is noted whether the patient can engage in activities of heavy intensity (jogging) or only light intensity (walking 10 to 15 steps). The patient is queried regarding changes in fatigue levels: Is fatigue unusual or persistent? Is the patient able to engage in usual activities or is he or she required to retire earlier? It is noted whether the patient has symptoms of fatigue, such as dyspnea on exertion, chest pain, palpitations, edema in the extremity, numbness, or leg pain or cramps. If pain or cramps are present, the nurse determines their onset (sudden or over a period of hours, days, weeks), duration, and character. Pain may be continuous, with a burning sensation or generalized aching; present only over a specific location (foot, calf, thigh, or buttocks); or sharp and burning, with numbness in the distal aspect of the affected extremity that wakes the patient from sleep. Such ischemic rest pain should be differentiated from night cramps, which are characteristically relieved by hanging the affected extremity in a dependent position or by a brief period of walking. With acute arterial embolism in extremities with poor collateral circulation, sudden pain may be accompanied by gradual sensory and motor loss; pain may be aggravated by movement of the extremity (Capasso & Coté, 1993). The medical history should be reviewed for evidence of chronic illnesses such as hypertension, hyperlipidemia, diabetes, heart disease or congenital heart defects, and bleeding disorders. The psychosocial history should include smoking or tobacco use, alcohol consumption, occupation (sedentary or active requirements), stressors, and related environmental factors. Conditions predisposing the patient to mural thrombi formation (rheumatic valvular disease, atrial fibrillation, previous cardiac surgery, left ventricular aneurysm, chronic congestive heart failure, and recent myocardial infarction) should be noted (Bowers & Thompson, 1992). The family history should be reviewed for similar disorders. Medications the patient is taking should be listed and analyzed for their relationship to intraoperative events. Review of current medications, prescribed and over the counter, should include antiinflammatory drugs, fibrinolytics, vasodilators, antihypertensives, digitalis preparations, anticoagulants, steroids, and birth control pills. Allergies to drugs, as well as to dyes, shellfish, and iodine, should be noted.

Box 16-1 *Key Assessment Points: Focused Assessment Guidelines*

Health Perception/Health Management

Patient's perception of problem, onset, characteristics, course since onset, related symptoms, alleviating factors, treatments, and response to treatments. Includes patient's perceived pattern of health and general well-being, associated problems, as well as risk factors and family history

Specific to vascular disorders: pain, discomfort, associated exercise intolerance, fatigue, family history of atherosclerosis, respiratory and cardiac risk factors (smoking; high-fat, high-cholesterol diet; sedentary life-style)

Nutrition/Metabolic

Dietary patterns; any special diet or restrictions; weight, food, and fluid consumption relative to metabolic need; food and fluid preferences; allergies.

Specific to vascular disorders: diet high in calories, fat, cholesterol, and salt; obesity; transient or ongoing difficulty in swallowing; may present with severe nutritional deficiencies related to multisystem vascular insufficiency or advanced age

Elimination

Elimination patterns (bowel and bladder); continent, frequency, nocturia; characteristics of stool and urine; use of laxatives or medications

Specific to vascular disorders: transient or ongoing bowel/bladder incontinence; sudden, severe onset of abdominal distress if ischemia associated with multiple emboli and infarcted mesenteric vessels; may report symptoms of acute renal failure: anuria, oliguria; constipation related to decreased physical activity

Activity/Exercise

Patterns of patient's exercise, leisure, and activity levels, including factors that interfere with patient's normal patterns

Specific to vascular disorders: May report intermittent claudication, pain at rest, shortness of breath, motor deficits, limited mobility related to onset of ischemic muscle pain with physical activities; leg muscle weakness associated with ischemic changes; may be unable to perform activities of daily living

Sexuality/Reproductive

Usual pattern of sexual activity

Specific to vascular disorders: may report impotence related to multisystem vascular disease

Sleep/Rest

Patient's usual patterns of sleep, rest, and relaxation

Specific to vascular disorders: may report sleep disturbance related to ischemic pain occurring at rest

Value/Belief

Patient's values, beliefs, and goals

Specific to vascular disorders: patient's values and beliefs may present conflicts related to planned medical management and surgery

Cognitive/Perceptual

Includes patient's cognitive function ability, insight regarding current situation, judgment ability; pain perception and management

Specific to vascular disorders: Pain, arterial: may describe pain as sharp, burning, constant, or intermittent. May have severe cramping pain after activity/exercise (intermittent claudication) or may have persistent pain at rest. Pain, venous: may describe pain as aching, heavy, or full feeling, or tenderness; pain intensifies with prolonged sitting or standing in one position

Role/Relationship

Includes patient's occupation; family, work, and social relationships, and patient's perception of responsibilities

Specific to vascular disorders: may report inability to perform usual roles; decreased social interaction due to inability to maintain usual activities

Coping/Stress

Patient's usual coping pattern and effectiveness of measures used; perceived ability to manage situation and stress

Specific to vascular disorders: may report history of smoking/tobacco use, chronic alcohol abuse. May express fear/anxiety about impending surgery; family support or lack of family and other support systems

Self-perception/Self-concept

Patient's attitude about self and perception of body image.

Specific to vascular disorders: may report altered self-concept, low self-esteem; low self-esteem may be a result of inability to perform usual activities or may be a result of the inability to control situation; may report depression

---

The patient with an abdominal aortic aneurysm may have a history of lower back pain or pain in the lower abdomen that radiates to the back or groin. The patient may complain of hearing his or her heart beating when lying down. Less common is the complaint of actually feeling an abdominal mass or abdominal throbbing. Complaints of dizziness or weakness may indicate that the aneurysm is leaking. Signs of rupturing abdominal aortic aneurysms include constant, intense back pain; falling blood

---

Box 16-2 Key Assessment Points: Physical Examination Guidelines

The general physical assessment should include the patient's age, height, weight, overall physical condition, mental status, and vital signs. The following physical assessment areas are focused to the circulatory system and for patients with vascular disorders.

Cardiovascular Assessment

Physical examination should include the following:
Heart rate and rhythm (dysrhythmias, tachycardia)
Auscultation of bruits (abdominal aortic, carotid, femoral, popliteal)
Heart sounds, murmurs, jugular vein distention
Blood pressure and any hypertension
Palpation of pulses (carotid, brachial, radial, femoral, popliteal, dorsalis pedis, and posterior tibial)
Note pulse rhythm, rate, quality, and contour; diminished, decreased, or absent pulses should be noted
Assess pain related to ischemic changes (intermittent claudication or pain at rest)
Palpate for pulsating mass at or above the umbilicus
Assess capillary refill time in extremities
Note dependent rubor or cyanosis in extremities

Neurologic Assessment

Assess mental status and level of consciousness (alert, oriented, disoriented)
Visual deficits
Speech (normal, difficult, slurred, hoarse)
Pupils (size and reaction to light, accommodation)
Motor status, any transient or permanent deficits (reflexes, weakness, paralysis, gait disturbances)
Sensory deficits (numbness, decreased sensitivity to pressure, temperature, or pain)
Any alterations in cognitive function
Headaches, dizziness, dysphagia, or unequal handgrips

Integumentary Assessment

Skin should be assessed for the following:
Color: cyanosis, pallor, rubor, blanching, redness
Temperature: cold/cool, warmth
Texture: increased pigmentation, thinning, mottling, edema

Hair distribution, thinning
Nails, thick or brittle
Evidence of skin breakdown: lesions, ulcerations, gangrene
Evidence of normal healing and approximation of wound edges
Signs and symptoms of infection: erythema, edema, undue tenderness, warmth, induration, foul odor, or purulent drainage

Respiratory Assessment

Assess respirations for rate and rhythm
Note symmetry of chest expansion
Auscultate breath sounds
Note any adventitious or abnormal breath sounds
Note any shallow or irregular breathing patterns, shortness of breath, and coughing; if cough productive, note sputum consistency, color, and quantity

Gastrointestinal Assessment

Assess for changes in normal bowel patterns
Note stools: color, consistency, presence of occult blood
Note any nausea, vomiting, or abdominal distention (paralytic ileus)
Note diarrhea or constipation, including onset and duration

Musculoskeletal Assessment

Assess activity level; any decreased or diminished ability in activity level, joint movement, or range of motion
Muscle tone and strength, muscle atrophy, weakness
Coordination, ability to perform activities of daily living

Renal Assessment

Assess urine output: color, character, and amount
Patient's weight
Anuria or oliguria

---

pressure; decreasing red blood cell count with increasing white blood cell count; and soft abdomen (Smeltzer & Bare, 1992).

The patient with carotid atherosclerosis may have a history of varying neurologic symptoms. Holloway (1993) identifies four important clinical manifestations that indicate the need for surgery. The most severe of these is a cerebral infarction or cerebral vascular accident (CVA), which is characterized by paralysis and sensory loss on the side of the body opposite the involved cerebral hemisphere. Not always responsive to surgical intervention, the patient with cerebral infarction may have mild or perma-

nent long-term neurologic deficits from the CVA. A second surgical indication is reversible ischemic neurologic deficits (RINDs) and transient ischemic attacks (TIAs). These are caused by temporary insufficient blood supply to focal areas of the brain. The extremity on the opposite side of the involved cerebral hemisphere is usually affected. With reversible ischemic neurologic deficits, symptoms persist for more than 24 hours, but completely resolve within 2 weeks; transient ischemic attacks resolve completely within 24 hours. TIAs may occur in a series and cause transient blindness if the retina is involved. Both of these conditions are responsive to surgical intervention. Two other indications for surgery include asymptomatic carotid bruits with severe stenosis of the internal carotid artery and recurrence of carotid stenosis after a previous endarterectomy.

Physical examination. Common nursing diagnostic techniques for the vascular system include inspection, auscultation, and palpation. Arterial occlusion results in circulatory insufficiency to the tissues; a variety of changes may be observed distal to the occlusion. The affected extremity may be pale or cyanotic; when vessels are unable to constrict and remain dilatated, the skin may be reddish blue (rubor). The skin may be cold to the touch. Temperature should be compared bilaterally and between the upper and lower extremities. Superficial veins may be collapsed, with delay in venous filling. Trophic changes in the skin may result in muscle atrophy, with thin, shiny, dry, hairless skin and thickened nails. Paresthesias may be present. There may be pain or tenderness; with long-term insufficiency, ulceration or gangrene may be present. Ischemic ulcerations usually occur in the distal aspect of the extremity or foot, involving areas exposed to trauma (toes, dorsum of the foot, or malleoli). These need to be distinguished from venous stasis ulcers, which usually occur on the medial aspect of the leg with a surrounding area of hyperpigmentation and stasis dermatitis (Bowers & Thompson, 1992). Gangrene usually affects the toes, foot, or distal leg. Gangrene may be pregangrenous (blue toes with palpable pulses), dry and uninfected, wet, or infected. Patients with vascular problems of the upper extremities should be examined for digital ischemia, fingertip ulcerations, and gangrene. The Allen test should reveal normal flow through the ulnar arteries.

Venous circulation should be similarly inspected. Venous insufficiency may be detected through observation of obvious thrombosis, edema, or varicosities. Pain usually intensifies with prolonged sitting or standing and is often described as an aching, tired, or full feeling in the legs. Redness, thickening, warm skin, and tenderness may be present along a superficial vein, indicating potential superficial vein thrombophlebitis. Deep vein thrombosis may cause swelling, tenderness, and pain; further diagnosis is required. A positive Homan's sign (pain on dorsiflexion of the foot) usually indicates thrombosis. Fever and tachycardia may be present; the patient should be observed for signs of pulmonary embolism.

Pulses may be diminished or impalpable distal to the occlusion. Pulses should be examined with the distal pads of the second, third, and fourth fingers; the thumbs should not be used. Firm but not hard palpation is necessary. Depending on the location of vascular disease, the carotid, brachial, radial, femoral, popliteal, dorsalis pedis, and posterior tibial pulses may be palpated. Pulses should be compared—the upper extremities with the lower extremities and the left with the right—for rate, rhythm, equality, amplitude, and contour. Different systems are used for grading pulses. Smeltzer and Bare (1992) suggest that pulse quality, or amplitude, be graded on a scale of 0 to 4: 0 is an absent pulse; +1 is marked impairment of pulsation; +2 is moderate impairment of pulsation; +3 is slight impairment of pulsation; and +4 is a normal pulsation. Holloway (1993) suggests a scale of 0 to 3: 0 is an absent pulse; +1 is detectable by Doppler ultrasound stethoscope only; +2 is weakly palpable; and +3 is a strong palpable pulse. It is not uncommon for pulses to be marked preoperatively for convenient assessment during and at the conclusion of surgical intervention.

Bruits are low-pitched, unexpected murmurs or sounds that may be difficult to hear. They usually occur over areas of local obstruction, produced by turbulent blood flow through a stenotic lumen or dilated segment of the vessel. They are auscultated with a stethoscope. Sites at which bruits may be encountered include the carotid, jugular, temporal, aortic, renal, and femoral arteries.

Physical examination of the patient with an abdominal aneurysm may reveal a pulsating mass in the area of the umbilicus to left of the midline. Blood pressure may differ between arms. The patient may have pallor, tachycardia, dizziness, or syncope and be hypertensive. Auscultation may reveal a systolic bruit over the mass.

REVIEWING THE DIAGNOSTIC WORKUP

Diagnostic studies provide information that complements and confirms the results of a patient history and physical examination. They are important in assisting to predict therapeutic results and in monitoring medical and surgical therapies. Information regarding lumen size and patency, aneurysm development, and blood flow can be critical to determining the type and timing of therapy. The following section is meant to help the perioperative nurse identify and interpret the results of common noninvasive and invasive vascular studies.

Noninvasive Diagnostic Studies

Noninvasive hemodynamic testing has become an essential component to evaluation of patients with vascular diseases. Peripheral vascular laboratory studies assist the surgeon before, during, and after surgical intervention with detecting, localizing, and quantifying vascular disease. Two common noninvasive diagnostic studies are Doppler ultrasound and plethysmography; duplex scanning is gaining popularity among vascular surgeons and radiologists.

Doppler ultrasound. Doppler ultrasound has proven to be the single most important modality to noninvasive evaluation of lower extremity ischemia. It detects shifts in sound reflected from moving blood cells. Depending on the type of device used, this information may be presented as an audible signal, recorded in waveforms, or generated as an image of the vessel lumen. Coupling Doppler ultrasound with a pneumatic tourniquet cuff enables measurement of lower extremity blood pressure. Venous Doppler ultrasound detects valve incompetence; directional Doppler flowmeters are preferred in determining forward and reverse flow.

Plethysmography. Plethysmography detects and records arterial pulsations indicating volume changes in the extremity, digit, or eye. Changes in pulse and leg size can be monitored with each heartbeat. Segmental blood pressures can be obtained, as can venous outflow or reflux. Indications for plethysmography include peripheral arterial, cerebrovascular, and venous disease.

Impedance plethysmography. Combined with Doppler flow detection, impedance plethysmography detects acute deep vein thrombosis through changes in venous volume. For chronic venous insufficiency, photoplethysmography may be used.

Photoplethysmography. Photoplethysmography (PPG) uses a photodetector to pick up back-scattered infrared light; cutaneous blood flow is continuously recorded in the capillary network. Qualitative information before, during, and after exercise is obtained by comparing the opacity of the underlying tissue caused by changes in the blood content of the skin (Porter, 1991). PPG is useful for evaluating both arterial and venous insufficiency in both the superficial and deep venous system.

Computed tomography. Computed tomography (CT) is useful for identifying true aneurysms and aortic dissection, which cannot be detected by ultrasound.

B-mode scan. B-mode scanning uses sound wave reflections from tissue to form a still image of an artery and visualize its pulsatile characteristics.

Duplex scan. Duplex scanning has been used for many years to examine the carotid artery. Recent advances have permitted the development of transducers that permit examination of the peripheral arteries from the aorta through the tibial vessels.

Combining techniques of both the B-mode scan and the Doppler ultrasound, duplex scanning allows visualization and examination of the artery under study. It precisely detects the location of hemody-namic, significant lesions and determines the length and origin (stenotic or occlusive) of intraluminal lesions (Porter, 1991).

Frequency spectral analyzer. The frequency spectral analyzer is often used in combination with B-mode or duplex scans to analyze the contours of the pulse and changes in its intensity during the cardiac cycle.

Magnetic resonance angiography. Magnetic resonance angiography (MRA) techniques are used in addition to or in the place of conventional x-ray angiography to determine blood vessel structure and to measure blood flow. MRA requires no exposure to ionizing radiation and circumvents systemic reactions sometimes caused by contrast media (AHCPR, 1994).

Invasive Diagnostic Studies

The increasingly sophisticated nature of noninvasive diagnostic studies has reduced the indications for formerly common invasive studies. Nonetheless, angiography continues to play a selective role in the delineation of arterial, aortic, and venous disease.

Arteriography. Arteriograms are indicated for patients undergoing vascular surgery, but not as a routine diagnostic measure. Using contrast media to provide radiographic images, arteriography plays an important role in specific diagnostic evaluation of aortic, peripheral arterial, and carotid artery disease. Vessel stenosis, occlusions, aneurysms, and collateral circulation can be demonstrated. Peripherally, arteriograms reveal detailed angiographic visualization of the entire lower extremity vascular system, including the pelvic arteries and the small vessels in the distal leg and foot. Intraoperatively, the results of an arteriogram are used for anatomic information regarding reconstruction of the involved vessel(s).

Digital subtraction angiography. Digital subtraction angiography (DSA) is somewhat less expensive and less risky than arteriography. However, it often produces less resolution than intraarterial angiography. Intravenous digital subtraction angiography is usually performed using a catheter introduced into the brachial vein (Porter, 1991). It is used in peripheral vascular disorders and to visualize pulmonary arterial circulation in the diagnosis of pulmonary embolism.

Aortography. Aortography defines and localizes the occlusive process in the aorta. The results of the aortogram will be reviewed to determine the involvement of the renal arteries, infrarenal aorta, and the common internal and external iliac arteries, as well as the superficial femoral and tibioperoneal arteries.

Venography. Venography delineates the precise nature of valvular incompetency. It may also be used to identify filling defects in the deep veins to confirm deep vein thrombosis.

Pulmonary angiography. Intraluminal filling defects in the pulmonary arteries detect pulmonary embolism. These are indicated either by an outline or a sudden cutoff of the artery. Pulmonary angiography is additionally useful because pulmonary artery pressures may be measured during the study.

Laboratory Studies

Laboratory studies will vary according to the patient's overall medical history and the specific diagnosis requiring surgery. In general, the perioperative nurse might expect to find results of a complete blood count, hemoglobin and hematocrit, coagulation studies, serum electrolytes, kidney functions (blood urea nitrogen and serum creatinine), arterial blood gases, serum cholesterol, triglycerides, and lipid levels, as well as results of type and screen or type and cross-match studies. These patients usually also have an electrocardiogram and chest x-ray film; the perioperative nurse should review these in addition to any procedure-specific vascular radiology studies.

NURSING DIAGNOSES

The most common and significant vascular disease requiring surgical correction is atherosclerosis. The physiologic process of atherosclerosis is characterized by focal changes, known as atheroma or plaque, on the intimal layer of the artery. Atherosclerosis evolves over a long time and is the most common cause of occlusive vascular disease. It is directly responsible for vessel lumen stenosis, obstruction by thrombosis, aneurysm development, and vessel wall ulcerations. Atherosclerosis has high morbidity and mortality and tends to be generalized throughout the vascular system. Consequently, patients admitted to the OR with occlusion of one vessel may have arterial insufficiency in other vessels. The arteries most commonly affected are the aorta, iliac, femoral, popliteal, renal, and carotid arteries.

Arteriosclerosis, or hardening of the arteries, involves a group of pathogenic processes that result in generalized vascular disease. Although the pathologic processes of arteriosclerosis and atherosclerosis differ, rarely does one occur without the other, and the terms are used interchangeably. Common surgical interventions for stenosed or occluded arteries include endarterectomy, segmental resection, and bypass grafting. Risk factors associated with atherogenesis need to be considered; these include lipid disorders, hypertension, smoking, stress, seden-

tary life-style, diabetes, and obesity. Surgery and perioperative nursing care can be complicated. The following discussion is based on nursing diagnoses that are generic to most surgical patients but apply particularly to vascular surgery patients.

Generic Nursing Diagnoses

Perioperative nursing is characteristically a team effort. One of the hallmarks of perioperative nursing is close mutual collaboration between the members of the patient care team. Collaboration requires an exchange of information, trust in team members' abilities, and respect for each other's role. The nursing literature has often delineated nursing diagnoses as independent, performed as a nursing initiative; dependent, performed at the request or "order" of other health care team members; and interdependent, performed together, with knowledge and care contributed by the involved care providers. Many patients in the vascular surgery OR clearly require both nursing and medical interventions, and the nursing diagnoses developed for perioperative care planning are interdependent and collaborative. Therefore no attempt has been made to characterize the following list of nursing diagnoses according to their independent or dependent nature; they are assumed, in most instances, to be collaborative. Nursing diagnoses vary according to the individual patient and the surgical procedure, but nursing diagnoses for selected vascular surgery procedures include the following:

1. Abdominal aortic aneurysm
   a. Cardiac output, decreased, high risk for (related to changes in intravascular volume, third space fluid shift, or an increase in systemic vascular resistance)
   b. Fear (related to severity of illness and fear of death)
   c. Fluid volume deficit, high risk for
   d. Injury, high risk for (related to surgical procedure, atherosclerosis, and anticoagulation therapy)
   e. Knowledge deficit, high risk for (regarding preoperative and postoperative care related to surgical intervention)
   f. Self-esteem disturbance, high risk for (related to dependence on prosthetic device)
   g. Skin integrity, impaired, high risk for
   h. Tissue perfusion, altered, high risk for (peripheral, renal, or gastrointestinal related to interruption of arterial blood flow)
   i. Pain (related to surgical tissue trauma or ischemia)
   j. Infection, high risk for (related to prosthetic arterial graft placement)

2. Carotid endarterectomy
   a. Fear (related to severity of illness, fear of death, and possible complications from surgical intervention)
   b. Injury, high risk for (related to surgical position, impairment of cranial nerves resulting from surgical trauma, blood accumulation, or edema in surgical area)
   c. Tissue perfusion, altered, high risk for (cerebral) (related to interruption of arterial blood flow)
3. Femoral-popliteal bypass
   a. Fear (related to severity of illness)
   b. Infection, high risk for (related to prosthetic arterial graft placement)
   c. Injury, high risk for (related to surgical procedure, atherosclerotic disease, or anticoagulant therapy)
   d. Knowledge deficit, high risk for (related to planned surgical intervention)
   e. Skin integrity, impaired (related to surgical incision, possible preexisting stasis ulcers, and decreased sensation)
   f. Tissue perfusion, altered, high risk for (peripheral)
   g. Mobility, impaired, high risk for (related to surgical procedure and possible preexisting disability)
   h. Pain (related to surgical incision and increased perfusion to previous ischemic tissue)
4. Venous thrombectomy/arterial embolectomy
   a. Fear (related to severity of illness and fear of death)
   b. Injury, high risk for (related to surgical procedure or anticoagulant therapy)
   c. Knowledge deficit, high risk for (related to planned surgical intervention)
   d. Tissue perfusion, altered, high risk for (peripheral)
   e. Skin integrity, impaired, high risk for
5. Laser-assisted peripheral angioplasty
   a. Injury, high risk for (related to surgical intervention, atherosclerosis, anticoagulant therapy or use of laser)
   b. Knowledge deficit, high risk for (related to planned surgical intervention)
   c. Mobility, impaired physical
   d. Pain (related to immobility or tissue ischemia)
6. Arteriovenous access
   a. Infection, high risk for (related to surgical intervention and preexisting physical condition)
   b. Knowledge deficit, high risk for (related to care of access site)
   c. Pain (related to surgical intervention)
   d. Skin integrity, impaired (related to surgical intervention and preexisting physical condition)
7. Vena cava filter insertion
   a. Fear (related to severity of illness and fear of death)
   b. Knowledge deficit, high risk for (related to planned surgical intervention)
   c. Mobility, impaired physical
   d. Pain (related to immobility during surgical procedure)
8. Varicose vein ligation
   a. Knowledge deficit, high risk for (related to planned surgical intervention)
   b. Tissue perfusion, altered, high risk for (peripheral)
   c. Self-esteem, situational low (related to cosmetic appearance of varicose veins and surgical incision[s])
   d. Pain (related to surgical incision[s])

Impaired skin integrity. The vascular surgery patient may have the high risk for or actual impairment of skin integrity (ulcerations or gangrene). Intact, patent blood vessels, necessary for the delivery of oxygen to tissues and removal of metabolic waste, are compromised because of the inherent nature of the disease process. Arterial stenosis or obstruction and reduction in venous flow result in inadequate tissue nutrition; ischemia, tissue breakdown, injury, infection, or death may occur. The desired patient outcome is that skin integrity will be maintained. To achieve this outcome, perioperative nursing interventions aim to maintain correct body alignment, to protect bony prominences and vulnerable areas with padding, to avoid shearing force when transferring the patient, to protect vulnerable neurovascular bundles from compromise, to place restraining straps snugly but not tightly, to keep bed sheets dry and wrinkle free, and to use cushioning devices on the OR bed (egg-crate or gel-filled mattress).

Altered tissue perfusion. The same etiologic factors that potentiate altered skin integrity influence alterations in tissue perfusion. Inadequate cellular nutrition and oxygenation, which result from the atherosclerotic process, lead to altered tissue perfusion. When using this nursing diagnosis, the perioperative nurse should specify whether the altered perfusion is peripheral, which is common to patients with vascular disease of the extremities; cerebral, which might be found in the patient with carotid disease; or renal or gastrointestinal, which might be found in the patient with abdominal aortic aneurysm. The risk for altered cardiopulmonary tissue perfusion exists in the patient with venous thrombosis because pulmonary embolism is a possible complication.

The desired outcome is that the patient will demonstrate improved tissue perfusion in the affected location. To achieve this outcome, perioperative nursing interventions are designed to monitor vital signs, assess and compare pulses bilaterally, assess skin color, temperature, and turgor; to check capillary refill, assess neurologic status including level of consciousness, orientation, pupils, speech, reflexes, strength, and mobility; and to monitor intake and output, pertinent laboratory values, and sensory and motor function.

Fluid volume deficit. Any interruption of the circulatory system carries the risk for blood loss. In addition, fluid volume is influenced by electrolyte balance. Potassium is an important electrolyte for patients with vascular disorders. Circulatory insufficiency, as well as treatment of hypertension with diuretics, may potentiate potassium imbalance. Sodium imbalances may similarly occur in hypertensive patients. If the patient is hypokalemic, there may be a consequent magnesium deficiency; magnesium plays an important role in maintaining stable cardiac rhythms. The desired patient outcome is that fluid and electrolyte balance will be maintained. To achieve this outcome, the perioperative nurse monitors intake of IV fluids, blood and blood products, and irrigation; monitors output, including blood loss and output from urinary, nasogastric, and any Penrose or other drainage device; monitors pertinent laboratory values; monitors vital signs; and monitors skin color, temperature, and turgor.

Pain. The reason for pain will vary according to the reason for surgery. With venous thrombosis, pain is related to the inflammatory process. With chronic arterial insufficiency, pain is related to peripheral tissue ischemia. The desired outcome is that the patient will be assisted in controlling pain. To achieve this outcome, the perioperative nurse includes interventions to monitor origin of pain, administer prescribed analgesics, and assist the patient with personally effective techniques to help control pain (Puntillo & Weiss, 1994).

Anxiety and fear. Emotional responses to disease and surgery vary from individual to individual. Nonetheless, the vascular surgery patient will likely experience some anxiety or fear related to diagnosis, prognosis, and surgical treatment. If there is the threat of loss of a limb or body part, anxiety and fear may be increased. These patients may additionally experience a *high risk for body image disturbance; ineffective coping; self-esteem disturbance;* or *altered role performance.* The desired outcome is that the patient will experience reduced anxiety or fear. To achieve this outcome, perioperative nursing interventions aim to provide clear, concise explanations; identify and reduce environmental stressors; assist the patient with personally effective techniques to reduce anxiety; encourage ventilation of concerns and fears; listen attentively, noting verbal and nonverbal communication; demonstrate warmth, calmness, and acceptance of the patient's anxiety; and use touch.

Knowledge deficit. Patients may not fully understand their disease process or may not have reasonable expectations of the results of surgery. The vascular surgery team's ability to intervene with lasers and prosthetic implants may overwhelm a patient who does not fully understand terminology or how a specific intervention works. Patients have the right to wish or not wish for full explanations. The perioperative nurse should ascertain that the patient has no serious misconceptions. Explanations of the expected sequence of perioperative events should be provided in simple, understandable terms. If the patient exhibits a serious lack of understanding, the perioperative nurse should communicate and refer the knowledge deficit to the surgeon, discharge unit nurse, or other health care team member as appropriate. The desired outcome is for the patient to demonstrate knowledge of the physiologic and psychologic responses to surgery.

The perioperative care plan should include a review of postoperative care and education regarding preventive health care measures (Engler & Engler, 1994). Patient teaching should include the following:

- Signs and symptoms of venous thrombosis (stiffness, soreness, redness, heat or edema over affected area, Homan's sign, elevated temperature, and tachycardia) and arterial insufficiency (color and temperature change, pain, skin breakdown, and loss of sensation)
- Keeping the extremities at the level of the heart while at rest (recommendations regarding elevation or slight dependency of the legs depend on whether arterial or venous disease is present)
- Proper application of antiembolism stockings (removing for 15 minutes every 8 hours and checking the skin for redness and irritation)
- Caution against vigorous rubbing or massaging extremities; use of hot-water bottles, heating pads, and hot foot soaks (unless specifically prescribed); and exposure to cold
- Explanation of the vasoconstrictive properties of nicotine; encouragement to quit smoking (with referral to self-help group as indicated)
- Encouraging the patient to drink adequate fluid each day to prevent dehydration, which can lead to blood concentration and clot formation
- Avoidance of restrictive clothing (garters, girdles, tight belts)

- Avoidance of prolonged periods of immobility, which can lead to venous stasis (sitting or standing)
- Avoidance of crossing legs or ankles; watching for and reporting edema
- Prevention of bruising or bleeding
- Development of an exercise plan that will fit into the patient's life-style; walking stimulates circulation and promotes tissue repair
- Maintenance of meticulous foot care (cleanliness, inspection, lubrication, care of toenails, proper shoes and socks, safety, activity)
- Review of dietary instructions, medications to be taken and avoided, and ways to prevent emotional upset and manage stress; avoidance of obesity
- Review of beginning skin breakdown signs and symptoms that require prompt attention: redness, blisters, discolorations, swelling, and pain

Hypothermia. Hypothermia may result from the length of the surgical procedure, vasoconstriction caused by the disease process or aging, or wide surgical exposure. Intraoperatively, the patient's temperature will be monitored. Thermia blankets are often used; the placement of the blanket will depend on whether intraoperative angiography will be performed. If angiography is done, a full thermia blanket would obstruct radiographic views; a pediatric blanket for the upper extremities might be selected instead. The desired outcome is that the patient will maintain normothermia. To achieve this outcome, the perioperative nurse limits physical exposure, exposing only body areas necessary for surgical preparation and intervention; places a warming device on the OR bed; uses intravenous fluid warmers and warm irrigation fluids; adds warm cotton blankets to unexposed parts; applies protective head coverings when needed; and provides warm blankets at the end of the procedure.

Impaired gas exchange. Patients with venous thrombosis have the risk for impaired gas exchange related to embolization of the thrombus. These patients need careful monitoring for signs of pulmonary embolism. The desired outcome is that the patient will maintain adequate ventilation. To achieve this outcome, the perioperative nurse monitors vital signs, establishes baseline values for respiratory assessment, auscultates breath sounds, assists with relaxation techniques, monitors level of consciousness and orientation, assesses skin color and temperature, monitors intake and output, positions the patient to facilitate chest expansion, monitors pertinent laboratory values, and monitors oxygen saturation level.

PLANNING PATIENT CARE

In addition to the generic nursing diagnoses presented earlier, the perioperative nurse should consider other factors when planning care for the patient undergoing vascular surgery. The vascular surgery patient is at high risk for various injuries. The risk for injury is increased by the use of small cardiovascular needles, pledgets and gauze dissectors, vessel loops, and clips. Constant observation of items that might be inadvertently retained is necessary; additional counts of these items may be required. The length of vascular procedures also increases the patient's risk for injury as these patients exhibit a general state of poor circulation and circulation is restricted distal to the area of arterial occlusion. Correct positioning is extremely important to prevent injury; proper skeletal alignment and padding of bony prominences are essential.

The nursing team needs to prepare necessary equipment and supplies, verify that they are in working order, and plan for additional items that might be requested. This is part of the quality assessment and risk management function of perioperative nursing. Prostheses need to be prepared properly and implants correctly documented. Medications must be prepared, labeled, and documented. The correct OR bed for the surgical intervention needs to be in the room. Numerous accessory items need to be obtained and dispensed to the surgical team. Diagnostic studies need to be available for intraoperative review. Laboratory results need to be on the medical record. Blood or blood products need to be checked and properly stored.

When the patient is admitted to the holding area or OR, the medical record is reviewed and evaluations by other health care team members noted. The patient is correctly identified, and the nurse introduces himself or herself. The patient is then interviewed and information for the primary, focused perioperative nursing assessment is obtained and/or validated. During this process, skin integrity is noted and the patient's anxiety and fear are assessed. The patient's level of understanding is determined, explanations are provided, and expected outcomes of perioperative nursing care are discussed. The circulatory system is assessed and baseline data are obtained and documented; these will be important for determining whether or not the patient achieves identified goals.

Anesthetic management of the vascular surgery patient may be difficult. Patients are often elderly, with multiple medical problems and numerous risk factors. The type of anesthesia may range from monitored anesthesia care with local anesthetic; regional anesthesia, either primary or as an adjunct to general anesthesia; or prolonged general anesthesia.

The perioperative nurse will need to collaborate closely with members of the anesthesia team during planning and implementing patient care.

CARE PLANS

To achieve successful patient outcomes, the perioperative nurse must organize and plan care skillfully. This is one of the strengths of the experienced perioperative nurse, who rapidly assimilates changing information and responds with forethought and prompt, precise nursing action. Communication must be maintained and priorities established with the perioperative team. Care of the vascular surgery patient is complex; efficiency and cooperation are demanded. The following procedure-specific care plans have been developed as guidelines for perioperative nurses who wish to develop similar plans for the surgical procedures in which they participate. The nursing diagnoses selected are not all-inclusive; instead, a common, priority nursing diagnosis is presented. Because it is expected that all perioperative patients will meet the generic patient outcomes, as applicable, these are referred to as such. The nursing actions are presented in a sequence that reflects actual care delivery. The Guide to Nursing Actions accompanying each care plan is meant to assist the perioperative nurse in carrying out actions. It is expected that these care plans will be modified for the individual patient and care setting.

GUIDES TO NURSING ACTIONS
Abdominal Aortic Aneurysm (Fig. 16-1)

1. Perioperative care planning depends on a careful, comprehensive assessment. Consideration needs to be given to the physiologic consequences of the disease process, because these patients are often elderly, have chronic medical conditions (generalized arteriosclerotic vascular disease, hypertension, renal dysfunction, and diabetes), and experience major stress from surgery (Chase, 1994). Perioperative nursing assessment is guided by the fact that the aneurysm might rupture and by recognition that the patient may have cardiovascular, cerebral, and pulmonary impairment caused by atherosclerosis. The patient will have numerous nursing diagnoses. For this care plan, *high risk for fluid volume deficit* and *altered tissue perfusion* have been selected. To determine if the patient achieves the identified outcomes, it will be necessary to review the baseline vital signs, central venous pressure measurements, blood chemistry results, and electrolyte levels, as well as to assess the lower extremities. Pulses should be assessed and graded. Any alterations in the lower extremities (cool, mottled, pale skin or absence of pulses) should be noted.

2. The patient may be anxious; a calm, efficient manner; minimal environmental stimulation; and simple, understandable explanations will assist in reducing anxiety. Family anxiety can be reduced through the provision of frequent perioperative nursing reports.

3. Verify operative procedure with the patient's statement and operative consent form. The patient's statement and operative consent form should correspond regarding procedure and site.

4. Verify all known allergies and document on the operative record.

5. General anesthesia will be used. Hemodynamic monitoring catheters (A-line, CVP, Swan-Ganz) will be placed to carefully monitor cardiac function, blood volume, and circulation. Assist anesthesia provider with placement of invasive catheters and with the administration of anesthesia; provide explanations and support to the patient.

6. An epidural catheter may be placed for postoperative pain control. The epidural provides for postoperative pain relief without sedation and allows the patient to cough more vigorously and effectively. Assist anesthesia provider with epidural catheter placement; provide explanations and support to the patient.

7. Determine that patient has correct knowledge and understanding of the planned anesthesia and catheter placements. Assess patient for any specific fears, concerns, or anxieties related to planned procedures and anesthesia. Provide explanations and support to the patient.

8. The supine position will be used. Assess the patient's skin and muscle mass; provide extra padding to bony prominences and vulnerable areas (elbows and heels). A thermia or reflective blanket may be used; sheepskin or foam padding may be placed on the OR bed. A foot cradle may be applied to keep the weight of the drapes off the extremities and to allow easier assessment of peripheral pulses. Maintain correct body alignment; place the safety strap appropriately.

9. Preoperative marking of peripheral pulses assists in easy location for intraoperative monitoring.

10. An indwelling urinary catheter will be inserted if one is not present. Use aseptic technique for catheter insertion. Keep the drainage bag off the floor; place so it is easily observable. Prevent kinks and stretching of the tubing. Document catheter insertion.

FIG. 16-1
CARE PLAN FOR ABDOMINAL AORTIC ANEURYSM

KEY ASSESSMENT POINTS

General physical and mental condition
Presence of chronic health problems
Baseline vital signs
Limitations in mobility
Pain (location—low back, abdomen, flank)
Color, warmth, skin turgor, skin condition (mottling), pulses, sensation and motor ability, capillary refill, edema in lower extremities
Lab values (clotting profiles, blood gases, electrolytes, CBC, blood urea nitrogen [BUN], creatinine)
Recent or sudden change in occurrence of pain
Knowledge assessment (risk factors, disease process, symptoms)
Understanding of procedure/anesthesia/ICU
Understanding of rehabilitation, self-care ability, support systems
Anxiety/fear

NURSING DIAGNOSIS:

All generic nursing diagnoses apply to this patient, with the addition of:
High risk for fluid volume deficit
High risk for altered peripheral tissue perfusion

PATIENT OUTCOMES:

All generic outcomes apply, with the addition of:
1. The patient will maintain hemodynamic stability as evidenced by:
   a. Vital signs will remain within baseline values
   b. Urine output will be 30 cc per hour
   c. Absence of peripheral or dependent edema
   d. Laboratory values will remain within normal limits
   e. Skin color, temperature, and turgor will remain within normal range
2. The patient will demonstrate adequate peripheral tissue perfusion as evidenced by:
   a. Lower extremities will be warm and dry to touch; pink
   b. Peripheral pulses will be normal/expected
   c. Capillary refill will be 2 to 3 seconds
   d. Sensation in the lower extremities will be intact
   e. Motor ability in the lower extremities will not be compromised

NURSING ACTIONS:

	Yes	No	N/A
1. Physical assessment performed?	☐	☐	☐
2. Psychosocial assessment performed?	☐	☐	☐
3. Verbal verification of operative site and consent signed correctly?	☐	☐	☐
4. Allergies verified and documented?	☐	☐	☐
5. Method of anesthesia explained?	☐	☐	☐
6. Epidural catheter explained?	☐	☐	☐
7. Patient understands planned anesthesia and catheter placements?	☐	☐	☐
8. Positioned correctly?	☐	☐	☐
9. Pulses marked?	☐	☐	☐
10. Catheter inserted?	☐	☐	☐
11. Nasogastric tube inserted?	☐	☐	☐
12. Prep per institutional protocol?	☐	☐	☐
13. Privacy maintained?	☐	☐	☐
14. Warm blankets added?	☐	☐	☐
15. Thermia unit?	☐	☐	☐
16. ESU used?	☐	☐	☐
17. Dispersive pad site checked?	☐	☐	☐
18. Irrigation/IV solutions warmed?	☐	☐	☐
19. Blood/blood products administered?	☐	☐	☐
20. Autotransfusion used?	☐	☐	☐
21. Doppler monitoring?	☐	☐	☐
22. Pulses palpated?	☐	☐	☐
23. Graft precautions initiated?	☐	☐	☐
24. Implants recorded?	☐	☐	☐
25. Intake and output recorded?	☐	☐	☐

NURSING ACTIONS—cont'd

	Yes	No	N/A
26. Specimens to lab?	☐	☐	☐
27. Counts performed and correct?	☐	☐	☐
28. Dressings applied?	☐	☐	☐
29. Medication documented? (Circle below)			
• Local anesthetic			
• Heparin			
• Topical hemostatics			
• Antibiotics			
• Contrast dye			
30. Report to postanesthesia care unit?	☐	☐	☐
31. Other generic care plans initiated? (specify)	☐	☐	☐

Document additional nursing actions/generic care plans initiated here:

_____

_____

_____

EVALUATION OF PATIENT OUTCOMES

	Outcome met	Outcome met with additional outcome criteria	Outcome met with revised nursing care plan	Outcome not met	Outcome met applicable to this patient
1. Hemodynamic stability was maintained.	☐	☐	☐	☐	☐
2. Peripheral tissue perfusion was adequate.	☐	☐	☐	☐	☐
3. The patient met outcomes for additional generic care plans as indicated.	☐	☐	☐	☐	☐

Signature: _____ Date: _____

11. A nasogastric tube may be inserted. Document tube insertion.

12. Follow institutional protocol for skin preparation. The area prepared will be wide and include access to the groin. Skin preparation should be gentle. Note the condition of the skin at the preparation site before and after skin preparation procedures. Note any nicks, abrasions, rashes, petechiae, purpura, or hematomas.

13. Maintain patient privacy during all preparatory and draping procedures.

14. Warm blankets may be added to the unexposed body parts to help maintain normothermia.

15. A thermia unit or reflective blanket may additionally be used. Follow institutional protocol for use of the thermia unit.

16. The electrosurgical unit (ESU) may be used. Follow institutional protocol for the safe use of electrical equipment.

17. Assess and document the skin condition at the site of dispersive pad placement before application and after removal.

18. Warming irrigating and intravenous solutions and controlling room temperature help maintain normothermia.

19. Follow institutional protocol for the identification and administration of blood or blood products. Document.

20. Autotransfusion may be used to reinfuse pooled collected blood. Follow institutional protocol.

21. Doppler monitoring may be used for peripheral pulses.

22. The results of pulse monitoring, by palpation and Doppler, should be documented.

23. If a knitted graft is used, it will need to be preclotted before systemic heparinization. Grafts sterilized with ethylene oxide must be adequately aerated. If a glutaraldehyde-stored graft is used, multiple rinsings are required.

24. Follow institutional protocol for documenting implants.

25. Accurately record intake and output (blood loss, urine drainage, nasogastric tube drainage).

26. Follow institutional protocol for and document the preservation and disposition of surgical and laboratory specimens (electrolytes, blood gases, plaque, or aneurysmal sac).

27. Follow institutional protocol for performing and recording sponge, sharp, and instrument counts. Vascular surgery requires vessel loops, umbilical tapes, double-armed sutures with small needles, cannulas, and gauze dissectors; this increases the risk for retained foreign objects.

28. Apply dressings aseptically. Remove excess preparation solution to prevent skin irritation. Apply tape to prevent "tape burns."

29. Record any medications administered intraoperatively. In addition to those listed, consider diuretics and vasopressors.

30. The report to the postanesthesia or intensive care unit should include perioperative patient care outcomes and their achievement.

Carotid Endarterectomy (Fig. 16-2)

1. Perioperative care planning depends on a careful, comprehensive assessment. Consideration needs to be given to the physiologic consequences of the disease process because these patients are often elderly, have additional medical conditions, and experience major stress from surgery. Preoperative nursing assessment is guided by the recognition that the patient may have preexisting cardiovascular, cerebral, and pulmonary impairments secondary to atherosclerosis. The patient will have numerous nursing diagnoses. For this care plan, the diagnosis of *high risk for altered cerebral tissue perfusion* has been selected. A focused neurologic assessment should be done for intraoperative and postoperative comparison. Note the following:
   a. Level of consciousness and mental status (clear, confused, disoriented)
   b. Speech (speaks clearly with normal tones, hoarseness, or slurred speech)
   c. Pupils (size and reaction to light)
   d. Sensory and motor function: movement, reflexes, hand grips
   e. Cranial nerves:
      III—Oculomotor: extraocular eye movements intact
      VII—Facial: face symmetric; ability to smile and clench teeth
      X—Vagus: swallow and gag reflex intact, no bradycardia
      XI—Spinal accessory: able to move arms and shoulders
      XII—Hypoglossal: ablility to protrude tongue, midline; swallow reflex
   A nerve stimulator may be used intraoperatively to identify or assess nerve function. Any alterations (cool, mottled, pale skin or absence of pulses) in the peripheral extremities should also be noted. Results of preoperative angiography should be available in the OR.

2. The patient may be anxious: a calm, efficient manner; minimal environmental stimulation; and simple, understandable explanations will assist with reducing anxiety. Family anxiety

FIG. 16-2
CARE PLAN FOR CAROTID ENDARTERECTOMY

KEY ASSESSMENT POINTS
General physical and mental condition
Presence of chronic health problems
Baseline vital signs
Limitations in mobility
Respiratory status (rate, rhythm, signs of respiratory distress)
Neurologic status (level of consciousness, mental status, speech, pupil size and reaction to light, sensory and motor function in all extremities, cranial nerve function)
Lab values (clotting profiles, blood gases, electrolytes, CBC, BUN, creatinine)
Knowledge assessment (risk factors, disease process, symptoms)
Understanding of procedure/anesthesia/ICU
Understanding of rehabilitation, self-care ability, support systems
Anxiety/fear

NURSING DIAGNOSIS:
All generic nursing diagnoses apply to this patient, with the addition of:
High risk for altered cerebral tissue perfusion related to interruption of arterial blood flow

PATIENT OUTCOMES:
All generic outcomes apply, with the addition of:
The patient will maintain adequate cerebral tissue perfusion as evidenced by intact neurologic status. The patient will:
1. Maintain/regain preoperative level of consciousness
2. Have clear speech
3. Have equal and full muscle strength and mobility
4. Experience no sensory/motor dysfunction
5. Have pupils that are equal and reactive
6. Have vital signs within baseline values

NURSING ACTIONS:

	Yes	No	N/a
1. Physical assessment performed?	☐	☐	☐
2. Psychosocial assessment performed?	☐	☐	☐
3. Verbal verification of operative site and consent signed correctly?	☐	☐	☐
4. Allergies verified and documented?	☐	☐	☐
5. Method of anesthesia explained?	☐	☐	☐
6. Patient understands planned anesthesia?	☐	☐	☐
7. Positioned correctly?	☐	☐	☐
8. Pulses marked?	☐	☐	☐
9. Catheter inserted?	☐	☐	☐
10. Prep per institutional protocol?	☐	☐	☐
11. Privacy maintained?	☐	☐	☐
12. Warm blankets added?	☐	☐	☐
13. ESU used?	☐	☐	☐
14. Dispersive pad site checked?	☐	☐	☐
15. Irrigation/IV solutions warmed?	☐	☐	☐
16. Doppler monitoring?	☐	☐	☐
17. Pulses palpated?	☐	☐	☐
18. Shunt devices used?	☐	☐	☐
19. Carotid stump pressure measured?	☐	☐	☐
20. Embolectomy catheter checked?	☐	☐	☐
21. Intake and output recorded?	☐	☐	☐
22. Specimens to lab?	☐	☐	☐
23. Counts performed and correct?	☐	☐	☐
24. Dressings applied?	☐	☐	☐
25. Medication documented? (circle below)			

- Local anesthetic
- Heparin
- Topical hemostatics
- Antibiotics
- Contrast dye

	Yes	No	N/a
26. Report to PACU?	☐	☐	☐
27. Other generic care plans initiated? (specify)	☐	☐	☐

Document additional nursing actions/generic care plans initiated here:

_____

_____

_____

EVALUATION OF PATIENT OUTCOMES

	Outcome met	Outcome met with additional outcome criteria	Outcome met with revised nursing care plan	Outcome not met	Outcome not applicable to this patient
1. The patient's neurologic status remained intact.	☐	☐	☐	☐	☐
2. The patient met outcomes for additional generic care plans as indicated	☐	☐	☐	☐	☐

Signature: _____ Date: _____

can be reduced through the provision of frequent perioperative nursing reports.

3. Verify operative procedure with the patient's statement and operative consent form. The patient's statement and operative consent form should correspond regarding procedure and site.

4. Verify all known allergies and document on the operative record.

5. General anesthesia or a cervical block may be used. With either method, anesthesia staff will be able to monitor reduced cerebral perfusion and neurologic deficits intraoperatively. With general anesthesia, the electroencephalogram is used; with cervical blocks, the patient is monitored through observation with conscious sedation. Assist anesthesia staff as needed; provide explanations and support to the patient.

6. Determine that the patient has correct knowledge and understanding of the planned anesthesia. Assess for any specific fears, concerns, or anxieties related to anesthesia. Provide explanations and support to the patient.

7. The supine position will be used. The head will be supported; the shoulders may be slightly elevated with a rolled sheet. Antiembolism devices may be applied to the legs. A footboard may be added. Assess the patient's skin and muscle mass; provide extra padding to bony prominences and vulnerable areas (elbows and heels). Maintain correct body alignment; place the safety strap appropriately.

8. Preoperative marking of peripheral pulses assists in easy location for intraoperative monitoring.

9. An indwelling urinary catheter may be inserted. Use aseptic technique for catheter insertion. Keep the drainage bag off the floor; place so it is easily observable. Prevent kinks and stretching of the tubing. Document catheter insertion.

10. Follow institutional protocol for anatomic landmarks for surgical preparation. Skin preparation should be gentle. Note the condition of the skin at the preparation site before and after skin preparation. Note any nicks, abrasions, rashes, petechiae, purpura, and hematomas.

11. Maintain patient privacy during all preparatory and draping procedures.

12. Warm blankets may be added to unexposed body parts to help maintain normothermia.

13. The electrosurgical unit may be used. Follow institutional protocols for safe use of electrical equipment.

14. Assess and document the condition of the skin at the dispersive pad site before application and on pad removal.

15. Warming irrigating and intravenous solutions and controlling the room temperature help maintain normothermia.

16. Doppler monitoring may be used for peripheral pulses.

17. The results of pulse monitoring, by palpation and Doppler, should be documented.

18. A shunt device should be available. Consideration should also be given to the possibility of a vein patch graft if arteriotomy closure appears to produce stenosis. Anticipate extra supply needs and preparation of a vein donor site.

19. Carotid stump pressure may be measured. Anticipate supply needs.

20. An embolectomy catheter may be required. The concentricity of the embolectomy catheter should be checked before catheter passage. Multiple inflations increase pliability and control of the balloon.

21. Accurately record intake and output.

22. Follow institutional protocol for and document the preservation and disposition of surgical and laboratory specimens (plaque, electrolytes, blood gases, and so on).

23. Follow institutional protocol for performing and recording sponge, sharp, and instrument counts. Vascular surgery requires vessel loops, umbilical tapes, double-armed sutures with small needles, cannulas, and gauze dissectors; this increases the risk for retained foreign objects.

24. Apply dressings aseptically. Remove excess preparation solution to prevent skin irritation. Apply tape to prevent "tape burns." Note whether any drains are incorporated in the dressing.

25. Record any medications administered intraoperatively.

26. The report to the postanesthesia or intensive care unit should include perioperative patient care outcomes and their achievement.

Femoral-Popliteal Bypass (Fig. 16-3)

1. Perioperative care planning depends on a careful, comprehensive assessment. Consideration needs to be given to the physiologic consequences of the disease process because these patients are often elderly, have additional medical conditions, and experience major stress from surgery. Preoperative nursing assessment is guided by the recognition that the patient may have preexisting cardiovascular, cerebral, and pulmonary impairments secondary to atherosclerosis. In addition to numerous nursing diagnoses, the patient undergoing femoral-popliteal bypass has *altered tissue perfusion* in the af-

FIG. 16-3
CARE PLAN FOR FEMORAL–POPLITEAL BYPASS

KEY ASSESSMENT POINTS

General physical and mental condition
Presence of chronic health problems
Baseline vital signs
Limitations in mobility
Pain (level/location)
Color, warmth, skin turgor, skin condition (sores, ulcers), pulses, sensation and motor ability, capillary refill, edema in affected extremity
Allergies (specific to contrast material)
Exercise status in affected limb
Recent or sudden change in exercise status or occurrence of pain
Knowledge assessment (risk factors, disease process, symptoms)
Understanding of procedure/anesthesia/ICU
Understanding of rehabilitation, self-care ability, support systems
Anxiety/fear

NURSING DIAGNOSIS:

All generic nursing diagnoses apply to this patient, with the addition of:
Altered peripheral tissue perfusion

PATIENT OUTCOMES:

All generic outcomes apply, with the addition of:
The patient will demonstrate adequate/improved peripheral tissue perfusion as evidenced by:
1. Lower extremities will be pink, warm, and dry
2. Peripheral pulses will be normal/expected
3. Capillary refill will be 2 to 3 seconds
4. Sensation in the lower extremities will be intact
5. Motor ability in the lower extremities will not be compromised
6. Ischemic pain will be relieved

NURSING ACTIONS:

	Yes	No	N/A
1. Physical assessment performed?	☐	☐	☐
2. Psychosocial assessment performed?	☐	☐	☐
3. Verbal verification of operative site and consent signed correctly?	☐	☐	☐
4. Allergies verified and documented?	☐	☐	☐
5. Method of anesthesia explained?	☐	☐	☐
6. Patient understands planned anesthesia?	☐	☐	☐
7. Fluoroscopy table?	☐	☐	☐
8. Positioned correctly?	☐	☐	☐
9. Pulses marked?	☐	☐	☐
10. Catheter inserted?	☐	☐	☐
11. Prep per institutional protocol?	☐	☐	☐
12. Privacy maintained?	☐	☐	☐
13. Warm blankets added?	☐	☐	☐
14. ESU used?	☐	☐	☐
15. Dispersive pad site checked?	☐	☐	☐
16. Irrigation/IV solutions warmed?	☐	☐	☐
17. Doppler monitoring?	☐	☐	☐
18. Pulses palpated?	☐	☐	☐
19. Graft precautions initiated?	☐	☐	☐
20. Implants recorded?	☐	☐	☐
21. Embolectomy catheter checked?	☐	☐	☐
22. Intake and output recorded?	☐	☐	☐
23. Specimens to lab?	☐	☐	☐
24. Counts performed and correct?	☐	☐	☐
25. Dressings applied?	☐	☐	☐
26. Medications documented? (circle below)			

• Local anesthetic
• Heparin
• Topical hemostatics
• Antibiotics
• Contrast dye

	Yes	No	N/A
27. Report to PACU?	☐	☐	☐
28. Other generic care plans initiated? (specify)	☐	☐	☐

Document additional nursing actions/generic care plans initiated here:

_____

_____

_____

_____

EVALUATION OF PATIENT OUTCOMES

	Outcome met	Outcome met with additional outcome criteria	Outcome met with revised nursing care plan	Outcome not met	Outcome not applicable to this patient
1. The patient had adequate/improved peripheral tissue perfusion.	☐	☐	☐	☐	☐
2. The patient met outcomes for additional generic care plans as indicated.	☐	☐	☐	☐	☐

Signature: _____ Date: _____

fected extremity due to chronic insufficient arterial blood flow in the diseased vessels. Assessment should include the integumentary system, noting skin color, temperature, hair distribution, and any ulcerations. Peripheral pulses should be assessed and graded. Sensation, mobility, capillary refill time, and the presence of pain should be noted. *Pain,* related to peripheral ischemia, may be reported as a burning, shocking, or cramping sensation and often intensifies with increased muscle activity and nocturnally, with the patient at rest. *Skin integrity* may be *impaired* from circulatory compromise.

Results of preoperative angiography should be available in the OR. In planning this patient's care, consider the need for intraoperative angiography and the types of grafting possible. In addition to the reversed saphenous vein, an in situ saphenous graft may be performed; instruments for incising the valves will be required. The angioscope may be used to monitor the lysis of valve leaflets; the angioscope, fiberoptic light, irrigation pump, camera, monitor, and videocassette recorder will be required. Because increased fluid volume is administered, patient assessment and collaboration with anesthesia regarding fluid volume status is important. If popliteal patency is compromised, tibial vessels may be used for lower anastomoses; microvascular instruments and sequential grafts may be required. Balloon angioplasty may be planned; appropriate calibers and catheters will be required.

2. The patient may be anxious: a calm, efficient manner; minimal environmental stimulation; and simple, understandable explanations will assist with reducing anxiety. Family anxiety can be reduced through the provision of frequent perioperative nursing reports.

3. Verify operative procedure with patient's statement and operative consent form. Patient's statement and operative consent form should correspond regarding procedure and site.

4. Verify all known allergies and document on the operative record.

5. Regional anesthesia, via an epidural catheter, may be used for the procedure and for postoperative pain control. Postoperatively, the epidural provides for pain relief without sedation and allows the patient to cough more vigorously and effectively. Assist anesthesia with epidural catheter placement; provide explanations and support to the patient.

6. Determine that the patient has correct knowledge and understanding of the planned anesthesia. Assess for any specific fears, concerns, or anxieties related to anesthesia. Provide explanations and support to the patient.

7. Consider the possibility of intraoperative angiography when selecting the OR bed. If this patient is being reoperated for occlusion, intraoperative angiography will be performed; a fluoroscopy table is often used.

8. The supine position will be used; the thigh will be externally rotated and abducted and the knee flexed. Assess the patient's skin and muscle mass; provide extra padding to bony prominences and vulnerable areas (elbows and heels). Maintain correct body alignment; place the safety strap appropriately.

9. Preoperative marking of peripheral pulses assists in easy location for intraoperative monitoring.

10. An indwelling urinary catheter may be inserted. Use aseptic technique for catheter insertion. Keep the drainage bag off the floor; place so it is readily observable. Prevent kinks and stretching of the tubing. Document catheter insertion.

11. Follow institutional protocol for anatomic landmarks for surgical preparation (entire leg and groin will be involved). Skin preparation should be gentle. Note the condition of the skin at the preparation site before and after skin preparation procedures. Note any nicks, abrasions, rashes, petechiae, purpura, hematomas, or ulcerations.

12. Maintain patient privacy during all preparatory and draping procedures.

13. Warm blankets may be added to the unexposed body parts to help maintain normothermia. Reflective blankets or a thermia unit may also be used.

14. The electrosurgical unit may be used. Follow institutional protocols for safe use of electrical equipment.

15. Assess and document the condition of the skin at the dispersive pad site before application and on pad removal. The dispersive pad should be placed on the unaffected extremity.

16. Warming irrigating and intravenous solutions and controlling room temperature help maintain normothermia.

17. Doppler monitoring may be used for peripheral pulses.

18. The results of pulse monitoring, by palpation and Doppler, should be documented.

19. A prosthetic graft may be used. Knitted grafts need to be preclotted before systemic heparinization; ethylene oxide sterilized grafts must be properly aerated; glutaraldehyde stored grafts must be multiply rinsed.

20. Follow institutional protocol for documenting implants.

21. An embolectomy catheter may be used. The concentricity of the embolectomy catheter should be checked before catheter passage. Multiple inflations increase the pliability and control of the balloon.
22. Accurately record intake and output.
23. Follow institutional protocol for and document the preservation and disposition of surgical and laboratory specimens (plaque, electrolytes, blood gases, and so on).
24. Follow institutional protocol for performing and recording sponge, sharp, and instrument counts. Vascular surgery requires vessel loops, umbilical tapes, double-armed sutures with small needles, cannulas, and gauze dissectors; this increases the risk for retained foreign objects.
25. Apply dressings aseptically. Remove excess preparation solution to prevent skin irritation. Note tightness of dressing to avoid occluding blood flow.
26. Record any medications administered intraoperatively.
27. The report to the postanesthesia or intensive care unit should include perioperative patient care outcomes and their achievement.

Thrombectomy/Embolectomy (Fig. 16-4)

1. Perioperative care planning depends on a careful, comprehensive assessment. Consideration needs to be given to the physiologic consequences of the disease process because these patients are often elderly, have additional medical conditions, and experience major stress from surgery. Preoperative nursing assessment is guided by the recognition that the patient may have preexisting cardiovascular, cerebral, and pulmonary impairments secondary to atherosclerosis. The patient undergoing venous thrombectomy or arterial embolectomy may be admitted to the OR on an emergency basis. The extensiveness of the assessment may be limited for the patient with an acutely ischemic extremity. The primary symptom of acute peripheral ischemia is usually severe, unrelenting pain that is aggravated by movement of and pressure on the extremity. There is a gradual loss of sensory and motor function. Pulses distal to the occlusion are usually absent; the extremity is pale and mottled in appearance. In addition to *altered tissue perfusion* in the affected extremity, there may be *anxiety* and *fear*. Modify the care plan for the individual patient. For this care plan, the outcome may not be measurable in the OR; arterial spasm may prevent detection of all of the criteria for determining improved peripheral tissue perfusion. In that event, nursing staff in the postanesthesia care or discharge unit will need to collaborate in determining achievement of the stated outcome. Alterations (cool, mottled, pale skin and absence of pulses) in the affected extremity should be noted. Results of preoperative angiography should be available in the OR.

2. The patient may be anxious: a calm, efficient manner; minimal environmental stimulation; and simple, understandable explanations will help reduce anxiety. Family anxiety can be reduced through the provision of frequent perioperative nursing reports.
3. Verify operative procedure with the patient's statement and operative consent form. The patient's statement and operative consent form should correspond regarding procedure and site.
4. Verify all known allergies and document on the operative record.
5. Local anesthesia may be used. Adhere to institutional protocols for monitoring local anesthesia patients if monitored anesthesia care is not provided by the anesthesia staff.
6. Determine that patient has correct knowledge and understanding of the planned anesthesia. Assess patient for any specific fears, concerns, or anxieties related to anesthesia. Provide explanations and support to the patient.
7. Consider the possibility of intraoperative angiography when selecting the OR bed. If the patient is being reoperated for occlusion, intraoperative angiography will be performed; a fluoroscopy table is usually required. Transfer and positioning should focus on protecting the affected extremity from physical trauma.
8. The supine position will be used. Assess the patient's skin and muscle mass; provide extra padding to bony prominences and vulnerable areas (elbows and heels). Maintain correct body alignment; place the safety strap appropriately.
9. Preoperative marking of peripheral pulses assists in easy location for intraoperative monitoring.
10. Follow institutional protocol for anatomic landmarks for surgical preparation. Skin preparation should be gentle. Note the condition of the skin at the preparation site before and after skin preparation procedures. Note any nicks, abrasions, rashes, petechiae, purpura, hematomas, or ulcerations.
11. Maintain patient privacy during all preparatory and draping procedures.
12. Warm blankets may be added to the unexposed body parts to help maintain normothermia.
13. The electrosurgical unit may be used. Follow institutional protocols for safe use of electrical equipment.

FIG. 16-4
CARE PLAN FOR THROMBECTOMY/EMBOLECTOMY

KEY ASSESSMENT POINTS
General physical and mental condition
Presence of chronic health problems
Baseline vital signs
Limitations in mobility
Pain (onset/location/quality/degree)
"Embolic syndrome"—pain, pallor, paresthesia, pulselessness (no distal arterial pulses), paralysis in affected extremity
Allergies (specific to contrast material)
Results of Homan's sign in affected limb
Lab results (partial thromboplastin time [PTT], Hb, Hct)
Knowledge assessment (risk factors, disease process, symptoms)
Understanding of procedure/anesthesia/ICU
Understanding of rehabilitation, self-care ability, anticoagulant therapy, support systems
Anxiety/fear

NURSING DIAGNOSIS:
All generic nursing diagnoses apply to this patient, with the addition of:
Altered peripheral tissue perfusion

PATIENT OUTCOMES:
All generic outcomes apply, with the addition of:
The patient will demonstrate adequate/improved peripheral tissue perfusion as evidenced by:
1. Lower extremities will be pink, warm, and dry
2. Peripheral pulses will be normal/expected
3. Capillary refill will be 2 to 3 seconds
4. Sensation in the lower extremities will be intact
5. Motor ability in the lower extremities will not be compromised

NURSING ACTIONS:

	Yes	No	N/A
1. Physical assessment performed?	☐	☐	☐
2. Psychosocial assessment performed?	☐	☐	☐
3. Verbal verification of operative site and consent signed correctly?	☐	☐	☐
4. Allergies verified and documented?	☐	☐	☐
5. Method of anesthesia explained?	☐	☐	☐
6. Patient understands planned anesthesia?	☐	☐	☐
7. Fluoroscopy table?	☐	☐	☐
8. Positioned correctly?	☐	☐	☐
9. Pulses marked?	☐	☐	☐
10. Prep per institutional protocol?	☐	☐	☐
11. Privacy maintained?	☐	☐	☐
12. Warm blankets added?	☐	☐	☐
13. ESU used?	☐	☐	☐
14. Dispersive pad site checked?	☐	☐	☐
15. Irrigation/IV solutions warmed?	☐	☐	☐
16. Doppler monitoring?	☐	☐	☐
17. Pulses palpated?	☐	☐	☐
18. Embolectomy catheter checked?	☐	☐	☐
19. Specimens to lab?	☐	☐	☐
20. Counts performed and correct?	☐	☐	☐
21. Dressings applied?	☐	☐	☐

22. Medications documented (circle below)
 • Local anesthetic
 • Heparin
 • Topical hemostatics
 • Antibiotics
 • Contrast dye

	Yes	No	N/A
23. Report to PACU?	☐	☐	☐
24. Other generic care plans initiated? (specify)	☐	☐	☐

Document additional nursing actions/generic care plans initiated here:

_____

_____

_____

EVALUATION OF PATIENT OUTCOMES
1. Peripheral tissue perfusion was improved.
2. The patient met outcomes for additional generic care plans as indicated.

	Outcome met	Outcome met with additional outcome criteria	Outcome met with revised nursing care plan	Outcome not met	Outcome not applicable to this patient
1.	☐	☐	☐	☐	☐
2.	☐	☐	☐	☐	☐

Signature: _____ Date: _____

14. Assess and document the condition of the skin at the dispersive pad site before application and on removal. The dispersive pad should be placed on the unaffected extremity.

15. Warming irrigating and intravenous solutions and controlling room temperature help maintain normothermia.

16. Doppler monitoring may be used for peripheral pulses.

17. The results of pulse monitoring, by palpation and Doppler, should be documented.

18. The concentricity of the embolectomy catheter should be checked before catheter passage. Multiple inflations increase pliability and control of the balloon.

19. Follow institutional protocol and document the preservation and disposition of surgical and laboratory specimens (thrombus, electrolytes, blood gases).

20. Follow institutional protocol for performing and recording sponge, sharp, and instrument counts. Vascular surgery requires vessel loops, umbilical tapes, double-armed sutures with small needles, cannulas, and gauze dissectors; this increases the risk for retained foreign objects.

21. Apply dressings aseptically. Remove excess preparation solution to prevent skin irritation. Note tightness of dressing to avoid occluding blood flow.

22. Record any medications administered intraoperatively.

23. The report to the postanesthesia or intensive care unit should include perioperative patient care outcomes and their achievement.

Laser-Assisted Angioplasty (Fig. 16-5)

1. Perioperative care planning depends on a careful, comprehensive assessment. Consideration needs to be given to the physiologic consequences of the disease process because these patients are often elderly, have additional medical conditions, and experience major stress from surgery. Preoperative nursing assessment is guided by the recognition that the patient may have preexisting cardiovascular, cerebral, and pulmonary impairments secondary to atherosclerosis. The patient undergoing laser-assisted angioplasty may have numerous nursing diagnoses. For this care plan, the diagnosis of *pain* (acute discomfort) related to enforced immobility on a hard OR bed has been selected. To help the patient minimize this discomfort, it is necessary to determine if there are any preexisting limitations to mobility. These should be considered in positioning. Determine how the patient deals with discomfort (for example, music, relaxation techniques, guided imagery, or meditation); assist and encourage the patient to use these. Contrast dye will be used; check for patient allergies. Coordination is necessary for this surgical procedure. Equipment needs (angioscope, laser, transluminal balloon catheter and accessories, intraoperative arteriograms, and image intensifier) require team planning. Pulses should be assessed and graded. Any alterations in the lower extremities (cool, mottled, pale skin and absence of pulses) should be noted.

2. The patient may be anxious: a calm, efficient manner; minimal environmental stimulation; and simple, understandable explanations will help the patient reduce anxiety. Family anxiety can be reduced through the provision of frequent perioperative nursing reports.

3. Verify operative procedure with patient's statement and consent form. The patient's statement and operative consent form should correspond regarding procedure and site. With calcified lesions, this consent should include provisions for an in situ bypass if the laser fails and for a vein graft if there is vessel perforation.

4. Verify all known allergies and document on the operative record.

5. Regional anesthesia, spinal or epidural, may be used.

6. Determine that patient has correct knowledge and understanding of the planned anesthesia. Assess for any specific fears, concerns, or anxieties related to anesthesia. Patients may need reassurance and explanations about the anesthesia and the sensations they may expect.

7. The fluoroscopy table is needed.

8. The supine position will be used. Assess the patient's skin and muscle mass; provide extra padding to bony prominences and vulnerable areas (elbows and heels). Maintain correct body alignment; place the safety strap appropriately.

9. Preoperative marking of peripheral pulses assists with easy location for intraoperative monitoring.

10. An indwelling urinary catheter may be inserted if one is not present. Use aseptic technique for catheter insertion. Keep the drainage bag off the floor; place so it is easily observable. Prevent kinks and stretching of the tubing. Document catheter insertion.

11. Follow institutional protocol for anatomic landmarks for the surgical preparation. The area will be wide and involve both legs. Skin preparation should be gentle. Note the condition of the skin at the preparation site before and after skin preparation procedures. Note any nicks, abra-

FIG. 16-5
CARE PLAN FOR LASER-ASSISTED ANGIOPLASTY

KEY ASSESSMENT POINTS

General physical and mental condition
Presence of chronic health problems
Baseline vital signs
Limitations in mobility
Pain (intermittent claudication/ischemic rest pain)
Color, warmth, skin turgor, skin condition (ulcerations), pulses, sensation and motor ability, capillary refill, edema in affected extremity
Allergies (specific to contrast material)
Exercise status in affected limb
Recent or sudden change in exercise status or occurrence of pain
Knowledge assessment (risk factors, disease process, symptoms)
Understanding of procedure/anesthesia/ICU
Understanding of rehabilitation, self-care ability, anticoagulant therapy, support systems
Anxiety/fear

NURSING DIAGNOSIS:

All generic nursing diagnoses apply to this patient, with the addition of:
Pain (acute discomfort)

PATIENT OUTCOMES:

All generic outcomes apply, with the addition of:
The patient will demonstrate minimized pain and discomfort related to immobility as evidenced by the patient's ability to:
1. Verbalize understanding of reasons for enforced mobility
2. Maintain immobility
3. Verbalize discomfort to perioperative nurse
4. Be assisted with comfort, relaxation measures

NURSING ACTIONS:

	Yes	No	N/A
1. Physical assessment performed?	☐	☐	☐
2. Psychosocial assessment performed?	☐	☐	☐
3. Verbal verification of operative site and consent signed correctly?	☐	☐	☐
4. Allergies verified and documented?	☐	☐	☐
5. Method of anesthesia explained?	☐	☐	☐
6. Patient understands planned anesthesia?	☐	☐	☐
7. Fluoroscopy table?	☐	☐	☐
8. Positioned correctly?	☐	☐	☐
9. Pulses marked?	☐	☐	☐
10. Catheter inserted?	☐	☐	☐
11. Prep per institutional protocol?	☐	☐	☐
12. Privacy maintained?	☐	☐	☐
13. Warm blankets added?	☐	☐	☐
14. Laser safety precautions initiated?	☐	☐	☐
15. X-ray personnel available?	☐	☐	☐
16. Radiation safety precautions initiated?	☐	☐	☐
17. Medications labeled/documented?	☐	☐	☐
18. Irrigation/IV solutions warmed?	☐	☐	☐
19. Doppler monitoring?	☐	☐	☐
20. Pulses palpated?	☐	☐	☐
21. Graft precautions initiated?	☐	☐	☐
22. Implants recorded?	☐	☐	☐
23. Angioplasty catheter checked?	☐	☐	☐
24. Input and output recorded?	☐	☐	☐
25. Specimens to lab?	☐	☐	☐
26. Counts performed and correct?	☐	☐	☐
27. Dressings applied?	☐	☐	☐

28. Medications documented (circle below)
   • Local anesthetic
   • Heparin
   • Topical hemostatics
   • Antibiotics
   • Contrast dye

	Yes	No	N/A
29. Report to PACU?	☐	☐	☐
30. Other generic care plans initiated? (specify)	☐	☐	☐

Document additional nursing actions/generic care plans initiated here:

_____

_____

_____

EVALUATION OF PATIENT OUTCOMES

	Outcome met	Outcome met with additional outcome criteria	Outcome met with revised nursing care plan	Outcome not met	Outcome not applicable to this patient
1. The patient's discomfort was minimized.	☐	☐	☐	☐	☐
2. The patient met outcomes for additional generic care plans as indicated.	☐	☐	☐	☐	☐

Signature: _____ Date: _____

sions, rashes, petechiae, purpura, hematomas, or ulcerations.

12. Maintain patient privacy during all preparatory and draping procedures.

13. Warm blankets may be added to the unexposed body parts to help maintain normothermia.

14. Follow institutional protocols for laser safety related to personnel, the unit, the patient, and the environment. Document the size of the laser probe and settings.

15. X-ray personnel need to be available.

16. Follow institutional protocols for radiation safety for personnel and the patient.

17. All medications on the sterile field (heparinized saline for irrigation and contrast dye for angiography) should be correctly labeled. Document intraoperative medications.

18. Warming irrigating and intravenous solutions and controlling room temperature help maintain normothermia.

19. Doppler monitoring may be used for peripheral pulses.

20. The results of pulse monitoring, by palpation and Doppler, should be documented.

21. A bypass graft may be necessary. If a knitted graft is used, it will need to be preclotted before systemic heparinization. Grafts sterilized with ethylene oxide must be adequately aerated. If a glutaraldehyde-stored graft is used, multiple rinsings are required.

22. Follow institutional protocol for documenting implants.

23. The concentricity of the angioplasty catheter should be checked before insertion.

24. Accurately record intake and output and amount of perfusate flush.

25. Follow institutional protocol for and document the preservation and disposition of surgical and laboratory specimens (electrolytes, blood gases, and so on).

26. Follow institutional protocol for performing and recording all sponge, sharp, and instrument counts. Vascular surgery requires vessel loops, umbilical tapes, double-armed sutures with small needles, cannulas, and gauze dissectors; this increases the risk for retained foreign objects.

27. Apply dressings aseptically. Remove excess preparation solution to prevent skin irritation. Note tightness of dressing to avoid occluding blood flow.

28. Record any medications administered intraoperatively.

29. The report to the postanesthesia or intensive care unit should include perioperative patient care outcomes and their achievement.

Arteriovenous Access Procedures (Fig. 16-6)

1. Perioperative care planning depends on a careful, comprehensive assessment. Consideration needs to be given to the physiologic consequences of the disease process because these patients are often in acute renal failure, have associated medical conditions, and experience major stress from surgery. Preoperative nursing assessment is guided by the recognition that the patient in acute renal failure will have numerous nursing diagnoses. These patients often have *altered nutritional status, impaired skin integrity,* and *impaired mobility.* All of these factors, along with the possible insertion of a prosthetic graft, contribute to the *high risk for infection* of these patients. Arteriovenous access may be accomplished by creating a direct arteriovenous fistula between the radial artery and the cephalic vein or by using a prosthetic graft or saphenous vein to join the brachial artery and cephalic vein.

2. The patient may be anxious: a calm, efficient manner; minimal environmental stimulation; and simple, understandable explanations will help reduce anxiety. Family anxiety can be reduced through the provision of frequent perioperative nursing reports.

3. Verify operative procedure with the patient's statement and operative consent form. The patient's statement and operative consent form should correspond regarding procedure and site.

4. Verify all known allergies and document on the operative record.

5. Local or regional anesthesia will likely be used. Assess for any specific fears, concerns, or anxieties related to anesthesia. Patients may need reassurance and explanations about the anesthesia and the sensations they may expect. Verify that the patient has emptied the bladder. Follow institutional protocol for perioperative monitoring of the patient receiving local anesthesia.

6. The supine position will be used; it may be modified to a "lawn chair" position with moderate Trendelenburg's to increase patient comfort. A hand table or armboard will be used to position the upper extremity; prevent hyperabduction of the arm. Assess the patient's skin and muscle mass; provide extra padding to bony prominences and vulnerable areas (elbows and heels). To help the patient minimize discomfort from enforced immobility, determine preexisting limitations; consider these in positioning and maintain correct body alignment. Place the safety strap appropriately. Assess and encourage the patient to use personally effective methods

FIG. 16-6
CARE PLAN FOR ARTERIOVENOUS ACCESS PROCEDURES

KEY ASSESSMENT POINTS
General physical and mental condition
Cause of renal failure
Presence of chronic health problems
Baseline vital signs
Limitations in mobility
Nutritional status
Skin integrity, color, warmth, turgor, pulses, sensation, capillary refill in affected extremity
Lab values (PTT; blood gases; electrolytes, especially potassium level; CBC; BUN; creatinine clearance; serum creatinine)
Allergies (specific to local anesthetics)
Knowledge assessment (infection risk factors, disease process, symptoms)
Understanding of procedure/anesthesia/ICU
Understanding of rehabilitation, access site care, self-care ability, dialysis protocols, signs of graft occlusion, support systems

Anxiety/fear
Coping mechanisms

NURSING DIAGNOSIS:
All generic nursing diagnoses apply to this patient, with the addition of:
High risk for infection

PATIENT OUTCOMES:
All generic outcomes apply, with the addition of:
The patient will be free of infection at the access site as evidenced by:
1. Temperature will be within normal limits
2. WBC and differential will be within normal range
3. There will be no redness or drainage at access site

NURSING ACTIONS:

	Yes	No	N/A
1. Physical assessment performed?	☐	☐	☐
2. Psychosocial assessment performed?	☐	☐	☐
3. Verbal verification of operative site and consent signed correctly?	☐	☐	☐
4. Allergies verified and documented?	☐	☐	☐
5. Method of anesthesia explained?	☐	☐	☐
6. Positioned correctly?	☐	☐	☐
7. Pulses marked?	☐	☐	☐
8. Prep per institutional protocol?	☐	☐	☐
9. Privacy maintained?	☐	☐	☐
10. Warm blankets added?	☐	☐	☐
11. ESU used?	☐	☐	☐
12. Dispersive pad site checked?	☐	☐	☐
13. Irrigation/IV solutions warmed?	☐	☐	☐
14. Doppler monitoring?	☐	☐	☐
15. Pulses palpated?	☐	☐	☐
16. Graft precautions initiated?	☐	☐	☐
17. Implants recorded?	☐	☐	☐
18. Prosthetic sterility checked?	☐	☐	☐
19. Patient teaching performed?	☐	☐	☐
20. Counts performed and correct?	☐	☐	☐
21. Dressings applied?	☐	☐	☐

22. Medications documented (circle below)
- Local anesthetic
- Heparin
- Topical hemostatics
- Antibiotics
- Contrast dye

	Yes	No	N/A
23. Report to PACU?	☐	☐	☐
24. Other generic care plans initiated? (specify)	☐	☐	☐

Document additional nursing actions/generic care plans initiated here:

_____

_____

_____

EVALUATION OF PATIENT OUTCOMES

	Outcome met	Outcome met with additional outcome criteria	Outcome met with revised nursing care plan	Outcome not met	Outcome not applicable to this patient
1. The patient showed no signs or symptoms of infection at the access site.	☐	☐	☐	☐	☐
2. The patient met outcomes for additional generic care plans as indicated.	☐	☐	☐	☐	☐

Signature: _____ Date: _____

(music, relaxation techniques, guided imagery, and meditation) to help deal with discomfort.

7. Preoperative marking of peripheral pulses assists in easy location for intraoperative monitoring.

8. Follow institutional protocol for anatomic landmarks for surgical preparation. Note the condition of the skin at the preparation site before and after skin preparation procedures. Note any nicks, abrasions, rashes, petechiae, purpura, hematomas, or ulcerations.

9. Maintain patient privacy during all preparatory and draping procedures.

10. Warm blankets may be added to the unexposed body parts to help maintain normothermia.

11. The electrosurgical unit may be used. Follow institutional protocol for the safe use of electrical equipment.

12. Assess and document the skin condition at the site of dispersive pad placement before application and after removal.

13. Warming irrigating and intravenous solutions and controlling room temperature help maintain normothermia.

14. Doppler monitoring may be used for peripheral pulses.

15. The results of pulse monitoring, by palpation and Doppler, should be documented.

16. A bypass graft may be necessary. If a knitted graft is used, it will need to be preclotted before systemic heparinization. Grafts sterilized with ethylene oxide must be adequately aerated. If a glutaraldehyde-stored graft is used, multiple rinsings are required.

17. Follow institutional protocol for documenting implants.

18. Note the integrity of the sterile package, sterile monitors, and expiration date before opening the shunt. There should be minimal handling of the prosthesis before insertion.

19. Patient teaching may include instructions on the care of the access graft: avoid restrictive clothing or jewelry on the affected extremity; avoid any pressure or application of cold to the access site; cushion the affected extremity and protect it from injury; keep a sterile dressing over the site; palpate for thrills over the site each day; do not take blood pressure or draw blood samples from the extremity with the access site; notify the physician if signs of infection or clotting at the access site are noted (explain these signs).

20. Follow institutional protocol for performing and recording all sponge, sharp, and instrument counts. Vascular surgery requires vessel loops, umbilical tapes, double-armed sutures with small needles, cannulas, and gauze dissectors; this increases the risk for retained foreign objects. Apply dressings aseptically. Remove excess preparation solution to prevent skin irritation. Dressings may be marked so the nurse in the discharge unit can identify the arterial and venous sites. Note tightness of dressing to avoid occluding blood flow.

21. Record any medications administered intraoperatively.

22. The report to the postanesthesia or intensive care unit should include perioperative patient care outcomes and their achievement.

Vena Cava Filter Insertion (Fig. 16-7)

1. Perioperative care planning depends on a careful, comprehensive assessment. Consideration needs to be given to the physiologic consequences of the disease process with patients undergoing vascular surgery. Circulatory compromise, inadequate tissue perfusion, and additional medical conditions may be present. The patient undergoing vena cava filter insertion, due to recurrent pulmonary emboli or trauma, may have numerous nursing diagnoses. For this care plan the diagnosis *high risk for altered pulmonary tissue perfusion* has been selected. The vena cava filter is inserted to prevent distal embolization of intraluminal thrombi. Potential complications include pulmonary embolism, myocardial infarction, and cerebrovascular accident. The patient may have received anticoagulant therapy, fibrinolytic agents, or antiplatelet agents. Assess the patient's vital signs, heart and lung sounds, and cardiac rhythm. Note the presence of any chest or abdominal pain, dyspnea, or cough. Check peripheral pulses and the color and temperature of the skin. Numerous laboratory results may be on the patient's medical record; check these for abnormalities. The patient may also have *pain* related to the inflammatory process. There may be *altered peripheral tissue perfusion* related to the interruption in venous flow, *impaired gas exchange* related to embolization of the thrombus, and *altered skin integrity* related to venous stasis. Modify the care plan for the individual patient.

2. The patient may be anxious: a calm, efficient manner; minimal environmental stimulation; and simple, understandable explanations will help reduce anxiety. Family anxiety can be reduced through the provision of frequent perioperative nursing reports.

3. Verify operative procedure with the patient's statement and operative consent form. The pa-

FIG. 16-7
CARE PLAN FOR VENA CAVA FILTER INSERTION

KEY ASSESSMENT POINTS
General physical and mental condition
Presence of additional health problems
Baseline vital signs
Limitations in mobility
Pain (sudden, severe, substernal)
Skin integrity, color, warmth, turgor, pulses, sensation, capillary refill in lower extremities
Lab values (clotting profiles, blood gases; lactate dehydrogenase [LDH], bilirubin)
Diagnostic study results (chest x-ray, ECG, lung scan, pulmonary angiogram)
Respiratory status (rate, rhythm, quality, dyspnea, shortness of breath, cough, lung sounds for decreased sounds, crackles, pleural friction rub)
Cardiac status (rate, rhythm, results of auscultation)
Knowledge assessment (infection risk factors, disease process, symptoms)
Understanding of procedure/anesthesia/ICU

Understanding of rehabilitation, anticoagulant therapy, self-care ability, use of antiembolism hose, support systems
Anxiety/fear
Coping mechanisms

NURSING DIAGNOSIS:
All generic nursing diagnoses apply to this patient, with the addition of:
High risk for altered pulmonary tissue perfusion

PATIENT OUTCOMES:
All generic outcomes apply, with the addition of:
The patient will demonstrate adequate pulmonary tissue perfusion as evidenced by:
1. Heart rate will remain greater than 60 and less than 100 beats per minute
2. S1 and S2 heart sounds will be normal
3. No chest pain, abdominal pain, cough, or dyspnea
4. Lung fields will remain clear to auscultation

NURSING ACTIONS:

	Yes	No	N/A
1. Physical assessment performed?	☐	☐	☐
2. Psychosocial assessment performed?	☐	☐	☐
3. Verbal verification of operative site and consent signed correctly?	☐	☐	☐
4. Allergies verified and documented?	☐	☐	☐
5. Method of anesthesia explained?	☐	☐	☐
6. Fluoroscopy table?	☐	☐	☐
7. Positioned correctly?	☐	☐	☐
8. Pulses marked?	☐	☐	☐
9. Prep per institutional protocol?	☐	☐	☐
10. Privacy maintained?	☐	☐	☐
11. Warm blankets added?	☐	☐	☐
12. ESU used?	☐	☐	☐
13. Dispersive pad site checked?	☐	☐	☐
14. Irrigation/IV solutions warmed?	☐	☐	☐
15. Doppler monitoring?	☐	☐	☐
16. Pulses palpated?	☐	☐	☐
17. Implants recorded?	☐	☐	☐
18. Input and output recorded?	☐	☐	☐
19. Specimen to lab?	☐	☐	☐
20. Counts performed and correct?	☐	☐	☐
21. Dressings applied?	☐	☐	☐
22. Medications documented (circle below) • Local anesthetic • Heparin • Topical hemostatics • Antibiotics • Contrast dye			
23. Report to PACU?	☐	☐	☐
24. Other generic care plans initiated? (specify)	☐	☐	☐

Document additional nursing actions/generic care plans initiated here:

_____

_____

_____

EVALUATION OF PATIENT OUTCOMES

1. Pulmonary tissue perfusion was adequate.
2. The patient met outcomes for additional generic care plans as indicated.

	Outcome met	Outcome met with additional outcome criteria	Outcome met with revised nursing care plan	Outcome not met	Outcome not applicable to this patient
1.	☐	☐	☐	☐	☐
2.	☐	☐	☐	☐	☐

Signature: _____ Date: _____

tient's statement and operative consent form should correspond regarding procedure and site.

4. Verify all known allergies and document on the operative record.
5. Local or monitored anesthesia may be used. Assess for any specific fears, concerns, or anxieties related to anesthesia. Patients need reassurance and explanations about the anesthesia and the sensations they may expect. Follow institutional protocol for perioperative monitoring of the patient receiving local anesthesia. Verify that the patient has emptied his or her bladder.
6. The fluoroscopy table is needed.
7. The supine position will be used. If jugular insertion is used, the head will be turned and supported; protect the dependent ear and eyes. Assess the patient's skin and muscle mass; provide extra padding to bony prominences and vulnerable areas (elbows and heels). To help minimize discomfort from the fluoroscopy table and enforced immobility, determine if there are any preexisting limitations to mobility; consider these in patient positioning. Maintain correct body alignment and place the safety strap appropriately. Assess and encourage the patient to use personally effective methods (music, relaxation techniques, guided imagery, or meditation) to assist in dealing with discomfort.
8. Preoperative marking of peripheral pulses assists in easy location for intraoperative monitoring.
9. Follow institutional protocol for anatomic landmarks for surgical preparation. The area will depend on whether a jugular or femoral insertion site is used. Skin preparation should be gentle. Note the condition of the skin at the preparation site before and after skin preparation procedures. Note any nicks, abrasions, rashes, petechiae, purpura, or hematomas.
10. Maintain patient privacy during all preparatory and draping procedures.
11. Warm blankets may be added to the unexposed body parts to help maintain normothermia.
12. The electrosurgical unit may be used. Follow institutional protocol for the safe use of electrical equipment.
13. Assess and document the skin condition at the site of dispersive pad placement before application and after pad removal.
14. Warming irrigating and intravenous solutions and controlling the room temperature help maintain normothermia.
15. Doppler monitoring may be used for peripheral pulses.
16. The results of pulse monitoring, by palpation and Doppler, should be documented.
17. X-ray personnel are required. Follow institutional protocol for radiation safety of personnel and the patient.
18. Follow institutional protocol for documenting implants.
19. Accurately record intake and output.
20. Follow institutional protocol for and document the preservation and disposition of surgical and laboratory specimens (electrolytes, blood gases, and so on).
21. Follow institutional protocol for performing and recording all sponge, sharp, and instrument counts.
22. Apply dressings aseptically. Remove excess preparation solution to prevent skin irritation. Apply tape to prevent "tape burns."
23. Record any medications administered intraoperatively.
24. The report to the postanesthesia or intensive care unit should include perioperative patient care outcomes and their achievement.

Varicose Vein Ligation (Fig. 16-8)

1. Perioperative care planning depends on a careful, comprehensive assessment. Varicose vein ligation is performed either due to the physiologic consequences of associated chronic venous stasis or for primary cosmetic reasons. Cosmetically, varicose veins are psychologically disturbing and often cause the patient to have *situational low self-esteem*. Physiologic consequences of the disease process can cause an increase in transmural venous pressure, edema, impaired cellular nutrition, and eventual tissue damage. Any patient undergoing varicose vein ligation has *altered peripheral tissue perfusion* in the affected extremity. Clinical assessment includes inspection of the extremity for color, temperature, edema, and any alterations in sensation. If venous stasis has been chronic, there may be increased skin pigmentation or ulcerations around the ankle of the affected extremity. Assess the patient's preoperative pain level (aching or heaviness) in the affected extremity. Pulses in the affected extremity should be present and there should be no loss of motor ability unless edema is severe.
2. The patient may be anxious: a calm, efficient manner; minimal environmental stimulation; and simple, understandable explanations will help reduce anxiety. Family anxiety can be reduced through the provision of frequent perioperative nursing reports.
3. Verify operative procedure with the patient's statement and operative consent form. The pa-

FIG. 16-8
CARE PLAN FOR VARICOSE VEIN LIGATION

KEY ASSESSMENT POINTS

General physical and mental condition
Presence of additional health problems
Baseline vital signs
Limitations in mobility
Pain (leg cramps when standing)
Skin integrity, color, warmth, sensation, in affected extremity
Edema, heaviness in affected extremity
Dilation of leg veins
Knowledge assessment (infection risk factors, disease process, symptoms)
Understanding of procedure/anesthesia/ICU
Understanding of rehabilitation, signs and symptoms of wound infection and bleeding, self-care ability, use of antiembolism hose, support systems
Anxiety/fear
Coping mechanisms

NURSING DIAGNOSIS:

All generic nursing diagnoses apply to this patient, with the addition of:
Altered peripheral tissue perfusion

PATIENT OUTCOMES:

The patient will demonstrate adequate peripheral tissue perfusion as evidenced by:
1. Lower extremities will be warm and dry to touch; pink
2. Peripheral pulses will be normal/expected
3. Capillary refill will be 2 to 3 seconds
4. Sensation in the lower extremities will be intact
5. Motor ability in the lower extremities will not be compromised

NURSING ACTIONS:

	Yes	No	N/A
1. Physical assessment performed?	☐	☐	☐
2. Psychosocial assessment performed?	☐	☐	☐
3. Verbal verification of operative site and consent signed correctly?	☐	☐	☐
4. Allergies verified and documented?	☐	☐	☐
5. Method of anesthesia explained?	☐	☐	☐
6. Positioned correctly?	☐	☐	☐
7. Prep per institutional protocol?	☐	☐	☐
8. Privacy maintained?	☐	☐	☐
9. Warm blankets added?	☐	☐	☐
10. ESU used?	☐	☐	☐
11. Dispersive pad site checked?	☐	☐	☐
12. Irrigation/IV solutions warmed?	☐	☐	☐
13. Specimen to lab?	☐	☐	☐
14. Counts performed and correct?	☐	☐	☐
15. Dressings applied?	☐	☐	☐
16. Medications documented (circle below)			
• Local anesthetic			
• Heparin			
• Topical hemostatics			
• Antibiotics			
• Contrast dye			
17. Report to PACU?	☐	☐	☐
18. Other generic care plans initiated? (specify)	☐	☐	☐

Document additional nursing actions/generic care plans initiated here:

_____

_____

_____

EVALUATION OF PATIENT OUTCOMES

	Outcome met	Outcome met with additional outcome criteria	Outcome met with revised nursing care plan	Outcome not met	Outcome not applicable to this patient
1. Peripheral tissue perfusion was improved.	☐	☐	☐	☐	☐
2. The patient met outcomes for additional generic care plans as indicated.	☐	☐	☐	☐	☐

Signature: _____ Date: _____

tient's statement and operative consent form should correspond regarding procedure and site.

4. Verify all known allergies and document on the operative record.

5. Regional or general anesthesia may be used. Assist anesthesia staff with the administration of anesthesia; assess patient for any specific fears, concerns, or anxieties related to anesthesia. Patients need reassurance and explanations about the anesthesia and any sensations they may expect.

6. The supine position, with the legs slightly abducted, will be used. (If the lesser saphenous veins are being stripped, prone position may be necessary.) Assess the patient's skin and muscle mass; provide extra padding to bony prominences and vulnerable areas (elbows and heels). Maintain correct body alignment; place the safety strap appropriately.

7. Follow institutional protocol for anatomic landmarks for surgical preparation. Skin preparation should be gentle. Note the condition of the skin at the preparation site before and after skin preparation procedures. Note any nicks, rashes, petechiae, purpura, or hematomas.

8. Maintain patient privacy during all preparatory and draping procedures.

9. Warm blankets may be added to the unexposed body parts to help maintain normothermia.

10. The electrosurgical unit may be used. Follow institutional protocols for safe use of electrical equipment. Dispersive pad should be applied to the unaffected extremity.

11. Assess and document the skin condition at the dispersive pad site before application and on removal.

12. Warming irrigating and intravenous solutions and controlling the room temperature help maintain normothermia.

13. Follow institutional protocol for and document the preservation and disposition of surgical specimens. Use universal precautions with any material received from the sterile field.

14. Follow institutional protocol for performing and recording all sponge, sharp, and instrument counts.

15. Apply incision dressings aseptically. Remove excess preparation solution to prevent skin irritation.

16. Apply compressive leg bandages. These are of paramount importance to preventing hematoma formation. The figure-of-eight wrapping technique delivers more pressure effectively, stays

on longer, and produces fewer tourniquet effects.

17. Record any medications administered intraoperatively.

18. The report to the postanesthesia or intensive care unit should include perioperative patient care outcomes and their achievement.

References

Agency for Health Care Policy and Research (AHCPR). (1994). *Magnetic resonance angiography—vascular and flow imaging.* AHCPR Publication No. 95-0004. Rockville, MD: The Agency.

Bergan JJ. (1991). What's new in peripheral vascular surgery. *ACS Bulletin, 76*(1), 63-65.

Bichat X. (1814). *Desault's surgery.* Philadelphia: Thomas Dobson.

Borgini L & Almgren CC. (1990). Peripheral vascular angioscopy. *AORN Journal, 52,* 543-550.

Bowers AC & Thompson JM (1992). *Clinical manual of health assessment.* (4th ed.). St. Louis: Mosby.

Capasso VC & Coté K. (1993). The management of patients undergoing arterial reconstructive surgery. *Medsurg Nursing, 2*(1), 11-20.

Chase CR. (1994). Development of a case management plan for aortoiliac bypass graft surgery patients. *Seminars in Perioperative Nursing, 3*(1), 16-21.

Engler MB & Engler MM (1994). Cardiovascular nurse interventionist: An emerging new role. *Nursing & Health Care, 15*(4), 198-202.

Fogarty AM (1991). Angioscopy: New developments in vascular surgery. *AORN Journal, 53*(3), 725-728.

Holloway NM, (1993). *Medical surgical care planning.* Springhouse, PA: Springhouse.

Johnson G. (1994). What's new in vascular surgery. *ACS Bulletin, 78*(3), 27-30.

Mannick JA, (1993). What's new in peripheral vascular surgery. *ACS Bulletin, 78*(3), 27-30.

Martin LC, et al. (1994). Management of lower extremity arterial injuries. *Journal of Trauma, 37,* 591-599.

Mathias JM (1994). Aortic aneurysm repair made less invasive. *OR Manager, 10*(9), 22-23.

Moss MT (1993). Outcomes management in perioperative nursing services. *Nursing Economics, 11,*364-369.

Naslund T. (1994). New aneurysm repair tested. *The Vanderbilt University Medical Center Reporter, 6*(vol. 1).

Polk HC Jr, Gardner TR, & Stone HL. (1993). *Basic Surgery.* St. Louis: Quality Medical Publishing.

Porter JM, (1991). Chronic lower-extremity ischemia. *Current problems in surgery, 28*(1), St. Louis: Mosby.

Puntillo K & Weiss SJ. (1994). Pain: Its mediators and associated morbidity in critically ill cardiovascular surgical patients. *Nursing Research, 43*(1), 31-36.

Schwartz SI, Shires CR, & Spencer LW. (1989). *Principles of surgery.* New York: McGraw-Hill.

Smeltzer SC & Bare BC. (1992). *Brunner and Suddarth's textbook of medical-surgical nursing* (7th ed.). Philadelphia: JB Lippincott.

Veith FJ. (1989). *Current critical problems in vascular surgery.* St. Louis: Quality Medical Publishing.

Zickler P. (1995). Balloon catheters. *Medical Device Research Report, 2*(1), 8-11.

Chapter 17

Plastic and Reconstructive Surgery

Sandra Smyth

We are indebted to the ancient physicians for the ingenious idea of applying, to the cure of the harelip, that property of living animal parts, by virtue of which a recent division, whose edges are brought in contact, unites and disappears at the end of a certain time. From this general principle, the treatment of all simple wounds proceeds; upon it rests the operation now to be examined . . . the cleft [of the harelip] must be reduced to the state of a recent division . . . the bloody edges of the division must be brought together and kept in contact. All surgeons have agreed upon this double indication; but they have not all pursued the same route to accomplish it.

Some have had recourse to cauteries of different kinds, and to active stimulants, to reduce the edges to a state of rawness. Others . . . have employed cutting instruments . . . in the approximation of the raw edges . . . dry or bloody sutures . . . have engaged the attention of practitioners.

BICHAT, 1814

"Plastic surgery is the surgical subspecialty concentrating on the restoration of function and form to body structures damaged by trauma, the aging process, disease processes . . . and congenital defects." (Black, 1993) The term "plastic" comes from the Greek "plastikos," to sculpt or mold.

HISTORICAL CONSIDERATIONS

Many advances in surgery depend on previous discoveries. Throughout history, humans have been concerned with restoration of wounded, disfigured, or unsightly parts of their bodies. The earliest evidence of plastic and reconstructive surgery appeared in Hindu medical records that described reconstruction of the amputated nose. In 600 BC, noses were amputated from criminals and adulterous women. Reconstruction was practiced by potters or bricklayers known as the Koomas. Noses were reconstructed using forehead flaps. In the sixteenth century Gaspara Tagliacozzi described the use of a delayed skin flap from the arm to reconstruct the nose (Wood & Jurkiewicz, 1994).

Many advances in surgical procedure are established during times of war. Skin grafting techniques were first described in the early nineteenth century. World Wars I and II produced a climate for the advancement of many surgical specialties to include plastic surgery.

In 1944 Bunnell described in detail his recommendations for primary suture of flexor tendons; previously, suture in this area had a high failure rate. Delayed tendon grafting was also tried, but primary suturing gave equally good results in a one-stage operation that allowed the patient to return to work in weeks rather than months. In 1973 dynamic splinting was introduced, improving postoperative patient management.

The work of McCraw, Vasconez, Bostwick, and others in the 1970s reintroduced muscle and muscle skin flaps previously described in the 1900s by Tanzini (Wood & Jurkiewicz, 1994). Microvascular free flaps are a standard of care in the 1990s for reconstruction of the head and neck, breast, extremities, and for defects of the muscle, subcutaneous tissue, and skin.

THE BROAD FIELD OF PLASTIC SURGERY

The ultimate goal of the plastic surgery team is to improve the quality of life of the patient. Plastic surgery is a rare subspecialty in that it encompasses all areas of the body. Surgical procedures performed by plastic surgeons fall into three categories: (1) congenital deformities, (2) traumatic or acquired deformities, and (3) aesthetic surgical procedures. Plastic surgery seeks to obtain primary wound healing with minimal scar formation of the skin and adjacent tissues.

Congenital deformities include deformities of the facial bones (facial clefts), soft tissue of the head (cleft lip, hemangiomas), the hand (supernumerary digits or syndactyly), the genitourinary or gynecologic systems (hypospadius or epispadius, absence of the vagina), or the body (giant hairy pigmented nevus). Congenital deformities often are both aesthetically and functionally problematic (McKenna & Black, 1994). A cleft lip, for example, may result in feeding problems for the infant's family, and the baby's appearance may inhibit bonding.

Traumatic or *acquired deformities* may be the result of an accident, gunshot wound, fall, or previous surgery. These include craniofacial, maxillofacial, and deficits of tissue or function (acute burns, pressure ulcers, tumors of the body, scars, and injuries of the extremities).

Reconstruction after cancer surgery may include stretching the skin with tissue expanders to provide more tissue coverage of a deficient area, as in postmastectomy breast reconstruction. Microvascular techniques can bring a segment of the jejunum into the throat to replace tissue lost to pharyngectomy or laryngectomy, or bone and soft tissue from the scapula to re-create a mandible or to augment soft tissue from the abdomen to shape into a new breast. Many of the most striking advances in plastic surgery have resulted from advanced microsurgical techniques.

Procedures dealing with a dissatisfaction of personal appearance are referred to as *aesthetic* procedures. These include facelift, blepharoplasty, brow lift, rhinoplasty, chemical peel, mentoplasty, abdominoplasty, breast augmentation, suction lipectomy, and gynecomastia.

ASSESSMENT CONSIDERATIONS

The majority of plastic surgical procedures are elective. This gives the perioperative nurse adequate time to do a thorough preoperative assessment. This assessment begins at the time the patient seeks the services of the plastic surgeon and should include general, psychosocial, and diagnostic assessments. It is important for the nurse to establish a rapport with the patient and to provide a comfortable and nonthreatening environment for the interview. The relationship established during the preoperative interview can influence the entire perioperative experience.

General Health

Questions related to the *general health* of the patient include age, weight, height, general appearance, allergies, recent weight gain or loss, history of infections, physical disabilities, prescribed and over-the-counter medications used, heart disease, diabetes, alcohol and tobacco use, history of drug use and abuse, and a family history of anesthesia reactions. These indicators will assist the perioperative nurse and physician with the patient's plan of care (Burden, 1993).

Psychosocial Assessment

Psychosocial assessment is a vital area of consideration. The patient's ability to understand and participate in the planning of perioperative care must be evaluated. The perioperative nurse must determine the patient's expectations of surgery and the support systems available during the recuperative period. The motivation for surgery should be discussed at length. Realistic expectations are a necessary part of a successful postoperative result (Spencer, 1994; Black, 1993).

Questions that should be included in the preoperative evaluation include the following:

- What is your understanding of the surgical procedure?
- What do you expect to achieve with this surgery?
- Are you comfortable with the decision to have this surgery?

- Do you have any concerns related to the procedure?
- Have you discussed your surgery with your [husband, wife, or significant other]?
- Have you arranged for family care while you are recovering?
- What kind of family support system do you have?
- Do you have an adequate support system for emotional and physical needs?
- How long do you expect to be out of work?
- Have you discussed your medical leave with your employer?
- Are you aware that all patients are different and that you may not be able to return to work at the projected time?
- How do you plan to pay for this procedure?
- Are there special matters you do not want disclosed to others?

Diagnostic Assessment

Diagnostic assessment is determined by the type of procedure to be performed and the patient's age and medical history. The adult patient undergoing general anesthesia for a major operation will have a complete blood count (CBC), electrolytes, electrocardiogram (ECG), and chest x-ray for patients over 40 (or with a history of heart or lung disease). In addition, autologous blood may be banked or the patient may be typed and screened for bank blood for procedures in which significant blood loss may occur.

Patients undergoing selected surgical procedures have special needs. Questions and plans for care should take these into consideration. Postoperative cancer patients may need special counseling to deal with their disease and disturbed self-image. Genetic counseling should be recommended to the family of a patient with congenital anomalies. Psychologic or psychiatric assistance may be needed by patients and their families to help them cope with the birth of a child who is less than "perfect." This option should be considered for the child as well to provide for maximal integration into society.

Assessment of Anomalies

Once the perioperative nurse has identified the patient's specific underlying problem and the patient's feelings and perceptions about it, assessment focuses on aspects of the present problem. Some aspects of congenital anomalies require careful integration with the medical and family history. The perioperative nurse tries to verify that the patient and the family understand the circumstance of the problem requiring surgical intervention, as well as the treatment planned.

Cleft lip and palate. Cleft lip and cleft palate, which occur in about 1 in 1000 births, are among the most common cleft defects (Table 17-1). There is a higher incidence in boys, and the left side of the face is involved more often than the right. The incidence is 2:1000 in Asians and less than 0.5:1000 in African Americans. (Wirt, Algren, & Arnold, 1992). The infant with a cleft lip (unilateral or bilateral) and/or cleft palate may have other anomalies that include clefting as part of a syndrome. The lip is closed first, and the infant must be of sufficient size to withstand the operative procedure. The "rule of 10s" may be used: weight greater than 10 pounds, hemoglobin level over 10 g/dl, and more than 10 weeks of age. Nutrition and maternal bonding are paramount in the care of these infants. Special feeding techniques and equipment may be necessary to ensure adequate calorie intake and prevent aspiration (Richards, 1994; Wirt, Algren, & Arnold, 1992). (Chapter 21 reviews important assessment considerations for pediatric patients.)

Craniofacial anomalies. Some craniofacial anomalies, resulting from abnormalities in the growth centers of the cranium and face, are severely disabling and disfiguring. Surgical correction requires interdisciplinary teams and extensive operation. Depending on the anomaly, the preoperative evaluation will include x-ray studies such as cephalometrography to ascertain bone development and position, magnetic resonance imaging (MRI) for soft tissue differentiation, and/or computed tomography (CT) for brain development. Three-dimensional imaging may also be done from CT data. Evaluations of airway patency and deglutition are essential. Infants with micrognathia (as seen in mandibulofacial dysostosis and Treacher Collins and Pierre Robin syndromes) may need a tracheostomy and feeding gastrostomy in the neonatal period.

Reconstruction is directed by the functional need. Prematurely closed cranial sutures must be released as soon as possible to permit normal brain growth. This release may be responsible for prevention of retardation, which is caused by the limiting of brain growth that increases intracranial pressure. In syndromes with midface retrusion (such as Crouzon's syndrome and Apert's syndrome), the eyes appear to protrude; in reality they are in normal position without the necessary support and protection by the orbits. Ophthalmic consultation for protection of the corneas may be necessary (Joganic & Reiff, 1994).

Despite the fact that surgical correction of craniofacial deformity often results in dramatic improvement in appearance, function, and social rehabilitation, assessment must include a sensitive consideration of physical and psychosocial parameters. The

Table 17-1 Comparison of cleft lip and cleft palate

Cleft lip	Cleft palate
Incidence	
1:800	1:200
Inheritance	
Multifactorial inheritance Male predominance	Associated with syndromes (chromosomal), environmental factors, and teratogens
Anatomy	
Unilateral/bilateral May involve external nose, nasal cartilages, nasal septum, maxillary alveolar ridges, and dental anomalies	Soft palate and/or hard palate Midline of posterior palate May involve nostril and absence of nasal septal development (communication with oral and nasal cavity)
Management	
Surgical—Z-plasty First few weeks of life if no respiratory, oral, or systemic infections occur	Delayed repair—12 to 18 months before development of speech
Short-term problems (before repair)	
Feeding, possibly	Feeding—aspiration
Special postoperative care	
Suture line protection and care Position—right side or upright in infant seat; avoid prone positioning to protect suture line Special feeding—Breck feeder or Asepto syringe, sometimes breast—until suture line heals	May be prone, supine, or side-lying Feeding cup, Breck feeder, or Asepto syringe; avoid spoon, fork (also tongue blade, toothbrush, and other objects that could damage suture line)
Long-term problems	
Social acceptance (depends on success of repair), orthodontic if associated with cleft palate	Speech, otitis media, possible hearing loss, upper respiratory tract infections Orthodontic Feeding Social acceptance (voice changes, facial appearance if with cleft lip)

From Wong DL. (1995). *Whaley and Wong's nursing care of infants and children* (5th ed.). St. Louis: Mosby.

timing of the surgical procedure will depend on the child's growth. Normal patterns of growth and development that consider the child's perceptions of separation from family, significance of body parts, and fears and anxieties are all part of perioperative care planning.

Ear deformities. Ear defects range from minor variations to total absence of the external and internal components. Microtia, or the absence of an external ear, is a severe deformity. Major total ear reconstruction is staged and includes carving and modeling of costal cartilage and its placement beneath the skin where the ear should be placed. Secondary procedures, several months later, lift the graft with its adherent soft tissue and place it to form the posterior side of the new ear. Tissue expansion may or may not be a part of this patient's lengthy treatment regimen. Minor external ear procedures include otoplasty for protruding ears. This ear deformity is an absence or variation in the cartilaginous folds, which are re-created to shape the ears more closely to the head; repair may be undertaken before the child begins school. Assessment includes psychosocial components as well as focused inquiry into associated problems with hearing or speech.

Maxillary and mandibular trauma or deformities. Maxillary defects, congenital or traumatic, are usually related to retrusion. The maxilla appears deficient, often causing the mandible to appear prominent (prognathic). Common fracture lines of the facial skeleton, described by LeFort, also delineate the lines used for surgical fracturing during reconstruction.

- LeFort I is a transverse fracture through the maxilla above the teeth
- LeFort II is a pyramidal fracture through the nasal bones and the inferior rim of the orbit

- LeFort III is also known as craniofacial dysostosis; the fracture separates the facial bones from the cranium

Treatment is by open reduction and internal fixation with interosseus wires, miniplates, intermaxillary fixation, and suspension wires from the mandible to the orbits or cranium. External fixation devices may be employed to maintain space in the mandible when bony segments are lost to trauma or extensive procedures and immediate definitive reconstruction is deemed inappropriate. Assessment includes planning for impaired verbal communication; inspecting the integrity of the oral mucosa; determining the patient's risk for and planning to prevent infection; assessing sensory and perceptual deficits, especially visual; and assisting with interventions aimed at maintaining effective airways and breathing patterns and preventing vomiting and possible aspiration on extubation in the OR. (Chapter 20 reviews important perioperative assessment and planning for the patient undergoing surgical intervention as a result of trauma.)

Eye and eyelid deformities. The position of the globe is discussed under craniofacial reconstruction. Eyelid deformities include excess skin, herniated fat pads, exposure of the sclera (ectropion), notching (coloboma is seen in some anomalies such as Treacher Collins syndrome), and partial or complete absence of the eyelashes.

Excess skin and bulging fat pads are treated by blepharoplasty. Ectropion is a complication of blepharoplasty as well as a looseness of the lower lid caused by aging (senile ectropion). Treatment is with a wedge excision of the edge of the lid (Kuhnt-Szymanowski procedure). Trauma may damage the lacrimal ducts or musculature. Care must be taken to protect the cornea during any procedure around the eye. Chapter 11 describes important perioperative considerations in caring for patients undergoing surgery of the eye.

Nasal fractures and deformities. Trauma to the nose results in bony deformity, airway obstruction, and deviation or collapse of the septum. Simple fractures do not require open reduction and are often treated in the emergency department. Open reduction and rhinoplasty procedures have similar operative requirements. Cosmetic rhinoplasty is performed to change the shape of the external nose, such as removing the dorsal hump or narrowing the bridge or tip. Focused assessment will involve determining the effectiveness of breathing patterns and airway clearance.

Oral procedures and neck dissection. Surgery on the tongue and oropharynx and into the neck is most often extirpative. The patient usually has undergone treatment of a carcinoma of the mouth, pharynx, larynx, nasal sinuses, and/or nasal cavities. Such surgery may result in major defects and deformities. Reconstruction may be accomplished either by local flaps and skin grafts or by distant flaps. The patient is often malnourished and emaciated. The risk of wound infection and compromised wound healing is significant. (Important perioperative assessment considerations for the patient undergoing head and neck surgery are presented in Chapter 10.)

Breast. Breast surgery may be entirely aesthetic, functional, or corrective. Breasts are symbolic of a woman's femininity and sexuality (Donahoe, 1995). The four procedures most often performed are augmentation, reduction mammoplasty, mastopexy, and postmastectomy reconstruction. Augmentation is usually performed on healthy, young adult women. Preoperative physical assessment findings are usually normal; psychosocial assessment and consideration of emotional needs will be important to perioperative care planning. Augmentation may be planned for a patient who has undergone subcutaneous mastectomy for chronic nodular breast disease or premalignant disease requiring multiple biopsies. Planning for emotional support remains a perioperative nursing priority.

The implants are silicone envelopes filled with saline. Capsular contraction (thickened scar formation around the implant) is the most frequent complication and may be reduced through the use of textured implants and submuscular placement of the implant (Wood & Jurkiewicz, 1994).

Reduction mammoplasty is performed to reduce the size and weight of breasts. The patient experiences pain in the back, neck, and shoulders from the weight of the breasts and has deep shoulder grooves. She may have difficulty breathing deeply and be unable to participate in active sports. Limited excursion of the lungs can lead to kyphosis and emphysema. The patient undergoing breast reduction may donate one or two autologous units of blood for intraoperative administration.

Mastopexy (breast lift) is performed for ptosis and will use tissue suture lines similar to those used in reduction. Mastopexy may also involve insertion of implants.

Postmastectomy reconstruction is two-staged and either begun as part of the mastectomy or performed as a delayed procedure. Depending on the amount of skin and muscle tissue remaining, a permanent implant or tissue expander may be inserted (alloplastic reconstruction). Larger defects may necessitate the use of a rotated muscle flap such as a transverse rectus abdominis musculocutaneous (TRAM) or latissimus dorsi (autogenous reconstruction). The TRAM flap may also be transferred as a free flap with a remaining pedicle on the inferior epigastric vessels. Secondary procedures include sculpting the mound and nipple reconstruction; this is often combined with contralateral breast reshaping. Special assessments include scheduling the surgery at a time appropriate for optimal healing in the chemotherapy cycle, the patient's nutritional and psychosocial status, and the integrity of the previous incision and surrounding skin (Cordeiro & Hidalgo, 1994).

Abdomen, trunk, and back. The most common aesthetic procedures are abdominoplasty and suction-assisted lipectomy (SAL), or liposuction. Abdominoplasty removes redundant abdominal skin and fat. Autologous blood is often given. Abdominoplasty may be done in conjunction with ventral hernia repair and/or as a panniculectomy for morbid obesity. SAL uses a variety of trocar-type cannulae and removes fat through small stab wounds easily hidden in natural creases. For every 150 ml of fat removed, a 1% drop in hematocrit may be expected. Fluids are replaced at a 3:1 ratio to prevent hypovolemia and fluid shifts. Autologous blood transfusion may be indicated for procedures removing more than 1500 ml of fat.

Pressure sores (or decubitus ulcers) are found over bony prominences and repaired according to the depth of the wound. Skin grafts may be used to close a superficial wound; massive myocutaneous flaps are necessary for extensive wounds. These patients are often malnourished, emaciated, and poorly equipped to prevent recurrence. Perioperative nursing assessment includes determining the reason for the grafting procedure, the cause and extent of the ulcer, the type of grafting procedure planned, expectations for successful graft adherence, and the resources available for home management during rehabilitation.

Upper extremity and hand. All bone injuries of the hand and soft tissue and nerve injuries of the upper extremity are in the purview of plastic surgery. These injuries are most often caused by trauma. Surgery ranges from simple repair of lacerations through tendon and nerve injuries to total amputation with replantation by microsurgical techniques. Congenital deformities such as syndactyly (fusion or webbing of fingers), extra digits, or absence of digits will require a variety of approaches. Focused assessment involves preoperative determination of sensory and perceptual alterations and deficits, as well as planning for mobility limitations.

Lower extremity. Surgery on the lower extremity may involve soft tissue injuries with or without concomitant bone injuries. Venous stasis ulcers are treated with skin grafts, local flap closures, or free tissue transfers. Medical assessment involves radiographic studies, noninvasive Doppler studies, and arteriography. Patients with chronic ulcers will often have other serious medical complications such as diabetes and cardiovascular disease; their workup is vastly different from the young trauma patient with open tibial fracture. The perioperative nurse's assessment will include determination of tissue perfusion, skin integrity, and sensory and perceptual alterations.

NURSING DIAGNOSES

After collection and organization of relevant data affecting perioperative nursing care, a list of potential and actual patient problems is developed. These problems are conceptualized as nursing diagnoses. Factors that influence perioperative nursing diagnoses are type of procedure to be performed, anesthesia requirements, special equipment and procedures, and the patient's general medical health. Perioperative nursing diagnoses should follow guidelines set by the North American Nursing Diagnosis Association (NANDA). These diagnoses should focus on the prevention of complications, preservation of the body's defenses, detection of changes in the body's regulatory systems, resocialization of the patient, implementing physician-prescribed or interdependent activities, and provision of comfort and safety. The nursing diagnoses that most commonly affect the plastic surgery patient are to be used in addition to the generic nursing diagnoses for perioperative patients presented in Chapter 7.

Activity Intolerance

Activity intolerance is defined by Carpenito (1993) as a state in which an individual is physiologically or psychologically unable to endure or tolerate an increase in activity. Preoperatively, activity intolerance may be related to interference with sleep patterns, depression, prolonged bed rest, pain, treatment schedules, diagnostic schedules, or stress. The presence of activity intolerance will vary according to the severity of the patient's medical condition. These patients may need special assistance in transfer procedures as well as positioning devices to help maintain body alignment during surgery. Elderly patients or those with prolonged immobility who require skin grafting for decubitus ulcers should be assessed for activity intolerance. This diagnosis also affects postoperative care regimens. Any surgical procedure causes tissue damage, and anesthetic medications leave a potential for pain, decreased range of motion of affected parts, and physical weakness. This improves over time but must be recognized by the patient and staff. Provisions for appropriate rest periods and elevation of the affected part (as in extremity surgery) are essential.

Ineffective Airway Clearance

Partial or complete airway obstruction leads to the real or potential inability to pass air through the respiratory tract. Airway management, critical for all patients, is of particular concern for those undergoing craniofacial or maxillofacial procedures. Observations of the respiratory rate and depth and airway patency must be made frequently. Intermaxillary fixation holds the teeth in occlusion. An order is obtained from the surgeon about when and where the wires should be cut to release the jaws in an emergency. Many surgeons perform a tracheostomy to eliminate this possibility. Facial edema, seroma, or hematomas may compromise the trachea in any procedure involving the jaw or neck, and all of these patients must be monitored. For a face-lift (rhytidectomy or meloplasty) patient, family members must observe the patient, especially during the first 24 hours. Often, despite extensive preoperative teaching, patients do not understand the extent of the surgery and the need for good postoperative care. Many surgeons keep the patient overnight in the hospital, but many patients go home. Descriptions of abnormal edema, bleeding, stridor, and increased respiratory rates must be given to family members, along with instructions to call the surgeon and/or return to the hospital if these signs are noted.

Anxiety

Any surgery provides the patient with new anxieties. Reconstructive patients are concerned about the defect and its correction, the amount of pain, and the ability to obtain appropriate and timely relief. Cosmetic surgery patients may feel guilty for wanting to have a new appearance and may but not want to appear vain. They will verbalize thoughts such as "I must be crazy to put myself through this," and will often go through a postoperative period of depression at having brought about this discomfort just to change or improve their looks. The perioperative nurse needs to come to terms with his or her own concepts of body image and accept the patient's wish to change his or her body. The cosmetic patient's pain and discomfort are as real as the cancer patient's and must be respected and treated appropriately. Anxiety can be eased by understanding comments and reassurance. The perioperative nurse may need to repeat explanations and instructions; cognitive function is often impaired by high levels of anxiety. It may be helpful to grade anxiety levels as low, moderate, or high. The patient should be assisted to identify coping strategies that have been personally effective in the past. If appropriate, these strategies can be facilitated by the perioperative nurse. Such strategies as meditation, guided imagery, touch, and music may be of benefit.

Altered Body Temperature

The patient's core temperature must be maintained at different levels depending on the type of surgery being performed. The craniofacial or maxillofacial patient may have exposed brain during the procedure, so warm irrigating fluids are needed. Sterile solution warmers may be used for this purpose. During microvascular procedures, chilling of the patient, the extremity undergoing the surgery, or the replanted or newly anastomosed tissue flap can lead to spasm of the small vessels and subsequent irreversible tissue death. The body temperature may be maintained by use of a thermia unit (warming blanket) or forced-air warming device (such as the Bair Hugger); anesthesia staff may use a humidifier to warm and moisten inspired gases. Intravenous fluids, blood, and blood products are warmed. The patient's temperature will be monitored with a probe; the core temperature should be greater than 36°C. It may be necessary to warm the room temperature to approximately 72°F. This is also essential for the burn patient, whose loss of skin integrity contributes to rapid body cooling and massive fluid loss through convection and radiation.

Pain

Trauma patients may be in pain before coming to the OR. Nursing care measures designed to support injured areas during transport and onto the OR bed are important. Older patients may have joint arthralgia, and immobility during long procedures can be very uncomfortable both intraoperatively and postoperatively. The variety of plastic surgical procedures causes the scope of comfort alterations to widen; they must be addressed according to the patient's perceptions and needs. Perioperative nursing actions that assess the level of discomfort and plan with the patient to minimize discomfort are important.

Ineffective Coping, Individual and/or Family

Ineffective coping results when patients have inadequate resources (physical, psychologic, or behavioral) to cope with internal or external stressors (Gulanik, et al., 1994). Changes in body image, inability to function normally, low self-esteem, and awareness of personal mortality are handled differently by every person. Patients whose coping mechanisms are compromised may or may not be able to verbalize their inabilities or to ask for help. Children with congenital deformities are especially at risk for psychologic problems because of society's emphasis on physical beauty (Richards, 1994). Preoperative screening of the cosmetic surgery patient should prevent surgery on those with unrealistic expectations, who will never be satisfied with the results. The perioperative nurse will need to plan assistive activities for patients with ineffective coping; referrals to other health team members may be required.

Impaired Verbal Communication

Dealing with speech and communication impairment may require the assistance of speech therapists. The perioperative nurse must be aware of the potential deficit that will be caused by extirpative surgery such as intraoral, maxillary, or mandibular resections. Provision of a pen and pencil, magic slate, or symbol board can help to maintain good communication with the patient and the staff. Mechanisms for communication should be planned with the patient before surgery.

Fluid Volume Deficit

All major procedures provide the possibility of volume depletion. High-risk patients must be identified, intravenous lines protected and kept patent, and the need for blood and blood products and their availability ascertained. The patient undergoing SAL will require replacement of fluid at a ratio of 3:1 to prevent fluid shifts and electrolyte imbalances. Debilitated patients may be accustomed to a decreased blood volume, which, when expanded during surgery to a level considered normal, will require unexpected transfusions. Patients undergoing major reconstruction will have arterial lines inserted; arterial blood gas, hemoglobin, and hematocrit levels will be frequently assessed. Perioperative nurses collaborate closely with the anesthesia and surgical team in planning to prevent or manage fluid volume deficits. Accurate estimations of fluid loss in suction canisters, on sponges and drapes, and in drainage collection devices should be communicated as frequently as needed. Recordings of total intake and output help the nursing staff on the discharge unit (postanesthesia care or other recovery unit) identify perioperative events that might affect fluid volume maintenance.

Fluid Volume Excess

Excess circulating fluid is dangerous for all patients and especially for those undergoing intracranial or extracranial procedures. Intracranial pressures can suddenly become elevated, leading to cellular compromise. The burn patient may receive excess fluid, as seen in those with massive edema. This can lead to cardiac overload. Monitoring of intake and output is critical. Careful and close collaboration with the anesthesia and surgical teams is required for patients at risk for fluid volume excess.

Risk for Infection

Any incision provides entry for bacteria. Care must be taken with the craniofacial patient because of the presence of real or potential openings into the dura and communication with the nasopharynx. Tracheal and oral suctioning should be performed with catheters separate from the intranasal catheter. Postoperative nasal secretions should be tested with Dextrostix to determine the presence of sugar. This indicates a spinal fluid leak and a real risk for meningitis or encephalitis. Oral and mucosal incisions have the risk for infection; good oral hygiene is imperative.

Patients undergoing vascularized tissue grafts are also at risk for infection. Draping for graft procedures may be complicated; close attention needs to be paid to maintaining aseptic technique during these maneuvers (Donahoe, 1995). Antimicrobial skin preparation is carried out to isolate graft and recipient sites. Instruments used on the recipient site may be considered contaminated; they may require isolation on a separate sterile field. Sterile x-ray film, used to make a pattern of the defect, may be resterilized before being moved to the instrument tray for the donor site. The perioperative team may change gowns and gloves when moving from the recipient to donor site to harvest the graft. Once the donor site is closed and dressings applied, additional sterile sheets may be placed over it. Prophylactic antibiotics will be administered intraoperatively. These are just some of the additional aseptic precautions the perioperative nurse uses to intervene in the patient's risk for infection.

Altered Nutrition: Less Than Body Requirements

Procedures involving the head and face decrease patient comfort and ease when eating. Postoperatively, patients may experience nausea and revulsion at the sight of certain foods. Those with intermaxillary fixation (IMF) need dietary consultation to teach adaptations to a blenderized diet to prevent weight loss of greater than 5 to 10 pounds. Burn patients require massive calorie intake, and stress itself increases caloric needs above what most patients would consider an "increased" caloric intake. Nutritionally compromised patients, especially those with malignancies, pose greater intraoperative and postoperative risks because their wounds will heal more slowly and their recovery will take longer. Chemotherapy also changes perceptions of taste and decreases appetites. These patients are often emaciated. The patient with decreased nutrition will have assessment of skin integrity and muscle mass as part of perioperative care planning. Bony prominences must be well protected at all times to maintain skin and tissue integrity. Depending on the length of the surgical procedure and the patient's status, egg-crate foam, gel-filled, or other special mattresses may be used to prevent dependent skin pressure.

Altered Tissue Perfusion

During microvascular grafting, vasospasm, ischemia, and direct tissue injury may lead to altered tissue perfusion. Perioperative nursing efforts are directed at collaborating with the surgical team to prevent clotting and occlusion of vessels during anastomoses. Dextran, heparin, and aspirin are agents used before and during the procedure to retard vessel thrombosis (Wood & Jurkiewicz, 1994). Local irrigation with heparinized saline to prevent clotting and lidocaine to prevent vasospasm may also be indicated. Careful labeling of all medications on the sterile field is required. In the immediate postoperative period, assessment of the donor and recipient sites in grafting procedures is important. Before transfer to the postanesthesia care unit, the perioperative nurse should check for any signs of swelling, increased drainage, or change in color or temperature of the graft tissue; this will continue to be monitored because hematoma formation beneath a skin graft is the most common cause of graft failure (Hidalgo, 1995). Doppler ultrasound measurements may be made, comparing preoperative and postoperative flow ranges in flaps; in addition, Doppler ultrasound may be used to identify major arteriovenous supply in vascularized pedicle free flaps perioperatively (Westlake, 1991).

Body Image Disturbance

The patient whose change in body image is the result of age, trauma, or extirpative surgery needs time to recognize and assimilate these changes and to form a new and integrated concept of self (Pruzinski, 1993). Understanding and acceptance are the keys to these changes and must be shown by the perioperative nursing staff and taught to the family and significant others. In more severe cases, professional counseling may be required. The perioperative nurse documents unusual comments and supports the patient's efforts to understand the procedures and resulting image changes.

Impaired Swallowing

Procedures about the face, mouth, and neck may impair swallowing. Cleft palate patients have nasal escape of air and food and are prone to aspiration. These patients, especially young children, have to be closely watched. Dietary restrictions are upheld, and care is taken not to damage any intraoral suture line with eating utensils, straws, or fingers. Elbow restraints for children must be applied before anesthesia is reversed. Adults find that difficulty in feeding oneself neatly is embarrassing. They often refuse to eat in the presence of others. Use of feeding syringes and ready access to oral suctioning is required in the early postoperative stage.

PLANNING

Planning for perioperative patient care necessarily revolves around the nursing diagnoses prioritized for the individual patient (Abbott, 1994). Nursing care for perioperative patients extends across the preoperative, intraoperative, and postoperative phases. Targeted nursing actions may become part of the nursing care plan. When caring for patients who are undergoing elective, aesthetic plastic and reconstructive surgery, the nurse may help the patient set realistic goals for nursing diagnoses. This takes into consideration the patient's wishes, aspirations, and capabilities. In other circumstances, as with trauma patients, the perioperative nurse uses his or her knowledge of selected nursing diagnoses and devises goals that are considered to be in the patient's best interest. This is part of the advocacy role of perioperative nursing.

Modifying Generic Care Plans

The generic care plans described in Chapter 7 can be applied with little modification to patients undergoing all types of plastic and reconstructive surgery.

Knowledge deficit. The plastic surgery nurse may wish to add specific items to the generic care plan for knowledge deficit. Issues to be addressed include those relating to changes in body image and postoperative appearance and the inability to eat normally or communicate effectively.

Freedom from infection. Specific risk factors depend on the type of procedure. However, cosmetic as well as reconstructive patients undergoing flap procedures of any type should be interviewed about their smoking status, vitamin and aspirin ingestion, nutrition, and whether they are undergoing chemotherapy or radiation therapy. In cancer reconstruction, proper classification of wounds is essential for accurate surgical site infection surveillance and predicting which patients are at greater risk for wound infection. These patients are at risk because their immune systems are under stress. Universal precautions and institutional protocols must be followed for confining and containing instrumentation on the surgical field that has been contaminated by tumor resection or transection of the respiratory or gastrointestinal tract or used on the recipient site or for endoscopy.

Maintaining skin integrity. Specific additions to the generic care plan for maintaining skin integrity may include notations on airway obstruction (as seen in nasal reconstruction, preoperatively as well as when the nasal vaults are packed postoperatively). If a procedure forces mouth breathing, appropriate nursing actions include lubrication of the lips and oral mucous membranes. Other observations include support and protection of the wound by appropriate dressings; securing the drains or tubings to the dressing; application of adhesive skin tapes (Steri-Strips) to take tension off the suture lines; use of Montgomery straps to preserve the skin if dressings need more than twice-daily changes; support of the operated limb in plaster splints during emergence from anesthesia so that the plaster does not bend or crack as it cures; and prevention of shearing forces across the wound when moving the patient from the OR bed to the transfer bed or stretcher.

Positioning injury. The perioperative nurse follows developed institutional protocols for positioning the patient before surgery. Patient position is determined through collaboration of the nurse, surgeon, and anesthesia provider. The team should move the patient in a way that prevents shearing forces during position changes.

Injury from retained foreign objects. In oral procedures, a gauze pack may be placed in the posterior pharynx around the endotracheal tube. The nurse notes the time of placement and removal. Microsurgical anastomoses of blood vessels provide the opportunity to retain miniature vessel loops and clamps, needles, and gauze dissectors. These should be included in the instrument and needle count and documented.

Injury from chemicals. The perioperative nurse adds to the generic care plan the types of medications commonly administered for local, topical, and sedative use, especially for ambulatory surgery. Medications commonly used in microvascular surgery may also be added.

Injury from physical hazards. Standard and special equipment used may be added to the generic care plan or the Guides to Nursing Actions section. The nurse considers adding the need for x-ray or other films (MRI, CT, and so on) to be kept in the room for review. Also considered are the microsurgical microscope, special air-powered drills, saws and abraders, lasers (including protective goggles for the patient), various dermatomes, stapling devices, cameras, and pulse oximeter and other monitoring devices such as the automatic blood pressure cuff. Laser vaporization of lesions may contaminate the air with plume containing particles of formaldehyde, benzene, cellular debris, and other contaminants. During laser procedures the staff should be protected by use of laser masks, goggles, and laser-rated smoke evacuation systems (Ball, 1995).

Electrical injury. The operating room of the 1990s is filled with electrical equipment. Precautions should be taken with electrically powered saws, ESU generators, monitors, and other equipment used during the procedure.

Maintaining fluid and electrolyte balance. Additional risk factors are added to the generic care plan for the trauma patient who receives massive transfusions (risk for hyperkalemia, hypomagnesemia, and hypocalcemia), the nutritionally deficient patient (risk for hypokalemia or hypocalcemia), and the SAL patient, whose fluid replacement ratio of 3:1 should be instituted as soon as surgery begins.

Participation in rehabilitation. The perioperative nurse in the outpatient surgical facility is most likely to assist the patient and family with learning to manage postoperative care. Demonstration of this knowledge is assisted by prepared, written instructions, which are signed after being explained to the patient or family member. A driver is necessary because the patient cannot be allowed to drive home after receiving sedation. Instructions to call the surgeon or come to the emergency department should be given for symptoms of hemorrhage, severe edema (leading to respiratory compromise in the facial surgery patient), or severe pain unrelieved by medication. It should be noted that many patients are users of drugs, legal and illegal, which may not be reported in the preoperative assessment. Patients' tolerance for the usual sedative and analgesic medications, compounded by anxiety, is often much higher than expected. The perioperative nurse should attempt to gain a report of medication use that is as honest as possible. Discussion of alternative pain control techniques is helpful with all patients. Patients are given an appointment with the surgeon within the next day or two, and follow-up telephone calls are made by one or more members of the surgical team.

CARE PLANS

Assessment, nursing diagnosis, and outcome identification all lead to a plan of care with prescribed nursing actions. The perioperative nurse may implement these actions independently or collaborate with other members of the surgical team. This chapter concludes with care plans devised for selected plastic and reconstructive surgical procedures. Like the other procedure-specific care plans in this book, they are guidelines for perioperative nurses who wish to establish care plans in their practice settings. These care plans have been designed to accommodate identification of nursing diagnoses, documentation of nursing actions, evaluation of patient outcomes, and modification of the plan to meet individual patient needs. The nursing actions are listed in the sequence with which they might be carried out in patient care settings. Each care plan is accompanied by a Guide to Nursing Actions, in which the actions are explained and their relevance to the specific patient procedure elaborated. In some of these guides, further explanation of the selected nursing diagnoses is offered. Nursing diagnoses are highly patient specific; in many instances, the perioperative nurse may find it necessary to develop alternative nursing diagnoses for individual patients.

Assessing and evaluating patient outcomes allows the perioperative nurse to determine if the plan was effective. It is helpful to develop criteria for evaluating outcomes; these are listed in the outcome section of the care plan. When outcomes are clearly established, evaluation of whether the patient met an outcome becomes a matter of looking at the success or failure of nursing actions in terms of the outcome criteria. Provision has been made for modification and change in outcomes to reflect the patient's changing status. Constant and continuous reassessment of the patient's status during surgery is a primary perioperative nursing consideration. The perioperative nurse plans for and anticipates changes in status during all surgical interventions. If outcomes are not met, the patient's status may have changed, and a new problem is identified. As new problems appear, they may take priority over former ones. Regardless of the reason, new outcomes, actions, and outcome criteria are established. The dynamic process of perioperative care planning moves forward to accommodate the patient's changing status.

GUIDES TO NURSING ACTIONS
Microvascular Surgery: Replantation and Free Tissue Transfers (Fig. 17-1)

1. Preoperative assessment of the replantation patient may be limited by the urgency of restoring a devascularized or severed body part. The severed part should arrive in the OR wrapped in saline-dampened gauze and in a container with ice to keep it cool. Ischemia time must be assessed.

   Physical assessment should include assessment of the injury or defect, level of discomfort, and tissues available for transfer. The patient's medical history should also be considered. Chronic illnesses such as diabetes, hypertension, bleeding disorders, and cardiac and respiratory pathology may increase morbidity. Nutritional status, drug and alcohol use, and smoking history are also considered.

   Preoperative testing, which includes noninvasive vascular studies, CT scan, MRI, and arteriography, may be performed on the patient facing elective free tissue transfers.

   Since reconstructive surgery requires a large commitment of time, resources, and emotional energy, *psychologic status* and *patient support systems* must be considered.

2. The perioperative nurse should verify the availability of blood for transfusion. All microsurgical patients should be typed and matched for blood. The elective patient may have autologous blood available.

3. Before taking the patient to the OR, special supplies and equipment must be obtained. These supplies include but are not limited to the following:
   - Instruments—soft tissue, orthopedic, micro
   - Sterile supplies—draping materials, gowns, gloves, sutures, sponges
   - Power equipment—drills, dermatomes
   - Microscope—lenses, loopes
   - Doppler—box and sterile probe
   - Tourniquet—cuff and padding
   - Nerve stimulator
   - Electrosurgical unit and cord
   - Bipolar unit and cord
   - Suction canisters
   - Warmers—fluid, warming blanket, Bair Hugger
   - Positioning aids—gel pads, egg-crate mattress, pillows, tape, Velcro straps
   - Ice—if severed part involved
   - Medications and solutions
   - In the case of replantation, two sterile setups may be needed, one table for the severed part and one for the replantation procedure. Iced saline in a basin may be used to keep the severed part cold until preparation for replantation.

4. A thermia blanket may be used to help maintain core temperature between 98.6° and 101° F. This blanket should be placed on the OR bed early enough to warm before patient positioning. Additional warmth may be obtained by using a Bair Hugger and warmed fluids.

5. Before patient transport to the OR the room temperature should be adjusted. Room temperature will be 75° to 80° F to prevent vasospasm and maintain the patient's core temperature of 98° F.

6. Patient positioning is determined by the type and length of procedure. All bony prominences should be well padded. A gel-type mattress is preferred for lengthy procedures. Patient comfort and safety are important. The staff should be prepared to reposition the patient as needed during the procedure, paying strict adherence to aseptic technique.

7. During the induction of anesthesia the perioperative nurse should be available to assist the anesthesia provider. Emergent cases may require central lines and rapid induction techniques. Suction should be readily available.

FIG. 17-1
CARE PLAN FOR MICROVASCULAR SURGERY: REPLANTATION AND FREE TISSUE TRANSFER

KEY ASSESSMENT POINTS

Nature of injury (acute reconstruction)
Prehospital emergency care given (acute reconstruction)
Condition of recipient/donor site
General health status (nutrition, systemic disease)
Mobility limitations/positioning requirements
Understanding of procedure, perioperative events

NURSING DIAGNOSIS

All generic nursing diagnosis apply to this patient, with the addition
of:
High risk for altered tissue perfusion

PATIENT OUTCOMES:

All generic outcomes apply, with the addition of:
The patient will maintain adequate tissue perfusion to the site. There
will be:
1. Evidence of warm skin temperature and good color (good capillary refill) at the operative site
2. No excess swelling, drainage, or unrelieved pain at operative site
3. Adequate Doppler flow measurements

NURSING ACTIONS:

	Yes	No	N/A
1. Preop assessment performed?	☐	☐	☐
2. Blood ordered/available?	☐	☐	☐
3. Special equipment/supplies available?	☐	☐	☐
4. Thermia blanket/Bair Hugger available?	☐	☐	☐
5. Room temperature adjusted?	☐	☐	☐
6. Patient positioned correctly?	☐	☐	☐
7. Assist with anesthesia induction?	☐	☐	☐
8. Urinary catheter inserted?	☐	☐	☐
9. ESU available/checked?	☐	☐	☐
10. Dispersive pad checked/applied?	☐	☐	☐
11. Operative site determined/marked?	☐	☐	☐
12. Skin prep per institutional protocol?	☐	☐	☐
13. Aseptic technique maintained?	☐	☐	☐
14. Perioperative monitoring?	☐	☐	☐
15. Blood loss monitored?	☐	☐	☐
16. Irrigation/IV solutions warmed?	☐	☐	☐
17. Monitor ischemia/tourniquet time?	☐	☐	☐
18. Medications administered/documented?	☐	☐	☐
19. Maintain contact with the family?	☐	☐	☐
20. Specimen(s) to lab?	☐	☐	☐
21. Counts performed/correct?	☐	☐	☐
22. Dispersive pad site checked?	☐	☐	☐
23. Dressings applied?	☐	☐	☐
24. Drains/catheters secured?	☐	☐	☐
25. Postop assessment?	☐	☐	☐
26. Postop teaching?	☐	☐	☐
27. Other generic care plans initiated?	☐	☐	☐

Document additional nursing actions/generic care plans initiated
here:

_____

_____

_____

EVALUATION OF PATIENT OUTCOMES:

	Outcome met	Outcome met with additional outcome criteria	Outcome met with revised nursing care plan	Outcome not met	Outcome not applicable to this patient
1. The patient's tissue perfusion was maintained/restored.	☐	☐	☐	☐	☐
2. The patient met outcomes for additional generic care plans.	☐	☐	☐	☐	☐

Signature: _____ Date: _____

8. Placement of a urinary catheter is necessary for accurate measurement of renal function and hydration. Microvascular surgical procedures frequently last more than 12 hours. A urimeter is the preferred collection device and should be placed in a location visible to both the perioperative nurse and the anesthesia provider.

9. The electrosurgical/bipolar unit should be checked.

10. Application of the dispersive (ESU) pad includes checking the site for appropriate placement and documentation of site location and condition.

11. Location of operative site will be determined by the primary surgeon. The operative site may be marked or outlined before surgery. Marking pens, rulers, tape measures, a camera, and background material may be required during the procedure. Doppler ultrasound may be used during the marking phase to locate vessels to be used during the procedure.

12. The surgical site should be cleansed with the preparatory solution of the physician's choice. Solutions should be warmed according to manufacturer's recommendations. Note the condition of the skin at the preparation site before and after skin preparation procedures. For replantation patients, note any signs of diminished circulation, such as color change or ecchymosis.

13. Strict aseptic technique is used. During free tissue transfers it may be necessary to turn the patient and repeat preparation and draping. Protection of the sterile field during this activity is essential. Special care is taken when moving from recipient to donor site (change gown and gloves and isolate instruments).

14. The perioperative nurse collaborates closely with anesthesia staff in monitoring the patient. Perioperative monitoring includes all vital signs, input and output, ischemia time of the severed part or free tissue transfer, tourniquet time, and maintenance of normothermia. Core temperature may be monitored with an esophageal thermometer or rectal probe. Decreased core temperature will predispose small vessels to vasospasm.

15. Blood loss is monitored by estimating loss on drapes, weighing sponges, and measuring suction canisters (allowing for irrigation fluids).

16. Irrigation and intravenous solution should be warmed to maintain normothermia and prevent vasospasm. A sterile fluid warmer may be used on the field to maintain the temperature of fluid used for moist sponges and irrigation.

17. When injury involves the arm or leg, a tourniquet may be used. Ischemia time (from the time of injury or removal of tissue from its circulation) and tourniquet time are measured and recorded. Once the tourniquet has been inflated, it should be released every 2 hours for 20 minutes if possible.

18. Medications used may include heparin (50,000 U in 500 ml normal saline) and lidocaine (Xylocaine 2%, without epinephrine). Type and dosages of medications are determined by the primary surgeon. All medications on the sterile field should be carefully labeled. Prophylactic antibiotics may also be administered intravenously and used as irrigation.

19. The perioperative nurse should provide periodic updates to the family. This greatly relieves their anxiety and deepens their faith in the ability of the surgical team.

20. Follow institutional protocol for preservation and disposition of surgical specimens. Use universal precautions with all materials and containers received from the sterile field. Document all specimens collected and their disposition.

21. In addition to routine counts of sponges, sharps, and instruments, counts of all extra instruments and microsurgical components, such as vessel loops, clips, and clamps, must be correct before closure of the wound.

22. The dispersive pad should be removed and the condition of the skin checked.

23. The dressings used are absorbent and supportive. Splints may be utilized as support for involved extremities. Protection of blood supply to newly vascularized tissue must be maintained. These areas may be lightly covered with an emollient gauze dressing. Bandaging should not preclude visual inspection during the postoperative period.

24. Note the placement of all tubes, drains, or catheters. Care should be taken to prevent pressure on revascularized areas by drains or tubes. This includes an oxygen mask and its elastic ties, tracheostomy tapes, and bandage materials. Even minimal pressure or weight can compromise the blood supply to the operative site.

25. Following replantation, postoperative assessment of tissue perfusion remains a nursing priority. If occlusion occurs in a vessel or artery of a reimplanted part and is not immediately corrected surgically, all or part of the area will die. Assessment may be determined via Doppler, temperature probe, measurement of tissue oxygen tension, and capillary refill of the affected area. Arterial clots cause the replanted or transplanted areas to appear pale in early stages and cyanotic in later stages. Capillary refill is slow,

Table 17-2 Assessment of vascular occlusion

	Arterial	Venous
Skin color	Pale, mottled blue	Cyanotic, blue
Capillary refill	Sluggish (>3 seconds)	Brisk (<3 seconds)
Tissue turgor	Prunelike, then hollow	Tense, swollen, distended
Temperature	Cool	Cool
Dermal bleeding	Scant amount of dark blood	Rapid bleeding, dark blood

From Beare PG & Myers JL. (1994), *Adult health nursing* (2nd ed.). St. Louis: Mosby.

over 3 to 4 seconds; the skin seems hollow and the temperature cool. Signs of venous occlusion include an immediate cyanotic appearance, brisk capillary refill, distention of the part, and cool temperature (Table 17-2). A baseline must be established for assessment of the tissues to ensure continuity of care within all disciplines. The surgeon must be notified at the first sign of compromised circulation. Postoperative medications include aspirin (usually by rectal suppository) and antibiotics. Dextran, a plasma expander, may be used to reduce blood viscosity and improve capillary blood flow.

26. Patient and family education is begun in the preoperative phase and continues throughout the recovery phase. Smoking by the patient or others in the patient's presence can compromise blood flow to the replanted part because of the vasoconstrictive effects of nicotine on small blood vessels. Signs to this effect on the patient's bed and door will help.

Craniofacial and Maxillofacial Reconstruction (Fig. 17-2)

1. Preoperative assessment is needed to establish a baseline for each patient. Physical assessment should include assessment of the injury or defect, level of discomfort, and tissues available for transfer. The patient's medical history should also be considered. Chronic illnesses such as diabetes, hypertension, bleeding disorders, and cardiac and respiratory pathologic conditions may increase morbidity. Nutritional status, drug and alcohol use, and smoking history are also considered. Preoperative teaching should include the patient and any significant others. Because reconstructive surgery requires a large commitment of time, resources, and emotional energy, psychologic status and patient support systems must be considered. During teaching the perioperative nurse has the op-

portunity to discuss the surgical procedure, the possible use of postoperative endotracheal or tracheostomy tubes, facial fixation devices and grafts, and required postoperative care.

2. The perioperative nurse should verify the availability of blood for transfusion. All patients undergoing lengthy procedures should be typed and matched for blood. The elective patient may have autologous blood available.

3. Before taking the patient to the OR, special supplies and equipment must be obtained. These supplies include but are not limited to the following:
   - Instruments—soft tissue, orthopedic, neurologic, and plastic surgical
   - Sterile supplies—draping materials, gowns, gloves, sutures, sponges, neurologic sponges
   - Tracheostomy tray and tubes
   - Power equipment—drills, craniotomes, saws
   - Plates, screws, arch bars, wires
   - Electrosurgical unit and cord
   - Bipolar unit and cord
   - Suction canisters
   - Warmers—fluid, warming blanket, Bair Hugger
   - Positioning aids—gel pads, egg-crate mattress, pillows, tape, Velcro straps
   - Medications and solutions

   In the case of multiple surgeons operating simultaneously, two sterile setups may be needed, one table for the oral procedure and one for the cranial procedure.

4. A thermia blanket may be used to help maintain core temperature between 98.6° and 101° F. This blanket should be placed on the OR bed early enough to warm before patient positioning. Additional warmth may be obtained by using a Bair Hugger and warmed fluids.

5. Patient positioning is determined by the type and length of procedure. All bony prominences should be well padded. A gel-type mattress is preferred for lengthy procedures. Patient comfort and safety are important. The staff should be prepared to reposition the patient as needed during the procedure, paying strict adherence to aseptic technique. Generally the patient will be in the supine position with the head on a cushioned support or neurologic head rest. If an iliac graft is to be obtained, the patient may need a roll under the affected hip.

6. During the induction of anesthesia the perioperative nurse should be available to assist the anesthesia provider. Emergent cases may require central lines and rapid induction techniques. Suction should be readily available. A tracheostomy setup should be available.

FIG. 17-2
CARE PLAN FOR CRANIOFACIAL/MAXILLOFACIAL RECONSTRUCTION

KEY ASSESSMENT POINTS

Type/location of fracture/injury
Skin integrity
Plan for communication
Hydration status
Oxygenation/airway
Nutritional status
Problems with vision
Understanding of procedure, perioperative events

NURSING DIAGNOSIS:

All generic nursing diagnoses apply to this patient, with the addition of:
Impaired verbal communication
Ineffective airway clearance

PATIENT OUTCOMES:

All generic outcomes apply, with the addition of:
The patient will be able to communicate via alternative methods.
The patient's airway will be maintained.

NURSING ACTIONS:

	Yes	No	N/A
1. Preop assessment performed?	☐	☐	☐
2. Blood ordered/available?	☐	☐	☐
3. Special equipment/supplies available?	☐	☐	☐
4. Thermia blanket/Bair Hugger available?	☐	☐	☐
5. Patient positioned correctly?	☐	☐	☐
6. Assist with anesthesia induction?	☐	☐	☐
7. Urinary catheter inserted?	☐	☐	☐
8. ESU available/checked?	☐	☐	☐
9. Dispersive pad checked/applied?	☐	☐	☐
10. Operative site determined/marked?	☐	☐	☐
11. Skin prep per institutional protocol?	☐	☐	☐
12. Perioperative monitoring?	☐	☐	☐
13. Blood loss monitored?	☐	☐	☐
14. Irrigation/IV solutions warmed?	☐	☐	☐
15. Medications administered/documented?	☐	☐	☐
16. Maintain contact with the family?	☐	☐	☐
17. Specimen(s) to lab?	☐	☐	☐
18. Counts performed/correct?	☐	☐	☐
19. Dispersive pad site checked?	☐	☐	☐
20. Drains/catheters secured?	☐	☐	☐
21. Dressings applied?	☐	☐	☐
22. Suction available until recovered?	☐	☐	☐
23. Wire cutters?	☐	☐	☐
24. Tracheostomy obturator?	☐	☐	☐
25. Postop teaching?	☐	☐	☐
26. Other generic care plans initiated?	☐	☐	☐

Document additional nursing actions/generic care plans initiated here:

_____

_____

_____

EVALUATION OF PATIENT OUTCOMES:

	Outcome met	Outcome met with additional outcome criteria	Outcome met with revised nursing care plan	Outcome not met	Outcome not applicable to this patient
1. The patient was able to communicate via alternative methods.	☐	☐	☐	☐	☐
2. The patient's airway was maintained.	☐	☐	☐	☐	☐
3. The patient met outcomes for additional generic care plans.	☐	☐	☐	☐	☐

Signature: _____ Date: _____

7. Placement of a urinary catheter is necessary for accurate measurement of renal function and hydration. Craniofacial procedures are frequently long. A urimeter is the preferred collection device and should be placed in a location visible to both the perioperative nurse and the anesthesia provider.

8. The electrosurgical/bipolar unit should be checked.

9. Application of the dispersive (ESU) pad includes checking the site for appropriate placement and documentation of site location and condition.

10. Location of operative site will be determined by the primary surgeon. The operative site may be marked or outlined before surgery. Marking pens, rulers, tape measures, a camera, and background material may be required during the procedure.

11. A shave preparation may be necessary using a dry electric razor or wet technique with a disposable razor. The surgical site should be cleansed with the preparatory solution of the physician's choice. Solutions should be warmed according to manufacturer's recommendations. Note the condition of the skin at the preparation site before and after skin preparation procedures, as well as the area shaved.

12. The perioperative nurse collaborates closely with anesthesia staff in monitoring the patient. Perioperative monitoring includes all vital signs, input and output, and maintenance of normothermia. Core temperature may be monitored with an esophageal thermometer or rectal probe.

13. Blood loss is monitored by estimating loss on drapes, weighing sponges, and measuring suction canisters (allowing for irrigation fluids). All output should be recorded in a timely manner and totaled at the end of the procedure with separate notations for nasogastric tube drainage and urinary output. Fluid balance is especially critical for young patients and the elderly.

14. Irrigation and intravenous solution should be warmed to maintain normothermia. A sterile fluid warmer may be used on the field to maintain the temperature of fluid used for moist sponges and irrigation.

15. Antibiotics are usually given immediately preoperatively and at 4- to 6-hour intervals. Obtain as needed, according to the physician's preference. Recheck the patient's allergy data.

16. The perioperative nurse should provide periodic updates to the family. This greatly relieves their anxiety and deepens their faith in the ability of the surgical team.

17. Follow institutional protocol for preservation and disposition of surgical specimens. Use universal precautions for all materials and containers received from the sterile field. Document all specimens and their disposition.

18. Count all special plates, screws, and gauze dissectors, in addition to routine sponge, sharp, and instrument counts. Record count results.

19. The dispersive pad should be removed and the condition of the skin checked.

20. Note the placement of all tubes, drains, or catheters.

21. Apply dressings to incision and drainage sites. Clean the skin around the dressing site before placing the dressing. To lessen shearing of superficial skin layers, do not stretch the tape where it touches the skin.

22. Keep suction available during anesthesia reversal and until patient leaves the OR. Have sterile suction catheters for intranasal suction. Keep them separate from tips used for oral or tracheostomy suctioning.

23. For patients with intermaxillary fixation, have wire cutters and written orders from the surgeon as to which wires may be cut in an emergency.

24. Patient with a tracheostomy tube. Secure the tracheostomy tube with twill tape, and use tracheostomy sponges (precut slits) for dressing the tube site. Support the tube when the patient is moved from the OR bed to the discharge vehicle. Oxygen or ventilator tubing attached to the tube should be positioned so that no traction is placed on the tube.

25. Patient and family teaching is begun in the preoperative phase and continues throughout the recovery phase. Smoking by the patient or others in the patient's presence can compromise blood flow to the surgical sites because of the vasoconstrictive effects of nicotine on small blood vessels. Signs to this effect on the patient's bed and door will help.

Suction-Assisted Lipectomy (SAL) (Fig. 17-3)

1. Preoperative assessment includes checking skin integrity and elasticity (good elastic tone is an important preoperative consideration for patient selection). Laboratory values should be evaluated with special consideration of hemoglobin and hematocrit. The patient's medical history should also be considered. Chronic illnesses such as diabetes, hypertension, and bleeding disorders may increase morbidity. There is a risk for fluid volume deficits. Neurovascular status should be assessed for postoperative comparison; blunt injury to motor nerves is a possible complication of the procedure (Pettis & Vogt,

FIG. 17-3
CARE PLAN FOR SUCTION-ASSISTED LIPECTOMY (SAL)

KEY ASSESSMENT POINTS

Rate/quality peripheral pulses
Use of anticoagulant medications (prescription/over the counter)
History anemia, diabetes, bleeding disorders
Preexisting numbness/paresthesia at site(s) to be suctioned
Cardiovascular status
Understanding of procedure, perioperative events, home care

NURSING DIAGNOSIS:

All generic nursing diagnoses apply to this patient, with the addition
  of:
High risk for fluid volume deficit

PATIENT OUTCOMES:

All generic outcomes apply, with the addition of:
The patient will maintain adequate fluid volume with hemodynamic
  stability.
1. Fluid balance will be maintained.
2. Vital signs will be within normal limits
3. Hemoglobin & hematocrit will be within normal limits.

NURSING ACTIONS:

	Yes	No	N/A
1. Preop assessment performed?	☐	☐	☐
2. Patient positioned correctly?	☐	☐	☐
3. Operative site determined/marked?	☐	☐	☐
4. Condition of operative site noted and recorded?	☐	☐	☐
5. ESU available/checked?	☐	☐	☐
6. Dispersive pad checked/applied?	☐	☐	☐
7. Special equipment/supplies available?	☐	☐	☐
8. Perioperative monitoring? (include blood loss)	☐	☐	☐
9. Asepsis maintained during procedure?	☐	☐	☐
10. Specimen(s) to lab?	☐	☐	☐
11. Counts performed/correct?	☐	☐	☐
12. Dispersive pad site checked?	☐	☐	☐
13. Dressings applied?	☐	☐	☐
14. Medications administered/documented?	☐	☐	☐
15. Postop garment applied?	☐	☐	☐
16. Other generic care plans initiated?	☐	☐	☐

Document additional nursing actions/generic care plans initiated
here:

_____

_____

_____

EVALUATION OF PATIENT OUTCOMES:

	Outcome met	Outcome met with additional outcome criteria	Outcome met with revised nursing care plan	Outcome not met	Outcome not applicable to this patient
1. The patient's fluid balance was maintained.	☐	☐	☐	☐	☐
2. The patient met outcomes for additional generic care plans.	☐	☐	☐	☐	☐

Signature: _____ Date: _____

1992). The perioperative nurse should verify with the patient that preoperative antimicrobial skin preparation was carried out (the patient may have been instructed to shower with an antimicrobial skin cleanser for a number of days) and that aspirin or aspirin-containing medications have not been used in the recent past (approximately 2 weeks). The patient's NPO status and consent should also be checked. The patient's expectations of the surgery should be elucidated.

2. Surgical position will vary. Supine, prone, lateral decubitus, or supine lateral decubitus position may be selected. In any of these positions, care needs to be taken to position the arms carefully; provide adequate support and accessory support devices (beanbags, rolls, and so on), pad dependent pressure areas, and correctly place safety straps.

3. The anatomic landmarks for surgical skin preparation will vary. The perioperative nurse may assist the surgeon in marking regions that will undergo SAL; an indelible marking pen is required. The area is then prepped with the antimicrobial agent of the surgeon's choice, taking care not to remove the skin markings.

4. The condition of the skin at the preparation site should be noted.

5. The electrosurgical unit may or may not be required, depending on the site and extent of the procedure.

6. The skin should be assessed at the site of application of the electrosurgical dispersive pad if the ESU is used.

7. A variety of suction machines are available for SAL. The perioperative nurse should be familiar with the proper operation of all equipment and the recommended pressure settings. Cannulas will vary in length, shape, and inner and outer diameters; a range of sizes will be necessary.

8. Monitoring is critical. SAL may be performed with the patient under local, regional, general, or spinal anesthesia. The extent of perioperative nursing monitoring will vary. Intravenous lines will be inserted; electrocardiogram, blood pressure, and pulse oximetry will be monitored. Careful monitoring of fluid volume is a primary responsibility. During the procedure, the surgeon is kept informed of lipid loss for each area suctioned; some suction machines automatically measure ratios of blood-to-fat loss. Fluid replacement therapy will take into account insensible losses, as well as intraoperative blood and fat loss. Depending on these volumes, lactated Ringer's solution, synthetic colloids, or blood replacement may be necessary.

9. Draping and movement of SAL areas (limbs or behind the knees) provide a challenge to maintaining asepsis.

10. Follow institutional protocol for the preservation and disposition of specimens.

11. Follow institutional protocol for counting sharps, sponges, and instruments.

12. The dispersive pad should be removed and the condition of the skin rechecked.

13. The suctioned site should be cleansed of blood and exudate. Dressings include small adhesive strips (Steri-Strips) or Band-Aids over the incision. Occasionally, extra padding with cushioning dressings (ABD pads) may be applied over the suctioned areas. These extra pads are removed after 24 to 36 hours.

14. Medications administered may include antibiotics and local anesthesia with epinephrine. All medications on the sterile field should be labeled and documented.

15. The postoperative garment, or a compression dressing with wide elastic tape, is placed immediately after surgery. The garments are specially ordered, and their availability must be ascertained in advance. They usually remain in place for a week postoperatively before they can be removed for bathing or showering. Thereafter they may be removed for bathing or for washing the garment, but they must be reapplied and worn day and night for up to 6 weeks.

Cosmetic Facial Surgery (Fig. 17-4)

1. Preoperative assessment of the cosmetic facial surgery patient is critical. The patient must be realistic about the reasons for the surgery. The effects of aging and/or weight loss lead to excess skin and soft tissue about the face and neck. The underlying musculature sags as well, and the fat pads about the eyes herniate, forming "bags." Surgery removes redundant tissue and tightens the supporting muscles. The patient's smoking history should be reviewed. Verify with the patient that he or she has not taken aspirin or medications containing aspirin during the 3 weeks before surgery. Antiinflammatory agents, some foods (Chinese foods and shellfish), and vitamin E alter bleeding patterns. Smokers have a much higher incidence of postoperative skin flap necrosis and therefore a longer healing period. Baseline vital signs should be checked. Review the medical history for evidence of allergies, hypertension, thyroid or cardiovascular disease, and diabetes. Blepharoplasty patients should be specifically queried regarding eye disorders (glaucoma, corneal abrasions, dry-eye syndrome). Visual field tests may have been per-

FIG. 17-4
CARE PLAN FOR COSMETIC FACIAL SURGERY (FACE-LIFT, BROW-LIFT, BLEPHAROPLASTY)

KEY ASSESSMENT POINTS

Preexisting eye disease, eyelid abnormality, vision problems (blepharoplasty)
Expectations of surgical outcome
Psychosocial status
History of anemia, bleeding disorders, hypertension, heart disease
Understanding of procedure, perioperative events, home care

NURSING DIAGNOSIS:

All generic nursing diagnoses apply to this patient, with the addition of:
High risk for fluid volume deficit
High risk for ineffective breathing pattern (face-lift)
High risk for injury related to altered vision (blepharoplasty)

PATIENT OUTCOMES:

All generic outcomes apply, with the addition of:
The patient will have adequate fluid volume.
The patient will demonstrate effective breathing.
The patient's vision will remain unaltered.
The patient will:
1. Have normal vital signs, oxygenation, laboratory values, and surgical site free of seroma, hematoma
2. Have respirations that remain regular in depth, rate, and quality
3. Maintain preoperative vision

NURSING ACTIONS:

	Yes	No	N/A
1. Preop assessment performed?	☐	☐	☐
2. Patient positioned correctly?	☐	☐	☐
3. Operative site determined/marked?	☐	☐	☐
4. Condition of operative site noted and recorded?	☐	☐	☐
5. ESU available/checked?	☐	☐	☐
6. Dispersive pad checked/applied?	☐	☐	☐
7. Special equipment/supplies available?	☐	☐	☐
8. Perioperative monitoring? (include blood loss)	☐	☐	☐
9. Laser safety protocol followed?	☐	☐	☐
10. Specimen(s) to lab?	☐	☐	☐
11. Counts performed/correct?	☐	☐	☐
12. Dispersive pad site checked?	☐	☐	☐
13. Dressings applied?	☐	☐	☐
14. Medications administered/documented?	☐	☐	☐
15. Postop instructions for family members?	☐	☐	☐
16. Other generic care plans initiated?	☐	☐	☐

Document additional nursing actions/generic care plans initiated here:

_____

_____

_____

EVALUATION OF PATIENT OUTCOMES:

	Outcome met	Outcome met with additional outcome criteria	Outcome met with revised nursing care plan	Outcome not met	Outcome not applicable to this patient
1. The patient's fluid balance was maintained.	☐	☐	☐	☐	☐
2. The patient maintained an effective airway.	☐	☐	☐	☐	☐
3. The patient maintained good visual acuity.	☐	☐	☐	☐	☐
4. The patient met outcomes for additional generic care plans.	☐	☐	☐	☐	☐

Signature: _____ Date: _____

formed for postoperative comparison. Consent should be checked for both the procedure and intraoperative photography.

2. Perioperative explanations should include intravenous sedation, use of local anesthetics, location of scars, and the need to relax during the procedure. Determine the patient's preferred relaxation technique (for example, music, imagery) and facilitate its use. The supine position is usually used; assist the patient to a position of comfort. Provide accessory devices as needed (pillow, cushioned head rest, and so on).

3. Anatomic landmarks will vary according to the procedure. Clear antimicrobial skin preparation agents will likely be used. Protect the eyes and ears (as applicable) from preparation solution.

4. The condition of the skin at the preparation site should be noted.

5. Depending on the surgical procedure, have the electrosurgical unit available.

6. If the electrosurgical unit is used, assess and note the condition of the skin at the site of dispersive pad application.

7. Special equipment will vary according to the surgeon's preference. However, the hair will need to be restrained as much as possible, for which small rubber bands may be used. Marking pens and accessories for local anesthesia will be required. The laser may be used; laser resurfacing may be performed for some wrinkles or superficial scars (Barbarich, 1995). Many surgeons incorporate SAL of the neck into the facelift. Check the availability of cannulas and aspirator. An operating headlight or lighted retractor may be requested.

8. Monitoring should include cardiac monitor and regular observations of respiratory rate. Pulse oximetry (attached to a fingertip) has proved to be an effective guide to tissue perfusion because it detects decreases before they are evident in the cardiac rate. Often the patient needs only to be reminded to breathe deeply to increase the perfusion rate to an acceptable level. This is especially important if sedatives or narcotics have been administered; frequently note the patient's level of consciousness. Any dyspnea, bradycardia, arrhythmias, hypotension, or hypertension should be noted and immediately reported; emergency drugs should be available.

9. If the laser is used, initiate laser safety precautions according to institutional protocol.

10. Follow institutional protocol for the preservation, documentation, and disposition of surgical specimens. Use universal precautions with all material and any containers received from the sterile field.

11. Follow institutional protocol for sponge, sharp, and instrument counts.

12. If the electrosurgical unit was used, the dispersive pad should be removed and the condition of the skin rechecked.

13. When the surgery is completed, the patient's hair should be washed immediately. Warm saline mixed with peroxide can be used to remove as much of the blood as possible. The hair should be rinsed with plain saline or water and towel-dried before the dressing is applied. Dressings for a face-lift patient will be extensive because the neck and cheek flaps must be kept in contact with the underlying tissue. Drains may be placed and connected to suction. The bulky head dressing remains in place and is changed on the first or second postoperative day. Application of cold during the first 12 to 24 hours decreases edema. The eyelids are not dressed but kept moist with cool compresses of iced saline to reduce edema. The astringent effect of cool tea bags often helps reduce eyelid swelling after the first day or so.

14. Medications should be documented (route, dose, time administered, and effect). These may include local anesthetics, sedatives, narcotics, and antibiotic ointment.

15. Because many cosmetic surgery patients do not stay in the institution overnight, the primary caregiver must be fully aware of the signs of postoperative complications. Any patient with surgery about the neck could develop a hematoma or seroma, which would compromise the trachea. The head of the bed should be raised because pillows alone can cause flexion of the neck and decreased circulation to the skin. Coughing, retching, or vomiting also cause bleeding and should be prevented with antitussive and antiemetic medications. The patient and family should be told to call the surgeon or come to the emergency department if excessive swelling occurs or the patient has increased shallow respirations, difficulty breathing, or stridor. The patient should not smoke. Care should be taken with hair dryers; they should be used where the hand can feel the air, set on a low temperature, and kept moving. Additional postoperative teaching will vary according to the procedure.

Cleft Lip and Palate (Fig. 17-5)

1. Preoperative assessment should take into consideration the child's stage of growth and development; patients vary in age according to the procedure. The child's fears should be considered and explanations geared toward the level of

FIG. 17-5
CARE PLAN FOR REPAIR OF CONGENITAL DEFORMITIES OF LIP AND/OR PALATE

KEY ASSESSMENT POINTS

Nutritional status/ability to take fluids via modified technique (if breastfeeding unsuccessful)
Age, weight, developmental status
History bleeding disorder
Family anxiety/coping mechanisms
Parental home care ability

NURSING DIAGNOSIS:

All generic nursing diagnoses apply to this patient, with the addition of:
High risk for infection at suture line
High risk for aspiration

PATIENT OUTCOMES:

All generic outcomes apply, with the addition of:
The patient will:
1. Have a suture line free of infection, bleeding, sloughing, or irritation
2. Manage secretions and formula/feedings without aspiration.

NURSING ACTIONS:

	Yes	No	N/A
1. Preop assessment performed?	☐	☐	☐
2. Patient positioned correctly?	☐	☐	☐
3. Thermia unit available?	☐	☐	☐
4. Skin preparation according to protocol?	☐	☐	☐
5. Condition of operative site noted and recorded?	☐	☐	☐
6. ESU available/checked?	☐	☐	☐
7. Dispersive pad checked/applied?	☐	☐	☐
8. Special equipment/supplies available?	☐	☐	☐
9. Perioperative monitoring? (include blood loss)	☐	☐	☐
10. Maintenance of aseptic technique?	☐	☐	☐
11. Specimen(s) to lab?	☐	☐	☐
12. Counts performed/correctly?	☐	☐	☐
13. Dispersive pad site checked?	☐	☐	☐
14. Dressings and restraints in place?	☐	☐	☐
15. Medications administered/documented?	☐	☐	☐
16. Other generic care plans initiated?	☐	☐	☐

Document additional nursing actions/generic care plans initiated here:

_____

_____

_____

EVALUATION OF PATIENT OUTCOMES;

	Outcome met	Outcome met with additional outcome criteria	Outcome met with revised nursing care plan	Outcome not met	Outcome not applicable to this patient
1. The patient's suture line was clean and intact.	☐	☐	☐	☐	☐
2. The patient maintained an effective airway.	☐	☐	☐	☐	☐
3. The patient met outcomes for additional generic care plans.	☐	☐	☐	☐	☐

Signature: _____ Date: _____

understanding. Security objects should be allowed to accompany the child to the OR. Skin integrity should be assessed, depending on the deformity (oral mucous membranes should be included). The child may have associated problems with the ears (fluid accumulation or otitis media), feeding, and speech. Parents should be allowed to stay with the child as long as possible, even during induction if permitted by institutional policy. Closure of the lip is performed at approximately 3 months of age and palate closure at 9 months to 2 years. Revisions of the lip, correction of nasal deformity, and pharyngeal flaps for velopharyngeal insufficiency are conducted during the preschool years and into adolescence as needed. Consent for surgery and photography (if appropriate) should be reviewed. Modify the care plan according to the individual patient's age and needs.

2. The supine position will be used, with the neck slightly extended. Special positioning precautions will depend on the child's age and size.

3. A thermia blanket should be used to maintain core temperature in a young child.

4. Skin preparation is done according to institutional protocol. Care must be taken to protect the eyes; ophthalmic lubricant and/or tape to keep the eyelids closed may be required. A bacteriostatic agent may be swabbed inside the mouth as part of preparation.

5. The condition of the skin at the preparation site should be noted.

6. An electrosurgical unit may be required.

7. If the electrosurgical unit is used, care must be taken to select an appropriate dispersive pad size and note the condition of the skin at the site of pad application.

8. Special instruments will vary according to the planned surgical intervention. A plastic surgery instrument set will be needed, with syringes and needles for local infiltration. Marking pens and instruments specific to the procedure will vary and must be added.

9. The perioperative nurse will need to collaborate with anesthesia staff during patient monitoring. In infants, blood loss will need to be measured and reported accurately.

10. Routine aseptic precautions will be in effect.

11. Follow institutional protocol for the preservation, documentation, and disposition of surgical specimens. Use universal precautions with all material and containers received from the sterile field.

12. Routine sharp, sponge, and instrument counts will be conducted; if a pharyngeal pack was placed, its removal should be ensured.

13. If the electrosurgical unit was used, the dispersive pad should be removed and the condition of the skin rechecked.

14. The reconstructed lip must be protected against tension. Often a Logan bow or other lip protective device is taped in place. The small child's elbows must be placed in restraints before reversal of anesthesia and kept restrained for 10 days to 2 weeks; the older infant may require a jacket restraint. It is sometimes difficult for parents to see the need for restraints; this teaching must be reinforced. Postoperatively the child should be placed in a side-lying position (an infant seat may be used) and observed for mechanical respiratory difficulty. Some surgeons leave a traction suture in the tongue until the child is fully recovered from anesthesia.

15. Medications need to be documented, particularly the amount and dilution of epinephrine, which is occasionally used as a hemostatic agent in the palate or pharynx.

Skin Grafting (Fig. 17-6)

1. Preoperative assessment of the patient undergoing skin grafting depends on the cause of the wound. Grafts are applied to burn patients and to those with unhealed wounds needing skin coverage. These wounds include secondarily healing surgical wounds, superficial leg ulcers, or pressure sores. Grafting may also be done to cover the surface of a microvascular free tissue transfer. The perioperative nurse will need to determine the reason for the grafting. Generally, assessment data should include nutritional information (may contribute to poor wound healing), baseline musculoskeletal and neurovascular data (for postoperative comparisons), and the condition of the graft site (there should be healthy granulation tissue). Note any areas of diminished sensation, poor skin turgor, ulcerated areas and their appearance, and limitations in mobility. Laboratory values reviewed should include white blood cell and complete blood counts, clotting profiles, and serum protein level. Culture results should also be reviewed (if applicable).

2. Positioning of the patient for the skin graft must allow relatively easy access to the donor and recipient sites. Accessories such as rolled sheets, sandbags, and other support devices may be required. Bony prominences should be padded and dependent skin areas protected.

3. Donor and recipient sites will need to be prepared. Anatomic landmarks for prepared areas will vary according to grafting site.

FIG. 17-6
CARE PLAN FOR SKIN GRAFTING

KEY ASSESSMENT POINTS

Reason for skin graft
Location/condition of recipient site
Donor tissue site
Age, weight, mental acuity
Medical condition (diabetes, anemia, etc.)
Mobility limitations
Circulatory status
Nutritional status
Understanding of procedure, perioperative events
Patient capability for prevention of recurrence, home management, self-care

NURSING DIAGNOSIS:

All generic nursing diagnoses apply to this patient, with the addition of:
Impaired skin integrity

PATIENT OUTCOMES:

All generic outcomes apply, with the addition of:
The patient's skin integrity will be restored. The graft site will:
1. Have adequate circulation (color, temperature, sensation, capillary refill and Doppler measurements satisfactory)
2. Heal without infection, hematoma, edema
3. Maintain intact approximation of skin edges

NURSING ACTIONS:

	Yes	No	N/A
1. Preop assessment performed?	☐	☐	☐
2. Patient positioned correctly?	☐	☐	☐
3. Skin preparation according to protocol?	☐	☐	☐
4. Condition of operative site noted and recorded?	☐	☐	☐
5. ESU available/checked?	☐	☐	☐
6. Dispersive pad checked/applied?	☐	☐	☐
7. Special equipment/supplies available?	☐	☐	☐
8. Perioperative monitoring?	☐	☐	☐
9. Maintenance of aseptic technique?	☐	☐	☐
10. Specimen(s) to lab?	☐	☐	☐
11. Counts performed/correct?	☐	☐	☐
12. Dispersive pad site checked?	☐	☐	☐
13. Dressings and splints in place?	☐	☐	☐
14. Medications administered/documented?	☐	☐	☐
15. Other generic care plans initiated?	☐	☐	☐

Document additional nursing actions/generic care plans initiated here:

_____

_____

_____

EVALUATION OF PATIENT OUTCOMES:

	Outcome met	Outcome met with additional outcome criteria	Outcome met with revised nursing care plan	Outcome not met	Outcome not applicable to this patient
1. The patient's skin integrity was restored.	☐	☐	☐	☐	☐
2. The patient met outcomes for additional generic care plans.	☐	☐	☐	☐	☐

Signature: _____ Date: _____

4. The condition of the skin at the donor and recipient sites should be noted (for example, reddened, draining, or necrotic).

5. Depending on the type of skin graft planned, the electrosurgical unit may be required.

6. If the electrosurgical unit is used, note the condition of the skin at the site of dispersive pad application.

7. Special equipment for skin grafting includes a dermatome or knife for harvesting the graft. Small grafts may be taken with a single-edged razor blade in a special handle (Weck knife). The dermatomes may be electric or manually powered. The Reese dermatome requires special adhesive tapes and blades that fit onto the machine as well as special adhesive for the skin itself. Skin preparation includes use of a degreaser. Care must be taken during assembly. The blade is inserted by the surgeon just before use. The Padgett dermatome works with a small motor and disposable blade. The skin is lubricated with mineral oil. Stents are made of cotton, Dacron, or foam rubber and function to press the graft gently but firmly onto the recipient bed. Spinal needles (3½ inches) are used to inject the donor sites (usually with 0.5% or 0.25% lidocaine (Xylocaine) with epinephrine). Skin grafts may be "meshed" with a device that makes preselected cuts, allowing the graft to be stretched over a larger area and providing slits for exudate. This type of graft is less aesthetic and is not used where it would be cosmetically unacceptable.

8. The perioperative nurse will need to collaborate with anesthesia staff in monitoring the patient. Some grafting procedures are extensive, and the patient may be debilitated or elderly with complicating medical conditions.

9. Draping procedures involve two sites; movement between sites should be carefully monitored. Gowns and gloves may be changed when moving between sites; instruments may be isolated from the donor site.

10. Follow institutional protocol for preservation, documentation, and disposition of specimens (or unused harvested skin). Use universal precautions with material or containers received from the sterile field. Document specimens or banking of harvested skin.

11. Follow institutional protocol for sponge, sharp, and instrument counts.

12. If the electrosurgical unit was used, the dispersive pad should be removed and the condition of the skin rechecked.

13. Dressings for skin grafts include an impregnated gauze over the graft, application of a stent with tie-over sutures or staples, and a bulky outer dressing. Applications of plaster splints or casts immobilize the extremity. Donor site dressings are applied with an oxygen-permeable membrane (Op-site or Tegaderm) and compressed with a circumferential wrap and Ace bandage for the first few days.

The skin graft survives by osmosis for the first few days after grafting and must remain in contact with the recipient bed. Loss of the graft is usually caused by disruption of the graft from the bed by fluid collection (seroma or hematoma) or shearing forces. The graft is held in place by fibrin and supported by the application of a stent or tie-over bolus and the dressing. The wound must be kept from any movement. When on an extremity, the wound is supported by a plaster splint or cast, which immobilizes the joint above and below the wound. Care must be taken when transferring the patient to the postoperative bed or transfer vehicle.

14. Depending on the type of grafting procedure, medications (local anesthetics or antibiotics) may have been administered. Document medications administered from the sterile field.

Breast Surgery: Postmastectomy Breast Reconstruction (Fig. 17-7)

With modifications, this care plan may be adapted to most breast surgeries. The emphasis of the nursing diagnosis should be broadened to include actual or the risk for *body image disturbance, self-esteem disturbance, anticipatory grieving, anxiety,* and *fear* expected in the patient undergoing breast surgery.

1. Preoperative assessment involves determining the patient's knowledge regarding the planned surgical intervention. The perioperative nurse also assesses the patient who has had chemotherapy for nutritional status, skin integrity, stomatitis, fluid volume status, coping strategies, and self-concept issues. The nursing diagnosis selected for this patient, *risk for altered tissue perfusion* after the implant procedure requires preoperative baseline assessment of perfusion adequacy at the implant site for postoperative comparison. Depending on the patient, modify the care plan according to prioritized needs.

2. Positioning will vary according to the type of reconstruction planned. For prosthesis insertion, the patient will be supine; the head of the OR bed may be slightly elevated, with the arm abducted 20 to 30 degrees (too much abduction will stretch the pectoralis muscles). For insertion of a combined tissue expander/prosthesis, the arm may be abducted to nearly 90 degrees

FIG. 17-7
CARE PLAN FOR BREAST SURGERY: POSTMASTECTOMY BREAST RECONSTRUCTION

KEY ASSESSMENT POINTS
Expectations of surgery
Feelings about diagnosis (breast cancer)
History/status chemotherapy or radiation
Nutritional status
Skin integrity
Support systems
Understanding of procedure, perioperative events, home care requirements

NURSING DIAGNOSIS:
All generic nursing diagnoses apply to this patient, with the addition of:
Impaired skin integrity

Body image disturbance
High risk for altered tissue perfusion

PATIENT OUTCOMES:
All generic outcomes apply, with the addition of:
The patient's tissue perfusion and skin integrity will be maintained at the reconstructed site. There will be adequate color, temperature, and capillary refill.
The patient will progress toward a positive integration of physical changes and sexuality concerns into the body image.

NURSING ACTIONS:

	Yes	No	N/A
1. Preop assessment performed?	☐	☐	☐
2. Patient positioned correctly?	☐	☐	☐
3. Skin preparation according to protocol?	☐	☐	☐
4. Condition of operative site noted and recorded?	☐	☐	☐
5. ESU available/checked?	☐	☐	☐
6. Dispersive pad checked/applied?	☐	☐	☐
7. Special equipment/supplies available?	☐	☐	☐
8. Perioperative monitoring?	☐	☐	☐
9. Maintenance of aseptic technique?	☐	☐	☐
10. Specimen(s) to lab?	☐	☐	☐
11. Counts performed/correct?	☐	☐	☐
12. Dispersive pad site checked?	☐	☐	☐
13. Dressings in place?	☐	☐	☐
14. Medications administered/documented?	☐	☐	☐
15. Document the use of implants following protocol?	☐	☐	☐
16. Other generic care plans initiated?	☐	☐	☐

Document additional nursing actions/generic care plans initiated here:

_____

_____

_____

EVALUATION OF PATIENT OUTCOMES:

	Outcome met	Outcome met with additional outcome criteria	Outcome met with revised nursing car plan	Outcome not met	Outcome not applicable to this patient
1. The patient's tissue perfusion and skin integrity was maintained at the reconstructed site.	☐	☐	☐	☐	☐
2. The patient verbalized problems, concerns, and resources for integrating a positive body image.	☐	☐	☐	☐	☐
3. The patient met outcomes for additional generic care plans.	☐	☐	☐	☐	☐

Signature: _____ Date: _____

(to allow tunneling for the reservoir conduit). For rotation flaps, the patient may be in a lateral position, with the OR bed tilted to bring the anterior chest slightly upward. Patient positioning needs to be coordinated with the surgical team.

3. Anatomic landmarks for skin preparation will also vary according to the planned reconstruction. For rectus abdominis myocutaneous flaps, skin preparation will include the breast and abdomen, from side to side and neck to groin. For tissue expander or implant placement, the lower portion of the preparation extends to the waist. Placement of absorbent pads underneath the torso will help keep the patient's back clean. Breast reconstruction may be accompanied by mastopexy (breast-lift) on the opposite side; skin preparation will then include that breast.

4. The condition of the skin at the preparation site(s) should be noted.

5. The electrosurgical unit should be available and checked. In some procedures, two units may be used. Documentation should include identification numbers of both units and pad placement sites.

6. The skin should be assessed before placement of electrosurgical dispersive pad(s). If an extensive skin preparation is done, the pads should be protected from preparation solution.

7. Special equipment needed for implant or tissue expander insertion includes a lighted retractor and/or headlight, uterine sounds for blunt dissection, and a malleable retractor or "fish" for the closure. Prostheses and trials are required. If the implant is also a tissue expander, be sure to save the magnetic locating device (to identify the injection port) for use in the office afterward. For rotation of a pedicle flap, the lighted retractor is used. Microvascular instruments may be needed if the flap is to be "supercharged" with a microvascular anastomosis at its distal end.

8. The perioperative nurse will need to collaborate with anesthesia staff during patient monitoring.

9. Follow manufacturer's recommendations for sterilizing all implanted materials.

10. Follow institutional protocol for the preservation, documentation, and disposition of surgical specimens. (If the care plan is modified for breast reduction, separately label and weigh tissue from each breast before laboratory disposition.)

11. Follow institutional protocol for sponge, sharp, and instrument counts.

12. The dispersive pad site(s) should be rechecked on pad removal.

13. Postoperative dressings include an emollient gauze or ointment over the incision and soft bulky dressings over the implant or tissue expander. The surgeon may prefer to wrap the patient circumferentially with Ace wraps or place her in an elastic brassiere. For flap reconstructions, the dressing is absorbent and bulky and does not occlude any pedicle or anastomotic site. Care should be taken to see that drains do not lie over the pedicle or place undue pressure on the reconstruction. Blood supply is assessed by color, temperature, tissue turgor, capillary refill, and arterial blood flow monitoring via Doppler (Giomuso & Suster, 1994).

14. Any perioperative medications administered from the sterile field should be documented.

15. Follow institutional protocol for documenting implants.

16. Note any drains that have been incorporated into the dressing.

References

Abbott C. (1994). Planning patient care: A functional health patterns approach. In M Phippen & M Wells, *Perioperative nursing practice.* Philadelphia: WB Saunders.

Ball K. (1995). Lasers. In M Meeker & J Rothrock, (Eds.). *Alexander's care of the patient in surgery,* (10th ed.). St. Louis: Mosby.

Barbarich S. (1995). Laser resurfacing offers new technique in plastic surgery. *Advanced Technology Newsletter, 2*(4), 3.

Bichat X. (1814). *Desault's surgery.* Philadelphia: Thomas Dobson.

Black J. (1993). Nursing care of patients having plastic surgery. In J Black & E Matassarin-Jacobs, (Eds.). *Luckman and Sorensen's medical surgical nursing.* Philadelphia: WB Saunders.

Burden N. (1993). *Ambulatory surgical nursing.* Philadelphia: WB Saunders.

Carpenito L. (1993). *Nursing diagnosis: Application to clinical practice* (5th ed.). Philadelphia: JB Lippincott.

Cordeiro PG & Hidalgo DA. (1994). Options for breast reconstruction after mastectomy. In *Care of the surgical patient.* New York: Scientific American.

Donahoe K. (1995). Plastic and reconstructive surgery. In M Meeker & J Rothrock, (Eds.). *Alexander's care of the patient in surgery* (10th ed.). St. Louis: Mosby.

Giomuso CB, & Suster V. (1994). Free flap breast reconstruction. *Medsurg Nursing, 3*(1), 9-23.

Gulanick M, et al. (1994). *Nursing care plans: Nursing diagnosis and intervention.* St. Louis: Mosby.

Hidalgo DA. (1995). Plastic surgical reconstruction. In *Care of the surgical patient.* New York: Scientific American.

Joganic EF & Reiff JL. (1994, March 14). *Nursing care of the craniofacial surgical patient.* Paper presented at the AORN Congress, New Orleans.

Kneedler J & Dodge G. (1994). *Perioperative patient care, the nursing perspective* (3rd. ed.). Boston: Jones and Bartlett.

McKenna C & Black J. (1994). Pediatric surgical nursing, plastic surgical nursing. *Nursing Clinics of North America, 30*(1), 701-738.

Pettis D & Vogt P. (1992). Complications of suction-assisted lipoplasty. *Plastic Surgical Nursing, 12*(4), 148-151.

Pruzinski T. (1993) Psychological factors in cosmetic plastic surgery: Recent developments in patient care, *Plastic Surgical Nursing, 13*(2), 64-71.

Richards M. (1994). Common pediatric craniofacial reconstructions. *Nursing Clinics of North America, 30*(1), 791-799.

Spencer K. (1994). Selection and preoperative preparation of plastic surgery patients. *Nursing Clinics of North America, 30*(1), 697-710.

Westlake C, (1991). Commitment to function: Microsurgical flaps. *Plastic Surgical Nursing, (11)*3, 95-100.

Wirt S, Algren C, & Arnold S. (1992). Cleft lips and palates: A multidisciplinary approach, *Plastic Surgical Nursing, 12*(4), 140-145.

Wood J & Jurkiewicz M. (1994). Plastic and reconstructive surgery. In S Schwartz (Ed.). *Principles of surgery*, (6th ed.). New York: McGraw-Hill.

Chapter 18

Genitourinary Surgery

Gratia M. Nagle

At the present time there is no more said of all the systems of the ancients and the moderns, respecting the formation of urinary stones. Faith no longer is placed in animal magnetism. In the fermentation of white and glutinous glairous matter, in its concretion by volatile alkali, etc.; but we know that the urine of the soundest man contains the rudiments of calculus, and that, when left at rest for some time, it deposits a larger or smaller quantity of crystals, concrete salts, and sand. . . . Researches have long been made for a remedy, capable of breaking down and dissolving the calculous concretions. Frequently it has been supposed to have been found, and its apparent success boasted of. Unhappily, experience has not confirmed the virtue of these pretended lithontriptics or stone-breakers. . . . The failure of lithontriptic remedies reduces the indications, which we may hope to accomplish with regard to calculi, to two only; to prevent and alleviate the symptoms . . . and to facilitate their expulsion or to extract them, when they are situated in places that are accessible to the surgeon's instruments.

BICHAT, 1814

Genitourinary surgery involves the management of diseases of the urogenital tract in males and the urinary tract in females. The urinary system, comprising the adrenal glands, kidneys, ureters, bladder, and urethra, is responsible for the formation, storage, transport, and elimination of urine. The kidneys play a major role in homeostasis, excreting the products of metabolism and controlling the concentration of most of the body's fluids. Embryologically, the genital and urinary tracts are closely related. Genitourinary tract developmental anomalies occur in more than 10% of the population and may predispose the patient to infection, stone formation, or chronic renal failure (McCance & Huether, 1994). Acquired lesions of the genitourinary tract include, but are not limited to, obstruction, stenosis, fibrosis, hyperplasia, strictures, infections, calculi, and tumors.

HISTORY

A number of forces affecting the development of genitourinary surgery continue to interest perioperative nurses and physicians caring for patients with genitourinary problems. Technology has allowed urology to offer an array of noninvasive surgical interventions for the problems that plagued early humankind.

Weyrauch (Kropp, 1987) has traced the history of prostatectomy to 460 BC. Removal of bladder stones through an incision is one of the earliest known surgeries; itinerant lithotomists flourished from the time of Hippocrates to the early eighteenth century. Kropp (1987) suggests that the term "lithotomy position" is derived from the position in which ancient lithotomists placed patients during bladder stone removal. Stone formation was variously attributed to temperament; sexual, dietary, and alcoholic indulgence; poor digestion; temperate climate; moist, thick stagnant air or marshes; indolence (laziness was thought to retard the evacuation of urine); well water; the presence of associated disease states (rheumatism, rickets, and arthritis); and familial tendency (Bichat, 1814).

A multitude of remedies (lithontriptics) were developed to dissolve urinary stones. Among these were the blood of a goat, petroleum, millipedes, the eyes of a lobster, lemon juice, lime with eggshells (to which soap was added to overcome the constipation produced by the lime), and onions (Bichat, 1814). When these remedies failed, as most did, surgical extraction of the stone was attempted. Stones were believed to be encapsulated; sounds were used to create gentle friction to separate the stone from its cystic membrane. Sounds of various types were developed for locating bladder stones; these were made of metal or gum elastica and were rigid or flexible, hollow or solid. Stone forceps were used, in which the stone was grasped and repeatedly squeezed. Various instruments for cutting stones were also developed.

Because any surgery, including stone extraction, presented dangers to the patient, interest in medicinal remedies for genitourinary ailments persisted. A 1909 book written by two physicians offered treatment suggestions for a number of problems (Wood & Ruddock, 1909). Bloody urine, determined often to be caused by small stones in the ureter or kidney, was to be treated by a strong brew of marshmallow tea, made from the leaves, buttons, or roots of the marshmallow; if ulceration was present, oil of turpentine was to be added to the cup of tea. Cystitis was thought to be cured by a tea of the pods or hulls of the common bean; parsley tea or tea of the trailing arbutus was also prescribed. Hot fomentations of hops and rest in the horizontal position were recommended for the pain accompanying cystitis, as was tepid bladder irrigation. Bright's disease of the kidneys was thought to be related to scarlet fever, exposure to wet and cold, and the irritating action of drugs and alcohol. Unfermented cider, tea made from peach leaves and queen-of-the-meadow, milk, tea from hops, or radishes the size of a finger eaten three times a day were variously prescribed.

Warmed or vapor baths were recommended to assist the bloodstream in carrying off deleterious materials when the kidneys were inactive.

A remedy for kidney stones, which Wood and Ruddock (1909) determined to be superior to any patent kidney cure sold, was to burn saltpeter to a coal, pulverize it, and take one fourth of a teaspoonful twice a day. Other remedies for kidney stones included essence of peppermint, carrots, and sheep sorrel tea. For the pain associated with kidney stones, local application of heat, cupping, and hot baths were recommended, along with diuretic therapy.

Wood and Ruddock (1909) also described various therapies for impotence. One remedy was the application of electricity to the affected part; if a battery could not be obtained for this purpose, they recommended toning the organs with a salt-water sponge bath. Proper nutrition, fresh air, and exercise were prescribed, along with avoiding tobacco and stimulants. Other remedies included unicorn root tea and hemp tea to increase sexual passion. The authors properly cautioned against too strong a dose of hemp tea, which could produce delirium.

For the hysteric retention of urine, which was attributed to women and thought more likely to occur during menstrual periods, a simple and prompt remedy was to place the hands in cold water. The authors recommended this treatment, possibly accompanied by forceful prevention of the patient's breathing for a certain time by holding the mouth and nose, as infinitely preferable to catheterization.

In the early nineteenth century, although instruments were inadequate and light sources were relegated to candles or lamps, attempts were made to visualize the inside of the bladder. In 1876, Nitze developed the instrument that became the basis of the modern cystoscope and urologic endoscopy (Walsh, et al., 1992). In 1902 the first renal grafting was performed, heralding dramatic advances in kidney transplant surgery (Shepherd, 1986). Improved endoscopic instrumentation and accessories, antibiotic and immunosuppressant therapies, diagnostic radiography and imaging, as well as scientific research discoveries paved the way for modern genitourinary surgery.

Advances in the treatment of urinary tract stones continue to characterize genitourinary surgery. Extracorporeal shock wave lithotripsy (ESWL), first introduced in 1980, has often supplanted both nephrolithotomy and percutaneous nephrolithotripsy (Gillenwater, 1996). Transurethral ureteroscopic electrohydraulic lithotripsy (EHL) is another surgical procedure for removing kidney stones. Procedures combining an endoscopic probe or ureteroscope to visualize the stones and lithotripsy to crush them have proven superior to conventional surgery for removing kidney stones (Cubler-Goodman, Devlin, & Dinatale, 1993). Such procedures include transurethral ureteroscopic lithotripsy, EHL, ESWL, and percutaneous and ultrasonic lithotripsy. Successful removal of stones by any of these procedures depends on the size, location, shape, and position of the stone. Transurethral ureteroscopic lithotripsy has the advantage of offering endoscopic access to the distal portion of the urinary tract and permitting direct fragmentation and removal of stones therein (Corriere, 1994). Changes in instrument design and alternative methods of generating shock waves have eliminated the need for water baths in the latest ESWL equipment. Because shock waves are less powerful in new units, a greater number of shock waves are generally required. Although less anesthesia may be needed due to the lower frequency of these units, and stones below the pelvic bone are now accessible, stone fragmentation has not proven to be adequate for the spontaneous passage of residual gravel.

Treatment of benign prostatic hypertrophy by prostatectomy has been effective in relieving symptoms of enlarged prostate; research indicates that it is important to evaluate benign prostatic hyperplasia (BPH) symptoms from the patient's perspective when assessing BPH treatment options (Fowler & Barry, 1993). Controversy continues, however, regarding open prostatectomy versus transurethral approaches, regarding "watchful waiting" versus surgical intervention, and regarding the incidence of urethral strictures and frequency of postoperative cystoscopy (Lu-Yao, Barry, & Chang, 1994). Balloon inflation under fluoroscopy to stretch the outside layer of the prostate, separating the lobes and widening the channels, has also been reported for benign enlargement of the prostate. Because of the high prevalence of BPH (one in every four men in the United States will require treatment for symptomatic BPH by the age of 80), the Agency for Health Care Policy and Research (AHCPR) published its eighth clinical practice guideline to recommend management of this condition. The decision diagram in Fig. 18-1 is the guideline's framework for diagnosis and treatment. Treatment of carcinoma of the prostate, a leading cause of cancer-related death of American men, has been improved by detection through transrectal prostatic aspiration, often guided by ultrasound. Developments in surgical resection by radical prostatectomy have placed emphasis on preventing impotency as a result of surgery. Of recent interest is cryoablation for prostate cancer, the second most common neoplasm in men over the age of 50 (see Box 18-1 for risk factors for prostate cancer). Primarily indicated in the treatment of localized tumors, supercooled nitrogen is introduced via a transrectal ultrasound, destroying cancerous tissue cells through freezing (Keetch, Moore, & Shea, 1995). This minimally invasive approach to prostatic carcinoma carries side effects of potential rectal injury and fistula, as well as risk for incontinence and impotence (Mathias, 1995).

A variety of implantable Silastic prostheses, splints, and implants have resulted from advances in biomedical engineering. Ureteral splints can be implanted to protect healing ureters or permanently implanted to protect ureteral compression by tumor. The development of testicular prostheses and penile implants has allowed male patients to experience more normal sexual functioning and appearance. For neurogenic bladder, inflatable sphincters may be inserted that ring the bladder neck; artificial urinary sphincters may also be used to treat postprostatectomy incontinence (Tiemann, et al., 1993).

The laser has shown some promise in the treatment of selected carcinomas of the genitourinary tract. The neodymium:yttrium-aluminum-garnet (Nd:YAG) laser has been widely used in endourology; the argon-pumped tunable dye laser has also been used in photodynamic treatment protocols for bladder cancer.

Renal transplantation has been firmly established as accepted therapy for selected cases of chronic renal failure; advances in immunosuppressive therapy have contributed significantly to both patient and graft survival. Extracorporeal renal surgery has allowed the correction of several pathologic conditions of the renal artery and kidney; vascular lesions and neoplasms have been treated by removing the kidney and cooling, repairing, and reimplanting it.

To demonstrate to physicians and administrators the need for the professional nurse in the operating room (OR), perioperative nurses must identify their unique focus and demonstrate accountability in terms of that focus. Nursing diagnosis is a mechanism for identifying the practice of perioperative nursing, whereas care planning is the mechanism to demonstrate accountability. Perioperative nursing care plans should extend to meet the needs of patients in each subspecialty of surgery. Therefore this chapter lists nursing diagnoses common to the patient undergoing genitourinary surgery. Furthermore, this chapter suggests modifications that can be made to the generic care plans for the genitourinary surgery patient population. Finally, prototype care plans will be offered for specific genitourinary surgical interventions.

ASSESSMENT CONSIDERATIONS

Assessment is the systematic collection and interpretation of data. The perioperative nurse continu-

Decision diagram: Management of BPH

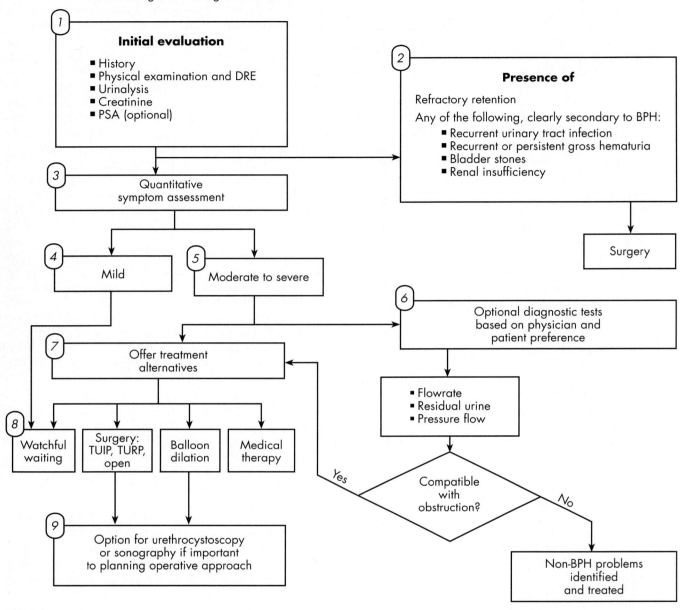

Fig. 18-1. Decision diagram: Management of BPH

ously gathers accurate data about the patient and the influencing environmental factors. This information is used to identify patient problems that relate to nursing care and to develop nursing diagnoses, the mainstay for the perioperative care plan. Assessment begins with a review of the patient's history. Because some genitourinary patients are elderly, recommendations for modifying perioperative assessments are presented in Box 18-2.

History

In reviewing the patient's health history, the perioperative nurse focuses on information related to genitourinary function. The history usually begins with the patient's chief concern or complaint; it is helpful to have patients validate in their own words the reason for seeking medical attention. Patients may be embarrassed by discussing problems associated with parts of their anatomy or physiologic functions they consider private. Seidel, et al. (1995) suggest that the nurse use language the patient can understand, without being condescending. Casual talk or jokes about the genitalia or sexual functions are inappropriate. An example of a focused history and physical examination for the genitourinary patient follows:

Box 18-1 Risk Factors for Prostate Cancer

Age over 50
Residence in the United States
Diet high in animal fat
Alcohol use
Family history of prostate cancer
Occupational exposure to cadmium, fertilizer, exhaust fumes, and rubber
Prostate-specific antigen (PSA) level >4 ng/ml

From Seidel HM, et al. (1995). *Mosby's guide to physical examination* (3rd ed.). St. Louis: Mosby.

Box 18-2 Geriatric Considerations in Renal/Urinary Assessment

General Approach
- Allow more time than for a younger adult
- Articulate clearly; the geriatric patient may be hearing impaired
- Impaired sight, comprehension, or mobility may result in less than optimum cooperation
- Provide clear, concise instructions

History Collection
- May need to repeat questions
- Be alert for answers that do not appear appropriate; the patient may not have understood the question correctly because of impaired hearing or impaired comprehension
- New-onset incontinence may be a manifestation of urinary tract infection

Physical Assessment
- The physical examination itself is not different, but the approach needs to be altered to ensure that the appropriate information is assessed without undue discomfort or embarrassment for the patient
- Maintain an environment with minimal noise, distractions, and interruption
- The glomerular filtration rate decreases with age
- Creatinine clearance decreases with age

From Beare PG & Meyers JL. (1994). *Principles and practices of adult health nursing*, (2nd ed.). St. Louis: Mosby.

I. History
   A. Family history (focus: hereditary and/or non-inherited renal disease)
      1. Hypertension
      2. Diabetes mellitus
      3. Gout
      4. Malignancy (family history of prostate cancer increases patient risk [Newton, Moore, & Gaehle, 1994])
      5. Polycystic kidney disease
      6. Hereditary nephritis (Alport's syndrome)
      7. Renal calculi
      8. Cardiovascular disease
      9. Disorders of related systems (neurologic, spinal cord, peripheral nervous system)
   B. Previous history (focus: predisposition to or presence of renal disease)
      1. Previous genitourinary surgery (and other surgery)
      2. Occupational hazards (exposure to toxins and chemicals)
      3. Genital lesions and sexually transmitted diseases
      4. Urinary history (infections, calculus, dysuria, hematuria, frequency)
      5. Weight loss and gain
      6. Fever and malaise
      7. History of infectious or chronic disease process (tuberculosis, pheochromocytoma)
   C. History of present illness (focus: signs and symptoms)
      1. Pain
      2. Altered voiding patterns
      3. Nausea, vomiting, or anorexia
      4. Altered bowel elimination
   D. Medication history (all of the following may alter genitourinary status and function) (Alfaro-Lefevre, et al. 1992)
      1. Antibiotics/antifungals
      2. Anticoagulants/antihypertensives/vasodilators
      3. Analgesics/nonsteroidals (include over-the-counter)
      4. Anticholinergics/cholinergics
      5. Diuretics
      6. Alpha and beta adrenergics/beta adrenergic blockers
      7. Antihistamines/histamines
      8. Antineoplastics/hormonals/androgens
      9. Adrenocorticosteroids
      10. Anticholinergics/cholinergics
      11. Anticonvulsants/antidepressants/antipsychotics
   E. Allergies (include shellfish, iodine, contrast dye, and tape)
II. Physical examination
   A. Inspection (observation)
      1. Level of consciousness and comprehension
         a. Through interview evaluate psychosocial needs

b. Alleviate fears and embarrassment as appropriate

c. Expand on knowledge deficit by assessing level of understanding regarding the proposed procedure. Patients should:

   (1) Know why they are having surgery

   (2) Be able to state what procedure involves in their own words

   (3) Verbalize any concerns about diagnosis, procedure, or expected outcome

d. If dealing with a pediatric patient, assess cognitive level and emotional maturity:

   (1) Security measures should be offered

   (2) Speak at child's level of understanding

2. General appearance

  a. Skin color, temperature, turgor, and texture

  b. Presence of edema, distention, or ecchymosis

  c. Joint mobility and range of motion

  d. Presence of any implanted prosthetics

3. Review and obtain baseline vital signs

  a. Observe adequacy of oxygen perfusion

  b. Note presence of costovertebral fullness

B. Auscultation (should always be the first step following inspection of the urology patient)

1. At the intercostal region of the anterior abdomen for aortic or renal bruits and murmurs, or; note rate and character of apical beats

2. Over abdomen, evaluate presence and character of bowel sounds

3. Across posterior thorax, evaluate presence and character of breath sounds

C. Palpation (will alter normal peristalsis)

1. With patient supine, lightly palpate abdomen to assess muscular resistance and tenderness in suprapubic region and at right and left upper quadrants

2. While patient is still supine, palpate again, deeply, to evaluate abdominal organs and detect masses

3. To assess kidneys, use deep palpation to locate outer aspects

  a. Normal kidney is firm, smooth, and nontender

  b. Use left hand for left kidney and right hand for right kidney

  c. Lift flank with one hand and place examining hand anteriorly at costal margin as supine patient inhales

  d. Left kidney is rarely palpable; neither are readily assessed except in thin adult

  e. Tenderness or pain may indicate renal abnormality

4. Evaluate the inguinal area for nodes, hernia, or varicocele

5. Include testes, penis, and prostate as indicated

  a. Testicles should be sensitive to pressure but not tender to light palpation

  b. Testicles should be oval shaped and have a smooth consistency

  c. Prostatic lobes should be symmetric and mobile with firm, smooth consistency; normally 4 cm in size

  d. Prostate diseases and common findings include:

   (1) BPH: boggy consistency with symmetric enlargement

   (2) Adenocarcinoma: discrete nodule or lobular induration with symmetric enlargement

   (3) Prostatitis: moderate to extreme tenderness with asymmetric enlargement

   (4) Neurologic impairment: unable to tighten anal sphincter

6. Assess radial and pedal pulses for quality and character

D. Percussion

1. At the costovertebral margins to determine kidney pain and tenderness

  a. Patient should be sitting

  b. Place palm over costovertebral angle and strike examining hand lightly with other fist

  c. Patient should feel a dull thud without tenderness or pain

2. Of the abdomen to determine ascites or bladder distention

  a. Evaluate tympany versus dullness over all quadrants

  b. Lower quadrants should be tympanic, and area of liver should denote dullness

  c. Dullness in suprapubic region generally reflects bladder distention

3. Assess lungs for resonance versus dullness

  a. Resonance normal over anterior aspects and apices and over posterior aspects to ninth rib

  b. Bases gradually develop dullness over borders

Pain. Genitourinary disorders may be accompanied by pain. Rea, et al. (1987) suggest the PQRST method for pain evaluation.

*P*rovocation refers to factors that aggravate pain. Renal pain may be aggravated by movement, percussion in the costovertebral margin, hydration, or traction on the renal pedicle, as in nephroptosis.

*Q*uality of pain is an important distinguishing feature. Pain from the kidney is usually noted as a dull ache in the flank; chronic prostatitis can cause a dull ache in the perineum or back. Bladder infection is often accompanied by a dull, continuous suprapubic pain. Ureteral obstruction often leads to colic; pain is felt in the flank and lower abdomen.

*R*adiation of pain and the primary region are similarly important. Patients with renal tumors or extensive infection may experience referred shoulder pain. Pain from ureteral obstruction may be referred to the lower abdomen, scrotum, and inner thigh. Because the testes and kidney have the same nerve supply, kidney disease may cause pain to be referred to the testis along the spermatic cord. Scrotal pain may represent referred pain from the ureter. Primary scrotal pain may result from epididymitis, orchitis, or testicular torsion. Most testicular tumors do not cause pain (Tanagho & McAniinch, 1991). Pain that originates in the flank or abdomen and moves progressively toward the groin may represent an acutely obstructing stone.

*S*evere flank pain may be present in the patient with a stone at the lower end of the ureter. Pain may also be severe and persistent with urinary retention.

*T*iming of pain, its onset, and duration should also be assessed in the genitourinary patient, especially whether pain is related to voiding and whether it occurs during or after urination.

Voiding patterns. Because genitourinary problems manifest themselves as voiding abnormalities, the patient should be queried specifically about problems with voiding patterns. These may include hesitancy, decreased caliber and force of the urinary stream, frequency, urgency, nocturia, dysuria, enuresis, polyuria, incontinence (stress versus urge incontinence should be noted), pyuria, pneumaturia, and hematuria. Changes in the color and odor of urine should also be noted.

In addition to specific focused inquiry about the genitourinary system, the perioperative nurse will be concerned about patient allergies to medications or contrast dye, current and significant past medical problems, psychosocial status, and educational needs. Anxiety, threats to body image, support systems, and sociocultural as well as psychosocial needs should also be evaluated for their relevance to perioperative care planning.

Physical Examination

The patient with genitourinary problems will have undergone a thorough physical examination. As part of the assessment data base, the perioperative nurse reviews the results of the general and focused physical examination. The nurse validates and confirms findings that relate to perioperative care planning. These were briefly reviewed earlier. Genitourinary patients may have altered levels of consciousness, changes in skin condition (edema, rashes, poor turgor, friability), altered peripheral vascular circulation, compromised cardiovascular status, muscle irritability, and areas of tenderness. All of these affect planning for the patient's care during surgery.

DIAGNOSTIC STUDIES

In the course of establishing a medical diagnosis, diagnostic studies may be performed to (1) identify the source of the disorder, (2) assess structural pathologic changes in the patient's body, (3) assess the patient's physiologic responses, and (4) assess the patient's functional impairments. The following list summarizes various diagnostic studies that may be conducted before a patient is scheduled for genitourinary surgery:

- Serum analyses (complete blood count, SMA_{12}, blood urea nitrogen level, serum creatinine, clotting profile, serum osmolality, PSA, follicle-stimulating hormone, luteinizing hormone)
- Urine examinations
- Kidney, ureters, and bladder (KUB) film
- Intravenous pyelography (IVP)
- Retrograde pyelography (RGP)
- Kidney function tests (clearance, concentration, and excretion)
- Cystogram
- Retrograde urethrogram
- Ultrasound
- Computed tomography (CT)
- Renal arteriography
- Cystoscopy
- Voiding studies (cystourethrography and radionuclide voiding studies)
- Magnetic resonance imaging (MRI)

Radiologic Evaluation

X-ray studies of the genitourinary tract often begin with a plain film of the abdomen. Sometimes referred to as the "control film," a KUB film is used to identify normal landmarks and assess significant alterations in the skeleton, soft tissue, gas pattern, or calcifications.

Kidney, ureters, and bladder (KUB) film. Radiographic study of the kidneys, ureters, and bladder is a preliminary step in urinary tract examination. The KUB film is completed before renal studies or intravenous pyelography. In preparation for this study, the patient is asked to lie on his or her back on an x-ray table. The test is like a simple abdominal flat plate and takes only a few minutes. Abnormal results that a KUB film may reveal include (1) calcium in blood vessels, lymph nodes, cysts, tumors, or stones; (2) calculi along the course of the ureters; (3) abnormal fluid or ascites; (4) abnormal size, shape, and position of a kidney; and (5) presence of foreign bodies.

Intravenous pyelogram. IVP is ordered for suspected renal disease or urinary tract dysfunction. Sequential films are taken as the kidneys concentrate and excrete intravenously injected contrast dye. Each phase of the process is reviewed during the study. IVP allows visualization of the size, shape, and structure of the kidneys, ureters, and bladder. Also detectable are ureteral or bladder stones, tumors, and kidney disease. In preparation for IVP, the nurse should explain to the patient the purpose and procedure of the test. It is important to include in teaching that the patient must remain NPO (nothing by mouth) 12 hours before the examination. In addition, IVP requires that a radiopaque iodine contrast substance, such as Hypaque or Conray, be injected intravenously. After injection of the contrast dye, x-ray films are taken. Abnormal results that an IVP may reveal include (1) altered size, form, and position of the kidneys, ureters, or bladder; (2) renal or ureteral calculi; (3) tumors; (4) presence of only one kidney; (5) hydronephrosis; (6) cystic disease; or (7) large kidneys, suggesting obstruction.

Retrograde pyelogram. Retrograde pyelography is an x-ray examination of the upper urinary tract. This study is generally conducted to confirm IVP findings or when IVP does not provide sufficient anatomic information, the patient is allergic to contrast dye, or there is renal insufficiency or obstruction. It is important that any renal function tests of blood and urine be completed before this diagnostic study. The retrograde pyelogram is usually performed in the surgical department with the patient sedated. The patient is placed in the lithotomy position. This position allows passage of a cystoscope to introduce catheters into the ureters to the level of the renal pelvis. Once the catheters are in place, iodine contrast dye is injected and films are taken. Abnormal retrograde pyelography findings include (1) intrinsic disease of the ureters and the pelvis of the kidney and (2) extrinsic disease of the ureters such as obstructive tumors or stones. *Retrograde urethrograms* provide information about strictures, diverticula, stones, or neoplastic disease.

Cystogram. In cystography, a catheter is placed in the bladder and the bladder is filled with contrast medium. Information about bladder anatomy and contour is obtained. Voiding cystograms examine the rate of emptying and caliber of the stream; reflux may be demonstrated. Postvoiding films yield evidence on the degree of bladder emptying.

Arteriogram. Arteriography defines the arterial supply of the kidneys. It may be indicated for trauma, to assess vascular integrity, for renovascular hypertension, to evaluate renal parenchymal lesions, to determine the nature of space-occupying lesions, to detect arteriovenous malformations, or to obtain precise anatomic information about renal arterial lesions. An arteriogram is always done before transplantation procedures.

Computed tomography and magnetic resonance imaging. CT of the kidney may be conducted to diagnose pathologic renal conditions such as tumors, cysts, obstructions, calculi, and congenital anomalies (Pagana & Pagana, 1995). Both CT and MRI are used to stage renal tumors. Location, extent of involvement of adjacent or more distant structures, and tumor size are evaluated. CT, in many instances, replaces the need for angiography.

Ultrasound. Ultrasonography is used to differentiate cystic from solid renal masses. It is also used to guide percutaneous needle aspiration biopsy of the kidney or prostate gland and to evaluate corporal cavernosal integrity (cavernosography) before procedures for erectile dysfunction.

Endoscopic Examination

Cystoscopy is one of the most important and precise of all urologic diagnostic methods. It allows visualization of the interior of the bladder, urethra, and prostatic urethra by means of a cystoscope. When performed as a diagnostic test, cystoscopy can be performed in the urologist's office or OR suite with the patient under local anesthesia. The patient is positioned in the lithotomy position before the external genitalia are cleansed. Abnormal cystoscopy findings include (1) cancer of the bladder; (2) bladder stones; (3) prostatitis; (4) urethral strictures; (5) and prostatic hyperplasia. Cystoscopy may be accompanied by ureteroscopy and by renal and ureteral brush biopsies.

Renal endoscopy (nephroscopy) may be performed percutaneously or through an incision. Introduction of the fiberscope into the renal pelvis allows diagnostic examination, removal of calculi, and biopsy of small lesions (Walsh, 1992).

Radioisotopes

Isotope renograms provide graphic representation of renal blood flow as well as of tubular secretion and the kidney's anatomy and function. The gamma radiation used has a short half-life, making it safe, and it is readily detectable. The distribution of the radioactive material is scanned or mapped. The resulting image provides information about the distribution of the radioisotope in the kidney. Various agents can be used for the scan; these are selected according to their ability to provide information about structure, perfusion, or excretory function of the kidney.

Laboratory Analyses

Laboratory studies will include both diagnostic evaluation of urine and selected blood chemistries.

Urinalysis. Routine urinalysis yields information about pH (normal is 4.6 to 8), specific gravity (normal is 1.005 to 1.030), protein (30 to 150 mg/day), sugar (0 to 0.5 g/day), ketones (negative), nitrites and leukocytes (negative), and microscopic sediment such as crystals and casts (negative) (Pagana & Pagana, 1995). The perioperative nurse should review the specific gravity; elevated specific gravity may indicate fluid volume deficits, and low specific gravity may indicate the potential risk for a fluid volume excess. Glycosuria may also indicate the potential for a fluid volume deficit. The presence of sugar and acetone in the urine needs medical follow-up; ketoacidosis may result. Ketones in the urine of a nondiabetic patient may indicate that the patient's nutritional status is less than body requirements for carbohydrates; nutritional and dietary counseling may be recommended. Twenty-four-hour collections of urine may be required to assess creatinine clearance, protein loss, and output of specific ions and amino acids.

Blood chemistry profiles. In addition to serum electrolyte levels, clotting profiles, blood type and crossmatch, serologic studies, and complete blood counts, a number of common blood chemistry studies may be found in the patient's medical record.

Blood urea nitrogen (BUN). The BUN test evaluates levels of urea nitrogen in the blood; the kidneys are responsible for excreting this waste of protein metabolism. For adults, the normal BUN level ranges from 10 to 20 mg/dl (Pagana & Pagana, 1995). Increased BUN levels may indicate kidney dysfunction. Shock, congestive heart failure, dehydration, high-protein tube feedings, and gastrointestinal bleeding may also elevate BUN levels.

Creatinine. Like urea nitrogen, creatinine is excreted by the kidneys. The creatinine level is less affected by the patient's nutritional and hydration status or the presence of liver disease than is BUN. The creatinine level may be directly measured (normal serum values are 0.5 to 1.2 mg/dl) or measured as a BUN/creatinine ratio. Normal ratios vary according to protein intake and mass of voluntary muscle; Pagana & Pagana (1995) suggest that a ratio of 20:1 is normal, although other sources suggest

other ranges. Creatinine clearance tests may also be conducted to assess glomerular filtration rates. In this test, the serum creatinine level is compared with the amount of creatinine excreted over 24 hours (shorter collection periods may be used). Normal reference values for creatinine clearance are 97 to 137 ml/min for males and 88 to 128 ml/min for females (Pagana & Pagana, 1995). Serum creatinine and creatinine clearance tests have proved to be more valuable for renal assessment than has BUN.

NURSING DIAGNOSES

The nursing process is a systematic way of identifying a patient's needs and then planning nursing actions to meet those needs. Perioperative nurses use a variety of ways to collect and review data about their patients. In analyzing the data obtained from the patient's medical record and the patient interview, the perioperative nurse is in a prime position to identify and develop nursing diagnoses that will help provide highly specialized and individually focused perioperative nursing care. After reviewing relevant data, the perioperative nurse makes a nursing diagnosis. Some of these nursing diagnoses will be amenable to independent nursing intervention; others require collaboration with the perioperative team. Perioperative nursing diagnoses focus on the care (emotional and physical) requirements of the patient, the patient's comfort and safety, and the support (emotional, physical, restorative, and educational) the patient requires. When identifying nursing diagnoses common to patients undergoing genitourinary surgery, the perioperative nurse may wish to consider the following.

Knowledge Deficit (Related to Planned Surgical Intervention and/or Postoperative Follow-up Care)

Perioperative nurses commonly intervene in knowledge deficits. Patients may not fully understand the nature of their diagnosis, the planned surgical intervention, or the anticipated postoperative course. At times, the perioperative nurse will provide explanations and clarify misunderstandings; at other times, the perioperative nurse will refer the patient to another health care professional (for example, unit nurse, physician, dietitian, home health care provider), depending on the patient's information and education needs (Box 18-3). The perioperative nurse verifies that the patient's surgical consent form is properly signed, that the planned surgical intervention on the consent form corresponds to the scheduled surgery and to the patient's statement about the surgery, and that the specific site is verified with the patient. The perioperative nurse then provides information about the sequence of perioperative events, explaining insertion of invasive lines and catheters, transport and positioning, anticipated length of surgery, postoperative discharge disposition (postanesthesia care unit, intensive care unit, or ambulatory recovery), plus methods of communicating with the patient's family or significant others. The perioperative nurse generally provides information about what will happen (procedural information) and what it will feel like (sensory information). Discharge planning may begin during discussion of anticipated postoperative events and the patient's self-care and home management abilities (Box 18-4).

Anxiety/Fear (Related to Lack of Understanding of Diagnostic Tests and Procedures and/or Fear of Planned Surgical Intervention)

Anxiety is probably a universal emotional response of surgical patients. A patient scheduled for diagnostic cystoscopy, a "minor" procedure on the OR schedule, may be anxious and embarrassed that sensitive areas of the body will be exposed. Men may worry about having an erection during handling of the genitals when they are examined or antiseptically prepared (Seidel, et al., 1995). Anxiety may also be related to the anticipated discomfort of urinary tract instrumentation, diagnostic outcomes, or complications from the procedure or anesthesia. Patients having local or regional anesthesia may fear pain. It is sometimes easier to intervene in a patient's fears because they are related to a specific event. Explanations and support can be targeted to fear-producing phenomena. Anxiety, although often associated with fear, is more diffuse. The patient may not be able to identify specifically the source of their vague feeling of disquiet. A calm, unhurried manner on the part of the nurse, allowing the patient to ask questions or verbalize feelings, and repeated explanations will help reduce anxiety. Attempt to discover if the patient has used specific anxiety-reducing strategies in the past. These might include meditation, relaxation techniques, or music. Kaempf and Amodei (1989) suggest that music might be beneficial for reducing anxiety if the music is selected according to the patient's preference. When possible and appropriate, the perioperative nurse helps the patient use personally effective anxiety-reducing strategies. If the patient is receptive to touch, hand holding, a simple pat on the arm, or stroking the brow is often useful for calming fears and anxieties (McNamara, 1995).

High Risk for Injury (Related to Positioning, Electrical Hazards, Lasers, or Foreign Body Left in Wound)

One of the primary functions of perioperative nursing is preventing patient injury. For patients undergoing genitourinary surgery, injury can occur during surgical positioning with the use of adjunctive electrical equipment and lasers, and during complicated procedures such as urinary diversion in which there is the potential for retained foreign objects.

Surgical positioning. The nursing diagnosis *high risk for injury related to positioning* addresses the patient at risk for injury from positioning during the surgical procedure. Each surgical patient needs to be assessed for positioning problems and appropriate preventive measures instituted. The focus of those interventions should be to minimize undesirable effects on circulation and respiration; to provide protective padding and support to prevent pressure necrosis, neuropathies, and musculoskeletal strains; and to make the conscious patient as comfortable as possible. When the perioperative nurse plans the execution of positioning maneuvers, he or she can prevent or minimize injuries associated with positioning. Five major surgical positions are used in genitourinary surgery: lithotomy, supine, hydraulic sling, prone, and lateral.

LITHOTOMY POSITION. The lithotomy position is employed in urologic procedures such as cystoscopy, ureteroscopy, transurethral resection, bladder neck suspensions, perineal prostatectomies, and artificial urinary sphincter procedures. Lithotomy position is particularly dangerous because it can cause pressure points and strains of the hips and lower back. When the lithotomy position is planned, the perioperative nurse may have the following positional aids available: pillow or headrest, padding for bony prominences (foam, sheepskin, pillows, gel-filled pads or blankets), armboards, safety strap, stirrups, protective padding and covering for the legs, and table attachments. Prolonged elevation of the legs in the lithotomy position can increase the patient's risk of vascular occlusion or thrombosis (Paschal & Strzelecki, 1992).

Various modifications of the lithotomy position are used for transurethral and perineal urologic surgery. As with any surgical position, adequate exposure of the surgical site is critical. In achieving this exposure, however, important physiologic functions may be compromised. Care must be taken to prevent extreme hip flexion. The peroneal nerve should be protected from compression against the stirrups by padding the area at the proximal end of the fibula (Paschal & Strzelecki, 1992). When the lithotomy and Trendelenburg's positions are combined, slow, deliberate, and gentle bed manipulation is required to prevent hemodynamic alterations, respiratory compromise, and shearing forces (Ronk & Kavitz, 1994). If shoulder braces are used for extreme Trendelenburg's position, they must be padded and placed over the acromial processes rather than more centrally, which would injure the brachial plexus (Rothrock & Sculthorpe, 1993). The following Guide to Nursing Actions is provided to accompany the nursing diagnosis *high risk for injury related to lithotomy position:*

1. Ensure that adequate padding is provided under the sacrum and across the pelvic brim.
2. Ensure that stirrups are properly positioned and padded. Pad knees and ankles that come in contact with metal stirrups. Apply antiembolism

stockings or alternating compression device as indicated (based on patient risk factors and the length and extent of the procedure).
3. Simultaneously raise and lower the legs, flexing both legs toward the abdomen first. When the patient is in the stirrups, check flexion of the knees and hips (avoid extreme flexion) and external rotation and abduction of the thigh (avoid extremes). Eliminate pressure points against the popliteal spaces, calves, and Achilles' areas.
4. Position and secure arms on armboards, at the patient's side, or across the chest. Arms positioned on armboards must not abduct beyond the patient's normal range of motion or greater than 90 degrees. Locking armboards are recommended. When adducting arms at the patient's side, protect the radial nerve from compression against the ether screen and the ulnar nerve from compression against the OR bed.
5. Visually check the patient's hand position before lowering or raising the foot of the surgical bed.
6. Assess the patient's respiratory status, vital signs, and radial/pedal pulses.
7. Compare preoperative and postoperative neurovascular status.

SUPINE POSITION. The supine position is employed for urologic procedures such as penile implants, hydrocelectomy, vasectomy, epididymectomy, orchiectomy, orchiopexy, and radical lymphadenectomy. When a patient is positioned supinely, pressure areas need to be assessed and padded as necessary. Areas in which pressure injuries are most likely include the occiput, spinous process of the first thoracic vertebra, scapula, medial and lateral epicondyles of the humerus, olecranon process, sacral region, styloid process of the ulna and radius, and calcaneus. The following Guide to Nursing Actions is provided to accompany the nursing diagnosis *high risk for injury related to supine position:*

1. Align the body in an anatomically appropriate position. Select positioning accessories according to the patient assessment (for example, use a small lumbar support for a patient with preexisting back pain).
2. Apply the safety strap above the knees without impeding circulation.
3. Position legs so that they are not crossed.
4. Pad the heels and ensure that they do not hang over the edge of the OR bed.
5. Assess and pad pressure areas as necessary. Select positioning accessories (for example, egg-crate foam mattress) according to patient risk factors and the length of the surgical procedure.
6. Position the patient with arms at side and palms turned toward the patient or downward. Position the arms so they do not come into contact with

the metal frame of the OR bed. Use elbow pads. Prevent overabduction of the arms on armboards.

7. When appropriate, consult with the surgical team regarding modification of traditional supine position to contoured supine "lawn chair" position.

8. If utilizing a hyperthermia blanket under the patient, avoid pooling of preparation solutions under the patient and potential burns by placing absorbent material beneath the patient before preparing and by removing it before draping.

HYDRAULIC SLING. The hydraulic sling is used as a positioning device with surgical patients undergoing extracorporeal shock wave lithotripsy (ESWL). During this noninvasive procedure, the perioperative nurse must ensure that the anesthetized patient is placed and positioned on the hydraulic sling safely. Once in position, the patient is hydraulically raised and positioned over and then partially submerged in a large tub of water. Newer lithotripters do not require water submersion. The following Guide to Nursing Actions is provided to accompany the nursing diagnosis *high risk for injury related to hydraulic sling position:*

1. Protect electrocardiogram leads, intravenous insertion site, and epidural catheter with adhesive plastic coverings.

2. Ensure availability of staff to transfer the patient from the stretcher to the hydraulic sling. If regional (epidural) anesthesia is used, the patient can assist with transfer and assume a position of comfort.

3. Position the patient so the back, from the scapula area up, is supported by the foam backrest.

4. Position the patient so the head is supported on a well-padded horseshoe headrest.

5. Secure the patient with padded straps across the upper chest, around each thigh, across the ankles, and diagonally across the abdomen and chest. Check for pressure points and undue stretch on muscles, ligaments, and joints.

6. Position the arms on padded rests or across the patient's chest as the hydraulic sling is raised and submerged into the tub of water.

PRONE POSITION. The prone position is often chosen for urologic procedures involving the adrenal glands and kidneys and for percutaneous endopyelotomy. This position is dangerous because of compromised respiratory exchange and pressure on the bony patellar, iliac, rib, and acromial prominences. The perioperative nurse should have the following positional aids available: pillow or headrest, axillary rolls, padding for bony prominences (foam, gel-filled pads, sheepskin, blankets, or pillows), elevated prone armboards, chest pads or rolls, padding for ankles to elevate feet from bed, and a safety strap. Antiembolism stockings or an alternating compres-

sion device should be employed to assist venous return. The perioperative nurse may wish to review the following Guide to Nursing Actions when using the nursing diagnosis *high risk for injury related to prone position:*

1. Turn patient onto chest pads, following endotracheal intubation, in a log roll fashion. Protect head with small support pillow or cushion. Protect the dependent ear because the head will be turned to the side.

2. Bring arms upward slowly by lateral extension, flexion at elbows, and gradual elevation toward the head. Secure the arms on padded prone-style armboards with the palms down.

3. Place axillary rolls to prevent pressure on the brachial plexus and to assist lung expansion.

4. Protect patellar, iliac, elbow, and ankle areas with foam or gel-filled pads.

5. Elevate feet on pillows or blankets to prevent pressure on the toes and foot drop.

6. Check male genitalia and female breasts to ensure freedom from compression.

7. If an alternating compression device is used, pad between patient ankles and electrical attachment to stockings.

8. Stabilize the patient with a safety strap and padded tape as appropriate. Avoid pressure on the scapulae if employing tape across the back.

LATERAL POSITION. The lateral position is employed for urologic procedures such as nephrectomy, nephroureterectomy, and percutaneous ultrasonic lithotripsy. The lateral position is particularly dangerous because of potential nerve damage, compromised respiratory perfusion, and decreased venous return. The perioperative nurse should have the following positional aids available: pillow or headrest, padding for bony prominences (foam, gel-filled pads, sheepskin, blankets, or pillows), armboards, safety strap, metal kidney rest attachments (optional), and a suction beanbag (optional). The perioperative nurse may wish to review the following Guide to Nursing Actions when using the nursing diagnosis *high risk for injury related to lateral position:*

1. Turn the shoulders and hips slowly and simultaneously to the lateral position (after the patient is anesthetized in the supine position). The lumbar area should be positioned to allow elevation of the kidney rest or flexion of the OR bed. Antiembolic stockings or an alternating compression device will help promote venous return.

2. Flex the lower leg at the hip and the knee.

3. Extend the upper leg.

4. Position pillows between the knees and feet. Pad under the dependent ankle and knee. If the alternating compression device is employed, pad be-

tween the ankle and electrical attachment on stockings.

5. Support the upper arm on an overbed armboard with the elbow flexed and palm down.

6. Position the lower arm on an armboard with the elbow slightly flexed and palm up.

7. Position the lower shoulder slightly forward and place an axillary roll to prevent compression of the scapula and brachial plexus. A small pillow may be placed under the head. Protect the dependent ear.

8. Check male genitalia and female breasts to be sure they are free from pressure.

9. Stabilize the patient in the lateral position by using a safety strap or padded tape across the hips. Avoid compressive pressure on the head of the uppermost femur when applying tape.

10. Assess vital signs, respiratory status, and radial/pedal pulses.

Laser. The nursing diagnosis *high risk for injury related to use of laser* addresses the surgical patient at risk of injury related to the use of laser equipment during a surgical procedure. Urologists commonly employ the Nd:YAG laser in treating carcinomas of the penis, small bladder tumors, and urethral strictures. Tunable dye lasers are also used in urology; the laser beam can be delivered through an endoscope or fiberoptic system. Responsibility for the care and management of the laser is often assumed by the perioperative nurse. This nurse should know about laser safety, laser beam characteristics, operational aspects of laser mechanics, and the hospital's protocol for laser use in the OR. Lasers differ in their wavelength, function, and required safety precautions. The following Guide to Nursing Actions has been developed for the nursing diagnosis *high risk for injury related to use of laser:*

1. Follow recommended safety precautions for each laser used. Eye protection, endoscopic lens covers, and window and port coverings will vary according to type of laser used.

2. Test the laser on the morning of surgery, before the patient is brought into the OR. A perioperative checklist is helpful.

3. Hang a sign on the OR door indicating that a laser is in use. This sign should have the word "Danger" on it, as well as "Laser in Use" and the type of laser being used.

4. Never use alcohol-based solutions to disinfect the patient's skin.

5. Surround the targeted tissue with moistened sponges or towels when using the CO_2 laser. Monitor moisture level during the procedure.

6. Wear safety glasses designed for the specific laser in use. When safety glasses are stored, protect them from scratching.

7. Place machine in "standby" setting when not in use.

8. Use nonreflective instruments in or near the beam.

9. Protect the eyes of the patient under general anesthesia with moistened eye pads, wet gauze, or towels. The eyes should be taped closed. Provide the awake patient with protective goggles appropriate to the laser being used.

10. If laser is being used near the rectal area, a wet pad may be inserted to tamponade the rectum. Account for the pad.

11. Identify the laser pedal to prevent accidental firing.

12. Establish fire protocols and have appropriate fire extinguishers immediately available.

13. Follow institutional protocol for documenting on the patient's record the surgeon, procedure, type of laser used, length of use, and wattage.

High Risk for Infection Related to Implanted Prosthesis

The nursing diagnosis *high risk for infection related to implanted prosthesis* addresses the surgical patient at risk of infection resulting from an implanted prosthesis. Genitourinary procedures requiring the use of a prosthesis include penile, artificial urinary sphincter, and testicular prosthesis implantations. The following Guide to Nursing Actions is provided to accompany the nursing diagnosis *high risk for infection related to implanted prosthesis:*

1. Read and follow the manufacturer's recommendations for all implants.

2. Check the structural integrity of each prosthesis before implantation.

3. Prevent surface contaminants (talc, lint, or skin oils) from coming in contact with the prosthesis.

4. Review the medical record and reassess the patient to determine if infection is present anywhere in the body, especially if urinary tract or genital infection is present. Report these findings; surgery may be canceled.

5. Verify the availability of antibiotics for intravenous administration and irrigation.

6. An antibiotic irrigation solution will be used. Check patient allergies, dose of antibiotic, solution for irrigation, solution concentration after mixture, and temperature of irrigating fluid. Label all solutions on the sterile field. Document medications administered from the sterile field.

7. Perform surgical scrub of operative area with Betadine scrub solution for 5 minutes.

8. Surgical team should double-glove during implant procedure.

9. Maintain meticulous aseptic technique. Isolate the anus with a plastic adhesive drape if the

perineal approach is used or the perineum is exposed during the procedure.

10. Keep room traffic to a minimum and keep doors to operating suite closed.

Fluid and Electrolyte Problems

In addition to their role in excreting waste products, the kidneys are responsible for electrolyte balance, acid-base balance, and balance of water and regulation of serum osmolality. The myriad genitourinary disorders that bring the patient to the OR have different effects on fluid and electrolyte balance. The patient with chronic renal insufficiency may have diminished ability to concentrate urine and regulate sodium, potassium, calcium, magnesium, chlorides, and phosphates. Fluid volume deficits from decreased renal perfusion may be accompanied by altered oral mucous membranes, decreased cardiac output, and decreased urinary output. Sodium and fluid retention may result in fluid volume excess accompanied by hypertension, edema, and ineffective breathing patterns. Manifestations of excess sodium may include seizures and altered thought processes. Patients in renal failure may also have metabolic acidosis, hyperkalemia, hyperphosphatemia, hypermagnesemia, and hypocalcemia. When relief of a partial or complete urinary obstruction occurs, as may be effected by surgical intervention, post-obstructive diuresis occurs. Hypovolemia and significant losses of sodium, potassium, calcium, magnesium, and carbonate may result (Walsh, et al., 1992). The perioperative nurse collaborates closely with anesthesia staff in the monitoring of fluid and electrolyte balance and fluid replacement therapies.

Potassium is the primary intracellular cation, playing a vital role in cell metabolism. The ratio of intracellular to extracellular potassium is balanced within a narrow range. The slightest alteration may adversely affect cardiac and neuromuscular function, and therefore serum levels must be closely monitored and maintained. Potassium is lost through the kidneys, the gastrointestinal tract, and the skin. An elevated serum potassium level does not usually occur without a corresponding reduction in renal function. The kidneys do not conserve potassium as readily as sodium, and they regulate potassium balance by adjusting the amount secreted in the urine. As the serum potassium level rises, so does the concentration within the renal tubular cell, favoring a shift into the renal tubule with a consequent excretory loss in the urine. Aldosterone increases potassium loss; corticosteroids and postsurgical stress cause aldosterone levels to rise. Hypokalemia may result from this shift into the cells. Other factors that increase the risk of hypokalemia

are congenital adrenal hyperplasia, long-term use of diuretics, abnormally elevated urinary output, and diaphoresis (Horne & Swearingen, 1993).

The patient developing hypokalemia may be managed with potassium replacement therapies, generally 40 to 80 mEq/day IV in divided doses at a slow rate of infusion. The patient should be placed on a cardiac monitor because hyperkalemia may easily result from too high a dosage. Other measures include potassium-sparing diuretics, potassium chloride salt substitutes, and, postoperatively, increased intake of potassium-rich foods (Horne & Swearingen, 1993).

High Risk for Fluid Volume Excess (During Endourology)

The nursing diagnosis *high risk for fluid volume excess* addresses the surgical patient at risk of vascular, cellular, or extracellular fluid overload. During cystoscopic examination and transurethral resection, the bladder must be distended. This is accomplished with the use of continuous irrigation. The perioperative nurse preparing for a transurethral resection must be careful to select a sterile isosmotic irrigating solution that is nonelectrolytic and nonhemolytic. Water should not be used because if a sufficient amount enters into the venous system it may hemolyze or break down red blood cells. Saline should not be used because it will dissipate the electrical current employed. Commonly used irrigation fluids include 1.5% glycine and 3% sorbitol.

In preparation for cystoscopy and procedures confined to the bladder, the nurse should use sterile water for irrigation. In preparation for ureteroscopy and nephroscopy, saline should be used. The following Guide to Nursing Actions is provided to accompany the nursing diagnosis *high risk for fluid volume excess:*

1. Hang a nonhemolytic, isotonic, nonelectrolytic irrigation solution, such as glycine 1.5% or sorbitol 3%, during transurethral resection of the prostate or bladder neck contracture. Use a sterile, closed irrigation system.
   a. Hyperabsorption will not change osmolarity but may produce hyponatremia.
   b. Osmolarity of irrigant is similar to circulation.
   c. Retroperitoneal space fluids are readily reabsorbed into vascular spaces and plasma volume, and composition may be altered.
2. Hang sterile, distilled water for cystoscopy or transurethral resection of bladder tumors. Use sterile, closed drainage system.
   a. Water is potentially the most dangerous irrigant due to hemolysis.
   b. Any signs of extravasation should be investigated.

3. Hang 0.9% saline solution for nephroscopic and ureteroscopic procedures. Use sterile, closed drainage system.
   a. Saline absorption will not change osmolarity or electrolyte composition but can cause fluid overload.
   b. Saline approximates a physiologic solution.
   c. Systemic absorption can occur from ureteral or collecting system perforation with extravasation and from pyelolymphatic, pyelorenal, or pyelovenous backflow.
   d. If electrosurgery is required, change irrigant to glycine or sorbitol.
4. Hang irrigation approximately 2½ to 3 feet above the cystoscopy table to maintain a pressure below 30 cm in the bladder.
5. Hang irrigation solutions in tandem ("piggy-backed") so that irrigation is continuous.
6. Monitor the return of irrigation.
7. Monitor vital signs.

Additional Nursing Diagnoses

Through assessment the perioperative nurse selects and prioritizes nursing diagnoses that reflect the patient's status and the problems to which he is most vulnerable. The following nursing diagnoses represent patient risks and clearly indicate the complexities and challenges of caring for patients undergoing genitourinary surgery. The perioperative nurse must decide if the diagnosis is appropriate to the patient for whom he or she is developing a plan of care.

1. *High risk for infection* related to impaired skin integrity or implanted prosthesis, vascular access site, invasive lines, catheters, immunosuppression (transplant patients)
2. *Ineffective breathing patterns* related to depressant effects of anesthesia, medications (narcotic analgesics, muscle relaxants), surgical positioning, and/or postoperative pain and splinting
3. *High risk for ineffective airway clearance* related to depressant effects of anesthesia; medications; thick, tenacious secretions; or postoperative pain and splinting
4. *Pain* related to tissue trauma and/or reflex muscle spasm, procedural manipulation, incision, or passage of urinary stones
5. *Impaired skin or tissue integrity* related to surgical incision
6. *High risk for impaired skin integrity* related to surgical positioning, electrical equipment, or presence of uremia. The patient with chronic renal failure may have decreased activity of oil and sweat glands, itching, capillary fragility, abnormal blood clotting, retention of pigments, and deposition of calcium phosphate on the skin (Thompson, et al., 1993). The patient undergoing ileal conduit urinary diversion is at risk of impaired skin integrity at the stoma site.
7. *High risk for altered peripheral and/or renal tissue perfusion* related to pooling of blood from decreased venous return secondary to loss of vasomotor tone associated with anesthesia. Peripheral tissue perfusion may also be altered by manipulation of large vessels during pelvic and retroperitoneal lymphadenectomies. Altered renal tissue perfusion is related to intraoperative manipulation of the kidney or adrenal gland, renal insufficiency, and alterations in renal regulatory mechanisms.
8. *High risk for fluid volume excess* related to renal insufficiency or endourologic infusions
9. *High risk for fluid volume deficit* related to surgical intervention, alteration in renal regulatory mechanisms, or structural and functional changes in the elderly patient's renal system (Larsen & Martin, 1994)
10. *High risk for sexual dysfunction, altered sexuality patterns, altered role performance, chronic low self-esteem, hopelessness or powerlessness, personal identity or self-esteem disturbances, impaired adjustment and impaired social interaction or social isolation* may all be related to aggressive surgical interventions or the psychosocial impact of disease states. Patients coping with the probability of impotence or an ostomy site will be those most likely affected with these potential problems. The perioperative team should strive to assist these patients with their coping mechanisms and seek professional psychologic caregivers to aid in postoperative adjustment.
11. *High risk for altered patterns of urinary elimination* related to surgical procedure, urinary catheterization, suprapubic catheter, nephrostomy tube, ureteral catheter, presence of artificial urinary sphincter, bladder spasms, or postoperative urinary retention
12. *High risk for injury or altered thought processes* related to weakness or possible confusion in patients with increased BUN
13. *High risk for activity intolerance and fatigue* related to the low hematocrit level that develops with chronic renal disease, altered sleep patterns, or nutritional deficits
14. *Body image disturbance* related to surgical procedure, fear of impotence, loss of sexual identity, presence of implant or catheter, loss of an organ or body function, or urinary diversion
15. *Decisional conflict* related to dialysis or renal transplant
16. *Ineffective individual or family coping and altered family processes* related to alterations in

life-style, chronic disease, prolonged hospitalization, or fear of organ rejection (transplant patient) or social rejection

17. *Anticipatory and/or dysfunctional grieving* related to loss of a body part or function, changes in life-style, or prognosis

18. *Altered nutrition: less than body requirements* related to disease state, side effects of dialysis, anorexia, nausea and vomiting, dietary restrictions, or oral ulcerations

19. *High risk for functional, stress or urge incontinence* related to surgical intervention such as with radical prostatectomy

PLANNING PATIENT CARE

Once nursing diagnoses have been identified and prioritized, outcomes and the criteria by which they will be measured are developed. Outcomes flow from the nursing diagnosis. Thus if the nursing diagnosis *high risk for fluid volume deficit* was selected, the desired outcome would be "The patient will experience normovolemia" (or "The patient will show no signs of fluid deficit"). Criteria to measure this outcome could include such parameters as maintenance of blood pressure within acceptable ranges, adequate skin turgor, adequate urinary output, and moist mucous membranes. These criteria can be assessed and evaluated intraoperatively to determine whether the patient met the stated outcome. Some nursing diagnoses and related outcome statements require criteria that may not be met while the patient is still in the OR. Depending on institutional practice, these criteria may be evaluated by the postanesthesia care unit nurse on the perioperative care plan; during a postoperative visit, chart audit, or follow-up patient surveys or telephone calls; or through collaboration with the physician who follows the patient postoperatively. As hospital stays become shorter and more patients are cared for in ambulatory surgery settings, the nursing profession will require creative ways of measuring outcomes. Evaluation of patient care is an important part of nursing accountability. The following nursing care plans have been developed to guide the perioperative nurse in using nursing diagnoses for patient care planning in the OR. The care plans are designed to accommodate the care planning process and allow documentation on one form. Each care plan has space for individualization and additions. The Guide to Nursing Actions accompanying each care plan provides more detailed information and rationales for the identified nursing actions. Repetition of information is deliberate to obviate the need for continuously referencing previous care plans. Perioperative nurses are invited to use aspects of the care plans that can be applied to a specific patient. The plans are individualized and added to as necessary. The perioperative care plan allows the perioperative nurse to demonstrate accountability for highly specialized OR care.

GUIDES TO NURSING ACTIONS

Extracorporeal Shock Wave Lithotripsy (Fig. 18-2)

1. Assessment should include a review of the patient's cardiac and respiratory status, clotting profiles, baseline vital signs, any signs of infection, the patient's height and weight, and a negative pregnancy test for females. There are specific height and weight limitations with the older ESWL units. Determine whether the patient has complied with restrictions (NPO, avoiding aspirin, and tapered anticoagulant therapy). Pain is a common nursing diagnosis for these patients. Assess the nature, intensity, location, and duration of pain. The patient may need to be monitored for syncopal episodes associated with intense pain (renal colic). Assist the patient with nonpharmacologic pain measures that have been personally effective in the past (for example, guided imagery or relaxation therapy). Provide music and headphones as appropriate (determine the patient's music preference). If preoperative medication has been ordered, assess its effectiveness.

2. Explanation of procedures can effectively eliminate fear and anxiety.

   a. Provide information about the following preoperative and intraoperative routines:
      - Blood work (bring results)
      - Electrocardiogram (bring results)
      - Chest x-ray film (bring results)
      - IVP (bring results)
      - NPO status
      - Preoperative medication
      - Preoperative waiting area
      - Scheduled time and estimated length of procedure
      - Body position during procedure
      - Presence of stents and catheters postoperatively
      - Possibility of postoperative facial swelling and/or bruising and why these may occur
      - Induction and type of anesthesia
      - Postanesthesia care unit

   b. Reinforce teaching and information provided by the anesthesia provider and urologist.

   c. Inform the patient of the anticipated postoperative care regimen and determine self-care management ability.

   d. Provide the following information about kidney stone disintegration by means of shock waves:

FIG. 18-2
CARE PLAN FOR EXTRACORPOREAL SHOCK WAVE LITHOTRIPSY (ESWL)

KEY ASSESSMENT POINTS

Weight and height
Cardiopulmonary status
Coagulation studies in normal range: (Activated partial thromboplas-
  tin time [APT], PT, bleeding time)
Negative urinalysis/urine cultures
Negative pregnancy test, if applicable

NURSING DIAGNOSIS

All generic nursing diagnoses apply to this patient, with the addition
  of:
High risk for infection

PATIENT OUTCOMES

All generic outcomes apply, with the addition of:
The patient will be free of infection.
There will be no:
Fever
Pyuria or bacteriuria
Dysuria

NURSING ACTIONS

	Yes	No	N/A
1. Patient assessment performed?	☐	☐	☐
2. Perioperative explanations provided?	☐	☐	☐
3. ESWL unit checked, functioning properly?	☐	☐	☐
4. Positioned correctly in sling?	☐	☐	☐
5. Water at correct temperature?	☐	☐	☐
6. Anesthesia explained?	☐	☐	☐
7. Privacy maintained?	☐	☐	☐
8. Special equipment/supplies available?	☐	☐	☐
9. Radiation safety precautions initiated?	☐	☐	☐
10. Protective ear plugs in place?	☐	☐	☐
11. Vaseline or similar substance applied?	☐	☐	☐
12. Specimen recorded/to lab in dry container?	☐	☐	☐
13. Perioperative medications administered/recorded?	☐	☐	☐
14. Warm blanket provided?	☐	☐	☐

Document additional nursing actions/generic care plans initiated
here:

_____

_____

_____

EVALUATION OF PATIENT OUTCOMES

	Outcome met	Outcome met with additional outcome criteria	Outcome met with revised nursing care plan	Outcome not met	Outcome not applicable to this patient
1. No signs or symptoms of infection are noted.	☐	☐	☐	☐	☐
2. The patient met outcomes for additional generic care plans as indicated	☐	☐	☐	☐	☐

Signature: _____ Date: _____

- What are shock waves?
- How are they generated?
- Shock wave characteristics
- Shock wave effects
- When and how stones will be passed

Patients undergoing ESWL are at high risk for infection. The perioperative nurse should refer to the care plan for *high risk for infection*. Precipitating factors for infection include, but are not limited to, the following:

a. Stasis of urine from blockage by calculi
b. Inadequate nutrition
c. Infectious stones (struvite calculi)
d. Previous recurrent infections and fever from long-term calculi
e. Instrumentation of urinary tract (includes stents/catheters)
f. Residual stone fragments

Some of the classic signs of early infection the perioperative nurse should be alert to include:

a. Low-grade fever (99° F)
b. Cloudy urine
c. Frequency
d. Suprapubic discomfort
e. Pain during and after voiding

Perioperative teaching includes care of stents/catheters, antibiotic therapy, fluid requirements (increase water), signs of infection, and early ambulation.

3. Important considerations in checking the ESWL unit daily include the following:
   a. Equipment in the treatment room checked for external damage?
   b. Power supply unit switched on with key switch?
   c. Patient positioning control switched on?
   d. Hydraulic system switched on and checked?
   e. Image intensifier adjustment checked?
   f. Diagonal control of patient positioning checked?
   g. Focus position of the electrode checked?
   h. Water supply system switched on and checked?
   i. Water supply to the tub opened and water temperature checked?
   j. X-ray unit switched on?
   k. Compressed air supply checked? (Pressure of 1.0 = 0.1 bar)
   l. Air pumped into x-ray window and checked?
   m. Air pumped into image intensifier cap and checked?
   n. Image intensifier adjustment function checked?
   o. Generator shock wave number checked and shock circuit plug-in units switched on?
   p. Shock wave generator moved backward and electrode checked? Shock wave generator moved forward?
   q. Flush gas supply checked?
      - Pressure of 1.4 bar
      - Flow rate of 151 per hr
   r. Individual pulse released?
   s. Patient positioning checked?
   t. Stretcher stops checked?
   u. Water in the tub checked?
      - Water in tub for 2 hr
      - Temperature 36° C

4. Refer to the Guide to Nursing Actions to prevent injury related to hydraulic sling positioning (p. 442). Have adequate personnel available to transfer patient to and from the sling. Special positioning techniques will be required for patients shorter than 4 feet, 5 inches; taller than 6 feet, 6 inches; or weighing more than 280 pounds.

5. Check the water temperature on the indicator at the column. Water temperature during treatment is to be about 36° C. When water temperature in the tub is less than 36° C, add warm water; if necessary, increase the target value. At a temperature of greater than 36° C, lower the target value and add cold water. Do not let the water stand in the tub for more than 2 hours. After this period, shock wave intensity is reduced because of gas absorption by the water.

6. Anesthesia may be general, regional (continuous epidural), or local. Explanation of the anticipated administration and effects of anesthesia can help reduce anxiety.

7. The patient's privacy should be maintained (a bathing suit is usually provided).

8. A cystoscopy room, with cystoscopy equipment, ultrasonic lithotripsy probe and ureteroscope, stone baskets, and so on, should be available. Patients often require stone manipulation for ESWL treatment. Occasionally a stone may need to be extracted from the lower ureter. A ureteral catheter with radiolucent markings should be available in the lithotripsy suite to aid in stone location.

9. Fluoroscopy is used to locate the stone on the lithotripter screen and to visualize the stone during treatment. Follow institutional protocols for radiation safety.

10. Over a period of 30 to 60 minutes, 500 to 1500 shock waves are administered. A loud sound occurs each time a spark is fired. Protective ear plugs should be worn by the patient and the personnel in the OR. Patients may wear protective headphones to protect the ears while listening to music.

11. Before the application of shock waves, ensure that no gas bubbles have accumulated on the patient's body in the shock wave entry and exit area. Vaseline or similar material applied to the kidney area helps prevent air bubbles. Bubbles reduce the shock wave effect in an uncontrollable way and may lead to unsatisfactory kidney stone disintegration. Bubbles can occur when the degassing unit does not work properly or the water is in the tub for more than 2 hours.

12. If a stone is extracted endoscopically, follow institutional protocol for the preservation and disposition of surgical specimens.

13. Any medication (sedative, antispasmodic, or narcotic) administered by the perioperative nurse should be documented. Assess vital signs before and after administration of pain medication. Monitor and document pain relief and medication side effects.

14. At the conclusion of the procedure, the patient should be transferred from the sling to the discharge vehicle. Warm blankets should be added.

15. Patient education regarding the prevention of kidney stones is important; 80% of patients with kidney stones are at risk for recurrence (Shellenbarger & Krouse, 1994). A sample teaching guideline is provided in Box 18-5.

Ureteroscopic Stone Extraction (Fig. 18-3)

1. Small stones, 5 mm or smaller, may be removed from the ureter using a basket introduced into the ureter during cystoscopy. Ureteral stones are accompanied by severe pain (renal/ureteral colic); hematuria, nausea, and vomiting may also be present. Help the patient use personally effective means of coping when assessment reveals the presence of pain. Ureteroscopic lithotripsy may also be used for these stones; modify the care plan accordingly. The results of preoperative diagnostics should be available (IVP and other films or scans). Pain may heighten anxiety; perioperative explanations should be slow and deliberate.

2. The perioperative nurse should determine the patient's learning needs and provide information that includes the following:
   a. Information regarding perioperative events and routines:
      • Intravenous line insertion
      • Electrocardiogram leads
      • Fluoroscopy or x-ray equipment
      • NPO status (confirm)
      • Preoperative medication (determine effectiveness)
      • Where family or significant other will wait
      • Estimated length of surgery
      • Body position during surgical procedure (determine if patient has any mobility limitations)
      • Type of anesthesia
      • Insertion of stents and catheters
      • Discharge unit (postanesthesia care unit or ambulatory recovery)
   b. Reinforce teaching and information provided by the anesthesia provider and urologist.

3. The patient will be in lithotomy position on the urology table. See the Guide to Nursing Actions for lithotomy position (p. 441).

4. Follow institutional protocol for antimicrobial skin preparation.

5. The use of warmed preparation solution may decrease patient discomfort. It is best to add a small amount of warmed sterile water to the preparation solution. Placing Betadine and other antimicrobials in a warming unit alters their chemical composition.

6. The potential for anxiety, embarrassment, and emotional distress may be present when the genitalia are exposed. A considerate, caring attitude is necessary. All attempts should be made to maintain privacy.

7. Supplies and equipment for cystoscopy are required in addition to ureteroscopes and basket extractors. Equipment should be checked before use. Important considerations in checking endoscopy instruments and accessories include the following:
   a. Inspection of the lens for scratches and clarity of vision
   b. Integrity of the sheath
   c. Mobility of all moving parts
   d. Ensuring that the obturator tip protrudes past the end of the sheath
   e. Integrity of the rubber tips ("nipples")
   f. Patency of channels through instruments
   NOTE: The perioperative nurse also needs to inspect the wires of the stone baskets. Basket wires that are broken or cracked at the end nearest the shaft may be passed into the ureter, but they may be impossible to withdraw without trauma. Newer baskets are disposable and arrive in sterile, double peel-pak containers.

8. Follow institutional protocol for radiation and laser safety. Laser disintegration of ureteral stones has become a common adjunct to ureteroscopic stone removal. The laser used is a pulse-dyed unit called the Candela laser. Special orange-tinted lens are required in the protective goggles. Laser protocol is similar to that for the Nd:YAG laser.

9. After sterilization of cystoscopes by ethylene oxide, aeration time is critical to prevent burns

---

Box 18-5 Preventing Recurrence of Kidney Stones

Passing a kidney stone can be a very painful experience. Anyone who has experienced the agony of passing a stone is eager never to endure such pain again. Fortunately, some measures can help prevent the recurrence of kidney stones.

What are Kidney Stones?

Just as the name implies, kidney stones are small, gravelly stones formed in the kidney. Kidney stones are usually made up of uric acid or calcium but sometimes may contain oxalate. After the stone matures in the kidney, it passes down the ureter into the bladder and then out the urethra. It is this movement that causes the pain. Sometimes the stone is too large to be passed through the urinary tract and must be removed surgically.

What Causes Kidney Stones?

A number of factors can cause kidney stones. These include:
- *Heredity.* If someone in your immediate family has had kidney stones, you have an increased chance of also having kidney stones.
- *Injury.* Sometimes an injury to the kidney can cause a stone to form.
- *Biochemical imbalances.* Some people have too much calcium in their bodies, and some of this calcium forms stones.
- *Diseases.* Diseases such as hyperparathyroidism, hyperthyroidism, and certain types of cancer can cause kidney stones. Patients with gout have too much uric acid in their blood and have a greater chance of forming uric acid kidney stones.
- *Gender and age.* Men have a greater chance of forming kidney stones than do women. Most men who get kidney stones are between 20 and 50 years of age.
- *Diet.* People who eat foods high in oxalate (such as okra) and calcium seem to have an increased risk of developing kidney stones. Too much salt may also be a factor.
- *Urine.* Some people's urine is very concentrated or alkaline; this can lead to kidney stone formation.
- *Not drinking enough water.* When you don't drink enough water, your urine becomes very concentrated,

which can lead to the formation of stones. People who live in an area with very hot summers or who have jobs in which they perspire a lot have an increased risk of developing stones.
- *Urinary tract infections.* People who have urinary tract infections are more likely to have kidney stones.
- *Medications.* Certain medications can cause kidney stones to form. Too much vitamin C has been found to enhance stone formation.
- *Postpregnancy.* Many women get kidney stones after giving birth. The reason has not been discovered yet, although some doctors suspect hormonal changes or the addition of calcium to the diet.

Sometimes it is a combination of these factors that is causing your kidney stones.

How do We Prevent Kidney Stones from Recurring?

The best treatment for kidney stones is to prevent them from recurring. If possible, your doctor will try to determine what kind of kidney stone you had. He or she will then explain to you how to best prevent any more stones from developing. Some of the preventions may include:
- *Drinking lots of fluids, especially water.* Keep your body well hydrated to prevent concentrated urine and stone formation. Drinking cranberry juice can help people whose urine is too alkaline.
- *Avoiding foods high in oxalate.* If your stones are formed of oxalates, you may need to cut out certain foods from your diet, such as tea, chocolate, nuts, and spinach.
- *Avoiding foods high in uric acid.* If your stones are caused by excess uric acid, you will need to reduce the foods you eat that ar high in uric acid such as organ meats, shrimp, and dried beans.
- *Restricting milk and milk products.* If your stones are formed from calcium, you may need to cut back on your calcium intake. Cutting back on milk and other products high in calcium may help prevent calcium stones.
- *Changing medication.* If a medication seems to be causing stones to form, you doctor may change your medication.

From *Mosby's patient teaching guidelines.* (1995). St. Louis: Mosby.

---

to patients or to those handling the equipment. Insufficiently aerated materials can cause skin irritation, burns of body tissue, and hemolysis of blood. In general, mechanical aeration of a cystoscope requires a temperature of 122° to 140° F for 8 to 12 hours. Cystoscopes aerated at room temperature require 7 days. If cold chemosterilization (soaking) is used, care must be taken to

ensure that items have been completely immersed in a properly concentrated amount of solution for the required time. Lids should be in place on containers used for soaking. Aseptic technique must be used for removing items. Adequate rinsing is necessary to ensure that no residual chemosterilant is on instruments, because this too can cause patient burns.

FIG. 18-3
CARE PLAN FOR URETEROSCOPIC STONE EXTRACTION

KEY ASSESSMENT POINTS

Patient understanding of planned intervention
Patient understanding of postop management
Serum sodium/potassium values
Negative urinalysis/urine cultures
Negative pregnancy test, if applicable

NURSING DIAGNOSIS

All generic nursing diagnoses apply to this patient, with the addition of:
Knowledge deficit related to procedure and postop management

PATIENT OUTCOMES

The patient will exhibit an understanding of proposed treatment and postop follow-up care by:
1. Restating proposed treatment in his or her own words
2. Confirming knowledge of required stents and/or catheters
3. Expressing awareness that hematuria may occur for up to 2 weeks
4. Verbalizing awareness of potential ureteral colic and availability of medication to manage discomfort

NURSING ACTIONS

	Yes	No	N/A
1. Patient assessment performed?	☐	☐	☐
2. Perioperative care explained?	☐	☐	☐
3. Positioned correctly?	☐	☐	☐
4. Prep per institutional protocol?	☐	☐	☐
5. Prep solution warmed?	☐	☐	☐
6. Privacy maintained?	☐	☐	☐
7. Special equipment/supplies available?	☐	☐	☐
8. Radiation/laser safety precautions initiated?	☐	☐	☐
9. Precautions taken to prevent chemical burns?	☐	☐	☐
10. Fiberoptic light system checked/functioning?	☐	☐	☐
11. Irrigation solution/system prepared?	☐	☐	☐
12. Return flow monitored?	☐	☐	☐
13. Medications documented?	☐	☐	☐
14. Specimen to lab in dry container?	☐	☐	☐
15. Catheters/stents recorded/labeled?	☐	☐	☐
16. Postop explanations provided?	☐	☐	☐

Document additional nursing actions/generic care plans initiated here:

_____

_____

_____

EVALUATION OF PATIENT OUTCOMES

	Outcome met	Outcome met with additional outcome criteria	Outcome met with revised nursing care plan	Outcome not met	Outcome not applicable to this patient
1. The patient expressed understanding of surgical and perioperative interventions.	☐	☐	☐	☐	☐
2. The patient met outcomes for additional generic care plans as indicated.	☐	☐	☐	☐	☐

Signature: _____ Date: _____

10. When checking the fiberoptic system, the perioperative nurse should inspect the light source to ensure that it is adjustable in intensity. Fiberoptic light bundles or cables should not be twisted or tangled.

11. Nonhemolytic irrigation solution should be used. The irrigation solution commonly used is sterile 0.9% saline. When it is necessary to employ electrosurgery, the irrigation is temporarily changed to sterile water, glycine, or sorbitol. The irrigation solution should be used at body temperature. Cold irrigation solutions may cause bladder spasms or hypothermia. Irrigation solutions hung approximately 2½ to 3 feet above the urology table will provide the correct pressure within the bladder. Irrigation solutions should be hung in tandem ("piggybacked") to maintain continuous irrigation.

12. Monitor return flow from irrigation system.

13. If local anesthetics are used, check for patient allergies before administration. Record medication, dose, and route of administration.

14. After the stone has been retrieved by the stone basket, the perioperative nurse should be prepared to send the specimen for surgical pathologic examination. Follow institutional protocol for the preservation and disposition of surgical specimens. Stone specimens should be sent in a dry container; formalin alters the chemical composition and will make chemical analysis impossible. Implement universal precautions for any container received from the sterile field. Record specimens.

15. An indwelling pigtail or J stent is generally placed in the operative ureter. These stents commonly have a nonabsorbable string attached to the distal end. The string extends out of the urethral meatus, allowing removal in the office setting. A two-way Foley catheter with a 5-ml balloon may also be aseptically connected to a large-volume (2000 ml) urinary drainage system. The large drainage system eliminates the need to empty the drainage bag frequently.

    NOTE: The stents are inserted utilizing fluoroscopy. One pigtail end is placed in the pelvis of the kidney and the other within the bladder. Following insertion, the string is securely, but lightly, taped to the male penis or female lateral perineum. If a Foley catheter is also inserted, the string may be taped to the catheter without tension.

16. Postoperative explanations may include fluid and dietary information, instructions to measure and strain urine and save any stones that are passed, stent and catheter care, and signs and symptoms to report to the physician (elevated temperature, dysuria or flank pain, urinary tract infection, persistent urine leakage, or hematuria). Box 18-5 may be reviewed with the patient.

    NOTE: Persistent leakage of urine through the meatus is a common indication of stent migration. This will often be accompanied by a feeling of pressure and urinary urgency.

Transurethral Resection of the Prostate (TURP)
(Fig. 18-4)

1. The patient undergoing TURP may be anxious about surgery and instrumentation of his genitalia. Explanations of perioperative routines, in language that the patient understands, may decrease anxiety. The patient's medical data base should be reviewed. Urinalysis may show evidence of infection; serum creatinine levels may be elevated in patients with prolonged, severe prostatic obstruction. The patient may have received alpha-adrenergic blockers to relax the urethral sphincter. Results of ultrasound (or cystogram) may be required in the OR. If the patient is elderly, antiembolic stockings or an alternating compression device may be indicated. Determine whether the patient has any limitations to mobility (for example, arthritis) that require special consideration during positioning, and assess skin integrity and muscle mass.

2. The patient will be positioned on a urology table in the lithotomy position. Pad bony prominences and prevent the skin from contact with hard surfaces (OR bed or stirrups). See the Guide to Nursing Actions for lithotomy position (p. 441).

3. Follow institutional protocol for antimicrobial skin preparation.

4. Warmed preparation solutions decrease patient discomfort. Follow manufacturer's recommendations for warming antimicrobial skin preparation solutions.

5. The potential for anxiety, embarrassment, and emotional distress may be present when the genitalia are exposed. A considerate, caring attitude is necessary. All attempts should be made to maintain privacy.

6. A nonhemolytic and nonelectrolytic irrigation solution should be used during TURP. Irrigating solutions commonly used are 1.5% glycine and 3% sorbitol. The irrigation solution should be used at body temperature because cold irrigation solution may cause bladder spasms or hypothermia. Special warming units for TURP irrigation are commonly employed. Irrigation solutions hung approximately 2½ to 3 feet above the urology table will provide the correct pressure in the bladder. Irrigation solutions should be hung in

FIG. 18-4
CARE PLAN FOR TRANSURETHRAL RESECTION OF THE PROSTATE

KEY ASSESSMENT POINTS
Serum sodium/potassium values
Pedal pulses
Urinalysis/urine culture
Preoperative urinary flow pattern

NURSING DIAGNOSIS
All generic nursing diagnoses apply to this patient, with the addition of:
Altered patterns of urinary elimination.

PATIENT OUTCOMES
All generic outcomes apply, with the addition of:
Urine flow through the indwelling catheter will be unobstructed:
1. Catheter will remain patent and drain tension free.
2. Collecting system will be below level of patient's bladder.
3. The catheter will be taped in place; connections will be secure.
4. There will be no complaints of dysuria.

NURSING ACTION:

	Yes	No	N/A
1. Patient assessment performed?	☐	☐	☐
2. Positioned correctly?	☐	☐	☐
3. Prep per institutional protocol?	☐	☐	☐
4. Prep solution warmed?	☐	☐	☐
5. Privacy maintained?	☐	☐	☐
6. Irrigation solution/warming system prepared?	☐	☐	☐
7. ESU checked/functioning?	☐	☐	☐
8. Dispersive pad site checked?	☐	☐	☐
9. Fiberoptic light system checked/functioning?	☐	☐	☐
10. Special equipment/supplies available?	☐	☐	☐
11. Equipment properly aerated or rinsed?	☐	☐	☐
12. Return flow monitored/patient observed for signs of TUR syndrome?	☐	☐	☐
13. Specimen to lab in formalin?	☐	☐	☐
14. Catheters secured and documented?	☐	☐	☐

Document additional nursing actions/generic care plans initiated here:

_____

_____

_____

EVALUATION OF PATIENT OUTCOMES

	Outcome met	Outcome met with additional outcome criteria	Outcome met with revised nursing care plan	Outcome not met	Outcome not applicable to this patient
1. Urinary flow through the catheter/drainage system was maintained.	☐	☐	☐	☐	☐
2. The patient met outcomes for additional generic care plans as indicated.	☐	☐	☐	☐	☐

Signature: _____ Date: _____

tandem ("piggybacked") to maintain continuous irrigation.

7. The electrosurgical unit will be used. Special considerations in using the electrosurgical unit during TURP include the following:
   a. The electrode of the cutting loop should be stabilized so that it retracts properly into the sheath after each cut.
   b. Insulation of the electrode should be intact.
   c. The cutting loop should not be broken.
   d. The sheath must be made of fiberglass or bakelite to prevent short circuiting of the electric current.
   e. Conductive lubricants that provide a pathway for electric current should not be used on the sheath.

8. The condition of the skin at the dispersive pad application site should be checked before application and after pad removal.

9. The fiberoptic light system should be checked before use.

10. Special equipment and supplies include resectoscopes (with working elements, sheath, obturator, and so on), telescopes, cutting loop, sounds, adapters, syringes, and lubricant. Important considerations in checking resectoscope instruments and accessories include the following:
    a. Inspection of the lens for scratches and clarity of vision
    b. Integrity of the sheath
    c. Mobility of all moving parts
    d. Obturator tip protrusion past the end of the sheath
    e. Integrity of the rubber tips
    f. Patency of channels through instruments

11. Instruments may be gas sterilized or cold chemosterilized (soaked). The use of chemical agents presents the risk for patient injury. After sterilization of resectoscopes with ethylene oxide, aeration time is critical to prevent burns to patients or to those handling the equipment. Insufficiently aerated materials can cause skin irritation, tissue burns, and hemolysis. In general, mechanical aeration of a resectoscope requires a temperature of 122° to 140° F for 8 to 12 hours. Resectoscopes aerated at room temperature require 7 days. If chemosterilization is used (soaking), instruments should be fully immersed in a closed container in a solution of the appropriate concentration for the required time. Aseptic technique in rinsing and transfer of soaked items to the sterile field must be ensured.

12. Return flow of irrigation solution must be monitored. The potential for irrigant extravasation into open venous sinuses or bladder perforation exists. This high risk for fluid volume ex-

cess related to transurethral resection syndrome is commonly referred to as TUR syndrome. This can be described as a shift of body fluids and electrolytes caused by decreased extracellular sodium. The patient should be observed for the following symptoms:
   a. Sudden restlessness
   b. Apprehension
   c. Irritability
   d. Slow pulse
   e. Rising blood pressure
   If these occur, the perioperative nurse needs to help obtain and send blood samples for serum electrolyte levels. If the laboratory results indicate a low serum sodium level, hypertonic sodium chloride may be added to intravenous solutions or a diuretic may be used. The rate of administration of fluid therapy will be slowed, and the pressure of irrigation fluid will be decreased.

13. The resected prostatic tissue specimen is removed by fitting an Ellik evacuator to the resectoscope sheath. The prostatic tissue is then removed by manual pulsatile pressure of the ellik evacuator. Tissue and solution from the evacuator are emptied over the wire mesh extending from the urology table. The perioperative nurse should have the following materials available for sending specimens for pathologic examination:
    a. One or two Ellik evacuators
    b. A spoon or other means to collect the prostatic tissue from the mesh
    c. A properly labeled specimen container
    d. A completed pathology slip

14. A three-way Foley catheter with a 30-ml balloon should be aseptically connected to a large-volume (4000 ml) urinary drainage system. The large drainage system eliminates the need to empty the drainage bag frequently. Maintain patency of the drainage system; avoid kinks or loops in the catheter or tubing. Secure the catheter to the patient with slight traction and secure connections. Keep the drainage system below the level of the patient's bladder. The perioperative nurse should consider *altered patterns of urinary elimination* related to the postdwelling urinary catheter and assess the patient for distention and discomfort. Document the presence and size of the indwelling urinary catheter.

Laser Ablation of Carcinoma of the Penis (Fig. 18-5)

1. Penile carcinoma, although rare, occurs primarily in uncircumcised males. Carcinoma in the preputial cavity may demonstrate symptoms of foul discharge, bleeding, or outlet obstruction.

FIG. 18-5
CARE PLAN FOR LASER ABLATION OF CARCINOMA OF THE PENIS

KEY ASSESSMENT POINTS

Patient understanding of laser therapy
Patient's psychosocial status toward disease
CBC (anemia common in this population)
Urinary flow pattern (obstruction common)

NURSING DIAGNOSIS

All generic nursing diagnoses apply to this patient, with the addition
   of:
Body image disturbance

PATIENT OUTCOMES

All generic outcomes apply, with the addition of:
The patient will have decreased disturbance in body image. The patient will:
1. Express feelings/concerns about genital surgery
2. Resolve fears and anxiety
3. Express constructive integration of body image

NURSING ACTIONS

	Yes	No	N/A
1. Assessment performed?	☐	☐	☐
2. Positioned correctly?	☐	☐	☐
3. Prep per institutional protocol?	☐	☐	☐
4. Prepping solution warmed?	☐	☐	☐
5. Condition of skin noted at prep site?	☐	☐	☐
6. Privacy maintained?	☐	☐	☐
7. Laser safety precautions initiated?	☐	☐	☐

Document additional nursing actions/generic care plans initiated here:

_____

_____

_____

EVALUATION OF PATIENT OUTCOMES

	Outcome met	Outcome met with additional outcome criteria	Outcome met with revised nursing care plan	Outcome not met	Outcome not applicable to this patient
1. The patient's disturbance in body image was decreased.	☐	☐	☐	☐	☐
2. The patient met outcomes for additional generic care plans as indicated.	☐	☐	☐	☐	☐

Signature: _____ Date: _____

Lesions on the glans may appear red and velvety or may be nodular, wartlike growths with secondary infection. The patient may be extremely embarrassed by penile lesions, as well as anxious about the surgical outcome and the use of a laser. The patient may have misconceptions about the cause of the lesions. It is important to allow the patient to express his feelings and concerns. A private environment for nursing assessment encourages the patient to ask questions. The perioperative nurse's acceptance of the patient's concerns and questions reassures the patient and facilitates learning and coping. The perioperative nurse will use the diagnosis of *body image disturbance* if the patient is experiencing, or is at risk of experiencing, a disruption in the way he perceives his body image. Provide information about events that will take place. Explanations about the laser are extremely important (regarding eye protection, sounds, and smells).

2. The supine position will be used. Assist the patient to assume a position of comfort on the OR bed.

3. Solutions for skin preparation must not have an alcohol base. Examples of alcohol-based preparation solutions are isopropyl alcohol, ethyl alcohol, and tincture of iodine. These are flammable and must not be used. Fumes may collect in the drapes and ignite when the laser unit is used. Follow laser protocol for antimicrobial skin preparation.

4. The use of warmed preparation solutions may decrease patient discomfort. Adhere to manufacturer's recommendations for warming antimicrobial solutions.

5. Note the condition of the penis and document lesions and infection.

6. The potential for anxiety, embarrassment, and emotional distress may be present when genitalia are exposed. A considerate, caring attitude is necessary. All attempts should be made to maintain privacy.

7. The laser should be prepared, checked, and tested before the patient is brought into the OR. A preoperative checklist is helpful. The perioperative nurse should report any malfunction of the laser immediately. Affix a warning sign to the outside of the OR door that says "Danger: Laser in use" and states the type of laser being employed. The CO_2 and Nd:YAG lasers are the most widely used, but the argon laser has also been effective for the treatment of this condition. Only personnel with appropriate eye protection should enter the OR suite. The eye is the organ most susceptible to laser injury. Each type of laser requires a specific type of safety glasses, because each affects the eye differently:

a. Argon laser: Amber-tinted lens
b. Carbon dioxide laser: Clear glass with side guards
c. Nd:YAG laser: Green-tinted lens
Refer to the Guide to Nursing Actions for laser safety (see p. 443).

Nephrectomy (Fig. 18-6)

1. The anticipated loss of a body part can be a source of grieving to a patient. The kidney is a major body organ; patients may have serious concerns about normal physiologic functioning following its removal. The perioperative nurse should attempt to assess the impact of the perceived loss. If the patient is donating a kidney, he or she may worry that the recipient's body will reject the kidney. Other patients may have concerns about diagnoses or postoperative complications. Explanations that address specific concerns should help the patient begin to resolve this grief. In addition, the perioperative nurse should determine if the patient has any mobility limitations, allergies, or other conditions that would affect intraoperative care.

2. The position selected depends on the renal disease, the need for exposure, and the patient's condition. In general, the lateral position for a flank (subcostal) or lumbodorsal approach is used. However, in cases of renal trauma or large tumors of the kidney, a transabdominal approach may be used. Sequential compression stockings are applied. For radical nephrectomy, a transthoracic approach may be used. Following nephrectomy, the patient often expresses pain. Because of this pain, many are prone to splint or guard the operative side to a degree that inhibits adequate airway clearance and pulmonary exchange. The perioperative nurse should consider the risk for *ineffective airway clearance* and review regimens to assist the patient with pulmonary toilet techniques. Suggesting a pillow to squeeze against the affected side during deep breathing and coughing exercises and encouraging early ambulation will increase mobilization of pulmonary secretions.

3. An indwelling urinary catheter will be inserted. Use aseptic technique for catheter insertion. Secure the catheter to the patient and secure connections. Place the bag where it is readily observable. During positional change (supine to lateral and lateral to supine), prevent undue tension on the catheter and kinks or loops. Document catheter insertion and size.

4. Follow institutional protocol for antimicrobial skin preparation.

FIG. 18-6
CARE PLAN FOR NEPHRECTOMY

KEY ASSESSMENT POINTS

Cardiopulmonary status
BUN/creatinine clearance/serum creatinine values
Radial/pedal pulses
Patient knowledge of pulmonary toilet technique

NURSING DIAGNOSIS

All generic nursing diagnoses apply to this patient, with the addition of:
Ineffective airway clearance

PATENT OUTCOMES

The patient will effectively mobilize pulmonary secretions:
1. The patient will exhibit satisfactory respiratory exchange as evidenced by O_2 saturation and spirometry
2. Arterial blood gas will be within normal range
3. Coughing will be effective

NURSING ACTIONS

	Yes	No	N/A
1. Patient assessment performed?	☐	☐	☐
2. Positioned correctly?	☐	☐	☐
3. Foley catheter inserted?	☐	☐	☐
4. Prep per institutional protocol?	☐	☐	☐
5. Condition of skin at prep site noted?	☐	☐	☐
6. ESU checked/functioning?	☐	☐	☐
7. Dispersive pad site checked?	☐	☐	☐
8. Special equipment/supplies available?	☐	☐	☐
9. Input/output documented?	☐	☐	☐
10. Specimen recorded?	☐	☐	☐
11. Counts performed; correct and documented?	☐	☐	☐
12. Catheters/drains secured and documented?	☐	☐	☐

Document additional nursing actions/generic care plans initiated here:

_____

_____

_____

EVALUATION OF PATIENT OUTCOMES

	Outcome met	Outcome met with additional outcome criteria	Outcome met with revised nursing care plan	Outcome not met	Outcome not applicable to this patient
1. Patient exhibited no signs/symptoms of ineffective airway clearance.	☐	☐	☐	☐	☐
2. The patient met outcomes for additional generic care plans as indicated.	☐	☐	☐	☐	☐

Signature: _____ Date: _____

5. Note the condition of the skin (scratches, nicks, or rashes) at the preparation site.

6. The electrosurgical unit should be available and checked.

7. Assess the skin at the site of application of the dispersive pad before pad placement and on removal.

8. Abdominal instruments and kidney instruments will be required; instruments for rib resection should be available. Chest instruments will need to be added if the thoracoabdominal approach is used.

9. Intake and output should be recorded and reported to the postanesthesia care unit nurse as part of the perioperative discharge report.

10. Follow institutional protocol for the preservation and disposition of surgical specimens. For donor kidneys, follow protocols for hypothermic preservation. Initiate universal precautions with containers received from the sterile field. Record specimens.

11. Follow institutional protocol for sponge, sharp, and instrument counts.

12. All tubes, drains, and catheters should be recorded. Use aseptic technique for dressing application and securing tube/drainage sites. Cleanse the area surrounding the dressing of exudate.

Kidney Transplant (Recipient) (Fig. 18-7)

1. Renal diseases treated by transplant include chronic glomerulonephritis, diabetic nephropathy, chronic pyelonephritis, malignant nephrosclerosis, and polycystic kidney disease. Patient assessment includes a focused inquiry on symptoms, general condition, and factors that will influence care planning, such as disabilities, allergies, and skin integrity. Histocompatibility, cross-match, and ABO compatibility testing will have been completed. Immunosuppressive drug therapy, necessary for graft survival, places the patient at risk for viral, fungal, and bacterial infection. There are three sources of donor kidneys: living related, cadaver, and nonrelated living donors. Patients may have deep individual feelings about organ donation from any of these sources. Patients will vary in age; consult Chapter 21 for care plan information about the pediatric patient and Chapter 22 for information about the aging patient. Patients may have a vascular access site or peritoneal dialysis catheter in place. The perioperative nurse should review the medical data base and validate that no local (angioaccess prosthesis) or systemic (peritonitis from peritoneal dialysis catheter) infection is present. The availability of blood and blood products should be checked; perioperative transfusion will likely be given (blood transfusions influence graft survival). In addition to the high risk for alterations in fluid volume status, the nursing diagnoses in Box 18-6 should be considered.

2. The supine position will be used. Preoperative neurovascular assessment is important for positioning. There may be peripheral neuropathies caused by underlying nutritional deficits and uremia. Protecting the patient from injury, and padding and protecting dependent pressure areas is essential. Invasive lines will be inserted for patient monitoring. Central venous pressure catheters are extremely useful for monitoring fluid replacement therapy. Protect all lines during positioning. Sequential compression hose will be applied.

3. Use strict aseptic technique in the insertion of the indwelling urinary catheter. Place the drainage bag where it is readily observable but keep it off the floor. Secure the catheter to the patient; secure connections. Prevent kinks and loops in the catheter or tubing. Document catheter insertion.

4. An antibiotic irrigant will be instilled into the bladder. Prepare solution at the correct concentration and document its administration.

5. Follow institutional protocol for antimicrobial skin preparation. The kidney is usually placed in the iliac fossa through an oblique or curvilinear lower abdominal incision. Skin preparation may extend from the nipples to the knees. The transplant recipient is vulnerable to poor wound healing due to longstanding nutritional depletion. Strict aseptic technique during skin preparation, as well as intraoperatively, is important to aid the healing process. Note and document the condition of the skin at the preparation site for rashes and nicks.

6. The electrosurgical unit will be used. Check the unit before use. Note the condition of the skin before application and after removal of the dispersive pad.

7. Abdominal and vascular instruments are required. Anticipate the need for meticulous dissection and multiple anastomoses, including vascular attachments, to establish urinary tract continuity. All instruments and equipment should be ready for the transplant procedure in advance. After removal of the kidney from the donor, warm ischemic time must be kept to a minimum. There are two techniques for short-term hypothermic preservation. Simple hypothermia is achieved by flushing with an appropriate solution (such as Collins' solution). Pulsatile perfusion may also be used. The current

FIG. 18-7
CARE PLAN FOR KIDNEY TRANSPLANT (RECIPIENT)

KEY ASSESSMENT POINTS

Urinalysis/urine culture
All hematologies
Cardiopulmonary status
Skin integrity
Presence of infection

NURSING DIAGNOSIS

All generic nursing diagnoses apply to this patient, with the addition of:
High risk for fluid volume deficit or excess

PATIENT OUTCOMES

The patient will exhibit balanced fluid volume by:
1. Laboratory studies within normal range
2. Balanced intake and output of fluids
3. Satisfactory cardiopulmonary status
4. Effective pulmonary toilet

NURSING ACTIONS

	Yes	No	N/A
1. Patient assessment performed?	□	□	□
2. Positioned correctly?	□	□	□
3. Foley catheter inserted?	□	□	□
4. Antibiotic bladder instillation performed?	□	□	□
5. Prep per institutional protocol?	□	□	□
6. Dispersive pad site inspected?	□	□	□
7. Special equipment available?	□	□	□
8. Input/output recorded?	□	□	□
9. Medications documented?	□	□	□
10. Specimens to lab?	□	□	□
11. Counts performed; correct and documented?	□	□	□
12. Dressings aseptically applied?	□	□	□
13. Catheters/drains secured/documented?	□	□	□
14. Postop expectations explained?	□	□	□

Document additional nursing actions/generic care plans initiated here:

_____

_____

_____

EVALUATION OF PATIENT OUTCOMES

	Outcome met	Outcome met with additional outcome criteria	Outcome met with revised nursing care plan	Outcome not met	Outcome not applicable to this patient
1. There was no evidence of altered fluid volume.	□	□	□	□	□
2. The patient met outcomes for additional generic care plans as indicated.	□	□	□	□	□

Signature: _____ Date: _____

Box 18-6 Nursing Diagnoses for the Kidney Transplant Recipient

Altered protection related to immunosuppression therapy

Alteration in urinary elimination related to possible impaired renal function

Anxiety related to possible rejection; procedure

High risk for infection related to use of immunosuppressive therapy to control rejection

Knowledge deficit related to specific nutritional needs; possible paralytic ileus, fluid, sodium restrictions

Impaired health maintenance related to long-term home treatment after transplantation; diet, signs of rejection, use of medications

Spiritual distress related to obtaining transplanted kidney from someone's traumatic loss

From Ackley BJ & Ladwig GB. (1993). *Nursing diagnosis handbook: A guide to planning care.* St. Louis: Mosby.

---

albumin perfusates allow the kidneys to be stored for up to 72 hours. The donor kidney is surrounded by saline slush in an insulated carrier during transport. The donor kidney is brought to the OR and placed in cold (4° C) saline solution on the sterile field. Once the donor kidney has been anastomosed, the graft should be observed. It should look pink and firm. Grafts with diminished flow are at risk for hyperacute rejection. This is evidenced by a blue, soft appearance and may begin immediately following anastomosis. If this occurs, prepare for removal of the transplanted kidney.

8. Intake and output and blood loss should be carefully monitored; collaborate with the anesthesia staff. The transplant recipient is at increased risk for fluid volume fluctuations. The perioperative nurse should consider the diagnosis *high risk for fluid volume deficit* or *excess* in caring for these patients.

9. Heparin irrigation will be used during vessel anastomoses. All medications on the sterile field should be carefully labeled and documented.

10. There is usually not a surgical specimen; the native kidney is left in place (unless contraindicated). The transplanted kidney is placed in the retroperitoneal space in either pelvic fossa. Document any specimens sent for blood or microbial analyses.

11. Follow institutional protocol for sharp, sponge, and instrument counts.

12. Apply surgical dressings aseptically. When securing dressings with tape, anticipate some postoperative edema. Do not place tape so tightly that it may cause postoperative "tape burns."

13. Document all catheters, tubes, and drains. A Silastic stenting catheter may be inserted and brought out the urethra with the urinary catheter.

14. Discharge planning and explanations of postoperative expectations may be initiated by the perioperative nurse on a transplant team. Box 18-7 provides a sample information sheet.

Penile Implant (Fig. 18-8)

1. Impotence is the inability to obtain and sustain an erection. There are various categories of impotence; not all will be treated with surgical implantation of a penile prosthesis. The patient is likely to have a great deal of anxiety; this may be related to embarrassment or fear that the implant will fail. The perioperative nurse's attitude will help the patient cope with this anxiety, and the nurse should assist the patient with personally effective coping mechanisms.

2. Either general or regional anesthesia may be used. Explanations and empathic responses to patient concerns about anesthesia help the patient cope with anxiety.

3. Either supine or lithotomy position may be used. Refer to the Guides to Nursing Actions for safe patient positioning (p. 441).

4. Follow institutional protocol for antimicrobial skin preparation. If the lithotomy position is used, the anus should be isolated with an adhesive drape to prevent the risk for infection.

5. Warmed preparation solutions decrease patient discomfort. Follow manufacturers' recommendations for warming antimicrobial solutions.

6. Note the condition of the skin at the preparation site.

7. Maintaining privacy during preparatory maneuvers helps the patient deal with embarrassment.

8. The electrosurgical unit should be available and checked.

9. The condition of the skin at the site of the dispersive pad should be assessed before and after application.

10. A minor instrument set with fine instruments and dilators will be required. Some inflatable penile prostheses require a filling solution. This solution is usually a radiopaque contrast material. The perioperative nurse will need to dilute two parts of Cysto-Conray II with one part of sterile water for drug diluent or, more com-

---

Box 18-7 *Going Home After a Kidney Transplant*

You will be allowed to go home 2 to 3 weeks after surgery. You should avoid any heavy lifting for the next 2 to 3 months. Avoid contact sports, but do make walking part of your daily routine. You should be able to return to your job about 6 weeks after surgery.

Although the drugs you will be taking can cause some undesirable side effects, your new kidney can return your life to near normal. Dialysis will no longer be needed, and you should have fewer dietary and fluid restrictions. Also, you will feel better and have more energy.

Your renal (kidney) trasplantation is over, and you've been discharged from the hospital. Your home care is now beginning, and there are some things you need to know about taking care of yourself and monitoring your new kidney's function.

Keeping Records

For the first 3 weeks after discharge, you will need to keep daily records on the following:
- *Daily urine output.* You need to measure and record how much urine you produce.
- *Daily fluid intake.* Measure and record all fluids, including ice.
- *Weight.* Weigh yourself every morning before eating and after urinating.
- *Temperature.* Take your temperature at the same time every afternoon. If you begin running a temperature higher than 100° F, call your doctor.
- *Blood pressure.* Take blood pressure readings every day at the same time and record the readings.

Diet and Medication

You should have fewer diet restrictions now than when you were undergoing dialysis, but the immunosuppressive medication you will be taking to prevent kidney rejection can cause some side effects that can be controlled by diet. *Cyclosporine* can raise potassium levels, and you may have to restrict your potassium intake. *Prednisone* can cause salt retention, increased appetite, and an increase in your blood sugar level. You may need to follow a low-sodium, low-calorie, and/or restricted-sugar diet.

Cyclosporine and prednisone have other side effects. Cyclosporine can cause flushing, hair growth on the face and body, gum swelling, headaches, high blood pressure, and kidney toxicity. Prednisone can cause rounding of the face and abdomen, increased sweating, easy bruising, acne, muscle weakness, cataracts, joint pain, delayed wound healing, and restlessness or moodiness.

Another immunosuppressive drug is *azathioprine.* Azathioprine can decrease your white blood cell count and cause temporary hair loss.

The side effects of these drugs are usually not too troublesome, and some can be controlled. After a few months, when the dosage is lowered, some of these side effects may decrease or disappear.

You must take your immunosuppressive medication for the rest of your life. If you stop, your body will reject your new kidney. Notify your doctor if you forget to take your medication.

If you are taking prednisone, your doctor may also tell you to take food or milk when you take the prednisone to help prevent stomach irritation.

You should never take aspirin, since it can cause stomach bleeding. You may take acetaminophen (Tylenol) for pain. Check with your doctor before you take any prescriptive or over-the-counter drug.

Health Habits

Personal hygiene is very important. Here are some health habits you should follow:
- Take a bath or shower every day.
- Use lotion to lubricate dry skin.
- Don't scratch bites or rashes, since this may lead to infection.
- Use topical antibiotics on minor skin wounds.
- Avoid people with colds.
- Wash your hands.
- Tell your dentist that you have had a kidney transplant and are taking immunosuppressive drugs. You may need to take antibiotics before undergoing any dental work.

You must take care of yourself and your new kidney. Avoid any contact sports such as football or hockey but do make walking part of your daily routine. Your doctor may recommend birth control for a period of time.

---

monly, 300 ml of Hypaque 25% to 360 ml of sterile water for drug diluent. If the patient is allergic to iodine or contrast media, normal saline solution may be used. The implant components must be free of all air bubbles. Only instruments shod with Silastic tubing should be used on the components or the connecting tubing.

11. Each prosthesis should be checked for structural integrity before implantation. Any inadvertent puncture or nick will present the potential for mechanical failure. Punctures or nicks can also serve as collection points for debris, which could cause foreign body reactions or be loci of infection. A damaged prosthesis should not be

FIG. 18-8
CARE PLAN FOR PENILE IMPLANT

KEY ASSESSMENT POINTS

Determine absence of arthritic condition
Establish absence of infection
Interview regarding immune system deficits
Assess psychosocial adjustment
Confirm understanding of procedure and postop management

NURSING DIAGNOSIS

All generic nursing diagnoses apply to this patient, with the addition
  of:
Anxiety

PATIENT OUTCOMES

All generic outcomes apply, with the addition of:
The patient's anxiety will be reduced. The patient will:
1. Describe anxiety and coping methods
2. Verbalize feelings of less anxiety to the perioperative nurse
3. Use personally effective coping mechanisms

NURSING ACTIONS

	Yes	No	N/A
1. Assessment performed?	☐	☐	☐
2. Method of anesthesia explained?	☐	☐	☐
3. Positioned correctly?	☐	☐	☐
4. Prep per institutional protocol?	☐	☐	☐
5. Warmed prep solution used?	☐	☐	☐
6. Condition of skin noted at prep site?	☐	☐	☐
7. Privacy maintained?	☐	☐	☐
8. ESU available/checked?	☐	☐	☐
9. Dispersive pad site checked?	☐	☐	☐
10. Special equipment/supplies available?	☐	☐	☐
11. Implant inspected?	☐	☐	☐
12. Implant precautions initiated?	☐	☐	☐
13. Implants recorded?	☐	☐	☐
14. Medications documented?	☐	☐	☐
15. Counts performed/correct?	☐	☐	☐
16. Catheter inserted?	☐	☐	☐
17. Dressings applied?	☐	☐	☐

Document additional nursing actions/generic care plans initiated
here:

_____

_____

_____

EVALUATION OF PATIENT OUTCOMES

1. The patient's anxiety was reduced.
2. The patient met outcomes for additional generic care plans as
   indicated.

	Outcome met	Outcome met with additional outcome criteria	Outcome met nursing care plan	Outcome not met	Outcome not applicable to this patient
1.	☐	☐	☐	☐	☐
2.	☐	☐	☐	☐	☐

Signature: _____ Date: _____

implanted. A new, undamaged, prosthesis should be available at the time of operation.

12. Lint, fingerprints, talc, and other surface contaminants can cause foreign body reactions. Utmost caution should be taken to avoid contaminants.

13. Follow institutional protocols for documenting implanted devices.

14. Antibiotic irrigant is recommended to reduce the potential complication of infection. All solutions on the sterile field should be labeled and all medications documented.

15. Follow institutional protocol for sharp, sponge, and instrument counts.

16. An indwelling urinary catheter is inserted preoperatively following preparation of the sterile field. The Foley catheter should be aseptically connected to a urinary drainage bag. Secure the catheter to the patient and secure connections. Prevent kinks and stress on the catheter site during patient transfer to the discharge vehicle. Keep the drainage bag below the level of the patient's bladder. Document catheter insertion and record intraoperative output.

17. Depending on the surgical approach, a petrolatum gauze, Kling dressing, Tegaderm, or a small gauze dressing may be used.

References

Alfaro-LeFevre R, et al. (1992). *Drug handbook: A nursing process approach*. Redwood City: Addison-Wesley Nursing, Benjamin/Cummings.

Bichat X. (1814). *Desault's surgery*. Philadelphia: Thomas Dobson.

Corriere JN. (1994). What's new in urology, *ACS Bulletin, 79*(1), 82-84.

Cubler-Goodman A, Devlin MA, & Dinatale R. (1993). Endoscopic lithotripsy for urinary calculi. *AORN Journal, 58*(5), 954-969.

Fowler FJ & Barry MJ. (1993). Quality of life assessment for evaluating benign prostatic hyperplasia treatments. *European Urology, 24*(1), 24-27.

Gillenwater JY, et al. (1996). *Adult and pediatric urology*. (3rd ed.). St. Louis: Mosby.

Horne MM & Swearingen PL. (1993). *Fluid, electrolytes, and acid-base balances*. St. Louis: Mosby.

Kaempf G & Amodei ME. (1989). The effect of music on anxiety. *AORN Journal. 50*, 112-118.

Keetch DW, Moore S, & Shea L. (1995). Cryosurgical ablation of the prostate. *AORN Journal, 61*(5), 807-813.

Kropp KA. (1987). The lithotomy position. In Martin JT (Ed.), *Positioning in anesthesia and surgery*. Philadelphia: JB Lippincott.

Larsen PD & Martin JH. (1994). Renal system changes in the elderly. *AORN Journal, 60*(3), 298-301.

Lu-Yao GL, Barry MJ, & Chang MS. (1994). Transurethral resection of the prostate among Medicare beneficiaries in the United States: Time trends and outcomes. *Urology, 44*(5), 692-699.

Mathias JM. (1995). New technology: Cryoablation for prostate cancer. *OR Manager, 11*(2), 8-9.

McCance KL & Huether SE. (1994). *Pathophysiology: The biologic basis for disease in adults and children* (2nd ed.). St. Louis: Mosby.

McNamara SA. (1995). Perioperative nurses' perceptions of caring practices. *AORN Journal, 61*(2), 377-388.

Newton M, Moore S & Gaehle KE. (1994). Prostate cancer: Staging through laparoscopic lymphadenectomy. *AORN Journal, 59*(4), 823-836.

Pagana KD & Pagana TJ. (1995) *Mosby's diagnostic and laboratory test reference* (2nd ed.). St Louis: Mosby.

Paschal CR & Strzelecki LR. (1992). Lithotomy positioning devices. *AORN Journal, 55*:4, 1011-1022.

Rea R, et al. (1987). *Emergency nursing core curriculum*. Philadelphia: WB Saunders.

Ronk LL & Kavitz JM. (1994). Perioperative nursing implications of radical perineal prostatectomy. *AORN Journal, 60*(3), 438-446.

Rothrock JC & Sculthorpe RH. (1993). Anesthesia and patient positioning. In JC Rothrock (Ed.), *The RN first assistant*. (2nd ed.). Philadelphia: JB Lippincott.

Seidel HM, et al. (1995). *Mosby's guide to physical examination* (3rd ed.). St Louis: Mosby.

Shellenbarger T & Krouse A. (1994). Treating and preventing kidney stones. *Medsurg Nursing, 3*(5), 389-394.

Shepherd RR. (1986). Urology. In JA McCradie, Burns GP, & Donner C (Eds), *Basic Surgery*. New York: MacMillan.

Tanagho EA & McAniinch JW. (1991). *Smith's general urology*. Norwalk, CT: Appleton & Lange.

Thompson JM, et al. (1993). *Mosby's clinical nursing* (3rd ed.). St. Louis: Mosby.

Tiemann D, et al. (1993). Artificial urinary sphincters: Treatment for postprostatectomy incontinence. *AORN Journal, 57*(6), 1366-1378.

Walsh PC, et al. (1992). *Campbell's urology*. Philadelphia: WB Saunders.

Wood GP & Ruddock EH. (1909). *Vitalogy*. Vitalogy Association.

Special Considerations in Care Planning

Chapter 19

Ambulatory Surgery

Jane Hershey Johnson

In a private house you will have to get the room ready as well as the patient. Have it thoroughly cleansed, well aired, and at a temperature of about 70° Fahr. There should be a long, firm table on which the patient can lie, so placed that a strong light falls upon it, plenty of basins, clean towels, hot and cold water, soap, and a nail-brush, ice, pins, needles, scissors, sponges, vaseline, and carbolic acid. The doctor will tell you what else will be needed, and what dressings he wishes you to prepare. But these he will usually provide himself.

WEEKS, 1890

OVERVIEW AND HISTORY

Before the 1900s, most surgery was performed in the home. Hospitals were rather primitive; infection and mortality led people to view hospitals as a place to go to die, not to get well. As knowledge was gained regarding asepsis, more complex surgery began to be conducted in hospitals. Eventually, hospitals became technologically superior and safer settings for surgery than the home. In 1909 a Scottish physician wrote about 8988 pediatric surgical procedures performed as outpatient surgery at the Glasgow Royal Hospital for Sick Children (Nicoll, 1909); in 1918 the first outpatient surgery clinic in the United States was established in Sioux City, Iowa (Waters, 1919). Problems with quality of care, insurance coverage, and anesthesia curtailed the early growth of ambulatory surgery. During the 1950s and 1960s, interest in ambulatory surgery grew. There was a lack of hospital beds, nurses, and physicians in the United States, as well as long waiting times for elective surgery. In 1961 the Butterworth Hospital in Grand Rapids, Michigan, started an ambulatory surgical program (Burden, 1993). The first successful free-standing ambulatory surgery center (FASC) was established in 1970 in Phoenix, Arizona.

Since then there has been a rapid increase in the number of surgeries conducted on an outpatient basis in both free-standing and hospital-based centers throughout the United States. The number of procedures performed increased from 30,523 in 1984 to 121,491 in 1986 (Lehr, 1988). In 1992 a total of 2,870,792 surgical operations were performed in outpatient surgery centers, which was an increase of 11.1% from 1991 (Henderson, 1993). Henderson predicted this figure would reach 4 million by the year 1995 as a result of consumer demand, advancing endoscopic technology, and the rapid acceptance by third-party payors. It is projected that 85% of all surgeries will be performed in outpatient centers by the end of the century (McBreen, 1993). Ambulatory services will be the hospital's principal product; inpatient care will be focused on multiorgan failure, trauma, and chronic illness.

In addition to the increased number of procedures performed every year, there has been tremendous growth in the number of ambulatory surgery centers established annually over the past decades. According to the Health Care Financing Administration (HCFA), the number of ambulatory surgery centers (ASCs) grew from 42 in 1982 to 851 in 1987. In 1992 there was a 9% increase in the number of outpatient surgery centers from 1587 in 1991 to 1696 in 1992 (Henderson, 1993). Currently ambulatory surgery is performed in the hospital, in free-standing facilities, and in physicians' offices. Hospital-based outpatient surgery has been the leader in the number of procedures performed each year. Free-standing surgery centers, which may be either hospital affiliated or independently owned and operated, are second according to the number of surgeries conducted. There has been a significant rise in the number of surgical procedures performed in physicians' offices. To survive the associated changes with reforming the health care delivery system, all three settings must keep a competitive edge.

Explanations for the dramatic increase in ambulatory surgery can be grouped into three categories: economics, technology, and consumerism. The primary factor influencing the growth of ambulatory surgery has been its cost-savings potential (Phillips & Hokans, 1994). The high cost of hospitalization prompted third-party payors to provide reimbursement incentives for alternative surgical settings. Ambulatory, or same-day, surgery has proved to be an efficient, cost-effective way to provide quality care for many surgical procedures. Developments in surgical endoscopic technology, laser and fiberoptic equipment, and anesthesia have resulted in less invasive surgical techniques with positive patient outcomes. A clear example of this is the change in operative techniques and length of stay for the patient undergoing cataract extraction. As recently as 1977, the cataract patient was admitted to the hospital the day before surgery, spent up to 2 hours in the operating room, and was confined postoperatively to a bed, with sandbags restricting head movement for several days. Currently the cataract patient arrives about 1 hour before the procedure, is in the operating room about 30 minutes, and after a short recovery period of 1 to 2 hours is discharged. Today's surgical patient is generally a well-informed, educated consumer who demands accessible, convenient, high-quality, and affordable health care. The influence of health maintenance organizations, managed care, and health care reform have required health care providers to make drastic changes in both surgical settings and patient care delivery systems.

Increased awareness of healthy life-styles has fostered an attitude of wellness, health maintenance, and self-help on the part of consumers. For many people, hospitalization connotes illness, loss of control, and disruption of their lives. Children may exhibit fear of the unknown during hospitalization; separation anxiety is greatly reduced when children are not required to spend the night in the hospital. Elderly people often view hospitalization as a more serious indication of their declining health than the condition actually warrants. Although no surgical procedure is stress free, the concept of ambulatory surgery is a significant complement to a philosophy of wellness.

In general, ambulatory surgery has numerous advantages for surgical patients and their families. These advantages include minimal interference with the patient's life-style; less restrictive routines and rules than a hospital; more consideration for individual patient needs; a decreasing length of time that the patient is separated from family; reduced cost; and decreased risk of nosocomial infection. On the other hand, there are inherent disadvantages, such as patients not having the knowledge or resources needed to perform self-care activities at home and noncompliance with preoperative or postoperative instructions (Lea & Phippen, 1992). Continuous quality improvement programs and appropriate patient assessment of educational needs can help reduce some of these disadvantages.

EXTERNAL REGULATORY INFLUENCES

Both federal and state regulatory agencies have an impact on how care is administered in ambulatory surgery centers. On the federal level, both HCFA and Medicare influence payment for services delivered in the ASC setting. Ongoing efforts to reform the health care delivery system continue to play an important role in determining changes in ambulatory surgery. The Department of Health on the state level publishes *Rules and Regulations for Ambulatory Surgical Facilities*. These regulations provide the foundation for administering care to the ASC patient and supply guidelines for establishing positive patient outcomes. Lack of compliance with federal and state regulations may result in closure of the facility and/or reduction of payment for services.

In 1989 regulatory changes introduced by HCFA had a significant effect on ambulatory surgery. The emphasis of these changes was to ensure that high-quality care was the underlying factor in the provision of outpatient surgery. Selected surgical procedures (such as cataract surgery, percutaneous transluminal coronary angioplasty, and pacemaker insertion) were required to be preauthorized regardless of whether they were performed as inpatient or outpatient procedures. As a result of these regulations, if preauthorization is not obtained, payment to the ASC may be denied or delayed for Medicare patients. In addition, the medical records of Medicare outpatient surgery patients are randomly audited. As in inpatient auditing procedures, generic screening indicators have been developed by the HCFA to measure the quality of patient care for ambulatory surgery.

HCFA Generic Quality Screening Guidelines

One of the ways quality is measured is through the review of the patient's medical record. The need for documentation in ambulatory surgery patient care is just as critical as in other settings. Records that do not contain adequate information/documentation can elicit questions about the quality of care provided in the ASC. To meet the HCFA's screen for quality, perioperative nurses working in the ASC setting need to document evidence of the following on the patient's record:

- *Adequate preoperative assessment.* An appropriate and timely history and physical examination should be completed and in the record. The surgeon should add an evaluating note including information about the operative site. Required diagnostic workup including laboratory, x-ray, and electrocardiogram (as appropriate for patient and procedure) results should be on the record. Vital signs must be taken and recorded preoperatively. Any abnormal results must be addressed and resolved before surgery.
- *Intraoperative interventions—patient monitoring.* Abnormal blood pressure (BP), pulse (P), O_2 saturation, temperature, blood loss, or respiratory difficulty should be monitored with documentation of appropriate intervention.
- *Postoperative care.* There should be evidence that the patient has been adequately monitored for abnormal temperature, BP, P, O_2 saturation, respiratory difficulty, bloody drainage, significant changes in physical or mental status, or adverse drug/transfusion reaction and/or medication error.
- *Discharge plan.* There should be an appropriate, documented discharge plan with provisions for follow-up; patient education should be appropriate for the individual patient's learning needs.

Joint Commission Standards for Ambulatory Care

As part of its "Agenda for Change," the Joint Commission on Accreditation of Healthcare Organizations has moved to performance-focused standards in its accreditation process. A performance-focused standard emphasizes what is to be done, how well it is done, and whether it is being improved. In order to meet standards, ambulatory surgery centers need to identify the essential activities in the patient care process being measured, the structures and resources required to successfully implement and perform the care process, the characteristics of the process when it is performed well, how the process is measured and what the dimensions of quality outcomes are, and how the performance of the care process and its outcomes can be improved. Some important questions for the ambulatory surgery center to address are the following:

- Are there written policies and procedures regarding the medical director, nursing administration, and nursing staff?
- Are there established protocols for responding to emergencies, for nurse credentialing, and for noncompliant patients?
- Is there a list of current, approved surgical procedures that may safely be performed in the ambulatory surgery setting?
- Is there a procedure identifying patient selection criteria (American Society of Anesthesiologists [ASA] Class I, II, III permissible)?
- Are there written procedures that ensure appropriate patient education before ambulatory surgery? At discharge?
- Is there a continuous quality improvement program that tracks and follows up on anesthesia complications, cancellations resulting from medical reasons, postprocedure hospital admission, postoperative infections, or unplanned return to surgery?

The Joint Commission is interested in issues pertaining to established standards. Standards of care for ASC patients need to be consistent if high-quality care is to be ensured. Some of the specific criteria that the Joint Commission uses in its scoring guidelines for operative procedures include selecting appropriate procedures, preparing the patient, monitoring the patient during and after procedures, and discharging the patient from the setting (JCAHO, 1994). Compliance with Joint Commission guidelines is critical for ASC accreditation, which is frequently linked to third-party reimbursement for services provided.

Accreditation Association for Ambulatory Health Care, Inc.

The Accreditation Association for Ambulatory Health Care, Inc. (AAAHC) has been providing evaluation, accreditation, and recognition of high-quality ambulatory health care organizations since 1979. An ASC may be accredited by either the Joint Commission and/or AAAHC. AAAHC's criteria for accreditation of ASC facilities and office surgical practices are outlined in the *Accreditation Handbook for Ambulatory Health Care,* in the chapter, "Surgical Services." The publication *Physical Environment Checklist for Ambulatory Surgical Centers,* which is available through AAAHC, should also be reviewed in preparation for the accreditation process. Accreditation can help ensure safe, consistent patient care.

STANDARDS OF CARE

A number of professional associations set standards of care. Three professional associations that have developed standards of care for ambulatory surgery are the American Society of Post Anesthesia Nurses (ASPAN), the American Society of Anesthesiologists (ASA), and the Association of Operating Room Nurses (AORN). These associations provide national standards of care as well as guidelines for nurses' clinical and professional actions.

ASPAN Standards of Nursing Practice

The ASPAN Standards of Nursing Practice (ASPAN, 1992) address the preanesthesia or preprocedural phase of patient care as well as postanesthesia care.

Preanesthesia care. Like the HCFA, the ASPAN recommends that assessment data be collected on ambulatory surgery patients. Relevant preoperative information should be gathered by a professional registered nurse through patient interview (or interview of the family or significant other), physical examination, review of radiology studies, electrocardiogram (ECG), laboratory values, and consultation. After assessing the patient, an appropriate plan of care is developed by the nurse.

Postanesthesia care. ASPAN identifies data required for the initial, ongoing, and discharge assessments for the following postanesthesia care unit (PACU) areas:

- Phase I (initial recovery from the effects of anesthesia)
- Phase II (transitional period until stable and ready to leave facility)

Discharge assessment and patient teaching are vital aspects of PACU care to ensure positive patient outcomes for ambulatory surgery.

ASA Postanesthesia Care Standards

The ASA has also established standards for postanesthesia care. Standard IV (1990) reads as follows:

The patient's condition shall be evaluated continually in the PACU.

1. The patient shall be observed and monitored by methods appropriate to the patient's medical condition. Particular attention should be given to monitoring oxygenation, ventilation, and circulation. During recovery from all anesthetics, a quantitative method of assessing oxygenation such as pulse oximetry shall be employed in the initial phase of recovery.
2. An accurate written report of the PACU period should be maintained. Use of an appropriate PACU scoring system is encouraged for each patient on admission, at appropriate intervals prior to discharge, and at the time of discharge.

3. General medical supervision and coordination of patient care in the PACU should be the responsibility of an anesthesiologist.
4. There shall be a policy to ensure the availability in the facility of a physician capable of managing complications and providing cardiopulmonary resuscitation for patients in PACU.

AORN Standards

The AORN publishes standards and recommended practices for perioperative nursing. Like other standards, the AORN standards have as their intent the provision of high-quality perioperative nursing services and measures by which perioperative nurses demonstrate competency. The standards of clinical practice are broad in scope and encompass the practice of perioperative nursing in all surgical settings. They are based on the nursing process and provide a holistic framework for the delivery of perioperative patient care. These standards may be found in Chapter 1.

ASSESSMENT CONSIDERATIONS

External regulations and standards of care provide criteria for the provision of high-quality ambulatory surgery care. The challenge to nurses in the ambulatory surgery setting is to apply the traditional standards and practices of perioperative nursing in a few short hours. Methods of patient assessment may range from meeting with the patient in person or by telephone to relying on information received from the surgeon's office staff. Frequently, the patient is seen by the anesthesia provider, interviewed by the perioperative nurse, and has required laboratory and preadmission diagnostic testing all in the same visit. This data will be critical in helping the anesthesiologist classify the physical status, or the ASA class, of the patient. Generally ASA Classes I, II, and III patients can be safely treated in a free-standing surgery unit or a hospital-based ASC.

Using a Health Questionnaire

Having the patient complete a health questionnaire at home saves time during the interview. This allows the perioperative nurse time to validate and further explore findings of direct significance to planning care and to answer patient questions. The patient is able to list current medications by referring directly to the medicine bottles. Information that might be included in a preadmission questionnaire follows:

1. Patient's name, sex, height, and weight
2. List of conditions for which the patient is currently under medical care
3. Smoking, alcohol and drug use

Box 19-1 Key Assessment Points

1. NPO (nothing by mouth) status
2. Illness since pre-admission testing (PAT)
3. Last menstrual period for females of childbearing age
4. Name/phone number of responsible adult to drive patient home
5. Availability of responsible adult to stay with patient the first 24 hours postoperatively
6. ASA classification
7. History of malignant hyperthermia and/or latex sensitivity or allergy
8. Patient's understanding of surgery to be performed and surgery center routine, learning needs, self-care and home management ability, and available support systems

4. List of all medications the patient is taking (prescription and over-the-counter), including dosage, number of times a day, and the reason medication is being taken
5. Allergies and type of reaction (include medications, food, environment, and latex)
6. Physical restrictions
7. Previous hospitalizations, surgeries, and anesthesia (request dates and any problems)

Nursing Assessment and Interview

The preoperative interview should provide data about the patient's health history. Questions are designed to identify problems that could affect optimal patient outcome. A holistic approach that incorporates physical and psychosocial elements includes assessment of the family support system, which could affect discharge planning and home care. The key assessment points for the ambulatory surgery patient are noted in Box 19-1. Other information that should be gathered includes the following:

1. Patient identification and mental status
2. Baseline vital signs, height, and weight
3. Skin assessment
4. Review of recent or current health problems (ask if pregnant and date of last menstrual period (LMP) when applicable)
5. Determination of the patient's understanding of the anesthesia, the procedure, recovery, and home health maintenance requirements
6. Verification of consent(s) and confirmation of side, site, and procedure
7. Confirmation of NPO status, other prescribed regimens (presurgical skin preparation and cessation of medications as determined by physician)
8. Review of required laboratory and diagnostic studies; abnormal values are noted and reported appropriately
9. Removal of prosthetics (dentures, glasses, contact lenses, hearing aid), makeup (only as required), jewelry
10. Notation that patient has voided before the surgical intervention
11. Confirm name and phone number of person driving patient home

A sample preoperative admission sheet is shown in Fig. 19-1.

The preoperative assessment and interview generally indicates the level of patient knowledge regarding the surgical intervention. The nurse working in the ASC must quickly assess the patient's learning needs. Patient education should contribute to the patient's understanding of the type of anesthetic to be administered, the surgical procedure, pain and nausea control, length of PACU stay, and postoperative health maintenance routines. Checklists regarding preoperative preparation, written preoperative instructions, telephone calls, demonstrations of postoperative routines, and written postoperative instructions are commonly used. Icenhour (1988) found that patients' perceived satisfaction with care related to the designation of a formal time for patient teaching. Patients who received only written instructions, with little formal reinforcement, were confused about their discharge instructions.

Assessment should result in relevant nursing diagnoses. These may include the following:
- Impaired physical mobility
- Sensory/perceptual alterations
- Decreased cardiac output
- Ineffective breathing patterns, ineffective airway clearance
- Fluid volume deficit, fluid volume excess
- Impaired skin integrity
- Altered tissue perfusion
- Anxiety and fear
- Knowledge deficit
- Ineffective coping
- Body image disturbance, anticipatory grieving

Nursing diagnoses are always based on identifiable patient data. Once they are established, nursing diagnoses are prioritized and incorporated into a plan of nursing care. That care plan should be documented and should incorporate patient outcomes (Fig. 19-2). Planning for patient safety requires that discharge teaching and home health maintenance, as well as transportation concerns, be reviewed with the patient and family or significant other.

SURGICENTER
PREOPERATIVE ADMISSION SHEET

SCHEDULED SURGERY:				OR CHECKLIST	Yes	No	N/A
Date:	Arrival Time:	Accompanied with:		History & Physical			
Driver (Same☐)		Driver's Phone Number:		Signed Permits			
Height:	Weight:	NPO Since:		Labs on Chart			
Admitting VS:	T:	P:	R:	BP:	Anesthesia Consent			
Sore Throat: ☐ Yes ☐ No	Cold: ☐ Yes ☐ No	Family MD:		Name Band Arm/Leg R/L			
Congestion: ☐ Yes ☐ No	Cough: ☐ Yes ☐ No			Dentures			

HISTORY OF PROBLEMS					Jewelry (Rings Taped)			
Heart	☐ Yes ☐ No	Kidney	☐ Yes ☐ No		Voided			
BP	☐ Yes ☐ No	Hepatitis	☐ Yes ☐ No		Pt. Confirm Site/Side			
Lung	☐ Yes ☐ No	Jaundice	☐ Yes ☐ No		Preop Teaching			
Seizures	☐ Yes ☐ No	Diabetes	☐ Yes ☐ No		Pt. Verbalizes Understanding			

Other: (Previous Surgery)

Other:

Last Menstrual Period:

MEDICATIONS TAKEN AT HOME:

Accucheck: Yes   No

Result:

MEDICATIONS GIVEN PREOP:

ALLERGIES:

Time	Medication	Site	Initials

Initials / Full Signature

NURSES' NOTES:

Fig. 19-1. Preoperative admission sheet. (Courtesy Delaware County Memorial Hospital, Surgicenter, Drexel Hill, PA.)

PATIENT CARE PLAN

Nursing Diagnosis	Pt. Goals/Expected Outcome	M	NM	N/A	Reevaluation/Comments
	The patient will:				
1. Anxiety: R/T operative procedure	1. Exhibit reduced anxiety responsive to pt. teaching & emotional support				
2. Anxiety: R/T pain/discomfort of operative site	2. Exhibit reduced anxiety responsive to pt. teaching				
3. Injury: Risk for R/T improper positioning or immobilization during OR procedure	3. Exhibit no musculoskeletal, circulatory, neurologic or respiratory compromise				
4. Skin integrity: Risk for impairment	4. Exhibit no breakdown in skin integrity				
5. Infection: Risk for R/T operative site	5. Experience no contamination of operative site				
6. Risk for loss of dignity: R/T disrobing, prepping, operative exposure, positioning, dressing checks	6. Maintain dignity				
7. Infection: Risk for: R/T indwelling catheters/drains	7. Experience no contamination of indwelling catheters/drains				
8. Thermal regulation: Risk for alteration in body temperature	8. Maintain normal body temp				
9. Risk for: knowledge deficit	9. Exhibit understanding of pt. teaching done at pt.'s level of understanding & pertaining to surgical procedure being done. Pt. verbalized comprehension of discharge instructions.				
10. Other:					
Note: In its original form this care plan used the term "potential for," which has been changed to "risk for" to reflect more current terminology.					Key: R/T = related to; M = met; NM = not met; N/A = not applicable for this patient

Fig. 19-2. Patient care plan. (Courtesy Delaware County Memorial Hospital, Surgicenter, Drexel Hill, PA.)

Focused Assessment

The basic premise is that the patients selected for ambulatory surgery meet certain criteria. They should be stable and functioning, free of infection, and able to participate in self-care, either on their own or with the support of family or significant others. After the general assessment, the perioperative nurse may proceed to focused assessments of systems of relevance to safe and effective outcomes from surgery and anesthesia.

Integumentary system. When observing and assessing the skin and appendages, note the color, turgor, integrity, and temperature of the skin. It is also important to note localized infections, rashes, abrasions, and bruises. Abnormalities may not become apparent until the patient is exposed to be preparped or to have the tourniquet or electrosurgical unit (ESU) dispersive pad applied before the planned surgical procedure. It is important to document abnormalities present before the surgery to avoid questions of quality of care postoperatively.

Respiratory system. Assessment of respiratory status is important for all patients. It is critical in planning for safe administration of and recovery from inhalation anesthetics. It is also important for the ambulatory patient when planning transportation into the OR and perioperative positioning. The perioperative nurse observes for signs of cyanosis and quality of perfusion to the extremities. A history of smoking and presence of a cough should be noted. The patient is questioned about dyspnea and orthopnea. If the cataract patient requires two or more pillows to sleep at night, the perioperative nurse anticipates the need for special planning to position the patient for surgery.

Cardiovascular system. During assessment the nurse will record baseline vital signs and have an opportunity to assess the quality, rate, and rhythm of the pulses. Perfusion to the extremities is concurrently noted by observation of skin color and temperature. The nails are observed for clubbing and thickening and the nail beds for cyanosis. The patient is asked about episodes of tachycardia, dysrhythmia, blood clots, or dyspnea. The list of current medications is reviewed to determine if the patient is taking any cardiac drugs. The health questionnaire should provide information about a history of peripheral edema, hypertension, syncopal episodes, angina, rheumatic fever, heart murmur, valve disease, and the presence of a pacemaker.

Neurologic system. Assessment of the patient's neurologic status may begin with an overall observation of the patient's general level of awareness and orientation, and it may then progress to identifying impairments. Verify visual acuity in both eyes and the presence of visual aids: glasses, contact lenses, or prostheses. Observe for unusual discharge, and note its color, consistency, and amount. If the patient is scheduled for eye surgery, the finding of discharge should be brought to the ophthalmologist's attention. If the patient has glaucoma, it is important to know the medication used and its potential systemic side effects and precautions. For instance, anesthesia staff would need to know if the patient was using an indirect-acting, irreversible anticholinesterase drug because of its interaction with succinylcholine; this could cause postanesthetic respiratory distress. Blind patients require special care in orientation to their surroundings to ensure safety and to reduce anxiety.

In assessing the patient's hearing acuity, note the presence of hearing aids. When the patient is severely hearing impaired, it may be beneficial to leave the hearing aid in place during surgery. If the patient is scheduled for local or regional anesthesia, this may facilitate communication during the procedure. If the patient is deaf and can lip read, nurses should leave their masks down as long as possible and explain that they will communicate on a magic slate or note pad while the mask is up. The patient who communicates by signing may need an interpreter.

Communication deficits, speech patterns, and speech quality should be assessed. The poststroke aphasic patient may require special communication methods. This should be anticipated and provided for whenever possible. Knowing that the patient has had a laryngectomy or tracheostomy is important for establishing communication and planning intraoperative care.

Alterations in the patient's tactile sensory perception, such as hyperesthesia, paresthesia, anesthesia, or pain, will require special planning and extreme care when moving or positioning, both to prevent injury and to provide comfort.

Musculoskeletal system. The focus is generally on mobility limitation when the musculoskeletal system is assessed. Knowledge of limited range of motion and amputations is important when planning for proper movement and positioning the patient in surgery. External fixation devices such as casts will require prior planning. The patient with contractures presents a special challenge, not only for positioning but often for assessment of the operative area. Prior knowledge of special limitations and conditions enables the perioperative nurse to assemble the necessary staff and/or equipment to satisfactorily accomplish the planned surgical intervention without delay.

Gastrointestinal system and nutritional status. In addition to recording the patient's height and weight, the perioperative nurse assesses the patient's nutritional status. This includes objective appraisal of the patient's overall body structure and size; both overweight and underweight patients require special considerations in positioning. The health questionnaire should provide information regarding indigestion, bowel changes, liver problems or jaundice, or bleeding tendencies and anemia. *Altered nutrition: less than body requirements* may predispose the patient to delayed wound healing or to increased risk of infection.

Gastrointestinal complaints of nausea and vomiting, gastritis, esophagitis, and the presence of gastrostomy, ileostomy, or colostomy should alert the nurse to the risk of actual or risk for disturbance in fluid and electrolyte balance. The use of laxatives and diuretics should be carefully queried.

Genitourinary status. Minor urologic and gynecologic procedures make up a significant percentage of ambulatory surgical procedures. Assessment begins with general kidney and bladder function and progresses to gender-specific concerns. The male patient should be questioned about prostate problems; weakened, slow, or delayed urine stream; swelling or pain in the testes; or unusual urethral discharge. Female patients should provide information about menstrual irregularities; date of last menstrual period, if applicable; date of last Papanicolaou smear; and any unusual vaginal discharge or itching. Other important information includes a history of breast lumps, date of last mammogram, and whether the patient is taking birth control pills or may be pregnant.

DIAGNOSTIC STUDIES

The number and type of preoperative diagnostic tests may vary from one institution to another. They are generally determined by the anesthesia department, with established criteria dependent on the patient's age, coexisting health problems, planned surgical procedure, and type of anesthesia. Additional information is gathered from the physician's office, the patient's completed health history questionnaire, old records from previous surgery, and the preoperative interview/nursing assessment.

The ASA physical status classification helps the anesthesia provider to determine patient selection, the best method of anesthesia, and the required preoperative testing. Patients who fall into Classes I, II, and III are candidates for the ambulatory surgery setting (Meeker & Rothrock, 1995). Class I patients are normal, healthy individuals. Class II patients may have mild to moderate systemic disturbances, such as mild diabetes controlled by diet or an oral hypoglycemic agent, mild essential hypertension, moderate obesity, or chronic bronchitis. Class III patients have more severe systemic disturbances such as insulin-dependent diabetes, severe hypertension, or angina.

The patient scheduled for monitored anesthesia care, regional anesthesia, or general anesthesia will usually have a complete blood count and urinalysis. The criteria for ordering a chest x-ray and ECG are individually determined but are frequently required for administration of anesthesia in adults over 40 years old. Additional chemistry profiles, including serum electrolyte and glucose levels, measurement of partial thromboplastin and prothrombin times, and urinalysis of human chorionic gonadotropin level, are ordered according to the type of procedure, the physician's order, and the patient assessment. For instance, serum electrolyte tests may be ordered to determine potassium levels for the patient taking diuretics. A fasting serum glucose level is ordered for diabetic patients. For some patients it is important to check for problems with normal clotting mechanisms by evaluating the partial thromboplastin and prothrombin times. Preoperative assessment should include questions regarding aspirin or anticoagulant therapy, as well as a history of medical conditions that may predispose the patient to bleeding abnormalities.

Urinalysis may reveal infection that requires treatment before elective surgery can be performed. An untreated respiratory infection may contribute to the development of a postoperative infection, or it may complicate the course of anesthesia as a result of impaired gas exchange or pulmonary obstruction and could result in rescheduling the planned surgery.

The perioperative nurse reviews the results of the preoperative tests and uses this information to formulate nursing diagnoses and plan appropriate care. Using the nursing diagnosis *high risk for infection* as an example, the perioperative nurse checks the complete blood count results for a decreased hematocrit level related to a decrease in red blood cells, which could indicate anemia. If there is an accompanying iron deficiency, immunologic defenses can be diminished and the risk for infection increased. When white blood cell and differential white blood cell counts are reviewed, an elevated neutrophil count alerts the nurse to the possibility of infection, whereas a decreased neutrophil count may leave the patient more susceptible to infection. High lymphocyte levels unrelated to malignancy may indicate infection, whereas a low lymphocyte count without other differential shifts may indicate immunodeficiency. If factors contributing to the risk for infection are identified, the perioperative nurse would institute appropriate nursing actions.

If ordered, chest x-ray results and ECGs with interpretations should be on the chart before the patient goes to surgery. Although this seems obvious, if results are waived, an undetected, asymptomatic partial pneumothorax or myocardial infarct could be present. These would require cancellation of the surgery.

MODIFICATIONS OF THE GENERIC CARE PLANS

The generic care plans found in Chapter 7 are directly applicable to the ambulatory surgery patient.

Modifications of the generic care plans should include considerations for monitoring the patient receiving local anesthesia, monitoring the patient receiving additional sedation, and patient discharge instruction whenever appropriate.

Care of the Patient Receiving Local Anesthesia

The patient selected for ambulatory surgery is generally healthy or may have a chronic but stable condition; therefore many surgical procedures may be completed with the use of only local anesthesia. The extent to which the perioperative nurse monitors the patient receiving local anesthesia depends on the individual policies and procedures of the institution and the anesthesia department. Recognizing that practice settings vary, the AORN has established *Recommended Practices for Monitoring the Patient Receiving Local Anesthesia* (AORN, 1996). These recommendations outline the perioperative nurse's responsibilities.

1. Monitoring the patient for reactions to drugs and changes in physiologic and/or behavioral states is accomplished by recording baseline vital signs before drug administration, continuously monitoring vital signs during the procedure, reporting changes to the physician, and evaluating the patient at the completion of the procedure. The perioperative nurse should monitor the following:
   - Blood pressure
   - Heart rate and rhythm
   - Respiratory rate
   - Oxygen saturation
   - Skin condition
   - Mental status
2. It is the responsibility of the perioperative nurse to possess the knowledge, skill, and ability both to use and to interpret information obtained from the monitoring equipment.
3. During the administration of a local anesthetic, the patient record should include documentation of continuous assessment, planning, implementation, and evaluation of patient care.
4. The institution should have written policies and procedures for monitoring the patient receiving local anesthesia that are reviewed annually and are readily available within the practice setting.

In addition to the needs demonstrated by surgical patients in general, the local anesthesia patient may exhibit increased anxiety. This may interfere with the patient's ability to cooperate with requests made by the perioperative nurse and the physician. Establishing rapport and encouraging the patient to ask questions or express concerns can help ensure a more favorable experience for the patient. The patient's coping mechanisms should be assessed. Many patients have developed methods of dealing with anxiety that are healthy and personally effective. Determine whether the patient has these strengths (for example, meditation, guided imagery, relaxation techniques, or music) and help the patient use his or her personal method of reducing anxiety. Box 19-2 offers some suggestions for this.

There are two chemically different types of local anesthetics, the amide group and the ester group. The most commonly used amide local anesthetic

---

Box 19-2 Assisting the Patient with Personally Effective Coping Techniques

Meditation

Focus your thoughts on one thing, such as your breathing, a sound, or a word. When your mind starts to wander, notice the thoughts and feelings that emerge, then return to observing your breathing or repeating the word you are focusing on.

Deep Breathing

Begin inhaling by filling your abdomen with air. Keep inhaling and allow air to fill your lower chest. Continue to breathe in until you feel your collar bone rise. To exhale, reverse the process. Allow air to escape from the top to the lower parts of your chest, then push the remaining air from your abdomen. Because exhaling is the most relaxing phase of breathing, take longer. You may count *1, 2* when you inhale, and *1, 2, 3, 4* when you exhale.

Visualization

Pick a place where you feel comfortable and relaxed. See the scene in your mind and engage your senses: try to smell (the flowers), hear (the birds), feel the things in the scene (the breeze).

Progressive Muscle Relaxation

Alternately tighten and relax each muscle group, starting with your face. Tighten these muscles, hold for a count of five, then release. Continue doing this with the muscles in your neck, shoulders, chest, arms, hands, abdomen, legs, and feet. As you relax each muscle group, imagine the tightness melting away.

Adapted from Sebastian LB. (1994). Adding relaxation techniques to your bag of tricks. *Nursing Spectrum, 3*(4), 17-18.

agents are lidocaine hydrochloride, available as Xylocaine in concentrations from 0.5% to 2%, alone or with epinephrine dilutions of 1:50,000, 1:100,000, and 1:200,000; bupivacaine hydrochloride, available as Sensorcaine or Marcaine in concentrations from 0.25% to 0.75%, alone or with epinephrine 1:200,000; and mepivacaine hydrochloride, available as Carbocaine, Cavacaine, Isocaine, or Polocaine in concentrations of 1% to 2%, is generally administered alone without a vasoconstrictor. Local anesthetics from the ester group include cocaine hydrochloride in concentrations of 4% and 10%; tetracaine, available as Pontocaine in 0.5% concentration; and procaine, available as Novocain or Unicaine.

Amide anesthetic drugs are metabolized by the liver and excreted by the kidneys. Patients may experience toxic reactions to these drugs, especially in the presence of hepatic disease. Allergic reactions are uncommon with the use of amide-type local anesthetics. Toxic reactions occur when there is a buildup of the drug concentration in the bloodstream. Adverse reactions can be prevented or reduced by carefully monitoring the amount of drug administered in relationship to the patient's weight, health status, vascularity of the injection site, and the addition of a vasoconstrictor such as epinephrine to the local anesthetic drug. Signs of a toxic reaction (Burden, 1994) include the following:

Minor signs
  Anxiety or a vague sense that something is wrong
  Slurred speech
  Tingling or numbness of tongue
  Blurred vision
  Tinnitus
  Nausea and vomiting
  Muscle twitching
Serious signs
  Drowsiness
  Confusion
  Dysrhythmia
  Cardiac depression or arrest
  Seizures
  Respiratory depression

For the patient experiencing minor signs of a toxic reaction to the local anesthetic agent, the perioperative nursing actions include monitoring the heart rhythm and vital signs, administration of oxygen, and continual assessment and evaluation of the patient's status. This information is communicated to the surgeon and other members of the OR team. If the toxic reaction becomes serious, emergency interventions may be required. Institutional policy for monitoring the patient receiving local anesthesia must include a protocol for toxic and allergic reactions.

Ester-type anesthetic agents are metabolized in the plasma by pseudocholinesterase enzymes. Although uncommon, some patients are allergic to para-aminobenzoic acid (PABA), which is the primary product of ester agent metabolism. The patient may experience the following allergic reactions to ester agents:

Mild allergic reaction
  Pruritus
  Erythema
  Small hives
Severe allergic reaction
  Bronchial constriction
  Cardiovascular collapse

The intervention for allergic reaction is to treat the symptoms with an antihistamine such as diphenhydramine (Benadryl) or cimetidine (Tagamet) for mild reactions and epinephrine or aminophylline for severe reactions. Patients can also develop allergic reactions to the preservative added to the local anesthetic. Patient education is extremely important in the event of an allergic response. The nurse should provide the patient with the generic and trade names of the agent as well as information on obtaining a medical alert bracelet. Emphasis should be placed on the importance for the patient to always communicate this allergy to health care professionals.

During the administration of a local anesthetic that contains epinephrine, the nurse should also observe for epinephrine reactions: nervousness, anxiety tremors, headache, pallor, nausea, and hypertension.

The primary goal of the management of local anesthetic reactions is, of course, prevention. This is accomplished by careful assessment of the patient preoperatively, including the patient's weight, mental status, history of liver disease, history of allergic reactions to ester agents, and the area for local infiltration. Monitoring the patient's vital signs, cardiac rhythm, and level of consciousness before and during the injection will immediately alert the perioperative nurse to any changes in the patient's status. If not already instituted, intravenous therapy should be initiated to provide a route for supportive drug treatment. In any emergency, emergency and resuscitative equipment and trained staff must be available.

Documentation on the intraoperative record should include but is not limited to preoperative assessment as stated above; baseline vital signs and patient status; name of agent used, including the use of a vasoconstrictor and its dilution; site of infiltration; time and dosage of agent administered; person administering agent; any untoward reactions to the agent, interventions, and response to those interventions; and the patient's status at the time of transfer to PACU and on discharge. Evidence of continuous monitoring, patient assessment, and interventions need to be documented on the patient's record.

Monitoring the Patient Receiving Intravenous (IV) Conscious Sedation

In addition to monitoring the patient receiving local anesthesia, the perioperative nurse may also be responsible for monitoring the patient receiving IV conscious sedation in the ambulatory surgery center. Criteria should be established by the anesthesiologists, certified registered nurse anesthetists (CRNAs), perioperative nurses, and surgeons outlining situations that are appropriate for the patient to be monitored by the perioperative nurse versus anesthesia personnel. The respective responsibility of the perioperative nurse and surgeon during the sedation period should be clearly identified. Each institution should have established criteria that specifically state the patient selection, NPO requirements, type of monitoring to be used, medications that may be administered by the RN, and determination of whether managing patients receiving IV conscious sedation is within each individual RN's scope of practice according to the State Board of Nursing. Many institutions require Advanced cardiac life support (ACLS) certification to monitor patients receiving IV conscious sedation. Watson (1992) recommends the development of competency-based education programs for nurse-monitored sedation.

AORN has established *Recommended Practices for Monitoring the Patient Receiving Intravenous Conscious Sedation* (AORN, 1996). The RN will complete a preoperative assessment that includes the following:
- Physical assessment
- Current medications
- Drug allergies/sensitivities
- Concurrent medical problems
- History of substance abuse
- Baseline vital signs and height/weight/age
- Level of consciousness
- Emotional state
- Ability to communicate
- Perceptions regarding procedure and sedation

Similar to monitoring the patient receiving local anesthesia, the perioperative nurse should not have any other responsibilities that would leave the patient unattended or interrupt continuous monitoring. In addition to the monitoring parameters established for the patient receiving local anesthesia, before administering IV conscious sedation, oxygen (Box 19-3) and an IV access line should be in place. It is the nurse's responsibility to be familiar with both the desirable and undesirable effects of the sedation being administered.

> ### Box 19-3 Preventing Fires in Oxygen-Enriched Atmospheres
>
> In a 1995 action alert, the Emergency Care Research Institute (ECRI) cautioned about fire risks for patients receiving supplemental oxygen from open sources such as masks and cannulas. This creates an oxygen-enriched atmosphere (OEA) in which tissue embers or vapor from the ESU pencil may ignite. Because supplemental oxygen is routinely used with patients undergoing IV conscious sedation (or local anesthesia, according to patient requirements), ECRI recommends the following during facial, head, and neck surgery:
> 1. When an open oxygen source (mask, cannula) is used, alert the surgeon.
> 2. Consider switching patient ventilation to air or low oxygen concentration at least 1 minute before use of heat-producing instruments (ESU, laser).
> 3. Tent surgical drapes to allow oxygen, which is heavier than air, to drain away from the patient's head to the floor. Untented surgical drapes covering the patient may direct excess oxygen into the surgical field.*
>
> Adapted from Health Devices Alerts. (1995, May 5). Number 1995-A18, Anesthesia Units, ECRI, 5200 Butler Pike, Plymouth Meeting, PA 19462.
> *In their discussion of similar dangers, Greco and his colleagues (1995) suggest open-face draping techniques or the use of compressed air beneath the drapes as a substitute for oxygen supplementation in unsedated patients in addition to the ECRI recommendations.

Desirable effects
    Intact protective reflexes
    Cooperation
    Diminished verbal communication
    Easy arousal from sleep
Undesirable effects
    Nystagmus
    Slurred speech
    Unarousable sleep
    Hypotension
    Agitation
    Combativeness
    Hypoventilation
    Respiratory depression
    Airway obstruction
    Apnea

An emergency cart with a defibrillator and resuscitative drugs must be immediately available in the event that untoward effects occur. The perioperative nurse monitoring the patient must be knowledgeable regarding the functions and proper use of the monitoring equipment and must be skilled in administering oxygen as well as managing the patient's airway.

The sedation may be administered immediately before the injection of a local anesthetic for its sedative and amnesic action or during the procedure for its analgesic effect. Diazepam (Valium) is administered to relieve anxiety. Intravenous administration of diazepam should be slow because of the drug's irritating properties at the venous injection site. Because diazepam has a central nervous system depressant effect, the nurse should observe for confusion, hypotension, and respiratory or cardiovascular depression. The patient may experience ataxia, vertigo, diplopia, or blurred vision and therefore must be warned against trying to ambulate alone postoperatively until the effects have worn off. There may be paradoxic reactions such as hyperexcited states, anxiety, hallucinations, or muscle spasticity; in the presence of any of these reactions the medication should be discontinued.

Fentanyl (Sublimaze), a narcotic analgesic, is used as a supplement to local anesthetics for its analgesic and sedative effects. The more common serious adverse reactions to fentanyl are respiratory depression, apnea, muscular rigidity, and bradycardia. These reactions can lead to respiratory arrest, circulatory depression, or cardiac arrest if left untreated. Other reactions include hypotension, dizziness, blurred vision, nausea and vomiting, laryngospasm, and diaphoresis. Secondary rebound respiratory depression may occur postoperatively, so the patient should be monitored closely.

One of the more frequently used drugs today is midazolam (Versed), which is a short-acting central nervous system depressant. Midazolam is used for its sedative effect with the added benefit of retrograde amnesia. When used for conscious sedation, midazolam should not be administered by rapid or single bolus intravenous method. Serious cardiorespiratory events have occurred, including respiratory depression, apnea, and respiratory or cardiac arrest. Midazolam can lower blood pressure, especially in patients who are extremely apprehensive or anxious or who have essential hypertension. Other less commonly seen side effects include hiccups, nausea and vomiting, headache, and oversedation. At the intravenous site, patients may experience tenderness and pain during infusion.

Emergency/resuscitative equipment and personnel must be readily available. Hypotension may need to be treated with vasopressors and fluid therapy. An Ambu-bag with oxygen and an anesthesia machine should be available.

Documentation on the intraoperative record of the patient receiving IV conscious sedation should include evidence of ongoing assessment, nursing diagnosis, outcome identification, planning, intervention, and evaluation of patient care according to AORN's *Recommended Practices*. The following should be included in the perioperative nurse's documentation:

- Name, dosage, route, time, effects of all drugs used
- Type and amount of fluids administered and equipment used
- Physiologic data from continuous monitoring documented at 5- to 15-minute intervals or at significant events
- Level of consciousness
- Interventions and patient's response
- Untoward or significant patient reaction and the resolution

Patients who receive IV conscious sedation should be monitored postoperatively in the PACU until they return to a safe physiologic level, at which time they can be discharged to the care of a responsible adult.

Patient Teaching

One of the major differences between the patient teaching for the ambulatory surgical patient and the in-hospital surgical patient is the short amount of time the nurse has with the patient. Patient teaching starts as soon as it is determined that the patient will be scheduled for a surgical procedure. Therefore, patient teaching becomes a collaborative effort among the surgeon's office staff, the preadmission testing staff, and the ambulatory surgical center staff. The development of a patient teaching sheet that has a medical record copy as well as a copy for the patient can be useful. A sample sheet is shown in Fig. 19-3. Another effective means of providing patient teaching is the use of a preoperative teaching video that the patient can either view while waiting to complete all segments of the preadmission testing or take home to view with family members or friends. Patient teaching is continued and reinforced throughout the entire ambulatory surgical process and is completed with the follow-up postoperative phone call by the ambulatory surgery center nurse a few days after surgery.

Discharge

Another difference in the care of the ambulatory surgical patient is the fact that within a few hours of surgery the patient is discharged. Immediately after surgery the patient is monitored carefully in the first-stage PACU, but as soon as the patient is stable and reactive from anesthesia, the patient is transferred to the second-stage PACU. In stage II the patient may be offered fluids and light nourishment.

PREOP INSTRUCTIONS

NAME:_____ DATE OF SURGERY:_____

In order to make your surgical experience a pleasant one,
please follow these basic guidelines.

The following things must be done before reporting for your surgery:

1. **DO NOT EAT ANY SOLID FOOD** or **DRINK** anything—including water—after 12 midnight proir to surgery.

2. You may brush your teeth and gargle on the morning of surgery, but DO NOT SWALLOW ANY WATER.

3. You MUST make arrangements for a responsible adult to take you home after your surgery. You will not be allowed to leave alone or drive yourself home. It is strongly suggested someone stay with you the first 24 hours.

4. A parent must accompany a child scheduled for surgery and plan to stay at the hospital until the child is discharged. Please do not bring other children with you.

5. Please wear simple, loose-fitting clothing to the hospital. Do not bring any valuables (money, credit cards, checkbooks, etc.) or wear any jewelry on day of surgery.

6. If you have dentures, they will be removed before going to the operating room. They will be kept in a container at your bedside.

7. If you wear contact lenses or glasses, please bring a case for them.

8. Please do not wear any make-up or nail polish on your fingernails or toenails.

9. Take the following pills with a SMALL SIP of water as soon as you wake up in the morning of surgery before you come to the hospital:

   _____

   _____

10. If you develop a cold, flu, or fever, please notify your physician and/or surgeon immediately.

11. All patients going to the operating room must wear a special cap on their head, so it is advisable to postpone any hairdressing appointments until after surgery.

   • Please call preadmission testing at 284-8446 or the Admissions Office at 284-8690 if you have any questions.

   • The day before surgery someone from DCMH will call you to review instructions. If you will not be at home, it is IMPORTANT that you call the Surgicenter at 222-0000 between 12:30pm–2:30pm or 4:00pm–5:00pm, for AM ADMIT call 555-1111 between 2:00pm–4:00pm.

   We look forward to seeing you on your day of surgery. Thank you for your cooperation and for using our facilities here at DCMH.

   I acknowledge receipt of the instructions indicated above.

   Date:_____ Signature:_____

Fig. 19-3. Preoperative instructions. (Courtesy Delaware County Memorial Hospital, Surgicenter, Drexel Hill, PA.)

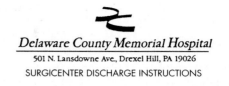

Delaware County Memorial Hospital

501 N. Lansdowne Ave., Drexel Hill, PA 19026

SURGICENTER DISCHARGE INSTRUCTIONS

_____ The anesthesia that you have received today may be acting in your body for the next several days; you may feel dizzy, sleepy, or lightheaded. Rest quietly for 12 to 24 hrs. and be careful of your activities.

_____ You have received local anesthesia only, the sensation in the area where you have had your surgery will return in a few hours.

ACTIVITIES

_____ You may resume normal activities.
_____ Do not drive a motor vehicle or operate hazardous machinery for 24 hours.
_____ Do not sign legal documents, or make important personal or business decisions for 24 hours.
_____ Limit your activities per physician's orders.

MEDICATIONS

_____ None _____ Prescriptions sent home with patient _____
_____ Take _____ for milder discomfort.
_____ Special medication instructions _____
_____

DIET

_____ Begin with clear liquids and then light foods (soups, jello, etc.).
_____ Progress to your normal diet if not nauseated.
_____ No alcoholic beverages for 24 hours.
_____ Special diet instructions _____

WOUND CARE

_____ Keep dressing dry.
_____ Do not remove the dressing until you see the doctor.
_____ Remove dressing _____ .
_____ You may shower _____ ; pat the wound dry and keep it clean and dry.
_____ Some bleeding is to be expected.
_____ You have sutures _____ that will dissolve.
               _____ that will be removed in the office.
_____ The white strips across the wound will fall off in a few days.

Call the surgeon if you have questions or problems such as:

_____ Pain not relieved by medication
_____ Excessive bleeding, swelling or redness around incision.
_____ Chills or fever over 100.4
_____ Affected extremity becomes cold, blue, tingly, or numb.
_____ Inability to urinate before you leave the Surgicenter and still unable to urinate in 4 hours.
_____ Repeated episodes of vomiting. Cannot keep clear liquids down 4 hours after discharge.

SPECIAL INSTRUCTIONS: _____
_____
_____

If you cannot reach your surgeon, go to the nearest emergency department.

FOLLOW-UP CARE:

You should see Dr. _____ in the office in _____ days, weeks.
Call soon for an appointment.

I understand these instructions given to me. ☐ If not: _____

_____   _____
Patient or Representative   Date

_____   _____
Physician Signature   Witness

Fig. 19-4. Surgicenter discharge instructions. (Courtesy Delaware County Memorial Hospital, Surgicenter, Drexel Hill, PA.)

PACU 2
OBSERVATION RECORDS

ARRIVAL TIME _____

IV: ☐yes ☐no   DRESSING: ☐yes ☐no   DRAINS: ☐yes ☐no   PAIN: ☐None   PREOP BP
                                                                  ☐Mild   _____
Site _____   Site _____   Type _____Amt _____   ☐Moderate
                                                                  ☐Severe

Edema: ☐Yes ☐No   DRAINAGE: ☐Yes ☐No   WOUND APPEARANCE: Up to Chair ☐Yes ☐No
Redness: ☐Yes ☐No   ☐Scant ☐Mod ☐Large   ☐D & I   ☐Other   With Family/Others ☐Yes ☐No
D/C Time _____   COLOR: ☐Serous   ☐Red   ☐N/A   Physician Visit ☐Yes ☐No
Signature _____   ☐Serosang   ☐Edematous
                             ☐Bright red

NURSES NOTES: _____

B.P. ∨ ∧ P U L S E R E S P	220 200 180 160 140 120 100 80 60 40 20 0		MEDICATIONS	TIME	RTE	SIGN

PADS: **TIME:**

V.S.
2 W/in ± 20% of Preop
1 20-40% of Preop
0 40% of Preop

AMBULATION
2 Steady Gait
1 With Assistance
0 Unable

NAUSEA/VOMITING
2 Minimal/No Nausea
1 Moderate
0 Vomiting

PAIN
2 Min/None
1 Moderate
0 Severe

SURG. BLEEDING
2 None/Expected
1 Minimal
0 Moderate to Severe

TOTAL:

INTAKE AND OUTPUT
Tolerated fluids ☐Yes ☐No ☐Refused
MENTAL STATUS
Approaches Preop   ☐Yes   ☐No
Voided   ☐Yes   ☐No
INTAKE & OUTPUT SUMMARY
         INTAKE   OUTPUT
ORAL _____   EMESIS _____
IV _____   OTHER _____
OTHER _____   URINE _____
TOTAL _____   TOTAL _____

DRESSING: DRAINS:
☐Yes ☐No   ☐N/A
DRAINAGE
☐Yes ☐No   TYPE   AMT
☐Scant ☐Mod
☐Large
COLOR   WOUND
☐Serous   ☐D & I
☐Serosang   ☐Red
☐Bright red   ☐Edematous

ANESTHESIOLOGIST ORDERS: _____

D/C INSTRUCTIONS
Reviewed with Pt.   ☐Yes   ☐No
VERBALIZES AND DEMONSTRATES
Understanding   ☐Yes   ☐No
Copy given to patient   ☐Yes   ☐No

Prescriptions given   ☐Yes   ☐No

MODE OF DISCHARGE ☐W/C ☐Walk
                      ☐Arms
☐Via Pt. Car   ☐Other: _____
Escorted By: _____
D/C to ☐Home   ☐Other _____

RELEASED BY _____   TIME _____

POSTOPERATIVE TELEPHONE FOLLOW-UP:
☐Yes   ☐No   ☐No Answer

Date _____ Time _____ Signature _____

COMMENTS: _____

Signature _____

Key: BP = blood pressure; D/C = discharge; D & I = dry and intact; V.S. = vital signs; W/C = wheelchair

Fig. 19-5. PACU 2 observation record. (Courtesy Delaware County Memorial Hospital, Surgicenter, Drexel Hill, PA.)

As soon as the patient reaches this area, a family member or friend is encouraged to be with him or her. If the patient is not experiencing nausea and/or vomiting, the IV will be removed. Postoperative instructions will be reviewed with the patient and family/friend; a written copy of the instructions is given to the patient. Fig. 19-4 includes sample instructions that should be given to the patient before discharge. Specific discharge instructions regarding medications for pain or antibiotics, activities, and wound care will vary according to the surgeon's preference and type of surgery performed.

In an exploratory study of patients having ambulatory surgery, Girard (1994) reported that recognition recall, free recall, and psychomotor performance were all reduced in the study population 2 hours after surgery, regardless of the length of time of anesthesia or number and kind of anesthetics used (these included general, IV narcotics, and IV barbiturates). Because many ambulatory surgery patients are discharged from 1 to 2 hours after surgery, the importance of written instructions that are reviewed with a responsible adult (family member, friend, significant other) as well as the patient cannot be underestimated in ambulatory surgery patients who receive general anesthesia.

In a small study that used a Delphi technique to reach consensus, nurses ranked in order the factors they considered most important in evaluating ambulatory surgery patients' discharge to home. Ranked first was adequacy of respiratory function, followed by stability of vital signs, level of orientation, swelling or drainage at the operative site, degree of pain, temperature, degree of vomiting, level of alertness, level of rehydration, skin color, ability to ambulate, clarity of vision, ability to void, and degree of nausea (Kitz, et al., 1988). These clinical criteria may be useful for establishing tools to quantitatively determine a patient's readiness for discharge. Fig. 19-5 illustrates a nursing record for Stage II PACU. In the center of the form, the postanesthesia discharge score (PADS) serves as criteria for determining if the patient is ready to be sent home. Each ambulatory surgery center must establish specific criteria for discharging patients and must determine which situations require the patient to be admitted to the hospital. Free-standing surgical centers generally have established which hospital patients would be transferred to in an emergency.

Postdischarge information is routinely collected from ambulatory surgery patients to determine both compliance and complications as well as satisfaction with care. Telephone follow-up, using a structured interview form, is one method of identifying opportunities for process improvement (Burney, 1994). Alternatively, mailed discharge surveys may be designed to capture similar important information (Williams & Brett, 1989). Although each survey method has benefits to recommend it, the underpinning effort is on developing a mechanism to identify problems early in recovery, to evaluate continuity of discharge planning and teaching, and to gather data for performance improvement (Petersen, 1992).

SUMMARY

Ambulatory surgery is a means of providing surgical intervention in a convenient, safe, and cost-effective setting. Ambulatory surgery has grown steadily in its availability and use over the past two decades. A major ambulatory surgery program can be a success for both the health care facility and the patient. Significant to this success is the provision of perioperative nursing care. Safe and effective patient outcomes require careful planning by the perioperative nurse. Perioperative nurses have always composed patient care plans; because of the brief, episodic, and intensive nature of the nurse-patient interaction in perioperative patient care units, these care plans were often articulated in the nurse's head and remained there. Accountability and renewed efforts to measure patient outcomes and quality of care dictate that care needs to be documented. The generic care plans in Chapter 7, the procedure-specific care plans, and the care plans for pediatric (Chapter 21) and aging (Chapter 22) patients should serve as useful guidelines for the development of care plans in ambulatory surgery units. Development of care plans to reflect individual institutional resources and policies should help provide the concentrated care required to meet patient needs for health, safety, comfort, and convenience.

References

American Society of Anesthesiologists. (1990). *Standards for postanesthesia care.* Park Ridge, IL: The Society.

American Society of Post Anesthesia Nurses. (1992). *Standards of nursing practice.* Richmond, VA: The Society.

Association of Operating Room Nurses. (1996). *Standards and recommended practices for perioperative nursing.* Denver: The Association.

Burden N. (1993). *Ambulatory surgical nursing.* Philadelphia: WB Saunders.

Burden N. (1994). Local anesthesia—and how it works. *Nursing Spectrum, 3*(1), 14-15.

Burney R. (1994). TQM in a surgery center. *Quality Progress, 27*(1), 97-100.

Dlugose D. (1994, June 22). *What's new in anesthesia for ambulatory surgery?* Paper presented at the Ambulatory Surgery Conference, Las Vegas, NV.

Girard N. (1994). Anesthesia and learning: The mind-body connection. *Seminars in Perioperative Nursing 3*(3), 121-132.

Greco RJ, et al. (1995). Potential dangers of oxygen supplementation during facial surgery. *Plastic and Reconstructive Surgery, 95*(6), 978-984.

Henderson J. (1993). Implications of outpatient surgery growth. *OR Manager, 9*(9), 24-26.

Icenhour ML. (1988). Quality interpersonal care: A study of ambulatory surgery patients' perspectives. *AORN Journal, 47*(6), 1414-1419.

Joint Commission Accreditation Manual for Healthcare Organizations. (1994). *Scoring guidelines* (Vol II). Oakbrook Terrace, IL: JCAHO.

Kitz DS, et al. (1988). Discharging outpatients: Factors nurses consider to determine readiness. *AORN Journal, 48*, 87-91.

Lea SG & Phippen ML. (1992). Client education in the ambulatory surgery setting. *Seminars in Perioperative Nursing 1*(4), 203-233.

Lehr PS. (1988). Ambulatory surgery conference highlights gains, problems facing industry. *AORN Journal, 48*, 194-199.

McBreen M. (1993). Best practices: Meeting the changing demands of ambulatory surgery. In Ambulatory Surgery, Symposium conducted in Washington, D.C.

Meeker M & Rothrock J. (1995). *Alexander's care of the patient in surgery*. St. Louis: Mosby.

Nicoll J. (1909). The surgery of infancy. *British Medical Journal, 2*, 753.

Petersen CA. (1992). Postoperative follow-up: Tracing compliance and complications. *Seminars in Perioperative Nursing, 1*(4), 255-260.

Phillips M & Hokans C. (1994). A review of ambulatory care analysis. *Nurs Econ, 12*(2), 88-92.

Sebastian LB. (1994). Adding relaxation techniques to your bag of tricks. *Nursing Spectrum, 3*(4), 17-18.

Summers S & Ebbert D. (1992). *Ambulatory surgical nursing: A nursing diagnosis approach*. Philadelphia: JB Lippincott.

Waters R. (1919). The downtown anesthesia clinic. *American Journal of Anesthesia, 33* (7), 71.

Watson DS. (1992). Developing a competency-based education program for nurse-monitored sedation. *Seminars in Perioperative Nursing, 1*(4), 224-231.

Weeks CS. (1890). *Textbook of nursing*. New York: D Appleton.

Williams M & Brett SP. (1989). Discharge surveys: A quality assurance method for ambulatory surgery. *AORN Journal, 49*(5), 1371-1380.

Chapter 20

Trauma Surgery

Jane C. Rothrock

In case of any accident, send a message to the doctor, describing as well as you can the nature and urgency of the case, so that he may come prepared with the necessary appliances; try to get rid of everybody who cannot be made useful, so as to secure plenty of fresh air and room to work. If respiration is suspended, or the danger imminent, treatment must be begun at once, on the spot, without loss of time, otherwise the patient may be carried to the nearest convenient house. . . . Have a warm bed to put him in. Remove the clothes with as little disturbance as may be, and do not cut anything that can be ripped . . . Take the clothes from the sound side first, . . . Special directions for undressing a woman are hardly needed; in case of a man, a point to be well remembered is to unfasten the suspenders behind as well as in front. All the clothing can then be easily removed under cover of a sheet.

WEEKS, 1890

$\mathcal{T}$he trauma operating room (OR) is an integral component in the delivery of emergency medical care. Life-threatening injuries are evaluated, explored, stabilized, and surgically repaired in a timely manner. This is not unlike treatment of the injured in the Mobile Army Surgical Hospital (MASH) units during the Korean War. The key to successful intervention in dealing with the multiply injured trauma patient is rapid mobilization for surgery, including concurrent multiple surgeries. This distinguishes the trauma OR from those in conventional facilities.

Trauma is the most common cause of death in the United States of persons 40 years of age or younger. It is the leading cause of death among people between 18 and 35 years of age. Of these, 75% are male. These fatalities result from five primary mechanisms of injury: motor vehicle accidents, falls, drownings, burns, and ingestions. Geriatric trauma continues to rise as the elderly are a rapidly increasing segment of the population. In addition, deaths from deliberate assaults and suicides must be considered. The resultant disabling injuries, aside from the loss of life, translate into an enormous economic burden on the U.S. health care system. The cost of accidental injuries, including accidents in which deaths or disabling injuries occur together with motor vehicle accidents and fires, is in the billions of dollars.

In many regions of the country, there are no formal systems of trauma care; because of the large economic burden on institutions, some previously existing trauma systems closed and efforts to develop new ones were unsuccessful (Eiseman, 1994). To revitalize the development of trauma systems and stem the closing of existing ones, Congress passed the Trauma Care Systems Planning and Development Act in 1990. First funded in 1992, the Act requires the development of a model trauma care system plan for states; offers grants to develop, implement, and monitor state trauma plans; and targets rural grants to improve emergency medical systems and trauma services. In 1993 the Division of Injury Control at the Centers for Disease Control and Prevention was advanced to center status and renamed the Center for Injury Prevention and Control (Lewis, 1994). The National Institutes of Health (NIH) has begun to develop more attention to trauma research. Although funding for programs like these has been a struggle during budgetary belt-tightening at the federal level, socioeconomic concerns in trauma care continue to focus on cost, reimbursement, access to care, and the application of registries and outcome analysis to define and improve quality of care.

In the last two decades, health care practitioners throughout the country have made a concerted effort to increase public awareness of this problem. Medical caregivers look to their own professions to encourage improvement in the health care delivery system in response to trauma. The members of the trauma OR team must remain well versed in mechanism of injury, critical care protocols, and treatment modalities. Such clinical competence affords the multiply injured trauma patient the highest quality of care while maintaining professional standards in perioperative practice.

ASSESSMENT CONSIDERATIONS

Preoperative nursing care of the trauma patient begins during the admission process. The perioperative nurse performs a rapid initial assessment in conjunction with the triage team's physical examination. Pertinent initial observations are made and data are documented for continuity of nursing care. The perioperative nurse is available for a potential emergency procedure if the need arises in the triage area.

The perioperative nurse performs a rapid systems assessment to establish the patient's potential for surgical priority using the following parameters:

A—Airway
B—Breathing
C—Circulation, cortex, and cord
Mechanism of injury

The patient's airway is assessed for patency. If the airway is not patent, rescue breathing will be initiated immediately to oxygenate the patient; mechanical control of the airway will require assistance with intubation. If the airway is patent, the assessment is conducted to verify that breathing and oxygen exchange are adequate. Circulation is assessed by verifying the presence of blood pressure and heart rate. The circulation of the brain's cortex is ascertained by the patient's level of awareness. Finally, circulation of the spinal cord is assessed by the patient's ability to recognize central and peripheral sensation and to move the extremities on command.

A high level of suspicion for overt injuries is necessary when the patient's mechanism of injury is determined.

Systems assessment is performed during the admission process (Fig. 20-1). The perioperative nurse does this assessment in a cephalocaudal order, beginning with the neurologic system.

Neurologic Assessment

The patient's level of consciousness is assessed by verifying the orientation parameters of person, place, and time. A confirmation of loss of consciousness at the scene of the accident is investigated. Pupil size, reactivity, and equality to light are noted. Unilateral dilatation of a patient's pupil may indicate intracranial pressure caused by a subdural or epidural lesion. Head injury occurs at a rate of 200 to 300 cases per 100,000 in the United States. The peak incidence of head trauma occurs in patients in their late teens. Males are more than twice as likely as females to sustain such injury. The most common cause of head injury is motor vehicle accidents. Trauma victims with a decreased level of consciousness or reported loss of consciousness are assessed by the neurosurgeon to ascertain potential intracranial injury. Subdural hematoma is suspected whenever the patient exhibits the following symptoms: ipsilateral pupillary enlargement, posturing, or deviation of eyes toward the affected hemisphere. Computed tomography (CT) or magnetic resonance imaging (MRI) is ordered to confirm this suspicion. A positive finding of subdural hematoma necessitates immediate surgical intervention for its evacuation.

Pupil dilatation should be assessed as one factor among other parameters, including widening of pulse pressure, bradycardia, tachypnea, abnormal posturing, and flexion or extension movements. Localized third cranial nerve damage caused by a facial fracture can also dilatate the pupils. This can be misinterpreted to indicate nonexistent intracranial lesion.

The perioperative nurse assesses the patient for symmetry of sensation, movement, and strength; asymmetry may indicate a brain or spinal cord lesion. Clinical descriptions of spinal cord lesions usually refer to deficits in the upper motor neuron (UMN) or lower motor neuron (LMN). UMN injuries involve the corticobulbar and corticospinal tracts, resulting in muscle spasticity and increased tendon reflexes. LMN injuries involve anterior horn cells or nerve fibers after their exit from the spinal cord, resulting in muscle flaccidity, loss of reflexes and tone, and muscle atrophy (Fig. 20-2). The exterior of the patient's head, scalp, and neck are examined for lacerations, abrasions, ecchymosis, and

DATE	MILITARY TIME	MICU	AMBULANCE	AIR	REFERRING M.D.

TRANSFERRING FACILITY	TYPENEX NUMBER	TRAUMA ALERT

TRAUMA C

TRAUMA ALERT ☐ YES ☐ NO MILITARY TIME:

FAMILY NOTIFIED ☐ YES ☐ NO PHONE #: _____ TIME:

BLOOD PRESSURE | **PULSE**

CARDIOVASCULAR
INVASIVE LINES (IV, A-LINE, CVP)

TYPE	GAUGE

PHARMACOLOGIC

TIME

200 190 180 170 160 150 140 130 120 110 100 90 80 70 60 50 40

200 190 180 170 160 150 140 130 120 110 100 90 80 70 60 50 40 30 25 20 15 10 5 0

HI-FLOW TUBING/RAPID INFUSER YES ☐ NO ☐
PERIPHERAL PULSES:
EKG TIME: RHYTHM:
MAST: FIELD TAA TIME
INFLATED ☐ YES ☐ NO ☐ LEGS ONLY
ARREST ☐ YES ☐ NO CPR ☐ YES ☐ NO
OPEN THORACOTOMY TIME:

GASTROINTESTINAL
SALEM SUMP: SIZE TIME:
DRAINAGE: COLOR AMT.
ABDOMEN: SOFT ☐ FIRM ☐
TENDER ☐ NON-TENDER ☐ UTO ☐
PERITONEAL LAVAGE: ☐ YES ☐ NO TIME:
AMT. INFUSED: AMT. DRAINED:
RECTAL EXAM: DR:
HEMETEST RESULTS: ☐ POS. ☐ NEG.

ALLERGIES:
CURRENT MEDS:

DRUGS	AMOUNT	ROUTE	TIME	INIT'S
1.				
2.				
3.				
4.				
5.				
6.				
7.				
8.				
9.				
10.				

TEMP:
TIME:

GCS/TS
Pulse OX
RESP

TETANUS TOX. 0.5 ml SQ LOT #
HYPER TET. 250 u IM LOT #
COMMENTS:

LIVING WILL: YES ☐ NO ☐ UTO ☐ N/A ☐

X-RAYS	DONE	TIME	LAB	DONE	TIME	GENITOURINARY
C-SPINE			Ua			FOLEY: SIZE: TIME
SKULL			T&S			CYSTO YES NO TIME
CHEST			T&X __ UNITS			HEMASTIX RESULTS TIME
PELVIS			ADULT PKT			**INTAKE** / **OUTPUT**
L SPINE			PEDI. PKT			CRYSTALLOID / URINE
T SPINE			CK/MB			BLOOD / N/G
OTHER:			DIC PROF.			COLLOID / CHEST TUBE
			PREGNANCY			MEDS / R:
			OTHER:			CT CONTRAST / L:
						OTHER / OTHER
			Drawn by:			
			Site:			TOTALS / TOTALS

NEUROLOGICAL
EXTREMITIES: PUPILS/REACT:
MAE YES ☐ NO ☐ O.D. O.S.
ADM. W/CERVICAL IMMOB. ☐ YES ☐ NO
CERVICAL PRECAUTION:

CATSCAN	TIME
HEAD	
SPINE	
ABD	
PELVIS	

RESPIRATORY
ADM. STATUS:
AMBU BAG N ETT O ETT MASK N/C
OXYGEN L/MIN
BREATH SOUNDS: PRESENT R L
CLEAR R L
DIMINISHED R L
ADVENTITIOUS SOUNDS:
TAA AIRWAY MASK N/C N ETT O ETT
ANESTHESIA INTUBATION: PULSE OX: CO$_2$:
VENTILATOR SETTING
CHEST TUBES: R# L#
AUTO TRANSFUSION: YES ☐ NO ☐
O$_2$/FIO$_2$ CHANGES: TIME:
TRACH/CRIC: ☐ YES ☐ NO TIME:

HISTORY

1. CONT. 2. BURN
3. FX DISLOC 4. ABR
5. LAC. 6. AVUL.
7. PUNCT. 8. GSW
9. CRUSH 10. AMP
11. HEMATOMA

FINAL DISPOSITION
TO: TIME: EXPIRED ☐ YES ☐ NO
TIME PRONOUNCED:

CONSULTANTS

KEY
CERVICAL IMMOBILIZATION
P.C = PHILADELPHIA COLLAR
SN = STIFF NECK
NL = NECK LOCK
L.B. = LONE BOARD
↑ = BP TAKEN IN ERECT POSITION
HID = HEAD IMMOB. DEVICE

RN SIGNATURE	INT.'S	TRAUMA SURGEON SIGNATURE	INT.'S
PRIMARY RN			
SECONDARY RN			

PLACE PATIENT
I.D. LABEL AND TYPENEX #
HERE

**COOPER HOSPITAL/
UNIVERSITY MEDICAL CENTER**

**SOUTHERN NEW JERSEY
REGIONAL TRAUMA CENTER**

TRAUMA ADMITTING RECORD

C642003 (Rev. 10/92)

Fig. 20-1. Trauma admitting record. (Courtesy Cooper Hospital/University Medical Center, Camden, NJ.)

NARRATIVE

TRAUMA SCORE FOR SOUTH JERSEY

		Value	Points
A.	Systolic Blood Pressure	>89	4
		76-89	3
		50-75	2
		1-49	1
		0	0
B.	Respiratory Rate	10-29	4
		>29	3
		6-9	2
		1-5	1
		0	0

C. Glasgow coma Scale

1. **Eye Opening**

Spontaneous	____ 4
To Voice	____ 3
To Pain	____ 2
None	____ 1

2. **Verbal response**

Oriented	____ 5
Confused	____ 4
Inappropriate words	____ 3
Incomprehensible words	____ 2
None	____ 1

3. **Motor response**

		Total GSC Points	Score
Obeys commands	____ 6		
Purposeful movement (pain)	____ 5	13-15 =	4
Withdraw (pain)	____ 4	9-12 =	3
Flexion (pain)	____ 3	6-8 =	2
Extension (pain)	____ 2	4-5 =	1
None	____ 1	3 =	0

TOTAL GCS POINTS
(1 + 2 + 3) _____

TRAUMA SCORE
(TOTAL POINTS = A + B + C) _____

VALUABLES

☐ TO SAFE   ☐ TO FAMILY   ☐ TO BEDSIDE

Fig. 20-1, cont'd. Trauma admitting record. (Courtesy Cooper Hospital/University Medical Center, Camden, NJ.)

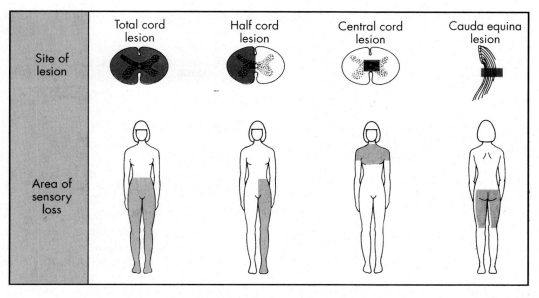

Fig. 20-2. Common patterns of sensory abnormality with cord lesions. *Upper diagrams,* site of lesion; *lower diagrams,* distribution of corresponding sensory loss. (From Thelan, LA, et al. [1994]. *Critical care nursing: Diagnosis and management* (2nd ed.). St. Louis: Mosby.)

crepitus. Ecchymosis below the eyes (raccoon's eyes) or behind the ear (Battle sign) may indicate a basal skull fracture (Fig. 20-3). Crepitus in the posterior cervical region along with abnormal movement and pain may indicate cervical spine injury. Any suspicion of spine injury is treated as such until proved otherwise. The cervical spine is immobilized with a rigid cervical collar. If intubation is required, the jaw-thrust method is used. Ear or nasal drainage is tested to rule out a cerebral spinal fluid (CSF) leak. This may be accomplished by testing for the appearance of a halo ring (a yellowing ring that appears around bloody drainage or a nasal or ear drip pad) or the presence of dextrose. The patient may complain of postnasal drip, which may also indicate a CSF leak.

Motor vehicle accidents account for 55% of spinal cord injuries. Approximately 11,000 persons sustain spinal cord injury each year; average lifetime care costs are estimated to be between $200,000 and $400,000. Spinal cord injury most frequently occurs in younger men, 80% under 40 years of age and 50% between 15 and 25. Anterior cervical plating is a method of stabilizing the cervical spine after traumatic, unstable cervical spine injury. The damaged cervical spine is fixed anteriorly through the insertion of an iliac crest cortical bone graft into the involved vertebral spaces; the graft is then secured with a metal plate and screws. Introduced in Germany in the 1950s, the anterior approach to the cervical spine allows greater visualization of the spinal cord and nerve roots, as well as preservation of the posterior spine stabilizing elements. This operation affords the patient greater flexion and extension of the neck than posterior cervical wiring and fusion historically did.

Respiratory Assessment

The patient's airway is reassessed periodically or more frequently if there is concern about patency. Adequate breathing is measured by observation of the chest for equal expansion and auscultation of both lung fields for clear breath sounds. The chest wall is visually examined for any evidence of trauma such as abrasions, contusions, tenderness, and ecchymosis. Manual inspection is performed for crepitus, flailing, or pain. Penetrating trauma wounds are closely examined to determine entrance and exit as well as the presence of impaled objects.

Chest trauma can arise from a variety of sources and accounts for 25% of all trauma deaths (Johnston & Johnston, 1994). Mechanisms of injury include motor vehicle accidents, gunshot wounds, rapid vertical deceleration from falls, crush injuries, and stab wounds. The trauma may be blunt (most often associated with motor vehicle accidents and crush injury) or penetrating (most often associated with gunshot or stab wounds). The perioperative nurse should assess the chest trauma patient for rib fractures, flail chest, hemothorax, and pneumothorax (Box 20-1). Other potential injuries include pulmonary or myocardial contusions, cardiac tamponade, and aortic tear. Ruptured thoracic descending aorta is seen as a result of a rapid deceleration motor vehicle accident or fall. The incidence of aortic rupture in persons thrown from a vehicle is more than

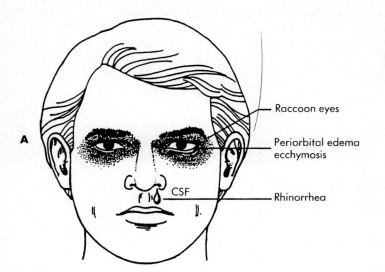

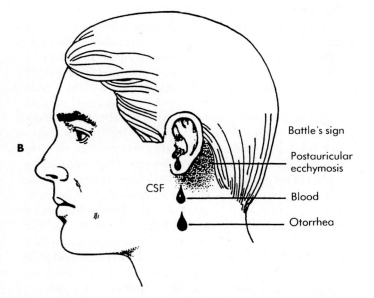

Fig. 20-3. **A,** Raccoon eyes, rhinorrhea, seen in anterior fossa fractures. **B,** Battle's sign with otorrhea, seen in middle fossa fractures. (From Barker E. [1994]. *Neuroscience nursing.* St. Louis: Mosby.)

twice that of persons who are not ejected. Aortic injury is caused by chest compression; the injury may occur at any location. Grade III descending aortic dissection occurs distal to the left subclavian artery.

Initial rapid assessment follows the same protocol as for all trauma patients (airway, breathing, circulation); definitive signs and symptoms often reveal tachypnea, tachycardia, chest pain, cyanosis and/or pallor, hemoptysis, and diaphoresis. The secondary assessment is more detailed, including full documentation of vital signs, a thorough history of the injury event, and subsequent head-to-toe examination.

Arterial blood gases are measured to determine adequate oxygenation. A chest x-ray film is done to rule out pneumothorax, hemopneumothorax, or pulmonary contusion. This x-ray film will also help determine treatment and length of the surgical procedure. The upright chest x-ray film is examined for the presence of the aortic knob or an acceptable width of the mediastinum to rule out a ruptured aorta. The chest x-ray film is then examined for rib, clavicle, or sternal fractures, which represent a high index of suspicion for underlying disease in the chest.

The patient's ability to sustain the airway is assessed to determine the capability of transport to the OR. Does the patient need a ventilator, or can spontaneous ventilation be maintained until general anesthesia is induced? Does the patient have a chest tube in place that will require special consideration in the OR?

Cardiovascular Assessment

After evaluation and restoration of the airway and breathing, massive external hemorrhage must be controlled if it is present. This is usually accomplished by applying direct manual pressure to the injured area. The patient's vital signs are assessed for trends to determine abnormalities. Hypotension and tachycardia are common significant findings in the trauma patient. A patient experiencing a hypotensive state may require fluid resuscitation, inotropic drugs, and vasopressor therapy to compensate for perfusion and ischemic conditions. Blood pressure measurement is very important for these patients, and continuous intraarterial blood pressure monitoring is the preferred method. Once the patient is stable, indirect methods of blood pressure assessment are appropriate; the focus is on individual blood pressure trends, not on absolute numbers or standardized blood pressure readings, to guide clinical judgment with stabilized trauma patients (Norman, Gadelta, & Griffin, 1991).

Bilateral peripheral pulses are checked for regularity, rhythm, quality, and strength. The patient's skin color is assessed for abrasions, lacerations, contusions, and eccyhmosis. Edema may indicate poor perfusion.

The perioperative nurse should document the type and location of the invasive lines inserted dur-

---

Box 20-1 Assessment/Finding of Tension Pneumothorax and Hemothorax

Tension Pneumothorax
Observations/findings

Respiratory distress: sudden, severe
Use of accessory muscles of respiration
Tachycardia
Cyanosis
Tachypnea
Hypotension
Chest pain
Restlessness and agitation
Paradoxic chest movement
Tracheal and mediastinal shift: toward unaffected side
Breath sounds
  Absent (affected side)
  Diminished (unaffected side)
Distant heart sounds
Subcutaneous emphysema

Laboratory/diagnostic studies

Chest x-ray examination: complete lung collapse, mediastinal or tracheal shift to unaffected side

Hemothorax
Observations/findings

Difficulty in breathing
Hyperresonance on percussion
Distant to absent breath sounds on affected side
Asymmetric chest movements
Hypovolemic shock if blood loss is severe
  Tachypnea
  Tachycardia
  Hypotension
  Anxiety
  Restlessness
  Pallor
  Pain

Laboratory/diagnostic studies

Chest x-ray examination
  Blunting of costophrenic angles
  Hazy appearance over lower chest
Hematocrit/hemoglobin

Adapted from Tucker SM, et al. (1996). *Patient care standards: Collaborative practice planning* (6th ed.). St. Louis: Mosby.

---

ing resuscitation. Typically these patients have large-bore intravenous lines, an arterial catheter, and a central venous pressure (CVP) and/or pulmonary artery line. Volume infusion of colloid or crystalloid is started, depending on the patient's vital signs. Research on shock continues to focus, in part, on the refinement of hypertonic saline and dextran (HSD) resuscitation in trauma patients; 7.5% NaCl and 12% dextran 70 solution has been studied for its superior cardiac output response. However, caution must be used when administering HSD to patients with a head injury, because the beneficial effects are not sustained and cerebral blood flow decreases 24 hours after surgery (Herndon, 1991). After initial infusion, subsequent treatment of volume depletion is often guided by CVP measurements; Stothert and Herndon (1995) suggest that CVP should be maintained between 5 and 10 mm Hg. The adequacy or inadequacy of invasive lines should be discussed with anesthesia personnel. If additional intravenous lines are needed for surgery, provisions should be made before the patient enters the OR suite. If the members of the team determine that blood transfusion is needed, preparations will be made at this time.

Gastrointestinal Assessment

The patient's abdomen is auscultated for the presence of bowel sounds. Palpation is performed for tenderness, guarding, firmness, and distention to determine potential pathologic conditions in one of the four quadrants of the abdomen. Pain referred to the left shoulder may indicate a ruptured diaphragm. Visual inspection is performed to locate any evidence of abrasions, ecchymosis, and penetrating wounds as indicators of organ involvement. Determination of penetrating wounds in the abdominal or thoracic cavity is done by using the nipple line as a division. Wounds at or above the nipple line are considered to be located in the thoracic cavity, and wounds below the nipple line in the abdominal cavity. Diagnostic peritoneal lavage results are used to confirm internal hemorrhage. Laparoscopy for evaluating abdominal trauma is often used, with excellent results. Exploratory laparotomy is indicated when the patient has any or all of the following symptoms: moderate to severe abdominal tenderness on palpation, rapidly falling hemoglobin and hematocrit levels, hypovolemia, positive diagnostic peritoneal lavage, and/or positive abdominal CT or MRI results. In blunt abdominal trauma, 90% of injuries are in the upper abdomen. The spleen is the most commonly involved organ.

All trauma patients should be considered to have a full stomach on admission (Hartsock & King, 1994). During induction of anesthesia the circulating nurse stands at the head of the OR bed to apply cricoid pressure for intubation. This lessens the possibility of regurgitation. Steady, firm pressure is exerted over the anterior throat at the cricoid ring until the endotracheal tube is passed. Placement is confirmed through auscultation of breath sounds in both lung fields. If there is a question of cervical spine integrity, in-line traction on the neck is maintained.

Genitourinary Assessment

The amount of urinary output, color, and method of urinary drainage is assessed. The urine should be tested by the perioperative nurse to determine the presence of glucose, protein, and blood. If hematuria is present, an intravenous pyelogram and voiding cystogram will be ordered to document renal and bladder function before surgery. An hourglass bladder formation on x-ray film indicates a contusion or retroperitoneal hematoma. If blood at the tip of the urinary meatus is seen, insertion of a urinary catheter is deferred until a urologist is available for consultation. This may indicate a ruptured urethra.

The anal reflex is tested for strength by digital examination. Decreased rectal tone may indicate a potential spinal cord lesion. Incomplete spinal cord injury necessitates immediate spinal decompression with the use of spinal column fixation instruments.

Integumentary Assessment

The patient's skin is noted for any alteration in skin integrity such as abrasion, laceration, ecchymosis, or burn. The extent, location, size, and description of the impairment should be documented preoperatively. Positioning on the OR bed is performed with utmost care because of the risk for decubitus ulcers in the patient with hypotension and tissue hypoperfusion. Liberal padding and protection from metal are among the many priorities in dealing with the trauma patient. Iatrogenic decubitus ulcers are preventable through awareness and education of the perioperative nursing staff.

Musculoskeletal Assessment

The patient is assessed for the presence of fractures and dislocations of the upper and lower extremities. In 1994 alone, the National Safety Council reported 890,000 cases of arm/hand/finger injury in the U.S.; the cost of a single injury is approximately $25,000 whereas serious upper extremity injury may be in excess of $375,000 per patient (Childs, 1995). During secondary assessment, mechanism of injury (blunt, penetrating, explosive, degloving, crush, amputation) is determined. The extremities are examined for absent or decreased pulse, capillary refill, pallor, generalized edema, deformity, ecchymosis, joint laxity, crepitus, decreased motion, and paresthesia. The perioperative nurse should attempt to estimate blood loss in the injured extremity(ies) and note the type of bleeding (pumping or squirting, which may indicate arterial injury or a slower oozing or dripping, which generally indicates venous damage). Documentation of fractures and dislocations is imperative in positioning to prevent further injury. Any fracture that is not being operated on should be elevated and iced to decrease edema. Pulses and capillary refill are reassessed periodically. The extremities are checked for the presence of compartmental syndrome, which is manifested by palpable tension, tenderness, decreased pulse, and motor weakness. These signs and symptoms indicate an ischemic episode, which if not treated may lead to amputation of the extremity.

Musculoskeletal injuries of the trauma patient frequently occur as a result of motor vehicle accidents. Persons who have sustained a rapid deceleration injury to the lower extremity as a result of motor vehicle accident, fall, or gunshot wound often have open fractures of the tibia or fibula. These fractures are classified by degree of increasing severity. A grade I open fracture is associated with a puncture wound and otherwise minimal soft tissue disruption. A grade II open fracture presents with a slightly larger area (2 cm) of soft tissue disturbance, whereas a grade III open fracture includes a larger skin wound (greater than 10 cm) with pronounced soft tissue and muscle tissue disruption, contamination, and fragmentation of wound periphery and fracture pattern. The method of stabilization of the open extremity fracture depends on its location, grade, and type. The external fixator is used when there is a significant soft tissue wound, severe bone loss, comminution, or when fasciotomy has been performed to relieve compartment syndrome (Fig. 20-4).

Trauma to the face results from motor vehicle accidents, falls, recreational events, or assaults. Motor vehicle accidents are the most common cause of injuries. 54% of facial injuries result from motor vehicle accidents. Maxillofacial trauma includes any injury to the bony structure, tissue, vessels, or nerves of the face. Patients who sustain blunt or penetrating trauma to the face will have fractures to the facial bones categorized by degrees of increasing severity, from LeFort I to III. LeFort I fracture involves a horizontal line separating the maxillary alveolus from the upper face. LeFort II fracture involves the nasomaxillary segments of the zygomatic or orbital portions of the midface in a pyramidal fracture. LeFort III fracture separates the facial bones from the cranium. The term "panfacial" includes these three categories. Patients with panfacial fractures present a special challenge to the trauma team. They must be prepared to undergo hours of recon-

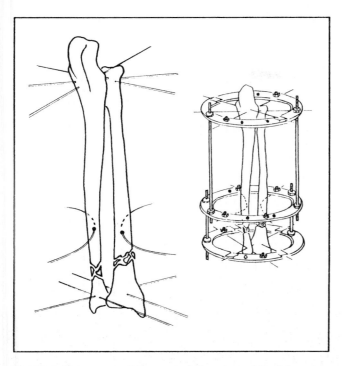

FIg. 20-4. Treatment of fracture of the ulna with dislocation of the head of the radius using Ilizarov external fixator. (From Ilizarov external fixator general surgical technique brochure, Richards Medical Co., Memphis, TN, 1990.)

structive surgery. Precautions must be taken to protect these patients from the complications of immobility and exposure caused by extensive operative repair; a procedure could continue for 12 to 24 hours at a time. Patients must receive the emotional support necessary to withstand the rigors of serial operations as well as the psychologic impact of potentially permanent disfigurement.

Psychosocial Assessment

As the perioperative nurse provides support and explanations, the patient's reactions to the trauma are noted. The patient may feel anxiety, denial, or anger. The anxious patient has a short attention span and may not be capable of understanding the injuries. Denial follows shortly after the injury. The patient has difficulty believing the situation and denies it until he or she can better cope with reality. The third stage is anger, in which the patient becomes furious about the situation and may react negatively to the support of the health care team, family, and friends. Social and psychologic counselors can assist the patient and family during transitional and stressful periods of acute and rehabilitative care.

Coping with loss, including the losses experienced during a life-threatening trauma, is multifaceted, involving physical, emotional, social, and spiritual dimensions. Coping can take many forms, and each form has advantages and disadvantages; the perioperative nurse cannot attribute "good" or "bad" qualities to a coping mechanism or expect it to manifest in stagelike progression. Instead, coping is highly individual, with each person and family coping in ways that are different from others. Coolican and her colleagues (1994) suggest that in life-threatening events, a wide circle of individuals is affected, including the family, however the patient may define that term. Anticipatory grief, which involves responding to and coping with impending loss (of the patient, the patient's function in the family or society, or other associated future losses) includes simultaneous holding onto, letting go, and drawing closer to the life-threatened patient. The perioperative nurse can assist the family and circle of friends by supporting them during their "grief work," a time when processing and working through the loss and grief are necessary to integrate them into ongoing living.

DIAGNOSTIC STUDIES

The trauma patient is managed by a priorities approach of systems assessment to evaluate, isolate, and treat injuries rapidly that could quickly lead to death. This approach is based on the concept of "treatment before diagnosis," and it provides the triage team with a structured procedure to detect and manage injuries relative to their severity.

Blood Work

The multiply injured patient requires several diagnostic tests before accurate medical diagnoses can be made. Routine blood studies in the trauma setting include the following: complete blood count (CBC) with hemoglobin and hematocrit levels, and chemistries, including electrolyte, blood urea nitrogen (BUN), creatinine, blood glucose, calcium, and amylase levels. Hepatitis B surface antigen is sought to determine the presence of hepatitis. Because many of these patients are on the threshold of shock, serum lactate is drawn to determine metabolic acidosis. Serum osmolality is measured to indicate either hypervolemia or hypovolemia. Persons with a serum osmolality of 300 or greater have ingested substantial amounts of alcohol before admission; a toxicology screen is drawn. This test, along with the serum osmolality, helps the trauma team plan care, especially for an unconscious or uncooperative patient.

Prothrombin time and partial prothrombin time are measured as determinants of blood clotting ability. Arterial blood gas is drawn to ascertain respiratory status. If an arterial line is not in place, the blood gas is taken directly from the femoral artery.

Blood for typing and screening is drawn on all patients; type and crossmatch will be done if the patient becomes hemodynamically unstable and requires transfusion. For patients who will be taken to the OR, a type and crossmatch for 6 units of packed cells is performed. In the trauma setting, where uncontrolled hypovolemia is often the precursor to circulatory collapse, volume infusion is imperative. The multiply injured patient will be given type-specific blood whenever possible; but when the circumstances require expediency, O-negative packed cells are infused until type-specific blood can be obtained.

Urinalysis

Urine specimens are obtained on all patients, preferably as clean-caught specimens. If the patient is unable to void, the specimen is obtained via a bladder catheter. Urinalysis includes tests for red and white blood cell counts, electrolytes, osmolality, and toxicology. Patients with blood at the urinary meatus have an intravenous pyelogram to rule out ureteral or urethral disruption. Patients suspected of having bladder injury, especially those with confirmed pelvic injury, have a cystogram. Both of these radiographic studies are performed in the resuscitation area.

Routine X-ray Studies

Routine x-ray studies are performed on all trauma patients. A lateral cervical spine x-ray film is taken, based on the assumption that the cervical spine is injured until proved otherwise. A supine chest x-ray film is taken as part of the respiratory assessment and to confirm intrathoracic catheter placement. An upright chest x-ray film is performed after stabilization of the cervical spine. Finally, a pelvis x-ray film is taken to determine the presence of fractures. Extremity x-ray films are taken as indicated; anterior/posterior and lateral views are ordinarily required, but oblique views and stress views of a joint may be necessary. If there is an amputated digit, it is also x-rayed. If the extremity is suspected of vascular compromise, a single-exposure, hand-injection angiography is performed in the triage area or OR. Onsite angiography is preferable to transporting the patient to the radiology department because transport to another department could worsen the injury and, if the vasculature requires surgical intervention, the OR suites are within a short distance of the triage area. The patient can be quickly mobilized for arterial repair. The extremity is temporarily fixed to facilitate vasculature surgical repair. Permanent fixation will be performed after the arterial repair has healed. Fractures confirmed by x-ray examination are reduced as soon as possible by closed reduction under radiographic control or by various methods of open reduction and internal fixation in the OR.

Computed Tomography and Magnetic Resonance Imaging

Trauma protocol requires that patients who lost consciousness at the scene of the accident, who present with overt brain or maxillofacial injury, or who offer an inconsistent history on admission have CT of the head. MRI is used for better definition of mass lesions, for visualization of the posterior fossa and brain stem, and to detect subtle changes in tissue water content (Barker, 1994). For patients with a spinal injury, a myelogram may be performed in the admitting area to assess level of cord compression or confirm reduction of the cervical spine fracture through traction.

Peritoneal Lavage

Because many factors during triage can render physical examination of the abdomen inconclusive, protocol delineates that diagnostic peritoneal lavage be performed if the patient complains of abdominal pain, the abdomen appears rigid or distended, or the patient exhibits rapidly falling hemoglobin and hematocrit levels. A catheter is inserted into the peritoneal cavity through a small incision just above the umbilicus. Normal saline (1000 ml) is infiltrated into the cavity by gravity drainage and removed in the same manner. Positive lavage necessitating an emergency exploratory laparotomy includes any of the following: bloody aspirate; erythrocytes greater than $100,000/mm^3$; leukocytes greater than $500/mm^3$; or presence of gastrointestinal contents, vegetable fiber, bile, or bacteria. If there is doubt as to these results, the patient will have abdominal CT.

Electrocardiogram

Patients who sustain blunt chest trauma are monitored for cardiac injury. Their management is comparable to that of a myocardial infarction patient. In addition to the aforementioned protocol, blood is drawn for serial cardiac isoenzyme measurement. A 12-lead electrocardiogram (ECG) is obtained on admission, and serial ECGs are performed up to 4 days after injury. Clinical manifestations of impending failure would be determined through pulmonary artery monitoring and with the results of cardioangiography.

Ice Water Caloric Test

If massive brain damage is suspected, the examining neurosurgeon performs an ice water caloric test. The head of the bed is elevated 30 degrees, and 60 to 100 ml of ice water is instilled into the patient's ear. Pupillary response is observed by opening the patient's eyelids. If the brain stem's basic reflex, the occulovestibular reflex, is functioning, the eyes will look away from the cold stimulus. As the water warms up, nystagmus may be observed. The eyes will deviate toward the ear with the water in it, confirming that the brain stem reflex is intact.

Following the trauma protocol and assimilating the information obtained into a comprehensive individualized treatment plan enable the perioperative nurse to provide the highest quality of care in the most demanding situations.

HIGH-RISK NURSING DIAGNOSES

The following discussion of nursing diagnoses is representative of patient problems commonly encountered in perioperative trauma settings. The use of the term *risk* with a nursing diagnosis reflects the perioperative nurse's clinical judgment that the individual patient (or family) is more vulnerable to developing this problem than other patients. The discussion is not all-inclusive; variations will depend on the individual patient's circumstances. Clusters of signs and symptoms, which are often associated with nursing diagnoses, have been omitted. Instead, possible etiologic factors and perioperative nursing interventions are briefly reviewed. A nursing diagnostic category may be related to one or to multiple etiologic factors. A plan of care should include desired patient outcomes derived from the nursing diagnoses. Outcome statements are included with each diagnostic category. However, the criteria for measuring outcome attainment must be added to assess outcomes. Examples of measurable criteria accompany the sample care plan at the end of this chapter.

Ineffective Airway Clearance

The multiply injured trauma patient may have an impaired airway caused by obstruction from the tongue, presence of a foreign body, decreased level of consciousness (LOC), cranial nerve deficits, or edema in the upper airway. If the patient sustains an injury to the upper torso or throat, ineffective airway should be suspected because of fractured larynx and accompanying soft tissue edema. The perioperative nurse should monitor respiratory rate and rhythm, auscultate the lungs to detect adventitious sounds, and assess cough, gag, and swallow reflexes frequently. The desired outcome is that the patient will maintain a patent airway.

Ineffective Breathing Pattern

The airway and breathing of a trauma patient are assessed for symptoms of inefficiency. The trauma patient with a neurologic deficit (such as a high level of quadriplegia) may experience respiratory muscle fatigue, which produces an ineffective breathing pattern. Pneumothorax or hemopneumothorax produces a loss of thoracic pressure, resulting in decreased air exchange. A patient with multiple rib fractures or sternal fracture with associated chest injuries has painful respiratory expansion, which produces splinted ineffective breathing. Postoperatively the surgical trauma patient is predisposed to develop a paralytic ileus or gastric distention as a result of elevation of the diaphragm. The desired outcome is that the patient will attain and subsequently maintain an effective breathing pattern.

Decreased Cardiac Output

Decreased cardiac output is suspected in the head injury patient with dysrhythmias. Cardiac dysrhythmias are common because of the heightened sympathetic vasomotor activity within the sensitized medulla. Vena cava compression or mediastinal shift evidenced by x-ray studies indicates decreased cardiac output caused by decreased diastolic filling of the heart. Hypovolemia and hemorrhage produce a decreased hematocrit level, which lowers the oxygen-carrying capacity of the blood. Evidence of chest trauma warrants a high level of suspicion for myocardial contusion; a less effective pump mechanism and electrical instability should be considered. Decreased cardiac output results from increased pulmonary pressure caused by the release of vasoactive substances or development of a pulmonary embolism. A ruptured diaphragm with abdominal contents in the chest will decrease the patient's cardiac output. The desired outcome is that the patient will maintain or demonstrate improved cardiac output.

Pain

Trauma patients experience various levels of discomfort related to the type, extent, and severity of their injuries. Examples of pain may range from myocardial contusion to abdominal pain to rib fractures or external genitalia injury. If the patient has sustained a neurologic injury, pain needs to be managed because of its effect on intracranial pressure, but pain management in this patient population is complicated. Barker (1994) notes that codeine and fentanyl allow for continued evaluation of the pupils while decreasing painful stimuli; morphine should be avoided because of its effects on the cerebral vasculature. In addition to pharmacologic pain relief, the perioperative nurse should consider nonpharmacologic pain reduction strategies such as guided imagery and relaxation; these may enhance the release of endogenous endorphins (Johnson, 1994). The desired outcome is that the patient's pain and discomfort will be relieved or minimized.

Impaired Verbal Communication

Once the patient is intubated (either for a surgical procedure or for injuries requiring prolonged ventilation), he or she will experience communication difficulties. The desired outcome is that an effective means of communication will be established with the patient who is intubated but responsive.

Fear

The trauma patient will experience many types of fear during the acute and rehabilitative episodes of care. Depending on the mechanism, type, and location of injury, patients may fear respiratory compromise from a laryngeal injury. The patient who experiences facial disfigurement or amputation will fear a disturbance in body image. The desired outcome is that the patient will utilize effective coping mechanisms to reduce or minimize fear.

Fluid Volume Deficit

Trauma patients commonly have fluid volume deficit as a result of the hypovolemia caused by uncontrolled hemorrhage. There may be a large traumatic wound, internal bleeding, disruption of an intraabdominal organ or vascular integrity, fractures, or facial trauma with moderate to severe blood loss. Fluid volume deficit will result from a volume shift into the extravascular space. Neurologically injured patients exhibit fluid volume deficit, but from a somewhat different cause. In the spinal cord injury patient the fluid volume deficit is related to peripheral vasodilatation that occurs with loss of sympathetic vasomotor tone. In the brain injury patient with increased intracranial pressure, fluid volume deficit is caused by coagulopathy from the release of thromboplastin within the damaged brain tissue. During surgery, autologous salvage may be initiated; whole blood collection, concentrated washed red blood cell collection, and plasma pheresis may be accomplished intraoperatively (Orr & Girard, 1994). The desired outcome is that the patient will attain and maintain adequate fluid volume.

Impaired Gas Exchange

A priority in airway management for the trauma patient is related to the nursing diagnosis of *impaired gas exchange.* There are many causes of impaired gas exchange: aspiration of foreign objects into the upper airway and lungs, lung collapse, pulmonary contusion, lower airway obstruction resulting in retained secretions, atelectasis, pulmonary embolism, barotrauma secondary to the use of high pulmonary end-expiratory pressure, and accumulation of fluid in the alveoli and pulmonary interstitium. Traumatic injuries predispose the patient to an impaired airway gas exchange: head injury that results in ineffective breathing patterns, cervical cord injury with decreased mechanical ventilatory control, pneumothorax, hemopneumothorax, other hemorrhagic thoracic and intraabdominal injuries, and tracheobronchial rupture. Frequent auscultation of breath sounds and monitoring arterial blood gas results are part of the perioperative interventions to maintain adequate oxygenation and perfusion. The desired outcome is that the patient will maintain adequate gas exchange.

Impaired Physical Mobility

The trauma patient experiences impaired physical mobility in varying degrees, ranging from a casted fractured extremity to a complete quadriplegic spinal cord injury. Patients with severe pulmonary injuries are chemically impaired because neuromuscular blocking agents are used to maintain maximal ventilation. Trauma patients undergoing surgery are physically impaired until all procedures are completed. During perioperative events, interventions for immobility include protective positioning and maintaining a safe environment. The desired outcome is that the patient will preserve physical mobility.

Risk for Infection

The risk for infection in a surgical patient is present whenever an incision is made into a previously intact skin surface. After a traumatic episode, that risk is increased when the patient undergoes multiple invasive procedures such as intravenous line insertions, urinary catheterization, and so on. Infection can be related to bacterial invasion from wound contamination from an open fracture, a large traumatic wound, or a traumatic amputation. In open cranial trauma, pathogens can be introduced into the dura through the lacerated skin or fractured bone. Mechanism of injury can predispose the patient to infection when there is penetration into the abdominal or thoracic cavity by a foreign object or spillage of bowel contents from a ruptured bowel caused by blunt trauma. The desired outcome is that the patient will be free from infection.

Altered Nutrition: Less Than Body Requirements

After traumatic injury there is a significant increase in the patient's caloric requirements and energy expenditure (hypermetabolism) as compared with actual intake. The patient is in a hypercatabolic state (increased protein degradation) from the traumatic injury and requires high intake. To meet these special metabolic and nutritional demands, nutritional consults and enteral feeding may be required. The desired outcome is that the patient will maintain adequate nutrition.

Self-Esteem Disturbance

The patient experiences many physical and psychologic changes after trauma. There may be a disturbance in the patient's body image as a result of multiple surgical procedures, including massive debridement or tissue transfer. The patient may experience the following disturbances in self-esteem: temporary, unexpected change in family role, with potential for permanent job or career role change; loss of earnings; and loss of emotional support as a result of the traumatic injury and hospitalization. Simple perioperative nursing interventions include talking with the patient and using touch for support and encouragement. The desired outcome is that the patient will cope effectively with disturbances in self-esteem.

Impaired Skin Integrity

Immobility predisposes the trauma patient to a variety of problems, including breakdown in skin integrity. Neurologic deficit and localized skin trauma can produce breakdown in skin integrity either from immobility or the injury itself. Researchers have reported that spinal cord injured patients whom were immobilized on boards during diagnosis and surgery can develop pressure ulcers within hours (Pressure sores on board, 1992). Grade III fractures have bone fragments protruding through the skin, resulting in breakdown in the skin barrier integrity. The perioperative nurse needs to institute measures to relieve pressure and improve circulation to dependent pressure sites. The desired outcome is that the patient's skin integrity will be maintained (without further impairments if some preexist).

Ineffective Thermoregulation

Alteration in thermoregulation should be suspected with head injury patients because of hypothalamic damage or posterior fossa syndrome. Spinal cord injury patients experience loss of function in the sympathetic nervous system with cord injury above the level T6, which will produce temperature regulation difficulties (hypothermia). During perioperative interventions, the nurse should prevent the head-injured patient from shivering; shivering increases the metabolic rate and may have a deleterious effect on intracranial pressure. Rectal and core temperature monitoring should be done, and palpation of skin surfaces to detect warmth, coolness, and moisture augment temperature monitoring. The desired outcome is that the patient will maintain normothermia.

Altered Tissue Perfusion

After traumatic injury there is often an alteration in tissue perfusion. A patient may experience a fluid volume deficit after a hemorrhagic episode or rapid intravenous fluid infusion. Thoracic hemorrhage such as a vascular insult or great vessel disruption will result in an alteration in tissue perfusion. Other common predisposing factors include sluggish venous return from loss of vasomotor control, peripheral vascular injury such as in amputation, pelvic trauma, and the presence of deep vein thrombosis. With cord-injured patients, spinal cord tissue perfusion is altered due to inflammatory response after injury, sympathetic blockade, and changes in tissue oxygenation (Barker, 1994). The perioperative nurse will assess blood pressure, PaO_2, cardiac output, and urinary output when determining the adequacy of the patient's hemodynamic status. The desired outcome is that the patient will maintain or improve tissue perfusion.

Ineffective Family Coping

Psychosocial support for the family is as important as psychosocial support for the patient. The acute nature of traumatic injury can rapidly put a family into crisis. Crisis support is one type of assistance aimed at helping people overcome the disequilibrium of a traumatic event, aiding in developing a realistic perception of the event, accessing adequate situational support, and effectively using their coping mechanisms (Hoffenburg & Buck, 1994). A body of nursing research on the needs of family members of critically ill or injured patients indicates that common family needs include being able to be with the patient, to do something for the patient, to know that the patient's comfort is being addressed, to have communication with members of the health care team that is honest, to have a caring attitude toward the injured family member, and to be kept informed (Smith, 1990). More recent studies support these findings. Johnson and her colleagues (1995) studied the effects of critical care hospitalization on family roles and responsibilities. The physical and emotional stress of families trying to pull together during a crisis while experiencing some family fragmentation and having increased responsibilities and changes in routines and feelings all underpin the need for the perioperative nurse to care for the family as they move from initial ineffective coping to drawing on inner strength and developing support systems.

CARE PLANS

Perioperative nurses are frequently engaged in caring for trauma patients, whether they work in designated trauma centers or acute care facilities. Trauma care requires perioperative nursing experts whose experience and knowledge allow them to assimilate large amounts of information rapidly and instantaneously and to react with precision and skill to changing patient circumstances. Caring for trauma patients requires a commitment to keep abreast of new advances and protocols for trauma care. The outcome of an injury depends not only on its severity, but also on how quickly the patient receives appropriate treatment. Perioperative nurses contribute to treatment interventions, collaborating with other health care professionals to ensure that high-quality care is available to prevent unnecessary death and disability. Continuous and systematic data collection is essential for planning and evaluating perioperative trauma care. Locsin (1995) has suggested that part of nursing's caring paradigm is the harmonious integration and coexistence of machine technology and caring technology. In the sophisticated perioperative trauma settings of the late 1990s, this is an apt description of the perioperative nursing role, where technologic competence is critical but not subservient to the element of humanistic caring for the patient, the family, and others affected by life-threatening injury.

GENERIC CARE PLAN

Perioperative trauma settings may wish to develop generic care plans for trauma patients. The following modifications and additions to the generic care plans presented in Chapter 7 are recommended as a beginning toward that end.

The Patient Demonstrates Knowledge of the Physiologic and Psychologic Responses to Surgery

In trauma patients, for whom surgery is urgent and unanticipated, modification of the patient outcome would include "The patient will have an advocate if unable to acknowledge the planned surgical intervention." Evaluation of the patient outcome should include a statement such as "Institutional protocol was followed with patients unable to acknowledge the planned surgical intervention." Under nursing actions, the trauma patient should be evaluated for motor as well as sensory impairments.

Additional entries in the Guide to Nursing Actions would include the following:

1. Verify the operative procedure with patient's physicians if the patient is unable to respond to preoperative assessment questions.
2. Verify that the operative consent form coincides with physician's response.
3. Verify that operative consent form and advanced directive are signed according to institutional protocol when patient is unable to sign.
4. Document the patient's appearance, method of ventilation, type and position of invasive lines, presence of cervical collar, position of extremity fixators and/or traction, and method of transport into the OR.

The Patient Is Free from Infection

For the generic care plan relating to freedom from infection, evaluation of the patient outcome should be modified to include the following additional parameters:

1. The patient's esophageal temperature remained below 100° F (or patient's rectal temperature remained below 101° F).
2. Wounds not approximated were cleaned and debrided to enhance circulatory perfusion.

The Guide to Nursing Actions for a generic care plan to prevent infection should include the following modifications:

1. Preoperative assessment should consider the patient's mechanism and extent of injury, arterial blood gas results, and CBC values.
2. Laboratory values should include arterial blood gas results that will indicate tissue oxygenation.

The Patient's Skin Integrity Is Maintained

Because the trauma patient is likely to have altered skin integrity, the patient outcome should be modified to "The patient's remaining intact skin (that is, not altered by trauma) remained intact."

Additional entries in the Guide to Nursing Actions should include the following:

1. Document the extent of degloving injury.
2. Check the patient's skin for the presence of foreign bodies such as gravel, dirt, and broken glass. Document the resultant wounds.
3. Document the presence of extremity fixators around which the surgical incision will be made.
4. Document the extent of systemic injury that will compromise skin integrity (for example, spinal fracture with neurologic deficit).
5. Check the patient's skin for the presence of edema.

The Patient Is Free from Injury
Related to Electrical Hazards

For the generic care plan relating to freedom from electrical injury, the Guide to Nursing Actions should include the following:

1. Monitor electrosurgical equipment. Note any appearance of skin reaction to the dispersive pad.
2. Monitor bipolar equipment. Follow manufacturer's recommendations when draping and securing the cord from the sterile field to the bipolar unit.

Box 20-2 Resuscitation Cart Supplies

"Patient Doe" addressograph	Central venous catheters
Blood pressure (BP) cuff	Cordis introducer
Doppler and gel	IV pressure pump tubing with large-capacity filter
Flashlight	Lactated Ringer's solution
Tape (nonallergic)	Pressure bags
Prep razors	IV extension tubing/IV dressings
Michel wound clips	Foley catheters with temperature probes
Lidocaine 1% with and without epinephrine	Catheter insertion trays and urine bags
Bacteriostatic saline and water	Nasogastric tubes
Advanced cardiac life support drugs	Diagnostic peritoneal lavage box
Mannitol 20%	Chest tube insertion box
Contrast dye	Pleurevacs/Pleurevacs with the autotransfusion system
Tetanus toxoid with diphtheria	Povidone-iodine swabs
Blood draw setup	Sterile prep trays
Blood tubes/arterial blood gas syringes	Sterile and clean gloves
Needles (assorted sizes)	Shield masks
Syringes (assorted sizes)	Alcohol swabs
IV catheters, #12 to #20	

Adapted from Hollingsworth-Fridlund P, Hall JB, & Dias JB. (1993). OR resuscitation for trauma patients. *Today's OR Nurse*, 15(4), 7-14.

The patient outcomes should allow for the trauma patient's neuromuscular damage. Consider adding a statement such as, "There was no evidence of neuromuscular damage other than that which resulted from the traumatic injury."

Additional entries to the Guide to Nursing Actions should include "Verify that electrical equipment has been approved by the facility's biomedical engineering department."

The Patient Is Free From Injury Related to Positioning

Additional entries to the Guide to Nursing Action should include "Document the presence of extremity fixators and/or traction."

Assessment of patient problems should include the presence of external fixators, which limit the degree of positioning.

The Patient Participates in Rehabilitation

Because the trauma patient might not be reasonably expected to participate in rehabilitation at the point of perioperative nursing intervention, the Guide to Nursing Action should include "If the patient cannot participate in discharge planning, modify to accommodate significant others and document same."

SAMPLE CARE PLAN AND GUIDE TO NURSING ACTIONS

The following sample care plan for the trauma surgery patient is meant to be the starting point for facility-specific plans of care. Trauma surgery often involves more than one body part, organ, or system;

complicated perioperative maneuvers are required for two or more teams operating simultaneously on injured areas. During initial resuscitation, communication and preparation for the patient's admission is critical; many trauma centers have resuscitation carts ready (Box 20-2). The primary survey is done rapidly once the patient is admitted, and vital signs, line insertion and laboratory studies, airway insertion and maintenance, respiratory monitoring, ECG, and hemodynamic monitoring consume the perioperative nurse's time with the patient. As definitive diagnostic test results are received, the patient is readied for transport and coordination of the trauma team in the OR is planned. Family support should be provided during this time, pain managed, and preparation for surgery accomplished. It has been recommended that reports between areas, such as trauma admitting and the OR, follow consistent and preestablished patterns (Nursing care of the trauma patient, 1992). Critical information needed for these patterns includes the patient's name (or means of identification), mechanism of injury, level of consciousness on arrival (the Glasgow Coma Scale is often used for this determination), history of substance abuse or toxicology screen results, prehospital history, the location and nature of the injuries, medication, blood/blood product and fluid resuscitation accomplished thus far, any surgeries performed in trauma admitting, and specific information related to injury management (e.g., traction, lines and their measurements, ventilator support). If specific information is available about positioning

---

Box 20-3 OR Resuscitation Supplies

Assorted suture
Vascular supplies box
Single-wrap instruments requested by trauma surgeons
Trauma surgeon's case pick list book
Towel clips
Sterile Doppler probes
Ligaclips with applicator set
Abdominal retractors (Balfour, extra wide Deaver, medium Harrington)
Major set
Abdominal vascular set
Chest set
Long instrument set
Electrosurgical unit (ESU) pencils
Assorted surgical drains
Assorted straight vascular grafts
Dressing supplies
Intravenous dye and supplies
Pleurevacs and autotransfusion Pleurevacs
Assorted size chest tubes
IV extension tubing
Minot instrument sets (resuscitation trays)
Felt pledgets and bolsters (full sheets for customizing size)
Assorted GI staplers

Adapted from Hollingsworth-Fridlund P, Hall JB, & Dias JB. (1993). OR resuscitation for trauma patients. *Today's OR Nurse,* *15*(4), 7-14.

---

requirements and devices needed in the OR, this is communicated, as is the anticipated time of arrival in the OR.

Because trauma patients average 3.5 surgeries per hospitalization (King, 1994), trauma ORs often have self-contained instrument sets as part of their OR resuscitation cart (Box 20-3). This allows rapid instrument preparation because no additional supplies are pulled until the extent or specific additional needs of the surgical intervention are known. This prevents opening unneeded supplies and instruments, streamlining initial care. The plan that follows is general, but also generalizable, to a broad framework in which to outline the essential elements of perioperative trauma care.

GUIDE TO NURSING ACTION
Caring for the Trauma Patient (Fig. 20-5)

1. Preoperatively assess the patient for proper identification, mechanism and extent of traumatic injury, respiratory compromise, allergies, sensory and motor function, location of indwelling lines, baseline laboratory results and vital signs, results of x-ray or CT/MRI examinations, and availability of blood and blood products. Check for surgical consent, advanced directive per institutional protocol. Despite the urgent nature of the surgical intervention, provide the patient and family with explanations and comfort. Establish time lines and means of communicating with the family at intervals during the surgery.

2. Facilitate the coordination of the surgical team members and determine the availability of an OR suite. Organize the preparation of the surgical instruments, including the procurement of cardiovascular instruments and suture ligatures. The OR suite is prepared for a catastrophic admission. Determine the availability of the following equipment: autotransfusion device, multiple suction canisters, electrosurgical unit, defibrillator unit and emergency medications, blood pressure infusion pumps, and blood and intravenous fluid warmers. Consider the need for warm isotonic irrigation, antibiotic irrigation, hemostatic agents, radiographic dye, neurosurgical sponges, bone wax, nonabsorbable dural suture, dural dissectors, low-volume cranial suction, irrigation and debridement supplies (irrigation is performed with large amounts of normal saline under pulsating pressure; the debridement of necrotic fascia, devitalized muscle tissue, and bone is necessary to decrease the risk of infection and promote wound healing), orthopedic instruments, bone-holding clamps, fracture-reduction clamps, pneumatic drill, etc. If the patient has compartment syndrome, the involved extremity is measured; an acceptable range of pressure is approximately 50 mm Hg. If the patient is not alert and the pressure is 30 to 60 mm Hg, a decision is made whether to perform fasciotomy. Provide adjunctive positioning equipment as required for the planned surgical intervention. Personal protective equipment should be donned by the trauma team.

3. Despite the emergency nature of the surgery, all attempts should be made to maintain sterility during preparation of the sterile field.

4. Follow institutional protocol for surgical counts during trauma surgery. Attempts should be made to initiate counts.

5. Determine the length of time for blood and blood product preparation; consult with the anesthesia team.

6. Provide induction support for anesthesia personnel. Assess and support in the identification of life-threatening dysrhythmias. Depending on the nature of the trauma, awake nasal intubation assistance may include the use of a local anesthetic agent, in-line traction of the patient's head, visualization of the epiglottis with a flex-

FIG. 20-5
CARE PLAN FOR THE TRAUMA SURGERY PATIENT

KEY ASSESSMENT POINTS

Airway, breathing, circulation
Mechanism of injury
Prehospital care
Lines inserted
Lab values
ECG/hemodynamic parameters
Definitive diagnostic results
Fluid resuscitation status
Level of consciousness
Patient/family coping/support available

NURSING DIAGNOSIS

All generic nursing diagnoses apply to this patient, with the addition
   of:
Anxiety/fear
Decreased cardiac output
Pain
Fluid volume deficit
Ineffective thermoregulation
Impaired gas exchange
Hypothermia
High risk for infection
Impaired skin integrity
Altered tissue perfusion

PATIENT OUTCOMES

All generic outcomes apply, with the addition of:
The patient will verbalize known sources of fear, anxiety, and discom-
   fort.
The patient will demonstrate maintenance and improvement of car-
   diac output.
The patient's fluid volume will be maintained and restored.
The patient's temperature will remain normothermic.
The patient will demonstrate normovolemia.
The patient will demonstrate a stable blood pressure, cardiac output,
   heart rate, pulmonary artery pressures, and adequate arterial blood
   gas values.
The patient's temperature will be normothermic.
The patient's hemoglobin and hematocrit will be maintained or im-
   proved from preoperative levels.
The patient's fluid and electrolyte level will be maintained or im-
   proved from preoperative levels.

NURSING ACTIONS

	Yes	No	N/A
1. Preoperative assessment?	☐	☐	☐
2. Appropriate instrumentation and equipment?	☐	☐	☐
3. Sterility maintained during preparation of operative field?	☐	☐	☐
4. Counts initiated?	☐	☐	☐
5. Blood/blood product availability?	☐	☐	☐
6. Assist with induction?	☐	☐	☐
7. Additional intravenous access?	☐	☐	☐
8. Patient properly positioned?	☐	☐	☐
9. Skin prep?	☐	☐	☐
10. Intraoperative documentation?	☐	☐	☐
11. Report communicated?	☐	☐	☐
12. Preparation for transport?	☐	☐	☐
13. Other generic care plans initiated? (specify)	☐	☐	☐

Document additional nursing actions/generic care plans initiated
here:

_____

_____

_____

EVALUATION OF PATIENT OUTCOMES

	Outcome met	Outcome met with additional outcome criteria	Outcome met with revised nursing care plan	Outcome not met	Outcome not applicable to this patient
1. The patient remained hemodynamically stable.	☐	☐	☐	☐	☐
2. The patient's anxiety/fear/discomfort was reduced.	☐	☐	☐	☐	☐
3. The patient met outcomes for additional generic care plans as indicated.	☐	☐	☐	☐	☐

Signature: _____ Date: _____

ible bronchoscope, or jaw-thrust method to protect the integrity of the patient's cervical spinal cord. Before induction the patient is asked to move all extremities to verify the integrity of the spinal cord. Assist with additional indwelling intravenous line and urinary bladder catheter placement. During this preparation phase, secure the patient on the OR bed with a safety strap applied across the thighs in a nonrestrictive manner.

7. Assist with and document the insertion of additional intravenous access lines and temperature monitoring devices.

8. The patient will be secured in a surgical position as required by the planned intervention. Protect dependent bony prominences from pressure injury with padding, and prevent alternate current pathways by securing the dispersive pad of the electrosurgical unit separately from the ECG leads. Reposition the safety strap and recheck adequacy of positioning devices and hemodynamic stability as the patient is repositioned. Some surgical procedures, such as repair of panfacial fractures, will require an air- or gel-filled mattress on the OR bed (these procedures may last up to 24 hours); a warming device (forced air or thermia unit) should be prepared for this patient.

9. Skin preparation will be carried out quickly and will cover a wide anatomic area. Confine fluids from extensive skin preparation so that they do not pool in dependent areas. If the patient's head is shaved in preparation for surgery, care is taken to limit contamination of the sterile field. Hair removed is the patient's personal property and must be contained and returned to the patient. The head is prepared according to institutional protocol.

10. In addition to routine perioperative documentation, intraoperative documentation should be made of procedure-specific events such as duration and position of aortic cross-clamping, use of tourniquet, and orthopedic devices. Also document the patient's position; method of intubation; medicated irrigations; time, type, and sequence of intraoperative x-ray films; results of counts; and the surgical procedure.

11. A complete systems report of the patient's injuries, surgery, and current hemodynamic status is communicated to the receiving care unit postoperatively. Include the following information: patient status and surgery(ies) performed, respiratory and other monitoring devices required in the unit; intravenous, intravascular, and drains/ catheters inserted; medications administered; and estimated time of arrival in the unit.

12. Organize equipment for patient transport; depending on the surgical intervention and the nature of the injury, this may include an oxygen tank, resuscitator bag (Ambu-bag), and a portable ECG oscilloscope with arterial line monitoring capacity.

References

Barker E. (1994). *Neuroscience nursing.* St. Louis: Mosby.

Childs SG. (1995). Hand trauma: Emergency measures to rehab. *Nursing Spectrum, 4*(15), 12-14.

Coolican MB, et al. (1994). Education about death, dying and bereavement in nursing programs. *Nurse Educator, 19*(6), 35-40.

Eiseman B. (1994). Our second responsibility in trauma care: A new clause in the social contract. *ACS Bulletin, 79*(3), 23-34.

Hartsock R & King CA. (1994, March 14). *Initial management of the critically injured patient: The resuscitative and perioperative nurses' roles.* Paper presented at the 1994 AORN Congress, New Orleans.

Herndon DN. (1991). What's new in trauma and burns. *ACS Bulletin, 76*(1), 56-58.

Hoffenburg JA & Buck DJ. (1994). Emergency support team. *Med-Surg Nursing, 3*(2), 142-143, 154.

Hollingsworth-Fridlund P, Hall JB, & Dias JB. (1993): OR resuscitation for trauma patients. *Today's OR Nurse, 15*(4), 7-14.

Johnson D. (1994). Advanced perioperative nursing: Selected physiological effects of trauma. *Seminars in Perioperative Nursing, 3*(4), 185-190.

Johnson SK, et al. (1995). Perceived changes in adult family members' roles and responsibilities during critical illness. *Image—the Journal of Nursing Scholarship, 27*(3), 238-243.

Johnston JS & Johnston C. (1994). A chest-trauma primer. *Nursing Spectrum, 3*(10), 14-16.

King CA. (1994). Coordination and collaboration of violent trauma care. *Seminars in Perioperative Nursing, 3*(4), 175-184.

Lewis FR. (1994). What's new in trauma. *ACS Bulletin, 79*(1), 78-80.

Locsin RC. (1995). Machine technologies and caring in nursing. *Image—the Journal of Nursing Scholarship, 27*(3), 201-203.

Norman E, Gadelta D, & Griffin CC. (1991). An evaluation of three blood pressure methods in a stabilized acute trauma population. *Nursing Research, 40*(2), 86-89.

Nursing care of the trauma patient. (1992). Trauma Nursing Coalition.

Orr MD & Girard N. (1994). Blood products replacements processed in the surgical field. *Seminars in Perioperative Nursing, 3*(4), 194-199.

Pressure sores on board. (1992). *AJN, 92*(10), 18.

Smith DA. (1990). The needs of family members of critically ill or injured patients. *Research Review: Studies for Nursing Practice, 7*(1), 2.

Stothert JC & Herndon DN. (1995). Evaluation and stabilization for emergency operation. In *Emergency care, care of the surgical patient.* New York: Scientific American Medicine.

Thelan LA, et al. (1994). *Critical care nursing: Diagnosis and management* (2nd ed). St. Louis: Mosby.

Tucker SM et al. (1996). *Patient care standards: Collaborative practice planning.* (6th ed). St. Louis: Mosby.

Weeks CS. (1890). *Textbook of nursing.* New York: D Appleton.

Chapter 21

Pediatric Surgery

Cheryl Nygren
Jane C. Rothrock

A very high degree of development of those qualities desirable in any nurse is requisite in the care of sick children. This calls for infinite tact, patience, and judgment, and especially is the habit of critical observation essential, for, with children too young to speak, the involuntary revelations of signs and gestures give often the only clew (sic) to the seat and kind of distress. The objective symptoms are, fortunately, very marked in children, and they respond to treatment with a readiness that makes them very interesting subjects.

WEEKS, 1890

*P*ediatric surgery is one of the most vigorously growing specialties within nursing and medicine. In addition to the surgical procedure itself, challenges include anesthetic management, respiratory support, infection control, fluid volume and electrolyte balance, and thermostasis, each with a comparatively narrower margin of error than that encountered in the adult operative patient.

GENERAL CONSIDERATIONS

Three physical characteristics make the care of pediatric surgical patients unique: the patient's size, age, and the fact that the requirement for surgery is most frequently dictated by a congenital rather than acquired problem. Many congenital defects requiring surgical intervention can now be detected before birth. Although some inherited anatomic malformations may be specifically sought, many are identified serendipitously when ultrasound is performed during the prenatal period. Depending on the type of malformation detected in utero, the fetus may be carried to term to achieve the most optimal surgical correction in the following situations:

- Small intact omphalocele, meningocele, or myelomeningocele
- Craniofacial, chest wall, or extremity deformities
- Esophageal, duodenal, jejunoileal, or anorectal atresias
- Cystic hygroma, small sacrococcygeal teratoma, or ovarian or enteric cysts

Some congenital defects may require an induced preterm delivery to achieve early ex utero correction. In each case the risk of premature delivery must be weighed against the risk of continued gestation, which would have a progressively ill effect on the fetus because of the defect. These defects include the following:

- Hydrops fetalis
- Obstructive hydronephrosis or hydrocephalus
- Gastroschisis or ruptured omphalocele
- Intestinal ischemia or necrosis caused by volvulus or meconium ileus

Preterm delivery with immediate surgical intervention may be the only method possible to maximize the subsequent growth and development of the child.

Congenital defects requiring surgical intervention are typically classified by their anatomic involvement, such as cardiac defects or defects of the abdominal or chest wall. Commonly, children with congenital defects undergo surgery soon after birth, and many may require multiple surgical procedures throughout their lifetime. Surgery requirements related to acquired conditions are most commonly caused by trauma (which is often orthopedic), an oncologic process, or infection, all of which can occur at any age.

Supportive Nursing

Perioperative management of the child requiring surgery also entails helping the parents and family manage significant levels of anxiety and stress. The concerns and reactions of parents often correlate with the age of the child, the reason for surgery, and the perceived potential outcome as it relates to the future of the family. Parents of a neonate born with a congenital defect often feel guilty and inadequate and may perceive themselves as failures, because the long-awaited baby is somehow imperfect. Defects, especially those that are physically visible, may embarrass the parents at a time when pride was the anticipated emotion. Occasionally, this disappointment may be directed toward the infant, resulting in an interrupted parent-child bonding process. Certainly the physical separation of parents from their child, regardless of the child's age, can create confusion regarding parental roles. Additional stresses faced by parents may include concerns for the care of other children at home, the financial impact on the family unit, lack of health care insurance, transportation, lodging, food, and time lost from work (Moon, 1993). Family problems that may have already existed can become greatly accentuated, particularly if one family member is blamed for the child's illness or injury. In a survey to determine satisfaction with care in pediatric hospitals, the sensitivity of the staff to the inconvenience and difficulties that the child's health problems and hospitalization cause the family was the most highly correlated variable with overall satisfaction ratings (What matters most, 1993).

A child old enough to understand separation from parents requires emotional support. The fear of strangers and the terror of physical harm are very real to children of all ages. Most children find it difficult to understand the concept of "good hurt," because all pain is greatly magnified, is perceived as purposeful, and is extremely frightening. Adolescents are concerned about pain, disfigurement, and prolonged separation from their peer group. The fact that they require hospitalization and surgery makes them "different" and possibly less valued by their friends.

Clear communication that is culturally sensitive and relatively free of medical rhetoric is essential to the successful perioperative management of pediatric patients and their families (Lewitt & Baker, 1994).

ASSESSMENT CONSIDERATIONS

Assessment of the pediatric surgical patient requires an understanding of normal growth and development processes related to the specific age group (Box 21-1). Basic evaluative criteria, such as vital signs, weight, neurologic status, and pain perception, depend greatly on the patient's age. An accurate evaluation of these criteria, with a recognition of abnormal findings, is essential to any preoperative assessment (Table 21-1).

Respiratory, Cardiovascular, and Neurologic Assessment

Evaluating respiratory, cardiovascular, and neurologic functions is an important perioperative assessment. A disturbance within one of these physiologic areas often causes abnormal symptoms in all three. It is also particularly common for children that fear and pain will have a significant impact on their physiologic status. For this reason, an understanding of the anatomic and physiologic differences between children and adults is critical.

Respiratory assessment. Accurate respiratory evaluation is of highest immediate priority because of the impact of ineffective ventilation on the cardiac function of the child. The vast majority of cardiac dysrhythmias and arrests are related to respiratory failure, which is extremely common in the critically ill infant. Primary anatomic differences are related to the child's upper airway structure, lung compliance, and use of diaphragmatic muscles for ventilation.

The posterior pharynx and the larynx of a young child are structurally different than those of the adult, which results in the glottis being much more cephalic and anterior. There is a normal narrowing of the trachea at the cricoid cartilage ring, providing an "anatomic cuff" whenever tracheal intubation is required. For this reason, cuffed endotracheal tubes are not used in children younger than 9 years of age because the tubes place pressure within the subglottic area, which could result in stenosis if intubation is traumatic or if use is prolonged. To eliminate this risk, an endotracheal tube that leaks at less than 30 cm of H_2O is placed.

Because the cross-sectional area of the child's airway is much smaller than that of the adult, any reduction in the airway radius may cause a tremendous increase in airflow resistance. A minimal amount of mucus or edema may cause enough airway obstruction to produce significant compromise of gas exchange. In addition, the cartilage of the larynx is easily compressed, and narrowing of the airway can occur with the neck either flexed or extended. Any decrease in the child's airway radius will increase airway resistance and will significantly increase the work of breathing (Wong, 1995). Similarly, compliance is a measure of the elasticity of the lung tissue and depends on surfactant for preventing alveolar collapse as the alveoli become smaller during expiration. Many infants requiring surgical intervention have decreased ventilatory compliance because of inadequate surfactant, causing atelectasis, pneumothorax, and pulmonary fibrosis or edema. The combination of increased airway resistance and decreased lung compliance may lead to severe respiratory failure in the young perioperative patient.

The configuration of a child's rib cage is more horizontal, with an intercostal musculature that is poorly developed compared with the rigid chest wall of the adult. Accessory muscles do not normally contribute to inspiration, causing the child to be much more dependent on the effective movement of the diaphragm for ventilation. Anything that may compromise the movement of the diaphragm can be a major source of rapid respiratory failure. Therefore correct positioning of the child throughout the operative procedure is essential (Cunningham, 1995). Research studies have shown that oxygenation in infants and young children is diminished when in a supine position as compared with a prone position. This results from enhanced ventilation and perfusion ratios, primarily from enhanced posterior chest wall expansion.

Congenital defects that involve the chest or abdominal wall can severely limit diaphragmatic excursion, which is one reason why surgery to correct

---

Box 21-1 Growth and Development with Related Issues for Pediatric Surgery

1. Infants
   Erikson's life stage—Trust versus basic mistrust
   Development
   4 weeks
   Motor: Gross—Head sags forward in sitting
   Fine—Hands clench on contact
   Adaptive—Regards object in line of vision only
   Language—Small throaty noises
   Personal-social—Stares indefinitely at surroundings
   16 weeks
   Motor: Gross—Head steady in sitting
   Fine—Reaches, grasps objects, brings to mouth
   Adaptive—Eyes follow slowly moving object well
   Language—Laughs aloud
   Personal-social—Spontaneous social smile
   28 weeks
   Motor: Gross—Rolls over
   Fine—Rakes at small pellet with whole hand
   Adaptive—Transfers toy from one hand to the other
   Language—Talks to toys
   Personal-social—Takes feet to mouth
   Relevant Issues to Surgery
   Distressing for the infant to be separated from mother or mother substitute. Separation may cause acute disturbances such as fretfulness and night wakenings. Patient should stay with mother until time of surgery. Patient can be distracted from separation from mother with pacifier, familiar toy, or cooing and singing. During induction of anesthesia the infant may be held until anesthetized.

2. Early Childhood
   Erikson's life stage—Autonomy versus shame and doubt
   Toddlers
   12 months
   Motor: Gross—Walks with one hand held
   Fine—Neat pincer grasp of pellet
   Adaptive—Tries to build tower of two cubes
   Language—Two words besides "mama" and "dada"
   Personal-social—Offers toy to image in mirror
   15 months
   Motor: Gross—Toddles independently
   Fine—Puts pellet into bottle
   Adaptive—Puts six cubes in and out of cup
   Language—Four to six words including names
   Personal-social—Points or vocalizes wants
   18 months
   Motor: Gross—Walks, seldom falling
   Fine—Turns two to three pages of book at once
   Adaptive—Builds tower of three to four cubes
   Language—Has 10 words
   Personal-social—Feeds self in part with spilling
   Relevant Issues to Surgery
   The toddler is at the stage of gaining self-confidence and begins to achieve mastery over self, others, and environment. The hospitalization process inhibits these goals from learning sphincter control to the ability to say "no." The toddler should stay with mother until time of surgery; if sleeping, toddler may be held during induction of anesthesia.

Condensed and modified from Korsch BM. (1975). The child and the operating room. *Anesthesiology,* 43(2) and Lowrey GH. (1986). *Growth and development of children* (8th ed.). Year Book Medical Publishers.

Continued.

Box 21-1 Growth and Development with Related Issues for Pediatric Surgery—cont'd

Preschool
2 years
Motor: Gross—Walks up and down stairs alone
Fine—Turns pages of book one at a time
Adaptive—Builds tower of six to seven cubes
Language—Three-word sentences, jargon discarded
Personal-social—Verbalizes toilet needs consistently
3 years
Motor: Gross—Rides tricycle, using pedals
Fine—Holds crayon with fingers
Adaptive—Copies circle and imitates cross
Language—Gives sex and full name
Personal-social—Feeds self well
4 years
Motor:—Hops on one foot
Adaptive—Picks longer of two lines
Language—Names one or more colors correctly
Personal-social—Washes and dries hands, brushes teeth
Relevant Issues to Surgery
Children between the ages of two and four have great sensitivity and are prone to a number of fears. For the first time they are aware and afraid of death. They interpret many unpleasant experiences as a form of punishment. The preschooler needs reassurance that he or she will be "O.K." and needs explanation of and preparation for hospital interventions. Be sure to speak in terms that a preschooler understands. For example, if a medication is described as bitter, associate it to a taste that would be familiar to the child. Introduce hospital monitoring equipment with nonthreatening examples. (Placement of pulse oximeter probe on index finger to ET's finger.) Allow the preschooler to use his or her imagination during induction of anesthesia by having one person tell a story as the child falls asleep.

3. Early School Age
Erikson's life stage—Initiative versus guilt
5 years
Motor—Skips, alternating feet
Adaptive—Counts 10 objects correctly
Language—Names penny, nickel, dime
Personal-social—Dresses and undresses without assistance
6 years
Motor—Stands on each foot alternately, eyes closed
Adaptive—Draws man with neck, hands, and clothes
Language—Defines words by function or composition; for example, "house is to live in"
Personal-social—Counts to 30
Relevant Issues to Surgery
The school-age child is interested in the hospital environment and is able to communicate needs to hospital personnel. The medical staff should encourage questions and offer choices of treatment (choice of anesthetic aromatic drops; that is, strawberry to mask smell of inhalation agent). During induction of anesthesia, one person should tell a story to the patient and questions should not be encouraged at this time, a tactic many school-age children use to delay induction time. If the school-age child is asleep on the stretcher, anesthesia should be induced on the stretcher and the patient moved to the OR bed after he or she is anesthetized.

Condensed and modified from Korsch BM. (1975). The child and the operating room. *Anesthesiology, 43*(2) and Lowrey GH. (1986). *Growth and development of children* (8th ed.). Year Book Medical Publishers.

---

congenital defects such as omphalocele, gastroschisis, and diaphragmatic hernia is performed soon after birth.

Assessment of the child's respiratory status should include evaluation of skin color, respiratory rate, pattern, depth, and quality of breath sounds. Signs of distress include visible use of accessory muscles and retractions, which involve the drawing in of the soft tissue around the thorax. Grunting, nasal flaring, shortness of breath, crowing sounds, and stridor also indicate increased respiratory effort (Menard, 1995). Wheezing may be heard during both the inspiratory and expiratory phases, accompanied with a cough that sounds "croupy" or "brassy." It is important to remember that breath sounds are easily referred from other areas of the lung and may be transmitted over an area of atelectasis or pneumothorax through the thin chest wall of the young child. Simple, rapid auscultation is best performed by initially listening to lung sounds with the stethoscope placed in the far lateral axillary line on each side. This type of auscultation provides the greatest possible distance between the opposite lung fields.

Cardiovascular assessment. Cyanosis and tachypnea can be signs of impending respiratory failure, but they also may be important indications of car-

Table 21-1 Pediatric vital sign values*

| Age | Weight (kg) | Pulse | Average rates | |
			Respiratory	Blood pressure (systolic)
Premature	.5-2.5	140-160	50-80	40-60
Birth-1 mo	2.5-4	130-140	40-60	50-70
1-6 mo	6-8	120-130	30-40	80-90
6 mo-1 yr	9	100-120	26-28	90
1-2 yr	11	100-110	26	90
2-4 yr	12-15	90-110	24	90-100
4-6 yr	16-21	80-100	24	90-100
6-8 yr	22-27	75-100	22	90-100
8-10 yr	28-32	75-100	22	100-110
10-12 yr	32-37	75-90	22	100-120
12-14 yr	38-44	70-85	20	110-125
14-16 yr	45-52	65-80	20	110-125

*Normal ranges of vital signs greatly depend on the age of the pediatric patient.

diovascular compromise and possible hemodynamic instability. Assessment of the cardiovascular status of a pediatric perioperative patient should be based on the understanding that the child's heart rate is usually higher and the stroke volume is less than in the adult. Tachycardia is the normal method of increasing cardiac output. However, tachycardia combined with an increased respiratory rate indicates either an unusually high oxygen consumption, such as with fever, or an inadequate systemic oxygenation. Bradycardia that remains prolonged for more than a few seconds is poorly tolerated by children and requires intervention. For transient bradycardia, administration of supplemental oxygen may be all that is required to increase heart rate. More prolonged bradycardia requires a combination of volume administration, inotropic agents, and afterload reduction to restore cardiac output.

General perioperative assessment of the pediatric cardiovascular system should include the evaluation of the child's heart rate, distal perfusion by palpation of peripheral pulses, and presence of a cardiac murmur. A much more specific and extensive assessment is required for the infant born with a congenital heart defect, depending on the type of cardiac defect. In addition, infants who require surgery within the first several days of life are likely to revert to fetal patterns of circulation such as shunting through the ductus arteriosus. All of these factors have a great deal of hemodynamic significance.

One additional important evaluation is the calculation of the normal circulating blood volume. Although a child's blood volume is higher per unit of body weight than that of the adult, the total volume is much less. For example, even though a 50-ml blood loss is small in an adult, a 50-ml blood loss in a 3-kg child results in a blood loss of greater than

Table 21-2 Circulating blood volume

Age group	ml/kg
Neonate—Birth to 1 month	85-90
Infant—1 to 12 months	75-80
Child—1 to 13 years	70-75
Adolescent—Adult	65-70

15% of the child's blood volume. Hypovolemia during any surgical procedure can occur with minimal blood loss, and blood replacement should be considered whenever losses exceed 7% of the child's circulating volume (Table 21-2).

Assessment for the clinical manifestations of shock in the young child is somewhat similar to that in the adult. Hypovolemic and cardiogenic shock can occur in the child both before and after surgery. Shock alone can become a major cause of death if it remains undiagnosed or if the child receives inadequate resuscitation. A child's blood pressure frequently remains within normal ranges during early to advanced shock processes; this is especially true of hypovolemic shock. The peripheral vascular system of a child is very responsive to central nervous system volume receptors. Peripheral vasculature constricts significantly, shunting blood more centrally to the heart and brain, thus maintaining an adequate blood pressure. A child who is hypotensive is already in an advanced shock process and requires aggressive resuscitative measures. Observing trends in blood pressure is typically more useful than attempting to determine the child's condition based on singular pressures. One simple method to calculate a normal systolic blood pressure is to take the child's age in years, multiply by 2, and add that figure to 80. (For example, a 5-year-old child: $5 \times 2 = 10$; $10 + 80 = 90$; 90 would be an acceptable systolic blood pressure for a 5-year-old child in most cases.) To correctly measure blood pressure, cuff size must be appropriate to both occlude the underlying artery and apply equal pressure to the artery. Menard and Park (1995) recommend the American Heart Association method: measure the circumference of the extremity and take 40% to 50% of the circumference in selecting the size of the cuff bladder. Cuff width then corresponds to approximately one-half the thickness of the arm.

Neurologic assessment. Children younger than 2 years are difficult to evaluate neurologically, whereas older children are evaluated using the same methods employed for adults. At any age the child's alertness and arousability are important to determine. The normal newborn has rapid, reflexive behavior as a typical, generalized response to any stimulus. In the preverbal child, an evaluation of behavior provides essential neurologic information, such as a delayed or lacking response to pain. Assessment of muscle tone is also useful. Infants and children demonstrate dominance of flexor muscles so that extremities will mildly resist manual extension, with quick recoil on release. Clinical manifestations of increased intracranial pressure in the young child include the following:

- High-pitched cry
- Bulging fontanel, which may be tense
- Separated cranial sutures with increased head circumference
- Distended scalp veins
- Irritability and resistance to being comforted

In the older child, neurologic examination should include assessment of arousability, orientation to place and person (time is occasionally too conceptual to be used with accuracy), and motor function, including pupil response. In regard to the unconscious child, all activities should be aimed at maintaining ventilation or hyperventilation and minimizing intracranial pressure. This includes elevating the head if possible and avoiding head positions other than the midline with the chin slightly lifted. Depending on the child's condition and level of unconsciousness, other tests that may be performed include the doll's eyes maneuver (oculocephalic reflex), caloric test, and funduscopic examination. Assessing the gag reflex is also important, with particular attention to protecting the airway if the gag is weak or absent. A full battery of additional examinations are conducted on a child who is an organ donor candidate to determine brain death.

The older child who is able to comprehend and verbalize normally may have difficulty responding appropriately because of anxiety and fear rather than as a result of a neurologic deficit. Determining the cause and effect of behavior is an important aspect of pediatric neurologic assessment. Speaking in a soft, calm voice; using simple language for commands; and explaining all activities going on around the child help alleviate some of his or her fears. Allowing the parents to remain with the child whenever possible has great positive effects.

Temperature

Evaluating the temperature of a child is also a critical assessment. Hypothermia can occur more rapidly in children because of a large surface area to-weight ratio, decreased mass, and lack of insulating subcutaneous fat. In addition, children less than 6 months of age lack an involuntary shivering mechanism, which normally helps generate central warming. As a result, infants break down brown fat in a process called "nonshivering thermogenesis," that depletes energy stores. Even minimal hypothermia can be dangerous in the young or very small child, causing increased oxygen consumption and increased vasoconstriction, with resulting hypoxemia, hypoglycemia, and increased lactic acid–producing metabolic acidosis. It can also deplete metabolic energy stores and cause fluid and electrolyte shifts. Pulmonary vasoconstriction may also occur, causing an increased right ventricular afterload and diminished cardiac output. For this reason, warming blankets under the child, overbed radiant warmers, and oxygen and anesthetic agent warmers are consistently used throughout many surgical procedures on children, as well as preoperatively and postoperatively. Fluids used both intravenously and for irrigation should also be warmed before use.

Fluid Balance

Critically ill children are susceptible to the development of fluid and solute imbalances, that can result in either body fluid depletion or overload. Symptoms may vary depending on the severity of the illness, the child's age, and individual physiologic response.

Volume depletion. Any condition that promotes excessive fluid loss or prevents the intake of adequate amounts of fluid predisposes the child to a volume depletion. Dehydration in the preoperative pediatric patient can be assessed through evaluation of body weight, vital signs, urinary output, skin turgor, mucous membranes, neurologic status, urine-specific gravity, plasma osmolarity, and plasma sodium concentration. Symptoms of circulatory shock may be evident in severe dehydration, including low blood pressure, tachycardia, and poor peripheral circulation resulting in cool, pale, mottled skin with poor capillary refill. The mucous membranes are dry

Table 21-3 Maintenance fluids requirements

Weight (kg)	Fluid requirement
0-10 kg	100 ml/kg/24 hours*
11-20 kg	1000 ml + 50 ml/kg over 10 kg/24 hours
>20 kg	1500 ml + 20 ml/kg over 20 kg/24 hours

*ml/kg is equivalent to cal/kg.

and cracked, and the anterior fontanel in infants is sunken.

Volume overload. Volume overload in the pediatric patient is most commonly related to the infusion of fluids and blood products rather than to a medical cause of fluid retention. Fluid replacement requirements must be based on the normal ongoing losses as well as on estimated additional losses, including caloric expenditure. Maintenance requirements for both fluid and calorie replacement in children are calculated on the body weight in kilograms (Table 21-3). The daily fluid requirement of children is more per kilogram of body weight than that of the adult because they have higher insensible water losses. This is the result of a greater surface area to-volume ratio and a higher metabolic rate.

All sources of fluid loss should be carefully monitored, totaled frequently, and compared with the absolute amount of fluids being received by the child. This must include all blood drawn, fluid lost in vomiting and diarrhea, and urine output. Intake should include all flushes administered, along with drugs and through monitoring lines, such as arterial, central venous pressure, or pulmonary arterial pressure lines.

Maintenance calculations may not necessarily apply to premature neonates or when the body is in an existing unbalanced state, that increases fluid and caloric requirements significantly.

Psychosocial Assessment

The final perioperative nursing assessment relates to evaluating the parent's and patient's (depending on age) understanding of the purpose and anticipated outcome of the surgery. It is important to determine the individual's perception of the event and the significance it holds within the family structure. For some families, surgery on a child may cause a situational crisis state, even if the surgery is minor.

If the surgery is elective, advanced preparation of the child and family for surgery can be the best method for supplying situational support. Books with color pictures, slide or videotape presentations, and tours of the preoperative and postoperative units are important and usually generate questions that

reveal concerns (Anderson, 1994). Children often have special fears that are specific to the word "sleep" as it is used when describing anesthesia. They may worry about not being able to sleep through the procedure and waking up in the middle of it. When explained that this is a "special sleep" that the physician controls, they may want to know if they will ever wake up and what happens if they do not (Squires, 1995). Many children fear that things other than what they are being told will be done to them while asleep; they will need reassurance. Older children and adolescents will fear death but may not express those fears because of a fantasy that "words spoken sometimes come true." Fear of pain also will be a major factor. In younger children, the greatest fear is frequently related to the shot that they may receive before going to the operating room. This is a familiar type of pain, and in and of itself can be almost overwhelmingly frightening to children. Some children, when learning that they will need an intravenous line and blood drawn, will be more upset about these procedures than about the surgery, especially if they have had previous hospitalizations with painful procedures. For all age groups, including adolescents, the separation of the child from the parents when entering the operating suite causes significant anxiety (Holden, 1995). Reassuring an early reunion is important.

Unanticipated surgery, such as with congenital defects requiring surgery soon after birth or because of traumatic injury, may further cause the parents to react in a highly stressful manner. The resulting behavior is manifested in individualized ways and can be easily misunderstood. Most commonly, the core emotion during these times is a sense of powerlessness and guilt, because they are unable to help their child. Responses can range from apathy to anger, from hysteria to depression. Honest, accurate information in clear, concise terms and decreasing time of separation between parent and child provide effective interventions for diminishing the negative effects of sudden surgery.

DIAGNOSTIC STUDIES

In general, children require the same diagnostic studies as adults. When a child is born with a congenital defect requiring surgical intervention, that was unknown before delivery, the defect is usually discovered shortly after birth during physical examination by the delivery room nurse, obstetrician, or pediatrician. Frequently, when a problem is not externally evident, the infant is discharged undiagnosed, and the mother will begin to have concerns related to her child's behavior. Routine blood work and radiologic examinations may be completed as a precursor to more specific testing.

Preoperatively, especially with preterm neonates, the use of arterial blood gases to monitor respiratory and acid-base status is common. With the advent of transcutaneous blood gas monitoring, continuous oxygen saturation monitoring, and carbon dioxide monitoring, invasive means are not as frequently required.

NURSING DIAGNOSES

Nursing diagnoses for the pediatric surgery patient depend on the specific operative procedure and on situational circumstances unique to each child. Nursing diagnoses and the nursing actions developed to intervene in the diagnoses effectively or to prevent their occurrence should include the parents, a significant adult, or the family. Family units can be significantly disrupted by surgery on a child, and those risks need consideration. The parent or significant adult can affect the child positively or negatively; psychosocial assessment and patient education strategies should focus on the patient and the parent/family/significant adult unit.

Physical Needs

Nursing diagnoses dealing with the physical needs of the pediatric patient may include the *risk for injury, risk for ineffective airway clearance* and *breathing pattern, risk for aspiration, risk for altered body temperature, risk for fluid volume deficit* or *excess,* and *risk for decreased cardiac output.*

Risk for injury. When the nursing diagnosis *risk for injury* is used, it is necessary to specify the potentially injurious event or circumstance. Chapter 7 identifies a number of potential injuries related to surgical positioning; chemical, electrical, and physical hazards; and retained foreign objects. Special attention needs to be paid to careful and safe surgical positioning. Skin condition, tissue integrity, and weight of the child are important when selecting the appropriate positioning accessories. The chronically ill, debilitated child requires additional padding to prevent skin injury to dependent body sites. Care needs to be taken to protect eyes and ears during positioning maneuvers. Additional restraints, such as body restraints, may be required.

Careful notation of the child's body weight is important in preventing injury from intraoperative local anesthetics. Davis and Crick (1988) suggest that pediatric dosages of lidocaine are safe up to 5 mg/kg; with Bupivacaine, which may be used for longer surgical procedures, dosages should not exceed 3 mg/kg. If epinephrine is added to local anesthetics, a 1:200,000 concentration may be preferred. It is important to label all medications on the sterile field and to document the drug, dosage, and route of administration.

Use of accessory equipment must be adjusted for pediatric patients. Appropriately sized electrosurgical dispersive pads need to be selected and application sites carefully assessed. Similarly, an appropriately sized tourniquet cuff is necessary. Protocols for tourniquet inflation levels differ for pediatric patients. Davis and Crick (1988) suggest that cuff pressures generally not exceed 100 mm/Hg above the systolic blood pressure. It is important to record the unit used, settings, inflation and deflation times and to monitor and frequently report inflation time.

Risk for ineffective airway clearance and ineffective breathing pattern. Infants are less able than adults to increase oxygen intake by increasing the depth of respiration. Instead, an infant will increase the rate of respiration to compensate for lack of oxygen; this is less efficient than increasing respiratory depth and involves considerable insensible heat and water loss. Oxygen content of the air will need to be increased to reduce respiratory effort; oxygen concentration, humidity, and temperature of inspired air will be controlled. Ineffective breathing patterns may be aggravated by certain surgical procedures (for example, thoracotomy and tight abdominal closures); these infants may need ventilatory support during transport to and while in the postanesthesia care unit (or longer). Young infants breathe primarily with their diaphragm; any surgical intervention that involves the chest or abdomen may interfere with respiratory excursion. Adequate ventilation may be further impaired by the infant's tiny air passages, which are easily occluded by edema or secretions. Monitoring is likely to include capnometry and oximetry; indwelling arterial lines may be preferentially placed into the umbilical or radial arteries.

Risk for aspiration. An infant or child's stomach is always considered full if the surgery is an emergency procedure. The perioperative nurse needs to assist the anesthesia provider with induction; rapid-sequence induction is most likely. Cricoid pressure should be applied as appropriate to prevent regurgitation and aspiration. The child's neck should be extended and the cricoid ring located before induction; then the perioperative nurse uses the index finger to apply firm but gentle pressure gradually on the ring. Two functioning suction lines and catheters should always be available to anesthesia.

Risk for altered body temperature. Infants and children have a greater body surface area, reduced lean body mass (required for generating and retaining heat), and thinner subcutaneous fat than adults; heat loss may be four times that of adults. The infant's response to hypothermia is mediated by a secretion of norepinephrine; this increases the metabolic rate, producing vasoconstriction with impaired tissue perfusion. Anesthetic drugs abolish the thermoregulatory response of the infant or child (deLorimier & Harrison, 1988); because environmental temperatures in the operating room are usually lower than body temperature, the body temperature falls.

There are many perioperative nursing interventions directed at preventing hypothermia. An overhead radiant heater over the OR bed an hour before the patient's admission to the OR may be used to maintain body temperature (Coran, 1995). Thermia units are commonly used; these may be padded warming blankets, reflective blankets, or heat-circulating water pads. The room temperature is usually increased before the infant or child's admission and returned to a comfortable operating temperature only if the child's temperature can be maintained at 36.5° C. Preparation solutions, intravenous solutions, blood, and irrigating solutions should be warmed to help prevent hypothermia. Temperature is monitored frequently by rectal or esophageal probes. Gases used during anesthesia are often heated and humidified. Perioperative nursing assessment and collaboration with anesthesia personnel are necessary both during and after the surgical procedure. When hypothermia is present, oxygen consumption decreases. As the infant emerges from anesthesia, the initiation of spontaneous respiration may be delayed until body temperature rises.

Risk for fluid volume deficit or fluid volume excess. Circulating blood volume levels are good indicators of whether an infant or child can safely tolerate the volume alterations of surgery. In the newborn, the limited blood volume creates a special threat; a few saturated sponges, each with about 20 ml of loss, may precipitate shock (Talbert, 1987). During surgery, dry sponges should be used and weighed shortly on discard from the field to minimize the error from evaporation (deLorimier & Harrison, 1988). Suction lines are often attached to calibrated canisters to determine loss more accurately. Tubing should be short to diminish the dead space and give more immediate estimates of loss with high-risk infants. When blood loss exceeds 10% of circulating blood volume, the perioperative nurse should anticipate the initiation of fluid volume therapy. Replacement fluids vary according to the hematocrit, the amount of blood lost, and the potential for depletion of clotting factors and platelets. Blood or blood products should be identified and documented according to institutional protocol, warmed, and carefully controlled for transfusion rate. Signs of decreased cardiac output from hypovolemic shock should be carefully monitored. Cyanosis and loss of pulse and blood pressure may develop rapidly, often without the warning signs of rising pulse and gradually falling blood pressure.

Psychosocial Needs

Children who require multiple corrective surgical procedures because of a congenital defect or to correct trauma are at risk for impaired growth and development related to the frequency of hospitalization and the isolation from the normal peer socialization process. Children having a noticeable congenital defect may not be accepted by their playmates, teachers, and even siblings, resulting in a risk for self-esteem disturbance. Some children, whose families are unable to accept less than a perfect child, are at great risk for child abuse simply because they are different from other children.

Anxiety and fear. Children may have greatly fantasized ideas of what surgery will be like. Such fantasy is likely to lead to misperceptions that cause heightened anxiety (Pauley, 1995). The threats posed by physical separation from parents, a significant adult, or family unit, and from anticipation of "needles," "going to sleep," "not awakening," and other painful interventions, may engender fear. Perioperative nurses need to be familiar with the rich and varied types of interventions reported by their colleagues to allay the anxieties and fears of pediatric patients.

Research on strategies to reduce anxiety has been frequently reported in nursing literature. In 1979 McGrath studied the effects of group instruction for pediatric patients. Her research indicated that group instruction was better than individual instruction for assisting children to display less upset behaviors and to cooperate during stressful interventions. Other researchers have been interested in group instruction. There is some consensus that instructing children in groups has the benefit of allowing role modeling and developing affiliative behaviors. Cooperation, which has been measured in a number of studies, can be perceived as an overt social response that can be directly influenced by imitation. When children are instructed in groups, a child can observe other children interacting during the instruction and interject a similar behavior into his or her own response. Additional benefits of group instruction are peer exposure and an opportunity to socialize with other children.

Smallwood (1988) described a hospital tour and simulation of the intraoperative experience for children. Intraoperative experiences were demonstrated on dolls. Children had the opportunity to get on an OR stretcher and play with an electrocardiogram (ECG) electrode, anesthesia masks, IV tubing, and other apparatus that may seem frightening until it is touched and experienced. Research on the beneficial effects of play have documented lower pulse rates and body movement posture that is less indicative of pain (Young and Fu, 1988).

Authors have stressed a careful use of words, such as "hospital sleep" rather than "put to sleep" when caring for pediatric surgical patients. Children are encouraged to bring security objects such as dolls or a treasured toy to the OR with them (Berry, 1993). Other authors have described the use of slide or tape programs to educate children before surgery (Abrams, 1982) and the use of surgery coloring books when it is difficult to schedule preoperative tours or education sessions (Doroshow & London, 1988). Table 21-4 presents suggestions for nursing interventions when planning preoperative education for pediatric patients.

Some of the research variables of interest to researchers in the determination of the most effective modalities for preoperative pediatric instruction are listed in Box 21-2.

There has been recent research on these variables. In their study of assessment of postoperative pain in children and adolescents, Savedra, et al. (1993) tested the adolescent pediatric pain tool. The results indicated that self-report measures using the tool were valid and reliable estimates of the location, intensity, and quality of postoperative pain. Vessey, Carlson, and McGill (1994) examined the use of distraction with children during the acute pain experience of venipuncture. The control group received comforting by touch and softly spoken words; the experimental group received a kaleidoscope as a distraction technique and were encouraged to look at the bright colors and patterns in it. Results confirmed that distraction was effective; the experimental group perceived less pain and demonstrated less behavioral distress. In 1995, Kirby explored factors that contribute to surgical anxiety in children. Of a list of possible anxiety-producing events, the noise level in the room was the single factor that consistently elicited negative reactions from children; they cited voices, beeping machines, radios, and other sounds as specific disturbers. These, along with future studies, should help perioperative nurses use research-based, innovative interventions in the pain and anxiety that accompany surgery in pediatric populations.

Intervening in Parental Needs

Parents (or significant adults) and siblings may be distraught when contemplating a child's hospitalization, surgery, and separation. They may feel powerlessness, because they increasingly feel that they have lost control over events and situations that affect their child and the family. There may be altered parenting if the child has undesirable characteristics or is terminally ill. Parents may have unrealistic expectations of themselves or of the child, developing an inability to provide a constructive and nurturing

---

> ### *Box 21-2 Effective Modalities for Preoperative Pediatric Instruction*
>
> 1. Common outcome measures
>   a. Behavioral (verbal and nonverbal body reactions)
>   b. Self-reports (child's verbal report of perceived pain and anxiety)
>   c. Physiologic measurements (biologic reactions such as heart rate, galvanic skin response, and cortisol levels)
> 2. Location of instruction (inpatient, outpatient, or home setting)
> 3. Presence of parent or significant adult
> 4. Intervener (nurse, physician, or other)
> 5. Pain/anxiety stimulus (treatment, painful intervention, and induction of anesthesia)
> 6. Type of intervention (cognitive or affective)
> 7. Group or individual instruction
> 8. Age of child
> 9. Timing of information (day before, few days before, or week before)
> 10. Duration of painful, anxiety-producing event (single or frequent episodes)
> 11. Classification of response as positive or negative; this is an important research question. Crying, loud verbalization, or increased activity during a painful or anxiety-producing intervention may not necessarily be a negative behavioral response, although it has often been characterized as such in research. The question remains, is the behavior a reflection of pain or anxiety, or is it a coping mechanism used by the child?
>
> From Broome ME, Lillis PP, & Smith MC. (1989). Pain interventions with children: A meta-analysis of research. *Nursing Research, 38,* 154-158.

---

environment. Altered family processes may occur as a normally supportive family faces challenges to its functioning integrity. Family communication may be impaired, and families may not seek or accept help appropriately. Ineffective family coping may result when resources (time, money, and emotions) become depleted as the family attempts to meet the stresses of a child's illness. A lack of knowledge (knowledge deficit) about what may realistically be expected and how to assist the child may exacerbate family needs.

The role of the family or significant adult in the child's hospitalization has been of interest to nurses and other researchers. In an early study by Hannallah and Rosales (1983), parents accompanied their children, who had not been premedicated, to an area adjacent to the operating room for anesthesia induction. A sleep dose of intravenous thiopental was ad-

Table 21-4 Preoperative teaching

Preoperative teaching consists of informing a child and parent(s) of necessary hospital routines and procedures. Its purpose is to help relieve anxiety and promote recovery from surgery and anesthesia.

Nursing diagnosis/patient problem	Defining characteristics	Nursing orders	Expected outcomes
Knowledge deficit: hospitalization *Etiology* Lack of prior experience	Verbalization of the problem Inaccurate follow-through of instruction Inappropriate or exaggerated behaviors: hysterical, hostile, agitated, apathetic Statement of misconception Request for information	To determine how much teaching will be necessary, ask whether family has taken a hospital surgery orientation tour and understands upcoming surgery Tour the nursing unit, playroom, and hospital room; show the family call lights, hospital gown, special surgical clothing, bedpan, urinal, and emesis basin; demonstrate how the bed works (inpatient only). For same day surgery, a short video of a child's experience in the surgical waiting area, the OR, recovery and discharge areas is helpful. Inform parents of the location of the surgical waiting room or other designated area where the physician may contact them after surgery If patient is going to the intensive care unit (ICU) after surgery, offer patient and parents the option of an ICU tour Explain admitting routine for checking vital signs; show blood pressure equipment and cup or bag for urine specimen Be honest about blood draws and "pokes;" every child will have at least one Explain the meaning and reason for "NPO" sign; it is helpful to place a sticker on the child a. Supervise the child carefully; separate those who can eat from those who cannot and arrange recreation for the latter b. Explain that the stomach also "goes to sleep" and that the postoperative diet will progress gradually from clear liquids to a general diet; observe for vomiting, bowel sounds, flatus, and stooling Explain that the child will be transported in a crib or on a stretcher (usually pertains to inpatient) Explain to the child that he will leave his parents during surgery but that they will be waiting for him when he returns Encourage the child to bring a special toy for security Show the family the surgical staff's clothing, particularly the masks, and allow the child to play with one Reemphasize where the parents should wait for their child and the availability of information at this waiting area Reemphasize the facts that the physician has given them; use drawings when appropriate It is especially important to describe the procedure in terms of what the child will feel, taste, see or smell Individualize the instruction to include any special tubes or equipment Stress to the child that the operation will include only the area of the body that has been discussed and indicated Arrange for instruction by clinical nurse specialists and consultants as necessary (ostomy, orthopedic, and so forth)	Patient and parents verbalize or demonstrate their understanding of the environment and of routine admitting procedures

Table 21-4 *Preoperative teaching—cont'd*

Nursing diagnosis/patient problem	Defining characteristics	Nursing orders	Expected outcomes
Anxiety *Etiology* Threat to or change in health status Threat to or change in environment	Sympathetic stimulation: • Cardiovascular excitation • Superficial vasoconstriction • Pupil dilatation Restlessness Insomnia Glancing about Poor eye contact Trembling; hand tremors Fear	Inform child and family that anesthesia is a special kind of sleep in which the child will not feel pain or remember the operation. *Caution:* The phrase "put to sleep" may be frightening to children, since their pets may have died that way Describe and show the family the anesthesia mask, emphasizing its pressure and smell Explain the function of intravenous feedings and the need for restraints	Patient and family indicate understanding and acceptance of anesthesia and IVs by verbalization
Ineffective breathing pattern *Etiology* Decreased energy and fatigue Pain Decreased lung expansion	Dyspnea Shortness of breath Tachypnea Cyanosis Cough Nasal flaring	Explain the need for deep breathing and coughing and for frequent turning while in bed Younger children may be given a bottle of bubbles to blow; paper bags and incentive spirometers may be used; blowing at balloons tied to bed also may be effective Explain that child will be encouraged to be out of bed and walking as soon as possible and will be medicated for discomfort as necessary	Patient's respiratory status is regular with no signs of complications
Anxiety *Etiology* Change in environment Change in health status	Sympathetic stimulation: • Cardiovascular excitation • Superficial vasoconstriction • Pupil dilatation Glancing about Poor eye contact Trembling; hand tremors	Show the child the oxygen equipment and explain that he may wake up with nasal sprays, a mask or oxygen hood over his head Inform parents of the estimated ½-2 hour stay in the postanesthesia care unit before the child is fully awake Describe the "wakeup" room to the child, including the presence of a nurse checking vital signs; also explain that side rails will be up on all beds to keep everyone safe Explain that an emesis basin will be available in case the child feels nauseous after the operation	Patient remains calm during postanesthesia care unit stay without fighting, trying to get up, or crying
Pain *Etiology* Surgical trauma	Communication (verbal or coded) of pain descriptors Guarding behavior; protective Self-focusing Distracted behavior (moaning, crying, restlessness) Facial mask of pain Autonomic responses not seen with chronic, stable pain (diaphoresis, blood pressure and pulse rate change, pupil dilatation, increased or decreased respiratory rate)	Warn the child to expect soreness after surgery. a. A preschooler can tell the nurse he hurts. A younger child will be watched for irritability; increased pulse, respiratory rate, and blood pressure and splinting respirations b. Explain that pain medications are available after most surgeries and usually are given through IV tubing c. Ensure the child that when he is in pain, medicine will be given.	Patient remains comfortable enough to eat, sleep, move in bed, and walk adequately
Anxiety (parental) *Etiology* Threat to or change in health status Threat to or change in environment Threat to or change in role	Expressed concern regarding changes in life events Anxiety Facial tension Voice quivering Glancing about Restlessness Insomnia	Encourage parents to support each other, taking turns staying with the child, knowing that it is all right to take breaks Encourage the family to express fears and fantasies and provide them with facts Encourage the parents to participate in the patient's care, as they wish Emphasize to the parent that the child "did nothing wrong" to necessitate surgery Build the child's self-esteem by supporting behaviors that show success in coping with the stress of hospitalization Warn parents of possible temporary postoperative behaviors such as withdrawal, regression, and nightmares	Parents are able to support their child through the hospitalization and positively reinforce mastery of difficult situations

Modified from NP & Beckel J. (1987). *Nursing care plans for the pediatric patient.* St. Louis: The CV Mosby Co.

ministered. When asleep, the child was immediately transferred onto the OR bed. In the control group, anesthesia induction was performed in the same manner but without the parents present. The mood of the children in both groups was comparable in the waiting area and the postanesthesia unit, but there was a significant decrease in the number of very upset and turbulent children in the parent-present group during preinduction and induction. Gauderer, Lorig, and Eastwood (1989) conducted a longitudinal study in which the parent was present in the operating room during mask intubation of anesthesia. In a 4-year period, 3086 parent-present inductions were performed, clearly demonstrating the feasibility, safety, and acceptance of this approach.

The importance of including parents (or significant adults) and siblings in preoperative preparation of the child is widely accepted in the 1990s. Parents attend tours and education sessions, participate in reinforcing and rehearsing taught behaviors, room-in, and are commonly present during the induction of anesthesia. Research has indicated that parents benefit from these activities in terms of both knowledge (Haskins, Merrill, & Bailey, 1988) and satisfaction (McGrath, 1979). Johnston, et al. (1988) were able to demonstrate a relationship between parental anxiety levels and the anxiety level of the child. This is an important consideration in planning for parental participation in events such as the induction of anesthesia. Careful assessment is necessary to achieve a positive effect. In Johnston's study, if the parent was anxious preoperatively and present during the induction, the child's anxiety level increased. In this study, however, the parents were not prepared for the events of anesthesia induction. Thus there is a need for more research on the effect of parental anxiety, the beneficial effects of parental education in reducing anxiety, and on the role of parents as interveners and coaches. As parents interact with the child to practice techniques, their supportive, nurturing role is reinforced. An interesting research variable that is difficult to control and measure when parental anxiety and satisfaction are being assessed is the "treatment" effect. It may be that, in part, the fact that something special is being conducted for the child increases the parental satisfaction with care and decreases anxiety; this may be communicated to the child, who similarly benefits. Nonetheless, the overall benefits of parental and family involvement in educational interventions have been well tested and supported. Accomplishing the goal of having a child sleeping or comfortable before separation from the parents varies in each practice setting. Parent-present induction requires perianesthesia and perioperative staffs trained in this approach, adequately prepared parents who

wish to be present, and space adjacent to or in the OR. If these variables are unable to be achieved, then the goal should be to have the child premedicated to enable a smooth separation from parents and facilitate induction of anesthesia.

CARE PLAN

Continuity of care has the potential of being improved when standardized approaches to nursing problems are used. In a benchmark study of best practices in children's hospitals, the use of clinical pathways to guide the expected preoperative and postoperative course of care were identified. It was suggested that these be used as parental guides also, outlining such events as when play may resume and return to school take place. (Pediatric hospitals identify best practices, 1995). Critical pathways combined with case management have been suggested as mechanisms for controlling costs while maintaining quality of care (Geeze, 1994). The generic care plan that concludes this chapter is not all inclusive, but may be considered one mechanism of streamlining care. It highlights important nursing actions for planning pediatric perioperative care. The Guide to Nursing Actions that accompanies the care plan provides more detailed explanations for the action. This care plan is a guideline; as nursing research continues to produce information on intervention effectiveness, the perioperative nurse will need to use these research findings to modify the plan (Barta, 1995). In addition, the care plan will need to be adapted to the individual patient. Nursing diagnoses that are likely to be relevant have been included. The outcomes and the criteria by which to measure them need to be validated through patient assessment and changed to meet the identified patient needs. The special challenge in pediatric surgery is in recognizing and meeting the broad spectrum of needs of the infant and child. That same challenge is the special reward of perioperative nurses who work in pediatric surgical settings.

GUIDE TO NURSING ACTIONS (Fig. 21-1)

1. Preoperative assessment of a pediatric patient should include evaluation of the child's physical and psychologic preparation for surgery. Growth and development standards should always be used when evaluating a child, with particular attention to areas where the child falls outside of a normal range, such as low weight, poor reflexive response, or abnormal feeding patterns. Immunizations should be up to date. Assessment includes discussing with the parents the child's typical behavior and any changes they have noticed as a result of the child's illness or injury. Assessment should also

FIG. 21-1
CARE PLAN FOR THE PEDIATRIC PATIENT

KEY ASSESSMENT POINTS
Growth and development stage
Adequacy of preparation, rehearsal, supportive care to child/family
Allergies (include latex)
Signed informed consent/advance directive
NPO for appropriate length of time
Lab tests, vital signs
Special considerations (respiratory/cardiac condition, learning or physical disability, cultural/ethnic needs, family history of malignant hyperthermia (MH)

NURSING DIAGNOSIS
All generic nursing diagnoses apply to this patient, with the addition of:
Knowledge deficit (specify)
High risk for injury (specify)
High risk for fluid volume deficit/excess
Anxiety/Fear
Altered body temperature

PATIENT OUTCOME
All generic outcomes apply, with the addition of:
Child and family will receive appropriate emotional support, with need for additional support identified and referrals made.
The child will remain safe from injury or harm.
The child will maintain normal body temperature and fluid volume.
The child will verbalize specific fears related to the surgical procedure, painful events, and hospitalization and separation from parents and will demonstrate minimum anxiety/insecurity.
The child will:
1. Remain free from injury
2. Exhibit an adequate hydration status
3. Remain normothermic
4. Have vital signs within expected limits for age
5. Respond to stimulation appropriately for age, without undue agitation, anxiety, fear, and behavioral regression

NURSING ACTIONS

	Yes	No	N/A
1. Preoperative assessment performed?	☐	☐	☐
2. Preoperative teaching to child/parent complete?	☐	☐	☐
3. Appropriate consent signed by parent/guardian/patient?	☐	☐	☐
4. Identification checked?	☐	☐	☐
5. Physical safety measures taken?	☐	☐	☐
6. Patient/family together as long as possible?	☐	☐	☐
7. Appropriate comfort measures taken?	☐	☐	☐
8. Appropriate-sized equipment for age available? (endotracheal tube [ETT], nasogastric tube, Foley, IV catheters and fluid apparatus, suction catheters, blood pressure cuffs, pneumatic tourniquet cuffs, ECG monitor leads, defib paddles, oximetry, arterial, central venous pressure, Pulmonary artery pressure [PAP], and other invasive monitoring equipment, ESU dispersive pad, thermia unit, instruments, etc.)	☐	☐	☐
9. Guidelines for pediatric CPR and drug doses available?	☐	☐	☐
10. Respiratory and cardiac status monitored?	☐	☐	☐
11. Patient's temperature monitored and maintained?	☐	☐	☐
12. All input and output documented?	☐	☐	☐
13. Family kept informed?	☐	☐	☐
14. Counts performed/correct?	☐	☐	☐
15. Specimen(s) to lab?	☐	☐	☐
16. Dressing applied/drains noted?	☐	☐	☐
17. Other generic care plans initiated? (specify)	☐	☐	☐

Document additional nursing actions/generic care plans initiated here:

_____

_____

_____

EVALUATION OF PATIENT OUTCOMES

	Outcome met	Outcome met with additional outcome criteria	Outcome met with revised nursing care plan	Outcome not met	Outcome not applicable to this patient
1. The child remained safe, attended at all times.	☐	☐	☐	☐	☐
2. The child remained well hydrated without signs of dehydration or fluid overload.	☐	☐	☐	☐	☐
3. Temperature remained between 36.8° C to 37.2° C (98.5° F to 98.9° F).	☐	☐	☐	☐	☐
4. Vital signs remained within anticipated boundaries.	☐	☐	☐	☐	☐
5. The child was accompanied by parents as far as possible, and significant objects or toys were allowed to accompany the child to the operating room. The child responded to comforting and reassurance.	☐	☐	☐	☐	☐
6. The child met outcomes for additional generic care plans as indicated.	☐	☐	☐	☐	☐

Signature: _____ Date: _____

include an evaluation of any previous hospitalizations and surgeries, including the child's response. Discussing the family's previous response and what they have told their child concerning this surgical event will also be helpful.

2. Teaching should provide both child and family with an opportunity to prepare for the surgical event. Age-appropriate play is usually the most effective teaching strategy and acts as an anxiety-reducing technique. Allowing the child to dress up in hospital garb, such as surgical scrubs, and to perform medical procedures on a doll can help the child "play out" fears. Tours or videos of the operating room, holding area, parent waiting area, postanesthesia care unit, and postoperative unit also help decrease the intimidation of both the parents and the child. Videos may be provided for viewing at home or in the surgeon's office.

3. For patients under the age of 18, appropriate permissions for diagnostic procedures and surgery are signed for by the parents or legal guardians, unless the patient is legally recognized as an emancipated minor who is living independently of a guardian. The policy on surgical permits and advance directives for minors will be different depending on the institution and local legal requirements; individual policies must be reviewed and adhered to.

4. Children should have an identification band securely fastened, and parents should remain with the child until identification is validated.

5. Safety measures should include using a body restraint or safety jacket on the premedicated child, which then secures to the stretcher at all times. Side rails must be in the up position, and the child should never be left unattended. For the same-day surgery patient, an infant or toddler may be carried to and held in the preinduction waiting area by the parent; when the OR is ready, a perianesthesia or perioperative team member will carry the child into the OR if parent-present induction is not planned. If an older ambulatory child has received premedication less than 10 minutes before entering the OR and shows no adverse effects, he or she may be permitted to ambulate into the OR accompanied by a perioperative staff member. This obviates the need for stretcher transfer, which may interfere with the older child's need for independence and some autonomy in participating in perioperative events.

6. The negative effects of parent-child separation are well known. If possible, parents should be allowed to remain with their child until induction of anesthesia is started, which will greatly minimize anxiety for both the child and family.

7. Comfort measures can mean multiple things, although the most significant include allowing children to remain with their parents as long as possible, permitting children to take a familiar toy or object with them, and keeping them away from a cold environment. Children will be much more relaxed if they remain very warm within their environment, with at least some familiar aspects, such as a toy or blanket from home. Even seemingly minor changes can cause major discomfort to young children, such as not being allowed to wear pajama bottoms or underwear to the operating room or having to adhere to NPO (nothing by mouth) requirements. Recent studies support the ingestion of clear liquids until 2 hours before anesthesia induction. Liberalization of fasting guidelines may make children less irritable at the time of induction. For premedicating pediatric patients, administration by mouth, nose, or rectum, rather than by injection, also decreases fear and the psychologic trauma of "needles."

8. The equipment required for any procedure depends on the type of procedure and the size of the child. The requirement for specialized equipment should be anticipated. As minimally invasive procedures, such as pediatric laparoscopy and thoracoscopy become more common, the use, maintenance, and placement of specialized equipment will require careful nursing consideration (Tkacz, 1994).

9. Standardized guidelines that provide a resource for all pediatric drug dosages based on the child's weight (which is usually calculated in kilograms) should be available. Should the child require cardiac resuscitation, information specifically addressing neonatal and pediatric resuscitation should be available.

10. All pediatric patients require close monitoring of cardiac and respiratory status throughout any operative procedure, because changes can occur rapidly, with subtle or no warning. Positioning of the patient, type and amount of anesthesia used, sudden or incipient blood loss, hypothermia, and overall stress reaction to the operative procedure can cause rapid changes in stability. The intubation process itself can cause severe bradycardia related to hypoxia and vagal stimulation, so the perioperative nurse should remain with the patient until the induction and intubation process has been accomplished; the child should not be stimulated until completely anesthetized to prevent possible laryngospasm (LeSaint & Hemmen, 1995). A recently recognized problem is children with latex allergy. A latex-

---

Box 21-3 Guidelines for Identifying Latex Allergy and Latex-Containing Products

Does the child have any symptoms, such as sneezing, coughing, rashes, or wheezing, when handling rubber products (balloons, tennis or Koosh balls, adhesive bandage strips) or when in contact with rubber hospital products, such as gloves or catheters?

Has your child ever had an allergic reaction during surgery?

Does the child have a history of rashes, asthma, or allergic reactions to medication or foods, especially milk, kiwi, bananas, or chestnuts?

How would you identify or recognize an allergic reaction in your child?

What would you do if an allergic reaction occurred?

Has anyone ever discussed latex or rubber allergy or sensitivity with you?

Has the child had any allergy testing?

When did the child last come in contact with any type of rubber product? Were you present?

From Wong DL. (1995). *Whaley & Wong's nursing care of infants and children* (5th ed.). St. Louis: Mosby.

---

free environment is required for both the induction of anesthesia and surgery. Because parents and children may be unaware of this allergy, the perioperative nurse should elicit information regarding untoward reactions (sneezing, coughing, rashes, or other symptoms) with any latex items, such as balloons, Koosh balls, or treatment-related items such as catheters, surgical gloves, or finger cots (Villareal & Johnson, 1995). Protocols for creating a latex-free environment and treating the undiagnosed latex-allergic child should be established in each perioperative practice setting. Boxes 21-3 and 21-4 suggest guidelines for identifying the latex-allergic child and latex-containing products. Continuous monitoring of ECG, transcutaneous oxygen, oximetry saturation, end-tidal carbon dioxide monitors, and blood pressure and other invasive pressure monitoring devices is required for pediatric surgical patients, along with measurement of input, output, and temperature. A rare but serious condition encountered with induction of anesthesia is malignant hyperthermia (MH). Halvey (1991) indicates that the incidence of MH in children is 1:15,000, compared with 1:50,000 in adults. In this poten-

tially fatal disorder, skeletal muscles increase their metabolic rate, causing an increase in O_2 consumption, in CO_2, lactate and heat production, respiratory and metabolic acidosis, and muscle rigidity (Ryan, 1993). Protocols for aggressive management of MH should also be determined in all perioperative practice settings.

11. The room temperature needs to be increased for a period of time before the patient's arrival; it can then be adjusted appropriately throughout the surgical procedure, because additional warming devices are used to maintain the child's temperature. Blood and fluid warmers should be used, along with oxygen and anesthetic warmers. Overbed radiant warmers are used, along with blanket warmers placed under the child. A rectal temperature probe should be placed immediately after induction so that the child's temperature can be continuously monitored. In addition, depending on the type of surgery, it may be possible to wrap the child's arms and legs with cast padding to preserve heat.

12. Fluid balance that maintains adequate hydration without fluid overload can be assessed with documentation of all fluid intake and losses.

13. Keeping the family aware of the surgical team's progress and the child's condition throughout the procedure provides enormous emotional reassurance and contributes to a more positive response postoperatively. Any delays that prolong the surgery should be promptly and honestly communicated. If the procedure is not proceeding as anticipated, or if the child becomes unstable and has a potentially poor outcome, the parents need this information before the end of the procedure so that they can begin to gather their own support mechanisms. Frequent updates on the child greatly enhance the parental and family response.

14. Perform sponge, sharp, and instrument counts according to institutional procedure. Document results.

15. Follow institutional protocol for the preservation and disposition of specimens. Use universal precautions with all materials and containers received from the sterile field. Document specimens (laboratory, tissue, culture).

16. Dressings should be applied aseptically. Benzoin may be applied to the skin to prevent inadvertent removal of dressings. Note the presence of any drains incorporated in the dressing.

17. Note the initiation of other generic care plans (for example, prevention of injury from surgical positioning, electrical hazards, and participation in effective home care management).

Box 21-4 Selected Items Possibly Containing Latex*

Medical Items

Adhesive bandage strips (Band-Aid brand)
Airways, masks
Anesthesia circuits
Blood pressure cuffs and tubing
Bulb syringe
Catheters
Chux (washable rubber)
Crutches (axillary, hand pads)
Dressings (moleskin, Coban[3M])
Elastic bandages (Ace wrap)
Electrode pads
Endotracheal tubes
Finger cots
Gloves (sterile and examining, surgical and medical)
Intravenous tubing, injection ports, bags, burets
Jobst spandex products
Medication vials
Nasogastric (NG) tubes
Penrose drains
PRN adapter (heparin lock)
Stethoscope tubing
Suction tubing
Syringes

Tape (cloth adhesive, paper)
Theraband strips and tubes
Tourniquet
Urodynamics rectal pressure catheters
Wheelchair cushions, tires

Nonmedical Items

Art supplies (paint, markers, glue)
Balloons (not Mylar)
Balls (Koosh, tennis)
Cleaning/kitchen gloves
Condoms
Dental dams
Diaphragms
Elastic exercisers
Elastic on legs, waist of clothing, rubber pants, possibly disposable diapers
Feeding nipples
Foam rubber lining on splints, braces
Infant toothbrush-massager
Pacifier
Racquet handles
Rubber bands
Water toys, swim, scuba equipment

*It is very difficult to obtain full and accurate information on the latex content of products, which may vary among companies and product series. Double-checking with suppliers before use with latex-allergic individuals is strongly recommended.
From Wong DL. (1995). *Whaley & Wong's nursing care of infants and children* (5th ed.). St. Louis: Mosby.

References

Abrams L. (1982). Resistance behaviors and teaching media for children in day surgery. *AORN Journal, 35,* 244-258.

Anderson S. (1994). Pediatric patient education for the operating room staff: The "Barney" phenomenon. *Seminars in Perioperative Nursing, 3*(3), 152-159.

Barta KM. (1995). Information-seeking, research utilization, and barriers to research utilization of pediatric nurse educators. *Journal of Professional Nursing, 11*(1), 49-57.

Berry RK. (1993). Effective patient education: Teaching children. *Nursing Spectrum, 2*(24), 14-15.

Broome ME, Lillis PP, & Smith MC. (1989). Pain interventions with children: A meta-analysis of research. *Nursing Research, 38,* 154-157.

Coran AG. (1995). The pediatric surgical patient. In *Care of the patient in surgery.* New York: Scientific American Medicine.

Cunningham SM. (1995). Positioning of infants and children for surgery. *Seminars in Perioperative Nursing, 4*(2), 112-116.

Davis JL & Crick JC. (1988). Pediatric hand injuries: Types and general treatment considerations. *AORN Journal, 48,* 237-249.

deLorimier AA & Harrison MR. (1988). Pediatric surgery. In LW Way (Ed.), *Current surgical diagnosis and treatment.* Norwalk, CT: Appleton & Lange.

Doroshow ML & London DL. (1988). Surgery and children: A colorful way to introduce children to surgery. *AORN Journal, 47,* 696-700.

Gauderer MWL, Lorig JL, & Eastwood D. (1989). Is there a place for parents in the operating room? *Journal of Pediatric Surgery, 24*(7), 705-707.

Geeze MA. (1994). Pediatric outpatient upper endoscopy: Perioperative case management. *Seminars in Perioperative Nursing, 3*(1), 27-39.

Halvey JD. (1991). Malignant hyperthermia. In C Bell (Ed.). *The pediatric anesthesia handbook.* St Louis: Mosby.

Hannallah RS & Rosales JK. (1983). Experience with parent presence during anesthesia induction in children. *Canadian Anaesthesiology Society Journal, 30*(3), 286-289.

Haskins DR, Merrill KD, & Bailey LR. (1989, February 21-23). Perioperative teaching of parents: A unit-based study. Abstract presented at the AORN Congress, Anaheim, CA.

Holden P. (1995). Psychosocial factors affecting a child's capacity to cope with surgery and recovery. *Seminars in Perioperative Nursing, 4*(2), 75-79.

Johnston CC, et al. (1988). Parental presence during anesthesia induction: A research study. *AORN Journal, 47,* 187-194.

Kirby V. (1995). Less noise = less anxiety for children's perioperative experience. *Nursing Quality Connection, 4*(6), 6.

LeSaint PW & Hemmen MS. (1995). Pediatric anesthesia. *Seminars in Perioperative Nursing, 4*(2), 117-119.

Lewitt EM & Baker LG. (1994). Race and ethnicity—Changes for children. *The Future of Children, 4*(3), 134-144.

McGrath MM. (1979). Group preparation of pediatric surgical patients. *Image—The Journal of Nursing Scholarship, 11,* 52-62.

Menard SW. (1995). Preoperative assessment of the infant, child and adolescent. *Seminars in Perioperative Nursing, 4*(2), 88-91.

Menard SW & Park MK. (1995). Blood pressure measurement in children: A brief review. *Seminars in Perioperative Nursing, 4*(2), 92-95.

Moon M. (1993). Overview: Setting the context for reform. *The Future of Children, 3*(2), 23-36.

Pauley B. (1995). Operation fascination. *Journal Postanesthesia Nursing, 10*(2), 89-93.

Pediatric hospitals identify best practices. (1995). *OR Manager, 11*(4), 13-15.

Ryan JF. (1993). Malignant hyperthermia. In CJ Cote (Ed.). *A practice of anesthesia for infants and children.* Philadelphia: WB Saunders.

Savedra MC, et al. (1993). Assessment of pain in children and adolescents using the adolescent pediatric pain tool. *Nursing Research, 42*(1), 5-9.

Smallwood SB. (1988). Preparing children for surgery: Learning through play. *AORN Journal, 47,* 177-185.

Squires VL. (1995). Child-focused perioperative education: Helping children understand and cope with surgery. *Seminars in Perioperative Nursing, 4*(2), 80-87.

Talbert JL. (1987). Pediatric surgery. In DC Sabiston, (Ed.). *Essentials of surgery.* Philadelphia: WB Saunders.

Tkacz NJ. (1994). Pediatric laparoscopy and thoracoscopy. *Pediatric Surgical Nursing, 29*(4), 671-679.

Vessey JA, Carlson KL, & McGill J. (1994). Use of distraction with children during an acute pain experience. *Nursing Research, 43*(6), 369-372.

Villareal P & Johnson CP. (1995). Nursing care of children with developmental disabilities having surgery. *Seminars in Perioperative Nursing, 4*(2), 96-111.

Weeks CS. (1890). *Textbook of nursing.* New York: D Appleton.

What matters most? (1993). *Nurse Extra, 1*(11), 16.

Wong DL. (1995). *Whaley and Wong's nursing care of infants and children* (5th ed.). St. Louis: Mosby.

Young MR & Fu VR. (1988). Influence of play and temperament on the young child's response to pain. *Children's Health Care, 16,* 209-215.

Chapter 22

The Aging Patient

Donna N. Hershey

I believe that not all heroic actions in health care take place in intensive care units or operating rooms. Gerontological nurses know and appreciate the smaller gains. The purpose of gerontological nursing is not to save lives, but to prevent untimely death and needless suffering. Both these goals include respect for human dignity—the preservation of personhood as long as life continues.

SCHWARTZ, 1989

*A*ging adults are the fastest growing segment of the population; half of all hospital admissions involve those over age 65 (Mikulencak, 1993). This increase in aging persons is expected to continue in the coming decade; the number of persons aged 65 to 74 will increase by 20%, the 75 to 84 year group will rise by 50%, and the 85 and older segment will increase by 120% (Capriotti, 1995). By the year 2025, 25% to 35% of the people in the U.S. will be older than 65 years (Pierce, 1995). The term "older" has become of limited use when describing the aging and aged. Social Security legislation of the 1930s, which established age 65 for retirement, fostered the use of this chronologic indicator as the beginning of old age. In current gerontologic frameworks, terms such as "young-old," "old-old," "frail elderly," and "chronologically gifted" are being used to differentiate the population of Americans who have reached the age of 65 and beyond. The perioperative nurse must recognize that age is multidimensional, with chronologic age being only one factor. Other dimensions of age include biologic, psychologic, functional, and social age (Rybash, Roodin, & Santrock, 1991).

The major causes of mortality in those 65 years and older include heart disease, cancer, stroke, chronic obstructive pulmonary disease, pneumonia, and influenza. There are various surgical interventions indicated for several of these conditions as well as for the following chronic problems faced by many elderly: arthritis, osteoporosis, incontinence, and visual and auditory impairments (Institute of Medicine, 1990). Surgery often improves the functional health status of the elderly, although not without risk, and should be considered a viable option. The decision to perform surgery on an older individual should not be based solely on age. Surgeries for which the elderly are most commonly hospitalized are listed in Box 22-1.

Advancements in the care and treatment of many illnesses have brought about dynamic changes in health care. One of these changes is in the reduction in length of stay (Table 22-1). This has implications for perioperative nurses as they seek to provide high-quality, individualized, cost-effective nursing care. Because patients are returning home sooner and often sicker, it is the perioperative nurse's responsibility to collaborate in assisting both the patient and the family with home care management. Participation in teaching concerning health care needs and discharge instruction and planning, as well as appropriate community referrals, is a way perioperative nurses can affect the elderly person's return to home and promote a return to optimal function.

Table 22-1 Average length of stay in non-federal short-stay hospitals, according to selected characteristics: United States, 1980 to 1990

	Average length of stay in days										
Total*	7.1	7.1	7.0	6.8	6.5	6.4	6.3	6.3	6.4	6.3	6.3
Sex*											
Male	7.7	7.6	7.5	7.3	7.0	6.8	6.7	6.9	7.0	6.9	6.8
Female	6.7	6.7	6.6	6.4	6.1	6.0	5.9	5.9	5.9	5.9	5.8
Age											
Under 15 years	4.4	4.6	4.6	4.6	4.5	4.6	4.6	4.7	5.0	4.9	4.8
15—44 years	5.2	5.2	5.1	5.0	4.9	4.8	4.8	4.8	4.7	4.7	4.6
45—64 years	8.3	8.0	7.9	7.6	7.2	7.0	6.8	6.8	6.8	6.7	6.7
65 years and over	10.7	10.5	10.1	9.7	8.9	8.7	8.5	8.6	8.9	8.9	8.7
65—74 years	10.0	9.9	9.6	9.2	8.5	8.2	8.0	8.2	8.4	8.2	8.0
75 years and over	11.4	11.1	10.6	10.2	9.3	9.2	9.0	9.1	9.3	9.4	9.2

*Age adjusted.
NOTES: Excludes newborn infants. Rates are based on the civilian population as of July 1.
SOURCE: Division of Health Care Statistics. (1992). National Center for Health Statistics: *Data from the National Health Discharge Survey.* Hyattsville, Maryland: Public Health Service.

Box 22-1 Common Operations Performed in the Elderly (65 Years and Older)

Women
Cardiac catheterization
Reduction of fracture (excludes skull, nose, and jaw)
Pacemaker insertion or replacement
Biopsies on the digestive system
Cholecystectomy
Extraction of lens
Insertion of prosthetic lens (pseudophakos)

Men
Prostatectomy
Cardiac catheterization
Direct heart revascularization (coronary bypass)
Pacemaker insertion or replacement
Repair of inguinal hernia
Biopsies on the digestive system
Extraction of lens

From Division of Health Care Statistics, National Center for Health Statistics. (1991). *Data from the National Hospital Discharge Survey.* National Center for Health Statistics. Health, United States. Hyattsville, MD: Public Health Service.

STANDARDS AND SCOPE OF GERONTOLOGIC NURSING PRACTICE

When devising and providing high-quality care to elderly persons, perioperative nurses may seek resources additional to their own knowledge and experience. The American Nurses Association's *Standards of Gerontological Practice* (ANA, 1987) is a useful guideline for tailoring nursing interventions to meet specialized patient needs. These standards may be used by the perioperative nurse for planning, implementing, and evaluating nursing care. In institutions where a nurse specialist, who possesses a master's degree and is an expert in gerontologic nursing, is available, consultation and collaboration are recommended in planning care. Although all of the standards include a rationale, structure criteria, and outcome criteria, the rationale and outcome criteria are shown only for ANA standard V, planning and continuity of care (Box 22-2). Although the standards do not prescribe or advocate any particular theoretic framework, they do establish the expectation that nursing activities will be based on theory. Theories contribute to and assist with increasing a general body of knowledge within a discipline. They are useful in interrelating concepts so that a different way of looking at a particular phenomenon is created. In gerontologic nursing, theories help crystallize a view of aging, guide and improve nursing practice, and are the basis for research designed to validate a particular theoretic perspective. Many potentially useful theories can be used to plan for and evaluate outcomes of nursing care of the aging patient.

Theory-Based Practice

Systems theory. Systems theory is concerned with change resulting from interactions among all of the various factors in a situation. This theoretic perspective takes into account the complexity and constant change of interactions between a person and the environment. Systems theory contributes to gerontologic nursing through its assessment of all the variables that affect the patient-environment interaction. Clearly a theory that recognizes the magnitude and complexity of this interaction has great use in providing care for aging patients.

Box 22-2 *Standards of Gerontological Nursing Practice*

Standard I. Organization of Gerontological Nursing Services

All gerontological nursing services are planned, organized, and directed by a nurse executive. The nurse executive has baccalaureate or master's preparation and has experience in gerontological nursing and administration of long-term care services for older clients.

Standard II. Theory

The nurse participates in the generation and testing of theory as a basis for clinical decisions. The nurse uses theoretical concepts to guide the effective practice of gerontological nursing.

Standard III. Data Collection

The health status of the older person is regularly assessed in a comprehensive, accurate, and systematic manner. The information obtained during the health assessment is accessible to and shared with appropriate members of the interdisciplinary health care team, including the older person and the family.

Standard IV. Nursing Diagnosis

The nurse uses health assessment data to determine nursing diagnoses.

Standard V. Planning and Continuity of Care

The nurse develops the plan of care in conjunction with the older person and appropriate others. Mutual goals, priorities, nursing approaches, and measures in the care plan address the therapeutic, preventive, restorative, and rehabilitative needs of the older person. The care plan helps the older person attain and maintain the highest level of health, well-being, and quality of life achievable, as well as a peaceful death. The plan of care facilitates continuity of care over time as the client moves to various care settings, and is revised as necessary.

Rationale

Planning guides nursing interventions and facilitates the achievement of desired outcomes. Plans are based on nursing diagnoses and contain goals and interventions with specific time frames for accomplishment.

Goals are a determination of the results to be achieved and are derived from the nursing diagnoses. Goals are directed toward maximizing the older person's state of well-being, health, and achievable independence in all activities of daily living. Goals are based on knowledge of the client's status, the desired outcomes, and current research findings to increase the probability of helping the client achieve maximum well-being.

Outcome criteria

1. The older person, the family, informal care givers, the physician, and other members of the health care team participate in the planning process as appropriate.
2. The plan of care reflects the nursing diagnoses.
3. The plan is initiated upon the older person's admission to the health care setting and accompanies the client upon discharge from the setting.
4. The plan exists in a concise, standardized, and retrievable form.
5. The plan is current and shows evidence of revision as goals and objectives are achieved or changed.

Standard VI. Intervention

The nurse, guided by the plan of care, intervenes to provide care to restore the older persons' functional capabilities and to prevent complications and excess disability. Nursing interventions are derived from nursing diagnoses and are based on gerontological nursing theory.

Standard VII. Evaluation

The nurse continually evaluates the client's and family's responses to interventions in order to determine progress toward goal attainment and to revise the data base, nursing diagnoses, and plan of care.

Standard VIII. Interdisciplinary Collaboration

The nurse collaborates with other members of the health care team in the various settings in which care is given to the older person. The team meets regularly to evaluate the effectiveness of the care plan for the client and family and to adjust the plan of care to accommodate changing needs.

Standard IX. Research

The nurse participates in research designed to generate an organized body of gerontological nursing knowledge, disseminates research findings, and uses them in practice.

Standard X. Ethics

The nurse uses the Code for Nurses established by the American Nurses' Association as a guide for ethical decision making in practice.

Standard XI. Professional Development

The nurse assumes responsibility for professional development and contributes to the professional growth of interdisciplinary team members. The nurse participates in peer review and other means of evaluation to assure the quality of nursing practice.

From American Nurses Association. (1987). *Standard of gerontological nursing practice*, Washington, DC: The Association.

Stress and adaptation theories. Stress and adaptation theories also have great promise as frameworks for providing professional nursing care to aging patients. The ability to adapt to changes has been posited as crucial to the adjustment to the physiologic and psychosocial aspects of aging. Adaptation is a response to these changes and can be seen as an attempt to maintain or reattain equilibrium. Adaptation theory focuses on effective or ineffective coping mechanisms that are developed in response to the stressors that accompany aging.

Growth and development theories. Growth and development theories are often developed with a linear, progressive, life-span direction. These theories have been applied to moral, psychosocial, cognitive, and interpersonal development. They are often recognized for their focus on progressive development, wherein it is postulated that each person passes through various fixed stages or levels; a passage may differ in quality but must be successfully completed before proceeding to the next stage. These theories have wide applicability to nursing. They do not necessarily reflect chronologic age or aging per se, but instead focus on the developmental progression from childhood to adulthood. Major theorists have identified developmental tasks of aging, and these are presented in Box 22-3. As the demographics of the aging population continue to change, future theorists may further refine these tasks by pondering whether the 65-year-old identifies the same priorities as the 80- or 95-year-old, or are their developmental needs and "tasks" different? Part of the lack of a clear answer to this question is the result of the more recent demographic changes in our society. In years past, life expectancy was much less, and as a result there was little reason to study segments of the aging population. This is one area that will, no doubt, expand as the population continues to age.

General goals for the aging person revolve around the central issues of maintaining dignity, managing one's financial affairs, obtaining proper health care, and engaging in meaningful activity (Eliopoulos, 1995). Satisfaction in old age can be impeded by physical transformation or disability, alteration in social roles and unmet expectations, loss of an optimal state of health and/or decline of external resources (Carnevali and Patrick, 1993). Losses in any of these areas can usually be handled well by an aging person. However, when losses occur in multiple areas or become cumulative and profound, intervention by a health care provider is often necessary to help the person regain a previous level of coping or functioning.

Nursing theories. Nursing theories similarly vary in their perspective on interrelationships between

---

> ## Box 22-3 Summary of Major Theorists' Views on the Developmental Tasks of Aging
>
> **Erikson** believes that individuals face stages of psychologic development as they age:
> - Trust vs. mistrust
> - Autonomy vs. shame
> - Initiative vs. guilt
> - Industry vs. inferiority
> - Identity vs. confusion
> - Intimacy vs. isolation
> - Generativity vs. stagnation
> - Ego integrity vs. despair
>
> The last stage, viewed as the major task in old age, is to accept one's life as having been whole and satisfying in order to achieve ego integrity. Dissatisfaction and regrets with the life one has lived can lead to a sense of despair and disgust.
>
> **Peck** identifies three tasks faced in old age:
> - *Ego differentiation vs. work-role preoccupation:* To develop satisfactions from one's self as a person rather than through the work role
> - *Body transcendence vs. body preoccupation:* To find psychologic pleasures rather than becoming absorbed with the health problems or physical limitations imposed by aging
> - *Ego transcendence vs. ego preoccupation:* To feel pleasure through reflecting on one's life rather than dwelling on the limited number of years left to live
>
> **Havighurst** described tasks of aging individuals to include the following:
> - Adjusting to decreased strength and health status
> - Maintaining involvement with friends and society
> - Establishing satisfactory living arrangement
> - Readjusting one's life-style to reduced income and retirement
> - Coping with the death of one's spouse
>
> **Ebersole** categorizes the developmental tasks of late life into three groups:
> - *Receptive tasks:* Power and capacity in physical, social, cultural, and intellectual realms are relinquished and a certain amount of dependency is accepted
> - *Expressive tasks:* A self-transcending philosophy is developed as older persons gain an appreciation for their place in life and the legacy they leave
> - *Dynamic tasks:* These tasks entail not only one's own physical and psychologic dying process but also helping others learn about death
>
> **Butler** and **Lewis** view the major tasks of late life as follows:
> - Adjusting to one's infirmities
> - Developing a sense of satisfaction with the life that has been lived
> - Preparing for death
>
> Modified from Eliopoulos C. (1991). Developmental tasks of aging. *Long-Term Care Educator*, 2(lesson 6):4.

the person who is the recipient of health care and the environment, health, and nursing. Simplistically put, they offer great explanatory value in planning nursing care and in providing rationales for selected nursing actions. These theories, like the theories of other disciplines, may be interpersonal, behavioral, interactional, or grounded in adaptation, self-care needs and deficits, or systems. All of these theories have implications for both gerontologic nursing and perioperative care of the aging patient.

ASSESSMENT CONSIDERATIONS

The effects of aging vary widely from individual to individual and do not progress at a uniform rate. The aging perioperative patient may exhibit a few or many physiologic and psychosocial characteristics of the aging process. One of the implicit challenges in caring for the aging patient is recognizing and working with individual variations. As in all patient care situations, the aging patient has the right to and the expectation of being treated with dignity and with respect for individual uniqueness. To guarantee appropriate, effective nursing care of aging patients, the perioperative nurse must base his or her interventions on a careful, deliberate assessment. The sequence of common physical examination findings that follows is not presented in the expectation that the perioperative nurse would actually conduct the entire examination. As with all assessment in collaborative nursing situations, the perioperative nurse reviews important assessment data on the patient's medical record, organizes and analyzes it according to importance to perioperative patient care, and verifies and validates findings that specifically relate to and affect the plan of care for the individual patient.

Physiologic Consequences of Aging

Physiologic changes related to chronologic age include general effects such as tissue deterioration, retarded cell division and atrophy, impaired cellular homeostasis, reduced efficiency of the immune system, and decreased neuromuscular response (Tortora & Grabowski, 1993). These structural changes at the cellular and extracellular levels affect changes in body function and appearance. Many of these age-related changes affect specific body systems in fairly typical ways. These are summarized in Table 22-2.

Physiologic aging may or may not have an impact on psychosocial aging; these are interrelated phenomena that are manifested to differing degrees in different patients. Negative stereotypes concerning the aging population do not adequately account for the individual differences in the ways people respond, physiologically or psychosocially, to becoming aged.

General Appearance

Physiologic changes. Decreases in height can occur as a result of multiple factors including a decrease in intervertebral disc height, an increase in spinal curvatures, and changes in the joints (Carnevali & Patrick, 1993). The ratio of lean-to-fat tissue changes with age, and fat tends to shift from the extremities to the center of the body, giving arms and legs a more angular appearance. Since basal metabolism declines with age, obesity is a serious problem for aging persons; however, the aging person who is overweight will not resemble his or her younger counterparts because of changes in fat distribution. In addition, "typical" characteristics of aging, such as gray or white hair and wrinkling of the skin, can further alter the appearance of aging patients.

Nursing implications. For perioperative nurses it is critical to validate whether the patient's height and weight as listed on the medical record are recent. Too often the patient's recollection of these measures is taken without objective verification. An accurate account of both measurements is needed for purposes of safe medication and anesthesia administration. The perioperative nurse should note any recent changes in the patient's energy level, which may indicate underlying systemic problems.

Integumentary System

Physiologic changes. As the activity of sebaceous and sweat glands decreases, skin becomes drier and less perspiration is produced. Natural oils in the outer skin layer may become trapped, resulting in seborrheic dermatitis or keratosis, in which dry, easily chapped, itching skin is not uncommon. Pigmentation may either increase or be absent in local or general skin areas, giving the skin a pale, anemic appearance. The epidermis loses its elasticity and the support previously provided by subcutaneous fat folds and wrinkles. Whereas a generalized dehydration process occurs in aging persons, the appearance of the skin is not a reliable measure of hydration because of age-related changes in the integument. These alterations in integrity can delay healing response and increase susceptibility to skin infections. Skin is more easily bruised, and small injuries may cause superficial hemorrhaging. Hyperkeratosis and skin tags are not uncommon; basal cell and squamous cell carcinomas may increase in incidence, and actinic keratoses and lentigines appear on skin surfaces. Vitamin deficiencies can also result in skin-related changes.

The rate and density of scalp hair declines, and baldness may occur in both men and women. Nail growth slows as a result of decreased peripheral circulation.

Table 22-2 Physiologic effects of aging, their significance to perioperative patients, and related nursing implications

Changes	Significance of changes	Nursing implications
Cardiovascular		
The number of elastic fibers in the heart decreases, resulting in rigidity. The cardiac wall stiffens. The endocardium thickens. The valves of the heart become rigid.	Cardiac output decreases; heart rate decreases and contractility of heart muscles is reduced. Cardiac reserve decreases.	Monitor patient for hypoxemia, shock, and cardiac failure. Minimize the number of stressors. Administer oxygen as needed.
In the arterial system, the concentration of collagen increases and individual fibers stiffen. The walls thicken, and calcium and cholesterol accumulate in the vascular walls.	Peripheral resistance increases and peripheral circulation decreases.	Monitor patient for signs and symptoms of thrombosis. Initiate measures for preventing venous thrombosis.
Sympathetic and parasympathetic nervous supply to heart decreases.	Ability to increase cardiac output decreases.	Monitor patient for signs and symptoms of hypotension and shock. Decrease the number of stressors and protect from falls from orthostatic hypotension.
Conduction of impulses may become blocked due to anatomic changes in conduction system and ischemia.	Interrupted conduction impulses causes dysrhythmias.	Monitor patient for signs and symptoms of cardiac dysrhythmias.
Respiratory		
Cross-linkage in collagen and elastic fibers around alveolar sacs increases; air spaces dilate; the number and size of alveolar pores increase, and lung tissue becomes less elastic.	Vital capacity of lung decreases about 25%; total lung capacity decreases minimally. Forced expiratory volumes and maximum breathing capacity decrease. Residual volume and functional residual capacity increase. Reduction in number of alveoli can result in decreased diffusion surface for oxygen and carbon dioxide.	Monitor patient's respiratory status for signs and symptoms of failure. Administer oxygen as needed. Encourage mobility, unless contraindicated.
	Blood oxygen level decreases; cerebral oxygenation decreases.	Institute patient safety measures.
	Inadequate elimination of carbon dioxide, combined with deterioration in renal and hormonal function, leads to electrolyte imbalances.	Monitor patient for electrolyte imbalances.
Costal cartilages calcify. Thoracic skeletal deformities occur, postural changes occur, and intervertebral discs of thoracic spine degenerate.	Rib mobility decreases; chest wall compliance decreases; anteroposterior diameter may increase, and the exchange of air between lungs and environment decreases.	Encourage pulmonary hygiene to prevent pulmonary infections. Monitor patient for signs and symptoms of pulmonary infection.
Muscle tone decreases as does sensitivity to stimuli.	Cough reflex diminishes.	Monitor patient for signs and symptoms of respiratory infection.
Epithelium dries and atrophies.	Ciliary mechanism becomes less effective.	Monitor patient for signs and symptoms of respiratory infection.
Neurologic		
The number of neurons decreases and they are infiltrated by lipofuscin and fat.	Losses occur in sensory functions, i.e., tactile sense decreases and pain tolerance increases. Intellectual ability remains stable.	Protect patient from pressure sores and other skin and joint damage. Talk with patient as an adult, not a child.
The nerve fibers degenerate and decrease in number.	Reaction time slows due to decrease of conduction velocity of impulse through peripheral nerves.	Institute safety measures. Give patient time to respond.

From McConnell, LC. (1987). *Clinical considerations in perioperative nursing.* JB Lippincott.

Table 22-2 Physiologic effects of aging, their significance to perioperative patients, and related nursing implications—cont'd

Changes	Significance of changes	Nursing implications
Renal		
Anatomic narrowing and loss of vessels occurs, and vasoconstriction is persistent.	Renal blood flow decreases.	Monitor patient for signs and symptoms of shock. Anesthesia and surgery significantly depress renal blood flow and glomerular filtration rate. Renal blood flow may not return to normal for 5 hours after surgery.
The amount of connective tissue between the apices of the pyramids of the kidney decreases; the number of functionally intact glomeruli diminishes.	Glomerular filtration decreases, effective plasma flow decreases, as does reabsorption time.	Monitor patient for side effects of drugs because drug excretion is often reduced.
	The ability of the kidney to form ammonia is impaired.	Monitor patient's fluid and electrolyte balance.
Gross anatomic change leads to retention and stasis of urine and loss of power to sterilize urine.	Bladder capacity decreases. The sensation of the need to void may be absent or occur only when the bladder is almost full to capacity. Urinary frequency occurs and the residual volume increases.	Monitor patient for signs and symptoms of urinary tract infection.
The prostate enlarges.	Normal urinary flow is obstructed.	Monitor patient for signs and symptoms of urinary tract infection.
Gastrointestinal		
Diminished taste buds, loss of teeth, and loss of the grinding surface of molars.	Poor appetite and inability to eat can lead to malnutrition.	Encourage intake of nutritious, appealing meals. Order soft or mechanical soft diet, as appropriate. Assist patient with meals. Monitor intake.
Hydrochloric production decreases.	Pernicious anemia develops due to absence of intrinsic factor in gastric secretions.	Monitor patient for signs and symptoms of pernicious anemia, i.e., anorexia, soreness of the tongue, and fatigue.
Gastric mobility decreases. Abdominal muscles lose elasticity.	Constipation occurs.	Encourage increased activity, fluid intake, and administer sedatives and narcotics judiciously. Monitor patient's bowel movements.
Blood flow to liver is reduced, decreasing drug detoxification.	Drug toxicity.	Be aware of effects of drugs in the elderly.
Musculoskeletal		
Bone resorption increases.	Brittleness of bone and tendency to fractures increases.	Carefully position patient on operating room table.
Muscle mass decreases.	Muscle strength, endurance, and agility decrease.	Move patient carefully and gently.
Joints degenerate.	Joints become stiff.	Carefully position patient on operating room table. Move patient carefully and gently.
Integumentary		
Epithelial cells thin, which leads to prominence of bony markings.	Risk of pressure sores increases.	Implement measures to prevent pressure sores.
Mitosis slows. Increased vascular fragility causes reduced vascularity.	Wound healing is delayed.	Promote wound healing via adequate nutrition and wound care.
Subcutaneous fatty layers thin; collagen and elastic fibers regress, and epithelial layer shrinks.	Skin becomes dry and inelastic; patient's susceptibility to cold environmental temperatures increases.	Avoid drying agents such as soaps; use lotion and moisturizers. Implement measures to prevent pressure sores. Do not use skin turgor as an indicator of hydrational status and keep the patient comfortably warm.

Table 22-2 Physiologic effects of aging, their significance to perioperative patients, and related nursing implications—cont'd

Changes	Significance of changes	Nursing implications
Sweat glands decrease in number, which prevents patient from sweating freely.	Susceptibility to heat exhaustion increases.	Monitor patient's temperature.
Melanocytes decrease	Caucasians become "more white."	Do not confuse pallor with anemia.
Sensory system		
Cochlea undergoes degenerative changes. Eardrum thickens, decreasing sound transmission.	Hearing is diminished. Difficulty hearing high-pitched sounds and gradual loss of hearing.	Speak clearly, slowly, and in a normal tone while standing in front of the patient. Shut out extraneous noise.
The elasticity of the lens decreases.	Eyesight is diminished.	Make sure patient has glasses. Focus high-intensity light on the area to be seen. Prevent patient from falling and sustaining injury.
Pupil size decreases due to increasing rigidity of the iris.	The ability to see in dim light diminishes.	Increase lighting to minimize falls. Keep a night light on in bathroom and along hallway.

Nursing implications. Because skin color may change with aging, it is not an accurate indicator of hemoglobin status. Likewise, skin turgor on the arms or extremities is not a good measure of hydration status because of the "tenting" effect that may occur normally. Examining the axillae for moisture has been suggested as one means of determining hydration status in aging persons; dry axillae are frequently correlated with dehydration (Simple assessment of dehydration in the elderly, 1994). Age-related skin changes such as thinning of epithelial layers, decreased local blood flow, and compromised thermoregulation, waste clearance, and nutrient transport put the patient at risk for skin tears, tape burns, and abrasions (Heyne, 1992); these have implications for transfer, positioning, and wound dressings with perioperative patients. Withholding oral fluids before surgery should be done with care because the aging patient is more prone to dehydration.

Aging patients are also at greater risk for developing hypothermia during the perioperative period. This can be attributed to factors such as the presence of neurologic and/or metabolic conditions including hypoglycemia, hypothyroidism, parkinsonism, and/or cerebrovascular accidents (CVAs). Both general and regional anesthesia affect thermoregulation in aging patients. Aging perioperative patients generally enter the postanesthesia care unit (PACU) with lower body temperatures and rewarm more slowly than younger patients. It is felt that this is caused by a lower intrinsic metabolic rate (Stevens, 1993) and a delayed and less intense shivering thermogenesis (Cory-Plett, 1995). An aging patient's skin may normally feel cooler because of the loss of

the protective padding of subcutaneous fat; therefore it is not a good estimator of basal temperature. The risk for impaired skin integrity should always be a nursing diagnosis of special concern for perioperative nurses, and care should be taken to prevent even seemingly minor traumas that can damage frail older skin.

Head, Neck, and Endocrine System

Physiologic changes. The same loss of bone density that leads to shortening of the spine can decrease the length of the neck and lead to a forward curvature. The carotid arteries may actually be easier to auscultate in aging patients because of the loss of subcutaneous fat. The size and shape of the head should not change as a result of the aging process.

Nursing implications. Thyroid problems, both hyperthyroidism and hypothyroidism, may have an atypical presentation in 25% to 40% of aging individuals (Rizzolo, 1992). The stress of surgery may make these abnormalities more apparent. The perioperative nurse should note any unusual cold intolerance, respiratory or blood pressure alterations, or lethargy, and he or she should carefully check relevant laboratory values contained on the medical record. Changes in the cervical spine can make intubation more difficult. Severe hyperextension can cause postoperative pain, thus the perioperative nurse should provide assistance to the anesthesia provider during the induction period.

Diabetes mellitus is a common problem with aging patients; diabetes occurs nearly 10 times more often in persons in the over-65 group than in persons in the 20- to 40-year-old group (LeMone, 1994). Pathophysiologic consequences of alterations in microcirculation and macrocirculation, impaired nerve conduction, and increased susceptibility to infection all present perioperative considerations for protecting the aging patient from injurious events. The stress of surgery often alters the insulin requirements for the aging diabetic patient, making monitoring of blood glucose levels a perioperative nursing priority.

Sensory Perceptual System

Physiologic changes. With advancing age, the lens of the eye becomes more rigid and the ciliary muscle weaker, resulting in lower visual acuity. Presbyopia (farsightedness), loss of clarity of the lens, and cataract formation are common. It is not uncommon for an aging person to have decreased pupil constriction and peripheral vision, and an increase in absolute light threshold, indicating an increase in the level of illumination necessary to see (Bates, 1991). Tear production may decrease, causing "dry eye."

Because of changes in the cochlea and hair cells, hearing loss may manifest itself initially with a loss of high-frequency tones, then progress to low-frequency tones. It is hypothesized that these same changes may also cause alterations in an aging person's sense of balance. If the tympanic membrane becomes more sclerotic and translucent, conduction hearing loss may occur. Ear cerumen may become very dry, sometimes totally obstructing the external auditory canal.

The aging patient may experience a loss of taste perception, and diminished salivation. A decline in the number of taste buds alters the sense of taste, which may lead to protein-calorie malnutrition (Blaylock, 1993). A decrease in saliva production not only can affect digestion, but can also make the mouth dry and prone to irritation from dentures or other equipment. Demineralization in the gums can lead to loss of teeth.

Nursing implications. Because many changes occur within the sensory perceptual systems of aging adults, perioperative nurses must take care to accommodate deficits. Glaring lights, shiny tile, and metallic equipment within the operating room will exacerbate an aging patient's visual problems. Likewise, before touching the patient unannounced, care should be taken to make sure that he or she can see persons approaching from either side. Protection of the eyes by lubricating and securing them with tape (in a closed position) should be done after the induction of a general anesthetic. If the patient wears a hearing aid, it should be brought to the OR to facilitate communication. Baseline assessments of pupil reaction and hearing ability should be obtained before administering anesthesia. With the insertion of airways or other equipment, a quick initial assessment of the mouth should be conducted to prevent dislodging teeth or causing injury.

Respiratory System

Physiologic changes. Significant bone mineral loss in the vertebrae may lead to "senile kyphosis," an exaggeration of normal spinal contours. This change in the curvature of the spine can also affect the respiratory system by limiting chest wall expansion. Weakening of the muscles of respiration in the chest wall and reduced effectiveness of respiratory cilia make coughing less vigorous in the aging adult. The lungs themselves undergo three changes: a decrease in elasticity, an increase in airway resistance, and a decrease in the number of functional alveoli (Seidel, et al., 1995). These changes can lead to some obvious deviations in the physical examination. Increased anteroposterior diameter, decreased respiratory excursion, and the presence of adventitious sounds in the lung bases may all be found in the older patient as a result of the aging process. In addition, Pao_2 and O_2 saturation rates are lower (Carnevali & Patrick, 1993).

Alterations in the respiratory pattern may also be found, with Cheyne-Stokes respirations normal during sleep (Bates, 1991) and a longer time needed for respirations to return to normal rates after exertion.

Nursing implications. An accurate baseline assessment of the aging patient's respiratory status is essential. The astute perioperative nurse will guarantee the availability of this information before induction to promote accurate intraoperative and postoperative monitoring. Because aging persons have an increased risk of respiratory infections, preoperative teaching on coughing and deep-breathing exercises is essential. The patient should be encouraged to practice these exercises both before surgery and during the early postoperative stage. Vigilant monitoring of oxygenation status should occur throughout the perioperative period. In the PACU, nurses should observe for confusion, often one of the signs of hypoxia in elderly individuals (Metzler & Fromm, 1993).

Breasts

Physiologic changes. In women, breasts appear pendulous, elongated, or flaccid as a result of loss of subcutaneous fat. Skin may be irritated under pendulous breasts. Men can experience gynecomastia, or enlargement of the breasts, because of changes in testosterone levels. Nipples become smaller, flatter, and less erectile. The skin may appear thin and dry, and loss of hair in the axillae may also occur.

Nursing implications. Support of the breasts and protection from injury are essential. Avoiding unnecessary exposure of the breasts in women is one way the perioperative and PACU nurses act as advocates for the aging patient.

Cardiovascular System

Physiologic changes. Because of a loss in cardiac elasticity and compliance, aging patients have a decreased resting heart rate, cardiac output, and stroke volume. Arterial walls also lose elasticity, and vasomotor tone and their lumen may be altered by either arteriosclerosis or atherosclerosis, thus increasing peripheral vascular resistance. Both systolic and diastolic blood pressure and pulse pressure may increase. In general, the heart does not tolerate stress as well and takes longer to return to baseline levels after exertion. The risk of developing dysrhythmias increases with age. Electrocardiographic changes include decreases in amplitude and lengthening of intervals (Carnevali & Patrick, 1993). Suspected changes in pain threshold may make an aging person's response to angina atypical.

Nursing implications. It is the perioperative nurse's responsibility to assess and validate baseline heart rate and blood pressure readings of aging patients and to monitor for subsequent changes. New dysrhythmias should be a sign for concern, as with any age group. Opinions differ on when to treat blood pressure elevations, because dropping the elevated blood pressure of an aging patient to normotensive levels can sometimes result in compromised cerebral circulation.

During the immediate postoperative period, attention should be paid to the relationship between position and blood pressure, because postural hypotension is more common in aged individuals.

Circulatory System

Physiologic changes. In general, the circulatory system is less efficient, creating a tendency for blood to pool in the extremities and an inclination toward dizziness and fainting during position changes. Although the loss of subcutaneous fat may make arteries and veins more prominent, pulses may be less palpable because of alterations in circulation. Vascular disease is not unusual, but it may be undetected because of the gradual changes that occur. The legs are a prime site for such problems. Hair growth, which slows with the aging process, may be markedly diminished or absent on the lower extremities.

Nursing implications. Patency in peripheral pulses should be documented in the patient's medical record. Preoperative teaching should include flexion and extension exercises for the lower extremities and general weight shifting to reduce the risk of postoperative thrombi or embolus. Prevention of injury to the extremities is also an important periop-

erative nursing responsibility during transfer and positioning maneuvers.

Gastrointestinal and Genitourinary Systems

Physiologic changes. Gastrointestinal changes are both general and specific. Overall atrophy and the loss of strength and tone of muscle tissue and supporting structures cause reduced gastrointestinal motility. Diminished secretion of gastric acid and changes in neurosensory feedback also affect the digestive process. Older patients may have related problems with flatulence, heartburn, indigestion, and feelings of abdominal or epigastric discomfort.

The abdomen may be more rounded because of a loss of muscle tone and also may have more fat deposition, despite fat loss in other areas of the body, such as the extremities. The decreased intestinal motility associated with aging may lead to complaints of constipation. Gastrointestinal carcinomas increase in incidence with age, yet pain may be less severe or absent in the same disease conditions that would elicit pain in a younger person. Intestinal obstruction or diverticulitis may also be problems with aging patients. Particular attention needs to be paid to patient complaints and related findings with regard to defining possible intestinal disorders.

Hypertrophy of the liver and atrophy of the kidney may occur, with the latter showing a marked decrease in function because of reduced numbers of functional nephrons. Bladder capacity is decreased by half, and loss of muscle integrity leads to incomplete emptying. Furthermore, the elderly patient may be unaware of the need to void. Incontinence, although not a normal consequence of aging, can be more common in aging women who have borne children and in older men with prostatic disease. Nocturia is another alteration in urinary function frequently reported in the later years.

Sexual changes. A number of age-specific changes in the reproductive system manifest themselves in both physical integrity and function. In men, the size of the prostate increases, the concentration of testosterone decreases, and the force and volume of ejaculation also decrease. The scrotum becomes more pendulous, pubic alopecia may occur, and erection develops more slowly.

Aging female patients experience a narrowing and shortening of the vagina, with accompanying diminished vaginal lubrication. The labia majora become flatter, and pubic hair turns gray and becomes more sparse. Atrophic vaginitis is not uncommon, a result of a thinning of the vaginal walls and a reduction in estrogen production.

Nursing implications. As a result of overall declines in gastrointestinal function, bowel sounds and the abdomen need to be assessed postoperatively. Medications may be poorly tolerated in normal doses because of a reduction in kidney function. Because the BUN level tends to rise in the later years, perioperative nurses should rely on the creatinine clearance test as a better measure of kidney function and screen anesthetics and other medications for potential nephrotoxicity (Carnevali & Patrick, 1993). The integrity of urinary function should be assessed preoperatively and postoperatively.

Because of the friability of tissue, gynecologic procedures may produce bleeding, irritation of mucosa, or both if a vaginal approach is used. Concerns related to sexual function need to be discussed openly with both male and female patients. Unless the normalcy of some of the physiologic changes that affect sexuality are understood, grave concerns about sexual activity may go undiscussed by the aging patient.

Musculoskeletal System

Physiologic changes. Loss of calcium leads to increased porosity and erosion of bones, making aging persons less able to tolerate stress on bones and increasing the risk of fractures. Joints are similarly affected, with deterioration at articulating surfaces and supportive structures. Joints most frequently affected are the hips, knees, hands, and lower spine. A majority of aging persons experience some degree of osteoarthritis, caused by natural bone demineralization, leading to frequent complaints of joint stiffness, soreness, and lack of joint flexibility and endurance. The first and most characteristic sign is pain in the weight-bearing joint. Although the spine may be involved, the hip and knee are primary sites. In the hip, range of motion is limited (especially internal rotation), and pain and crepitation are experienced during movement. Irregular enlargement of the bones of the joint, pain, and crepitation on movement may also be present in the knees.

In general, the muscular system is affected by loss of cell mass and muscle size, although previous levels of physical fitness may alter this process. Loss of muscle mass is usually associated with loss of muscle strength, tone, speed of movements, and endurance. Tasks take longer to complete, and muscle reflexes are less efficient. These changes in physical capability may induce the aging patient to reduce physical activity to preserve strength and functioning; this may further exacerbate effects on the musculoskeletal system. Kyphosis, with a compensation flexion of the hips and knees, may be noticeable. The stance is often broad based, and patients may need to hold their arms away from the body to achieve balance (Carnevali & Patrick, 1993).

Osteoporosis, which occurs more frequently in white and Asian postmenopausal women, may manifest itself in fractures of the wrist, vertebrae, and hip. Osteoporosis represents a category of disorders characterized by a loss of bone mass. Before actual injury, the decrease in bone density may cause a persistent, nonradiating pain at the affected site.

Nursing implications. The fragility of an aging person's skeletal system warrants extra care during the perioperative period. Special attention should be paid to preventing sudden or sharp movements during transfers or positioning, because these could fracture or injure frail bones. Body alignment that promotes comfort also requires perioperative nurses' attention in the operating room and PACU. Prolonged lying on narrow stretchers can aggravate the discomfort of arthritis; therefore the patient's comfort level should be assessed frequently, and measures to enhance comfort in positioning should be taken routinely with aging patients.

Central Nervous System

Physiologic changes. Concomitant with aging is a decrease in conduction velocity of some nerves, leading to delayed response and reaction times. Many neurologic changes associated with aging are part of the chronologic process, involving diminished reaction times, reduced motor skill ability, and age-related memory deficiencies. Degenerative losses in the receptor sites of the peripheral nervous system are thought to diminish sensitivity to pain. It should be noted that little research exists concerning pain in the elderly. Some decline occurs in tactile sensitivity, which affects the ability to localize and respond to stimuli. Difficulties with kinesthetic sense may lead to a pattern of increased stumbling, falls, or decreased agility. Tremors, which are exacerbated by anxiety, may develop. Many of these changes are gradual, minimal, or remedial, and individual differences and the role of environmental stresses may exacerbate them. From a general neurologic standpoint, there is less ability to adapt to alterations in the environment.

Deterioration of intellectual function is not common; however, losses in short-term memory do occur in the later years. Medications can also interfere with central nervous system function, causing slowed reaction time, disorientation, confusion, loss of memory, tremors, and anxiety. Alzheimer's disease increases proportionately with age, leading to behavioral manifestations such as agitation and inappropriate behavior (Antai-Otong, 1993).

Crystallized intelligence, which is derived from lifelong knowledge, remains stable, but fluid intelligence, the ability to abstract and learn new information, shows a decline. However, adjusted teaching strategies frequently can offset these changes.

What the patient already knows (crystallized intelligence) should be determined and teaching started at this point, with new information linked to old by following it with what is already known (Theis & Merritt, 1994). Senility or confusion is not a normal consequence of the aging process and should always be investigated carefully. Cognitive impairment is marked by impaired short- and long-term memory, personality changes, lack of initiative, and impaired performance and level of functioning; seeming confusion may actually be depression, anxiety, or related to medication (Antai-Otong, 1993). Of special concern is the appearance of new confusion, because in aging persons this can be a sign of an underlying disease process, such as dementia or delirium (Kane & Kurlowicz, 1994). However, a recent study of postoperative medications identified that patients given meperidine (especially by an epidural route) or benzodiazepines (particularly those that are long acting) were three times more likely to become delirious after surgery than patients not given these medications (Marcantonio, Juarez, & Goldman, 1994). These researchers suggested around-the-clock dosing with acetaminophen or nonsteroidal antiinflammatory agents to reduce narcotic requirements while maintaining adequate analgesia in aging patients.

Nursing implications. Perioperative nurses must take care to allow older persons adequate time to respond to environmental stimuli. Rushing aging patients or ignoring them can increase stress and further impair the ability to respond. Likewise, sudden, unexpected stimuli, such as touching the patient without speaking first, should be avoided. Careful assessment of the aging patient's mental status should be undertaken preoperatively so that accurate evaluation is available postoperatively. Confusion should not be considered "normal," but should be seen as a symptom of other underlying problems that warrant investigation.

Although little research exists regarding pain control in the aging population, many misconceptions continue to abound.

Misconception: Pain is a natural part of aging.

Reality: Although aging persons are at greater risk for developing disorders that may result in pain, the presence of pain is not inevitable with aging.

Misconception: Sensitivity to pain decreases with age.

Reality: The research that has been done in this area does not consistently substantiate this claim. The aging person may experience atypical presentations of pain, but this cannot be generalized for all conditions.

Misconception: Narcotics are too dangerous to give to the aging patient.

Reality: Careful monitoring of the response to pain medications, including narcotics, is essential. Dosages and time intervals need to be carefully titrated so that pain relief is achieved.

Misconception: If the aging person does not complain, he or she does not have pain.

Reality: People may not acknowledge pain for a variety of reasons, including fear of appearing weak, fear of losing decision-making control, and fear of becoming addicted to medications (McCaffery & Beebe, 1989).

Cognitively impaired aging persons present a challenge to the health care team in regard to pain reporting and control. Astute assessment of pain with attention to physical and other nonverbal cues is a skill the perioperative nurse needs to develop. The most common pain control intervention is the use of medications (Thomas, 1990). Physiologic changes that occur with aging affect the distribution, metabolism, and excretion of medications, making it a challenge to predict a patient's response to a particular pharmacologic pain agent. Pain medications should be encouraged in the postoperative period, because a preventive approach will help relieve pain before it becomes too severe. Careful titration of dosages and appropriate use of adjuvant analgesic therapy for each individual is imperative if pain control without harmful side effects is to be achieved. Nonpharmacologic interventions such as relaxation or music therapy should also be attempted.

Functional Ability and Self-Care

In summary, a number of normal age-related changes can affect individuals during their later years. Assessment of these changes and their effect on health status is a perioperative nursing responsibility of utmost priority. Most important, however, is not the number of changes present, but an evaluation of their effect on the individual's everyday existence. Most aging adults seek to preserve independence while adapting to the aging process. Studies have been conducted to investigate the relationship between self-concept and self-care (Smits & Kee, 1992). A significant correlation was found between functional health status and self-concept. Functional health status represents one's ability to fulfill roles and be involved in his or her environment. Despite the presence of at least one chronic condition in 80% of noninstitutionalized aging persons, the majority of people 65 and older describe their health as good or excellent (Carnevali & Patrick, 1993). Functional health can be viewed as a component of self-care. Aging increases self-care demands and their complexity. Orem's (1991) theory of self-care is based on the premise that adults have the right and responsibility to care for themselves to maintain rational life and health. Components of the model include self-care agency, therapeutic self-care demands, self-care deficits, and nursing agency. Self-care agency is the ability of an individual to engage in those activities necessary to maintain and promote healthy patterns of behavior. Therapeutic self-care demands refer to the measures to be done by or for an individual to achieve better health. Self-care deficits exist when therapeutic self-care demands exceed self-care agency. Nursing agency is used to intervene in response to identified self-care deficits (Smits & Kee, 1992).

Perioperative nurses can enhance the well-being of their aging patients by ensuring that they possess the knowledge and competence necessary to engage in health-promoting, self-care activities. Preoperative and postoperative instruction regarding activities, limitations, medications, and wound management help provide patients with a sense of control and responsibility for their own health. The patient's wishes and values regarding treatment options and the meaning of a high-quality life should be ascertained. The perioperative nurse should ask the patient about an advance directive, such as a living will or durable power of attorney. These sensitive questions can be posed by asking questions suggested by Bosek and Baker (1995): "If you were unable to make your own decisions, is there someone who best understands your beliefs and values about your care and could discuss your beliefs during decision making?" Patients deserve to be allowed to share and make known their beliefs and values, and these need to be considered when designing plans of care.

PERIOPERATIVE TEACHING

For aging patients, perioperative teaching requires modification of traditional approaches. The variety of sensory perceptual changes that occur with aging may make the use of audiovisual materials impossible or inappropriate. A one-to-one approach is recommended in conjunction with a quiet, private environment conducive to effective communication. Because families are the chief source of out-of-hospital care for elderly persons, important caregiver family members should be included in processes of patient education. Assessing the patient's ability to see and hear, and his or her previous experience with surgery, is an important first step in the teaching process. Obtaining frequent feedback on key teaching points is essential throughout the process. Demonstration and rehearsal of techniques, such as coughing and deep-breathing techniques, and frequent reminders to practice these, will facilitate the aging individual's ability to retain this information.

In an analysis of teaching practices for aging patients, Theis and Merritt (1994) identified the following preferences: a structured teaching session, use of visual material to enhance content taught, detailed rather than general information, individual rather than group settings for men, the affiliation of a group for women, a close relationship with the one teaching, and a high preference for the teacher to be a figure of authority with expertise.

In a study of aging patients' discharge experience, Congdon (1994) identified incongruities in the discharge process that caused struggles for patients and their families. Four essential areas of problematic categories emerged: (1) readiness for discharge (patients were ready but families were not); (2) family support (families supported patients, but perceived no support for themselves); (3) decision making (patients and families felt they were not involved); and (4) multidisciplinary teams (both patients and families experienced confusion and distress by the lack of coordination among providers). Perioperative nurses, especially those who provide care to aging patients in ambulatory settings, need to carefully consider standards for discharge preparation and initiate efforts to evaluate and improve them. This implies, in part, strong advocacy roles for aging patients and their families.

NURSING ROLES

The human body is remarkably made, with each organ system having a reserve capacity with a wide range of adaptive responses. This adaptive ability to meet stressors diminishes with age, especially in the old-old (older than 85 years). This results in a narrower range in homeostasis, which can be quickly compromised in the presence of psychophysiologic insults to the person. An operative experience can make these changes visible very quickly in the aging patient (Carnevali & Patrick, 1993).

Although surgical intervention for many previously fatal disease processes holds great promise for aging patients, safe surgical outcomes depend on the collaboration of the surgical team. The astute perioperative nurse who is aware of the special risks an aging patient is subject to is in the best position to plan for collaborative perioperative care in an effort to prevent or minimize complications. Perioperative nurses who are aware of the changes of aging that may alter the surgical course for aging patients can implement a variety of preventive actions. For example, knowing that pulmonary complications are the most common cause of postoperative death in the elderly, the perioperative nurse will take special care to monitor respiratory status and promote oxygenation in aging patients. Likewise, perioperative nurses who are concerned with the well-being of aging surgical patients will take action to protect their dignity and self-worth throughout the surgical experience. Through these interventions, the optimal health status of aging patients will be promoted, and perioperative nurses will act in accord with professional standards and ethics. The perioperative nurse needs to develop a comprehensive approach to the increasing numbers of aging patients who will be cared for in the perioperative practice settings of tomorrow.

LOOKING AT THE FUTURE

The National Institute on Aging (NIA) of the National Institutes of Health was established by Congress in 1974. The NIA has been given responsibility for "biomedical, social, and behavioral research and training related to the aging process and diseases and other special problems and needs of the aged" (HSR Reports, 1988). To meet this responsibility, NIA has a broad, multidisciplinary research agenda.

Behavioral and social research programs primarily support investigations into the social and behavioral aspects of aging. This program includes research foci that examine relationships between formal health care services and the physiologic, social, and psychologic aspects of aging, provider-patient behaviors and interactions, long-term institutional care of the elderly, institutional and noninstitutional care needs, and aspects of care for Alzheimer's patients and their caregivers.

Research topics of interest in adult psychologic development include the diverse influences of aging on cognitive function, personality, attitudes, and interpersonal relations over the entire life course. Social science research addresses the social conditions that influence health, well-being, and functioning in the middle and later years.

Health-related behaviors and attitudes of both aging patients and their families and significant others are important components of these research efforts. Much of the work of the NIA will help health caregivers to describe and know the evolving aging society in this country and to set the basis for examination of research issues for the future.

According to George (described in Gueldner, 1994), barriers persist in health care provisions to older adults; she notes that, although some improvement in access to care has been realized, older adults often obtain health care of poorer quality and with more delay than younger adults. The 1995 White House Conference on Aging had six primary purposes (ANA, 1995):

1. To increase public awareness of the interdependence of generations and the essential contributions of older individuals to society for the well-being of all generations.

Table 22-3 Possible alterations in laboratory reference values for the aged

Name of test	Possible change in value
Alkaline phosphatase	Increase
Amylase	Increase
Antinuclear antibodies (ANA)	May be present
Blood sugar, fasting and 2 hr pc	Increase
Blood urea nitrogen (BUN)	Increase
C_3C_4	Increase
Calcium	May lower, but this is not well documented?
Cholesterol	Increase until after 70
Cold agglutinins	Increase
Creatinine clearance	Decrease
Glucose tolerance test (GTT)	Change in curve
Gonadotropins (LH, FSH)	Eventually decrease, but increase postmenopausal
Immunoglobulins	Decreases and alterations
Lymphocytes	May decrease
17-ketosteroids	Decrease
PO_2	Decrease
Phosphorus	May lower with age
Pregnanediol	Decrease in women
Rheumatic factor (RF)	May be present
Sedimentation rate (ESR)	Increase
T_3 RIA	Decrease?
Triglycerides	Increase except very elderly
Transaminases (SGOT, SGPT)	Slight increase
Uric acid	Slightly higher values
Venereal Disease Research Laboratory (VDRL)	May become reactive?

From Corbett JV. (1987). *Laboratory tests and diagnostic procedures with nursing diagnoses.* Appleton & Lange.
Note that the effect of age on many tests is not known. The figures used for normals may sometimes be more reflective of the common underlying chronic diseases of the elderly rather than of a normal healthy stage. For example, hypertension affects many elderly clients, and it can cause some renal changes that in turn can change the values of various laboratory tests.

2. To identify the problems facing older individuals and the commonalities of the problems with problems of younger generations.
3. To examine the well-being of older individuals including the impact that wellness of older individuals has on our society.
4. To develop such specific and comprehensive recommendations for executive and legislative action as may be appropriate for maintaining and improving the well-being of the aging.
5. To develop recommendations for the coordination of federal policy with state and local needs and the implementation of such recommendations.

Box 22-4 Nursing Diagnoses Pertinent to the Aging Patient

Activity intolerance
Airway clearance, ineffective
Anxiety
Body image disturbance
Breathing pattern, ineffective
Cardiac output, decreased
Communication, impaired verbal
Constipation
Coping, ineffective individual
Diversional activity deficit
Fatigue
Gas exchange, impaired
Grieving, anticipatory
Health maintenance, altered
Health seeking behaviors (specify)
Incontinence (may be functional, stress, total, or urge)
Injury, risk for (related to perioperative events)
Knowledge deficit (related to perioperative events)
Mobility, impaired physical
Noncompliance (specify)

Nutrition, altered (likely to be less than body requirements)
Oral mucousmembrane, altered
Pain (may be chronic)
Personal identity disturbance
Powerlessness
Role performance, altered
Self-care deficit(s)
Self-esteem disturbance
Sensory/perceptual alteration (specify) (visual, auditory, kinesthetic, gustatory, tactile, olfactory)
Sexual dysfunction
Skin integrity, impaired
Skin integrity, impaired, risk for
Sleep pattern disturbance
Social isolation
Tissue perfusion, altered (specify type) (renal, cerebral, cardiopulmonary, gastrointestinal, peripheral)
Urinary elimination, altered patterns
Violence, risk for: self-directed or directed at others

---

6. To review the status and multigenerational value of recommendations adopted at the previous White House Conferences on Aging.

Clearly, further legislative and social policy will continue to examine the aging population and their health care needs. Perioperative nurses and their colleagues are already caring for an aging patient population, and there is much more information nurses need in order to provide effective, cost-efficient, high-quality care now and in the future.

CARE PLAN

Aging patients present a special challenge when organizing information from a history and physical to plan perioperative patient care. The interrelationship of physiologic and psychosocial dimensions has to be considered carefully. Laboratory values, which are one of the sources of data about the aging patient, may be altered. Whereas the effect of age on many laboratory values is not known, there are some indications that values change with age; these are summarized in Table 22-3.

Sensory losses, in terms of both perception and reception, need to be assessed. Sufficient time must be allotted for the patient to understand and comply with nursing requests. Explanations need to be offered slowly, may need to be repeated, and should be articulated clearly. Hearing loss may be present, which requires modifications of the speaking voice, or a hearing aid may need to accompany the patient to the OR. Significant others should be included in perioperative teaching activities. Impaired visual

perception may distort the patient's view of the OR or the ability to see what the nurse is demonstrating. Assistance may need to be provided because of impaired vision or limitations in mobility. Mobility limitations become critical indicators when planning safe transfer and surgical positioning. Fragile, dry, thin skin needs to be protected. Multiple nursing diagnoses may be derived in the care planning process (Box 22-4). These nursing diagnoses have been identified by known physiologic and psychosocial effects or through selected validation studies. They are not all-inclusive and are only selectively applicable to the individual patient.

In developing a generic care plan for aging patients, the perioperative nurse must recognize that the heterogeneity of the aging population makes it important to consider individual differences. The generic care plan offered here is based on some of the fairly universal characteristics that these patients bring to the perioperative settings. These characteristics challenge the knowledge and skills of the perioperative nurse when planning for a perioperative experience that is safe, effective, and individualized for the patient. The American Nurses Association (1987) has identified the following important elements of gerontologic nursing practice and the role of the nurse at the generalist level:

Gerontologic nursing practice involves assessing the health and functional status of older adults, planning and providing appropriate nursing and other health care services, and evaluating the effectiveness of such care.

Emphasis is placed on maximizing functional ability in the activities of daily living; promoting, maintaining, and restoring health, including mental health; preventing and minimizing the disabilities of acute and chronic illness; and maintaining life in dignity and comfort until death. Gerontologic nursing may be practiced in any setting, for example, the nursing home, the hospital, the client's home, the clinic, and the community. Gerontologic nursing focuses on the client and family (in this document, the term "family" refers to family members and significant others).

The generalist is involved in direct patient care in a variety of settings. The professional nurse who practices as a generalist is expected to develop, implement, and evaluate the plan of care for the aging patient. This plan of care should be established in collaboration with the patient and family and based on a recognition of age-related changes that affect the patient physiologically, culturally, socially, psychologically, and spiritually.

Familiarity with this statement can help the perioperative nurse establish desired outcomes of patient care. The generic care plan and the Guide to Nursing Actions that follow are only a small part of the interdisciplinary effort required for applying the existing body of knowledge about gerontology to perioperative nursing practice.

GUIDE TO NURSING ACTIONS
Care Plan for The Aging Patient (Fig. 22-1)

1. Assessment data should include physical, psychosocial, cultural, and spiritual status, results of functional assessment, communication patterns, coping patterns, and results of laboratory and diagnostic studies.

2. The sequence of perioperative events should be explained to the patient (and family if teaching is conducted before admission to the OR). Describe any sensory stimulation the patient will receive. Use common, basic teaching and communication skills. Explanation decreases anxiety. Use touch, realistic verbal reassurance, and eye contact during explanations.

3. Dentures, partial plates, and so forth may accompany the aging patient to the OR to reduce discomfort regarding physical appearance. These may be removed in the OR for anesthesia induction or in case of the need to intubate the awake patient. Follow institutional protocol for disposition of patient's belongings.

4. Aging patients often experience auditory alterations. Hearing aids may accompany the patient to the OR to diminish the potential for sensory/perceptual disturbance and to allow the patient to hear explanations and cooperate with requests. Follow institutional protocol for dispo-

sition of hearing aids once anesthesia has been induced. Otherwise, the hearing aid should remain in place.

5. Aging patients often experience visual perceptual deficits. Interference with clear vision or ability to see is confusing and potentially dangerous. Eye glasses or lenses may be present before induction to compensate for potential sensory/perceptual alterations. Follow institutional protocol for disposition of glasses or lenses immediately before induction of anesthesia.

6. The potential for decreased physical mobility increases with aging. The perioperative nurse will need to help the patient compensate for mobility limitations, decreased muscle tone and strength, limited range of motion and flexibility in joints, and impaired coordination. Spatial relationships are often impaired; this presents the potential for untoward outcomes (falls) during transfer procedures. The patient will need assistance, guidance, and supervision when moving to or from the OR bed.

7. Careful positioning is extremely important. Assist the patient into good body alignment. Although all of the patient's joints are susceptible to the structural changes of aging, the hip, knee, and ankle are most frequently affected. There may be only partial flexion in these joints. Elevation of the head of the OR bed, pillows placed close to the popliteal space but not directly under the knee, or elevation of the foot of the OR bed may assist with the safe positioning of joints. A footboard should be applied, especially where a footdrop already exists, to keep the weight of the drapes off the feet. Pressure is most severe in body areas over bony prominences; pad these carefully. Shearing force and friction are mechanical factors implicated in pressure sore formation. Shearing forces occur when tissue layers slide on one another, causing the subcutaneous vessels to kink or stretch; blood flow is consequently interrupted. During positioning and positional changes, move the patient carefully, lifting rather than sliding or pulling.

8. Aging patients are more susceptible to changes in temperature. Provide warm blankets, thermia unit, forced-air warmers, reflective blankets, or other devices to maintain normothermia. Expose only that portion of the patient's body surface that is necessary during skin preparation procedures.

9. Factors that contribute to impaired skin integrity in the aging patient include decreased activity, immobility, incontinence, poor nutritional

FIG. 22-1
CARE PLAN FOR THE AGING PATIENT

KEY ASSESSMENT POINTS

Functional
  Adaptation to current status
  Limitations in mobility
  Medications (include over-the-counter)
  Patterns of sleep/rest
  Home care ability/needs
Physical
  Skin integrity
  Nutritional status
  Problems with elimination
  Consequences of physiologic aging processes (review systems)
  Sensory alterations (communication, vision, hearing, taste, smell, kinesthetic)
Psychosocial status
  Cognitive status
  Family support
  Understanding of planned perioperative events, learning needs
Spiritual/cultural/religious/ethnic values/beliefs/needs

NURSING DIAGNOSIS:

All generic nursing diagnoses apply to this patient, with the addition of:
Risk for injury related to perioperative events
Risk for impaired skin integrity.
Knowledge deficit related to perioperative events

PATIENT OUTCOMES:

All generic outcomes apply, with the addition of:
The patient will be free of injury during the perioperative period.
Skin integrity will be maintained.
The patient and family will be able to describe perioperative events.
The patient will:
1. Not fall, sustain injury, or have any tingling sensations, numbness, edema, cramping, pain, ache, or swelling in joints that was not present preoperatively.
2. Have no pressure sores or other impairments to skin integrity that were not present preoperatively.
3. Be able to describe anticipated perioperative events.

NURSING ACTIONS

	Yes	No	N/A
1. Preoperative assessment performed?	☐	☐	☐
2. Preoperative teaching performed?	☐	☐	☐
3. Dentures removed?	☐	☐	☐
4. Hearing aid to OR?	☐	☐	☐
5. Eye glasses/lenses to OR?	☐	☐	☐
6. Assistance provided during patient transfer?	☐	☐	☐
7. Patient positioned carefully?	☐	☐	☐
8. Warm blankets/extra covering provided?	☐	☐	☐
9. Skin integrity assessed?	☐	☐	☐
10. External stimuli reduced?	☐	☐	☐
11. Antiembolism stockings applied?	☐	☐	☐
12. ESU pad site checked?	☐	☐	☐
13. Irrigating solutions warmed?	☐	☐	☐
14. Tissue handled carefully?	☐	☐	☐
15. Nonirritating tape used?	☐	☐	☐
16. Other generic care plans initiated? (specify)	☐	☐	☐

Document additional nursing actions/generic care plans initiated here:

_____

_____

_____

EVALUATION OF PATIENT OUTCOMES

	Outcome met	Outcome met with additional outcome criteria	OUtcome met with revised nursing care plan	Outcome not met	Outcome not applicable to this patient
1. The patient was free of musculoskeletal injury/limitations that were not present preoperatively.	☐	☐	☐	☐	☐
2. The patient's skin remained intact.	☐	☐	☐	☐	☐
3. The patient/family described perioperative events.	☐	☐	☐	☐	☐
4. The patient met outcomes for additional generic care plans as indicated.	☐	☐	☐	☐	☐

Signature: _____ Date: _____

status, presence of chronic disease states, fever, and infection. Assess the skin for rashes, erythema, lesions, pressure sores, or any disruption of skin layers, especially over sacrum, ischial tuberosities, trochanter area of the leg, heel, and the malleolus of the ankle. Document findings. If a pressure sore is present, note size, depth, and amount and color of any exudate; presence of pain; odor; and color of exposed tissue.

10. External stimuli interfere with sensory perception. Keep the OR lights off until it is necessary to illuminate the operative site. Keep extraneous conversation to a minimum so the patient can hear communications directed to him or her. Only one person should communicate with the patient at a time. Speak slowly and carefully; many aging patients compensate for hearing loss by lip reading. OR masks interfere with this compensatory mechanism. Use short sentences. Present one thought at a time; pause to allow the patient to respond.

11. Aging patients have an increased risk for thrombophlebitis. Antiembolism stockings or sequential compression hose may be used, depending on risk factors and anticipated operating time.

12. In placing the electrosurgical unit (ESU) dispersive pad, select a site that has an adequate amount of underlying tissue.

13. Warmed irrigating solutions help maintain normothermia.

14. The scrub nurse or registered nurse first assistant should handle all tissue carefully. Aging patients have a reduced vascular supply, with an accompanying reduction in ability to heal and regenerate tissue.

15. Aging patients often have frail and fragile skin. A minimal amount of a nonirritating tape should be used on the dressing. If a large amount of tape is needed, Montgomery straps should be considered.

SUMMARY

The aging patient who is in need of perioperative care may be frail elderly or functionally and physiologically well; chronically ill or experiencing an episodic dysfunction requiring surgical intervention. These patients represent both a challenge and diversity of perioperative nursing considerations. Possible effects of physiologic aging are not unilateral effects; aging patients do not fit into tight diagnostic categories and treatment regimens. Many aging patients characteristically are hardy, resilient, and have great emotional and attitudinal endurance. They require careful perioperative nursing assessment and planning to prevent potentially common problems. In providing this care, both perioperative nurses and their interdisciplinary team colleagues are well reminded that "sick old people are sick because they are sick, not because they are old."

References

American Nurses Association. (1987). *Standards of gerontologic nursing practice.* Washington, DC: The Association.

American Nurses Association. (1995). *Report to the House of Delegates on the White House Conference on Aging.* Washington, DC: The Association.

Antai-Otong, D. (1993). Cognitive and affective assessment of the geriatric patient. *Medsurg Nursing, 2*(1), 70-74.

Bates B. (1991). *A guide to physical examination and history taking.* (5th ed.). Philadelphia: JB Lippincott.

Blaylock B. (1993). Factors contributing to protein-calorie malnutrition in older adults. *Medsurg Nursing, 2*(5), 397-401.

Bosek MS & Baker TPH. (1995). Commentary: Rationing trauma care to the elderly. *Medsurg Nursing, 4*(3), 217-219.

Capriotti T. (1995). Unrecognized depression in the elderly: A nursing assessment challenge. *Medsurg Nursing, 4*(1), 47-54.

Carnevali D & Patrick M. (1993). Nursing management for the elderly. (3rd ed.). Philadelphia: JB Lippincott.

Congdon JG. (1994). Managing the incongruities: The hospital discharge experience for elderly patients, their families, and nurses. *Applied Nursing Research, 7*(3), 125-131.

Cory-Plett P. (1995). Special considerations of the elderly patient requiring anesthesia. *Canadian Operating Room Nursing Journal, 13*(1), 20-28.

Eliopoulos C. (1995). *Manual of gerontologic nursing.* St. Louis: Mosby.

Gueldner S. (1994). Complex clinical problems within the context of aging. *Reflections, 20*(3), 12.

Heyne C. (1992). Wound care in the elderly. *Reflections, 18*(4), 8.

National Institute on Aging. (1988). *How to keep current.* HSR Reports Washington DC.

Institute of Medicine. (1990). *The second fifty years: Promoting health and preventing disability.* Washington, DC: National Academy Press.

Kane AM & Kurlowicz LH. (1994). Improving the postoperative care of acutely confused older adults. *Medsurg Nursing, 3*(6), 453-458.

LeMone P. (1994). Responses of the older adult to the effects and management of diabetes mellitus. *Medsurg Nursing, 3*(2), 122-126.

Marcantonio ER, Juarez G & Goldman L. (1994). The relationship of postoperative delirium with psychoactive medications. *Journal of the American Medical Association, 272*(9), 1518-1522.

McCaffery M & Beebe A. (1989). *Pain: Clinical manual for nursing practice.* St. Louis: Mosby–Year Book.

Metzler DJ & Fromm CG. (1993). Laying out a plan of care for the elderly postoperative patient. *Nursing 93, 93*(4), 67-74.

Mikulencak M. (1993). The graying of America—changing what nurses need to know. *American Nurse, 25*(7), 1, 12.

Orem D. (1991). *Nursing: Concepts of practice* (4th ed.). St. Louis: Mosby–Year Book.

Pierce JR. (1995). Rationing trauma care to the elderly: An ethical dilemma. *Medsurg Nursing, 4*(3), 189-192, 215.

Rizzolo P. (1992). Thyroid. In R Ham & P Sloane (Eds.). *Primary care geriatrics* (2nd ed.). St. Louis: Mosby.

Rybash J, Roodin P, & Santrock J. (1991). *Adult development and aging* (2nd ed.). Dubuque, IA: WC Brown.

Seidel HM, et al. (1995). *Mosby's guide to physical examination* (3rd ed.). St. Louis: Mosby.

Simple assessment of dehydration in the elderly. (1994). *Nurse Extra, 11*(21), 5.

Smits M & Kee C. (1992). Correlations of self-care among the independent elderly: Self-concept affects well being. *Journal of Gerontological Nursing, 18*(9), 13-18.

Stevens T. (1993). Managing postoperative hypothermia, rewarming, and its complications. *Critical Care Nursing Quarterly, 16*(1), 60-77.

Theis SL & Merritt SL. (1994). A learning model to guide research and practice for teaching of elder clients. *Nursing & Health Care, 15*(9), 464-468.

Thomas B. (1990). Pain management for the elderly: Alternative interventions. *AORN Journal, 52,* 1268-1272.

Tortora G & Grabowski S. (1993). *Principles of anatomy & physiology* (7th ed). New York: Harper Collins.

Chapter 23

Multiculturally Diverse Clients

Gloria J. McNeal
Elizabeth Wing Kee Gonzalez
Elizabeth Petit de Mange
Iris Gautier Perez

It was told to me by our forefathers that we should never move east of the Rio Grande or west of the San Juan River. I thought at one time that the whole world was the same as my country, but I got fooled in it. Outside my own country we cannot raise a crop, our families and stock there increase, here they decrease, we know this land does not like us.

NAVAJO TREATY, 1868

Nurses have been and continue to be concerned with providing culturally specific and culturally sensitive care to culturally, racially, and ethnically diverse groups of people. As early as the 1960s, the Division of Nursing of the U.S. Department of Health supported nurses obtaining doctoral degrees in anthropology; Leininger, a nurse anthropologist, formalized the study and practice of the field of transcultural nursing in the 1980s (Outlaw, 1994). Recognizing the importance of understanding cultural diversity as one of the elements in reforming the health care system, the American Academy of Nursing (AAN) convened an expert panel on culturally competent nursing care in 1992. Part of the purpose of this panel was to identify issues affecting the provision of sensitive and competent nursing care; to examine research, education, and care delivery strategies and models that reflect the provision of that care; and to set a research and education agenda that would move the nursing profession forward in its mission to provide culturally competent care (AAN, 1992). Certainly perioperative nurses are aware of the change in demographics in the United States. The heterogeneity of perioperative populations is increasing. Like their nursing colleagues, perioperative nurses need to continue to become informed and sensitive to the cultural differences of the clients for whom they design and provide care (Gioiella, 1994). Those who practice, teach, and research the specialty of perioperative nursing must find innovative ways to recognize the diversities and complexities created by cultural heritage, race, and ethnicity. As we expand the philosophical basis of providing care, new opportunities will embrace culturally diverse populations who have historically been limited in their access to health care (Jezewski, 1993; Porter & Villarruel, 1993). Marketplace reforms, with their focus on cost containment and out-of-hospital care, will reposition the geographic location of the traditional perioperative practice setting.

A more community-based focus will take emergent tertiary health care delivery services to more accessible sites: same-day surgicenters, birthing rooms, free-standing invasive diagnostic laboratories, etc. Indeed, fiberoptic and telecommunication technologies will link inaccessible rural and inner city areas to large health care educational complexes and bring the latest technologic methodologies to the most remote regions of the nation. To address urgent care needs, the perioperative nurse will easily move between the tertiary and primary care settings, interfacing daily with clients who represent the nation's underserved populations.

This chapter addresses the cultural health care considerations for those clients* who are classified as members of the four federally defined minority populations: Black American, Asian American, Hispanic American, and Native American and Alaskan Native.† Although it is recognized that a whole host of other subgroups comprise the cultural mix of this nation, the health care literature of the United States has been especially inadequate in identifying, from a holistic viewpoint, the cultural health care needs of ethnic people of color. This chapter progresses from a broad consideration of the concepts of acculturation, culture, society, and perioperative nursing to a descriptive analysis of the four federally defined minority groups. Six categories are used to describe each minority population: demographic composition,‡ family structure, religion and spirituality, communication, health problems, and health beliefs. The transcultural nursing care theory will serve as the conceptual framework for the development of culturally congruent plans of care.

---

*The term "client," as opposed to "patient," will be used to connote the collaborative, holistic approach to nursing care, which includes as relevant entities the family and the extended community. Collaborative nursing care practice addresses the need to engage the multicultural consumer as an integral component of the nursing process. The authors perceive this approach to be a prerequisite to the identification of mutually established goals, interventions, and outcomes.

†While researching the subject matter herein presented, the authors have noted arguments both for and against the capitalization of the cultural subclassifications of the Caucasoid, Negroid, and Mongoloid populations. In an effort to be conscious of multicultural sensitivities and to maintain consistency in presentation, all ethnic designations and subcategorizations used throughout this chapter will be capitalized, regardless of the broadness of the category. The authors are fully cognizant of the sociopolitical/anthropologic opposition that may be raised with regard to this approach. However, the overall purpose of this work is to heighten perioperative nurses' awareness and to enhance their appreciation for the richness of the diversity inherent within the four federally defined minority populations.

ACCULTURATION

Historically, the "melting pot" description of the United States has connoted the harmonious presence of people of varying cultural orientations who have desired to mesh, blend, and assume the values and beliefs of the dominant societal group. The concept of acculturation, the assimilation of behavioral and cultural belief systems of the host group by the resident subcultural populations (Spector, 1985), has long been endorsed by the current health care delivery system and considered to be a desirable outcome. However, when it is recognized that annually an estimated 1 million persons, legally and illegally, enter this country (Lantz, 1989) in search of sociopolitical freedom and economic security, then a more realistic appreciation for the numbers of fundamentally different cultures that reside as distinct entities within the nation's boundaries must be brought to a heightened social awareness.

Indeed, what is presently in place in this nation is not a melting pot, but rather a richly diverse collection of people who, in varying degrees, seek to maintain their cultural and ethnic identities. Already evident in the pediatric subset of the population, especially in the southeastern and southwestern parts of the nation, is a gradual "browning of America." In these demographic areas, two out of every five children are classified as minorities. By the year 2000, two out of every three children will be ethnic children of color (Malone, 1993), and by the year 2080, majority status will not be held by any single ethnic population (Nickens, 1995).

CULTURE, SOCIETY, AND PERIOPERATIVE NURSING

Culture is the sum total of values, beliefs, mores, folkways, and so on learned from one's elders during the process of socialization (Giger & Davidhizar, 1991). It is a multifaceted construct, influenced by society, education, economics, experience, and values (Branch & Paxton, 1976; Schaefer, 1986; Reiskin & Haussler, 1994). More profoundly, it is a reference point that shapes and guides actions and reactions (Kotecki, 1990). Elements within a culture that af-

---

‡Generalized physical characteristics associated with each racial designation will not be presented in this chapter. Exceptions will be made when a physical finding specific to the racial subgroup under discussion is relevant to the delivery of health care. It is well recognized that the four federally defined minority populations are, in actuality, sociopolitical designations with variant representation. As such, these designations are not subject to the scientific rigor of anthropologic classification, but rather are loosely defined cultural orientations derived from the political climate of the nation at a given time. It is both grossly misleading and culturally insensitive to assign concrete physical characteristics to such fluid definitions; placement within these racial designations is as much self-selected as federally appointed.

Box 23-1 Ways to Develop Cultural Sensitivity

1. Recognize that cultural diversity exists.
2. Demonstrate respect for people as unique individuals, with culture as one factor that contributes to their uniqueness.
3. Respect the unfamiliar.
4. Identify and examine your own cultural beliefs.
5. Recognize that some cultural groups have definitions of health and illness, as well as practices that attempt to promote health and cure illness, that may differ from yours.
6. Be willing to modify health care delivery in keeping with the client's cultural background.
7. Do not expect all members of one cultural group to behave in exactly the same way.
8. Appreciate that each person's cultural values are ingrained and therefore very difficult to change.

From Stule P. (1996). In Cookfair JN (Eds). *Nursing care in the community* (2nd ed.). St. Louis: Mosby.

---

fect the nursing profession may have all or any number of the following components of society: family orientation; care during birth, sickness, and death; age- and sex-related values; language; time orientation; sleep and hygiene habits; modesty; communication of satisfaction and dissatisfaction; value of personal accomplishment; food habits; and religious orientation (Kotecki, 1990). Cultures in the United States are dynamic and continuously evolving; broad principles for developing culturally sensitive attitudes are presented in Box 23-1.

In many respects the perioperative setting has been visionary in its efforts to encompass cultural healing practices, and it is to be commended for its willingness to borrow knowledge of treatment methods from other world cultures. Biofeedback, biorhythm, acupuncture, relaxation techniques, therapeutic touch, and hypnosis have been perioperative methodologic approaches used in this country for decades (Branch & Paxton, 1976).

To help the perioperative nurse develop a culturally congruent plan of care—that is, one that enables clients to maintain their cultural identity—a sample culturologic nursing care plan appears at the end of this chapter. Key culturologic assessment data for use in the care plan are listed in Box 23-2 later in this chapter. The implementation of such a plan of care can be effectively accomplished using the concept of cultural relativism, the process by which the nurse seeks to view, nonjudgmentally, the client's behavior from the perspective of the client's cultural orientation (Kotecki, 1990). More specifically, it is

the process by which the perioperative nurse endeavors to evaluate, situationally, the impact of relevant subcultural norms, values, and customs upon the perioperative environment. Transcultural nursing care theory serves as the conceptual framework supporting the development of culturally competent plans of care.

TRANSCULTURAL NURSING THEORY

Holistic frameworks of care that address the concepts of cultural health and healing are based on traditions that have evolved over centuries. These cultural frameworks explore the physical and spiritual relationships among the man-earth-universe triad. Many cultural subgroups hold belief systems that view the disruption of harmony among the triad as the creation of imbalances that can result in illness of the mind, body, and spirit. These cultures believe that all healing modalities must seek to reestablish the human organism's innate balancing mechanisms (Branch & Paxton, 1976).

Defining care as the essence of nursing practice, transcultural care theory (Leininger, 1991) asserts the existence of measurable, elemental entities comprising care and caring behaviors that (1) are specific to human cultures and subcultures; (2) are inextricably bound to values, belief systems, and health care practices held by the ethnic group under consideration; and (3) contain transcultural similarities and differences. Leininger (1994) maintains that as the world of nursing and health care becomes culturally more complex, it is imperative that the nursing profession begin to examine the nature, essence, meanings, expressions, and forms of human caring.

Conceptual frameworks for the development of culturally competent plans of care are grounded in transcultural nursing theory. Although most nursing theorists identify man as a biopsychosocial, spiritual being, it is Leininger's (1991) theory of cultural care diversity and universality that emphasizes man's cultural dimension. The Leininger Sunrise Model (Fig. 23-1) provides the nurse with a theoretic foundation to support the development of cultural relativism and the implementation of its methodologic constructs. Additionally, it is important to understand that the model does not adhere to the traditional nursing metaparadigmatic (person-health-nursing-environment) framework. Indeed, from a sociolinguistic perspective, Leininger (1991) points out that in some non-Western cultures, the entity "person" has no meaning, especially in those societies in which the concepts of family and community take precedence over the concept of individual. Leininger (1991) stresses the need for the nurse to view the client as a member of the family

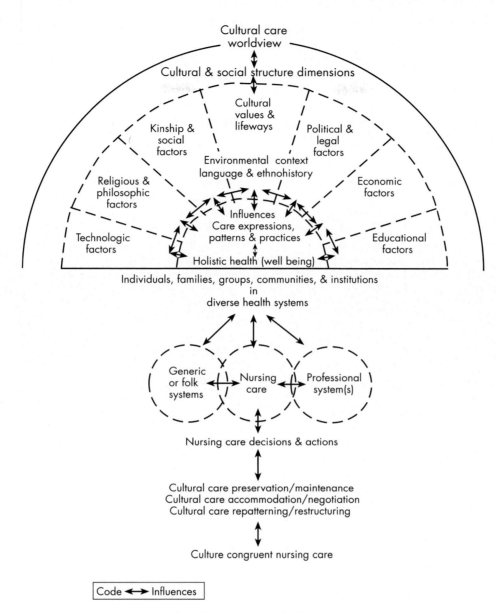

Fig. 23-1. The Leininger Sunrise Model.

or community unit and to serve as a coparticipant in the mutual development of the nursing plan of care.

From a holistic, worldview stance, the Sunrise Model serves as a cognitive map depicting the influencing cultural, social, and environmental dimensions affecting individuals, families, communities, and institutions. The model's conceptual framework identifies the rendering of culturally competent nursing care through a blending of folk and professional systems that are influenced by the larger world structural dimensions. The model lists the following three nursing decision action modalities as methodologic approaches to providing culturally congruent care: preservation/ maintenance, accommodation/negotiation, and repatterning/restructuring. Each nursing decision action modality and its use within the perioperative setting are described below.

Cultural Care Preservation/Maintenance

In Leininger's (1991) culture care preservation/maintenance nursing decision action modality, the perioperative nurse would seek to use relevant generic or folk health care practices to render culturally sensitive care. For example, the use of the hypnotic state of mind, as a behavioral technique, is not new in the perioperative setting. Indeed, it is recognized as a healing art and borrowed from Eastern health care theories. Part of a perioperative culturally relevant care plan might appropriately include the use of self-induced hypnosis as a nursing intervention in the management and control of pain. Such an approach would be of particular value for those Eastern cultural subgroups that engage in hypnosis as an act of devotion and would nicely blend folk and professional health care systems.

Cultural Care Accommodation/Negotiation

In Leininger's (1991) culture care accommodation/negotiation nursing decision action modality, the perioperative nurse would endeavor to alter a professional nursing practice to accommodate the client's cultural needs. For example, the religious teachings of the client and his or her family might necessitate omitting the use of volume replacement solutions that are derivatives of blood or blood products. The nurse would inform all members of the perioperative team, and appropriate adjustments would be made both to the fluid resuscitation phase of the intraoperative plan of care and to the fluid maintenance phase of the postoperative plan of care.

Cultural Care Repatterning/Restructuring

In Leininger's (1991) culture care repatterning/restructuring nursing decision action modality, the perioperative nurse would seek to collaborate with the client and his or her family to arrive mutually at life-style changes that promote health. For example, geophagy (the eating of clay or dirt) is a practice that was brought to this country by African slaves. More contemporary African Americans substituted laundry starch for clay when the family moved from the rural South to the more industrialized cities of the North. Although the eating of clay provided a rich source of iron, its substitute, laundry starch, did not. As a result, those African Americans who consumed laundry starch in large quantities became anemic (Spector, 1985).

Anemia and low iron stores pose serious perioperative risks. To help the client and his family maintain aspects of the practice of geophagy while adhering to health promotion tenets, the perioperative nurse would help the client/family unit to determine other ways the practice might be conducted without need for the actual consumption of laundry starch or clay. Safer substitute starchy food sources high in iron might be suggested by the perioperative nurse for both the preoperative and postoperative phases with appropriate explanations provided, thereby effecting more long-term life-style changes.

THE PERIOPERATIVE TRANSCULTURAL PLAN OF CARE

Culturologic Assessment

To use transcultural nursing theory as the framework for the development of the culturally competent perioperative plan of care, the nursing assessment form would need to be formatted as a checklist to facilitate the gathering of culturologic data. Given the reality of time constraints in the emergent phase of care, the form would contain categories that could be quickly marked and would address such concepts as ethnicity, place of birth, English fluency level, health beliefs and folk practices, religious considerations in health and illness, family structure, family role in decision making, cultural orientation, economic status, food preferences/avoidances, and educational level (Box 23-2). After the initial gathering of data during the assessment phase of care, the perioperative nurse would move on to mutually establish the nursing diagnoses, outcome criteria, and culturally relevant nursing interventions.

Nursing Diagnosis

Culturally relevant perioperative nursing diagnostic statements might include, but not be limited to, the following:

Powerlessness related to perceived hostile health care environment secondary to discontinuation of folk health care practices.

Anxiety related to ineffective coping mechanisms secondary to separation from cultural ties.

Social isolation related to ineffective communication secondary to language barrier. See Box 23-3 for a review of cultural variables in communication.

Spiritual distress related to cessation of religious practice secondary to separation from religious representatives.

Care should be taken by the nurse to seek corroboration from the client and family before assuming these diagnoses to be accurate. It must be remembered that many nursing diagnoses reflect the values of the dominant society (Geissler, 1991) and expect the client to be self-reliant, a concept that is not part of many cultural subgroups.

Interventions and Outcomes

Nursing interventions and expected outcomes for each diagnosis should generally provide for a continuation of cultural practices and beliefs, encourage the use of family as support, and match the client/family expectations of care. Where possible the perioperative nurse should collaborate with the transcultural nurse specialist, who can serve as a consultant in the development of the culturally sen-

---

Box 23-2 *Culturologic Assessment/Data Collection*

Ethnicity and Race
- What is the client's self-reported racial affiliation?
- What is the client's self-reported ethnic group affiliation?

Birthplace
- Where was the client born?
- Where has the client resided?

Communicative Competencies
- Is the client's language available in written form?
- What language is spoken in the home?
- Are health-related materials available in the client's spoken language?
- What is the client's English fluency level?
- Does the client require an interpreter?

Health Beliefs and Fold Practices
- What folk medicine/home remedies are practiced by the client?
- Does the client rely on cultural healers?
- What are the client's health promotion beliefs?
- What feelings are held by the client regarding Western health care delivery services?

Religious and Spiritual Considerations
- To what cause does the client attribute his or her illness?
- What is the client's religious affiliation?
- How are death, dying, and grieving perceived?
- What are the client's religious sanctions and restrictions?
- Do religious beliefs and practices influence the client's diet?
- Does the client's religion mandate fasting during certain times?

- How is "fasting" defined?
- What is the role of the client's religious beliefs and practices during health and illness?
- What is the role of the religious representative?
- Does the client's religious practice include inhalation/ingestion of substances used for sensory enhancement?

Food Preferences/Avoidances
- What foods are eaten or avoided in the home?
- Is the food specially prepared?
- What cultural meanings are ascribed to the act of eating?
- How does the client define food?

Socioeconomic Considerations
- What type of health insurance is carried by the client?
- Are there other sources of financial support?
- What socioeconomic level is held by the client's family?

Family Structure/Role and Social Network
- What is the role played by family members during health and illness?
- How does the client define family?
- Who are the family decision makers in the assessment of the client's health care needs?
- Who comprises the client's overall social support network?
- How is "caring" defined by the client's social support network?

Educational Level
- What is the client's highest educational level?
- What style of learning best meets the client's needs: demonstration, written, or oral presentations?

---

sitive plan of care (Leininger, 1989). A sample Culturologic Perioperative Plan of Care is presented in Fig. 23-2.

The remainder of this chapter addresses the culturologic considerations specific to each of the four federally defined minority populations. The reader is cautioned to remember that the following accounts are rather broad overviews of each cultural subgroup and are meant (1) to provide a beginning appreciation for the many cultural variations found within these rather diverse populations and (2) to demonstrate how these differences might affect the perioperative experience. An extensive list of citations appears at the conclusion of the chapter to guide the reader in the selection of references that provide a more in-depth accounting.

BLACK AMERICANS
Demographic Composition

The members of the Black American community make up a richly diverse composite, having their origins in Africa, the West Indies, and South America. More specifically, the Black American racial designation includes, but is not limited to, American citizens of anthropologic Negroid ancestry, whose *society of origin* determines membership in any of the following cultural subgroup categories: South African American, Ethiopian American, Trinidadian American, Jamaican American, Haitian American, Brazilian American, Cuban American, and the nation's indigenous African American, to name a few. However, by and large, the predominant ancestral heritage of the members of this American cultural

---

Box 23-3 Guidelines for Relating to Clients from Different Cultures

Assess your personal beliefs surrounding persons from different cultures:
- Review your personal beliefs and past experiences
- Set aside any values, biases, ideas, and attitudes that are judgmental and may negatively affect care

Assess communication variables from a cultural perspective:
- Determine the ethnic identity of the client, including generation in America
- Use the client as a source of information when possible
- Assess cultural factors that may affect your relationship with the client and respond appropriately

Plan care based on communicated needs and cultural background:
- Learn as much as possible about the client's cultural customs and beliefs
- Encourage the client to reveal cultural interpretation of health, illness, and health care
- Be sensitive to the uniqueness of the client
- Identify sources of discrepancy between the client's and your own conceptions of health and illness
- Communicate at the client's personal level of functioning
- Evaluate effectiveness of nursing actions and modify nursing care plan when necessary

Modify communication approaches to meet cultural needs:
- Be attentive to signs of fear, anxiety, and confusion in the client
- Respond in a reassuring manner in keeping with the client's cultural orientation
- Be aware that in some cultural groups discussion concerning the client with others may be offensive and may impede the nursing process

Understand that respect for the client and communicated needs is central to the therapeutic relationship:
- Communicate respect by using a kind and attentive approach
- Learn how listening is communicated in the client's culture
- Use appropriate active listening techniques
- Adopt an attitude of flexibility, respect, and interest to help bridge barriers imposed by culture

Communicate in a nonthreatening manner:
- Conduct the interview in an unhurried manner
- Follow acceptable social and cultural amenities
- Ask general questions during the information-gathering stage
- Be patient with a respondent who gives information that may seem unrelated to client's health problem
- Develop a trusting relationship by listening carefully, allowing time, and giving the client your full attention

Use validating techniques in communication:
- Be alert for feedback that the client is not understanding
- Do not assume meaning is interpreted without distortion

Be considerate of reluctance to talk when the subject involves sexual matters:
- Be aware that in some cultures sexual matters are not discussed freely with members of the opposite sex

Adopt special approaches when the client speaks a different language:
- Use a caring tone of voice and facial expressions to help alleviate the client's fears
- Speak slowly and distinctly, but not loudly
- Use gestures, pictures, and play acting to help the client understand
- Repeat the message in different ways if necessary
- Be alert to words the client seems to understand, and use them frequently
- Keep messages simple, and repeat them frequently
- Avoid using medical terms and abbreviations that the client may not understand
- Use an appropriate language dictionary

Use interpreters to improve communication:
- Ask the interpreter to translate the message, not just the individual words
- Obtain feedback to confirm understanding
- Use an interpreter who is culturally sensitive

From Giger JN & Davidhizar RE. (1995). *Transcultural nursing: Assessment and intervention* (2nd ed.). St. Louis: Mosby–Year Book.

---

subgroup is derived from the Black tribesmen of the African continent (Spector, 1985); hence the designation "African American" is ascribed to the majority of the members of this cultural subgroup. Until more recent times, Black Americans constituted less than 10% of the nation's population. It is predicted that by the year 2000, Blacks will increase their proportions from 12.4% to 13.1% of the American populace (U.S. Department of Health and Human Services, 1990b).

The role that socioeconomic factors play in health maintenance and disease prevention is well understood. Educational attainment, family configuration, median income, and rates of employment significantly affect the health status of all cultural groups. For Black Americans and other minorities, the impact is even more profound (Rosella, Regan-Kubinski, & Albrecht, 1994). These factors must be taken into consideration by the perioperative nurse both in the rendering of acute nursing care and in planning for discharge teaching and follow-up. Perioperative nurses must also develop the ability to assess the skin dark-skinned individuals; this information should be used to

FIG. 23-2
SAMPLE CULTUROLOGIC PERIOPERATIVE NURSING CARE PLAN

KEY ASSESSMENT POINTS

Racial and ethnic group membership
Communicative competencies
Health beliefs and folk practices
Religion and spirituality
Dietary sanctions/restriction
Family structure and social networks
Educational background
Socioeconomic considerations

NURSING DIAGNOSIS

Powerlessness related to perceived hostile health care environment
  secondary to discontinuation of folk health care practices.

CLIENT OUTCOMES

The client/family unit will:
Relate folk care practices and beliefs
Participate in planning/implementation phases of care
State that decisions regarding health regimen were supported
Express satisfaction with treatment modalities

NURSING ACTIONS

	Yes	No	N/A
1. Encourage use of alternative methods of therapy	☐	☐	☐
2. Support client/family unit making informed decisions	☐	☐	☐
3. When possible, delay treatment until culturologic needs are met	☐	☐	☐
4. When possible, permit cultural healers to enter perioperative suite to implement health care practices	☐	☐	☐
5. Allow client/family unit to ventilate feelings	☐	☐	☐
6. Permit client/family unit to participate in the planning and implementation of health care	☐	☐	☐

Document additional nursing actions/generic care plans initiated here:

_____

_____

_____

EVALUATION OF CLIENT OUTCOMES

The client/family unit:

	Outcome met	Outcome met with additional outcome criteria	Outcome met with revised nursing care plan	Outcome not met	Outcome not applicable to this patient
1. Related folk care practices and beliefs	☐	☐	☐	☐	☐
2. Participated in planning/implementation phases of care	☐	☐	☐	☐	☐
3. Stated that decisions regarding health regimen were supported	☐	☐	☐	☐	☐
4. Expressed satisfaction with treatment modalities	☐	☐	☐	☐	☐

Signature: _____ Date: _____

Box 23-4 Assessment of Skin in Dark-Skinned Individuals

1. Inspection and palpation are equally important in assessing the dark-skinned client. Skin color changes are best observed in the sclera, conjunctiva, oral mucosa, tongue, lips, nail beds, palms, and soles. Normal variations in pigmentation should be considered when assessing for skin color changes. The oral mucosa may have areas of darker pigmentation in the gums, the cheeks, and borders of the tongue. The lips may have a normal dark blue color. The presence of edema may cause dark skin to appear lighter in color. Changes in skin texture assessed by palpation may be the only indication of the presence of skin rashes.
2. In dark-skinned clients, pallor results in the loss of normal red tones in the skin. The brown-skinned person may have yellow-tinged skin when pallor is present. In the black-skinned client, pallor produces an ashen-gray color.
3. Jaundice is best observed in the sclera closest to the center of the eye. The dark-skinned client may have normal yellow pigmentation present in the sclera. Inspection of the hard palate for a yellow color can confirm the presence of jaundice.
4. Cyanosis may be difficult to detect in the dark-skinned client. Inspection in areas of lightest pigmentation will often indicate the presence of cyanosis, such as the nail beds, conjunctiva, palms, and soles.
5. Petechiae are best observed in the conjunctiva and oral mucosa. They may also be seen in areas of lighter pigmentation over the abdomen, gluteal folds, or inner aspect of the forearm.
6. Erythema is determined by palpating for increased skin temperature that is usually associated with conditions that produce this skin color change.

From Beare PG & Myers JL. (1994). *Principles and practice of adult health nursing* (2nd ed.). St. Louis: Mosby.

---

modify the generic care plan for skin integrity (Box 23-4) in Chapter 7.

Education. In 1987, one fourth of all Americans over the age of 25 had not completed high school. Broken out by race, the data are quite alarming: 36% of Blacks versus 23% of Whites had not graduated from the twelfth grade in that same year. The differences between the races become even more pronounced when the percentages of college graduates are compared. In 1987, Whites were twice as likely to graduate from college as were Blacks, 20.7% and 10.7%, respectively (U.S. Department of Health and Human Services, 1990a). The fact that educational attainment significantly affects health status is well documented, because better educated citizens are more likely to seek health care early and to follow prescribed treatment plans.

Median income. In 1987, 33% of all Blacks across the nation lived below the poverty level. In that same year, regionally, Blacks appeared to live in more impoverished conditions in the Midwest, and seemed to fare better, with respect to income, in the far West. The median income for Blacks in 1987 was $17,604 versus $30,809 for Whites. Educational attainment significantly narrowed the gap between the two races. Of married-couple families with 13 to 15 years of education, the median income was $40,448 for Whites and $35,692 for Blacks. For those who had completed 16 or more years of education, the median incomes rose to $57,674 for Whites and $51,641 for Blacks (U.S. Department of Health and Human Services, 1990a). Economic status is directly proportional to the incidence of disease and illness, as middle and upper income level families have greater resources with which to engage in preventive health care.

Unemployment. The unemployment rate in 1987 for Blacks was 13% as compared with Whites, who fared better at 5.3%. In that year, Blacks were more than twice as likely as Whites to be unemployed (U.S. Department of Health and Human Services, 1990a). Rates of employment directly relate to level of family income, and, for reasons already cited, significantly affect health status.

Family configuration. In 1987, almost 33% of all Black families consisted of female heads of household with children under 18 years of age. Although the percent are of all married Americans has significantly decreased since 1970, there remain striking differences between the White and Black races. In 1987, 67.4% of the White male population was married, compared with 50.9% of the Black male population. Divorce rates indicate the same respective disparities (U.S. Department of Health and Human Services, 1990a). Married-couple households, especially of dual income, are more likely to enjoy a lower incidence of disease and illness directly as a result of their higher annual incomes.

Cultural History. According to early historical documents, Black Americans voluntarily arrived on the North American continent 1 year before the docking of the Pilgrims at Plymouth Rock and well before the arrival of the first slave ships (Branch & Paxton, 1976). However, by 1860 the flourishing slave trade market had brought, involuntarily, more than 4 million Black Africans to the nation's shores. As a result, the majority of the current members of the Black American community are the direct descendents of slaves (Spector, 1985). Given this predominance, however, the perioperative nurse must be cautioned against perceiving the members of this multicultural population as a homogenous cohort.

In the rendering of culturally competent care, it is important for the perioperative nurse to consider the society of origin of the Black American for whom care is being delivered. Although it is beyond the scope of this chapter to provide an in-depth analysis of the various ethnic orientations of this multicultural group, the social histories of the West Indian American and African American populations serve as examples of the multifaceted challenges associated with the provision of culturally congruent care in the Black American community.

The Black West Indian American. The West Indies comprise many small islands under various governmental controls: Guadeloupe and Martinique belong to France; Bermuda, part of the Virgin Islands, and several other smaller islands belong to Great Britain; and the Commonwealth of the Bahamas, Barbados, Cuba, the Dominican Republic, Haiti, Jamaica, Trinidad, and Tobago are independent. British, French, Spanish, and Dutch explorers settled the West Indies. As a result, all four languages are spoken by the Blacks who reside on these islands. Additionally, Blacks comprise 50% to 85% of the population, depending on the island. The minority groups on these islands include the East Indian, Chinese, and White subethnic populations. The islanders are predominantly Protestant; however, some practice the Catholic, Jewish, Muslim, and folk/tribal religions (Brice, 1982).

Emancipation of the slave populations came to the West Indies much earlier than it did to the United States. Land ownership afforded the Black West Indian the opportunity to become upwardly mobile. In addition, the illegitimate Black West Indian children of the White plantation owner, called Mulattos, were recognized among the islanders for their mixed ancestry and elevated to middle class status. Together with their greater numbers, Black West Indians were able to enjoy a wealthier life-style very early on (Brice, 1982). Black West Indian who choose to immigrate to the United States bring this rich cultural history with them. Phenomenologically, Black West Indian Americans should not be perceived to share the same civil rights' experiences as African Americans, because the latter group can document descendants, dating back 400 years, whose place of birth was the United States.

The African American. Separate and apart from the West Indian Black American heritage is the historicity of the African American. The members of this cultural subgroup, by and large, did not choose to voluntarily immigrate to this nation; rather they were brought to this country as African slaves. Although the American institution of slavery ravaged the Black American family, it did permit the practice of religion and the formation of strong religious underground networks, by which many escaped to freedom (Hines & Boyd-Franklin, 1982). The oppressive, historical perspective of slavery, as it was practiced in the United States, is well documented elsewhere, and is not presented here.

For many decades after the Emancipation Proclamation, African Americans predominantly lived in the South. Between 1940 and 1970, over 1.5 million African Americans migrated to the North and West. In search of greater job opportunities, they settled in large American cities. Unfortunately, with limited income, restricted housing practices, and more overt racism, most were relegated to ghetto residences. Also, the majority lacked the technologic skills needed to advance in the more industrialized cities of the North. Relying heavily upon the Black Church to serve as an extended network of support, Black Americans slowly lifted some of the social and political injustices of the times (Hines & Boyd-Franklin, 1982; Mays, 1968). Although the literature is replete with information that emphasizes the deficits of the African American population, little is written about the resourcefulness of this group. Black Americans have learned to utilize their adaptive strengths to transcend social, political, educational, and cultural barriers (Hines & Boyd-Franklin, 1982).

Family Structure

The Black American nuclear family composition may differ significantly from that of the traditional White American nuclear family. Owing to the history of slavery and its major disruption of family ties and kinship, different kinds of Black American family relationships evolved to maintain the importance of family life (Spector, 1985). Reliance on an extended kinship network, not necessarily related to blood line, was and continues to be a major mode of coping with the oppression of the larger society. Black American nuclear family boundaries are elastic, multigenerational, and tend to link multiple domestic units. Extended family systems operate both in and out of the Black American home (Hines & Boyd-Franklin, 1982).

The Black American man's role of husband/father varies. Severe societal pressures placed on the family unit may negatively affect the family relationship. Black fathers are many times disillusioned by the realities of the work world. They usually have the highest job loss rates and, when employed, hold the lowest positions. These conditions cause Black men to expend great time and energy on providing the most basic needs for his family (Hines & Boyd-Franklin, 1982).

Because Black women are more likely to be the employed spouse, the traditional husband/wife role may be reversed. The Black man may assume child-rearing and housekeeping functions while the Black woman works outside the home. As a result, relationships between Black couples have been more egalitarian, historically, than have been relationships between mainstream American couples. Black men may not feel as threatened by having an employed spouse as their White counterparts might be, who are just now beginning to feel the conflicts surrounding dual-income marriages (Hines & Boyd-Franklin, 1982).

Complex extended kinship networks characterize the Black American family. Grandparents, aunts and uncles, and other nonrelated adults may assume positions of importance within the Black American family home. Unofficial adoption of children is a common practice, as parents may willingly permit their children to be "adopted" by extended or non-related family members to expose the child to better educational or economic resources (Hines & Boyd-Franklin, 1982).

Religion and Spirituality

Religion has played a strong role in the lives of Black Americans both during and after the slavery era. The Church often provided information about the escape to freedom. Hidden messages were contained in the spirituals that were sung during religious ceremonies. Some Negro spirituals described escape routes along the underground railroad (Hines & Boyd-Franklin, 1982); others promised a greater existence in the afterworld. Death was viewed as a passage to another state of existence, and the funeral was often a joyous occasion where the deceased was celebrated (Mays, 1968).

In more modern times religion provides rituals of great therapeutic value for Black Americans, whose membership can be found among many religious sects and denominations, including, but not limited to Baptist, Methodist, Jehovah's Witness, Church of God in Christ, Seventh Day Adventist, Pentocostal Churches, Nation of Islam, Presbyterianism, Lutheranism, Episcopalianism, Roman Catholicism (Hines & Boyd-Franklin, 1982), and Judaism.

The church was, and continues to be, the place where Black Americans are given a sense of pride and self-esteem. Many hold positions of prominence within the church, and, as a result, are well-respected members of the Black American community. The sociopolitical impact of the Black American religious sector on the larger society was at no time more evident, in recent years, than during the civil rights' marches of the sixties. Black American religious leaders continue to greatly influence larger society.

Communication

Members of the Black American community, depending on the number of years that they have resided in America, may speak any one of many languages and dialects, such as Dutch, French, Spanish, Swahili, Portuguese, and English. Here again, the society of origin is the deciding factor in helping the perioperative nurse understand the spoken language of the Black American for whom care is being rendered. It is important to note that for many Black Americans, English may be a second language and sometimes is not the language that is spoken in the home. In those instances in which English is not the spoken language, it will be necessary for the nurse to have an English-speaking family member serve as interpreter.

For Black Americans educated in the American or British school systems, English will be the spoken language. As in the larger society, dialects vary within geographic location and educational level.

Health Problems

Morbidity. The point of crossover, from morbidity to mortality, is often gradual and difficult to define (U.S. Department of Health and Human Services, 1990a). This fact is especially evident when applying the health-illness continuum to minority aggregates, because states of health and illness tend to be more culturally defined among these populations. Nevertheless, major health problems among the Black American community can be identified and include hypertension, malnutrition, periodontal disease, drug and alcohol abuse, and psychiatric disturbance (Spector, 1985). Adding to the severity of these health problems is the major prevalence of four important risk factors associated with general health status, which include cigarette smoking, elevated blood pressure, elevated serum cholesterol levels, and obesity.

Mortality. For all causes of death in 1987, Black American death rates were found to be 52% higher than the death rates of White Americans. Furthermore, when these data were disaggregated, it was demonstrated that Black Americans died from homocide and legal intervention at a rate six times that of Whites; for four of the fifteen leading causes of death (nephritis and allied conditions, diabetes mellitus, septicemia, and perinatal conditions), Black American death rates were twice those of White America. Comparing life expectancy for both groups in 1987, the numbers remained quite disparate: 72.2 years for White men and 65.2 years for Black men (U.S. Department of Health and Human Services, 1990a).

Health Beliefs and Practices

Black Americans, depending on the degree of acculturation, may or may not adhere to some of the health beliefs and practices discussed in this section. The more traditional beliefs about health stem from the African concept of life and the nature of being. All things, whether living or dead, influence life forces. As with many Euro-African culturally diverse populations, African American traditional beliefs about health do not separate mind, body and spirit. Health was believed to be a state of harmony, whereas illness was a state of disequilibrium (Branch & Paxton, 1976; Spector, 1985). Environmentally, the role of the community in health and illness was, and continues to be, viewed as essential to the Black American. In health, the community acts to maintain and prevent disability; whereas in illness, the community acts as a restorative agent (Branch & Paxton, 1976).

Disharmonious forces were believed to be dispelled from the body using voodoo, faith healing, or other folk medical practices. Voodoo is a belief system that uses the concept of magic to effect healing. Two forms of magic are described in the old literature: a harmless white magic and a more dangerous black magic. It is not known whether voodoo is practiced in its original form in more contemporary times (Spector, 1985).

The traditional faith healers were usually women, who possessed extensive training in the use of herbs and roots to treat illness. In fact, an early form of smallpox immunization was practiced by cultural healers, who would place a crust of cowpox upon a child's arm to effectively inoculate the child against the smallpox virus. Prayer was, and continues to be, the most common method of treating illness. The laying on of hands was also frequently described as a treatment modality (Spector, 1985).

It is generally believed that health is maintained with proper diet, rest, and the regular employment of laxatives to keep the system open. Asafetida, rotten flesh resembling a dried-out sponge, may be worn around the neck to ward off contagious disease. Cod liver oil may be used to prevent colds, and a sulfur-and-molasses preparation, applied to the back, may be used each spring to combat disease. Copper or silver bracelets may be worn around the wrists of children to protect them as they grow to maturity. The bracelets may be believed to warn of impending illness; when the skin beneath the bracelet turns black, extra precautions are to be taken. These precautions may be in the form of increased prayer, extra rest, and consuming a more nutritious diet (Spector, 1985).

Since it is known that access to and use of existing health care services are indicators of health status, the rate-of-use index can serve to indirectly measure health beliefs and practices of members of the Black American community. Trending data show that Black American rates of use of the health care delivery system vary with socioeconomic levels, years of schooling, and reported barriers to access (U.S. Department of Health and Human Services, 1990a).

ASIAN AMERICANS AND PACIFIC ISLANDERS
Demographic Composition
According to the U.S. Census Bureau (1992), Asian and Pacific Islander Americans reached 8,451,000 or 3.3% of the total U.S. population in 1992. By the year 2050, this group is expected to make up almost 11% of the total population. Yet today, Asian Americans and Pacific Islanders remain one of the most poorly understood and neglected ethnic groups, paying a heavy price for the myth of a model minority.

Although classified together in the census data and in most other statistics, Asian Americans and Pacific Islanders include a large, diverse number of subpopulations with differing languages and cultural traditions (Austin, Schoenrock, & Roberts, 1991). Under this single category are persons originating from 28 Asian countries and 25 identified Pacific Islands (U.S. Bureau of the Census, 1990).

Asian Americans include Chinese, Filipinos, Japanese, Asian Indians, Koreans, and Vietnamese. Pacific Islander Americans include Hawaiians, Samoans, Guamanians, and Tongans. Each subgroup has its own unique history, culture, language, religion, and history of immigration to the United States. For example, Japanese, Chinese, and Filipinos are represented by both new immigrants and descendants of persons who migrated to the United States several generations earlier. Others, such as the Vietnamese, Laotian, Hmong, and Cambodians, were virtually nonexistent in the United States until the influx of refugees from Southeast Asia began in 1975. Still others, such as the Hawaiians, Samoans, and Guamanians, are born U.S. citizens (U.S. General Accounting Office, 1990). Despite the diversity among Asian Americans and Pacific Islander Americans, there appear to be areas of similarity in Asian cultural values (Kinzie, 1985; Sue & Sue, 1990).

Family Structure
The structure of families among Asian Americans and Pacific Islanders is traditionally patriarchal. The father's behavior in relation to other family members is generally authoritative, distant, and aloof. Sons are generally valued. Most Asian women are expected to carry on the domestic duties, to marry, to become obedient helpers to their mothers-in-law, and to bear children, especially males. However, differences in the family structure among Asian American groups exist and may be attributed to the degree of assimilation of Western culture by family members, leading to changes in family life-style patterns.

Many Asians and Pacific Islander Americans live in extended family settings. The welfare of the family often has priority over individual needs (Sue & Sue, 1990). Interdependence and dependence are key concepts valued in many Asian countries. Because of the extended family kinship, when an Asian client is scheduled for surgery, consent may involve more than a traditional consent protocol. A husband may need to sign for a wife or a godfather for a child.

Allegiance to the parents or filial piety is a strong value found among many members of this cultural group (Sue & Sue, 1990). Even after marriage, there is an overriding sense of duty that is owed to the respective parents of the two spouses. Consequently, conflict often arises when the dominant American society expects Asian and Pacific Islander Americans to demonstrate spousal allegiance after entering the state of matrimony, when, in fact, their cultural norm is to maintain primary allegiance with the former family unit of the married partners.

The family structure is so arranged that conflicts within the family are kept to a minimum. Family harmony is highly valued, even at the expense of causing family members to repress their feelings, especially when expression of such feelings could potentially lead to family disruption.

Respect and formality in social relationships are important in the Asian culture (Shon & Ja, 1982). Addressing Asian American clients by their proper names, as a way of showing respect, will enhance the perioperative nurse's social relationship with these clients. It should be noted that Asian American clients may hesitate to ask questions, especially if they perceive the nurse or physician as authority figures, for fear of being considered discourteous.

Because Asian Americans value time differently than Anglo-Americans, promptness in meeting appointments may be a problem. The perioperative nurse must consider the client's perception of time when planning for same-day surgery or treatment procedures.

In summary, traditional Asian values emphasize respect and formality in social relationships, restraint and inhibition of strong feelings, obedience to authority, and obligations to the family. These cultural values have significant impact on the health behavior of Asian Americans.

Religion and Spirituality

Religious beliefs of Asian Americans and Pacific Islanders are very diverse. For example, the largest Muslim populations are found in Indonesia, Malaysia, and Pakistan, whereas the largest population of Catholics is found in the Philippines. Filipino Americans, who are Catholics, may be fatalistic in their attitudes and view death as a way to salvation. Asians and Pacific Islanders may also practice the Buddhist and Hindu religions. The largest populations of Buddhists are found in China, Korea, Cambodia, and Vietnam. Hinduism is predominantly practiced in India. As has been stated for all cultural and ethnic subgroups, the client's religious beliefs have significant implications for health care delivery. For example, for the Asian American client who practices the Muslim faith, the perioperative plan of care will need to address the dietary sanctions and restrictions mandated by the teachings of this religion. When possible, religious practice should be maintained.

While a consumer of health care services, the Asian and Pacific Islander American should be encouraged to pray and should be allowed to see spiritual leaders for comfort. Religious articles, artifacts, and symbols such as amulets are important and, when possible, should be permitted in the perioperative suite.

Communication

Asians are nonconfrontational and indirect when expressing themselves. They will not volunteer information because self-expression is discouraged within their culture. Consequently, most will not share feelings or emotions in public. Asian Americans may appear unconcerned when presented with a grave diagnosis or situation because of the emphasis their culture places on stoicism and the restraint of emotional public display (Lin-Fu, 1988; Uba, 1992). For the Pacific Islanders, topics regarding sexual intercourse, genitalia, venereal disease, and mental health problems are considered shameful or "taboo" to discuss. The perioperative nurse needs to understand that asking questions concerning sensitive topics may offend the client. Therefore, it is important to acknowledge that these questions may cause discomfort, and that it is perfectly acceptable for the client to decline to provide answers to sensitive issues.

Some Asian Americans may not speak the English language. Because of diversity in the languages used by Asian Americans and Pacific Islanders, the perioperative nurse needs to ascertain what specific language the client speaks. This assessment is important in the selection of the appropriate interpreter or translator to facilitate communication.

In many cases, the hospital situation tends to hinder effective and therapeutic communication with culturally diverse clients. Because the hospital experience is so foreign and intrusive, the perioperative nurse must be cognizant of the anxiety and alienation fostered by such environments and must anticipate the need for appropriate intervention.

Health Beliefs

In addition to understanding cultural values, perioperative nurses caring for Asian Americans and Pacific Islander Americans need to understand their traditional health beliefs and world views. Several paradigms of health, derived from the Chinese, dominate traditional Chinese, Japanese, Korean, and Southeast Asian beliefs and practices. Each reflects the central concept of balance between the person, society, and the universe. Asian Americans believe that there are forces, natural or supernatural, that disturb the balance or equilibrium, and those that restore it (Campbell & Chang, 1981). Yin and Yang, cold and hot, are forces that must be in balance. The balance can be upset by a disease, which may be restored by specific foods and practices that address the imbalance. Certain conditions, such as pregnancy and old age, are believed to shift an individual in a particular direction, suggesting the need to avoid certain foods and habits. The theory of "hot" and "cold" embraced by many Asian Americans often influences their perception of the nature of their illness and judgment regarding the appropriateness of the treatment prescribed (Louie, 1985). Such perceptions and judgments may, in turn, affect client compliance and help-seeking behavior.

Asian American clients who are scheduled for a cesarean section may request acupuncture in lieu of anesthesia. The practice of acupuncture is based upon the concept of *chi*, or energy, that moves through the body, which can be disturbed by other negative forces and rebalanced by use of these methods at specific points (or meridians) on the body (Chan & Chang, 1976).

Asian Americans believe that certain illnesses are caused by "bad wind" and people are vulnerable at different times because they are out of harmony with the universe. Fever, headache, arthritis, gastric pain, bruises, and paralysis are conditions attributed to "bad wind" (Louie, 1985). Headaches and fever are treated using coining. Coining is a form of treatment using manual pressure to remove "bad wind." This is done by rubbing a coin up and down the client's body until red marks appear. Arthritis, stomachaches, and paralysis are treated by cupping. To remove the "bad wind," a cup filled with heat is put on the skin, which creates a negative pressure inside the cup, resulting in the formation of bruises. Such folk practices command the need for astute assessment skills, especially with respect to altered skin integrity; marks on the skin due to coining or cupping must be validated and documented and may need to be closely monitored in the perioperative setting.

Some Asian Americans believe that human suffering is part of life; therefore they delay seeking help until symptoms of illness become unbearable. Formal health services are sought when they are in the acute phase of illness.

Familiarity with culturally influenced expectations and behaviors can enhance the perioperative nurse's interaction with Asian American clients. For example, in the Japanese culture emphasis is placed on respect and politeness. To avoid being considered disrespectful or impolite, the Japanese American client may display behaviors of deference toward authority figures, such as physicians, or may demonstrate behaviors of stoicism, leading to underreporting or failure to report serious symptoms of illness. Along the same line of thought, in an endeavor to maintain respectful behavior, an older Filipino American may avoid disagreement with health professionals as a way to maintain "face," despite the fact that he may be harboring negative feelings (Peterson, 1978).

Older Chinese American clients may maintain flexibility and a positive outlook using a traditional Chinese exercise called Tai Chi Chuan (Adler, 1983). If this is practiced, the client should be offered a room in which to perform the exercises while in the hospital. Older Filipino Americans may adhere to traditional belief of fatalism about life or illness as a curse for sins. These beliefs may influence their choice of whether or not to seek help. Knowledge about these beliefs and behaviors, when placed in a cultural context, can facilitate the interaction between the perioperative nurse and the client (D'Avonzo, Frye, & Froman, 1994).

During hospitalization, the Asian American client may be surrounded by family and friends, who will supply food and herbs to help the client get better. Asian American clients who are capable of self-care may allow others to feed and bathe them, so that they can conserve energy needed for the healing process. Without understanding the reason for this behavior, a perioperative nurse may perceive this behavior of dependency as a pathologic condition and may attempt to intervene, creating conflict with the client.

Health Problems

Recently it has been suggested that Asian Americans have different susceptibility to particular diseases as well as different physiologic responses to medications. For example, Zhou and associates (1989) reported that the Chinese had greater sensitivity to the effects of beta blockers in lowering blood pressure and a more rapid metabolism of the drug compared with Anglo-American clients. Similarly, Tien (1984) and Lin-Fu (1988) reported that Asian American clients manifest side effects readily and require lower dosages of neuroleptic medications than non-Asian clients.

In cataract surgery, it has been reported that lens implantation has been found to be more difficult in Asian clients because of the narrow eye fissures, tight eyelids, and shallow orbit (Lin-Fu, 1988). In laser surgery for narrow-angle glaucoma (iridotomy)—

because the iris is more pigmented and thicker in Asian Americans and Pacific Islanders than it is in most Anglo-Americans—the instrument setting standardized for Anglo-Americans does not result in adequate penetration (Lee, 1982). Perioperative nurses, therefore, may anticipate modifications in preoperative medication and operative procedures.

Members of Japanese, Chinese, and Filipino ethnic groups in the United States have lower death rates than Anglo-Americans (Liu & Yu, 1985). Death rates for members of these ethnic groups who are foreign-born are significantly higher than for counterparts born in the United States (Yu, 1986). Despite overall death rates, immigration to this country and the adoption of the American life-style and diet appear to increase the risk for certain diseases. An increased incidence of heart disease is seen in Chinese and Japanese Americans (Chen, 1993; Morioka-Douglas & Yeo, 1990) of colon cancer in Chinese Americans (Whitemore, 1989) and of diabetes in Japanese Americans (Fujimoto, Leonetti, & Kinyoun, 1987). Chinese Americans have a higher incidence of liver, esophageal, and pancreatic cancer (Morioka-Douglas & Yeo, 1990). Hypertension is common among Filipino women more than 50 years of age (Stavig, Igra, & Leonard, 1988).

In the rendering of culturally competent care for the Asian American client, the perioperative nurse will need to have knowledge of the client's culture, level of acculturation, and physiologic response to drugs. Furthermore, the guidelines for facilitating healthy adaptation and functioning must contextually view the client as a member of both the larger American society and the specific cultural entity to which he or she claims membership.

AMERICAN INDIANS AND ALASKA NATIVES
Demographic Composition

The United States federal government presently recognizes more than 500 American Indian and Alaska Native tribes, bands, pueblos, and villages (U.S. Department of Health and Human Services, 1993a). Approximately one third of tribal members live on reservations in 33 states, and 50% reside in urban centers throughout the 50 states. In 1990, the median annual family income for American Indians on reservations or tribal lands was approximately $13,700 (U.S. Department of Health and Human Services, 1993a).

Alaska Natives are considered to be the people of Athabascan, Tsimpsian, Tlingit, Haida, Eskimo, and Aleut descent (U.S. Department of Health and Human Services, 1993a). However, the reported membership of American Indian and Alaska Native tribes may not accurately reflect the total membership, for some may choose to affiliate with other ethnic

groups. The misclassification of American Indians has resulted in a gross underestimation of mortality and morbidity. Examples of underreported data, resulting from such misclassification, include data sets related to end-stage renal disease, infant mortality, and injury rates (Sugarman, et al., 1993). Although cultural differences exist among the numerous American Indian tribes, several authors (Buehler, 1993; Mail, McKay, & Katz, 1989) have noted commonalities in both history and philosophy. Mail, McKay, and Katz (1989) identified the following commonalities among the various tribal subgroups: "spiritual attachment to their land, sharing with others, a lack of materialism, a belief that inanimate and animate objects can have supernatural powers, strong family connections, and a desire to maintain their traditional culture and language."

Buehler (1993) contends that in order to develop a culturally sensitive plan of care for the American Indian client, the nurse needs to be aware of two considerations. The first is that the mistrust of Anglo-American society by American Indians has been fueled by the "historical and contemporary oppression by the dominant white society" (Buehler, 1993), a situation that poses a serious challenge for the perioperative nurse in the establishment of trusting relationships. The second consideration addresses the notion that for the American Indian client, as with many other culturally diverse groups, health is defined as the harmony that exists along several dimensions: mind, body, spirit, and environment (Bell, 1994). These dimensional entities are so intricately interwoven that the possibility of a cognitive separation is not even to be contemplated if a homeostatic balance is to be maintained. When developing culturally sensitive plans of care, these considerations must be kept in mind.

Historically, most Americans have been exposed to inaccurate accounts of American Indian history. The media have stereotyped, romanticized, and caricatured the life-style of American Indian tribes and individuals. American Indians have been portrayed as alcoholics, unreliable, and supernaturally intuitive. These biases have contributed to the development of the erroneous conclusion that American Indians are unable to make an intelligent choice between Western medicine and traditional healing practices.

Religion and Spirituality

The concepts of spirituality, religion, and health are intertwined in the daily life of American Indian cultures (Harris, 1993; U.S. Department of Health and Human Services, 1993a). Although an in-depth discussion of these concepts is beyond the scope of this chapter, to facilitate the delivery of appropriate health care, an awareness of the interrelationship of mind, body, spirit, and environment in American Indian philosophy is fundamental. In addition to those who adhere to the tenets of traditional American Indian philosophies, there are others who are members of organized Christian faiths. American Indians and Alaska Natives may hold membership in the following religious groups: the Church of Jesus Christ of Latter Day Saints, Seventh Day Adventists, Jehovah's Witnesses, Roman Catholic, Methodist, and Baptist. Additionally, one might find that the American Indian client may subscribe to both traditional beliefs and practices and to those beliefs and practices that are dictated by his or her religious affiliation. To uncover the subtle nuances related to religiosity and spirituality, interviewing questions regarding clients' religious and spiritual beliefs and practices are provided in Box 23-2.

Family Structure

The structure of American Indian families has several unique qualities that must be considered in the development of a culturally sensitive plan of nursing care. Although many tribes are matrilineal, that is, the state in which the distribution and ownership of name and property are determined by maternal lineage, the households are not necessarily matriarchal. American Indian families are usually extended families. The concept of extended family may include clan and tribal members as well as blood relatives. Although these members may or may not share the same household, they may participate in many family decisions, including those choices related to health care services.

As a practicing public health nurse for the Navajo Nation, one of the authors witnessed several examples of the family unit serving as the decision-making body for one of its members.

CASE STUDY *Traditional folkways and values*

M.B., a 48-year-old Navajo man diagnosed with coronary artery disease, was bilingual and lived in a remote area on the Navajo Reservation in the northeast corner of Arizona. He was informed by his provider of the need for bypass surgery and initially agreed to the scheduling of the procedure. M.B. "did not show" on the scheduled date. Several weeks later M.B. requested that the procedure be rescheduled. He explained that he could not keep the previous appointment because his adult children wanted to consult with a medicine man and have a ceremony before the surgery.

As a result of the focus on time management and cost containment, the provider and institution viewed this behavior as inconsiderate, uncooperative, and noncompliant. In actuality, the family culture had not been considered in this client's plan of care. As discussed earlier, the American Indian concept of health does not separate the body and the spirit. The perceived need for a traditional ceremony may outweigh the perceived benefits of a surgical procedure. The client might choose to use traditional healing alone or in conjunction with a medical procedure; however, in any case, it would not be uncommon for the family decision to take precedence. A positive approach, to benefit both the client and the institution, would be accomplished with the establishment of a nursing protocol, that affords American Indian clients the opportunity to consult with their families and traditional healers before scheduling health care interventions. It is important for the perioperative nurse to remember that American Indian clients hold the right to refuse, postpone, or cancel a procedure regardless of need, even when the reason for refusal is grounded in traditional folkways and values.

Communication

American Indians are often bilingual, able to speak both English and their native language. There are estimated to be more than 200 distinct indigenous languages spoken in North America (Cook & Petit de Mange, 1995). However, even though many might be bilingual, a client may not feel comfortable discussing, in English, certain issues with the health care provider who has not already established a trusting relationship. Typically, it was the public health nursing practice of the co-author, who worked with the clients of the Navajo Indian tribe, to engage the services of a translator while conducting home health visits. When, on several occasions, an attempt was made to converse with elderly Navajo Indian clients without benefit of a translator, the interviews were inadequate largely because the Navajo language lacks points of reference for many health care concepts.

For the Native American client whose primary language is not English, the employment of a professional translator is a strategy that can enable the nurse to develop culturally sensitive plans of care. The Navajo Nation employs and trains community health representatives to assist in translation. These individuals are required to be members of the Navajo tribe and members of the community in which they are employed. In addition to translation skills, they are trained in many health screening and health education concepts. When used, their assistance was found to be invaluable and facilitated effective communication with Navajo-speaking clients. Because, as stated above, many Western health-related concepts are not represented in native languages, the rehearsing of concepts with the translator before meeting with the client and family was found to be extremely beneficial. This strategy afforded the translator the opportunity to reflect on and select the most appropriate manner by which the information could be conveyed from client to nurse and vice versa.

At times a professional translator may not be available, and the use of a family member or other lay person may be the only choice. There are, however, many ethical questions to be considered in this situation. Among many things at issue is the concept of informed consent, especially in situations where the client has little or no knowledge of the health concepts and procedures of the dominant culture. One must also be cognizant of the ability to elicit family and client cooperation in the preoperative, postoperative, and discharge phases of care, where clarity of the translated information is of utmost importance.

Consideration should also be given to the appropriateness of specific interview questions. Higgins and Dicharry (1990) studied the reliability and validity of the Coopersmith Self-Esteem Inventory with Navajo women. These researchers found that questions addressing personal feelings and family relationships were considered rude, insulting, or irrelevant by some of the participants. Additionally, it was found that questions constructed in a positive framework more closely paralleled the American Indian concept of harmony and augmented the communication process.

**CASE
STUDY** *Assessing client needs and abilities*

T.W. is a 60-year-old Navajo-speaking client scheduled for same-day surgery. The day before the scheduled surgery, the perioperative nurse used a Navajo bystander to translate information about the procedure to the client. The nurse also gave the client written preoperative instructions in both English and Navajo. After the client was admitted to the hospital, the perioperative nurse learned that the client had eaten a large breakfast that morning. The procedure was cancelled.

A more thorough assessment of T.W.'s learning needs could have prevented this inconvenience for the client, the provider, and the facility. Although this client could speak Navajo, she could not read.

Many native languages are quite complex in written form. Although Navajo "words" are pronounced exactly as they are "spelled" (Wilson, 1989), a knowledge of markings is necessary. Vowels, for example, can be pronounced orally by letting air pass through the oral cavity or nasally by letting the air pass through the nose as well as the mouth (Wilson, 1989). The meaning of the word is determined by its pronunciation. Nasal markings are used in text to indicate correct pronunciations. The Navajo word "shi" is translated "I" when pronounced orally. When pronounced nasally, which is indicated by a nasal mark in text, "shi" is translated as "summer." The Navajo language was not codified until the 1900s. Other native languages, such as Tewa, the language spoken by the Indians of the Taos Pueblo, remain unwritten (Taos Pueblo representative, personal communication, July, 1991).

According to Harris (1993), American Indian children learn by observing demonstrations, whereas the children of non-Indian cultures tend to learn by trial and error. One of the co-authors of this chapter found, in working with Navajo Indian clients, the demonstration method of learning to be highly successful with Navajo-speaking adults, whose therapy included use of oxygen equipment. With minimal supervision, clients were expected to safely manage their oxygen therapies while residing in various types of non–fire retardant homes. The typical American Indian homestead includes trailers, wood frame houses, and traditional timber and clay hogans.* All of these homes have a central coal- or wood-fired heat source in the central living area. After observing a demonstration of correct procedure, clients were able to successfully maintain the oxygen tank, read the gauge, fill a portable tank, and creatively position the oxygen tubing away from all heat sources. The Literacy Volunteers of America, in the handbook *Do You Understand* (1989), recommends the use of cultural and gender-appropriate diagrams or stick figure drawings as another way to communicate with non–English speaking clients.

Communication patterns, such as extended pauses or periods of silence, are often used by the American Indian client. These patterns of speech may sometimes be confusing to the perioperative nurse, who may prematurely initiate closure during an extended period of silence, when in actuality the client wishes to continue the dialogue. Furthermore, the perioperative nurse may erroneously believe that the client either does not comprehend or is reluctant to provide answers to questions. Harris

---

*A "hogan" is a traditional round structure made of logs and mud. The structure may be used as a home or for ceremonial purposes.

(1993) observed that, in the learning situation, Navajo teachers allow a much longer period of time to elapse before expecting a response from Navajo children than is customarily permitted by the Anglo classroom teachers of the dominant society. Harris' (1993) study suggests that some American Indian cultural rules may indicate use of the deliberate pause as a linguistic act of contemplation and respect. During the interviewing phase of the health history, the perioperative nurse will need to be cognizant of the this style of communication.

Misinterpretation of body language is another common problem. As has been noted in the Asian American discussion, in the dominant American culture, lack of eye contact indicates avoidance behavior or the presence of low self-esteem. However, within the American Indian cultures, absence of eye contact indicates respect (Harris, 1993). In the perioperative setting, the nurse will need to consider all cultural behaviors before interpreting the true meaning of a client's avoidance of direct eye gaze.

Health Problems

A composite profile of American Indians and Alaska Natives is contained in the collection of data compiled by the federal government in the 33 states where the Indian Health Service delivers health care. The median age on the reservations is 23 years, with more than 25% of the total reservation residents living below the poverty level (U.S. Department of Health and Human Services, 1990). *Healthy People 2000* (U.S. Department of Health and Human Services, 1990) identifies two categories of health problems. The first lists the leading causes of death for American Indians that exceed the rate of death in the general population. For this problem area six causes have been identified: unintentional injuries, cirrhosis, homicide, suicide, pneumonia, and complications of diabetes. The second category considers the leading causes of death for American Indians in reservation states. The ranked causes are heart disease, cancers, injuries, stroke, liver disease, diabetes, pneumonia, influenza, suicide, homicide, and chronic lung disease. Although alcohol use is considered a factor in the rates associated with injuries, homicide, suicide, liver diseases, and complications of diabetes (U.S. Department of Health and Human Services, 1990), the reader is cautioned not to interpret this information to mean that all American Indians are alcoholics or use alcohol. Although current statistics (U.S. Department of Health and Human Services, 1990) indicate that approximately "95% of American Indian families are either directly or indirectly affected by a family member's abuse of alcohol," many Navajo Indians do not use alcohol,

owing to restrictions imposed by adherence to both traditional and religious values.

As was indicated above, cirrhosis and diabetes mellitus are two chronic diseases that occur in higher incidence among American Indians than among other American populations. In one governmental report it was found that diabetes occurred in approximately 20% of the members of many tribes, with a 40% incidence reported in two tribes in the state of Arizona (U.S. Department of Health and Human Services, 1990). In addition to diabetes and cirrhosis, there now is evidence of an increasing prevalence of obesity among American Indian groups, contributing significantly to the development of hypertension and cardiovascular disease. Other reported health problems include otitis media, poor nutrition, poor dental health, mental health problems, maternal child health needs, problems associated with aging, and unhealthy environmental conditions (U.S. Department of Health and Human Services, 1993a).

As with many other culturally diverse groups that reside in remote areas, access to primary health care is difficult for American Indians. Physician availability in many of these areas is "about half of the national average" (U.S. Department of Health and Human Services, 1990). Additionally, only members of federally recognized tribes are eligible for the health care provided by the Indian Health Service (U.S. Department of Health and Human Services, 1993a).* Others who live in areas not serviced by either the Indian Health Service or the various tribal programs must depend on local health care systems. These clients must obtain health care coverage through private insurance, public assistance, or self-pay. Studies indicated that, when hospitalized, clients tended to be admitted for the following diseases and complicating sequelae: obstetric complications, diseases of the respiratory system, digestive system diseases, injuries and poisonings, and circulatory system diseases (U.S. Department of Health and Human Services, 1993b).

In light of the higher incidence of serious health problems for the American Indian, it is imperative that a thorough physical examination and history be obtained. More information on successful interventions, such as education and treatment modalities related to specific tribes, can be obtained by contacting the Indian Health Service.†

*Indian Health Service provides assistance to members of federally recognized tribes. The classification of federal recognition was determined by the tribes that signed treaties with the federal government earlier in the nation's history.
†Indian Health Service Headquarters; Rockville, MD 20852; 301/443-4242

HISPANIC AMERICANS
Demographic Composition

The cultural classification of Hispanic Americans is a broad description of a richly diverse, heterogeneous group of people holding ancestral ties to Spain. Included are Mexican Americans; Cuban Americans; members of Spanish, Mexican, and Indian populations; Puerto Ricans; and other Spanish-speaking Caribbean Islanders (Statistical abstract, 1992). Because of the variety of subpopulations among Hispanic Americans, there are several other terms, such as "Latino" and "Raza," that are often used to identify this cultural subgroup (Griffin, 1992; Novello, Wise, & Kleinman, 1991).

Currently, there are 22 million Hispanic Americans in the United States. Hispanic Americans constitute approximately 9% of the total American population (U.S. Bureau of the Census, 1990). It is estimated that by the year 2000, there will be 31 million Hispanic Americans in this country; by 2050, Hispanics will be the largest ethnic group in the country (Rojas, 1994). Hispanic Americans live in every state, with the majority found in New Mexico, California, Texas, New York, Florida, New Jersey, and Illinois (Ginzberg, 1991; Griffin, 1992).

Although linked by ancestral ties to Spain, Hispanic Americans are a diverse group of people. The cultural classification encompasses both the more recent first- generation families and the second-, third-, and fourth-generation families, many of whom have become well acculturated members of dominant American society. The skin color of Hispanic Americans varies, ranging from all shades of black, brown, tan, and olive to white.

Ginzberg (1991) reports that socioeconomic considerations, in particular levels of education, occupation, and income, all influence the quality of health care available to this culturally diverse group. When compared with the dominant society, differences in levels of education, occupation, and income are found to exist (Juarbe, 1995). Conditions of less education, higher unemployment rates, and lower income predispose Hispanic Americans to poverty. Poverty, in turn, results in below-average health status and a higher incidence of specific diseases.

According to the U.S. Census report (1990), the median school years completed by the Hispanic American adult is 12.1 years, compared with the Anglo-American population of 12.7 years. Only 10% of the Hispanic American population completes a college education. The average income for Hispanic Americans has been reported to range from $15,000 to $25,000 per year, with 25% of Hispanic families living below the poverty level.

As a group, Hispanic Americans are more likely to lack health insurance, which negatively affects their access to the health care delivery system (Trevino, et al., 1991). The *Statistical Abstract of the U.S.* (1992) reports that 31.4% of Hispanics, compared with 12.7% of the Anglo-American population, are not covered by health insurance. These socioeconomic characteristics, coupled with a lack of fluency in English, subject this population to higher mortality and morbidity.

Family Structure

The Hispanic American family structure ranges from nuclear to extended. In the nuclear family structure the man is considered the head of the household. In the extended family structure the following blood-related and non–blood-related members may be included: grandparents, uncles, aunts, cousins, "church family" friends, neighbors, and "compadres" (godparents). Many decisions regarding health care are family decisions. Therefore, the Hispanic American client may need time to discuss health care options with significant others. Allowing time for clients to discuss health care issues with their relatives is of utmost importance in the development of mutual goals and expectations; Hispanic Americans value and need the presence of their family support system during their hospitalizations (Adams, Briones, & Rentfro, 1992: Arrunda, Larson, & Meleis, 1992). As with the other culturally diverse groups discussed in this chapter, it is important for the perioperative nurse to be aware of this interdependence within the Hispanic American family structure when planning and implementing perioperative care. Relaxing visitation restrictions and allowing the family to participate as an active support system could reduce stress during perioperative care events.

Religion and Spirituality

Catholicism is practiced by the majority of Hispanic Americans. However, many are also members of other faiths such as Jehovah's Witness, Protestant, and Evangelical. When perception of illness is influenced by religion, many use prayer for peace and comfort. Many Evangelicals believe in the "laying on of hands" for healing. Hispanic Americans may request the presence of their ministers or fellow church members to "lay on hands" for healing and recovery. Although there is little research at present to describe the impact of religion on illness, it is thought that religion may play a vital role in the healing process (Mickely & Soeken, 1992).

Communication

There are many Hispanic Americans who do not speak, read, or understand the English language (Bond & Jones, 1994). For the Spanish-speaking client to understand his or her perioperative care, it is essential for the perioperative nurse to provide the client with information and literature in Spanish. Although the Hispanic American client may be accompanied by family or friends during hospitalization, it is not always appropriate to use these individuals to translate sensitive information. The client's privacy may be violated, and the accuracy of the assessment may be encumbered (Smart & Smart, 1992). In such situations, the use of a Spanish-speaking health care provider to facilitate the communication process is preferred. Many hospitals have developed a roster of bilingual employees and volunteers to help communicate with non–English-speaking clients. In a study by Arrunda, Larson, and Meleis (1992), it was concluded that the meaning of comfort for Hispanic American cancer clients was closely associated with both the need to be listened to and the need to communicate with those providing the care.

Hispanic Americans place a high value on *respecto* (respect). The perioperative nurse will need to be sensitive to behaviors that might be practiced by members of the dominant society, which may, inadvertently, convey meanings of disrespect. This is particularly evident in how the client may be addressed. The perioperative nurse should approach the client in a formal manner, avoiding the use of familiar terms such as "honey," "sweetie," "grandma," and the like. The surname should be used to address the client until permission is granted to speak on a first-name basis. Closely associated with the high value placed on the demonstration of respectful behavior is the strong sense of pride held by the members of this cultural subgroup. Many, especially the elderly, are intensely proud, *probre pero orgulloso* (poor but proud) and interpret a lack of privacy as evidence of insensitivity. The perioperative nurse should take care to provide privacy when assessing, teaching, or implementing care; communication is seriously hindered when the client perceives a lack of respect on the part of the perioperative nurse or other health care providers.

Health Beliefs and Practices

Hispanic American views on health and illness are quite diverse, ranging from the sole practice of folk remedies to the sole reliance on scientific, modern medical practices (Higginbotham, Trevino, & Ray, 1990; Marsh & Hentges, 1988). Some believe illness to be the result of fate (*que sea, lo que Dios quea* [let it be God's will]) and health to be the result of good fortune; others view illness in a religious context (*una prueba* [a trial]), as that which is caused by a deity in punishment for a sin (Mickley & Soeken, 1992). Occasionally a Hispanic American will have no conflict in consulting both the folk practitioner *(curandero)*/spiritualist/herbalist and the modern Western medical health care provider. Ailinger (1988), in a study of Hispanic Americans and hypertension, reported 90% of the respondents believed in the efficacy of both folk practice and modern medical treatment.

The most common folk conditions include *empacho, susto,* and *male de ojo. Empacho,* a blocked intestine, is believed to be caused by a bolus of food that becomes lodged along the intestinal wall. This occurs by eating certain foods at the wrong times (for example, bananas late at night) or by eating improperly cooked food. Symptoms include bloating of the stomach, indigestion, nausea, vomiting, constipation, and diarrhea. Treatment includes massage of the abdomen and the ingestion of a variety of teas and olive or cooking oil by mouth.

Susto, a frightful event a person has no control over (for example, car accident or earthquake), results in a loss of the person's spirit or soul. Symptoms include insomnia, depression, anxiety, or nervousness. The goal of treatment is to return the lost spirit by using a ceremonial sweep with herbs and prayer or by use of relaxation techniques (Marsh & Hentges, 1988).

Mal de ojo, "evil eye," is thought to be caused by an individual with a strong power (or strong eye) who looks at or admires a person without the use of touch. Resulting symptoms include fever, irritability, headaches, diarrhea, and loss of weight. The cure is achieved either by permitting the person, who is the source of this evil eye or power, to touch the individual, thereby removing the evil eye, or by engaging in ceremonial sweeping and prayer.

Imbalances between "hot" and "cold" are believed to cause illness. The "hot-cold" theory originates from the Hippocratic humoral theories of disease. According to this theory, the body humors (blood, phlegm, bile) vary in temperatures. A harmony must exist between hot and cold elements to maintain health and prevent illness. Illnesses are categorized as being either hot or cold (Table 23-1); foods, herbs, and medications are also classified as hot or cold (Table 23-1) and used therapeutically to correct the disease state and restore the body to its harmony or balance. According to this theory, when treating a "hot" disease such as ulcers, a cure is effected with the administration of "cold" foods, herbs, or medications. Many of these foods, herbs, and medicines are easily accessible to the Hispanic American client. They are usually found in the *bodega* (a neighborhood Spanish store) or *botanica* (a local herbal store owned and operated by Hispanic Americans).

Table 23-1 Hot-cold conditions and their corresponding treatment*

Variable	Hot	Cold
Conditions	Fever, infections, diarrhea, kidney problems, rashes, skin ailments, sore throat, liver problems, ulcers, constipation	Cancer, pneumonia, malaria, joint pain, menstrual period, teething, earache, rheumatism, tuberculosis, colds, headache, paralysis, stomach cramps
Foods	Chocolate, cheese, temperate-zone fruits, eggs, peas, onions, aromatic beverages, hard liquor, oils, meats such as beef, waterfowl, or mutton, goat's milk, cereal grains, chili peppers	Fresh vegetables; tropical fruits; dairy products; meats such as goat; fish or chicken; honey; cod; raisins; bottled milk; barley water
Medicines and herbs	Penicillin, tobacco, ginger root, garlic, cinnamon, anise, vitamins, iron preparations, cod-liver oil, castor oil, aspirin	Orange-flower water, linden, sage, milk of magnesia, bicarbonate of soda

From Barkauskas VH, et al. (1994). *Health and physical assessment.* St. Louis: Mosby.
*Those who believe that illnesses result from an imbalance further believe that righting the imbalance leads to health. When there is too much of one extreme, the opposite extreme is applied with food or medicine to achieve a healthy balance. Therefore to treat the "hot" conditions listed here, one would apply a "cold" medicine or food, and vice versa.

Health Problems

The Council on Scientific Affairs (1991) reports disproportionate mortality and morbidity among Hispanic Americans. Rates of diabetes, hypertension, tuberculosis, and cancer are found to be higher for Hispanic Americans than for Anglo-Americans. Hispanic American populations tend to have three times the rate of incidence of diabetes mellitus when compared with other American groups. Furthermore, the incidence of diabetes tends to occur in the younger Hispanic American age groups, resulting in more serious long-term complications. With respect to cancerous conditions, the incidence of death from stomach cancer was found to be twice that of other populations, and, in Hispanic American women, the rate of cervical cancer doubled the rate of other groups.

CONCLUSION

In the provision of care for culturally diverse aggregates, perioperative nurses will be challenged to consider their own values, biases, and beliefs in the rendering of culturally relevant health care interventions. The development of culturally sensitive plans of care in the perioperative setting is predicated upon the recognition of, and appreciation for, the inherent differences found among the dominant American society's culturally diverse populations. By incorporating culturologic considerations into the professional plan of care, the perioperative nurse will effect the development of client-centered outcome criteria arrived at through a collaborative process, which addresses the needs of the client-family unit and considers the mind-body-spirit dimension.

References

AAN expert panel report on culturally competent health care. (1992). *Nursing Outlook, 40*(6), 277-283.

Adams R, Briones EH, & Rentfro AR. (1992). Cultural considerations: Developing a nursing care delivery system for a Hispanic community. *Nursing Clinics of North America, 27*(1), 107-116.

Adler S. (1983). Seeking stillness in motion: An introduction to Tai Chi for seniors. *Activities, Adaptation & Aging, 10*(3), 1-4.

Ailinger RL. (1988). Folk beliefs about high blood pressure in Hispanic immigrants. *Western Journal of Nursing Research, 10*(5), 629-636.

Arrunda EM, Larson PJ, & Meleis AI. (1992). Comfort immigrant Hispanic cancer client views. *Cancer Nursing, 15*(6), 387-394.

Austin B, Schoenrock S, & Roberts J. (1991). *Asian and Pacific Islander Elderly Bibliography.* San Diego: Resource Center in Minority Aging Populations, San Diego State University.

Barkauskas VH et al. (1994). *Health and physical assessment.* St. Louis: Mosby.

Beare PG & Myers JL. (1994). *Principles and Practice of Adult Health Nursing* (2nd ed.). St. Louis: Mosby.

Bell R. (1994). Prominence of women in Navajo healing beliefs and values. *Nursing and Health Care, 15*(5), 232-240.

Bond ML & Jones ME. (1994). Short-term cultural immersion in Mexico. *Nursing and Health Care, 15*(5), 248-253.

Branch MF & Paxton PP. (1976). *Providing safe nursing care for ethnic people of color.* New York: Appleton-Century-Crofts.

Brice J. (1982). West Indian families. In M McGoldrick, J Pearce, J Giordano, (Eds.), *Ethnicity and family therapy.* New York: Guilford Press.

Buehler J. (1993). Nursing in rural Native American communities. *Nursing Clinics of North America, 28*(1), 211-217.

Campbell T & Chang B. (1981). Health care of the Chinese in America. In G Henderson & M Primeaux (Eds.). *Transcultural health care,* Menlo Park, CA: Addison-Wesley.

Chan C & Chang J. (1976). The role of Chinese medicine in New York City's Chinatown, *American Journal of Chinese Medicine, 4,* 31-45.

Chen W. (1993). Cardiovascular health among Asian Americans/Pacific Islanders: An examination of health status and intervention approaches, *American Journal of Health Promotion, 7*(3), 199-207.

Cook LS & Petit de Mange B. (1995). Gaining access to non–

Native American cultures by non–Native American nurse researchers. *Nursing Forum, 30*(1), 5-10.

Council on Scientific Affairs. (1991). Hispanic health in the United States. *Journal of the American Medical Association, 26*(2), 248-252.

D'Avanzo CE, Frye B, & Froman R. (1994). Stress in Cambodian refugee families. *Image—the Journal of Nursing Scholarship, 26*(2), 101-105.

Eliason MJ. (1993). Ethics and transcultural nursing care. *Nursing Outlook, 41*(5), 225-228.

Fujimoto W, Leonetti J, & Kinyoun J. (1987). Prevalence of diabetes mellitus and impaired glucose tolerance among second generation Japanese American men. *Diabetes, 36,* 730-739.

Geissler EM. (1991). Transcultural nursing and nursing diagnoses. *Nursing & Health Care, 12,* 190-192; 203.

Giger J & Davidhizar R. (1991). *Transcultural nursing: Assessment and interventions.* St. Louis: Mosby.

Ginzberg E. (1991). Access to health care for Hispanics. *Journal of the Amrican Medical Association, 265*(2), 238-241.

Gioiella EC. (1994). Culturally competent care and the school environment. *Journal of Professional Nursing, 10*(1), 6.

Gonzalez EW, Gitlin LN, & Lyons KJ. (1995). Review of the literature on African American caregivers of individuals with dementia. *Journal of Cultural Diversity, 2*(2), 40-48.

Green NL. (1995). Development of the perceptions of racism scale. *Image—the Journal of Nursing Scholarship, 27*(2), 141-146.

Griffin RD. (1992). Hispanic Americans. *Congressional Quarterly Researcher, 2*(40), 929-952.

Harris G. (1993). American Indian cultures: A lesson in diversity. In DE Battle (Ed.), *Communication disorders in multicultural populations* (pp. 78-113). Boston: Andover Medical Publishers.

Higginbotham JC, Trevino FM, & Ray LA. (1990). Utilization of curanderos by Mexican Americans: Prevalence and predictors findings from HHANES 1982-194. *American Journal of Public Health, 80*(suppl), 32-35.

Higgins PG & Dicharry EK. (1990). Measurement issues in the use of the Coopersmith Self-Esteem Inventory with the Navajo women. *Health Care International 11*(3), 251-262.

Hines PM & Boyd-Franklin N. (1982). Black families. In M McGoldrick, J Pearce, J Giordano, (Eds.), *Ethnicity and family therapy.* New York: Guilford.

Jezewski MA. (1993). Culture brokering as a model for advocacy. *Nursing and Health Care, 14*(2), 78-84.

Juarbe TC. (1995). Access to health care for Hispanic women: A primary health care perspective. *Nursing Outlook, 43*(1), 23-28.

Kinzie J. (1985). Overview of clinical issues in the treatment of Southeast Asia refugees. In TC Owan (Ed.), *Southeast Asian mental health* (pp. 91-112), Rockville, MD: NIMH.

Kotecki CN. (1990). Communication. In M Kinney, D Packa, & S Dunbar (Eds.), *AACN's clinical reference for critical care nursing* (3rd Ed.). St. Louis: Mosby.

Lantz JM. (1989). Family culture and ethnicity. In PJ Bomar (Ed.), *Nurses and family health promotion concepts, assessment and interventions.* Baltimore: Williams & Wilkins.

Lee H. (1982). The anatomy of the Mongolian eyes and its relation to complication in cataract extraction and lens implantation. In Proceedings of the Conference on Health Problems Related to the Chinese in America, May 1982, San Francisco.

Leininger MM. (1989). The transcultural nurse specialist: Imperative in today's world. *Nursing Health Care, 10,* 251-256.

Leininger MM. (1991). *Culture care diversity and universality: A theory of nursing.* New York: National League for Nursing Press.

Leininger M. (1994). Transcultural nursing education: A worldwide imperative. *Nursing Health Care, 15*(5), 254-257.

Lin-Fu J. (1988). Population characteristics and health care needs of Asian Pacific Americans, *Public Health Reports, 103,* 18-27.

Liu W & Yu E. (1985). Asian/Pacific elderly: Mortality differentials, health status, and use of health services. *Journal of Applied Gerontology, (4),* 35-64.

Louie K. (1985). Providing health care to Chinese clients, *Transcultural Nursing, 7,* 18-21.

Mail PD, McKay RB, & Katz M. (1989). Expanding practice horizons: Learning from American Indian clients: Client educaton for special populations. *Patient Education and Counseling, 13* (2), 91-102.

Malone B. (1993). Shouldering the responsibility for culturally sensitive and competent health care. *Imprint, 40,* 53-54.

Marsh WW & Hentges K. (1988). Mexican folk remedies and conventional medical care. *American Family Physician, 37*(3), 257-262.

Mays BE. (1968). *The Negro's God: As Reflected in His Literature.* New York: Atheunum.

Mickley J & Soeken K. (1992). Religiousness and hope in Hispanic and Anglo-American women with breast cancer. *Oncology Nursing Forum, 20*(8), 1171-1177.

Morganthau T. (1993). The Clinton solution. *Newsweek,* September 20, 1993, 30-35.

Morioka-Douglas N & Yeo G. (1990). *Aging and health: Asian/Pacific Island American elders,* SGEC Working Paper Series, 3, Stanford, CA: Stanford Geriatric Center.

Navajo Treaty, 1868. In R Bell. (1994). Prominence of women in Navajo healing beliefs and values. *Nursing Health Care, 15*(5), 232-240.

Nickens HW. (1995). Race/ethnicity as a factor in health and health care. *Health Services Research, 30*(1), 151-162.

Novello AC, Wise PH, & Kleinman DV. (1991). Hispanic health: Time for data, time for action. *Journal of the American Medical Asociation 265,*(2), 253-255.

Outlaw FH. (1994). A reformulation of the meaning of culture and ethnicity for nurses delivering care. *Medsurg Nursing, 3*(2), 108-111.

Peterson R. (1978). *The elder Filipino.* San Diego: Center on Aging.

Porter CP, & Villarruel AM. (1993). Nursing research with African American and Hispanic people: Guidelines for action. *Nursing Outlook, 41*(2), 59-66.

Reiskin H & Haussler SC. (1994). Multicultural students' perceptions of nursing as a career. *Image—the Journal of Nursing Scholarship, 26*(1), 61-64.

Rojas D. (1994). Leadership in a multicultural society: A case in role development. *Nursing and Health Care, 15*(5), 258-261.

Rosella JD, Regan-Kubinski MJ, & Albrecht SA. (1994). The need for multicultural diversity among health professionals. *Nursing and Health Care, 15*(5), 242-246.

Schaefer RT. (1986). *Sociology.* New York: McGraw-Hill.

Shon S & Ja D. (1982). Asian families. In M McGoldrick, J Pearce, & J Giordano (Eds.), *Ethnicity and family therapy* (pp 208-228), New York: Guilford.

Smart JD & Smart DW. (1992). Cultural issues in the rehabilitation of Hispanics. *Journal of Rehabilitation, 58*(2), 29-3.

Spector RE. (1985). *Cultural diversity in health and illness.* Norwalk: Appleton-Century-Crofts.

Statistical Abstract of the United States (1992). Washington, DC: U.S. Bureau of the Census.

Stavig G, Igra A, & Leanard A. (1988). Hypertension and related health issues among Asians and Pacific Islanders in California. *Public Health Reports, 103,* 28-37.

Stule P. (1996). In Cookfair JN (Eds). *Nursing care in the community* (2nd ed.). St. Louis: Mosby.

Sue D & Sue D. (1990). *Counseling the culturally different.* New York: John Wiley.

Sugarman JR, et al. (1993). Racial misclassification of American Indians: Its effect on injury rate in Oregon, 1989 through 1990. *American Journal of Public Health. 83*(5), 681-684.

Tien J. (1984). Do Asians need less medicine? *Journal of Psychosocial Nursing, 22,* 19-22.

Trevino FM, et al. (1991). Health insurance coverage and utilization of health services by Mexican Americans, mainland Puerto Ricans, and Cuban Americans. *Journal of the American Medical Association 265*(2), 233-237.

Uba L. (1992). Cultural barriers to health care of Southeast Asian refugees. *Public Health Reports, 107,* 544-548.

U.S. Bureau of the Census. (1990). *Current population reports, population characteristics: The Asian and Pacific Islander population in the United States.* Washington, DC: U.S. Government Printing Office.

U.S. Bureau of the Census. (1992). *Statistical abstract of the United States* (112th ed.). Washington, DC: U.S. Government Printing Office.

U.S. Department of Health and Human Services. Public Health Service. (DHHS PHS, 1990a). *Health status of minority and low-income groups* (3rd ed.). Washington DC: U.S. Government Printing Office.

U.S. Department of Health and Human Services Public Health Service. (DHHS PHS, 1990b). *Healthy people 2000.* (DHHS Publication) No. (PHS) 91-50212. Washington: U.S. Government Printing Office.

U.S. Department of Health and Human Services Public Health Service. (DHHS PHS 1993a) Indian Health Service, *Comprehensive health care program for American Indians and Alaska Natives.* (DHHS Publication) Washington DC: U.S. Government Printing Office.

U.S. Department of Health and Human Services Public Health Service Indian Health Service. (DHHS PHS, 1993b). *Regional differences in Indian health.* (DHHS Publication). Washington DC: U.S. Government Printing Office.

U.S. General Accounting Office (1990). *Asian Americans, a status report.* GAO/HRD-90-36 FS. Washington DC: General Accounting Office.

Whitemore A. (1989). Colorectal cancer incidence among Chinese in North America and People's Republic of China: Variations in sex, age, and anatomical site, *International Journal of Epidemiology, 18,* 563-568.

Wilson GA. (1989). *Conversational Navajo dictionary English to Navajo.* Blanding, UT.

Yu E. (1986). Health of the Chinese elderly in America, *Research on Aging, 8,* 84-109.

Zhou H, et al. (1989). Racial differences in drug response: Altered sensitivity to and clearance of propranolol in men of Chinese descent as compared with American whites, *New England Journal of Medicine, 320,* 565-570.

Chapter 24

Planning for Unexpected Outcomes

Jane C. Rothrock

A celebrated man, though celebrated only for foolish things, has told us that one of his main objects in the education of his son was to give him a ready habit of accurate observation, a certainty of perception, and that for this purpose one of his means was a month's course as follows: he took the boy rapidly past a toy-shop; the father and son then described to each other as many of the objects as they could, which they had seen in the passing windows, noting them down with pencil and paper, and returning afterwards to verify their own accuracy. . . . I have often thought how wise a piece of education this would be for much higher objects; and in our calling of nurses the thing is essential. For it may be safely said, not that the habit of ready and correct observation will by itself make us useful nurses, but that without it we shall be useless with all our devotion.

NIGHTINGALE, 1860

*T*he prevention and management of untoward events in perioperative practice settings is the responsibility of the surgeon, anesthesia personnel, and perioperative nurse. The perioperative nurse assumes a collaborative role in patient assessment, intervention, and evaluation to facilitate team management of intraoperative emergencies. Advances in medical technology and increased patient acuity levels underscore the need for perioperative nurses to ensure patient safety during intraoperative emergencies such as cardiac arrest, shock, hemorrhage, and malignant hyperthermia (MH).

ETIOLOGIC AND ASSESSMENT CONSIDERATIONS

Identifying a patient at risk for intraoperative emergencies is the first step to planning nursing care. Nursing assessment helps the perioperative nurse anticipate and prioritize nursing activities during intraoperative emergencies.

Hemorrhage

Hemorrhage is a potential intraoperative emergency for each surgical patient. Hemorrhage lowers blood volume and decreases the flow of blood into the heart. If not corrected, hemorrhage leads to further compromise of the circulatory and respiratory sys-

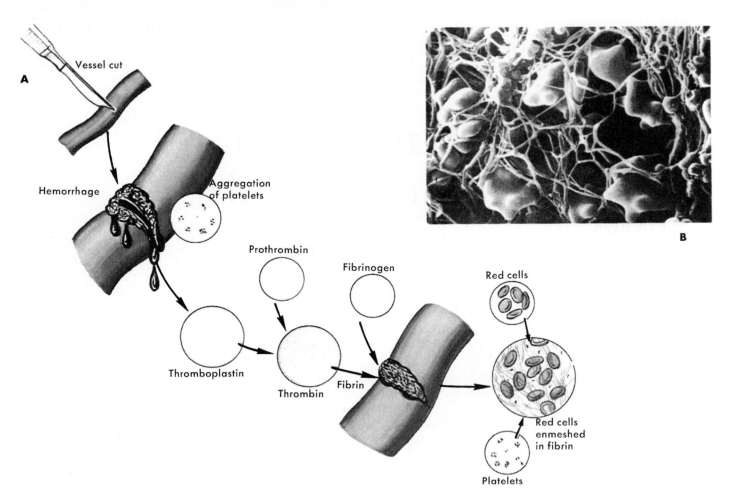

Fig. 24-1. Main steps in blood clotting. **A,** Platelet aggregation at site of injury, formation of thrombin from prothrombin, and fibrin clot with trapped red cells. **B,** Mesh of fibrin forming a clot. (**A,** from Thibodeau, 1987; **B,** Raven, P. H., & Johnson. (i, B. (1989), *Biology,* (2nd ed.). St. Louis: Mosby.)

tems, which may lead to shock and cardiac arrest. The perioperative nurse must identify patients at risk preoperatively to prepare for potential blood volume loss in case an intraoperative emergency arises.

Trauma patients. Trauma patients often have alterations in fluid volume before surgery. Preoperative fluid volume deficits may be caused by hemorrhage resulting from blunt or penetrating wounds, as seen in motor vehicle accidents, gunshot wounds, stabbings, fractured femurs, and compound injuries. Traumatic injuries such as automobile accidents often injure the chest and abdomen, whereas motorcycle accidents result in long bone fractures. The perioperative nurse prepares for intraoperative internal bleeding based on the type of traumatic injury incurred; close interdepartmental coordination and preparation for fluid replacement should be a priority for the perioperative nurse to facilitate correction of a fluid volume deficit. A full discussion of peri-

operative care of the trauma patient can be found in Chapter 20.

Interference with coagulation. Preoperative pharmaceutical, platelet, and coagulation disorders predispose the patient to alterations in normal mechanisms of hemostasis (Fig. 24-1). Patients taking aspirin, antihistamines, antiinflammatory drugs, chemotherapeutic agents, antibiotics, and anticoagulant therapy (that is, heparin or sodium warfarin) are predisposed to hemorrhage. Platelet disorders to screen for include (1) thrombocytopenia, (2) presence of disseminated intravascular coagulation (DIC), and (3) defects in the coagulation pathway such as vitamin K deficiency (Price & Wilson, 1992). These platelet disorders induce hemorrhage in the surgical patient. Inherited coagulation disorders such as hemophilia predispose patients to massive fluid loss if preventive replacement measures are ineffective.

Blood loss. Blood loss of 750 to 1300 ml results in a 15% to 25% blood deficit in an adult with normal circulating volume (Lewis & Collier, 1996). This volume deficit results in a reduction in cardiac output if replacement measures are ineffective; either rapid bleeding (25% to 35% of total blood volume) or slow bleeding (40% to 50% over a period of an hour) will reduce the cardiac output to zero (McFarland & McFarlane, 1993). Physical clues to this loss include tachycardia (over 100 beats per minute for adults), a rise in diastolic pressure (although blood pressure is not a good indicator of early hypovolemic shock), slight central nervous system changes (anxiety, hostility, fright), which may be the first early signs of impending hypovolemic shock, and positive capillary blanch test (Gulanick, et al., 1994).

Uncorrected loss of 2000 ml of blood results in a 30% to 40% loss in total volume. This volume deficit results in tachycardia and decreased systolic blood pressure, although the supine position may maintain normal ranges of pulse and blood pressure. Additional signs of decreased fluid volume include decreased pulse pressure, hyperventilation, oliguria, thirst, apprehension, and cool, pale skin.

Blood loss greater than 2000 ml is a 40% loss in fluid volume. Physical signs are exaggerated and include (1) increased tachycardia, (2) severe thirst, (3) narrow pulse pressure, (4) obscure diastolic pressure, and (5) no urinary output. The patient is lethargic and has depressed mental status.

Hypovolemic Shock

Shock has many causes, but in perioperative patients it is commonly caused by hemorrhage. Hemorrhage diminishes circulatory fluid volume to the extent that the body's metabolic needs are not met. This phenomenon is known as hypovolemic shock (Holcroft & Robinson, 1992). Patients at risk for hypovolemic shock include those experiencing (1) hemothorax, (2) ectopic pregnancy, (3) recent (less than 36 hours) childbirth, (4) hemophilia trait, (5) DIC, (7) aortic aneurysm, (8) trauma, and (9) invasive surgical procedures such as vascular bypass, abdominal perineal resection, or pneumonectomy. Loss of interstitial fluid causes hypovolemic shock indirectly; diffusion of plasma is from the intravascular space to the extravascular space. When the intravascular volume is decreased by approximately 15%, hypovolemic shock begins to develop. The progressive cascade begun by a decreased intravascular volume leads to reduced venous return, incomplete filling of the heart's ventricular chambers, decreased stroke volume, decreased cardiac output, reduced arterial blood pressure, and inadequate tissue perfusion. Capillary blood flow is diminished and oxygen delivery to the cells is inadequate. The consequences of hypovolemic shock are shown in Table 24-1. Patients at risk for hypovolemia resulting from an in-

Table 24-1 Nursing assessment of hypovolemic shock

Area of concern	Hypovolemic shock
General appearance	Anxiety, restlessness
Level of consciousness	Lethargy, stupor, or coma
Temperature	Increased or decreased
Heart rate	Increased, pulse thready
Auscultation	
Blood pressure	
Early	Pulse pressure decreased; diastolic pressure increased
Late	Systolic pressure decreased
Skin temperature and texture	Cool, moist, clammy, pale
Capillary refill time	Decreased
Peripheral pulses	Absent or diminished
Jugular venous distention	Absent or flat
Hemodynamic findings	
Central venous pressure	Decreased
Pulmonary capillary wedge pressure	Decreased
Cardiac output	Decreased
Peripheral vascular resistance	Decreased
Pulmonary function	
Respiratory rate	Increased; shallow or Cheyne-Stokes respirations
Auscultation	Early: clear; late: rales
Acid-base changes	
Early	Respiratory alkalosis
Late	Metabolic (lactic) acidosis
Urine output	
Early	Decreased (<20 ml/mm)
Late	Anuria
Urine sodium concentration	Decreased
Urine osmolality	Increased

From Thompson JM, et al. (1993). *Mosby's clinical nursing* (3rd ed.). St. Louis: Mosby–Year Book.

direct cause include those experiencing diarrhea, extensive diaphoresis, aldosterone deficiency (Addison's disease), diabetes mellitus, diabetes insipidus, emesis, extensive thermal injuries, ascites, gastrointestinal (GI) tract losses via ostomies, fistulas, or nasogastric (NG) tube, and those on diuretics (Beare & Meyers, 1994). Hypovolemia is initially handled by compensatory mechanisms (Fig. 24-2), but as these fail, progressive shock occurs.

Cardiac Arrest

Cardiac arrest is the sudden cessation of breathing and circulation in a patient who is not expected to die (Lowenstein, 1990); it results in permanent tissue damage and death if not successfully managed. Patients at risk for alterations in cardiac output include those with a history of atherosclerosis, hyper-

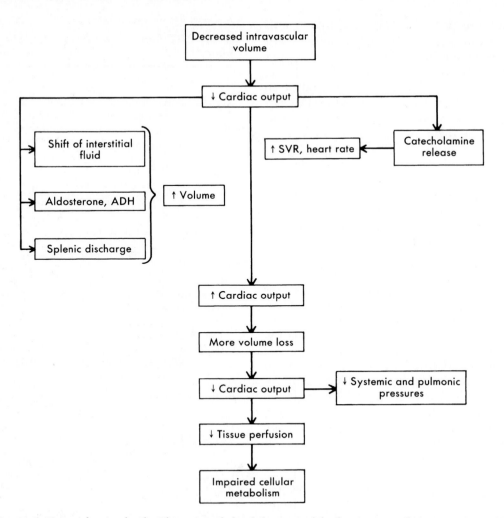

Fig. 24-2. Hypovolemic shock. This type of shock becomes life threatening when compensatory mechanisms are overwhelmed by continued loss of intravascular volume.

tension, diabetes mellitus, elevated cholesterol level, smoking, and sedentary life-style. Preoperative signs of potential alterations in cardiac output include shortness of breath, chest pain described as pressure, diaphoresis, hypertension followed by hypotension, and restlessness. Gastrointestinal signs include nausea, vomiting, and indigestion.

Intraoperative risk factors. Intraoperative risk factors imposed from the environment during surgery increase the potential for alterations in cardiac output. Environmental surgical stressors include intubation, extubation, tracheal suction, and manipulation of the bile duct and gallbladder. These surgical stressors alter cardiac output by activating the parasympathetic and sympathetic nervous systems.

The parasympathetic nervous system releases acetylcholine, which decreases cardiac electrical conduction and contractility. The sympathetic nervous system releases norepinephrine, which increases contractility, heart rate, and cardiac electri-

cal conduction. Additional situations altering the balance of the parasympathetic and sympathetic nervous systems during the intraoperative phase include (1) measurement of intraocular pressure with tonometer, (2) injection of dye during angiography, (3) positioning of cardiac catheters in the outflow pathway of the right ventricle, and (4) closure of the peritoneum during abdominal and thoracic procedures. These environmentally induced surgical stressors predispose the patient to alterations in cardiac output and cardiac arrest. The increase or decrease in cardiac contractility and cardiac output depends on whether the parasympathetic or sympathetic nervous system is stimulated.

Malignant Hyperthermia

Malignant hyperthermia is a hypermetabolic disorder of skeletal muscle. This phenomenon is precipitated by certain inhalation anesthetic agents and depolarizing neuromuscular blocking agents (muscle relaxants) used during general anesthesia (succinylcholine). The hypermetabolic condition of malignant hyperthermia results in a continuous release of calcium from individual muscle cells. This increase in intracellular calcium triggers the cascade of events associated with malignant hyperthermia.

The muscle cell is composed of a cell membrane surrounding an inner fluid sarcoplasm known as myoplasm. Intracellular calcium is stored in small sacs known as the sarcoplasmic reticulum. The sarcoplasmic reticulum stores 3000 times the amount of calcium normally found in the myoplasm. Before the muscle cell can respond to nervous stimulation, the sarcoplasmic reticulum must release calcium into the myoplasm. The muscle cell relaxes by pumping calcium back into the sarcoplasmic reticulum in normal muscle physiology.

In malignant hyperthermia, there is an abnormal reabsorption process or increased release of calcium by the sarcoplasmic reticulum (McCance & Huether, 1994). Increased calcium levels cause continuous and uncoordinated contractions, resulting in muscle rigidity or fasciculation. Sustained muscle contractions significantly increase the requirement for oxygen, resulting in increased heat, energy, carbon dioxide, and lactic acid production (Young & Kindred, 1993). This hypermetabolic state results in metabolic and respiratory acidosis. Acidosis affects the cell membrane permeability, resulting in a shift of potassium, calcium, creatine kinase (CK), and myoglobins to extracellular fluid (Pagana & Pagana, 1995). Thus the signs and symptoms of hypermetabolism and malignant hyperthermia are manifested in the musculoskeletal, respiratory, and cardiovascular systems when susceptible patients undergo anesthesia.

Patients at risk. Identifying patients at risk before anesthesia induction is important, because malignant hyperthermia may be fatal if corrective measures are not immediately initiated. The patient population in which malignant hyperthermia occurs most commonly is older children and young adults. Although both sexes are at risk, the incidence is higher in males (Donnelly, 1994). Once a patient has an identified susceptibility to malignant hyperthermia, subsequent episodes are prevented by initiating anesthesia protocols for malignant hyperthermia–susceptible patients. Patient education requires that basic principles of malignant hyperthermia are reviewed with the adult patient or with the child patient and family. Principles of preventing future episodes are then reviewed, such as alerting anesthesia personnel of the patient's anesthesia history so that appropriate decisions about the type of anesthetic (regional, local, conscious sedation, or general with nontriggering agents) can be determined. Prophylac-

---

Box 24-1 *Preoperative Screening for MH Susceptibility*

The following questions may be asked when the perioperative nurse is assessing the preoperative patient to screen for risk for malignant hyperthermia:
1. Is there a family history of MH?
2. Has there been an unexpected death or complication from anesthesia, including in the dentist's office, in the family?
3. Is there a family history or personal history of muscle disorders such as muscle weakness, unexpected muscle cramps (such as while resting), Duchenne muscular dystrophy, or central core disease (a syndrome characterized by undescended testes, pigeon breast, high forehead, and low-set ears)?
4. Is there a personal history of MH, dark (cola-colored) urine, or unexplained high fever following anesthesia or surgery?
5. Does the patient have certain physical characteristics, such as eye muscle abnormalities (droopy lids, crossed eyes), frequent joint dislocation, or spinal deformities such as scoliosis?

Although these questions are important to ask, the perioperative nurse should also understand that the family/personal history may be normal. Certain physical characteristics are believed to occur more frequently in MH- susceptible patients, but MH cannot be predicted solely on these characteristics. For that reason, all surgery settings should have an established MH protocol in place.

---

tic dantrolene sodium may be advised for the patient who has previously experienced a malignant hyperthermia episode if the surgical procedure will last more than 4 hours, will be stressful, or if the patient has an underlying disease that would be worsened by a hypermetabolic state.

Patients at risk for a malignant hyperthermia episode include those with a familial history of malignant hyperthermia, muscle disorders, or adverse anesthesia experiences or death during surgery, as well as those who have a personal history of malignant hyperthermia or anesthesia-related complications. A personal history of unexplained fever or dark (cola-colored) urine following anesthesia or muscle disease is also part of preoperative patient assessment (Box 24-1).

Signs and symptoms. Signs and symptoms of malignant hyperthermia appear in the cardiovascular, respiratory, musculoskeletal, integumentary, and genitourinary systems. Signs of malignant hyperthermia in the cardiovascular system include tachycardia, which may be a first sign of an acute episode of malignant hyperthermia. Symptoms can progress to ventricular fibrillation, ventricular tachycardia, and premature ventricular contractions. Blood pressure becomes unstable. Cardiac symptoms result from increased circulating catecholamines and hyperkalemia. The respiratory system's initial response to increased energy and oxygen expenditures is tachypnea. Tachypnea results from high CO_2 production arising from the hypermetabolic state. An increase in end-tidal CO_2 is the most sensitive indicator of malignant hyperthermia. Evidence of high CO_2 production may appear in the soda lime canister of the anesthesia machine, as the soda lime becomes discolored and warm to touch. The respiratory system may also be affected by masseter muscle rigidity (MMR) during intubation.

Masseter muscle rigidity or intense muscle fasciculations are triggered by administration of succinylcholine or volatile anesthetic agents during the induction process. Masseter muscle rigidity makes extension of the jaw, visualization of the vocal cords, and intubation difficult. Generalized muscle rigidity sets in during the later phase of malignant hyperthermia.

The skin is flushed and mottled in the initial phases of malignant hyperthermia. Mucous membranes and skin may or may not be cyanotic. Skin surface is warm from the hypermetabolic state. Diaphoresis may occur in the body's attempt to cool. Fevers associated with malignant hyperthermia may rise at a rate of 1° to 2° C (1.8° to 3.6° F) every 5 minutes (Barash, Cullen, & Stoeling, 1992). Temperatures of 43° C (109.4° F) are possible.

The genitourinary system initially responds with a reddish-brown urine (myoglobinuria) within 4 to 8 hours; anuria occurs as hypovolemia, inadequate tissue perfusion, and decreased cardiac output affect renal function.

Identification of patients at risk for malignant hyperthermia, cardiac arrest, shock, and hemorrhage is a necessary part of the perioperative nurse's role in anticipating and preparing for possible intraoperative emergencies. The perioperative nurse must be able to anticipate the potential for intraoperative emergencies to plan and intervene effectively. Diagnostic studies also provide data alerting the perioperative nurse to the patient's potential for untoward events.

DIAGNOSTIC STUDIES

Various diagnostic studies are used to determine patients' risk for hemorrhage (Table 24-2), shock (Table 24-3), cardiac arrest, and malignant hyperthermia. The diagnostic studies for hemorrhage, shock, and cardiac arrest are presented with the nursing diagnosis associated with each of the aforementioned intraoperative emergencies. Diagnostic studies used to identify malignant hyperthermia are reviewed under

malignant hyperthermia because the nursing diagnosis *hyperthermia* is a latent manifestation.

Confirming Nursing Diagnoses

Preoperative laboratory studies indicating *altered tissue perfusion* include abnormal platelet number (complete blood count), platelet function (Ivy bleeding time), and coagulation studies of the prothrombin and partial thromboplastin times. Hematocrit level is used to assess blood loss, hydration, and hematologic disorders. Blood hemoglobin level also reflects blood loss, anemias, and dehydration.

Arterial blood gas measurements are used to determine the degree of *impaired gas exchange*. This diagnostic test measures respiratory status and acid-base balance. Laboratory results may reflect decreased oxygen (Pao_2), increased carbon dioxide ($Paco_2$), and decreased pH values in the patient's arterial blood, confirming the nursing diagnosis and leading the perioperative nurse to collaborate in the intervention of respiratory acidosis.

Blood and urine evaluations indicate *alterations in fluid volume*. Serum electrolyte values such as calcium, chloride, potassium, sodium, and magnesium reflect the patient's acid-base balance. Blood urea nitrogen (BUN) levels are used to assess renal function and hydration status (McFarland & McFarlane, 1993). Increased BUN level, creatinine urine osmolarity, and polymorphonuclear leukocyte count reveal alterations in fluid shifts. In addition, hyperglycemia, hypochloremia, and decreased urine sodium level reflect shifts in interstitial fluid. If alterations in fluid shifts and volume remain uncorrected, alterations in cardiac output may develop.

Decreased cardiac output is reflected in many of the tests used for alterations in tissue perfusion, gas exchange, and fluid volume. An electrocardiogram (ECG) is performed preoperatively on patients with a history of heart disease. The ECG indicates the rhythm and conductivity of the heart and its ability to pump blood. Pulse pressure is another hemodynamic parameter the perioperative nurse can use to assess the patient's cardiac output. Pulse pressure is determined by stroke volume and vascular compliance (elasticity). Pulse pressure is the difference between systolic and diastolic pressures; a narrow pulse pressure in hypovolemic shock and hemorrhage reflects a low stroke volume and reflexive vasoconstriction (Christensen, 1992). Hypovolemia and shunting of blood to the body's core limits the blood circulating in the extremities; therefore changes in cardiac output may not be discernible until significant adjustments in tissue perfusion occur.

Malignant Hyperthermia

Currently, one preoperative diagnostic study can conclusively determine the patient's risk for malig-

Table 24-2 Coagulation studies

Study	Purpose	Normal values	Clinical significance
Bleeding time	Measures platelet and vascular function	2-9½ minutes	Prolonged in thrombocytopenia, thrombocytopathy, von Willebrand's disease, aspirin ingestion, anticoagulant therapy, and uremia
Platelet count	Assesses platelet concentration	150,000-400,000/mm^3	Decreased in idiopathic thrombocytopenic purpura (ITP) and bone marrow malignancies Drugs, especially chemotherapeutic agents, may cause prolonged bleeding Elevated in early myeloproliferative disorders After splenectomy, may predispose to later thrombotic episodes
Clot reaction	Assesses platelet adequacy to form fibrin clot	Clot retracts to one-half size in 1 hour, firm clot in 24 hours if undisturbed	Poor clot retraction in thrombocytopenia and polycythemia; lysis of clot in fibrinolysis
Lee-White clotting time (coagulation)	Assesses coagulation mechanism—time required for blood to form a solid clot after exposure to glass	6-12 minutes	Relatively insensitive test Prolonged with severe deficiencies of coagulation factors, in excessive anticoagulant therapy, and with selected antibiotics Decreased with corticosteroid therapy
Prothrombin time (PT)	Measures extrinsic and common coagulation pathway	11-16 seconds	Prolonged in deficiencies of factors VII and X and fibrinogen, excess dicumarol therapy, severe liver disease and DIC, and vitamin K deficiency
Activated partial thromboplastin time (APTT)	Measures intrinsic and common coagulation pathway	26-42 seconds	Prolonged in deficiencies of factors VIII to XII and fibrinogen, with circulating anticoagulant therapy, in liver disease and DIC, and in vitamin K deficiency Shortened in malignancies (except liver)
Thrombin time (TT) or thrombin clotting time	Measures fibrinogen to fibrin formation	10-13 seconds	Prolonged with low fibrinogen levels, inhibitors, DIC and liver disease, anticoagulant therapy, and in dysproteinemias
Thromboplastin generation test (TGT)	Measures ability to form thromboplastin	12 seconds or less	Prolonged in thrombocytopenia, with deficiencies of factors VIII to XII, and with circulating anticoagulants
D-Dimer test	Measures breakdown products of plasma fibrin clots	—	Elevated in DIC, pulmonary emboli, infarcts, thrombolytic therapy, surgery, trauma
Platelet aggregation test	Tests platelet function	Platelets aggregate within a specified time when exposed to substances such as adenosine diphosphate (ADP) collagen, epinephrine	Decreased or absent aggregation in thrombasthenia, aspirin ingestion, myeloproliferative disorders, severe liver disease, dysproteinemias, von Willebrand's disease

From Price SA & Wilson LM. (1992). *Pathophysiology: Clinical concepts of disease processes* (4th ed.). St. Louis: Mosby.

nant hyperthermia: the halothane-caffeine contracture test (CHCT) performed on biopsied muscle. This test is performed in a few medical centers across the nation, which means definitive diagnosis is not immediately available for many perioperative patients.

Intraoperative diagnostic studies performed during and after malignant hyperthermia crisis include urine and blood analyses. Arterial blood and central mixed venous blood gas levels and serum electrolyte studies indicate the presence of hyperkalemia and tissue hypoxia as well as respiratory and metabolic acidosis. In addition, blood and urine samples will be obtained for CK, lactate dehydrogenase (LDH), serum glutamic oxaloacetic transaminase (SGOT), myoglobin, coagulation studies, and myoglobinuria (Corkhill, 1993).

After patients at risk for intraoperative emergencies are identified according to diagnostic studies and the signs and symptoms associated with hem-

Table 24-3 Diagnostic study abnormalities in shock syndrome

Diagnostic study	Abnormal finding	Significance of abnormality
Blood		
Red blood cell count, hematocrit, hemoglobin	Normal	Remains within normal limits in shock because of relative hypovolemia and pump failure and in hemorrhagic shock before fluid restoration
	Decrease	Decreases in hemorrhagic shock after fluid resuscitation when fluids other than blood are used
	Increase	Increases in nonhemorrhagic shock due to actual hypovolemia because fluid lost does not contain erythrocytes
White blood cell count with differential	Leukopenia	Occurs in severe shock, especially when caused by gram-negative sepsis
	Leukocytosis with increased neutrophils	Is common in all forms of shock, especially hemorrhagic shock; neutrophils increase in response to tissue injury
Erythrocyte sedimentation rate	Increase	Is nonspecific, increases are in response to tissue injury
Blood urea nitrogen (BUN)	Increase	Usually indicates impaired kidney function due to hypoperfusion as a result of severe vasoconstriction
Serum creatinine	Increase	Usually indicates impaired kidney function due to hypoperfusion as a result of severe vasoconstriction, is more sensitive indicator of renal function than BUN
Blood sugar	Increase	Occurs in early shock because of release of liver glycogen stores in response to catecholamines
	Decrease	Occurs because of depleted glycogen stores with hepatocellular dysfunction possible as shock progresses
Serum electrolytes		
Sodium	Increase	Occurs early in shock because of increased secretion of aldosterone, causing renal retention of sodium
	Decrease	May occur iatrogenically when excess hypotonic fluid is administered after fluid loss
Potassium	Increase	Occurs when cellular death liberates intracellular potassium; also occurs in acute renal failure, after red blood cell hemolysis in transfusion reactions, and in the presence of acidosis
	Decrease	Occurs early in shock because of increased secretion of aldosterone, causing renal excretion of potassium
Calcium	Decrease	Sometimes occurs after rapid infusion of large amounts of citrated blood, also occurs secondary to respiratory alkalosis of early shock
	Increase	Occurs secondary to lactic acidosis, permitting increased ionization of calcium
Arterial blood gases	Respiratory alkalosis	Occurs early in shock secondary to hyperventilation
	Metabolic acidosis	Occurs later in shock when organic acids, such as lactic acid, accumulate in blood from anaerobic metabolism
Blood cultures	Growth of one organism (usually)	Grow gram-negative organisms most frequently in clients who are in septic shock
Urine		
Specific gravity	Increase	Occurs secondary to the action of antidiuretic hormone
	Fixed at 1.010	Occurs in acute tubular necrosis

From Lewis LM, Collier IC, & Heitkemper MM. (1996). *Medical-surgical nursing: Assessment and management of clinical problems* (4th ed.). St. Louis: Mosby.

orrhage, shock, cardiac arrest, and malignant hyperthermia, nursing diagnoses for the patient are identified.

NURSING DIAGNOSES

A fluid imbalance, or *fluid volume deficit,* is significant to patients experiencing intraoperative emer-

gencies. The patient with an uncorrected blood loss is at risk for *altered tissue perfusion* and *decreased cardiac output.* The patient with inadequate tissue perfusion related to hemorrhage requires fluid replacement with crystalloid and colloid solutions. Later, whole blood, blood components, or plasma expanders are used to supplement fluid volume deficit. The patient with inadequate tissue perfusion related to dehydration or diaphoresis requires administration of an appropriate electrolyte solution to correct the fluid volume imbalance. Understanding the cause of fluid imbalance enables the perioperative nurse to collaborate with other surgical team members effectively to correct fluid and electrolyte imbalances.

Altered tissue perfusion and tissue injury result from static circulation and pooled blood in the peripheral tissues, as seen in the shock phenomenon. Metabolic acidosis develops from the accumulation of cellular wastes and inadequate tissue perfusion. As cellular wastes increase because of inadequate circulation and gas exchange, insufficient oxygenation is available for normal cellular function. Therefore the risk for injury related to altered tissue perfusion becomes a problem if systemic circulation and cardiac output are not restored.

Decreased cardiac output is related to changes in myocardial contractility. Tissue damage from previous myocardial infarctions, temporary cardiac failure, myocardial contusions, and dysrhythmias alter the effectiveness of myocardial contraction. This decrease in cardiac output and circulation augments the problem of altered tissue perfusion and impaired gas exchange.

Dysrhythmias and tachycardia decrease the effectiveness of cardiac output. Tachycardia combined with vasodilatation and hypotension prevents adequate gas exchange and tissue perfusion. This cycle must be broken to prevent left heart failure, pulmonary edema, hypoxemia, and death.

Hyperthermia results from increased body metabolism in malignant hyperthermia. Elevated body metabolism increases cellular oxygen requirements and produces heat. The body attempts to reduce heat through vasodilatation and diaphoresis. However, vasodilatation may not cool peripheral circulation adequately, as seen in malignant hyperthermia crises. Continued hyperthermia, diaphoresis, and vasodilatation result in multisystem complications.

Profuse diaphoresis and vasodilatation soon lead to hypovolemia and fluid volume deficit. Hypovolemia increases respiratory and metabolic acidosis generated by the lactate produced from continuous muscle contractions. Increased lactate and carbon dioxide lead to altered tissue perfusion, impaired gas exchange of oxygen and carbon dioxide, decreased cardiac output, and tissue injury. Understanding the circuitous relationships of temperature regulation (that is, hyperthermia), fluid volume, gas exchange, tissue perfusion, and cardiac output is necessary for the perioperative nurse to prioritize nursing actions and interventions during intraoperative emergencies.

INTERVENTIONS

Nursing actions from the generic care plans for preventing patient injury, fluid and electrolyte imbalances, and alterations in patient safety and comfort apply to intraoperative emergencies. In addition, the care plan for hemorrhage includes nursing actions to manage hemostasis, fluid replacement, and protection from hypothermia.

Managing Hemorrhage

To manage hemorrhage, the perioperative nurse provides the tools needed for achieving hemostasis. Cardiovascular suture and fine-tipped instruments or a cardiovascular set should be immediately available to clamp and ligate bleeding vessels. Additional sponges appropriate to the wound size are needed to apply pressure to the bleeding vessel and maintain visualization of the site by removing pooled blood; suction will be needed immediately. Hemostatic agents such as epinephrine, thrombin, cellulose, or collagen should be available to assist in vasoconstriction and clot formation; the electrosurgical unit (ESU) should be readied.

The focus of fluid replacement in hemorrhage is to replace lost fluid volume rapidly (Table 24-4). Positive pressure sets, pressure cuffs, and macropore filters assist with rapid fluid administration. The perioperative nurse assists anesthesia staff with the calculation of blood loss by weighing sponges, calculating the amount of irrigation used on the sterile field, estimating the amount of blood loss in the suction canister, and monitoring reactions to transfusion of blood or blood components (Table 24-5). The patient's response to rapid fluid replacement will be monitored by processing electrolyte and arterial blood values and monitoring central venous pressure. Autotransfusion will be considered unless personnel limitations prohibit its use. Autotransfusion, a safe method for sustaining red blood cell mass, may be contraindicated in trauma (and other situations) where there is bacterial contamination and in patients with malignancy unless no other red cell source is available and the patient is in a life-threatening situation.

The final objective for hemorrhage management by the perioperative nurse is to promote temperature regulation and prevent hypothermia. Anesthesia often decreases the patient's metabolism and temperature. Invasive surgical procedures promote evaporative fluid and thermal losses from internal tissues. In addition, the heat contained within an intact body cavity is released by large incisions, extensive retraction, and frequent irrigation; this further reduces the patient's core body temperature. The cool OR environment promotes external cooling of the patient's core temperature and increases the

Table 24-4 Blood and blood components

Product	Description	Indication(s)	Action	Administration
Red blood cells, packed (PRC)	Concentrated red blood cells that remain after plasma is separated	To improve oxygen-carrying capacity of the blood (hemolytic anemia in aplastic crisis, chronic hypoplastic anemia, leukemia, lymphoma, and other malignant diseases with bone marrow failure; exchange transfusions; surgery; shock; conditions in which sudden changes in blood volume are not tolerated)	Increases oxygen-carrying capacity; elevates Hct (3% if unit of PRC has Hct of 70% to 80%)	See blood administration standard; administer through a filter; regulate flow to 25 ml/hr for 15 min; remain with patient; observe for reaction; if no reaction, regulate flow to 100 to 200 ml/hr in adult with no cardiac failure or elevated CVP and in infants and children regulate flow to 2 to 6 ml/kg/hr; add sodium chloride to PRC before administration when ordered; *no other solution or medication may be added to red cells*
Red blood cells, leukocyte poor	Concentrated red cells with leukocytes removed, usually by continuous flow centrifuge or washing	See PRC; severe febrile transfusion reactions caused by antileukocyte or antiplatelet antibodies; candidates for transplantation	See PRC	See PRC
Red blood cells, frozen	Glycerol added to red cells to protect cell from hemolysis while suspended in hypertonic solution when frozen; glycerol is removed before administration	See PRC; hypersensitivity reactions to plasma components such as IgA	See PRC	See PRC
Whole blood	Plasma and red blood cells; may or may not contain other cells and factors; dependent on length of time transpired after collection; unit usually contains 520 ± 45 ml of anticoagulated blood with Hct of about 40%	Restoration of decreased blood volume caused by hemorrhage or trauma in which more than 25% of volume is lost	Restores blood volume and increases oxygen-carrying capacity	Administer through a filter; remain with patient until 25 to 50 ml transfused, usually 15 to 30 min; observe for transfusion reactions; if no reaction, adjust flow rate to administer complete unit within 4 hr; warm unit no higher than 37° C using special coils when refrigerated blood needs to be administered quickly
Whole blood, modified		Hypovolemic shock	Increases oxygen-carrying capacity and provides volume without adding platelets, which release serotonin (a vasoconstrictor)	See whole blood
Whole blood with antihemophilic factor (factor VIII) removed	Prepared by removing factor VIII, using heparin in initial collection, or converting a previously collected unit of blood containing a citrate anticoagulant	Exchange transfusion in the adult	Provides volume without contributing to coagulation ability	See whole blood

Table 24-4 Blood and blood components—cont'd

Product	Description	Indication(s)	Action	Administration
Plasma	Plasma prepared from single donor unit of fresh blood	Burns; traumatic shock; replacement of certain coagulation factors	Provides plasma coagulation factors	Administer unit in less than 1 hr in hypovolemic patient; in normovolemic patient, administer at rate of 5 to 20 ml/kg
Plasma, fresh-frozen	Plasma prepared from single donor unit of fresh blood; it is frozen within 6 hr of collection	Source of fibrinogen and factors V and VIII	See plasma; 1 U usually contains approximately 400 mg fibrinogen, 200 U factors VIII and IX, and other stable and labile coagulation factors	Thaw frozen plasma in 37° C water bath with gentle agitation; *do not warm*; administer through a filter; *never add* medications or fluids
Plasma, liquid	Plasma prepared from single donor unit within 5 days after collection; stored frozen	Factor VII, IX, X, XI, and XIII deficiencies or abnormalities	Replacement of factors VII, IX, X, XI, or XIII	See plasma, fresh-frozen
Cryoprecipitated antihemophilic factor (factor VIII)	Preparation containing factor VIII is obtained from a single unit of blood; contains approximately 80 U factor VIII, and 200 mg fibrinogen in 15 ml of plasma	Hemophilia A; von Willebrand's disease (factor VIII deficiency)	Provides high concentrations of factor VIII and fibrinogen	Thaw in warm water bath at 37° C with gentle agitation; administer through filter rapidly within 6 hr after thawing if container not entered; 2 hr after thawing if container entered
Leukocyte concentrate	Leukocytes, platelets, and erythrocytes in varying amounts in 200 to 500 ml of plasma collected by apheresis; a compatible HLA donor is usually preferred (not identical donor whose use as a tissue donor is anticipated)	Bacterial sepsis not responsive to antibiotic therapy in presence of neutropenia; chronic granulomatous disease when bone marrow recovery is foreseen and temperature elevated for 24 to 48 hours	Provides granulocytes to more effectively control infection	Administer irradiated leukocytes to prevent engraphment and possible GVHD; regulate rate of flow to give 250 to 850 granulocytes/μl/ M^2, usually 1 U/day is ordered; slow rate of transfusion at appearance of elevated T wave, chills, and urticaria; stop transfusion when symptoms of transient pulmonary infiltrate appear
Platelet concentrate (random or single donor)	Platelets separated from whole blood suspended in plasma; collection from single donor preferred	Hemorrhage caused by thrombocytopenia; prevention of potential hemorrhage in bone marrow suppression caused by chemotherapy; abnormalities in platelet function	Corrects hemostatic deficit in thrombocytopenia and abnormally functioning platelets; I U usually increases platelet count 5000/ml in 70 kg adult	Administer through a filter (*never* a microaggregate filter); regulate flow rate to assure administration of total unit in less than 20 min

Table 24-4 Blood and blood components—cont'd

Product	Description	Indication(s)	Action	Administration
Normal serum albumin, USP 25% solution hyperoncotic (Note: 5% solution is osmotically equal to plasma)	Derived from pooled venous plasma; contains 25 g normal serum albumin/100 ml	Hypoproteinemia; burns; shock caused by trauma, hemorrhage	Increases oncotic pressure; increases circulating volume by drawing 5 times the infused volume of albumin into circulation unless patient is dehydrated; reduces hemoconcentration and blood viscosity	Administer at flow rate <2 to 3 ml/min to prevent rapid rise in blood pressure (BP), circulatory embarrassment, or pulmonary edema
Hespan, Hetastarch	A synthetic colloid derived from a waxy starch composed of amylopectin; it has a molecular weight suitable for use as a plasma expander; Hespan is 6% Hetastarch in 0.9% sodium chloride injection	An adjunct in treatment of hemorrhagic shock, burns, and septic shock	Volume expansion resulting from albumin-like properties Increases ESR when added to whole blood, thereby improving efficacy of granulocyte collection	For hemorrhagic shock, administer at 20 ml/kg/hr, slower rate usually ordered for other indications; contraindications; severe bleeding disorders, severe congestive heart failure (CHF), renal failure, increased PT or PTT times

likelihood of hypothermia. As blood loss continues, rapid fluid replacement is initiated to replace fluid volume deficit. Fluid replacement with unwarmed or room-temperature fluids further reduces the temperature of circulating blood. Replacement fluids may be warmed as they are being administered or kept in a warmer before administration to help with temperature maintenance. Warm blankets or towels placed on the patient's head, arms, shoulders, and feet provide external warmth and help retain body heat. In addition, the use of hyperthermia blankets for patients who do not require intraoperative anteroposterior x-ray films is a nursing action that assists in temperature regulation for the patient with fluid volume deficit related to hemorrhage.

Managing Hypovolemic Shock

The generic care plan at the end of this chapter for *shock* includes nursing actions to promote adequate tissue perfusion and temperature regulation. The first group of nursing actions should ensure establishment of an adequate airway. After the rate of breathing is assessed according to the patient's norms, bilateral lung expansion is assessed and oxygen is administered; oxygen saturation should be monitored continuously (Ackley & Ludwig, 1993). Airway management, evaluation of lung expansion, and administration of oxygen are often managed by anesthesia personnel when the patient receives general or spinal anesthesia. The perioperative nurse is responsible for providing these nursing actions when monitoring the patient's condition during local or intravenous conscious sedation anesthesia. These nursing actions promote adequate gas exchange, which is a prerequisite to adequate tissue perfusion.

To ensure adequate tissue perfusion, an adequate circulatory volume must be present. Shunting of blood to the body core results in pooled blood in peripheral tissues such as the extremities. Waste products accumulate, and insufficient nutrients reach peripheral tissues. Impaired exchange of carbon dioxide for oxygen results in tissue injury if not corrected. Rapid fluid replacement is the nursing activity implemented to correct hemorrhagic shock, to increase circulating fluid volume, and to reactivate the removal of cellular wastes from tissues. In addition to two established peripheral lines, prepare for additional peripheral lines and cutdowns. Replacement therapy will require infusing 3 ml of IV fluid per estimated milliliter of blood loss (Gulanick, et al., 1994).

During shock, much of the body's blood volume is shunted to the core. Shunting of peripheral blood is the body's mechanism of supplying sufficient nutrients to continue vital organ functions. Shunting also cools peripheral tissues. Therefore, another perioperative nursing objective when dealing with

Table 24-5 Reactions to transfusion of blood and blood components

Type of reaction	Onset	Observations	Nursing actions
Red blood cells (RBCs), all preparations			
Febrile nonhemolytic	Initiation of transfusion to 24 hr posttransfusion	Chills, elevated temperature, headache, nausea, vomiting	Check and record baseline T, P, R, and BP; slow infusion; notify physician; administer antipyretic or antihistamines as ordered; check and record T, P, and R every 15 min; saline-washed RBCs: frozen, thawed, washed RBCs or leukocyte filter may be ordered to decrease reaction
Febrile hemolytic	Immediately to 30 min after initiation of transfusion or when 25 to 50 ml infused	Restlessness, anxiety, precordial oppression, elevated T to 105° F (40.6° C), tachycardia, tachypnea, flushed face, back and thigh pain, generalized tingling, chills, nausea, vomiting, shock, DIC, renal failure, oliguria, hematuria, anuria	Stop transfusion immediately; change IV tubing; initiate normal saline at 4 to 6 ml/hr; cap blood tubing with sterile needle or cap; report symptoms to physician and blood bank; recheck identifying blood numbers with patient's numbers; monitor and record T, R, and cardiac rate and rhythm every 10 to 15 min; measure and record urine output with each voiding or every ½ hr; send first specimen to lab for testing; report output less than 15 ml/30 min or presence of bleeding; ensure that blood samples are drawn for testing; the following are usually ordered: Hgb, haptoglobin level, methemalbumin, bilirubin, differential agglutination, serologic studies, renal function tests, and aerobic and anaerobic cultures; complete transfusion record, send discontinued blood, tubing, and record to lab for testing; administer medications and fluids IV as ordered; diuretics, oxygen, electrolytes, and heparin may be ordered; prepare for dialysis
Whole blood			
Allergic reaction to plasma proteins	Within 30 min after initiating transfusion	Mild reaction; chills, elevated temperature, backache, pain in legs	Check and record baseline T, P, R, and BP; stop infusion; initiate slow (4 to 6 ml/hr) infusion of saline using new sterile IV tubing; notify physician and blood bank; monitor T, P, R, and BP every 10 to 15 min; ensure that blood specimen is drawn for testing; return remainder of blood product, tubing, and transfusion record to blood bank; indicate observations on transfusion record; usually red cells without IgA will be ordered for administration; oxygen, steroids, vasopressors, or epinephrine may be ordered for anaphylactic shock; prepare for resuscitation
	Immediately to 30 min after initiation of transfusion	Moderate-to-severe reaction: erythematous rash, urticaria, dyspnea, wheezing, hypotension, intestinal hyperperistalsis, anaphylactic shock	
	During transfusion to several days after	Urticaria, swelling of lymph nodes, sore throat	Slow transfusion rate; report observations to physician; administer antihistamines as ordered; blood obtained from a fasting donor may be ordered if reaction is severe
Circulatory overload	During transfusion to 24 hr after	Sharp cough, precordial pain, back pain, dyspnea, cyanosis, increased venous pressure, distended neck veins, productive cough, frothy sputum, pleural rales	Slow transfusion rate; report observations to physician; continue rate of flow as ordered; usually 2 ml/kg/hr; monitor T, P, R, BP, and central venous pressure (CVP) every 15 to 30 min

Table 24-5 Reactions to transfusion of blood and blood components—cont'd

Type of reaction	Onset	Observations	Nursing actions
Whole blood—cont'd			
Febrile (hemolytic)	See RBC	See RBC	See RBC
Febrile (WBC and/or platelet antibodies)	See leukocyte concentrate	See leukocyte concentrate	See leukocyte concentrate
Massive transfusions of red blood cells or whole blood			
Metabolic hyperkalemia and citrate toxicity with acid citrate dextrose (ACD) anticoagulant	Citric acid elevations of 100 mg/100 ml	Tremors, prolonged QT segment on ECG, hypocalcemia, acidosis then alkalosis, cardiac arrest if citric acid levels higher	When massive transfusions required, transfusion products with citratephosphate dextrose (CPD) anticoagulant usually ordered; monitor and record T, R, and cardiac function every 10 to 15 min; ensure that blood samples are drawn for electrolytes, calcium, pH, CO_2, bicarbonate levels; administer calcium gluconate IV as ordered; administer oral or rectal cation exchange resins as ordered for hyperkalemia
Pulmonary infiltrates	During transfusion	Chills, elevated temperature, tachycardia, nonproductive cough, dyspnea, respiratory distress syndrome	Stop blood immediately; change tubing; institute normal saline IV at 4 to 6 ml/hr; monitor and record T, P, R, and BP; auscultate chest for breath and heart sounds; report observations to physician
Bleeding tendency caused by dilutional effect	Transfusion volume equal to blood volume of patient	Bleeding in any body system, thrombocytopenia, coagulation abnormalities	Report observations to physician immediately; check and record T, P, R, and BP every 10 to 15 min; monitor cardiac function continuously; auscultate chest for heart and breath sounds every 15 to 30 min; administer platelet concentrate, fluids, and medications as ordered; manage hemorrhage as indicated and ordered
Pulmonary air embolus	During transfusion	Shortness of breath, chest pain, cyanosis, syncope, hypotension, shock	Stop transfusion immediately; place patient on left side; administer oxygen as ordered; monitor vital signs, CVP every 15 min
Leukocyte concentrate			
Acute reaction	Immediately	Elevated temperature, chills	Slow transfusion; monitor and record T, P, R, and BP every 15 to 30 min; auscultate chest for breath and heart sounds every 15 to 30 min; report observations to physician; medicate with Demerol when ordered
Transient pulmonary infiltrate		Retrosternal constriction, pallor, cyanosis, tachycardia, cough	
GVHD			Usually only irradiated leukocytes are administered for prevention of graft versus host disease (GVHD)
Platelets			
Febrile; usually caused by infusion of incompatible leukocytes contaminating platelet preparations	Immediately to 12 to 24 hr post-transfusion	Chills, hives, flushing	Check and record T, P, R, and BP every 15 to 30 min; administer medications when ordered; reaction usually self-limiting; patient may develop antibodies and destroy platelets in subsequent transfusions; check platelet count 1 hr after transfusion

Table 24-5 Reactions to transfusion of blood and blood components—cont'd

Type of reaction	Onset	Observations	Nursing actions
Plasma			
Similar to whole blood	Similar to whole blood	Similar to whole blood	Similar to whole blood
Whole blood with factor VIII removed			
Bleeding caused by heparin used as anticoagulant; reactions as in whole blood	During and after transfusion when large volumes administered; see whole blood	Bleeding in any body system See whole blood	Report observations to physician immediately, check and record T, P, R, and BP; monitor cardiac status continuously; administer protamine sulfate as ordered; measure and record urinary output See whole blood
Normal serum albumin			
Reactions are rare	During administration	Chills, elevated temperature, nausea	Slow transfusion rate; report observations to physician; check and record T, P, R, and BP every 15 to 30 min
Circulatory overload/bleeding during rapid infusion	During transfusion	Rising or elevated BP, circulatory overload, pulmonary edema; new areas of bleeding appear in hemorrhagic shock	Monitor rate of infusion carefully; slow rate of transfusion; report observations to physician; check and record T, P, R, and BP every 10 to 15 min; monitor cardiac status continuously; auscultate chest for heart and breath sounds every 15 to 30 min; observe closely for new sites of bleeding

shock is to help regulate the patient's body temperature and prevent hypothermia.

Perioperative nursing actions for shock include those previously cited for temperature regulation and the following additional interventions. Irrigating solutions should be warmed before they are used to irrigate a body cavity. Warm solutions are also used to moisten lap packs. Warm solutions prevent direct cooling of internal tissues. Warm blankets, sheets, or bath towels are applied to the head, across the shoulders and arms, and to the feet to prevent further heat loss and promote warming of the extremities. Additional nursing actions performed during shock include monitoring of tissue perfusion. Tissue perfusion assessment includes an evaluation of the warmth or coolness and the dryness or dampness of the skin. The perioperative nurse assesses tissue perfusion of the extremities by checking the rate and color of the patient's nail bed flush. Radial and pedal pulses are assessed for rhythm and strength. In addition, a Doppler flow meter should be available to assess the return of peripheral pulses for patients with inadequate peripheral tissue perfusion.

Managing Cardiac Arrest

Nursing actions performed during intraoperative *cardiac arrest* include the generic care plans for fluid and electrolyte balance, freedom from injury related to physical hazards, and shock, along with the following additions. The surgical team's priority is to move the patient to the supine position to administer cardiac resuscitation. The circulator requests additional personnel if needed to move the patient into the supine position (for example, from upright sitting or prone position). The scrub nurse provides a sterile drape or towel to cover the surgical incision. Next, the perioperative nurse prepares for open or closed chest resuscitation by (1) activating the defibrillator and ECG monitor, (2) passing the internal paddles to the sterile field for open chest resuscitation or preparing the external paddles for closed chest resuscitation, (3) performing a voltage check in accordance with the manufacturer's instructions, and (4) preparing cardiac medications for administration as requested by anesthesia personnel (Table 24-6). If the patient arrests before the insertion of IV access lines, certain drugs (such as epinephrine, atropine, and lidocaine) may be given via the endotracheal tube. CPR compression is halted during endotracheal installation. Drug doses are higher than the normal IV dose; the medication should be diluted in 5 to 10 ml of normal saline, vigorous positive pressure ventilation administered following instillation to promote bronchial absorption, then compressions resumed (Gleason, 1994).

Perioperative nurses should work with the hospital pharmacy department to develop logical setups of intraoperative code carts and use ACLS algorithms as a guide for stocking drugs on the cart (Saver, 1994). Standardized protocols attached to the cart can help prevent adverse drug events (Confer-

Table 24-6 Drugs commonly used in cardiac resuscitation

Drug	Route and dosage	Actions and indications
Atropine sulfate	0.5 to 1 mg by IV bolus; may be repeated at 3 to 5 min intervals up to a total of 0.04 mg/kg	Reduces vagal tone; enhances atrioventricular (AV) conduction; accelerates heart rate in cases of pronounced sinus bradycardia
Bretylium tosylate (Bretylol)	5 mg/kg IV bolus followed by defibrillation; may be increased to 10 mg/kg and repeated at 15 to 30-min intervals until maximal dose of 30 mg/kg has been given	For ventricular fibrillation and tachycardias that have not responded to other forms of therapy
Calcium chloride, 10% solution	2 to 4 mg/kg by IV bolus; may repeat at 10-min intervals	To increase myocardial contractile function; no significant beneficial effect during CPR; use during resuscitation limited to treat calcium channel blocker toxicity and acute hyperkalemia or hypocalcemia
Dobutamine hydrochloride (Dobutrex)	2.5 to 20 μg^*/kg/min by IV	Used to treat refractory pump failure; direct receptor stimulating agent; increases myocardial contractility
Dopamine hydrochloride (Intropin)	5 μg/kg/min by IV drip; may be increased up to 20 μg/kg/min; add norepinephrine if dopamine is >20 μg/kg/min	Actions depend on dosage; 2 to 10 μg/kg/min generally has beta-receptor–stimulating action on heart, with resultant increase in cardiac output; >10 μg/kg/min has alpha-receptor–stimulating action, with resultant peripheral vasoconstriction
Epinephrine hydrochloride (Adrenalin), 1:10,000 solution	Recommended 1.0 mg IV push; repeat every 3 to 5 min as needed; if used endotracheally, use full 1 mg Intermediate: 2 to 5-mg IV push, every 3 to 5 min High: 0.1 mg/kg IV push; every 3 to 5 min	Positive inotropic and chronotropic action; peripheral vasoconstrictor; causes ventricular fibrillation Pulseless ventricular tachycardia more amenable to defibrillation; increases perfusion pressure of cardiac compressions
Isoproterenol hydrochloride (Isuprel)	2 to 10 μg/min by IV bolus or intracardiac; dosage should be titrated to heart rate and blood pressure response Should be used, if at all, with *extreme* caution	Potent inotropic and chronotropic agent; may induce or exacerbate myocardial ischemia caused by greatly increased myocardial oxygen requirements; no appreciable effect on cardiac arrest from asystole or electromechanical dissociation; recommended only in hemodynamically significant and atropine-refractory bradycardia on temporary basis until pacemaker can be implanted
Norepinephrine bitartrate (Levophed)	0.5 to 1 μg/min as initial dose; average adult dose, 2 to 12 μg/min; should be titrated to blood pressure response; patients with refractory shock may required 8 to 30 μg/min	Potent vasopressor and positive inotropic effects; increases peripheral resistance; used in severe hypotension with low total peripheral resistance
Sodium bicarbonate (50 mEq)	1 mEq/kg by IV bolus; may repeat maximum of one half this dose; further doses governed by arterial blood gas and pH determinations	To counteract metabolic acidosis
Lidocaine hydrochloride (Xylocaine)	Initial bolus 1 to 1.5 mg/kg; additional boluses of 0.5 mg/kg may be given at 3 to 5-min intervals up to total of 3 mg/kg if needed	Antiarrhythmic; shortens refractory period and suppresses automaticity of ectopic foci; useful in treatment of both ventricular tachycardia and fibrillation
Magnesium sulfate	1 to 2 g IV over 15 min, then 1 g IM every 4 to 6 hr	Torsades de pointes, suspected hypomagnesemic state, or severe refractory ventricular fibrillation
Procainamide	20 to 30 mg/min (maximum 17 mg/kg)	Refractory ventricular fibrillation
Nitroglycerine	10 to 20 μg/min IV (if blood pressure >100 mm Hg)	Myocardial ischemia, hypotension/shock, acute pulmonary edema
Nitroprusside	0.1 to 5.0 μg/kg/min IV (if blood pressure >100 mm Hg)	Hypotensive agent

*μg (Micrograms) sometimes is written *mcg*.

From Phipps WJ, et al. (1995). *Medical-surgical nursing: concepts and clinical practice* (5th ed.). St Louis: Mosby.

ence on understanding and preventing drug misadventures, 1994).

Managing Malignant Hyperthermia

Nursing actions performed during a malignant hyperthermia crisis include those of the generic care plans for fluid and electrolyte balance and freedom from injury related to physical and electrical hazards. The perioperative nurse helps anesthesia personnel to discontinue the triggering anesthesia agents and to switch to nontriggering anesthetic techniques if the patient is stable and the surgical procedure will continue. The nurse also helps to cool the patient before thermal injury and assists in the administration of dantrolene sodium.

Dantrolene sodium is the definitive pharmacologic treatment for malignant hyperthermia. Dantrolene produces skeletal muscle relaxation by inhibiting the continued release of intracellular calcium. As the intracellular calcium decreases, the muscle cells return to normal metabolic function. The initial intravenous dose is a 2- to 3-mg/kg bolus in a continuous push. This dose may be repeated every 5 to 10 minutes until the maximum dosage of 10 mg/kg is reached or until the malignant hyperthermia is controlled. Pharmacologic control is evidenced by decreasing temperature, decreasing muscle rigidity, and improving acid-base balance.

As the perioperative nurse identifies an impending malignant hyperthermia crisis, additional personnel are requested to assist with documentation, icing of intravenous and irrigating fluids, and mixing of dantrolene. The perfusion team may be alerted; their objective is to lower the patient's temperature by cycling and cooling the patient's blood. The team is needed when the patient's temperature rises above 40° C (104° F) (Beck, 1994). The circulating nurse assists anesthesia personnel in three ways. First, the perioperative nurse obtains a prepared malignant hyperthermia tray or cart stocked with supplies and equipment needed for treating hyperthermia. Supplies include dantrolene sodium (up to 36 vials may be required), preservative-free sterile water in 500-ml containers, dextrose 50%, mannitol and furosemide, insulin, standard antiarrhythmic drugs, heparin, needles, syringes, tubing, a Foley catheter and urimeter, an NG tube, central and peripheral temperature probes, blood collection tubes, and a CVP and arterial blood line set.

The perioperative nurse assists anesthesia staff as anesthesia is stopped; the patient is hyperventilated with 100% oxygen at high gas flows (at least 10 L/min). The 1995 emergency protocol of the Malignant Hypothermia Association of the U.S. (MHAUS) suggests the circle system and CO_2 need not be changed. Dantrolene sodium requires vigorous shaking after dilution with preservative-free sterile water and is administered in timed intervals. When perioperative nurses help anesthesia personnel prepare dantrolene sodium, the time required to administer this vital medication and the risk for injury to the patient are decreased.

The perioperative nurse helps cool the patient in numerous ways. Surgical drapes are removed when doing so will not compromise sterility (Wilmore, 1994). Hypothermia blankets are placed on the patient's dorsal and ventral sides if possible. Ice packs placed in the groin and brachial plexus also help to cool the patient because major vessels to the extremities pass superficially at these sites. A nasogastric tube or rectal tube may be inserted and iced lavages performed to lower body temperature. Iced intravenous fluids help cool circulating blood. In addition, the scrub nurse prepares to conclude the surgical procedure as quickly as possible. If the malignant hyperthermia crisis arises during an open procedure, iced saline solution should be readily available for open-cavity irrigation (Golinski, 1995). If not in place, an indwelling urinary catheter will be inserted.

The perioperative nurse assesses the needs of the patient, surgeon, and scrub and anesthesia personnel to set priorities for nursing actions during intraoperative emergencies. Intraoperative emergencies occur in ambulatory surgery settings, preoperative holding areas, inpatient surgery settings, and postanesthesia care units. Each of these settings involves different priorities for nursing actions. The extent to which nursing actions are independent or interdependent depends on the surgical milieu and the role relationships between anesthesia personnel and the perioperative nurse. Many nursing actions performed during intraoperative emergencies are interdependent and are performed in collaboration with surgeons and anesthesia personnel.

GENERIC CARE PLANS

Initiating a plan of care during an unexpected outcome requires quick and rapid assessment, which is focused on the emergency. The results of assessment guide the setting of priorities. In most instances the perioperative nurse will collaborate with the surgical team during patient management. However, it is possible that the perioperative nurse will initiate the emergency care plan. In the evening or night, when a patient scheduled for surgery arrives in the OR before the arrival of the rest of the team, the perioperative nurse may first detect abnormalities indicating an impending emergency. Assessment results lead to nursing diagnoses, the establishment of desired patient outcomes and some criteria by which to measure them, and the implementation of the plan; all of these activities may take place in a few moments. Priorities are set and reordered based on changes in assessment data. The following four generic care plans address the unexpected outcomes reviewed in this chapter. Each care plan lists a number of potential nursing diagnoses; the most important ones will need to be selected. The plan of care is presented in a sequence that might be similar to real life, with the expectation that ordering of nursing actions will be first and foremost in response to the patient's situation and the coordination of team activities. The Guide to Nursing Actions accompanying each care plan begins with the desired outcome(s) of patient care. More detailed information is provided in directing the activities listed on the care plan. Many of the generic care plans in Chapter 7 will be in effect at the time of the unexpected event; a provision is made to identify these. Because of the critical and intensive nature of perioperative nursing, planning steps for the care plans are actually integrated with the nursing actions. Perioperative nurses traditionally respond to patient care needs with an almost simultaneous synthesis of assessment, planning, and implementation; this is a hallmark of the perioperative nurse's expertise and skill.

GUIDES TO NURSING ACTIONS
Malignant Hyperthermia (MH) (Fig. 24-3)
The desired outcome of intraoperative malignant hyperthermia is that the patient remains free from thermal injury, with adequate oxygenation and stable cardiovascular, acid-base, fluid and electrolyte, and coagulation status. The following Guide to Nursing Actions and the suggested care plan are based on the MHAUS 1995 Emergency Therapy for Malignant Hyperthermia protocol.

1. Call for additional personnel; eight to ten people may be required. Obtain cooling equipment, fluids, the MH cart, and other resuscitative supplies. All volatile inhalation anesthetics and succinylcholine are discontinued and the patient is hyperventilated with 100% oxygen at high gas flows. Load suture and prepare for rapid closure if the procedure is to be terminated. If the procedure is to continue, it will be completed as quickly as possible.

2. Assign personnel to mix dantrolene sodium. Up to 36 vials (for the average 70-kg adult) may be required. Each vial contains 20 mg of dantrolene and 3 g of mannitol and should be mixed with 60 ml of sterile water for injection (USP without a bacteriostatic agent). Dantrolene sodium requires vigorous shaking to mix the solution after reconstitution; it may take 5 minutes to prepare the initial dose. The initial intravenous dose is 2 to 3 mg/kg; this dose is repeated every 5 to 10 minutes (until signs of MH subside) up to a 10 mg/kg maximum.

3. Metabolic acidosis will be corrected as guided by blood gas analysis. In the absence of blood gas analysis, sodium bicarbonate, 1 to 2 mEq/kg, IV, should be given.

4. Simultaneously with the above, active measures are taken to cool the patient. Surface cool the patient with a hypothermia blanket and ice. Provide iced normal saline solution for stomach, rectal, bladder, and direct open-cavity lavage (such as in a laparotomy or thoracotomy procedure) and for IV administration (15 ml/kg every 15 minutes times three). Take appropriate precautions to prevent frostbite and hypothermic tissue injury. Cooling measures are usually terminated when the patient's temperature reaches 38° C (100° F to prevent hypothermia.

5. Dysrhythmias usually respond to treatment initiated to correct acidosis and hyperkalemia (see number 7 below). If they persist or are life-threatening, prepare to administer standard antiarrhythmic agents (calcium channel blockers are not used). Document drugs given.

6. Vigorous monitoring will be done, including end-tidal CO_2, arterial, central, and mixed venous blood gases; serum potassium; calcium; clotting studies; and urine output.

7. Hyperkalemia will be treated with hyperventilation, bicarbonate, and intravenous glucose and insulin therapy. Calcium (for example, 2 to 5 mg/kg $CaCl_2$) may be required to correct life-threatening hyperkalemia.

8. Urine output should be maintained at 2 ml/kg/hr.

9. It is recommended that the MHAUS hotline be called during the MH episode. This hotline provides 24-hour coverage by anesthesia consultants.

10. The patient is transferred to the postanesthesia care unit (PACU) or the intensive care unit (ICU) on the intended recovery bed with a hypothermia blanket. During transfer to the unit, monitor vital signs and continue administration of oxygen. The MH cart should accompany the patient to the unit. A comprehensive report is required. An MH episode may reoccur up to 48 hours after the initial episode; in the PACU or ICU, continued nursing interventions will focus on alterations in cardiac output, thermoregulation, ventilation, and fluid and electrolyte status (Saleh, 1992).

11. An Adverse Metabolic Reaction to Anesthesia (AMRA) report should be completed (past patient/family consent) and sent to the North

FIG. 24-3
CARE PLAN FOR MALIGNANT HYPERTHERMIA (MH)

KEY ASSESSMENT POINTS

Risk factors for MH susceptibility
Problems during intubation (MMR)
High end-tidal CO_2
Unstable BP
Rising temperature
Cardiac dysrhythmias/tachycardia

NURSING DIAGNOSIS

All generic nursing diagnoses apply to this patient, with the addition of:
Hyperthermia related to increased muscle contraction and metabolism
High risk for altered fluid and electrolyte imbalance related to hypermetabolism
High risk for altered tissue perfusion related to hyperthermia

PATIENT OUTCOMES

All generic outcomes apply, with the addition of:
The patient will maintain a core body temperature below 37.8° C (100 ° F)
Fluid & electrolyte balance will be achieved
Adequate oxygenation will be delivered to tissue

OUTCOME CRITERIA

1. Core body temperature will be maintained; there will be no diaphoresis, shivering, or tachycardia.
2. Fluid and electrolyte status will be maintained; there will be no evidence of respiratory or metabolic acidosis, serum electrolytes will be WNL, urine output will be adequate, and coagulation studies WNL.
3. Tissue perfusion will be adequate; O_2 saturation, ABGs, respiratory and cardiovascular status, mental status, vital signs will be WNL; skin integrity will be maintained under hypothermia cooling devices.

NURSING ACTIONS

	Yes	No	N/A
1. Additional personnel summoned?	☐	☐	☐
2. Dantrolene administered?	☐	☐	☐
3. Acidosis corrected?	☐	☐	☐
4. Active cooling measures initiated?	☐	☐	☐
5. Dysrhythmias treated?	☐	☐	☐
6. Patient monitored?	☐	☐	☐
7. Hyperkalemia treated?	☐	☐	☐
8. Urine output maintained?	☐	☐	☐
9. MH hotline called?	☐	☐	☐
10. Patient transferred safely?	☐	☐	☐
11. Adverse metabolic reaction form completed?	☐	☐	☐

Document additional nursing actions/generic care plans initiated here:

_____

_____

_____

EVALUATION OF PATIENT OUTCOMES

	Outcome met	Outcome met with additional outcome criteria	Outcome met with revised nursing care plan	Outcome not met	Outcome not applicable to this patient
1. Core body temperature was maintained below 37.8°.	☐	☐	☐	☐	☐
2. Acid-base, fluid, electrolyte, and coagulation studies returned to normal.	☐	☐	☐	☐	☐
3. Adequate tissue perfusion was achieved.	☐	☐	☐	☐	☐
4. The patient met outcomes for additional generic care plans as indicated.	☐	☐	☐	☐	☐

Signature: _____ Date: _____

American MH Registry, which collects and analyzes clinical and laboratory data from suspected and confirmed MH patients and researches the epidemiology, diagnosis, and treatment of MH. The patient and family should be counseled regarding MH and further precautions and referred to MHAUS.

Hemorrhage (Fig. 24-4)

The desired outcome in intraoperative hemorrhage is that the patient's fluid volume is maintained. Refer to the generic care plans for fluid and electrolyte balance and freedom from injury related to physical and electrical hazards (Chapter 7). Modifications to these care plans are as follows:

1. Provide cardiovascular suture or appropriate-sized stick ties for vessel ligature. Ensure that fine-tipped instruments such as right angles and vascular-like needle holders or a cardiovascular set are readily available.
2. Provide additional sponges appropriate to the wound size to the sterile field to apply pressure to the bleeding vessel. Use sponges to remove pooled blood at the site to enhance visualization. Keep suction available; obtain additional suction if necessary.
3. Provide topical hemostatic agents such as epinephrine, thrombin, cellulose, or collagen, as requested or planned, to facilitate clot formation.
4. Obtain fluid warmer/rapid fluid infuser and macropore blood filters for rapid fluid administration. Two IV lines will be maintained. Be prepared to assist in administration of crystalloid and colloid solutions. Prepare to initiate autotransfusion system. These may be either a reinfusion system (salvage-anticoagulate-filter-reinfuse) or washed systems (salvage-anticoagulate - filter - hemoconcentrate - wash-collect-reinfuse). The perioperative nurse must be proficient in the use of either type of system if he or she is to be the operator. Davis (1993) suggests the following activities for the scrub nurse:
   - Receive autotransfusion disposables from the operator onto the sterile field and hand off appropriate end to be connected to suction
   - Suction from pooled blood whenever possible; keep suction from fat layers and skin edges to a minimum
   - Keep tally of irrigation usage
   - Use large-bore, plastic suction tips whenever possible
   - Notify autotransfusion operator when introducing substances into the wound
5. Assist the anesthesia team with blood loss calculation by weighing bloody surgical sponges, calculating the amount of fluid used to irrigate the wound, and estimating the amount of blood loss in the suction canister.
6. Provide warm intravenous solutions during blood and isotonic fluid administration to prevent further reduction of circulating blood temperature.
7. Assist anesthesia personnel with verification of blood unit with the patient's identity to ensure blood compatibility. Coordinate collection and transfer of empty blood bags and blood component containers to the blood bank for analysis.
8. Provide hyperthermia blankets for patients not requiring intraoperative anteroposterior x-ray films. Provide warm blankets or towels across the patient's arms and shoulders, feet, and head to provide warmth externally and retain body heat.
9. Help monitor patient's hydration status by processing hematocrit, hemoglobin, arterial blood gas, prothrombin and partial thromboplastin times, and electrolyte blood samples to the laboratory; monitor results. Assist with the insertion of central lines and the monitoring of blood pressure, CVP, and pulmonary artery pressures. Sympathomimetics (Aramine, Vasoxyl, Neo-Synephrine) may be required; observe for cardiac dysrhythmias, especially bradycardia, with the administration of these drugs.

Cardiac Arrest (Fig. 24-5)

The desired outcome in intraoperative cardiac arrest is that the patient's hemodynamic stability will be restored. Refer to the generic care plans for fluid and electrolyte balance and freedom from injury related to physical and electrical hazards (Chapter 7). Modifications to these care plans are as follows:

1. Help to move the patient to the supine position to administer open- or closed-chest resuscitation. Call for help. Diagnose rhythm (quick-look paddles). If ventricular fibrillation (VF) or pulseless ventricular tachycardia, prepare to countershock (200 joules initially).
2. Conceal the surgical incision with a sterile drape to protect the wound. Remove drapes to expose the chest before countershock or for closed-chest resuscitation when rhythm not VF.
3. Assist with closed- or open-chest resuscitation by (a) lowering the OR bed to its lowest position, (b) providing the resuscitator with a standing stool to deliver compressions effectively, (c) activating the defibrillator and ECG monitor, (d) passing the internal paddles to the sterile field for open-chest resuscitation or preparing the external paddles for closed-chest resuscitation, (e) performing a voltage check in accordance with manufacturer's instructions, and (f) preparing cardiac medications for administration as requested by anesthesia personnel.

FIG. 24-4
CARE PLAN FOR INTRAOPERATIVE HEMORRHAGE

KEY ASSESSMENT POINTS

Increased systolic, decreased diastolic BP
Low CVP, PCWP
Tachycardia
Weak, thready pulse
Flat neck veins
Decreased urinary output (<30 ml/hr)
Dysrhythmias
Tachypnea
Hypoxemia (O_2 saturation <90%)
Pallor/cyanosis
Cool, clammy skin
In the awake patient: altered mentation

NURSING DIAGNOSIS

All generic nursing diagnoses apply to this patient, with the addition
  of:
Fluid volume deficit related to bleeding
High risk for altered tissue perfusion related to a fluid volume deficit

PATIENT OUTCOMES

All generic outcomes apply, with the addition of:
The patient's fluid volume will be maintained.
The patient will be free of injury related to a fluid volume deficit.
The patient will be free of fluid and electrolyte imbalances.

OUTCOME CRITERIA

1. The patient's mental orientation will be consistent with levels before fluid volume loss.
2. Fluid and electrolyte values will be consistent with preoperative status.
   - Serum electrolytes WNL
   - Arterial blood gases WNL
   - Absence of signs of imbalances
   - CVP WNL
   - Urinary output 30 ml per hour
   - O_2 saturation >90%
3. Vital signs will be consistent with preoperative measurement.
4. Fluid resuscitation will take place without transfusion reaction
5. Nail bed flush, skin temperature, and dryness will be consistent with preoperative measurement.

NURSING ACTIONS	Yes	No	N/A
1. Cardiovascular suture/instruments available?	☐	☐	☐
2. Assist with hemostasis at the field (sponges/suction)?	☐	☐	☐
3. Topical hemostatics used? (list these)	☐	☐	☐
4. Assist with fluid resuscitation? (document fluids infused, IV insertion, use of autotransfusion)	☐	☐	☐
5. Blood loss calculated? (document sources, amounts)	☐	☐	☐
6. Resuscitation fluids warmed?	☐	☐	☐
7. Safety measures to prevent transfusion reaction taken?	☐	☐	☐
8. Methods to keep patient warm initiated?	☐	☐	☐
9. Fluid volume status monitored? (document studies done, results, lines inserted, drugs administered as a result of monitoring)	☐	☐	☐

Document additional nursing actions/generic care plans initiated here:

_____

_____

_____

EVALUATION OF PATIENT OUTCOMES	Outcome met	Outcome met with additional outcome criteria	Outcome met with revised nursing care plan	Outcome not met	Outcome not applicable to this patient
1. The patient's mental status was consistent with preoperative status.	☐	☐	☐	☐	☐
2. Fluid and electrolyte balance was consistent with the patient's preoperative levels.	☐	☐	☐	☐	☐
3. Vital signs were consistent with preoperative measurements.	☐	☐	☐	☐	☐
4. There was no evidence of a transfusion reaction.	☐	☐	☐	☐	☐
5. Nail bed flush, skin temperature, and dryness were consistent with preoperative measurement.	☐	☐	☐	☐	☐
6. The patient met outcomes for additional generic care plans as indicated.	☐	☐	☐	☐	☐

Signature: _____ Date: _____

FIG. 24-5
CARE PLAN FOR INTRAOPERATIVE CARDIAC ARREST

KEY ASSESSMENT POINTS

Patient risk factors
Verification of cardiac arrest
Type of rhythm; assess whether ventricular fibrillation (VF) or pulse-less ventricular tachycardia (VT) **or** not VF
Results of countershock (if VF or pulseless VT)
ECG monitoring results (continuous)
Results of CPR, drug therapy

NURSING DIAGNOSIS

All generic nursing diagnoses apply to this patient, with the addition of:
Decreased cardiac output
Impaired gas exchange

PATIENT OUTCOMES

All generic outcomes apply, with the addition of:
The patient will achieve adequate cardiac output.
The patient will maintain adequate oxygenation.

OUTCOME CRITERIA

1. Cardiac output will be adequate, as evidenced by:
   - Strong peripheral pulses
   - Normal vital signs
   - Urine output >30 ml/hr
   - Warm, dry skin
   - Alert, responsive mentation
2. Gas exchange will be maintained, as evidenced by:
   - Respiratory rate <20/min
   - pO_2 >80 mm
   - Baseline heart rate for patient

NURSING ACTIONS

	Yes	No	N/A
1. Type of arrest diagnosed? (document initial rhythm and initial measures such as counter-shock, airway insertion, etc.)	☐	☐	☐
2. Surgical wound protected?	☐	☐	☐
3. Closed/open resuscitation? (extensive documentation will be required as the events of CPR unfold)	☐	☐	☐
4. Fluids administered? (document route, type, amount, patient response)	☐	☐	☐
5. Results of lab studies and hemodynamic monitoring noted? (numerous labs and results of CVP, PAP, PCWP, CO will need to be noted)	☐	☐	☐
6. Infusion/irrigation solutions warmed?	☐	☐	☐
7. Thermoregulation measures for patient initiated?	☐	☐	☐
8. Peripheral perfusion assessed?	☐	☐	☐
9. Venous pooling reduced? (the need for mechanical assistance in pump failure may require counterpulsation with intraaortic balloon pump (IAPB) or a ventricular assist device (VAD) may be indicated. Anticipate also the need for pacing or thoracotomy, and document additional nursing actions as appropriate).	☐	☐	☐

Document additional nursing actions/generic care plans initiated here:

_____

_____

_____

EVALUATION OF PATIENT OUTCOMES

	Outcome met	Outcome met with additional outcome criteria	Outcome met with revised nursing care plan	Outcome not met	Outcome not applicable to this patient
1. Cardiac output was adequate.	☐	☐	☐	☐	☐
2. Adequate oxygenation was maintained.	☐	☐	☐	☐	☐
3. The patient met outcomes for additional generic care plans as indicated.	☐	☐	☐	☐	☐

Signature: _____ Date: _____

FIG. 24-6
CARE PLAN FOR HYPOVOLEMIC SHOCK

KEY ASSESSMENT POINTS

Patient risk factors
Type/extent bleeding
Vital signs, pulse pressure
Laboratory results (Hct, coagulation studies, blood gases)
Capillary refill
Urine output
Peripheral pulses
Cool, clammy skin
CVP, ECG

NURSING DIAGNOSIS

All generic nursing diagnoses apply to this patient, with the addition
  of:
Fluid volume deficit
Decreased cardiac output
Ineffective breathing pattern

PATIENT OUTCOMES

All generic outcomes apply, with the addition of:
The patient will experience adequate fluid volume.
The patient will experience adequate cardiac output.
The patient's breathing pattern will be maintained.
1. Adequate fluid volume will be evidenced by:
   • Urine output >30 ml/hr
   • Normotensive BP
   • Heart rate <100/min
   • Warm and dry skin
2. Adequate cardiac output will be evidenced by:
   • Strong peripheral pulses
   • Alert mentation
3. Effective breathing patterns will be evidenced by:
   • Eupnea
   • Regular respiratory rate/rhythm
   • Verbal expression of comfort with breathing

NURSING ACTIONS

	Yes	No	N/A
1. Patient monitored?	☐	☐	☐
2. Skin/peripheral pulses assessed?	☐	☐	☐
3. IV/irrigation solutions warmed?	☐	☐	☐
4. Thermoregulation precautions initiated?	☐	☐	☐
5. Resuscitative fluids administered?	☐	☐	☐
6. Transfusion precautions implemented?	☐	☐	☐
7. Continuous reevaluation based on lab results, CVP, PAP, PCWP, CO, urinary output?	☐	☐	☐

Document additional nursing actions/generic care plans initiated
here:

_____

_____

_____

EVALUATION OF PATIENT OUTCOMES

	Outcome met	Outcome met with additional outcome criteria	Outcome met with revised nursing care plan	Outcome not met	Outcome not applicable to this patient
1. The patient's fluid volume was adequate.	☐	☐	☐	☐	☐
2. The patient achieved adequate cardiac output.	☐	☐	☐	☐	☐
3. The patient maintained effective breathing pattern.	☐	☐	☐	☐	☐
4. The patient met outcomes for additional generic care plans as indicated.	☐	☐	☐	☐	☐

Signature: _____ Date: _____

4. After cardiac arrest, obtain fluid warmer/rapid fluid infuser and macropore blood filters for rapid fluid administration.

5. Help anesthesia personnel to process hematocrit, hemoglobin, arterial blood gas, prothrombin and partial thromboplastin times, pH, chemistry, and electrolyte blood samples to the laboratory; monitor results. Assist with insertion of central lines, continuous monitoring of ECG, rhythm rechecks.

6. Provide warm saline for intracavity irrigation and to moisten lap packs.

7. Extend warm sheets or towels across shoulders, head, and feet to provide heat and retain body warmth in the cool OR environment.

8. Assess and document skin condition, peripheral pulses, and nail bed flush to determine peripheral tissue perfusion. Provide a Doppler flow meter to assess weak peripheral pulses.

9. Apply antithromboembolism device or bandages to correct venous pooling in the extremities resulting from a reduction of venous pressure. Anticipate need for pacer, thoracotomy, IAPB, VAD.

Hypovolemic Shock (Fig. 24-6)

The desired outcome in hypovolemic shock is that the patient achieves adequate fluid volume, cardiac output, and breathing patterns. Refer to the generic care plans for fluid and electrolyte balance and freedom from injury related to physical and electrical hazards (Chapter 7). Modifications to these care plans are as follows:

1. Assess and document the status of the patient's airway, respiratory rate, and equality of bilateral lung expansion to ensure the patient's airway and breathing are adequate during local anesthesia or intravenous conscious sedation. Mild to moderate anxiety may be the first sign of impending hypovolemic shock in the awake patient. Provide and document administration of oxygen per nasal cannula. Monitor blood pressure, heart rate, level of consciousness, urinary output, oxygen saturation, and ECG; report and document results.

2. Assess and document (a) the warmth or coolness and dryness or dampness of the skin, (b) the rate of return and color of nail bed flush, and (c) the rate and rhythm of radial and pedal pulses to assess peripheral tissue perfusion. Provide a Doppler flow meter to assess weak peripheral pulses.

3. Provide warm saline for intracavity irrigation and to moisten lap packs. Provide warm intravenous solutions during fluid replacement to prevent further cooling of internal fluid and tissues.

4. Extend warm sheets or towels across the patient's shoulders and feet. Wrap a warm towel around the patient's head to prevent further heat loss and to promote warming of extremities. Provide hyperthermia blankets for patients not requiring intraoperative anteroposterior x-ray films.

5. Obtain fluid warmer/rapid fluid infusers and macropore blood filters for rapid fluid administration. Start two large-bore, short-length peripheral IVs; the amount of volume that can be infused is inversely affected by the length of the IV catheter. If hypotension is present, be prepared to bolus with 1 to 2 L of IV fluid in the normal adult. If blood loss is mild (less than 20%), blood pressure may rapidly return to normal. However, if loss continues or is between 20% and 40%, the bolus will initially return BP to normal, but it will deteriorate when fluids are slowed (Gulanick, et al., 1994).

6. Ensure blood product (packed red cells, fresh frozen plasma, platelets) compatibility by verifying blood unit identification with the patient's identity. Coordinate collection and transfer of empty blood bags and blood component containers to the blood bank for analysis.

7. Assist with monitoring of the patient's hydration status by processing hematocrit, hemoglobin, arterial blood gas, prothrombin and partial thromboplastin times, and electrolyte blood sample to the laboratory; monitor results. Assist with insertion of central lines for a continuing shock state; CVP (to obtain information on filling pressures of right side of heart) and PAP and PCWP (to determine left-sided filling volumes) will be hemodynamically monitored, along with cardiac output. Urinary output will be assessed frequently, because oliguria is a classic sign of renal failure.

References

Ackley BJ & Ludwig GB. (1993). *Nursing diagnosis handbook: A guide to planning care.* St. Louis: Mosby.

Barash PG, Cullen BF, & Stoeling RK. (1992). *Clinical anesthesia.* Philadelphia: JB Lippincott.

Beare PG & Meyers JL. (1994). *Adult health nursing* (2nd ed.). St. Louis: Mosby.

Beck CF. (1994). Malignant hyperthermia: Are you prepared? *AORN Journal, 59*(2), 367-390.

Christensen B. (1992). Hemodynamic monitoring: What it tells you and what it doesn't, Part I. *Journal of Postanesthesia Nursing, 7*(5), 330-337.

Conference on understanding and preventing drug misadventures. (1994, October 21-23). Washington, DC.

Corkhill MS. (1993, March 3). *Malignant hyperthermia.* Paper presented at the AORN Congress, Anaheim, CA.

Davis VL. (1993, October). *The nurses' role in intraoperative blood retrieval and transfusion.* Paper presented at the Contemporary Forums' Perioperative Nursing Conference, New Orleans, LA.

Donnelly AJ. (1994). Malignant hyperthermia: Epidemiology, pathophysiology, treatment. *AORN Journal, 59*(2), 393-405.

Gleason C. (1994). Emergency drug therapy update. *Nursing Spectrum, 3*(24). 12-14.

Golinski M. (1995). Malignant hypothermia: A review. *Plastic Surgical Nurse, 15*(1), 30-35.

Gulanick M, et al. (1994). *Nursing care plans: Nursing diagnosis and intervention* (3rd ed.). St. Louis: Mosby.

Holcroft JW & Robinson MK. (1992). Shock. In DW Wilmore, et al. (Eds.). *Care of the surgical patient: Critical care.* New York: Scientific American Medicine.

Lewis SM & Collier IC. (1996). *Medical-surgical nursing: Assessment and management of clinical problems* (4th ed.). St. Louis: Mosby.

Lowenstein SR. (1990). Cardiopulmonary resuscitation in noninjured patients. In DW Wilmore, et al. (Eds.). *Care of the surgical patient: Critical care.* NY: Scientific American Medicine.

Malignant Hyperthermia Association of the United States. (1995). *Emergency therapy for malignant hyperthermia.* Sherburne, NY: MHAUS.

McCance KL & Huether SE. (1994). *Pathophysiology: The bio-logic basis for disease in adults and children* (2nd ed.). St. Louis: Mosby–Year Book.

McFarland GK & McFarlane EA. (1993). *Nursing diagnosis and intervention: Planning for patient care.* (2nd ed.). St. Louis: Mosby.

Nightingale F. (1860). *Notes on nursing.* London: Harrison & Sons.

Pagana KD & Pagana TJ. (1995). *Mosby's diagnostic and laboratory test reference* (2nd ed.). St. Louis: Mosby.

Price SA & Wilson LM. (1992). *Pathophysiology: Clinical concepts of disease processes.* St. Louis: Mosby.

Saleh KL. (1992). Practical points in the management of malignant hyperthermia. *Journal of Postanesthesia Nursing, 7*(5), 327-329.

Saver CL. (1994). Decoding the ACLS algorithms. *American Journal of Nursing, 94*(1), 27-36.

Wilmore DW. (1994). Fever, hyperpyrexia, and hypothermia. In DW Wilmore, et al. (Eds.). *Care of the surgical patient: Critical care.* New York: Scientific American Medicine.

Young MS & Kindred D. (1993). Malignant hyperthermia: Not just an operating room emergency. *Medsurg Nursing, 2*(1), 41-46.

Chapter 25

The Perioperative Nurse in the Postanesthesia Care Unit

Denise D. O'Brien

To decide as to the existence of disease, of course belongs solely to the doctor, but he will be largely guided by the observations of the attentive nurse, and she herself will often be called upon to judge as to the urgency of special indications. Shall she send for the doctor in the middle of the night, or apply her own resources? shall she give or withhold the medicine left to be used only in emergency? shall she alter or let alone an arrangement which has proved unexpectedly uncomfortable? are questions constantly arising. The nurse needs to be able to discriminate between the important symptoms, and those which are merely incidental—to recognize those which call for immediate action, and to know what kind of action on her part is called for.

WEEKS, 1890

*T*he perioperative nurse's responsibilities do not end with the closure of the incision and application of dressings. Safety measures and nursing actions must continue during the postoperative phase. This phase begins with the admission of the patient to the postanesthesia care unit (PACU) and ends with evaluation of the extent to which the patient s needs have been met (Association of Operating Room Nurses [AORN], 1996). The scope of perioperative nursing practice during the postoperative phase varies widely. It ranges from accompanying the patient to the PACU and giving a nursing report to the PACU nurse, to caring for patients in a postanesthesia recovery area in ambulatory surgery settings, to follow-up nursing evaluation during a postoperative visit, by phone, or even in the patient's home. Despite variations in scope of practice, the perioperative nurse will participate with members of the surgical, anesthesia, and perianesthesia nursing teams to ensure that the patient's physiologic equilibrium is monitored and complications are prevented. Activities directed toward these goals begin in the operating room (OR).

DISCHARGING THE PATIENT FROM THE OR

When the surgical incision is closed and dressings are applied, the site around the dressings should be cleaned of any blood, preparation solution, or other exudate. A clean gown is applied; even if the patient is still in an altered state of consciousness, the nurse maintains the dignity and privacy of the patient by preventing undue exposure of the body. Dependent pressure sites should be assessed for redness, bruising, rashes, or other alterations in skin integrity. If an electrosurgery unit (ESU) was used, the dispersive pad is removed and the condition of the skin at the pad site noted. All skin should be assessed for any alterations from the preoperative condition. A warm, clean blanket should be applied. The safety strap on the OR bed should be kept in position until the patient is ready for transfer to the postoperative bed or stretcher.

Transfer procedures must be carried out carefully. The patency of the airway and of intravascular monitoring lines, tubes, and drains must be protected. Undue stress on the incision site should be prevented. Adequate numbers of personnel or use of transfer devices are necessary to prevent shearing forces from pulling rather than lifting the patient. Transfer is usually carried out under the direction of the anesthesia team; alterations in circulating blood volume may precipitate hypotensive episodes during movement. With sophisticated anesthesia techniques, many patients will begin to emerge from anesthesia while they are still on the OR bed. It is important for the perioperative nurse to assess, along with the anesthesia team, the patient's ability to participate in "stir-up" activities, such as response to name and commands, raising of the head, strength of grasp, movement of extremities, coughing and deep breathing, and swallowing. These are important indices of recovery from anesthetic drugs, especially neuromuscular blocking agents, and will be a part of the report given to the PACU nursing staff. During preparation for transfer and discharge from the OR, vital signs will continue to be monitored.

After transfer to the postoperative bed or stretcher, the siderails are raised. Drainage tubes and apparatus, intravenous solutions, oxygen tubing, and so on need to be placed appropriately for transport. The patient's position on the bed or stretcher will be collaboratively determined by the perioperative nurse and anesthesia team; level of consciousness, airway patency, and patient comfort are all considerations. If the patient needs ventilation during transport to the PACU or other intensive nursing care unit, manual resuscitation bags will probably be used. Attention needs to be paid to the patency of the valves in these bags. Careful monitoring is necessary in case of vomiting into the mask with subsequent aspiration. Pulse oximetry monitoring and supplemental oxygen therapy may continue during transport. Institutional protocol will determine who accompanies the patient to PACU. If the patient received general or monitored anesthesia, a member of the anesthesia care team, surgical team, and the perioperative nurse may accompany the patient. The nurse and a member of the surgical team will probably accompany the patient who received local anesthesia or intravenous conscious sedation monitored by the perioperative nurse. Decisions about patient transport should consider the patient's status. Once the patient is ready for transport, it should be accomplished expeditiously.

ADMISSION TO THE PACU

As soon as the patient is received in the PACU, nursing admission procedures are initiated and a verbal report is given to the PACU nurse.

Baseline Admission Assessment

The PACU nurse will immediately assess the patient to establish baseline status. This may be done jointly with a member of the perioperative team, or results may be reported to a team member, often the anesthesia care team. The criteria recommended by the American Society of Post Anesthesia Nurses (ASPAN, 1995) are as follows:

Assessment

The assessment includes, but is not limited to, the patient s relevant preoperative status: electrocardiogram (ECG), vital signs and oxygen saturation, radiology findings, laboratory values, allergies, disabilities, substance abuse, physical and mental impairments, mobility limitations, and prostheses. In the pediatric patient, include the birth history, development stages, and parent/child interactions. Initial physical assessment includes documentation of the following:

1. Integration of data received at transfer of care.
2. Vital signs
   a. Airway patent, respiratory rate and competency, breath sounds, type of artificial airway, mechanical ventilator settings, and oxygen saturation
   b. Blood pressure—cuff or arterial line
   c. Pulse—apical, peripheral
   d. Temperature—oral, rectal, axillary, digital through dermal sensors, tympanic
3. Level of consciousness
4. Pressure readings—central venous, arterial blood, pulmonary artery wedge, and intracranial pressure if indicated
5. Position of patient

6. Condition and color of skin
7. Patient safety needs
8. Neurovascular—peripheral pulses and sensation of extremity(ies) as applicable
9. Condition of dressings
10. Condition of suture line, if dressing absent
11. Type, patency, and securement of drainage tubes, catheters, and receptacle
12. Amount and type of drainage
13. Muscular response and strength
14. Pupillary response as indicated
15. Fluid therapy, location of lines, condition of IV site and securement and amount of solution infusing (including blood)
16. Level of physical comfort and emotional support
17. Numeric score if used

Vital signs are recorded. General visual assessment is conducted and the patient's color, intravenous infusions, airway status, and level of consciousness are noted. The patient will be safely positioned and assigned a numeric score if a scoring system is used. Many PACUs use scoring systems to monitor the patient's progress and readiness for PACU discharge. These guides include objective criteria evaluated at specified intervals during the patient's PACU stay. The most commonly used are Aldrete, REACT, or a modification of these. As soon as the immediate patient assessment is performed, a verbal report is received.

Perioperative Patient Report

The PACU nurse will depend on an accurate patient report as part of the data base for postoperative care planning. This report is usually given by a member of the anesthesia care team; the perioperative nurse should collaborate and add, validate, and verify important information about the patient. The report should include the patient's name and age, preoperative and postoperative diagnoses, operative procedure(s) performed, information about the anesthetic technique and agents, and information about the intraoperative course (vital signs, fluid balance, length of operative procedure; any intraoperative complications, such as airway trauma or laryngospasm, shock, hemorrhage, dysrhythmias, significant shifts in vital signs). Any medications given during the intraoperative phase, such as steroids, antibiotics, insulin, or pressors, are reported to the PACU nurse. General information about language barriers, preoperative level of consciousness, pertinent medical history, allergies, or other preoperative alterations and limitations (physical, mental, emotional, visual, auditory, or expressive) should be reviewed to establish baseline patient information. The status of the airway and the presence of tubes, drains, and cath-

eters; intravascular lines; and infusions should be reviewed. The postoperative orders, any diagnostic or therapeutic studies or treatments to be initiated in the PACU, special symptoms or sequelae to observe for, and other special considerations are usually jointly reviewed by the PACU nurse and a member of the perioperative team. During report activities, the PACU nurse continues to assess the patient and report to the perioperative team. A member of the anesthesia care team remains with the patient as long as the patient's condition requires and until the PACU nurse assumes responsibility for the patient's care.

ONGOING PACU NURSING CARE

After the initial nursing assessment and perioperative patient report, the PACU nurse engages in planning and implementing patient care. Using the nursing process, the PACU nurse begins care planning by identifying relevant nursing diagnoses.

Nursing Diagnoses

The North American Nursing Diagnosis Association (NANDA) defines nursing diagnosis as a clinical judgment about individual, family, or community responses to actual or potential health problems/life processes. Nursing diagnoses provide the basis for selection of nursing interventions to achieve outcomes for which the nurse is accountable (NANDA, 1994). Nursing diagnoses that are applicable to patients in the post-anesthesia phase of care include, but are not limited to, the following (Carpenito, 1995; NANDA, 1994):

1. Pain
2. Anxiety
3. Decreased cardiac output
4. Alterations in fluid volume (both excess and deficit)
5. Impaired physical mobility
6. Risk for injury
7. Impaired gas exchange
8. Ineffective airway clearance
9. Ineffective breathing pattern
10. Risk for aspiration
11. Impaired skin integrity
12. Altered tissue perfusion
13. Altered patterns of urinary elimination
14. Risk for altered body temperature
15. Risk for infection
16. Knowledge deficit

These diagnoses have been incorporated into the generic care plan that concludes this chapter and modified according to the 1994 North American Nursing Diagnosis Association–approved nursing diagnoses. Nursing diagnoses are incorporated in the following discussion of common elements of postanesthesia nursing care.

Airway and respiratory management. Patients may be admitted to the PACU with endotracheal tubes or laryngeal mask airways (LMAs) still in place or already removed. Sophisticated anesthesia delivery commonly allows extubation or LMA removal in the OR as the patient begins to emerge from anesthesia, to regain reflexes, and to respond to verbal stimuli. Despite extubation or LMA removal, patients who have undergone general anesthesia have the risk for *ineffective airway clearance, aspiration, impaired gas exchange,* and *ineffective breathing patterns.* Many of these risks result from the possibility of airway obstruction. A common cause of upper airway obstruction is relaxation of the tongue on the posterior pharyngeal wall. The residual effects of anesthetic agents and adjunctive muscle relaxant drugs affect muscle control over the tongue and jaw and may dampen cough and gag reflexes. A patent airway can be maintained by repositioning the patient or the patient's airway or by inserting an artificial (oropharyngeal or nasopharyngeal) airway. If the patient is responsive, effective airway clearance through coughing and deep breathing, yawning, and inspiratory holding should be encouraged; guidance or assistance with incisional splinting may be required. If the patient is not responsive enough to generate deep breaths, is in too much pain, has an endotracheal tube, an oral or nasal airway, or has undergone a surgical intervention in which coughing is contraindicated, suctioning may be necessary. Suctioning may also be indicated for airway obstruction caused by bleeding or vomitus. If the patient has an LMA in place, suctioning should not be performed unless an anesthesia provider is present because of the possibility of stimulating laryngospasm (Brimacombe, 1993). Nursing assessment includes determination of the location and type of secretions and selection of appropriate suctioning techniques. Airway obstruction caused by laryngospasm, trauma-induced laryngeal edema, aspirated secretions, foreign body obstruction, or persistent hypoventilation may require reintubation and mechanical ventilation.

Once airway patency is established, respirations are assessed for rate, rhythm, depth, and character. The use of accessory respiratory muscles, intercostal retractions, bulging, or nasal flaring may indicate respiratory distress. Shallow respirations may indicate continuing respiratory depression from anesthesia. Hypoventilation may be caused by obesity, chronic lung disease, incisional pain, or residual effects of anesthetic, analgesic, or sedative drugs. Placing a hand in front of the patient's airway is a useful way of feeling the amount of exhaled air (Smelt-zer & Bare, 1996). Breath sounds are auscultated and their quality is noted. Supportive oxygen therapy should be documented according to device used, flow rate, and measurements of effectiveness. Display readouts from pulse oximetry should be monitored and recorded according to institutional protocol. If the patient is on a mechanical ventilator, the rate, fraction of inspired oxygen, tidal volume, vital capacity, and positive end expiratory pressure should be noted, along with other parameters on the specific unit's control panel.

Management of the patient during altered states of consciousness. Residual effects from anesthesia and intraoperative drug therapy often persist in the initial phases of recovery from anesthesia. The patient may have *impaired verbal communication, knowledge deficit* (that is, confusion and disorientation), *impaired physical mobility, risk for injury,* and *altered thought processes* in early recovery. Drowsiness, confusion, disorientation, or other sensory disturbances may be compounded by anxiety; pain; administration of narcotics or other sensory-altering drugs; or sensory overload from the noise, lights, traffic, and activities in the PACU. Assessing the patient's level of consciousness includes common measures such as asking the patient to identify the location, day, and time, or to respond to simple questions about his or her name or date of birth, the name of the health care facility, or current events. The nurse may need to reorient the patient to the location in the PACU and to the time of day. Speaking directly to the patient at regular intervals, engaging the patient in short conversations, offering explanations about procedures and sequences of events, providing privacy, preventing sensory overload while providing enough stimulation, and promoting active participation in recovery maneuvers are all nursing interventions that help the patient to gain and maintain orientation. The patient should be instructed to follow simple commands such as coughing and deep breathing, lifting the head, moving the extremities, making a fist, or squeezing a hand. The patient's ability to perform and comply with instructions should be progressively monitored. Pain and discomfort can be allayed by helping the patient assume a position of comfort unless contraindicated. Baseline preoperative information regarding sensory status is critical to determining if alterations in sensory perception relate to emergence from anesthesia or to complications of the anesthetic or surgical intervention. Persistent disorientation, abnormal emotional responses, or inability to comply with or perform simple commands requires careful nursing assessment and action. Documentation should include level of consciousness; presence of protective cough and gag reflexes;

activity level; oxygen saturation; and color of nail beds, lips, and oral mucosa.

Management of fluid balance. Alterations in fluid volume may present as a risk for or actual *fluid volume deficit* or *excess.* The perioperative patient depends on fluid therapy to maintain fluid and electrolyte balance. Prescribed fluid replacement therapy may be simple or complex, depending on the patient's preoperative status, intraoperative course, and anticipated postoperative recovery (Fakhry & Sheldon, 1995). Fluid lines need to be protected and kept patent. Careful attention should be paid to the infusion solution, rate, and site. Intraoperative fluid replacement and estimated blood loss should be reviewed. Although fluid replacement therapy aims to correct or prevent volume deficits, the risk for fluid volume excess is present in the postoperative patient. This relates to common effects of the surgical stress response and a normal, transitory postoperative oliguria.

Surgical stress response is hormonally mediated. One of the corticosteroid hormones, vasopressin (also called antidiuretic hormone [ADH]), is released in response to diminished renal blood flow. Renal blood flow may be reduced as a result of certain anesthetic agents or true hypovolemia. In either instance, ADH release may cause *altered renal tissue perfusion* with an accompanying period of reduced urinary output (Black & Matassarin-Jacobs, 1993). Surgical oliguria is further compounded by the effects of the mineralocorticoid aldosterone, which influences sodium retention. If fluid administration exceeds the kidneys' ability to excrete it, fluid volume excess may occur. If the patient has low urinary output, physiologic oliguria should be suspected as an underlying cause. Large volumes of fluid should be avoided. Nursing assessment should include a review of indices of hypovolemia when decreased urinary output is present. The presence of cool, clammy skin; tachycardia; low central venous pressure; and hypotension associated with decreased urinary output may indicate hypovolemia. Elevated central venous pressure, dyspnea, wet lung sounds, elevated blood pressure, and tachycardia may be signs of fluid volume excess. The color, amount, and concentration of urine should be correlated with the patient's general condition when renal function is assessed. Skin turgor should be assessed (the skin should be elastic) as should the oral mucous membranes (they should be moist). If the patient has not voided, nursing measures to assist independent voiding should be initiated. Assessment of the bladder by palpating the lower abdomen to ascertain distention, especially for patients who have received spinal or epidural anesthesia or undergone urinary tract instrumentation, is an important observation

and useful for determining nursing actions. Urinary catheterization should be a last resort for the patient who has *altered patterns of urinary elimination.*

Intake and output need to be measured carefully in the PACU. Replacement fluids should be calculated based on the patient s NPO (nothing by mouth) status and duration, operative time and losses, and weight. Intravenous fluids need to be regulated carefully, lines kept patent and protected, and amount of fluid intake recorded. The location (central or peripheral) of all fluid lines and the type and rate of infusion of each line should be documented. In determining output, urine, drainage from nasogastric and other tubes (for example, chest, nephrostomy, gastrostomy, T tube), blood loss, and wound drainage need to be considered. The presence or absence of nausea; time, amount, color, and consistency of emesis; results of laboratory analyses (urine specific gravity, electrolyte levels); and suction settings for nasogastric, chest, or intestinal tubes should be noted.

Wound and invasive site management. Surgical site infections are serious complications that interfere with the normal process of wound healing, increase patient discomfort, and lead to prolonged and costly length of stay. The first 24 to 48 hours after surgery are critical, because normal processes of inflammation and repair begin to seal the wound and destroy any bacteria deposited while the wound was open in the OR. In clean wounds, a platelet aggregate is formed almost immediately to stop the flow of blood at the wounded site. A protein and fibrin clot closes off the wound, and epithelial cells begin to migrate across the wound edges. Within 48 hours, an epithelial bridge is formed, new blood vessels are growing, tissue granulation begins, and collagen synthesis is initiated. Despite rigorous preoperative skin preparation, judicious use of prophylactic antibiotics, and strict implementation of perioperative asepsis, surgical site infections do occur.

In the PACU, the patient's medical record should be reviewed to identify patients at high risk for surgical site infection. The classification of the surgical procedure is important to predicting the risk for infection (see Chapter 7). Other risk factors include age, cardiovascular status, nutritional status, metabolic or systemic disease, history of smoking, and other immune system alterations. The nature and character of all wound drainage need to be noted. Dressings should be checked to determine that they are clean and dry. If it is necessary to remove a dressing to check for bleeding, to verify that a drainage tube is anchored, or because the edges have become unsealed, aseptic technique should be used. Drainage sites should be assessed; tubes need to be kept patent and connections secure. Drainage collected in closed wound suction devices should be measured; the character and amount of drainage should also be recorded. Attention should be paid to the infusion site. The risk for *infection* and *altered peripheral tissue perfusion* at the site, related to infiltration or thromboembolic events, should be considered. Intravenous and intravascular access sites, as well as the incision site, should be assessed for pain, redness, swelling, and temperature. Dressings should be intact at intravenous and intravascular sites. Skin integrity should be assessed at the site of intraoperative electrosurgical dispersive pad placement, at ECG electrode sites, and in dependent pressure areas.

Management of pain and anxiety. Pain and anxiety are not uncommon, and either may exacerbate the other. *Anxiety* may be present for all the reasons indicated in earlier chapters of this book: fear of the surgery, its outcome, anesthesia, a sense of powerlessness and loss of control, concerns about family and job responsibilities, home maintenance, and cost of health care. Anxiety is individual in both its underlying cause and its outward manifestations. The postanesthesia nurse, like the perioperative nurse, needs to be sensitive to changes in facial expression and mood and to verbalization of anxious feelings. Comfort measures, the use of touch, allowing time for the patient to verbalize or cry, providing explanations and clarifying information, and displaying a calm, reassuring manner are effective nursing measures to help patients cope with anxiety.

Patients may have *pain* in the PACU. Like anxiety, pain is personal. It may or may not be verbalized. Cultural or even religious significance may be attached to the pain. Subjective and objective evaluation should be conducted by the PACU nurse. The onset, site, duration, intensity, associated aggravating and alleviating factors, and patient's description of pain should be noted. A pain intensity or pain distress scale can be used for patient self-reporting of pain (Acute Pain Management Guideline Panel, 1992) (Box 25-1). The patient should be encouraged and assisted to use pain-control techniques that have been personally effective in the past, such as relaxation, guided imagery, or meditation. If a transcutaneous electrical nerve stimulation (TENS) unit or patient-controlled analgesia system has been prescribed, the patient will need to be instructed on its proper use. If environmental and positional changes are not effective in controlling pain, pharmacologic intervention should be considered. If pain medication is ordered on a dosage scale, the PACU nurse should review the patient s history of medication use or abuse, the preoperative and intraoperative medications given, and consult with the patient when selecting an appropriate dose. The time,

amount, type, route, and effectiveness of medication should be recorded.

Management of altered body temperature. The presence of *hypothermia* may be evident from temperature recordings, shivering, agitation, or complaints of being cold. Peripheral perfusion should be assessed. The color and temperature of the extremities, capillary refill, and presence or absence of pulses or paresthesias should be noted, as should body temperature and route. Warm blankets can be applied to the body, reinforced around the feet, and perhaps wrapped around the patient's head to rewarm and dilate blood vessels. If more aggressive measures are required to bring the patient's temperature up to 36° C, convective warming devices may be used. Hypothermia may be caused by intraoperative room temperatures, exposure of large areas of tissue, intraoperative drug therapy (that is, halothane or isoflurane), systemic hypertension, or impaired peripheral perfusion.

Postanesthesia patients may shiver or shake. Studies continue in an attempt to understand the physiologic mechanisms behind the phenomenon of postanesthetic shivering (Crossley, 1992). Drain (1994) states that exposure to the cold intraoperative environment and anesthetic CNS depressant and vasodilatation effects cause postanesthesia shivering. Treatment of shivering or shaking may include not only warming but also small doses of opioids (Crossley, 1992).

Hyperthermia may relate to a preexisting infection or sepsis or may indicate the untoward crisis of malignant hyperthermia. Chapter 24 discusses this potential perioperative complication. In the PACU, nursing interventions will be similarly directed at returning the patient to a normal metabolic state. Immediate monitoring of temperature and arterial blood gas and electrolyte levels will be initiated. Dantrolene will be administered intravenously, often at intervals until the total dose has been achieved. Sodium bicarbonate, diuretics, antiarrhythmic drugs, and drugs to treat metabolic imbalances will be prescribed. Both external and internal cooling measures will be attempted. The ECG will require close monitoring. An indwelling urinary catheter, an arterial line, and a central line will probably be inserted if they are not already present. Oxygen therapy will be initiated. Unless a malignant hyperthermia crisis is promptly recognized and treated, it will lead to death.

Management of alterations in cardiac status. Maintenance of adequate tissue perfusion depends primarily on satisfactory cardiac output. Cardiac output is the amount of blood ejected by the heart, measured in liters per minute. It is the product of the stroke volume (the amount of blood ejected per beat)

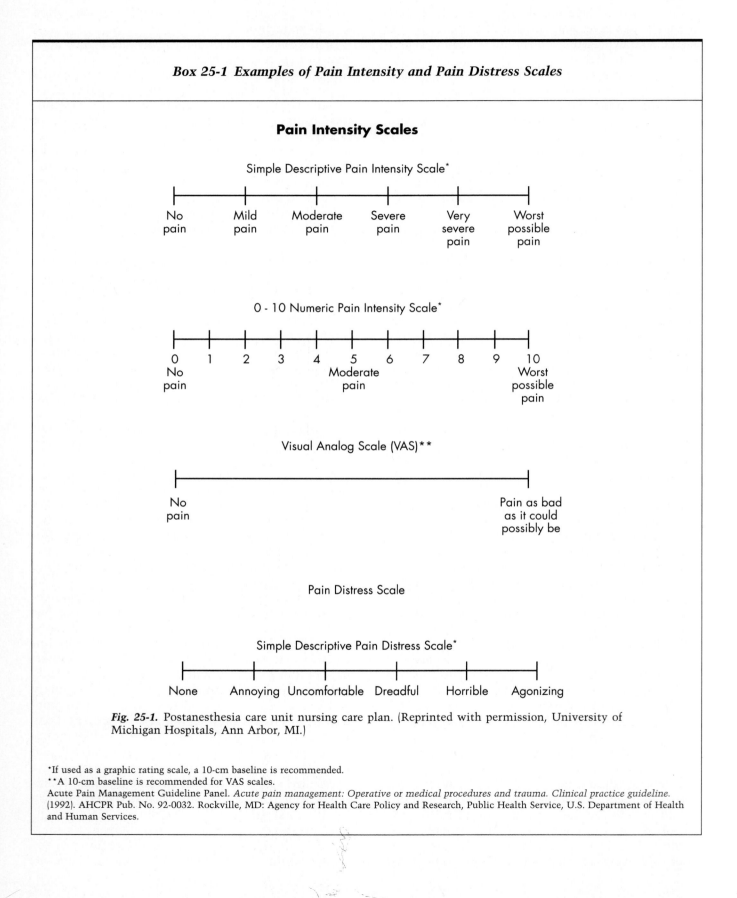

Box 25-1 Examples of Pain Intensity and Pain Distress Scales

Pain Intensity Scales

Simple Descriptive Pain Intensity Scale*

No pain	Mild pain	Moderate pain	Severe pain	Very severe pain	Worst possible pain

0 - 10 Numeric Pain Intensity Scale*

0 1 2 3 4 5 6 7 8 9 10
No pain   Moderate pain   Worst possible pain

Visual Analog Scale (VAS)**

No pain   Pain as bad as it could possibly be

Pain Distress Scale

Simple Descriptive Pain Distress Scale*

None Annoying Uncomfortable Dreadful Horrible Agonizing

Fig. 25-1. Postanesthesia care unit nursing care plan. (Reprinted with permission, University of Michigan Hospitals, Ann Arbor, MI.)

*If used as a graphic rating scale, a 10-cm baseline is recommended.
**A 10-cm baseline is recommended for VAS scales.
Acute Pain Management Guideline Panel. *Acute pain management: Operative or medical procedures and trauma. Clinical practice guideline.* (1992). AHCPR Pub. No. 92-0032. Rockville, MD: Agency for Health Care Policy and Research, Public Health Service, U.S. Department of Health and Human Services.

and the heart rate. Cardiac output may be measured by balloon-tipped flow-directed thermodilution catheters in critically ill patients. More often, it is assessed in terms of its general relationship and effect on the vascular system. Frequent blood pressure readings are obtained and compared with baseline and intraoperative values. Residual hypotension from anesthesia, preoperative medications, or peripheral pooling of blood may be counteracted by stir-up measures. Hypertension may be transient, caused by retained carbon dioxide in a patient who is hypoventilating. Changes in blood pressure must be correlated to the patient's overall condition and other parameters of assessment, such as level of consciousness, heart and respiratory rate, oxygen saturation, skin color and temperature, apprehension, restlessness, and urine output. Significant hypotensive changes in blood pressure, coupled with the signs and symptoms mentioned, may indicate hemorrhage or shock.

Blood pressure may be measured directly via intraarterial catheters (A lines). With this type of monitoring system, a characteristic waveform is displayed. Systolic readings, normally peaking at 100 to 140 mm Hg; diastolic readings, normally peaking at 60 to 90 mm Hg; pulse pressure; and mean arterial pressure (MAP) are obtained. MAP is the average pressure within the cardiovascular system throughout one cardiac cycle; it represents the average blood pressure. Central venous pressure (CVP) provides a means of assessing cardiac function (right ventricular filling pressure, or preload) and the status of intravascular volume. Used with patients who have normal, healthy cardiopulmonary function, CVP yields an adequate correlation between central venous and left ventricular end-diastolic pressures. In these patients, it may be an adequate guide to fluid replacement therapy. In many circumstances, however, CVP may not be an accurate index of cardiac function or intravascular volume status. In the critically ill patient, it is important to assess left ventricular function; CVP changes are late in reflecting left ventricular dysfunction. Instead, it is more likely that pulmonary artery pressure (PAP) monitoring will be used with cardiac surgery patients, patients experiencing shock, trauma patients, or perioperative patients with major system dysfunction. PAP monitoring yields important information about pulmonary artery wedge pressures, as well as pulmonary artery systolic and diastolic pressures; results of these readings allow precise, intensive management to maximize cardiac output and tissue oxygenation and to relieve or prevent pulmonary abnormalities (Darovic, 1995).

Changes in heart rate may profoundly affect myocardial performance. The rate, rhythm, and equality of pulses are assessed by the PACU nurse. Careful attention to the ECG monitor displays allows the nurse to correlate changes in heart rate with potential myocardial dysfunction. Tachycardia, over 100 beats per minute, may be associated with diminished stroke volume and cardiac output; because diastolic interval is shortened, ventricular filling time is diminished (Drain, 1994). Bradycardia, less than 60 beats per minute, may result in a severe drop in cardiac output if stroke volume is limited by cardiac disease or venous return is diminished.

Decreased cardiac output can precipitate cardiac dysrhythmias, as can fluid and electrolyte imbalances. The ECG must be observed closely for abnormal beats, as well as for rate, rhythm, and electrical waves and intervals. Premature ventricular contractions (PVCs) may be caused by prolonged bradycardia, blood gas alterations (especially hypoxemia), electrolyte disturbances (especially hypokalemia), drug toxicity, and coronary artery disease. They may occur with a normal heart rate or with bradycardia or tachycardia. PVCs can occur as a rare beat even in normal individuals. However, when they occur frequently, they are serious. According to Black and Matassarin-Jacobs (1993), PVCs are dangerous when they occur in pairs, are frequent (more than six times a minute), multiform, fall on a T wave, as bigeminy (after every normal QRS complex), or as a result of an acute myocardial infarction. PVCs can rapidly progress to ventricular tachycardia or fibrillation. Drug therapy (lidocaine) and oxygen therapy are usually indicated.

Nursing assessment and documentation of cardiac status should include results and means (noninvasive, A line, Doppler) of blood pressure readings, rate, quality, volume, and character of pulses (apical, carotid, femoral, peripheral, as appropriate), results of rates and rhythms from cardiac monitor readings, and results of other invasive monitoring.

The PACU Care Plan

The PACU nurse uses physical assessment skills, physiologic monitoring, the preoperative and intraoperative patient data base, results of laboratory and other diagnostic results, consultation with other members of the health care team, and subjective and objective patient data to devise a plan of care for the patient's PACU stay. This plan of nursing care offers the postanesthesia nurse a systematic method to help the patient return to optimum physiologic status after anesthesia. ASPAN guidelines for ongoing assessment incorporated into the PACU care plan follow (ASPAN, 1995).

The plan of ongoing assessment includes, but is not limited to, the following nursing actions:

1. Monitor, maintain, and/or improve respiratory function.
2. Monitor, maintain, and/or improve circulatory function.
3. Promote and maintain physical and emotional comfort.
4. Monitor surgical site.
5. Interpret and document data obtained during assessment.
6. Document nursing action and/or interventions with outcome.
7. Notify patient care unit of any needed equipment.
8. Include parent/legal guardian/significant other in care of patient as indicated.
9. Notify patient care unit when patient is ready for discharge from PACU and provide report of all operating and PACU significant happenings.
10. Document numeric score, if used.

Implementation

Figure 25-1 depicts a postanesthesia care unit record. A generic care plan for the postanesthesia patient is found at the end of this chapter. As with the other care plans presented in this book, it will need to be modified to meet institutional policies and protocols.

DISCHARGING THE PATIENT FROM PACU

Patients are ready for discharge from the PACU when they have recovered from the effects of anesthesia, have stable vital signs, minimal wound or other drainage, are alert and conscious (or have returned to their preoperative level of consciousness), have no unresolved or ongoing acute problems, and have a patent airway and adequate urinary output. ASPAN standards state that the the professional nurse continuously measures the patient s progress toward the desired outcomes and revises the plan of care and interventions as necessary (ASPAN, 1995). ASPAN assessment factors for evaluation and patient discharge follow (ASPAN, 1995).

Data collected and recorded to evaluate the patient s status for discharge:

1. Airway patency, respiratory function, and oxygen saturation
2. Stability of vital signs, including temperature
3. Level of consciousness and muscular strength
4. Mobility
5. Patency of tubes, catheters, drains, and intravenous lines
6. Skin color and condition
7. Condition of dressing and/or surgical site
8. Intake and output
9. Comfort

10. Anxiety
11. Child-parent/significant others interactions
12. Numeric score, if used

Discharge

Following documentation of a final nursing assessment and evaluation of the patient's condition, the postanesthesia nurse discharges the patient according to written policies and discharge criteria (approved by the medical staff). When a numeric scoring system is used, the discharge score is recorded, reflecting the patient s status. The postanesthesia nurse arranges for the patient s safe transport from the PACU.

Evaluation for Discharge

In 1987, Borchardt and Fraulini suggested that the initial PACU assessment be duplicated as the discharge assessment so that the same parameters are assessed and important changes noted. This continues to guide patient care today. The patient may be discharged by the anesthesiologist or by the use of medical staff–approved criteria (JCAHO, 1995). The Joint Commission on Accreditation of Healthcare Organizations has issued interpretations of its anesthesia standards for PACU discharge. According to the Joint Commission, the decision for PACU discharge is the responsibility of a licensed independent practitioner who has appropriate clinical privileges and is familiar with or has participated in the care of the patient. The intent of the standard may be met in one of two ways. The licensed independent practitioner may be present and write and sign a discharge order, or relevant discharge criteria may be used to determine if the patient is ready for discharge. Discharge criteria may be developed by the medical staff or delegated to anesthesia services for development. Discharge criteria may include the requirement that the licensed independent practitioner be contacted by telephone to make the discharge decision. The nursing staff may discharge the patient based on the telephone order or on the discharge criteria. If a scoring system is used, the patient is discharged when his or her evaluation score meets the discharge criteria.

Transfer of the Patient from PACU

The general safety considerations that apply to transporting the patient in any situation apply to transport from the PACU. It may be a nursing decision as to whether the patient is accompanied to the patient care unit by a PACU nurse; in some institutions, all patients may be accompanied to the clinical unit by a PACU nurse. Before the actual transfer, the receiving unit is called so that the assigned nurse has time to prepare the patient's room and organize special equipment that may be needed. A report may be given over the phone or a written transfer summary may be sent with the patient if a PACU nurse does not accompany the patient. The report, whether verbal or written, should include the operative procedure performed; anesthesia and reversal agents given; the patient's general condition and postanesthesia course; and information about dressings, drains, monitoring devices, medications administered, level of comfort, intake and output, and other information dictated by institutional protocol or patient safety (O Brien, 1994).

THE PERIOPERATIVE NURSE IN THE PACU

The perioperative nurse who cares for patients in the PACU, in either an acute care facility or an ambulatory surgery setting, should complete an orientation to the specialty care unit. It is not uncommon for perioperative staff to be cross-trained for PACU. Such cross-training allows for continuity of patient care and flexible staffing patterns. After PACU orientation, the perioperative nurse may rotate to the postanesthesia care unit on a regularly scheduled or need-identified basis. In either case, completion of an orientation program, the ability to function in emergency situations, and acquisition and maintenance of the skills required in caring for patients recovering from anesthesia are essential prerequisites for any nurse assigned to the PACU. ASPAN (1995) has identified perianesthesia competency-based practice for nurses. This includes, but is not limited to, airway management with respiratory equipment, ACLS or equivalent; neurologic assessment, intervention and evaluation; circulation (including cardiac rhythms), hemodynamic monitoring, neurovascular and renal monitoring; knowledge of anesthesia agents and adjuncts; patient comfort, including pain management and management of nausea and vomiting; thermal regulation; patient and professional nursing education; and documentation and legal issues. These elements require in-depth knowledge and complex skills. Mamaril (1993) states the following:

> "The PACU is a highly technical nursing unit in which nurses apply critical care nursing skills. The PACU provides specialized nursing care to diverse patient populations in an environment of constant activity, high volume, rapid turnover, and intense pressure. This creates a unique challenge because it requires quick response when emergencies occur."

Clearly, postanesthesia care requires the knowledge and skill of professional nursing.

GUIDE TO NURSING ACTIONS
Caring for the Patient in the PACU (Fig. 25-2)

1. The initial assessment is a rapid, precise review of the patient's overall condition. It may be performed independently by the PACU nurse or jointly with the anesthesia provider or other member of the perioperative team. It usually includes airway, level of consciousness, respirations, breath sounds, pulse, heart rate, temperature, oxygen saturation, skin color, presence of supplemental oxygen, tubes, invasive lines, and surgical site. Record the results.
2. Postanesthesia scoring systems may be used for initial patient assessment. The patient may be scored independently by the PACU nurse or jointly with the anesthesia care team or perioperative team. Record the score.
3. Check the patency of the airway. Reposition the airway, reposition the patient, or insert the artificial (oropharyngeal or nasopharyngeal) airway as necessary. Assess for return of swallow and gag reflexes.
4. Note the presence and adequacy of the artificial airway.
5. Administer or continue supplemental oxygen therapy as needed or ordered.
6. If the initial assessment was performed independently, it will be reported to the anesthesia or perioperative team member.
7. A report of important preoperative and intraoperative information should be received.
8. Pressure readings should be obtained. These may include blood pressure (invasive or noninvasive), intracranial pressure, and other pressures. Record, compare with baselines, and report significant changes.
9. Assess rate, depth, quality of respirations. Auscultate breath sounds. Review the patient history for at-risk conditions. Record each assessment; report significant changes. Encourage coughing, deep breathing, yawning, and inspiratory holding. Instruct and assist in incisional splinting.
10. Monitor heart rate (pulse or cardiac monitor). Record, compare with baselines, and report significant changes.
11. The patient's temperature is taken at admission and discharge, and when thermic treatment is in use. Record temperature and measurement route, compare with preoperative and intraoperative measurements, and report significant changes. Institute thermia unit as applicable.
12. Monitor oxygen saturation. Assess results of pulse oximetry. Initiate or discontinue oxygen therapy according to institutional policies.
13. Initiate or see that prescribed respiratory therapy (humidity and aerosol therapy, hyperinflation therapy [incentive spirometry], or chest physiotherapy) is carried out. Record these measures.
14. If ventilator assistance is required, set the panel controls as prescribed or with respiratory

FIG. 25-2
CARE PLAN FOR THE PATIENT IN THE PACU

KEY ASSESSMENT POINTS
Respiratory status
Circulatory status
Vital signs
Level of consciousness (LOC)/arousability
Tissue perfusion
Sensory/motor status
Level of pain/comfort

NURSING DIAGNOSIS
All generic nursing diagnoses apply to this patient, with the addition of:
The patient has the risk for:
Pain
Anxiety
Decreased cardiac output
Fluid volume deficit/excess
Impaired physical mobility
Injury
Impaired gas exchange/ineffective breathing patterns and/or airway clearance
Aspiration
Impaired skin integrity
Altered tissue perfusion
Altered patterns of urinary elimination
Altered body temperature: hypothermia/hyperthermia
Infection
Knowledge deficit

PATIENT OUTCOMES
All generic outcomes apply, with the addition of:
The patient's respiratory status will be maintained by:
* Respiratory rate depth, lung sounds, oxygen saturation/blood gas levels compatible with preoperative status
* Mechanical ventilatory support until the patient has adequate self-ventilation
* A patent airway
The patient's circulatory status will be maintained by:
* Blood pressure, pulse, and cardiac rhythm within acceptable parameters
* Adequate tissue perfusion
The patient will be free of preventable complications with:
* Temperature compatible with preoperative levels
* No signs/symptoms of infections/wound complications
* Dressings dry and intact
* Minimal/normal drainage from drainage sites
* No injury
The patient will verbalize minimal physical and emotional comfort.
The patient will regain and maintain sensory equilibrium as evidenced by:
* Orientation, with reflexes and mobility within preoperative levels
The patient's fluid and electrolyte balance will be maintained with:
* Serum electrolyte values, urinary output, other indices evidencing adequate fluid hydration

NURSING ACTIONS

	Yes	No	N/A
1. Initial assessment performed?	☐	☐	☐
2. Scoring system used?	☐	☐	☐
3. Airway patent?	☐	☐	☐
4. Artificial airway?	☐	☐	☐
5. Oxygen therapy?	☐	☐	☐
6. Initial assessment reported?	☐	☐	☐
7. Patient report received?	☐	☐	☐
8. Invasive/noninvasive pressures monitored?	☐	☐	☐
9. Respirations monitored?	☐	☐	☐
10. Heart rate monitored?	☐	☐	☐
11. Temperature monitored?	☐	☐	☐
12. Oxygen saturation monitored?	☐	☐	☐
13. Respiratory therapy?	☐	☐	☐
14. Ventilator assistance?	☐	☐	☐
15. Patient positioned per status?	☐	☐	☐
16. Skin assessed?	☐	☐	☐
17. Circulation assessed?	☐	☐	☐
18. Dressings dry/intact?	☐	☐	☐
19. Condition suture line noted?	☐	☐	☐
20. Drains/tubes/catheters patent?	☐	☐	☐
21. Drainage observed/recorded?	☐	☐	☐
22. Muscle strength/response assessed?	☐	☐	☐
23. Pupils checked?	☐	☐	☐
24. Fluid infusions regulated?	☐	☐	☐
25. Level of consciousness monitored?	☐	☐	☐

NURSING ACTIONS—cont'd

	Yes	No	N/A
26. Patient safety measures initiated?	☐	☐	☐
27. Comfort measures (physical/emotional) provided?	☐	☐	☐
28. Emergency equipment available?	☐	☐	☐
29. Patient complications?	☐	☐	☐
30. Medications given?	☐	☐	☐
31. Communication with patient's family/significant other?	☐	☐	☐
32. Prescribed treatments/tests done?	☐	☐	☐
33. Intake/output summarized?	☐	☐	☐
34. Discharged by whom?	☐	☐	☐
35. Scoring system used?	☐	☐	☐
36. Report given?	☐	☐	☐
37. Discharged to (record):	☐	☐	☐

Document additional nursing actions/generic care plans initiated here:

_____

_____

_____

EVALUATION OF PATIENT OUTCOMES

	Outcome met	Outcome met with additional outcome criteria	Outcome met with revised nursing care plan	Outcome not met	Outcome not applicable to this patient
1. Respiratory status was maintained.	☐	☐	☐	☐	☐
2. Circulatory status was maintained.	☐	☐	☐	☐	☐
3. Complications were prevented.	☐	☐	☐	☐	☐
4. The patient verbalized physical and emotional comfort.	☐	☐	☐	☐	☐
5. Sensory equilibrium was regained and maintained.	☐	☐	☐	☐	☐
6. Fluid and electrolyte balance was maintained.	☐	☐	☐	☐	☐

Signature: _____ Date: _____

therapy staff assistance, assess breath sounds, offer reassurance, suction as necessary, and assess the patient's readiness for extubation.

15. Positioning will be determined by the patient's status, the surgery performed, the presence of invasive lines, and the equipment. Note position and positional changes.

16. Assess the color, temperature, and turgor of the skin, nail beds, lips, and oral mucosa. Assess the condition of the skin at ECG and electroencephalogram electrodes and at the site of the intraoperative electrosurgical dispersive pad. Record, compare with preoperative condition, and report significant changes.

17. Assess peripheral pulses, color, temperature, and capillary refill in extremities. Record, compare with baselines, and report significant changes.

18. Dressings should be dry or have minimal drainage. The edges of the dressing should remain sealed. If dressing change is required, use aseptic technique. Document the condition of dressings.

19. If dressings are absent, clear (for example, skin tapes), or changed, inspect the suture line. Note and record approximation of wound edges, color, and presence of drainage or exudate.

20. Check the patency and connections of all tubes, drains, and catheters. Prevent undue strain and kinking.

21. Observe and record the amount, quality, and consistency of all drainage. Ascertain from surgeon expected or anticipated drainage from incisions, drains, or catheters/tubes.

22. Assess the patient's muscle strength and response and mobility of all extremities.

23. Check pupils if appropriate.

24. Regulate the rate of all infusions. Check the infusion site for infiltration, inflammation, and sterile dressing. Maintain the patency of infusion lines. Assess the patient for signs of fluid and electrolyte balance (intake and output, skin turgor, mucous membranes, and laboratory results).

25. Monitor the patient's level of consciousness. Determine orientation, ability to follow and participate in simple commands and short conversations. Stimulate the patient verbally and physically as appropriate (positional changes, movement of extremities, and so on). Record level of consciousness, compare with baseline, and report significant changes.

26. Initiate appropriate patient safety measures. Avoid sudden, rapid positional changes. Keep side rails up. Restrain only if necessary to prevent injury. Initiate electrical safety measures.

27. Provide physical and emotional comfort. Position the patient comfortably (as appropriate), provide privacy, reduce environmental stimuli, and objectively and subjectively evaluate discomfort. Administer pain medication according to nursing assessment. Evaluate and record the effectiveness of pain medication. Explain PACU interventions. Allow the patient time to verbalize; clarify misconceptions. Assist and encourage the patient with effective coping mechanisms. Provide warm blankets and other measures (convective warming device, thermal blankets, radiant warmers) for shaking or complaints of hypothermia. Offer compresses or lubricant for dry lips. Offer mouth rinse or swabs and ice chips/oral fluids as applicable.

28. Emergency equipment should be available in anticipation of possible shock, hemorrhage, cardiac dysrhythmias, cardiac arrest, airway emergencies (laryngospasm, bronchospasm, obstruction, respiratory arrest), malignant hyperthermia, untoward effects of anesthetic agents or drugs, hypertensive crisis, thromboembolic events, or reintubation.

29. Document any patient complications, treatments instituted, and patient response.

30. Record all medications given, including time, route, and patient response (if appropriate for the medication).

31. Communicate with the patient's family or significant other on patient arrival and discharge. Allow visitors according to institutional protocol.

32. Record all prescribed treatments and tests initiated in PACU.

33. Summarize intake and output. Note any emesis, irrigation and intravenous fluids, and all drainage. If the patient is unable to void, palpate the bladder for distention. Catheterize only as necessary.

34. Note by whom the patient is discharged (PACU nurse, physician, or telephone order).

35. If a scoring system is used, record the patient's discharge score.

36. A report should be given regarding important intraoperative and PACU patient parameters, patient condition, required equipment, and so on (in person, by phone, or in writing) to the nurse on the receiving unit.

37. Record to whom the patient was discharged (receiving unit nurse, family, or significant other), means of discharge (stretcher, wheelchair, or ambulatory), and accompanied by whom. If the patient is ambulatory, record discharge teaching, planning, referrals, and written discharge instructions given to patient/significant other.

SUMMARY

Careful, comprehensive care planning is necessary if the goal of returning the patient to a safe physiologic level after anesthesia is to be achieved. Care plans provide systematic methods for ensuring that safe, individualized, knowledgeable care is initiated for the patient in the PACU. Patients in the PACU can experience complications of varying severity while recovering from anesthesia. Common problems range from pain and agitation to failure to awaken, hypovolemia, and cardiac dysrhythmias. Hines, et al. (1992) studied nearly 18,500 consecutive patients entering a university teaching hospital PACU to identify the incidence of intraoperative and PACU complications. A combined complication rate of 26.7% (23.7% PACU complication rate versus 5.1% overall intraoperative complication rate) was found. Nausea and vomiting (9.8%), need for upper airway support (6.9%), and hypotension requiring treatment (2.7%) were the most commonly encountered PACU complications. Careful and vigilant nursing care to identify and treat such physiologic alterations becomes part of the nursing care plan to maintain the patient's safety, privacy, comfort, and dignity.

References

Acute Pain Management Guideline Panel. *Acute pain management: Operative or medical procedures and trauma. Clinical practice guideline.* AHCPR Pub. No. 92-0032. Rockville, MD: Agency for Health Care Policy and Research, Public Health Service, U.S. Department of Health and Human Services.

American Society of Post Anesthesia Nurses. (1995). *Standards of perianesthesia nursing practice.* Thorofare, NJ: The Society.

Association of Operating Room Nurses. (1996). A model for perioperative nursing practice. In *Standards and recommended practices* (pp 69-71). Denver: The Association.

Black JM & Matassarin-Jacobs E. (1993). *Luckmann & Sorensen s medical-surgical nursing: A psychophysiologic approach.* Philadelphia: WB Saunders.

Borchardt AC & Fraulini KE. (1987). Postanesthetic problems. In KE Fraulini, (Ed). *After anesthesia: A guide for PACU, ICU, and medical-surgical nurses.* Norwalk, CT: Appleton & Lange.

Brimacombe J. (1993). The laryngeal mask airway: Tool for airway management. *Journal of Post Anesthesia Nursing* 8:88-95.

Carpenito LJ. (1995). *Nursing care plans and documentation* (2nd ed.). Philadelphia: JB Lippincott.

Crossley AWA. (1992). Peri-operative shivering (editorial). *Anaesthesia* 47:193-5.

Darovic GO. (1995). *Hemodynamic monitoring: Invasive and noninvasive clinical application.* Philadelphia: WB Saunders.

Drain CB. (1994). *The post anesthesia care unit.* Philadelphia: WB Saunders.

Fakhry SA & Sheldon GF. (1995). Postoperative management. In *Care of the surgical patient.* New York: Scientific American.

Hines R, et al. (1992). Complications occurring in the postanesthesia care unit: A survey. *Anesthesia and Analgesia* 74(4):503-9.

Joint Commission for Accreditation of Healthcare Organizations. (1995). *Comprehensive accreditation manual for hospitals.* Oakbrook Terrace, IL: JCAHO.

Mamaril M. (1993). Standard of care: Legal implications in the postanesthesia care unit. *Journal of Post Anesthesia Nursing* 8:13-20.

North American Nursing Diagnosis Association. (1994). *NANDA Nursing diagnosis: Definitions and classification 1995-96.* Philadelphia: The Association.

O'Brien DD. (1994). Care of the post anesthesia patient. In CB Drain (Ed). *The post anesthesia care unit.* Philadelphia: WB Saunders.

Smeltzer SC & Bare BG. (1996). *Brunner & Suddarth's textbook of medical-surgical nursing* (7th ed.). Philadelphia: JB Lippincott.

Weeks CS. (1890). *Textbook of nursing.* New York: D Appleton.

Chapter 26

Research Considerations

Karen L. Ritchey

If nursing is ever to justify its name as an applied science, if it is ever to free itself from those old superficial, haphazard methods, some way must be found to submit all our practices as rapidly as possible to the most searching tests which modern science can devise.

STEWART, 1944

*T*he ultimate goal of any profession is to improve the practice of its members so that the clients have the greatest benefit. Perioperative nurses may attempt to solve practice problems through inherited information (rituals, traditions, sacred cows), authority sources (books, a professional association) or expert colleagues, their own experience, trial and error, logical reasoning, or research. Research may be conducted for a variety of reasons, but a major focus of nursing research is to improve the practice of nursing and patient care. The perioperative nurse has two important contributions to make in the realm of research: identifying pertinent practice and patient care questions for research and using research findings to improve that practice and patient care (Mayhew, 1993).

THE ACQUISITION OF KNOWLEDGE

The product of knowing is knowledge, and nursing knowledge has evolved into three general classifications. These have been identified by Kidd and Morrison (1988), Schultz and Meleis (1988), and Ziegler, Vaugh-Wrobel, & Erlen (1986) as follows:
- Practice wisdom
- Conceptual knowledge
- Empirically researched information

Practice Wisdom
Practice wisdom develops from repeatedly assessing, planning for, intervening with, and evaluating the clinical patient using tradition, personal experience, authority, intuition, role-modeling, and trial and error. Historically, knowledge based on practice wisdom has guided the perioperative nurse through anticipated and unanticipated circumstances. Decision making is focused on one patient and on what has worked in the past; rationales may be difficult for the perioperative nurse to articulate. Although this silent art of nursing was viewed as less important and credible than the formal empiric foundations of practice (nursing science), it has regained legitimacy as a necessary component of humane care. As the essential and often crucial nature of nurses' caring functions in promoting the health and well-being of their patients has gained research importance and become recognized by scholarly nurses and other health care providers, perioperative researchers have begun to study the phenomena and construct of caring.

Perioperative exemplar. Using Watson's theory of nursing as a caring science, McNamara (1995) undertook a qualitative analysis of the perceptions of caring behaviors of perioperative nurses. From a broad range of behaviors that were identified, key elements included recognizing the unique worth of individual patients, communicating by touch and word to establish relationships, and being aware of and sensitive to the patient's experience and feelings. Caring was also perceived as protection of patients from risks for injury and supporting them psychologically and spiritually. These behaviors may be broadly classified into the themes of caring touch, protective touch, and task touch identified by Watson (1994).

Conceptual Knowledge

Conceptual knowledge is constructed from the analysis of patterns or relationships among several patients, settings, or observations. The focus is on groups of patients and their responses to intervention, technology, or situations. This knowledge seeks to define concepts, to categorize facts, and to inspect "what is" through logical reasoning and/or problem solving.

Perioperative exemplar. Inadvertent hypothermia is a well-documented event in perioperative patient populations. The concept of physiologic thermal regulation is fairly well understood. Through a literature review, Dennison (1995) analyzed what is known about the incidence of inadvertent hypothermia and the patient populations at risk, and then went on to recommend eight perioperative nursing interventions to prevent hypothermia problems.

Empiric Knowledge

Empiric knowledge is derived from research. Research is the systematic formal testing of ideas, questions, and concepts in an effort to discover, expand, or verify knowledge. The term "research" designates the application of the scientific approach to a question of interest. Empiricism, the search for knowledge based entirely on what is seen, heard, smelled, or touched during an experiment, imposes a certain degree of objectivity because the study ideas are exposed to testing in the real world. Empiric research can validate hunches or correct misconceptions. It can provide data to argue for or against an issue. Empiric knowledge that has survived the scrutiny of replication and application to clinical practice contributes to the scientific base necessary to improve the practice of perioperative nursing (Beck, 1994).

Perioperative exemplar. The attributes of antimicrobial agents used in surgical hand scrubs have been quantified and studied for a number of years. As new products are introduced into the marketplace, research that compares their efficacy must be undertaken to validate product claims and guide product selection (Janken, Rudisill, & Benfield, 1992). Using criteria set forth in the Association of

Operating Room Nurses' (AORN) recommended practice for the purpose of the surgical hand scrub, Paulson (1994) examined five products and their ability to remove transient microorganisms, to reduce microbial recolonization, and to provide cumulative protection. His results supported the results of previous research on the attributes of chlorhexidine gluconate (CHG), suggested its use in either 2% or 4% concentration, and recommended an iodophor as the antimicrobial agent of choice for persons sensitive to CHG.

CLINICAL RESEARCH

The purpose of conducting and using clinical research is to improve patient care. Perioperative nurses have long been involved in quality assurance, quality improvement, and performance assessment; their concern with quality of care is well documented. Clinical research is one way to improve or to validate quality (Horn, 1995). It is important, worthwhile work. If clinical practice is based on research findings, questions about which perioperative nursing interventions work best for which patients can be determined, and patient outcomes should improve. Patients, however, are not the only beneficiaries of involvement with clinical research.

Benefits of Clinical Research

The integration of practice wisdom and empiric knowledge through research will benefit the patient, the perioperative nurse, the profession, the practice setting, and society as a whole. It begins with an atmosphere created by the imagination, study, and reflection required to identify and conduct a research project. When growth is stimulated, all of the participants benefit.

The patient. Although patients have similarities, no two are alike. Perioperative nurses cannot assume that the success of a particular intervention for one patient confirms that it will be successful for all patients. Perioperative nurses need to ask which interventions work best for which patients; what idiosyncrasies of one patient will make a response differ from that of another patient. Clinical research could ask whether all patients benefit equally from aseptic practices, or if some expensive techniques are selected because of tradition. Another question concerns whether we can identify a method of preoperative instruction that can be accomplished in a limited length of time and understood by persons who are either illiterate or have low reading levels. Research investigating patient care and outcomes will move the patient closer to individualized care and expeditious recovery.

PERIOPERATIVE EXEMPLAR. The effects of psychoeducational interventions with perioperative patient populations have been extensively reported and with confounding results. Preoperative instruction and its effect on coping with various aspects of the surgical experience leave many unanswered questions and suggestions for further research. Based on previous mixed results, Oetker-Black and Taunton (1994) sought to develop a measurement instrument that would enable perioperative nurses to more effectively assess the need of the patient for preoperative instruction and evaluate the effectiveness of that instruction. Their work was based on the theory that patients' own abilities to judge and describe what course of action was personally necessary to achieve an outcome, and their perceptions of whether they had the abilities to carry out the course of action (Bandura's self-efficacy theory), would affect the relationship between preoperative instruction and subsequent performance of taught behaviors. Use of the measurement instrument would, then, enable improved design of preoperative patient education strategies.

The perioperative nurse. Clinical research can benefit the practitioner by ensuring confidence in selected nursing actions. For example, a patient is admitted to the operating room (OR) with a fractured hip complicated by acute urinary retention. Medical-surgical textbooks recommend clamping the catheter after 1000 ml of urine is released from the bladder. The patient is in pain and will be anesthetized as soon as the urinary bladder is safely emptied. Must the perioperative nurse wait 5 minutes after the first 1000 ml of urine is drained to prevent bladder decompression and hypotension, or is it safe to empty the bladder completely without intermittent clamping? Results from an investigation by Bristoll, et al. (1989) suggest that the clamping rule may be a misconception made into a rule over time. Based on this clinical research, the perioperative nurse could decide, with some degree of confidence, that complete emptying of the urinary bladder would not cause any bladder wall injury in this fractured hip patient. In fact, it could expedite the anesthesia and thus the pain relief.

PERIOPERATIVE EXEMPLAR. Since the advent of universal precautions, the protective barriers afforded by surgical gloves has been a topic of interest to perioperative care providers. If the perioperative nurse needs a glove in an unsterile situation that he or she feels confident will provide protection, is a pair of examination gloves adequate or should a surgical glove be selected? Examination gloves are less costly, but do they provide adequate barrier protection? To answer this question, Zinner (1994) examined protective barrier properties of sterile surgical gloves and unsterile examination gloves. Her findings, which are similar to previous findings, led her to suggest that, when glove integrity is essential in an unscrubbed situation (a situation the circulator

might be in), sterile surgical gloves offer better protection. She also recommended, based on her findings and the findings of other studies, that failure rates occur in both types of glove, reinforcing the need to wash the hands past glove removal.

The profession. Perioperative nurses who use research have the potential to improve their critical thinking skills, to expand the ways in which they view patient situations, to assess patient care problems, and to plan patient care more effectively. This enhances perioperative nurses' perceptions of themselves as professionals, and their work may become more interesting and satisfying. Critical appraisal of published perioperative research serves to educate nursing colleagues outside the specialty and within the interdisciplinary team for the goal of providing safe, effective, high-quality nursing care. Efforts to build a scientific data base reinforce credibility as a nursing specialty. Clinical research measuring the effect of perioperative nursing on patient outcomes is difficult but necessary to demonstrate that perioperative nurses are essential surgical care providers. Empiric data on the strength of perioperative nursing's influence on patient outcomes is essential for health policy-making as resources for care diminish.

PERIOPERATIVE EXEMPLAR. As changes in health care increasingly move the patient from in-hospital to out-of-hospital care settings, what is the effect on patient recovery? Kleinbeck and Hoffart (1994) studied patients who underwent laparoscopic cholecystectomy in an outpatient surgical setting with discharge within 24 hours of surgery. Their qualitative analysis revealed that patients felt vulnerable without the presence of a nurse to answer questions; there were many activities that posed problems for patients in their progression toward resumption of normal routines that additional instruction and explanation would have alleviated. This finding was also supported in another study of same-day surgery concerns conducted by Oberle, Allen, & Lynkowski (1994). As a result of these studies, the researchers made many pragmatic recommendations for perioperative nurses to improve the outcomes and perceived recovery process for this patient population.

The department. When clinical research is conducted within a health care facility, the study results will readily apply to that department's patient population. A manager does not have to try to extrapolate a good result from elsewhere and wonder whether it will work in his or her clinical setting. Quebbeman and his colleagues (1992) studied how frequently blood penetrates surgical gowns during perioperative procedures and the factors that may cause gowns to fail as a barrier to blood strike-through. Three perioperative nurses observed how frequently the gown barrier protected surgeons and assistants-at-surgery during 234 operations. Findings of the study identified factors influencing the protective reliability of surgical gowns in surgery: the amount of time the gown is worn, characteristics of the gown, and the location of blood contact with the gown. It was also found that a single-layer gown had a higher risk of strike-through than a reinforced gown, including the reusable gown and a plastic-lined gown. The department manager could use the findings to support purchasing of reusable gowns, thus adequately protecting the surgical team members and the patient.

ANOTHER PERIOPERATIVE EXEMPLAR. Perioperative nurses perform many activities to intervene in the nursing diagnosis *high risk for infection*. With patients undergoing joint replacement, this risk is controlled, in part, through traffic patterns and environmental control of the aseptic environment. To determine compliance with traffic control patterns, Ratkowski (1994) explored a number of variables that influenced activity in joint replacement operating rooms in her surgical services department. The results of this study led to recommendations for departmental changes, which were implemented and then re-evaluated through follow-up surveys.

Society. Value, or worth, of an entity is assigned based on its definition. The worth of perioperative nurses as educated care providers integrating complex technical skill, judgment, and experience to accomplish a positive health result is strengthened through clinical research. Empiric data generated from rigorous methods help to indicate to society and health policy makers that (1) perioperative nurses are unequivocally willing and able to be accountable for their practice and (2) perioperative nurses can systematically demonstrate that their influence positively affects the public's welfare. Evidence of scientific clinical studies advances the value of perioperative nursing care and serves as a powerful argument for independent nursing roles as well as adequate compensation.

PERIOPERATIVE EXEMPLAR. As a professional association, AORN has taken seriously the need to identify priorities in perioperative nursing research. Through a Delphi technique, which works to achieve group consensus through repeated measurement, the Association has recently identified the top 10 priorities for current research (AORN priorities, 1994). Measurement of perioperative nursing contributions to patient outcomes was the first priority-ranked area for research; other areas of outcome measurement included the determination of cost-effective nursing interventions, the development of instruments to measure patient outcomes, more study of the effect of preoperative preparation on patient outcomes, the use of recommended practices (as op-

posed to ritual or tradition) on patient outcomes, and the determination of clinical indicators for measuring patient outcomes. Clearly, the profession of perioperative nursing has assumed an accountability for providing care to society that is underpinned by high quality, cost-effectiveness, and improved patient outcomes.

INCORPORATING RESEARCH AND PRACTICE ROLES

For the benefits of research to be realized, practicing perioperative nurses and researchers must be committed to advancing the science of nursing. The link between the two is dissemination and utilization of research results. The responsibilities of the researcher and the practicing perioperative nurse are interdependent (Fig. 26-1). Applying and using research findings in the practice setting is important to improved patient outcomes, to enhancing the professional practice environment, and to controlling the costs of delivering patient care (Titler, et al, 1994). The extensive literature that exists related to dissemination of research findings and their utilization in nursing practice suggests that a number of issues and perceived barriers remain to be overcome.

Barriers to Research Utilization

The current perioperative practice environment, characterized by cost-containment efforts, rapid development of new technology, and the restructuring of the delivery of perioperative care systems, compels perioperative nurses to provide care that is both efficient and effective. Therefore, research that contributes to the efficiency and effectiveness of perioperative patient care must be disseminated, understood, utilized, and evaluated on an ongoing basis (Nolan, et al., 1994). Barriers to achieving these four goals include the way research is communicated, the accessibility of the research findings, the quality and relevance of the research, the research values and skills of the practicing perioperative nurse, the time to read and implement research findings, and organizational and workplace limitations (Funk, et al., 1991).

Publishing research results. The implications of research can be realized only with dissemination of results. Nurse researchers can facilitate the utilization of new knowledge by doing the following (Lambo, 1995):

- Establishing a communication link with practicing nurses and a way to interact with them
- Disseminating data in clinical and research journals and to segments of the nursing population that target practitioners, such as in poster sessions and presentations at meetings of specialty nursing associations

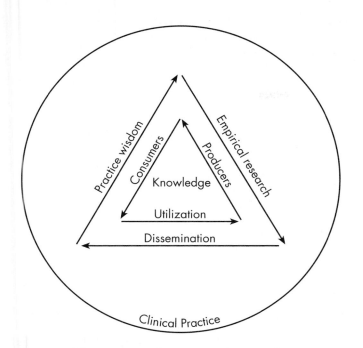

Fig. 26-1. The interaction between producers and consumers of research in the perpetual search for knowledge.

- Providing external assistance with implementing changes called for by research results
- Interpreting study results with an eye to clinical application
- Writing reports that are relatively free of technical jargon

"Dissemination" is defined as a process of scattering far and wide, as if sowing seed. Publishing a study only in a prominent research journal does not facilitate the "scattering" of the study results. Practicing perioperative nurses may not regularly read the research literature, and they generally spurn the complex analyses that another nurse scientist might require. To facilitate dissemination, researchers should consider writing a minimum of two research reports. The primary account should be written in a research journal with sufficient replication detail to meet the expectations of fellow investigators. The second article should appear in a clinical journal with a section titled "utilization" or "clinical importance" that suggests steps to follow before the applicable findings can be implemented clinically. In their study of factors that encourage and discourage practicing nurses to use nursing research findings, Pettengill, Gillies, and Clark (1994) discovered that a research newsletter was perceived as more helpful than either continuing education programs or computer networks for keeping up with research. Nurse researchers must focus more on providing sufficient information for the practicing nurse to determine whether a particular approach investigated might be helpful for specific patient populations.

Reading Research Reports

Nursing literature abounds with suggestions for nurses who read research. A research report should be critiqued by reviewing the statement of the problem or research question and looking at the literature review, hypotheses, methods and design, results of data analysis, limitations, and implications. Begin by determining whether the journal in which the article is published is a refereed one, meaning that the article was sent out for review before it was published. The title of the research report should tell you what was studied. In the beginning of the report, look for a clearly stated purpose or aim of the research. The problem statement describes what has been studied. The literature review describes what is already known about the problem and why the study is important. It often provides the theoretic framework that underlies the study; these may be nursing or nonnursing theories. Research questions and hypotheses differ in that the former are usually used when little is known about the topic (for example, "Does the room temperature affect thermoregulation in pediatric surgical patients?") and the latter are used when enough is known to draw tentative conclusions (such as, "Warmer room temperatures result in less hypothermia in pediatric surgical patients.").

Studies with small sample sizes may be clinically relevant and have statistical significance. However, if the research is the basis for recommending a change in a perioperative practice, a larger sample size and research that have been conducted before (replicated) with similar results should characterize the study. There are many ways to design a research study (Box 26-1). The data collection/measurement instrument (tool) should fit with the theoretic framework of the study and provide information on reliability (consistency and accuracy in collecting data) and validity (whether it measures what it is supposed to measure) (Reineck, 1991). Moreover, issues related to the clinical limitations of the measurement tool(s) should be addressed in the methodology section of the research report (LeFort, 1993). Taken together, the perioperative nurse should ask himself or herself whether the study's characteristics and findings fit with the setting the perioperative nurse practices in, whether it provides information relevant for current practice, and whether the information has value in solving a problem, making a decision, or changing a standard of care or a perioperative practice (Stetler, 1994).

Perioperative exemplar. Johnson (1994) explored the relationship between an on-site satellite laboratory and the frequency of delays in surgery for same-day surgery patients. Her study is well reported, with clearly identified nursing importance and an

---

Box 26-1 Types of Research Used in Nursing Studies

Applied

Research that concentrates on finding a solution to an immediate practical problem

Basic

Research designed to extend the base of knowledge in a discipline for the sake of knowledge production or theory construction, rather than for solving an immediate problem

Case Study

A research method that involves a thorough, in-depth analysis of an individual, group, institution, or other social unit

Clinical

Research designed to generate knowledge to guide nursing practice

Correlational

Investigations that explore the interrelationships among variables of interest without any active intervention on the part of the researcher

Descriptive

Research studies that have as their main objective the accurate portrayal of the characteristics of persons, situations, or groups, and the frequency with which certain phenomena occur

Ethnography

Method used to develop theories of culture that also produces descriptions of the ways of life in cultures or subcultures (LoBiondo-Wood & Haber, 1994)

Evaluation

Research that investigates how well a program, practice, or policy is working

Ex Post Facto

Research conducted after the variations in the independent variable have occurred in the natural course of events; a form of nonexperimental research in which causal explanations are inferred after the fact

Exploratory

A preliminary study designed to develop or refine hypotheses or to test and refine the data collection methods

Historical

Systematic studies designed to establish facts and relationships concerning past events

Methodologic

Research designed to develop or refine procedures for obtaining, organizing, or analyzing data

Nonexperimental

Studies in which the researcher collects data without introducing any new treatments or changes

Observational

Studies in which the data are collected by means of observing and recording behaviors or activities of interest

Philosophic

Method based on the investigation of the truths and principles of existence, knowledge, and conduct (LoBiondo-Wood & Haber, 1994)

Qualitative

Descriptive, subjective, naturalistic study that aims to generalize directly from the research situation to the informants' everyday lives by imposing as little structure as possible on the research situation and concentration on letting the informants' own words be heard (Mateo & Kirchhoff, 1991)

Quantitative

Research that seeks facts or causes in an objective and controlled way. Primary commitment to reliable and generalizable description and/or the testing of hypotheses (Mateo & Kirchhoff, 1991)

Survey

A type of nonexperimental research that focuses on obtaining information regarding the status quo of a situation, often via direct questioning of a sample of respondents

Unless otherwise indicated, information obtained from Polit & Hungler (1987). *Nursing research: Principles and methods.* Philadelphia: JB Lippincott.

---

understanding of clinical relevance versus pure statistical significance. In her discussion of delays, she reviews the impact of any delay in terms of lost time and lost revenue, as well as the impact on patients, nurses, and physicians.

FUTURE RESEARCH AGENDAS

It is fairly evident that the remainder of the decade will be devoted to some compelling research issues. These include various outcome measures, quality initiatives, patient satisfaction, testing and refining perioperative nursing diagnoses, and technology assessment. Despite the methodologic issues in measuring outcomes, perioperative nurses must accumulate a body of research that examines factors that influence perioperative patient outcomes and the selection of critical outcomes, health promotion with perioperative patients, and ways of measuring them. The questions of which parameters, measures, or observable outcomes are important and relevant will need to be answered. Part of this determination should focus on clinical outcomes (Hadorn, et al., 1994), and these may need to be further subdivided into immediate, intermediate, and ultimate outcomes (Gillis, 1995). The inclusion of patient self-reports as part of outcome determination leads to issues in question design and selection, modes for data collection, and study design (Fowler, et al., 1994). As the health care system becomes more integrated, it will be increasingly difficult to separate and segregate nursing contributions to patient outcomes from the full effect of the interdisciplinary team; perioperative nursing must be part of the data that is collected in new systems approaches by identifying data elements that quantify professional perioperative nursing care and their relationship to identified outcomes. Accepting these research challenges will, in part, enable the perioperative nursing profession to participate in a meaningful way in reshaping the health care system.

References

AORN priorities for perioperative nursing research. (1994). *AORN Journal, 60*(6), 914-924.

Beck CT. (1994). Replication strategies for nursing research. *Image—the Journal of Nursing Scholarship, 26*(3), 191-194.

Bristoll SL, et al. (1989). The mythical danger of rapid urinary drainage. *American Journal of Nursing, 89*, 344-345.

Dennison D. (1995). Thermal regulation of patients during the perioperative period. *AORN Journal, 61*(5), 827-832.

Fowler FJ, et al. (1994). Methodological issues in measuring patient-reported outcomes: The agenda of the work group on outcomes assessment. *Medical Care, 32*(7), 65-76.

Funk SG, et al. (1991). BARRIERS: The barriers to research utilization scale. *Applied Nursing Research, 4*(1), 39-45.

Gillis A. (1995). Exploring nursing outcomes for health promotion. *Nursing Forum, 30*(2), 5-12.

Hadorn D, et al. (1994). Making judgments about treatment effectiveness based on health outcomes: Theoretical and practical issues. *Journal of Quality Improvement, 20*(10), 547-554.

Horn S. (1995). Using clinical practice improvement. *Journal of Quality Improvement, 21*(6), 301-308.

Janken JK, Rudisill P, & Benfield L. (1992). Product evaluation as a research utilization strategy. *Applied Nursing Research, 5*(4), 188-201.

Johnson KF. (1994). Does an on-site satellite laboratory reduce surgical delay: A study of delays in a same-day surgical center. *AORN Journal, 59*(6), 1275-1290.

Kidd P & Morrison EF. (1988). The progression of knowledge in nursing: A search for meaning. *Image—the Journal of Nursing Scholarship, 20*, 222-224.

Kleinbeck SVM & Hoffart N. (1994). Outpatient recovery after laparoscopic cholecystectomy. *AORN Journal, 60*(3), 394-402.

Lambo EE. (1995). Enhancing the utilization of research reports. *Bridge, 14*, 1-3.

LeFort SM. (1993). The statistical versus clinical significance debate. *Image—the Journal of Nursing Scholarship, 25*(1), 57-62.

LoBiondo-Wood G & Haber J. (1994). *Nursing research: Methods, critical appraisal, and utilization* (4th ed.). St Louis: Mosby.

Mateo MA & Kirchoff KT. (1991). *Conducting and using nursing research in the clinical setting.* Baltimore: Williams & Wilkins.

Mayhew PA. (1993). The importance of the practicing nurse in nursing research. *Medsurg Nursing, 2*(3), 210-211, 246.

McNamara SA. (1995). Perioperative nurses' perceptions of caring. *AORN Journal, 61*(2), 377-388.

Nolan MT, et al. (1994). A review of approaches to integrating research and practice. *Applied Nursing Research, 7*(4), 199-208.

Oberle K, Allen M, & Lynkowski P. (1994). Follow-up of same day surgery patients: A study of patient concerns. *AORN Journal, 59*(5), 1016-1025.

Oetker-Black SL & Taunton RL. (1994). Evaluation of a self-efficacy scale for preoperative patients. *AORN Journal, 60*(1), 43-50.

Paulson DS. (1994). Comparative evaluation of five surgical hand scrub preparations. *AORN Journal, 60*(2), 246-256.

Pettengill MM, Gillies DA, & Clark CC. (1994). Factors encouraging and discouraging the use of nursing research findings. *Image—the Journal of Nursing Scholarship, 26*(2), 143-147.

Polit DF & Hungler BP. (1987). *Nursing research: Principles and methods.* Philadelphia: JB Lippincott.

Quebbeman EJ, et al. (1992). In-use evaluation of surgical gowns. *Surg Gynecol Obstet, 174*, 369-375.

Ratkowski P. (1994). Traffic control: A study of traffic control in total joint replacement procedures. *AORN Journal, 59*(2), 439-448.

Reineck C. (1991). Nursing research instruments: Pathway to resources. *Applied Nursing Research, 4*(1), 34-38.

Schlotfeldt RM. (1988). Structuring nursing knowledge: A priority for creating nursing's future. *Nursing Science, 1*, 35-38.

Shultz PR & Meleis AI. (1988). Nursing epistemology: Traditions, insights, questions. *Image—the Journal of Nursing Scholarship, 20*, 217-221.

Stetler CB. (1994). Refinement of the Stetler/Marran model for application of research findings to practice. *Nursing Outlook, 42*(1), 15-25.

Stewart I. (1944). In PR Cook Lessons from the past: Isabel Stewart, nursing education leader. *Nursing & Health Care, 16*(1), Jan/Feb, 1995, 20-23.

Titler MG, et al. (1994). Infusing research into practice to promote quality care. *Nursing Research, 43*(5), 307-312.

Watson MJ. (1994, March 15). *Caring in a world of technology.* Paper presented at the AORN Congress, New Orleans, LA.

Ziegler SM, Vaugh-Wrobel BC, & Erlen JA. (1986). *Nursing process, nursing diagnosis, nursing knowledge.* Norwalk, CT: Appleton-Century-Crofts.

Zinner NL. (1994). How safe are your gloves? A study of protective barrier properties of gloves. *AORN Journal, 59*(4), 876-882.

Index

Custom titles for your specialty.
The Perioperative Nursing Series. From Mosby.

*T*his exciting new series provides nurses with thorough coverage of the foundations of the different perioperative specialties. Individual titles outline pre-, intra-, and postoperative nursing responsibilities. Hundreds of full-color photographs clearly illustrate the key steps in surgical procedures. Overviews of the surgical team, musculoskeletal structures, perioperative nursing care, and instruments and equipment provide essential information applicable to all interventions and specialties. Patient teaching is highlighted to emphasize the importance of self-care.

Now available.

ORTHOPAEDIC SURGERY
Brenda Gregory
1994 (0-8016-6552-3)

CARDIAC SURGERY
Patricia Seifert
1994 (0-8016-6542-6)

Upcoming titles.

GASTROINTESTINAL SURGERY
Lynda Petty
November 1996 (0-8151-6814-4)

GENITOURINARY SURGERY
Gratia Nagle
December 1996 (0-8151-7029-7)

ENDOSCOPIC SURGERY
Kay Ball
January 1997 (0-8151-0600-9)

GYNECOLOGIC & OBSTETRIC SURGERY
Kevin Kauffman
February 1997 (0-8151-4987-5)

NEUROLOGIC SURGERY
Brenda G. Dawes
March 1997 (0-8016-2194-1)

VASCULAR SURGERY
Beth Ann MacVittie
August 1997 (0-8151-7031-9)

PLASTIC SURGERY
Nancy Marie Fortunato, Susan McCullough
October 1997 (0-8151-3305-7)

THORACIC SURGERY
Vicki J. Fox
December 1997 (0-8151-3320-0)

OPHTHALMIC SURGERY
Mary Ann Mawhinney
January 1998 (0-8016-1951-3)

ORAL & MAXILLOFACIAL SURGERY
Katie Steuer
March 1998 (0-8151-4646-9)

ENT SURGERY
James Laubert
November 1998 (0-8151-3167-4)

TRAUMA SURGERY
Vicki J. Fox
January 1999 (0-8151-3171-2)

For more information on these upcoming titles, contact your bookstore manager. To order currently available titles, call toll-free 800-426-4545. In Canada call 800-268-4178. We look forward to hearing from you soon!

PMA014

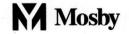